MASTER TECHNIQUES IN OTOLARYNGOLOGY

Head and Neck Surgery

FACIAL PLASTIC SURGERY

MASTER TECHNIQUES IN OTOLARYNGOLOGY

Head and Neck Surgery

FACIAL PLASTIC SURGERY

Series Editor

Eugene N. Myers, MD, FACS, FRCS Edin (Hon)

Distinguished Professor and Chairman Emeritus
Department of Otolaryngology
University of Pittsburgh School of Medicine
Professor
Department of Maxillofacial Surgery
University of Pittsburgh School of Dental Medicine
Pittsburgh, Pennsylvania

Editors

Wayne F. Larrabee Jr, MD, MSH, FACS

Director
Larrabee Center for Plastic Surgery
Clinical Professor
University of Washington
Seattle, Washington

James M. Ridgway, MD, FACS

Director
Facial Plastic and Reconstructive Surgery
Newvue Plastic Surgery
Bellevue, Washington

Sapna A. Patel, MD

Assistant
Larrabee Center for Plastic Surgery
Clinical Assistant Professor
Department of Otolaryngology—Head and Neck Surgery
University of Washington
Surgery Service
Department of Veterans Affairs Medical Center
Seattle, Washington

Wolters Kluwer

Philadelphia • Baltimore • New York • London
Buenos Aires • Hong Kong • Sydney • Tokyo

Acquisitions Editor: Ryan Shaw
Development Editor: Brendan Huffman
Editorial Coordinator: Alexis Pozonsky
Marketing Manager: Dan Dressler
Senior Production Project Manager: Alicia Jackson
Design Coordinator: Holly McLaughlin
Artist/Illustrator: Bernie Kida
Manufacturing Coordinator: Beth Welsh
Prepress Vendor: SPi Global

9 8 7 6 5 4 3 2 1

Printed in China

Library of Congress Cataloging-in-Publication Data
Names: Larrabee, Wayne F., Jr., editor. | Ridgway, James M. MD, editor. | Patel, Sapna, 1985- editor.
Title: Head and neck surgery. Facial plastic surgery / editors, Wayne F. Larrabee Jr, James M. Ridgway, Sapna Patel.
Other titles: Facial plastic surgery | Master techniques in otolaryngology.
Description: Philadelphia : Wolters Kluwer, [2018] | Series: Master techniques in otolaryngology | Includes bibliographical references and index.
Identifiers: LCCN 2017032190 | ISBN 9781451173703
Subjects: | MESH: Face—surgery | Reconstructive Surgical Procedures—methods
Classification: LCC RD523 | NLM WE 705 | DDC 617.5/20592—dc23 LC record available at https://lccn.loc.gov/2017032190

LWW.com

CCS1117

It is my honor to dedicate ***Master Techniques in Facial Plastic Surgery*** *to a true master of our specialty Claus D. Walter, MD. Claus Walter was an immensely talented and innovative surgeon, a dedicated teacher, and a mentor to me, Rich Holt, Ritchie Younger, and countless others. His life was a celebration of all aspects of facial plastic and reconstructive surgery. He died September 11, 2016, and will be missed very much.*

Contributors

Kofi Boahene, MD
Associate Professor
Department of Otolaryngology—Head and Neck Surgery
Johns Hopkins University School of Medicine
Baltimore, Maryland

Jacob O. Boeckmann, MD
Clinical Assistant Professor
Department of Otolaryngology—Head and Neck Surgery
University of California Medical Center
Orange, California

Jonathan W. Boyd, MD
Assistant Clinical Professor
Department of Otolaryngology—Head and Neck Surgery
University of California, Irvine
Orange, California
Chief
Department of Otolaryngology—Head and Neck Surgery
VA Long Beach Healthcare System
Long Beach, California

Patrick Byrne, MD, MBA
Professor and Director
Division of Facial Plastic and Reconstructive Surgery
The Johns Hopkins School of Medicine
Baltimore, Maryland

Michael A. Carron, MD
Associate Professor
Department of Otolaryngology
Wayne State University
Detroit, Michigan

Edward W. Chang, MD, FACS
Adjunct Professor
Department of Surgery
Touro University
Vallejo, California
Senior Physician
Department of Cosmetic Services
Kaiser Permanente
Santa Rosa, California

William P. Chen, MD, FACS
Clinical Professor of Ophthalmology
Department of Ophthalmology
UCLA School of Medicine
Los Angeles, California
Senior Surgical Attending
Eye Plastic Surgery Service
Harbor-UCLA Medical Center
Torrance, California

Christian P. Conderman, MD
Assistant Professor
Division of Facial Plastic & Reconstructive Surgery
Department of Otorhinolaryngology—Head and Neck Surgery
University of Texas—McGovern Medical School
Houston, Texas

Minas Constantinides, MD, FACS
Plastic Surgeon
Westlake Dermatology
Austin, Texas

Paul J. Donald, MD, FACS, FRCS(C)
Professor Emeritus
Department of Otolaryngology—Head and Neck Surgery
University of California, Davis
Surgeon
Department of Otolaryngology—Head and Neck Surgery
University of California Davis Medical Center
Sacramento, California

Charles East, FRCS
Consultant Surgeon
University College London Hospitals
Rhinoplasty London
London, United Kingdom

Jeffrey S. Epstein, MD, FACS
Assistant Volunteer Professor
Department of Otolaryngology
University of Miami, College of Medicine
Miami, Florida

Edward H. Farrior, MD
Associate Clinical Professor
Department of Otolaryngology
University of South Florida
Tampa, Florida

Hossam M.T. Foda, MD
Professor and Chief of Facial Plastic Surgery Division
Department of Otolaryngology
Faculty of Medicine, Alexandria Medical School
Alexandria, Egypt

John L. Frodel Jr, MD
Director, Facial Plastic Surgery
Department of Otolaryngology—Head and Neck Surgery
Geisinger Medical Center
Danville, Pennsylvania

Richard A. Gangnes, MD
Professor of Surgery
Department of Otolaryngology—Head and Neck Surgery
University of California, Irvine
Irvine, California; Orange, California
Attending Surgeon
Saddleback Memorial Hospital
Laguna Hills, California

Marc H. Hohman, MD
Assistant Professor
Department of Surgery
Uniformed Services University of the Health Sciences
Bethesda, Maryland
Facial Plastic and Reconstructive Surgeon
Residency Program Director
Department of Otolaryngology—Head and Neck Surgery
Madigan Army Medical Center
Tacoma, Washington

John B. Holds, MD, FACS
Clinical Professor
Department of Ophthalmology and Otolaryngology—Head and Neck Surgery
Saint Louis University School of Medicine
St. Louis, Missouri

G. Richard Holt, MD, MSE, MPH, MABE, DBioethics
Professor
Department of Otolaryngology—Head and Neck Surgery
The University of Texas Health Science Center
San Antonio, Texas

Yong Ju Jang, MD, PhD
Professor
Department of Otolaryngology
Asan Medical Center, University of Ulsan
Seoul, Korea

Gregory S. Keller, MD
Clinical Professor and Attending
Department of Head and Neck Surgery
University of California, Los Angeles
Los Angeles, California

Robert M. Kellman, MD
Professor and Chair
Otolaryngology and Communication Sciences
SUNY Upstate Medical University
Syracuse, New York

Jason H. Kim, MD, FACS
Otolaryngologist
St. Joseph Hospital
Fullerton, California

Russell W.H. Kridel, MD, FACS
Clinical Professor
Division of Facial Plastic Surgery
Department of Otorhinolaryngology—Head and Neck Surgery
University of Texas Health Science Center
Houston, Texas

Keith A. LaFerriere, MD, FACS
Adjunct Professor
Department of Otolaryngology—Head and Neck Surgery
University of Missouri
Columbia, Missouri

Richard D. Lisman, MD, FACS
Professor
Department of Ophthalmology and Ophthalmic Plastic Surgery
New York University School of Medicine
Director of Ophthalmic Plastic Surgery
NYU Medical Center
Institute of Reconstructive Plastic Surgery
Manhattan Eye, Ear and Throat Hospital—Lenox Hill
New York, New York

Corey S. Maas, MD, FACS
Founder and Director
The Maas Clinic
San Francisco, California

Devinder S. Mangat, MD, FACS
Surgical Director
Mangat Plastic Surgery
Vail, Colorado

E. Gaylon McCollough, MD, FACS
CEO, Founder
Department of Plastic Surgery
The McCullough Institute for Appearance and Health
Gulf Shores, Alabama

Dirk Jan Menger, MD, PhD
Rhinologist—Facial Plastic Surgeon
Department of Otorhinolaryngology
University Medical Center Utrecht
Utrecht, The Netherlands

Frederick J. Menick, MD
Private Practice
Plastic Surgery
St. Joseph's Hospital
Tucson, Arizona

Harry Mittelman, MD
Facial Plastic Surgeon
Mittelman Plastic Surgery
Los Altos, California

Mary Lynn Moran, MD
Private Practice
Franklin, Tennessee

Andrew H. Murr, MD, FACS
Professor and Chairman
Department of Otolaryngology—Head and Neck Surgery
University of California, San Francisco School of Medicine
San Francisco, California

Pietro Palma, MD, FACS
Clinical Professor
Department Otorhinolaryngology—Head and Neck Surgery
University of Insubria
Varese, Italy
Chief
YOUnique Rhinoplasty
Clinica del Viso—Milan Face Clinic
Milano, Italy

Ira Papel, MD
Professor
Division of Facial Plastic Surgery
Department of Otolaryngology—Head and Neck Surgery
The Johns Hopkins School of Medicine
Facial Plastic Surgicenter, Ltd.
Baltimore, Maryland

Stephen S. Park, MD
Professor
Department of Otolaryngology and Head and Neck Surgery
University of Virginia
Charlottesville, Virginia

Stephen W. Perkins, MD
Clinical Associate Professor
Department of Otolaryngology—Head and Neck Surgery
Indiana University, School of Medicine
Indianapolis, Indiana

Allen M. Putterman, MD
Professor of Ophthalmology and Co-director Oculofacial Plastic Surgery
Department of Ophthalmology
University of Illinois, College of Medicine
Attending Physician
Department of Ophthalmology
St. Joseph Hospital
Chicago, Illinois

Daniel E. Rousso, MD, FACS
Facial Plastic Surgeon
Rousso Facial Plastic Surgery and Aesthetic Medical Spa
Birmingham, Alabama

Julian M. Rowe-Jones, FRCS (ORL)
Director and Consultant Facial Plastic Surgeon
The Nose Clinic
Guildford, United Kingdom

James D. Sidman, MD
Professor
Department of Otolaryngology and Pediatrics
University of Minnesota
Director of Research and Academic Strategy
Children's ENT and Facial Plastic Surgery
Children's Minnesota
Minneapolis, Minnesota

Kathleen C.Y. Sie, MD
Professor
Department of Otolaryngology—Head and Neck Surgery
University of Washington
Division Chief
Pediatric Otolaryngology
Seattle Children's Hospital
Seattle, Washington

Bryan Sires, MD, PhD
Clinical Professor
Department of Ophthalmology
University of Washington
Seattle, Washington
Medical Director
Oculofacial Plastic Surgery
Allure Facial Laser Center
Kirkland, Washington

Jonathan M. Sykes, MD, FACS
Professor and Director
Division of Facial Plastic and Reconstructive Surgery
Department of Otolaryngology—Head and Neck Surgery
University of California, Davis
Sacramento, California

Edward O. Terino, MD, FACS
Medical Director
Plastic Surgery Institute of Southern California
Agoura Hills, California

J. Regan Thomas, MD
Mansueto Professor and Chairman
Department of Otolaryngology—Head and Neck Surgery
University of Illinois at Chicago
Chicago, Illinois

Travis T. Tollefson, MD, MPH, FACS
Professor and Director
Facial Plastic and Reconstructive Surgery
Department of Otolaryngology—Head and Neck Surgery
University of California, Davis
Sacramento, California

Dean M. Toriumi, MD
Professor
Division of Facial Plastic and Reconstructive Surgery
Department of Otolaryngology—Head and Neck Surgery
University of Illinois at Chicago
Chicago, Illinois

Claus Walter, MD*
Clinical Professor
Department of Otolaryngology—Head and Neck Surgery
The University of Texas Health Science Center at San Antonio
San Antonio, Texas

Tom D. Wang, MD
Professor
Department of Otolaryngology—Head and Neck Surgery
Oregon Health and Science University
Portland, Oregon

Edwin F. Williams, MD
Clinical Professor of Surgery
Department of Surgery—ENT
Albany Medical College
Albany, New York

Ritchie A.L. Younger, MD, FRCSC
Professor
Department of Surgery
University of British Columbia
Department of Otolaryngology
Vancouver Hospital
Vancouver, British Columbia, Canada

John A. Zitelli, MD
Adjunct Clinical Associate Professor
Department of Dermatology, Otolaryngology, and Plastic Surgery
University of Pittsburgh Medical Center
Pittsburgh, Pennsylvania

*Deceased

Preface

I would like to thank Wolters Kluwer publishers for undertaking this immensely complex project. I am grateful to Eugene N. Myers, MD, for providing the opportunity to edit this challenging and rewarding addition to the "Master" series. Most importantly I would like to thank the authors. Each agreed to take time from busy clinical practices and personal lives to share their wisdom with colleagues and fellow surgeons. Each author wrote his or her own chapter to provide our readers the most accurate clinical descriptions of their procedures.

We selected the authors with one simple criterion, which was to identify a surgeon who was a true master of his or her procedure—regardless of specialty or geographic background. We thus have specialists from facial plastic surgery, oculoplastic surgery, plastic surgery, and dermatologic surgery. We also have authors from around the world who are members of our global facial plastic surgery family. We were unable to include every procedure in the specialty but strove to select those we thought most important and relevant in reconstructive surgery, trauma, oculoplastic surgery, rhinoplasty, and cosmetic surgery to include aging face surgery. Some important areas such as laser surgery and various nonablative treatments are not represented simply due to rapidly changing and company-specific technologies. There are many talented surgeons and interesting procedures we regret not being able to include in this edition.

Thank you to the editorial staff, Dr. Myers, my associate editors, and the ever-patient families for their excellent contributions to *Master Techniques of Facial Plastic Surgery*.

Wayne F. Larrabee Jr, MD, MSH, FACS
Director, Larrabee Center for Plastic Surgery
Clinical Professor, University of Washington
Director, Global Surgical Outreach

Contents

PART VIII: TRAUMA 587

1 UPPER BLEPHAROPLASTY AND APONEURОTIC PTOSIS REPAIR

John B. Holds

INTRODUCTION

Blepharoplasty surgery is the central component of any midfacial restoration or rejuvenation. The procedure is often combined with brow lift surgery, ptosis repair, or other facial aesthetic procedures to enhance or achieve an appropriate aesthetic result. Upper eyelid blepharoplasty is also performed for aesthetic reasons to reduce and redrape excess skin, redefine the eyelid crease and supratarsal platform, and decrease overall fullness. In comparison, ptosis repair is a finely tuned and challenging surgical procedure that requires correct diagnosis, thoughtful planning, impeccable surgical technique, experience, and a thorough understanding of the anatomy of the eyelid. The patient's ocular, medical, and surgical history help determine whether surgical repair of ptosis is appropriate for that individual.

Ptosis or blepharoptosis is an abnormal sagging of the upper eyelid margin. The vast majority of cases of acquired ptosis are due to a dehiscence of the levator aponeurosis. Nevertheless, the causes of acquired ptosis are diverse, and it is helpful in evaluation and treatment to classify acquired ptosis into the following: aponeurogenic, from involutional or other disinsertional changes in the levator aponeurosis; myogenic, associated with decreased levator muscle function, as seen in myasthenia gravis (MG) or congenital progressive external ophthalmoplegia (CPEO); neurogenic, as seen in third nerve palsy or Horner's syndrome; and mechanical, associated with eyelid masses or scarring of the eyelid lamellae. Traumatic ptosis, sometimes considered a separate category, is more properly a subcategory of each of the foregoing categories.

Ptosis that causes significant superior visual field loss or difficulty with reading is considered to be a functional problem, and correction of this defect often improves a patient's ability to perform the activities of daily living. Ptosis is considered to be a cosmetic issue when it causes a tired or sleepy appearance in the absence of a significant visual function deficit. It is particularly important for the surgeon to have a preoperative discussion with the patient to communicate the alternatives, potential risks, and benefits of surgery.

HISTORY

In evaluating the patient for upper blepharoplasty and/or ptosis repair, it is important to consider the patient's goals and desires. An older patient with visual obstruction symptoms and no cosmetic desires is a very different patient from the patient who wants a cosmetic blepharoplasty. Both upper blepharoplasty and ptosis repair are sometimes deemed "medically necessary" as a covered service by insurance companies to decrease overhanging skin and improve superior visual fields. Patients pursuing blepharoplasty surgery should report their perception of issues including overhanging skin, prolapse of adipose tissue, and other facial aesthetic issues. All patients having eyelid surgery should be questioned about their coagulation status. Other pertinent historical queries should include the presence of thyroid eye disease, previous eye or eyelid surgery, and prior periorbital trauma. Complaints about dry eye seldom present an absolute contraindication to upper eyelid surgery but require additional assessment, counseling, and modification of surgical technique. All patients should be queried regarding dry eye symptoms as well as other ocular history and complaints.

In the patient with ptosis, one must begin with a careful history, with attention to duration and progression of ptosis, daily variation in the severity of ptosis, use of contact lenses, and any history of dry eye. The patient's history usually distinguishes congenital from acquired ptosis. Patients with congenital or acquired blepharoptosis may be aware of a family history of the condition. Marked variability in the degree of ptosis during the day and complaints of diplopia should trigger an evaluation for ocular MG.

PHYSICAL EXAMINATION

Eyebrow position is very important, as most prospective patients considering upper blepharoplasty have some degree of brow ptosis and might benefit from a brow lift. Brow ptosis commonly worsens somewhat following blepharoplasty surgery. Attempt to define how blepharoplasty and/or brow lifting will appear postoperatively and proceed with acknowledgment from the patient of the expected outcome. Blepharoptosis or ptosis is common in patients presenting for blepharoplasty and often requires concomitant repair.

Preoperative counseling must realistically inform the patient of the ability of surgery to modify all of these features as well as the risk of more common complications. Evaluation of the patient presenting for eyelid surgery should, if possible, include a slitlamp examination. A careful reporting of ocular and dry eye symptoms along with notations regarding eyelid position and function are a basic minimum. A basic Schirmer's secretion test (after anesthetic) is simple to perform and may be worthwhile to document. In preoperative examination and counseling, it is helpful to demonstrate to the patient with a mirror the degree to which the surgeon believes overhanging skin will be improved with blepharoplasty surgery (or worsened with ptosis repair without blepharoplasty surgery) and to note and point to adipose tissue pads that can be reduced. The limits of upper blepharoplasty are stressed, especially in regard to medial and lateral skin redundancy, which is often noted postoperatively and commonly requires a brow lift to improve. Patients undergoing surgery for medical indications require specific documentation of visual complaints, a desire for surgery, and reversible superior visual field loss on standardized perimetry. All patients must have facial photography with multiple views.

Physical examination of the patient with ptosis includes five clinical measurements. Although it is ideal to record these numbers in all patients considering blepharoplasty, these are critical measurements in evaluating the patient with ptosis:

- Margin reflex distance
- Vertical palpebral fissure height
- Position of the upper eyelid crease
- Levator function (upper eyelid excursion)
- Presence of lagophthalmos

The physician can record these data by using a drawing showing the cornea, the pupil size, and the position of the upper and lower eyelids in relation to these structures (Fig. 1.1). The margin reflex distance (MRD1) is the distance from the upper eyelid margin to the corneal light reflex from a penlight held at the level of the examiner's eye on which the patient is fixating in primary position. MRD1 is single most important measurement in describing the amount or severity of a ptosis. In severe ptosis, the light reflex may be obstructed by the eyelid and therefore have a zero or negative value. Retraction of the lower eyelid (scleral show) should be noted separately as the margin reflex distance 2 (MRD2). The MRD2 is the distance from the corneal light reflex to the lower eyelid margin. The sum of the MRD1 and the MRD2 should equal the vertical height of the interpalpebral fissure.

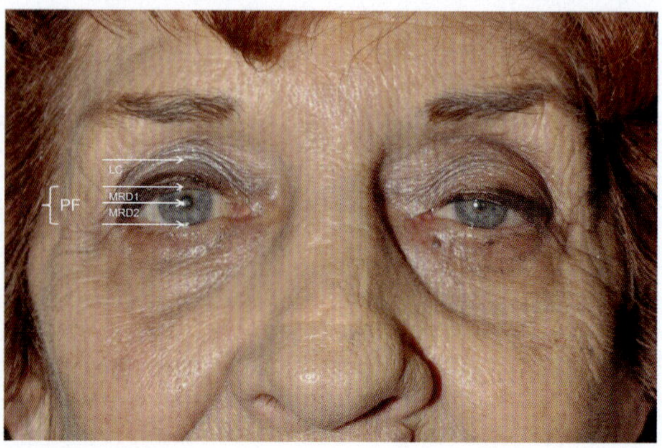

FIGURE 1.1
Important measurements in ptosis surgery: MRD1, margin reflex distance 1 from papillary light reflex to the upper eyelid margin; MRD2, margin reflex distance 2 from papillary light reflex to the lower eyelid margin; PF, palpebral fissure, sum of MRD1 and MRD2; LC, eyelid crease, often measured in downgaze, as overhanging upper eyelid skin may cover the true eyelid crease.

The distance from the upper eyelid crease to the eyelid margin is measured. Because the insertion of fibers from the levator muscle into the skin contributes to formation of the upper eyelid crease, high, duplicated, or asymmetric creases may indicate an abnormal position of the levator aponeurosis. In the typical Caucasian eyelid, the upper eyelid crease is 8 to 9 mm in males and 9 to 11 mm in females. The crease is usually elevated in patients with involutional ptosis and is often shallow or absent in patients with congenital ptosis. The upper eyelid crease is lower or obscured in the Asian eyelid, with or without ptosis. Levator function is estimated by measuring the upper eyelid excursion from downgaze to upgaze with frontalis muscle function negated. Finally, the patient should be evaluated for lagophthalmos.

Clinical features of a patient with acquired aponeurosis disinsertion consist of good levator function, higher than normal eyelid crease, and a ptotic eyelid that assumes a lower position on down gaze. If a history consistent with MG is obtained, tests for fatigability as well as an edrophonium (tensilon or enlon) test should be performed. The examiner should be cognizant of the frequency of bilateral ptosis that is more apparent on one side. Because of the equal innervation to both levator muscles, correcting only one upper lid may result in worsening the appearance of ptosis on the opposite side. This phenomenon follows Hering's law and is especially frequent in aponeurogenic ptosis.

INDICATIONS

Upper eyelid blepharoplasty indications

- Reduce the overhanging skin causing visual obstruction or cosmesis
- Define the supratarsal fold and eyelid crease
- Smooth contour and reduce prolapsed adipose tissue

Lid ptosis, secondary to aponeurosis compromise

- Raise the eyelid margin to a visually functional position
- Correct asymmetry of the lid height
- Improve symmetry of the eyelid crease and supratarsal fold

If blepharoplasty or ptosis repair is being performed for functional indications, it is vital to document the severity of ptosis with office notes and measurements, facial photographs, and formal visual field testing, showing the superior visual field constriction produced by the ptosis. It is also helpful to have photographs and notes available for reference at the time of surgery. After trauma, it is prudent to wait 6 months before eyelid surgery, as function may improve during that time. In MG, or any medical or neurologic condition that may undergo remission with therapy, it is wise to delay surgery until the condition is stable and optimally controlled.

CONTRAINDICATIONS

Surgical contraindications in upper eyelid surgery include the patient with inappropriate expectations, medically unstable patients including patients with recent (within 6 months) placement of a heart stent whose anticoagulation cannot be held for any period of time, and prior surgery and co-existing medical or ocular conditions that create unnecessary and unacceptable surgical risk. Dry eye syndrome or the patient prone to exposure keratopathy due to impaired protective mechanisms must be seen as relative or absolute contraindications to blepharoplasty and/or ptosis repair, depending on the severity of the clinical findings and the indication for surgery.

PREOPERATIVE PLANNING

Patients should discontinue aspirin and other anticoagulants, herbal medications, and antiplatelet agents 3 to 7 days preoperatively. This is best done in consultation with the patient's primary care physician and offers an excellent opportunity to ensure that no acute or chronic medical condition poses an issue with surgery. The vast majority of patients undergoing blepharoplasty or ptosis surgery can be done under a local or sedated local anesthetic. Four lid blepharoplasty or additional procedures, such as brow or face lift, may require a general anesthetic.

SURGICAL TECHNIQUE

Upper Blepharoplasty

With the patient sitting upright, mark the incision with a fine-tipped surgical marker before entering the operating room. The eyelid crease is first marked, extending medially and laterally. An appropriate amount of skin

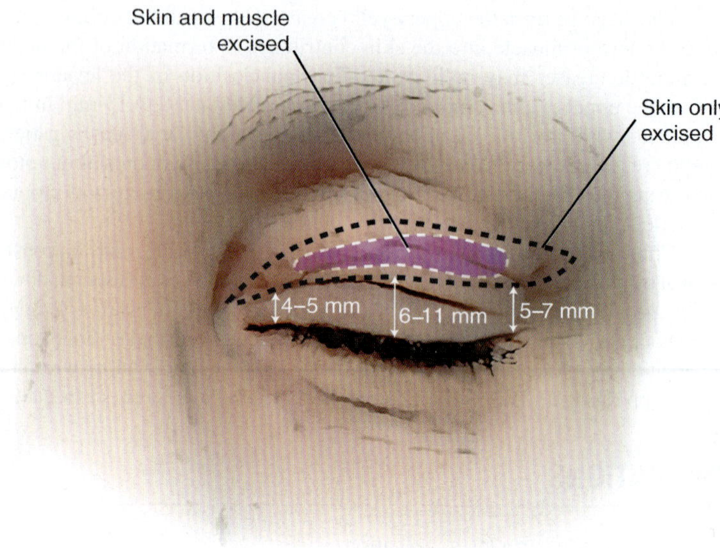

FIGURE 1.2
Marking of the eyelid crease and proposed skin excision. Hatching shows portion of the excision over which skin only is excised, versus skin and muscle.

for excision is then marked. Asymmetry in the amount of overhanging skin or the total amount of upper eyelid skin are more apparent with the patient upright and can be compensated with asymmetric excision. If brow lift surgery is to be performed, one should first perform the brow lift and then recheck the blepharoplasty excision intraoperatively after the brow lift to ensure excessive excision is not performed. Use the patient's natural eyelid crease to guide the positioning of the lid crease incision. The highest point in the central eyelid is generally at 8 to 11 mm height near the nasal aspect of the pupil (Fig. 1.2). The patient's desires also guide positioning of the lid crease, with the female crease generally 1 to 2 mm higher than the male crease. After marking the highest point in the eyelid crease centrally, a smooth downward curve is made to 4 to 5 mm above the upper punctum medially and 5 to 7 mm above the lateral canthal angle. Medial to the medial mark a smooth upward curve may be made, never extending medial to the canthal angle. Laterally, the incision never extends beyond the orbital rim where the skin thickens 12 to 16 mm lateral to the canthal angle. Amounts of skin for excision vary from a few mm up to 2 cm vertically. If attempting to maximize the effect of blepharoplasty, a good guide is to ensure that at least 20 mm of skin (pretarsal plus infrabrow vertical extent) remains postoperatively between the lashes and the inferior aspect of the eyebrow. Marks can be made 10 to 15 mm inferior to the inferior aspect of the brow laterally, smoothly tapering toward the medial and lateral ends of the lid crease incision. It is reasonable to use a smooth forceps to gently pinch together the skin proposed for excision. A slight degree of induced lagophthalmos and eversion of the lashes when gently pinching the eyelid skin together is generally desirable, and a significant degree of lagophthalmos suggests an overly aggressive excision.

In the operating room, it is helpful to inject the eyelid prior to the prep and drape with 1 mL/eyelid of lidocaine 2% with epinephrine 1:100,000 that is diluted 1:5 with normal saline (final epinephrine concentration 1:600,000). Given slowly, this injection is painless, except for the initial needle stick, and will give complete anesthesia with excellent vasoconstriction while the patient is being sterilely prepped. After carefully draping to ensure the drapes do not induce a brow malposition distorting the surgical effect, the incision is reinfiltrated with 2% lidocaine with epinephrine 1:100,000. The instillation of topical anesthetic and placement of metallic eye shields that completely cover the anterior globe protects the eyes from injury and will prevent startling the sedated patient with bright surgical lights.

A no. 15C Bard-Parker blade is used to incise the skin. Skin only is removed temporal to the lateral canthus. Skin and muscle are removed over the central eyelid using Westcott or Kaye scissors (Fig. 1.2). Skin only is also removed in the medial 5 to 6 mm of the incision. A skin-only excision lateral to the lateral canthus and medial to the upper punctum minimizes necessary cautery, limiting scar formation at the medial and lateral extent of the incision where it is most noticeable postoperatively. Over the central eyelid, a strip of orbicularis muscle is excised, exposing the orbital septum. Elderly patients or those with dry eye benefit from preservation of the orbicularis muscle and require no muscle or only a small central strip of muscle to be excised.

After cautery for hemostasis, the local anesthetic is injected beneath the orbital septum centrally (if it is to be opened) and directly into the medial adipose tissue pad. Surgical indications and individual preferences and variations will determine whether the septum is left intact or adipose tissue is excised almost flush with the orbital rim. Gentle pressure on the globe causes the preaponeurotic adipose tissue to bulge, facilitating medial and central opening of the orbital septum. Freeing the adipose tissue from the orbital septum and levator aponeurosis that it borders helps to prolapse the adipose tissue. The base of the adipose tissue to be removed is then cauterized, paralleling the incision, leaving a cuff of undisturbed adipose tissue anterior to the orbital rim (Fig. 1.3). Bipolar cautery or CO_2 laser cause minimal discomfort, with monopolar (Bovie) cautery requiring

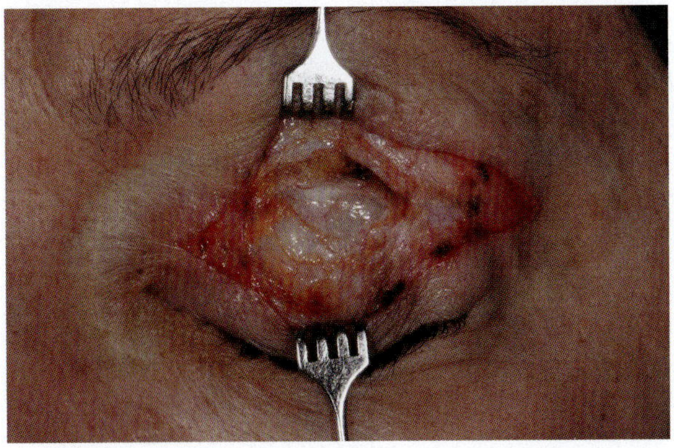

FIGURE 1.3
Upper eyelid following excision of a roll of central adipose tissue.

sedation. Adipose tissue is excised across the width of the eyelid with attention to the medial and lateral aspects, avoiding the excision of excessive adipose tissue centrally where it is most accessible. Laterally avoid the lacrimal gland. The medial adipose tissue pad requires careful exposure as it is inferior and medial to the central (preaponeurotic) adipose tissue. Retracting the skin and muscle away, pressure is applied, and the capsule of the medial adipose tissue pad is incised avoiding blood vessels encircling the base of the adipose tissue (Fig. 1.4). Pressure is applied with cautery and graded excision of the adipose tissue. In the lateral subbrow area, cautery shrinkage or a modest excision of the most inferior brow adipose tissue may lighten the lateral brow enhancing the result.

The incision is closed after achieving meticulous hemostasis. A simple running skin closure with 7-0 Polypropylene suture is efficient. It is helpful with large excisions to place an interrupted suture laterally where the lid crease incision angles upward above the lateral canthus. Centrally, supratarsal fixation of the pretarsal skin and lid crease may be helpful (Fig. 1.5). This is done with interrupted sutures or as part of the running suture to ensure the final position of the eyelid crease. Concomitant surgery for aponeurotic ptosis or aggressive excision of the orbicularis muscle destabilizes the pretarsal orbicularis muscle, making eyelid crease fixation important to prevent an unpredictable position of the lid crease. Sutures are more closely spaced laterally where the thicker skin is under more tension and tends to gape.

Alternative Approach

Excess redundancy of skin medially along the upper incision may require a W-plasty excision of an additional triangle of tissue at a 60-degree angle superior to the medial tip of the excision. It is possible to perform internal lifting of the eyebrow through the blepharoplasty incision. Both suture and Endotine (MicroAire, Charlottesville, VA) fixation are performed. Most surgeons find the results of these internal brow lift techniques to be temporary and unreliable. Asian upper blepharoplasty is described in Chapter 6.

Ptosis Repair

With few exceptions, acquired ptosis can be treated by an aponeurotic resection or repair. An external aponeurotic approach directly treats the most common cause for acquired ptosis, aponeurotic rarefaction, or disinsertion. Aponeurotic surgery is also the preferred approach in myogenic or neurogenic ptosis with adequate levator function. Only the aponeurotic approach to ptosis is to be covered in this text. Aponeurotic approaches to ptosis repair are ideally performed in combination with blepharoplasty surgery. The Mullerectomy procedure described by Urist and Putterman provides predictable correction of ptosis based on response to a

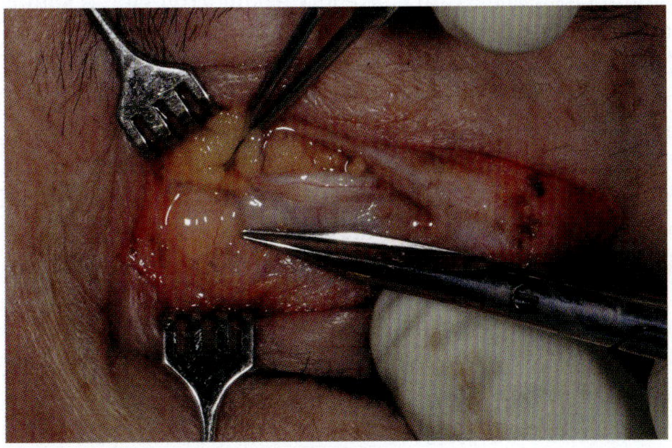

FIGURE 1.4
The whiter medial adipose tissue pad seen inferomedial to the central adipose tissue.

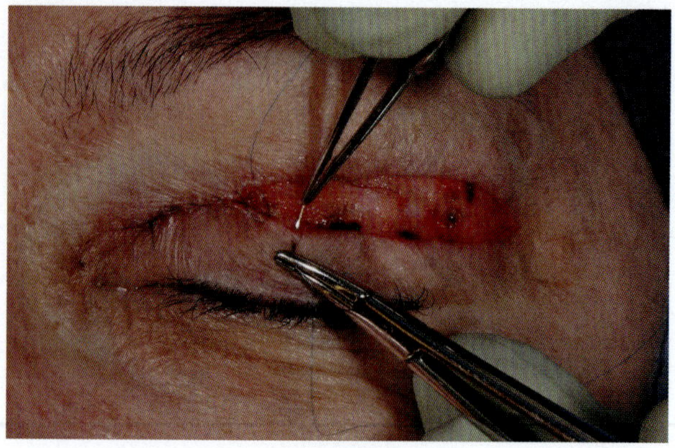

FIGURE 1.5
Running closure with supratarsal bite to the edge of the levator aponeurosis. Three such central bites at the height of the eyelid crease fixate and stabilize the crease height.

phenylephrine test in the ptotic eyelid. The simplicity of this procedure and ability to perform formulaic surgery predicted by a pharmacologic test make this technique popular. It is well described in Suggested Readings.

The eyelid crease is generally marked along the entire eyelid to correspond with the lid crease of the opposite upper lid. In patients undergoing bilateral surgery or ptosis repair combined with blepharoplasty, a natural position for the eyelid crease is created as described above in Upper Blepharoplasty. In adult patients with good levator function requiring no blepharoplasty, ptosis repair can be accomplished through a central 8- to 12-mm eyelid crease incision. Anesthesia is obtained by subcutaneous infiltration along the preplaced skin marking with 1.0 mL or less of 2% lidocaine with 1:100,000 dilution of epinephrine. It is important not to inject deeper than the skin, as this can influence intraoperative lid height adjustments. Topical tetracaine or proparacaine is instilled into the eye.

The skin is incised. If a blepharoplasty is to be performed, it is done at this point. In the blepharoplasty, avoid any local anesthetic injection underneath the levator aponeurosis or deep into the adipose tissue. The superior edge of the incision is retracted upward with a skin hook, and the disinserted edge of the levator aponeurosis is often identified through the translucent postorbicular fascia. While retracting the superior edge of the incision with a skin hook or Desmarres retractor, gentle pressure is applied on the globe. With retrograde orbital pressure, the preaponeurotic adipose tissue pad bulges forward to tent up the orbital septum. The orbital septum is buttonholed above its fusion with the aponeurosis. The incision should be directed superiorly into the adipose tissue. This allows the preaponeurotic adipose tissue to herniate (Fig. 1.6). The orbital septum is then further opened by placing one blade of the scissors behind the orbital septum and extending the incision medially and laterally. This maneuver is important to identify the preaponeurotic adipose tissue pad and the levator aponeurosis. The skin and orbicularis muscle are retracted with a forceps. The preaponeurotic adipose tissue pad is an anatomic landmark in this surgery, since the levator aponeurosis is located immediately beneath this structure. Mueller's muscle lies immediately under the levator aponeurosis. In cases of repeated operation, trauma, or in eyelids infiltrated by tumor, such as neurofibroma, the preaponeurotic adipose tissue pad may be the only identifiable structure.

The disinserted edge of the levator aponeurosis may be grasped with forceps and the patient asked to look superiorly. The surgeon can then feel the force generated against the forceps, confirming the structure to be the aponeurosis. Whitnall's ligament is often seen at the superior limit of the aponeurosis.

A Westcott scissors is used to excise a central strip of thinned levator aponeurosis (Fig. 1.7). over the upper central tarsus, baring the anterior surface of the tarsal plate (Fig. 1.8). If the levator aponeurosis is intact, the appropriate amount of aponeurosis is resected. If thinning of the aponeurosis is present, excise the thinned area to expose the distinct aponeurotic edge for anchoring onto the tarsal plate.

The levator aponeurosis is reattached to the central tarsal plate with a 5-0 polyglactin 910 (Vicryl) suture on a spatula needle (Fig. 1.9). The eyelid should always be everted to confirm that full-thickness passes have not occurred. The first suture is placed just medial to the pupil, which is the highest point of the normal eyelid 1.5 to 2 mm below the upper edge of the tarsus. A temporary tie with a bow knot will allow some loosening of the suture if it overcorrects the eyelid height. If the aponeurosis is advanced too inferiorly on the tarsal plate, the eyelid margin may evert. After the central suture is adequately placed, one to two sutures are placed medial and lateral to adjust eyelid height and contour (Fig. 1.10). The lid height should be overcorrected about 1 to 1.5 mm at surgery to compensate for anesthetic paralysis of the orbicularis muscle and to counteract a slight postoperative fall. When local anesthesia is used, the lid height and contour should be evaluated while the patient sits upright on the operating table.

In unilateral cases, it is often necessary to excise excess skin and orbicularis as a small blepharoplasty. However, one must be conservative with skin removal unless a blepharoplasty is to be performed on the contralateral eyelid as well. The skin incision is closed with a running 6-0 or 7-0 monofilament suture or 6-0 plain gut sutures. Antibiotic ointment is placed onto the incision and into the eye, and an ice pack is applied to reduce swelling.

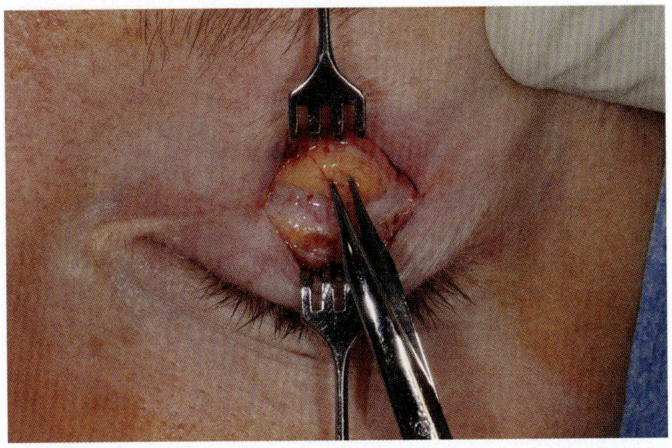

FIGURE 1.6
The orbital septum is exposed and buttonholed, exposing the levator aponeurosis.

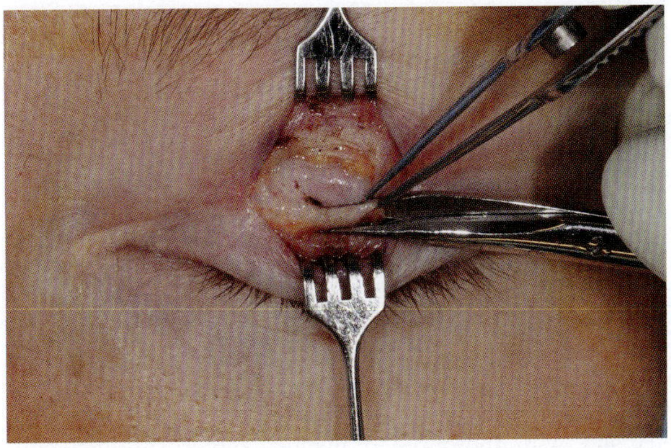

FIGURE 1.7
Exposed levator aponeurosis with distinct edge grasped by forceps. The preaponeurotic adipose tissue is retracted exposing Whitnall's ligament in the superior levator aponeurosis.

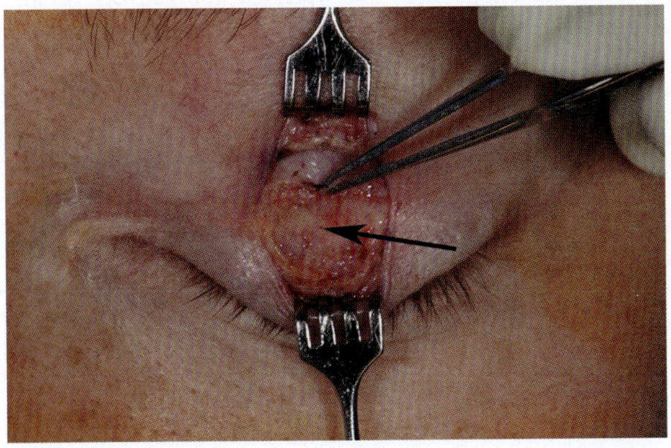

FIGURE 1.8
A Westcott scissors is used to excise thinned tissues exposing the central tarsal plate and creating a distinct cut edge of the levator aponeurosis.

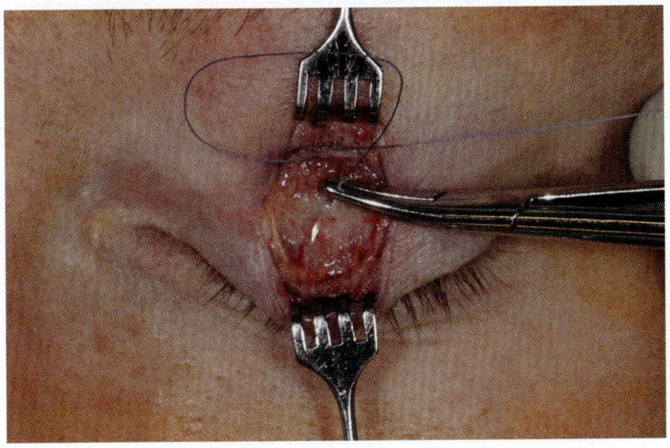

FIGURE 1.9
The levator aponeurosis is sutured to the upper tarsus with a 5-0 polyglactin 910 (Vicryl) suture. The initial suture bite is placed in line with the normal peak of the eyelid height.

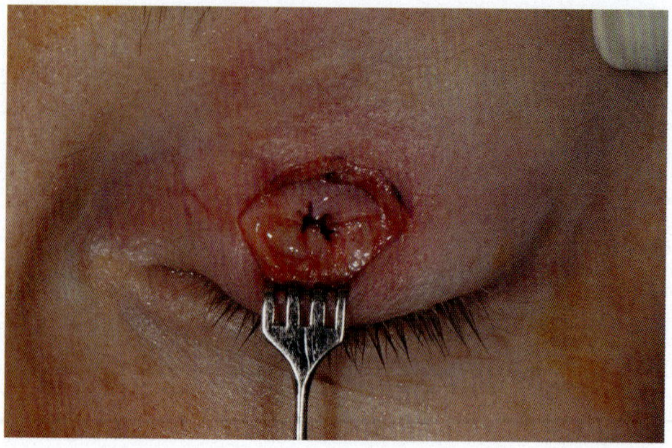

FIGURE 1.10
Additional sutures are placed medial and/or lateral to the first aponeurotic suture. Two to three such sutures generally suffice for the repair of involutional ptosis.

POSTOPERATIVE CARE

Elevation of the head and ice applied to the eyes for 24 to 48 hours limits postoperative ecchymosis and discomfort. A mild analgesic is helpful in the first few hours or days postoperatively.

Most patients undergoing only blepharoplasty or ptosis repair can drive a vehicle again and otherwise function pretty well within 24 to 48 hours. Antibiotic ointment applied to the incisions at bedtime is continued for 7 to 14 days, and sutures are generally removed within 6 to 10 days. Progress is assessed at follow-up visits, with patients generally able to resume all preoperative activities by 2 weeks after surgery.

COMPLICATIONS

The most common issues after upper blepharoplasty and ptosis repair are early minor asymmetries and concerns relating to edema, mild hypertrophic scarring, and a relative anesthesia of the lashes and pretarsal skin. Minor asymmetries often relate to brow asymmetry and, with appropriately planned surgery, are generally less severe than in preoperative photographs. A preoperative discussion of asymmetry, especially relating to brow position, and reference postoperatively to photographs is helpful. Normal wound healing induces a mild hypertrophy and contracture of surgical wounds, generally most apparent 4 to 6 weeks postoperatively. As this resolves over weeks to months, reassurance and temporizing are generally curative. The injection of 0.05 to 0.2 mL of diluted triamcinolone acetonide (Kenalog 10) along the incision will speed resolution of this thickening. A mild anesthesia of the pretarsal skin and lashes is apparent on placing eyeliner or mascara. This is normal and will resolve within a few months. Complaints of dry eye are generally mild in patients under good control preoperatively and who respond well to topical tear drops and punctual plugs or other treatments as needed. Severely overdone blepharoplasty may require skin grafting to the eyelid or adipose tissue or dermis adipose tissue grafting to the superior sulcus or lower eyelids. Careful preoperative counseling and attention to surgical technique are essential in treating these cases. Ptosis is an uncommon complication of blepharoplasty surgery and generally resolves over weeks to months. Review of preoperative photographs may reveal a ptosis missed on preoperative examination, which is now apparent with the lid margin visible.

During the first 3 weeks after ptosis surgery, if overcorrection or undercorrection is apparent that is unrelated to eyelid edema, an adjustment may be performed. The eyelid crease incision is anesthetized, bluntly opened, and eyelid height adjusted by advancing or recessing the levator aponeurosis.

RESULTS

Upper blepharoplasty and ptosis repair are common and often associated procedures for the treatment of common upper eyelid complaints. A patient with brow ptosis, dermatochalasis, and mild right ptosis is shown in Figure 1.11. It appears unlikely that the excellent symmetry and improvement in the upper eyelids seen postoperatively would have been achieved without a careful ptosis repair and judicious blepharoplasty.

PEARLS

- Upper blepharoplasty and ptosis repair require appropriate patient evaluation and surgical planning. Fitting these procedures into the overall picture of the patient's surgical rehabilitation is important.
- Evaluate the patient's needs as to cosmetic appearance. Educating the patient regarding postoperative appearance and possible complications is critical.

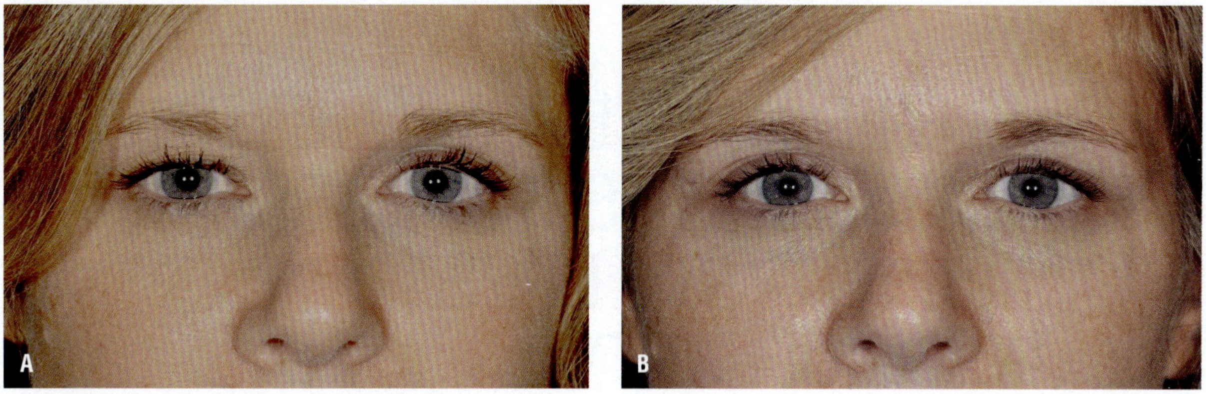

FIGURE 1.11 **A, B:** Pre- and postoperative imaging.

- Mark the upper blepharoplasty with the patient in the upright position prior to infiltration of local anesthetic, rechecking intraoperatively if a brow lift is performed first.
- Perform ptosis repair when necessary after appropriate evaluation.
- The aponeurotic repair of ptosis is done with the utmost care on a lightly sedated patient who can provide feedback on the operating room table as aponeurotic sutures are adjusted.
- Avoid high-risk patients with severe dry eyes and poor protective mechanisms.
- Provide instructions for postoperative lubrication so the patient can prevent complications.

PITFALLS

- Concomitant surgery for aponeurotic ptosis or aggressive excision of the orbicularis muscle destabilizes the pretarsal orbicularis muscle can cause eyelid crease fixation and unpredictable placement.
- If the brow lift procedure is performed first, considerable swelling of the upper eyelid tissues will be present and can complicate the accuracy of blepharoplasty and ptosis repair.
- Overaggressive tissue removal is much more difficult to correct than being too conservative.
- Unwanted eversion of the eyelid margin can occur if the aponeurosis is advanced too inferiorly on the tarsal plate.
- Injury to the levator aponeurosis is always preceded by failure to identify the preaponeurotic adipose tissue pad.
- Lid height should be overcorrected about 1 to 1.5 mm at surgery to compensate for anesthetic paralysis.

INSTRUMENTS TO HAVE AVAILABLE

- Standard oculoplasty surgical tray
- Steven's tenotomy scissors
- 0.5 Castroviejo forceps

SUGGESTED READING

Dresner SC. Further modifications of the Müller's muscle-conjunctival resection procedure for blepharoptosis. *Ophthal Plast Reconstr Surg* 1991;7(2):114–122.

Fagien S. *Putterman's cosmetic oculoplastic surgery with DVD*, 4th ed. New York: Elsevier, 2007.

Holds JB. Blepharoplasty. In: Levine MR, ed. *Manual of oculoplastic surgery, Chapter 10*, 4th ed. Thorofare, NJ: Slack Inc., 2010:75–82.

Holds JB, Anderson RL. Blepharoptosis. In: Tse DT, ed. *Color atlas of oculoplastic surgery, Chapter 9*, 2nd ed. Philadelphia, PA: Wolters Kluwer/Lippincott Williams & Wilkins, 2011:82–101.

Putterman AM, Urist MJ. Müller muscle-conjunctiva resection. Technique for treatment of blepharoptosis. *Arch Ophthalmol* 1975;93(8):619–623.

2 MÜLLER'S MUSCLE–CONJUNCTIVAL RESECTION–PTOSIS PROCEDURE COMBINED WITH UPPER BLEPHAROPLASTY

Allen M. Putterman

INTRODUCTION

Often, patients who present for cosmetic rejuvenation of the upper periorbita are found on physical examination to have both dermatochalasis and upper eyelid ptosis. In these situations, it is both possible and preferable to combine an upper blepharoplasty with ptosis surgery. Although this technique is commonly performed through an external approach with levator aponeurosis advancement or resection, many cosmetic surgeons do not appreciate the possibility of combining an internal Müller's muscle–conjunctival resection with an external upper blepharoplasty, especially when the skin and orbicularis oculi muscle are excised and an eyelid crease is reconstructed.

The Müller's muscle–conjunctival resection–ptosis procedure is a technique in which Müller's muscle in the upper eyelid is partially resected and advanced. The mechanism by which the correction of ptosis is achieved is probably due to a number of effects that include resection and advancement of Müller's muscle as well as the secondary effects of advancing the levator aponeurosis to the superior tarsal border. The classic approach to the treatment of a variety of ptosis presentations has been mostly through variations of an external (skin–muscle incision) approach through the upper eyelid crease whereby the anatomic "defect" is visualized and presumably repaired. This approach, however, more often requires the cooperation of the patient during the surgical procedure and heralds a host of potential variables that include, but are not limited to, sedative effects, local anesthetic effects, edema, and performance anxiety on the part of both the patient and the surgeon. On the contrary, the Müller's muscle conjunctival resection can be performed with continuous IV sedation or even general anesthesia as it does not require the intraoperative cooperation of the patient. The procedure is used to treat a variety of upper eyelid ptosis and can be combined with an upper blepharoplasty with or without crease reconstruction via a skin flap or a skin–muscle flap approach. This technique has many advantages over other "posterior approach" lid ptosis procedures and the external approaches, which includes the preservation of upper eyelid tarsus (which creates less risk of suture-induced keratopathy and theoretically preserves structural and functional aspects of the upper eyelid), repositioning of the elevated (involutional) eyelid crease to a lower positioned and more youthful level, and can more predictably improve upper eyelid position (margin reflex distance, MRD) and contour. In addition, the excision of skin–muscle and adipose tissue that is performed for a host of reasons, including adequate exposure of the levator aponeurosis (that can be volume depleting to the upper eyelid), can be avoided if desired. This procedure can be applied in most types of ptosis presentations, and there is rarely any need for additional surgery to treat residual ptosis or overcorrections.

Simply stated, I have found that this combined procedure produces both superior results compared with the levator aponeurosis procedure with upper blepharoplasty, especially in the patients who desire a lower positioned upper eyelid crease and/or whose upper eyelids elevate to normal levels after administration of phenylephrine.

HISTORY

The surgeon should question the patient about illnesses, medications, allergies, and edema. Emphasis is placed on ruling out thyroid disease, heart failure, hypertension, bleeding tendencies, glaucoma, and unusual swelling. Patients with thyroid disease may look as if they need cosmetic surgery, but the treatment is frequently medical—not surgical. Side effects, such as myocardial infarction and hypertension, have been reported on rare occasion after instillation of phenylephrine drops. Therefore, it is important to determine the presence of any significant cardiac risk factors. If such elements are of significant concern, the patient's primary care physician or cardiologist should be consulted as these issues will reemerge during consultation for surgery. Additionally, if there is a history of glaucoma, it may be prudent to contact their ophthalmologist regarding any concerns of pupillary dilation prior to a phenylephrine test.

A focused history with regard to the presence of lid ptosis is of considerable importance. Various classification models have been developed with reference to acquired, neurogenic, mechanical, and congenital origins. Each can help to organize one's approach in an evaluation. With all patients, I inquire about any history of trauma, previous surgeries, chronic ocular conditions, contact lens use, and lid fatigue.

Patients should also be questioned about intake of medications, in particular aspirin or anti-inflammatory medications such as ibuprofen, vitamin E, anticoagulants, and herbal remedies. These drugs must be discontinued for several weeks preoperatively to avoid the possibility of complications of bleeding during and after surgery.

PHYSICAL EXAMINATION

In the physical examination, multiple anatomic elements must be considered in the evaluation to ensure ocular rejuvenation and functional restoration. The mindful surgeon must assess the presence of brow ptosis, excessive upper eyelid skin, herniated orbital adipose tissue, abnormal creases, lid retraction, ptosis, and lacrimal gland herniation in each patient undergoing evaluation for surgery. Additionally, asymmetries of the eyebrows, eyelids, and possible dystopia should be reviewed with the patient while the patient is holding a mirror.

The evaluation of brow ptosis is important, as this condition is responsible for excessive eyelid folds created by brow descent into the infraorbital region. Often patients present with complaints of excess eyelid skin that is impairing the visual field or creating an aged appearance. Brow ptosis must be excluded as surgical excision of the upper eyelid skin only minimally improves eyelid appearance and visual fields.

Examination of the upper eyelid and the amount of excess skin and adipose tissue present is a subtle, but very important part of the clinical exam. It is important not only to determine the amount of excess eyelid skin but also to determine which regions have greater redundancy. Uniform skin redundancy is not a common rule in the aging periocular complex. Additionally, the evaluation of herniated adipose tissue is also performed at this time with notations in upper eyelid fullness. Confirmation of adipose tissue herniation is performed with manual elevation of the brow and pressure upon the lower eyelid. Herniation of adipose tissue worsens with this maneuver, while lid edema remains unchanged.

Evaluation of the eyelid crease is performed by elevating the brow complex and having the patient look downward. At this point, the surgeon evaluates the distance from the observed crease at the central point of the eyelid to that of the lid/lash margin. This marginal crease distance (MCD) is 9 to 11 mm in average patient. Measurements of much higher dimension should raise suspicion of levator aponeurosis disinsertion and concomitant eyelid ptosis. This is different from retraction of the upper eyelid, commonly seen in thyroid ophthalmopathy, in which the MRD1 is excessive (see Preoperative Planning).

If fullness is discovered along the lateral aspect of the upper eyelid, the examiner should consider the possibility of a prolapsed lacrimal gland as there is no notable orbital fat that occupies the temporal region of the upper eyelids. As with the examination of herniation of adipose tissue, elevation of the brow and pressure on the lower eyelid helps to determine the presence of this condition and aid in surgical planning.

INDICATIONS

This procedure is primarily used to treat blepharoptosis in patients whose upper eyelids elevate after administration of phenylephrine. Candidates commonly have minimal congenital contribution to their ptosis, may present with varying degrees of acquired unilateral or bilateral ptosis, and may have had a prior external approach to surgically correct their lid ptosis. The procedure is especially useful in those individuals who have had upper blepharoplasty where the correction of the ptosis was unsuccessful or not addressed and where additional external approach surgery may be both difficult and/or risky. In rare situations, this procedure can be performed with good results in those people who respond poorly to phenylephrine.

CONTRAINDICATIONS

Surgically speaking, this procedure is contraindicated in patients whose upper eyelids do not elevate closely to a normal level with the phenylephrine test and in patients who have had a previous levator resection. Holistically speaking, the surgeon should also try to find out why the patient wants surgery now. In this way, the surgeon can differentiate patients who have realistic, mature reasons for requesting surgery from those who do not.

PREOPERATIVE PLANNING

Two tests are done preoperatively to determine optimal candidates for the Müller's muscle–conjunctival resection procedure:

- Margin reflex distance 1 (MRD1) measurement
- Phenylephrine test

MRD1 Test

The MRD1 measurement is used to assess the upper eyelid levels (Fig. 2.1). It should be performed both before and during the phenylephrine test. The difference in MRD1 between the normal and ptotic sides indicates the degree of ptosis. The normal MRD1 ranges from approximately 3.0 to 4.5 mm, and this value is used as a reference in bilateral cases. The MRD1 measurement has the advantage of being able to quantify the ptosis alone without the palpebral fissure width. This is preferred because there is a Müller's muscle in the lower eyelid that can also respond to phenylephrine. Measuring the palpebral fissure width would lead to an erroneous interpretation of the upper eyelid level after instillation of phenylephrine.

Phenylephrine Test

In patients with ptosis that is 2 mm or less, a phenylephrine test is an important tool in evaluating for the presence of an active Müller's muscle. The MRD1 is measured before and after the instillation of 2.5% or 10% phenylephrine drops. The patient can be partially reclined, and their head is tilted backward, the upper eyelid is lifted, and the patient is instructed to gaze downward. Several drops of phenylephrine are dripped between the upper eyelid and the globe. To minimize the entry of phenylephrine into the nasal cavity, the examiner may digitally compress the canaliculi for 10 seconds. Topical anesthetic is often useful to reduce or avoid the stinging that can occur with application of neosynephrine. This step may be repeated immediately two more times. Three to five minutes after instillation of the phenylephrine, the MRD1 is measured. If the MRD1 increases by 1.5 mm or more, an active Müller's muscle (positive test) is present and the patient is a candidate for a Müller's muscle–conjunctival resection–ptosis procedure. During this process, the contralateral eye should also be evaluated in patients with unilateral ptosis. The development of ptosis in the nontest eye commonly relates to the presence of bilateral ptosis and a clinical confirmation of Herring's law.

Patients should be warned about pupillary dilation after this test, which may yield transient photophobia and visual blurring. It is also not uncommon for patients to experience transient ocular irritation that might relate to dryness or exposure symptoms and indicate to the surgeon the possibility of dry eye symptoms after surgery.

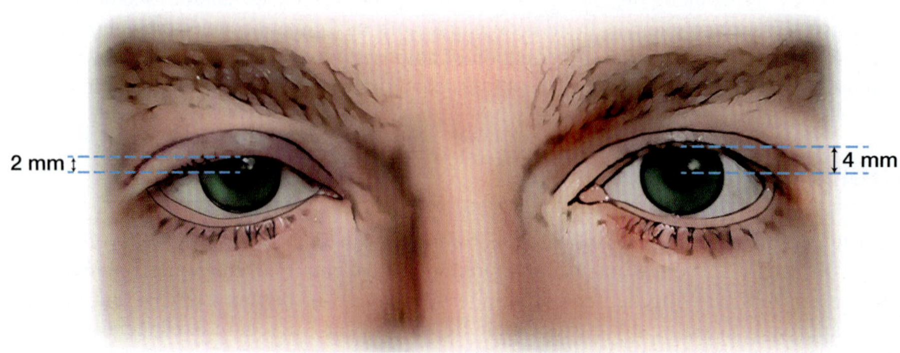

FIGURE 2.1 The margin reflex distance 1 (MRD1) is useful for determining the amount of ptosis. This is the distance from the light reflex on the patient's cornea to the central upper eyelid as the patient gazes in the primary position. The difference in MRD1 between the normal and ptotic lid determines the amount of ptosis.

SURGICAL TECHNIQUE

Anesthesia

Local anesthesia is preferred in adults. The upper eyelid skin to be removed is marked. A line is drawn with a methylene blue marking pen, beginning at the lateral canthus and extending in a horizontal direction of approximately 1 cm. This line marks the site of the lower lateral canthal incision. The site of the predetermined eyelid crease is then marked. When the surgeon is drawing the eyelid crease marks, the eyebrow must be elevated to reduce the excess upper eyelid skin fold and to make the upper eyelid skin taut and the lashes slightly everted. If this is not done, the crease may result in being much higher than desired because the skin is usually loose before it is marked.

The temporal, central, and nasal crease sites are marked by placing a millimeter ruler so that the zero line is at the eyelid margin. The distances above the eyelid margin can then be viewed and marked with a specially designed marking instrument. In women, the temporal mark usually is placed 10 mm above the upper eyelid margin; the central mark, 11 mm above the margin; and the nasal mark, 9 mm above the margin. In men, the marks are usually 9 mm temporally, 10 mm centrally, and 8 mm nasally. The temporal, central, and nasal marks are then connected and are extended with a line, which begins at the punctum and ends at the lateral canthus. The line sweeps laterally approximately 1 cm temporally to the lateral canthus in a slightly upward direction. There should be at least 5 mm of skin between this line and the line placed for the lower lateral incision.

A smooth forceps is used to grasp the crease line at the center of the eyelid with one blade. The other blade is used to pinch upper eyelid skin at various positions until, when the forceps is closed, all the redundant upper eyelid skin is eliminated and there is no eversion of the lashes and no lifting of the eyelid from its apposition to the lower eyelid margin. Once this position is determined, a dot is made with the marking pen at the top blade of the forceps. Similar marks are made nasally and temporally after the amounts of extra skin are determined in these positions. The three superior dots are connected and joined with the nasal and temporal ends of the eyelid crease line. The opposite eyelid is marked in the same manner. To ensure symmetry, the surgeon then compares the measurements of the eyelid crease and the amount of skin to be excised temporally, nasally, and centrally in the two eyelids (Fig. 2.2A).

A frontal nerve block is used with local anesthesia to avoid swelling and bruising of the upper eyelid by local infiltration, which would make the operation more difficult and inexact. After the upper eyelid is marked for blepharoplasty and the chosen sedative is administered, a 23-gauge retrobulbar needle is inserted into the superior orbit, entering just under the midsuperior orbital rim lateral to the supraorbital notch (Fig. 2.2B). The needle hugs the roof of the orbit during insertion until a depth of up to 4 cm is reached; then, 1.5 mL of 2% lidocaine (Xylocaine) with epinephrine is injected. Alternately, bupivacaine (Marcaine) may be used to prolong the anesthetic effect. Another 0.5 mL of the anesthetic solution is injected subcutaneously over the central upper eyelid just above the lid margin (where a traction suture of 4-0 silk is placed), and a small amount may be injected under the lines marked on the upper eyelid.

Marking Areas of Excision and Resection

A scratch incision is made over the marked upper blepharoplasty demarcations. A 4-0 black silk traction suture is inserted through skin, orbicularis muscle, and superficial tarsus 2 mm above the lashes at the center of the upper eyelid. Care must be taken to avoid a full-thickness penetration with this maneuver and injury to the corneal surface. A medium- or large-sized Desmarres lid retractor is used to evert the upper eyelid and to expose the palpebral conjunctiva from the superior tarsal border to the superior fornix. Topical tetracaine drops may be applied over the upper palpebral conjunctiva especially when light or no sedation is administered.

A caliper set at the determined amount of resection (i.e., 8.5 mm in a unilateral repair in those whose neosynephrine test restored the upper eyelid to the desired position), with one arm at the superior tarsal border, facilitates insertion of a 6-0 black silk suture through the conjunctiva 8.5 mm above the superior tarsal border (Fig. 2.2C). One suture bite centrally and two others approximately 7 mm nasal and temporal to the center mark the site. The preferred placement of the 6-0 black silk marking suture is 8.5 mm above the superior tarsal border (in those individuals with unilateral ptosis whose neosynephrine test brings them to a symmetric and satisfactory position), but the suture may be placed 6.0 to 9.5 mm above the border if the response of the upper eyelid level to the phenylephrine test is slightly greater or less than desired. The smaller resections (6.0 to 6.5 mm range) are typically more technically difficult to administer using the prescribed clamp, described below. The placement of this marking suture should be through conjunctiva only as penetration into or through Müller's muscle may cause significant bleeding.

Separation of Müller's Muscle from the Levator Aponeurosis

A toothed forceps is used to grasp conjunctiva and Müller's muscle between the superior tarsal border and the marking suture and to separate Müller's muscle from its loose attachment to the levator aponeurosis. This maneuver is possible because Müller's muscle is firmly attached to conjunctiva but only loosely attached to the levator aponeurosis.

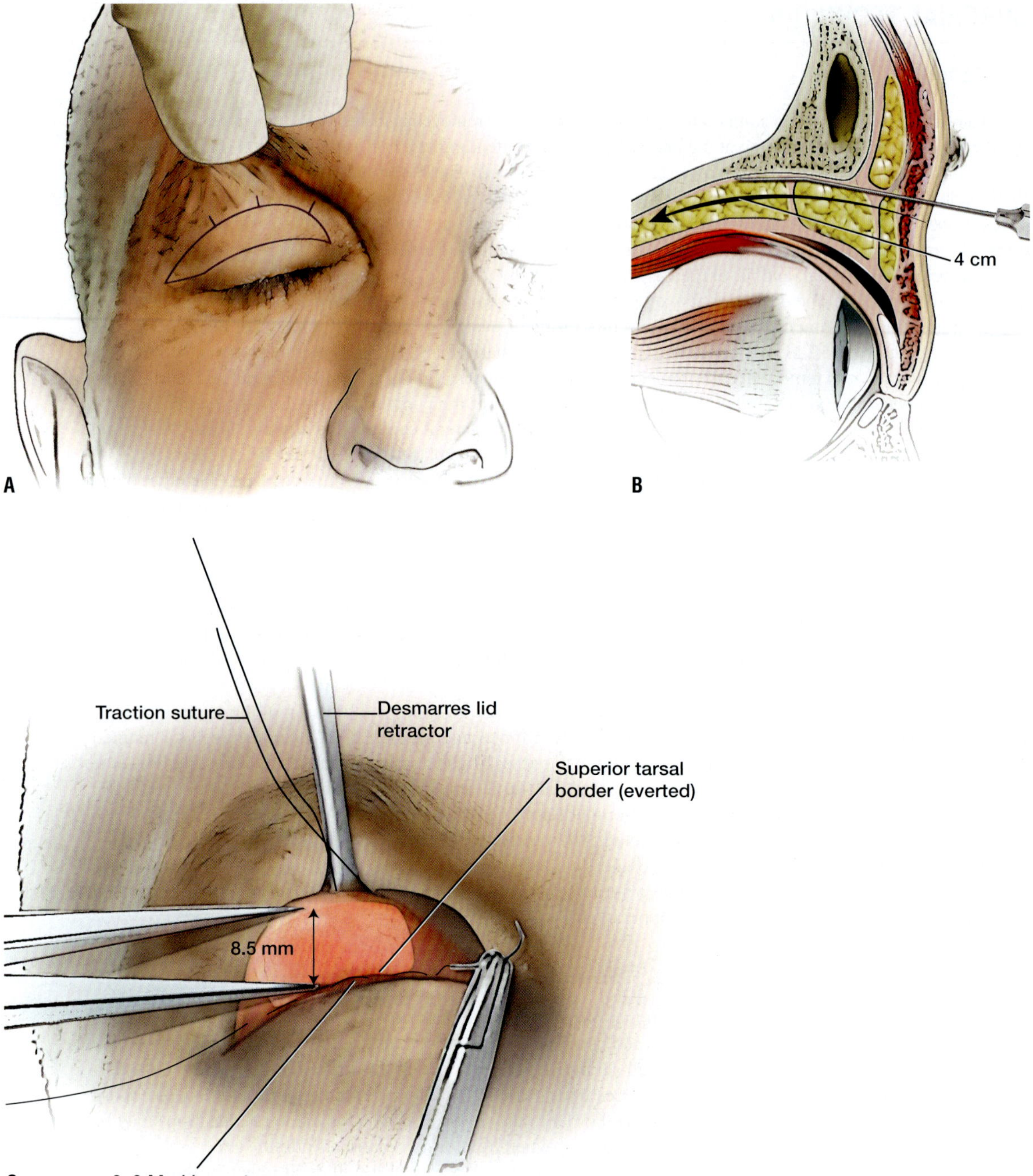

FIGURE 2.2 **A:** Outline of skin or skin and orbicularis oculi muscle to be excised. **B:** Administration of anesthesia before the Müller's muscle–conjunctival resection. A 4-cm, 23-gauge retrobulbar needle is inserted along the central orbital roof to its full length. An injection of 1.5 mL of 2% lidocaine with epinephrine achieves a frontal nerve block and avoids infiltration of the eyelid. **C:** The upper eyelid is everted over a Desmarres retractor, and a 6-0 black silk marking suture is placed through conjunctiva 6 to 9.5 mm above the superior tarsal border. One suture bite is taken centrally, and one bite is made 7 mm nasal and temporal to the central bite.

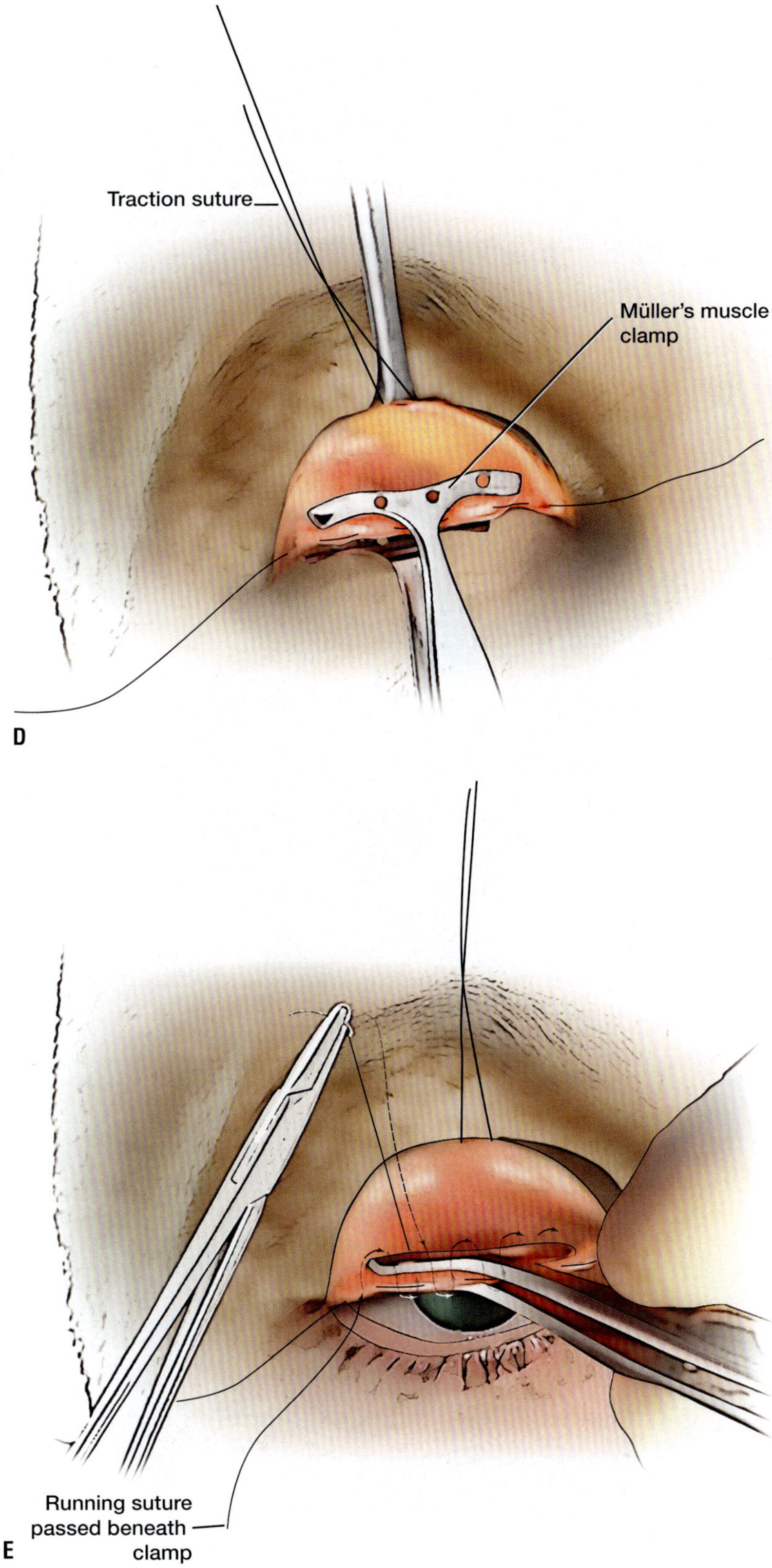

FIGURE 2.2 (*Continued*) **D:** A clamp is positioned so that each tooth of one blade engages each site of the marking suture; the other blade is above the superior tarsal border. **E:** As the Desmarres retractor is gradually released through rotation, the other clamp blade slides over tarsus as its teeth engage conjunctiva and Müller's muscle above the superior tarsal border.

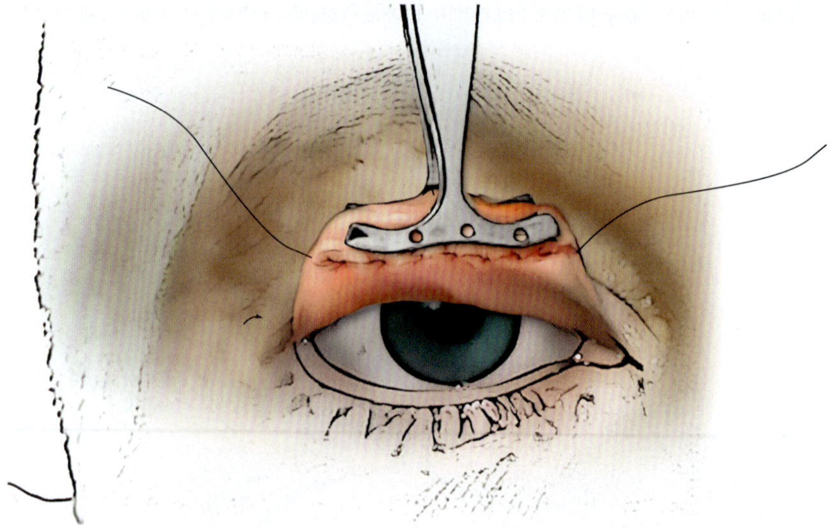

F

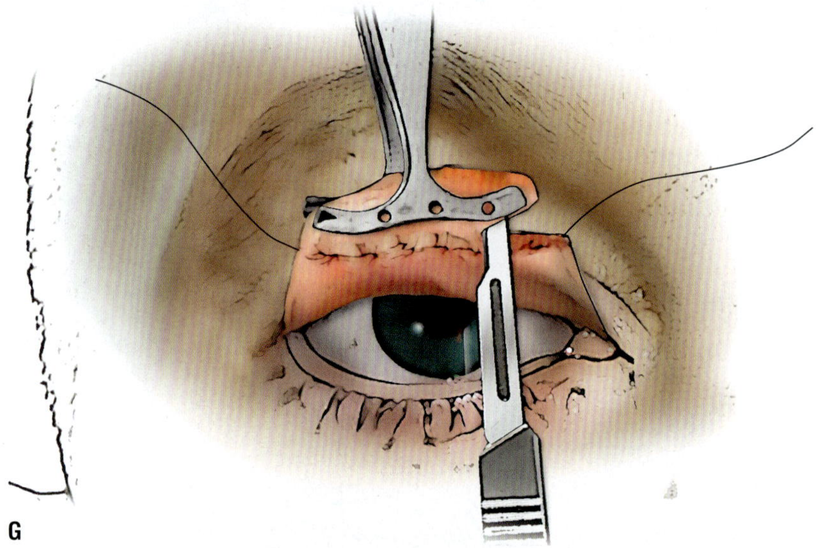

G

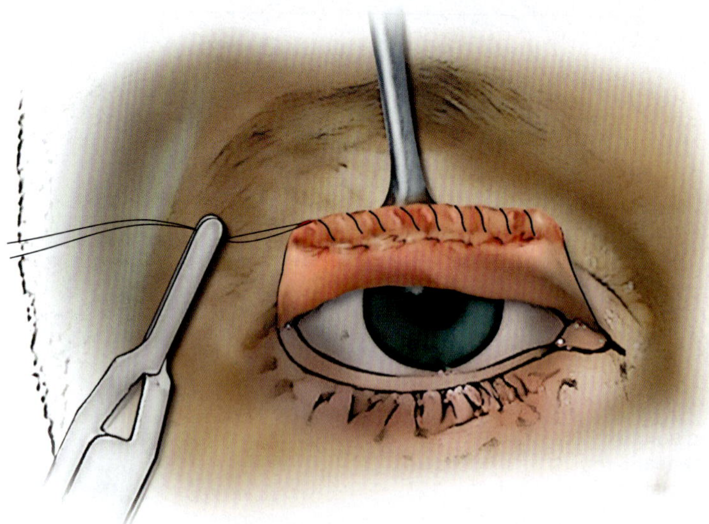

H

FIGURE 2.2 (*Continued*) **F:** A 5-0 plain catgut mattress suture runs in a temporal-to-nasal direction about 1.5 mm distal to the clamp; each suture bite includes upper tarsus, Müller's muscle, and conjunctiva. **G:** Conjunctiva–Müller's muscle is excised by running a no. 15 surgical blade against the edge of the clamp. **H:** The nasal suture arm runs continuously in a nasal-to-temporal direction through the edges of conjunctiva, Müller's muscle, and tarsus. Each arm of the suture passes through conjunctiva and Müller's muscle and exits through the temporal incision; the suture arms are tied.

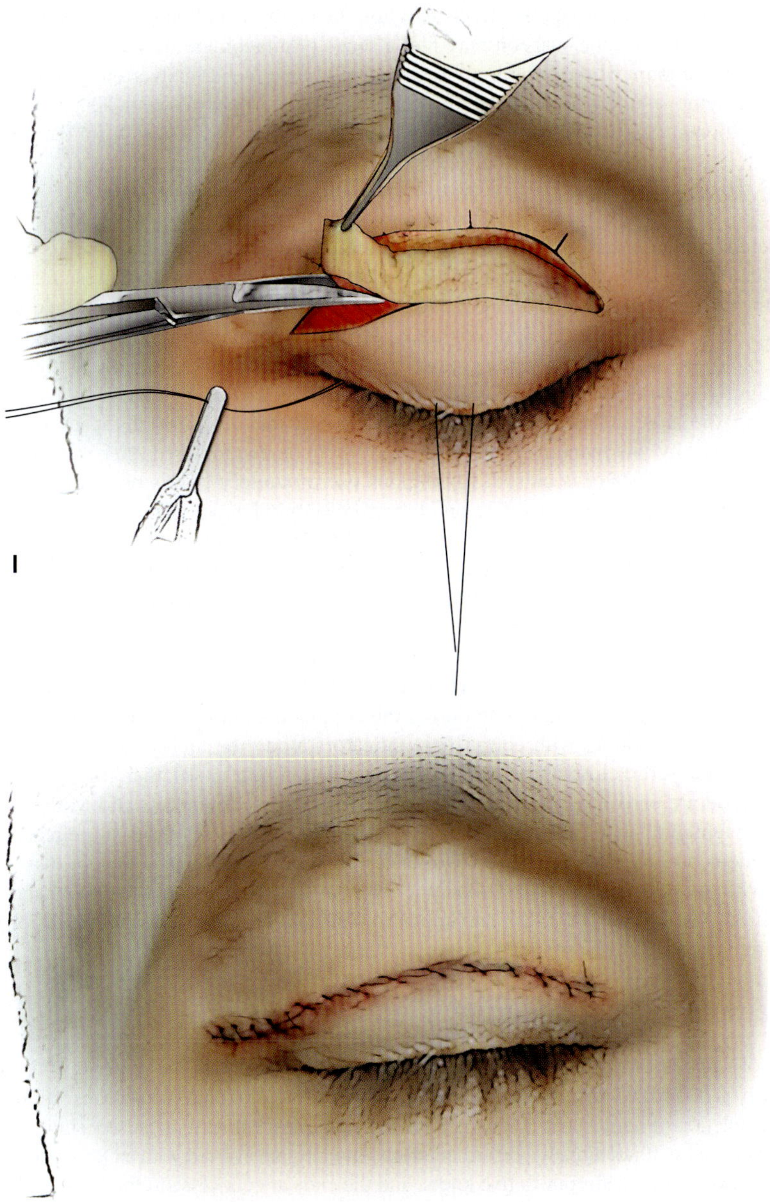

I

J

FIGURE 2.2 (*Continued*) **I:** Excision of outline ellipse of the skin and orbicularis muscle with a disposable cautery. **J:** Placement of three 6-0 polyglactin (Vicryl) sutures uniting the skin and levator aponeurosis. A 6-0 continuous silk suture closes the skin.

Clamp Application

Although this procedure can be performed with a variety of clamps and other instruments, it is much more easily and precisely performed with a particular instrument made for this procedure. One blade of this specially designed Müller's muscle–conjunctival resection–ptosis clamp (Bausch & Lomb, Storz Company, Manchester, MO) should be placed at the level of the marking suture. Each tooth of this blade engages each suture bite that passes through the palpebral conjunctiva (Fig. 2.2D). The Desmarres retractor is then slowly released (with the handle of the retractor brought from the resting cephalad position to a caudal position) as the other blade of the clamp engages conjunctiva and Müller's muscle adjacent to the superior tarsal border (Fig. 2.2E). Any entrapped tarsus is then released from the clamp with the surgeon's finger. The clamp is compressed, and the handle is locked. This leads to the incorporation of conjunctiva and Müller's muscle between the superior tarsal border and the marking suture.

The upper eyelid skin is pulled in one direction while the clamp is pulled simultaneously in the opposite direction. During this maneuver, the surgeon may feel a sense of attachment between the skin and the clamp. If this occurs, a greater amount of the levator aponeurosis may have been inadvertently trapped in the clamp. In this situation, the clamp should be released and reapplied into its proper position. This maneuver is possible because the levator aponeurosis sends extensions to orbicularis muscle and skin to form the lid crease.

Suturing and Resection of Conjunctiva and Müller's Muscle

With the clamp held straight up/vertically, a 5-0 double-armed plain catgut mattress suture is run 1.5 mm below the clamp along its entire width in a temporal-to-nasal direction in a horizontal mattress fashion, through the upper margin of the tarsus on one side and through Müller's muscle and conjunctiva on the other side and vice versa (Fig. 2.2F). The sutures are placed approximately 2 to 3 mm from each other. The surgeon uses a no. 15 surgical blade to excise the tissues held in the clamp by cutting between the sutures and the clamp. The knife blade is rotated slightly, with its sharp edge hugging the clamp (Fig. 2.2G). As the tissues are incised and separated from the clamp, the surgeon and the assistant watch to ensure that the plain catgut sutures on each side are not inadvertently severed by this maneuver. Bleeding will likely be encountered after this incision and almost always ceases once the conjunctiva is closed. Injudicious use of cautery at this point might also result in an inadvertent disruption of the plain catgut suture and therefore should be avoided.

The Desmarres retractor is used again to evert the eyelid while gentle traction is applied to the 4-0 black silk centering suture. The nasal end of the suture is then run continuously in a temporal direction; the suture passes should be about 2 mm apart and through the edge of superior tarsal border, Müller's muscle, and conjunctiva (Fig. 2.2H). Commonly, this suture just connects the edges of conjunctiva. During continuous closure with the 5-0 plain catgut suture, the surgeon must be careful to avoid cutting the original mattress suture. This is facilitated by the surgeon's using a small suture needle (S-14 Spatula, Ethicon) in addition to observing the mattress suture position during each suture bite during the conjunctival closure. The assistant should be applying continuous suction or swabbing with cotton-tip applicators along the incision edges. If the original horizontal mattress placement is too close to the clamp edge (within 1.5 mm or so), then this will be more difficult. The 5-0 plain catgut suture ends are passed through each side of the conjunctiva and Müller's muscle before they exit through the temporal end of the incision (Fig. 2.2H). Once each arm of the suture reaches the temporal end of the eyelid, the suture ends are connected with a serrefine clamp. This is to ensure that the suture is not inadvertently cut with the skin–muscle flap of the upper blepharoplasty procedure to follow and, if so, it can be more easily identified. Alternatively, if a skin flap upper blepharoplasty (without muscle excision) is performed, the suture can be tied (described below) at this time.

Upper Blepharoplasty

Several milliliters of same anesthetic solution is injected subcutaneously over the upper eyelids. Then, an upper eyelid blepharoplasty is performed through the steps of skin or skin and orbicularis muscle resection, excision of adipose tissue, and completion of hemostasis (Fig. 2.2I). Once again, please note that cautery should be minimized to avoid cutting the plain suture. If not already performed, the eyelid is again everted with a Desmarres retractor, the 5-0 plain catgut suture arms are tied with four to five knots, and the ends are cut close to the knot. In this way, the knot can be buried subconjunctivally, lessening postoperative keratopathy and surface irritation. After this step, the crease sutures are placed, and the skin is closed (Fig. 2.2J). If no crease is reconstructed, the skin is sutured at this time.

POSTOPERATIVE MANAGEMENT

Patients are observed postoperatively, as with blepharoplasty in general, to make sure that there is no excessive bleeding or possibility of retrobulbar hemorrhage, which has the potential for causing blindness. The patient applies cold compresses to the eyelids for the first 24 hours postoperatively. A topical antibiotic such as gentamicin (Garamycin) or a combination antibiotic/corticosteroid (TobraDex) ophthalmic ointment on the eye can be used once or twice a day for the first week or two. The patient may also use a sterile eyewash applied to cotton pads to wipe over the eyelids twice a day for 2 weeks after surgery. Patients are instructed for the first 2 weeks after surgery to bathe or shower only from the neck down and to wash their hair so that an abundant contact of soap and water with the eyes is avoided.

COMPLICATIONS

As with any surgery, there are a wide range of complications ranging from suboptimal to catastrophic. In each of these circumstances, it is important for the clinician to remain mindful of any symptoms or clues that indicate the early stages of a more advanced condition.

- Bleeding: Bleeding can range across a spectrum from simple bruising to a retrobulbar hemorrhage.
  - Soft tissue bruising: A common event, and under normal circumstances, this is very limited. Supportive patient counseling and warm compresses are helpful in resolving this problem.
  - Eyelid hematoma: This is a rare event and often indicates some degree of coagulopathy. If bleeding is continuous despite gentle pressure therapy (very rare), the wound should be opened, the hematoma removed, and hemostasis obtained.
  - Retrobulbar hematoma: This is a true medical emergency with a significant risk for loss of vision due to the development of an orbital compartment syndrome. All patients who complain of eye pain (not incisional pain), decreased visual acuity, proptosis, and marked difference in globe compressibility should be immediately evaluated. In the event of this acute circumstance, a lateral canthotomy and inferior catholysis can save vision as it releases the orbital compartment. Surgical exploration will be required for evacuation of the clot and repair of the canthus.
- Ocular Injury:
  - Corneal abrasion: Causes are numerous, and symptoms are often expressed by the patient in recovery after anesthesia has worn off and relate a foreign body sensation. Supportive measures of erythromycin ointment and drops are given. Consultation with an ophthalmologist is also prudent.
  - Globe trauma: Injury to the globe can occur in nearly any surgery and at any stage. The first measure is prevention. This is also a true ophthalmic emergency and requires immediate attention by a specialist.
- Asymmetry: This is commonly observed in the postoperative period and, to some degree, is expected. True evaluation for long-standing asymmetries should be performed after all swelling and bruising has resolved.
- Lagophthalmos: The incomplete closure of the eyelids can occur when the appropriate amount of soft tissues have been removed. Such a condition resolves over time. However, aggressive resection of soft tissues or suture placement into the orbital septum can limit eyelid motion. If conservative measures of massage and emollient therapy are unsuccessful, one may need to surgically explore the site with the subsequent removal of any restrictive scarring or suture. In the worst of circumstances, skin grafting may be necessary.
- Dry eyes: Patients with dry eyes will convey a history of continual, and even painful, ocular irritation. Treatment involves ocular hydration with ointment and artificial tear solutions. Punctal plugs may be necessary in patients with persistent symptomology.
- Scarring: With any surgical procedure, there is the risk for unfavorable scarring. Risks for unfavorable scarring in blepharoplasty include infection, hypertrophic or keloid history, wound dehiscence, suture retention, and tension. Scars in the eyelid region often heal in excellent fashion as long as the surgical incisions are appropriately placed. Conservative treatments involving massage, steroid injections, and taping are very helpful.
- Overcorrection of ptosis: Occasionally, the upper eyelid is too high (overcorrection). If this elevation occurs, the patient massages the upper eyelid downward while simultaneously fixating the brow two to four times each day for 1 to 4 weeks. If a gross overcorrection is encountered in the first 7 to 10 days, the plain suture can either simply cut or cut *and* excised followed by massage until the satisfactory eyelid position is achieved. If massage is ultimately ineffective or does not bring the upper lid to an optimum level, an external levator recession may be performed.

RESULTS

The average follow-up is 3.3 months but varies from 2 weeks to 7 years. Follow-up generally lasts until the patient's eyelids cease to change. The MRD1 at stabilization of lid levels is considered the final result.

In most patients with acquired ptosis (90% in my experience), the final eyelid level after treatment is within 2 mm of the opposite eyelid. In 88% of these treated eyelids, an MRD1 of 1.5 to 5 mm is achieved (Figs. 2.3 and 2.4). Patients with congenital ptosis have a final eyelid level after treatment within 1.5 mm of the opposite eyelid. In 84% of these treated eyelids, an MRD1 of 2.5 to 5 mm is achieved.

Rarely, in less than 2% of patients, additional surgery may be required to treat residual ptosis. This is most often achieved with a levator aponeurosis procedure. However, in rare situations, an internal approach resection may be repeated.

PEARLS

- A toothed forceps is used to grasp conjunctiva and Müller's muscle to separate Müller's muscle from its loose attachment to the levator aponeurosis.
- If there is a sense of attachment between the skin and the clamp, the levator aponeurosis may have been inadvertently trapped and needs to be released.
- Exiting the temporal wound with each arm of the suture allows the suture knot to slip subconjunctivally and avoids suture keratopathy.

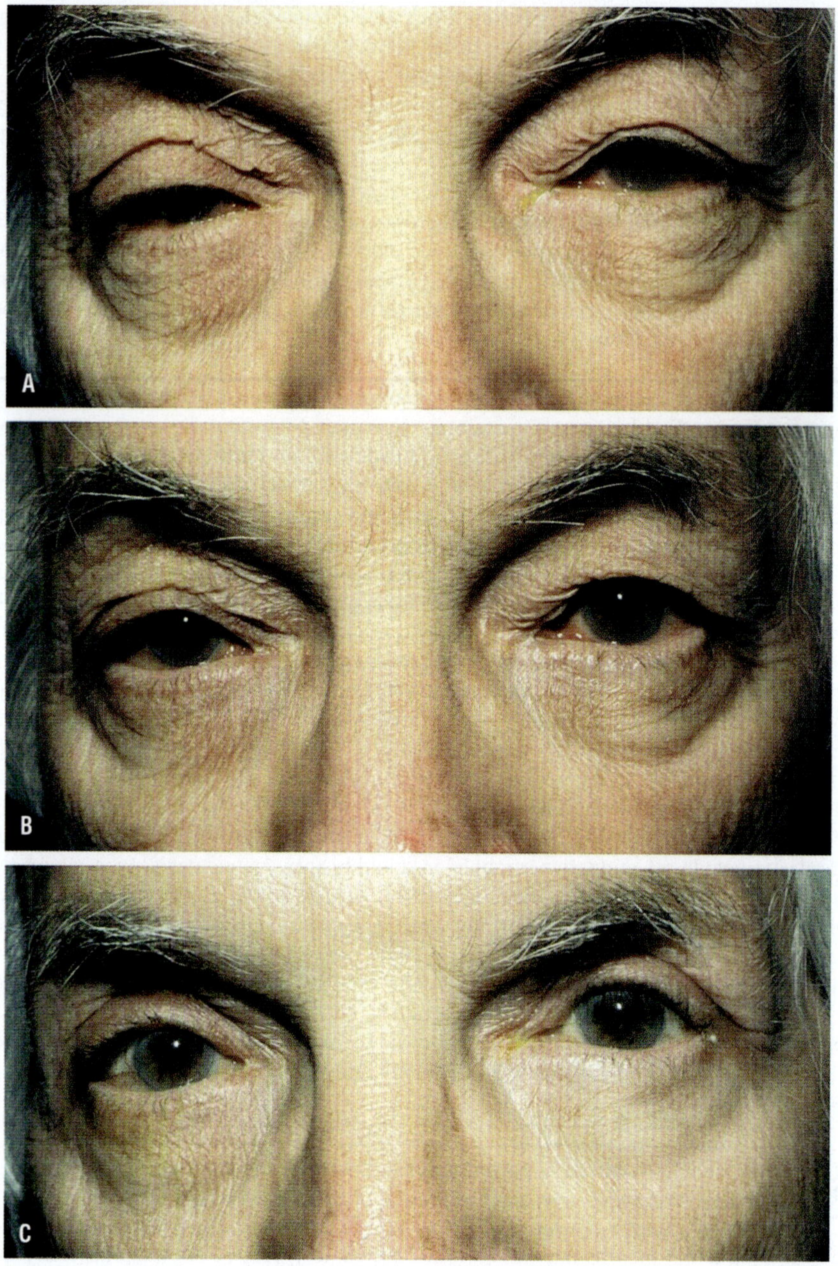

FIGURE 2.3 A: Preoperative appearance of a patient with bilateral upper eyelid ptosis associated with dermatochalasis (excessive skin) and herniated adipose tissue of all four eyelids. **B:** After instillation of phenylephrine in both upper fornices with elevation of both upper eyelids. **C:** After a bilateral Müller's muscle–conjunctival resection–ptosis procedure and excision of skin, orbicularis muscle, and orbital adipose tissue from both upper eyelids with eyelid crease reconstruction.

PITFALLS

- Accidental injury to Müller's muscle with a marking suture could lead to a subconjunctival hemorrhage. This can distort the muscle–conjunctival interface and lead to a conjunctival resection only.
- Engaging the teeth of the Müller's muscle clamp into each of the marking suture sites avoids the clamp not engaging Müller's muscle.
- Keeping the 5-0 plain mattress suture 1.5 mm from the distal end of the clamp avoids cutting the suture inadvertently.
- Place frontal nerve blocks in the center of the orbital roof. This avoids hitting the supraorbital artery, which could lead to a retrobulbar hemorrhage.

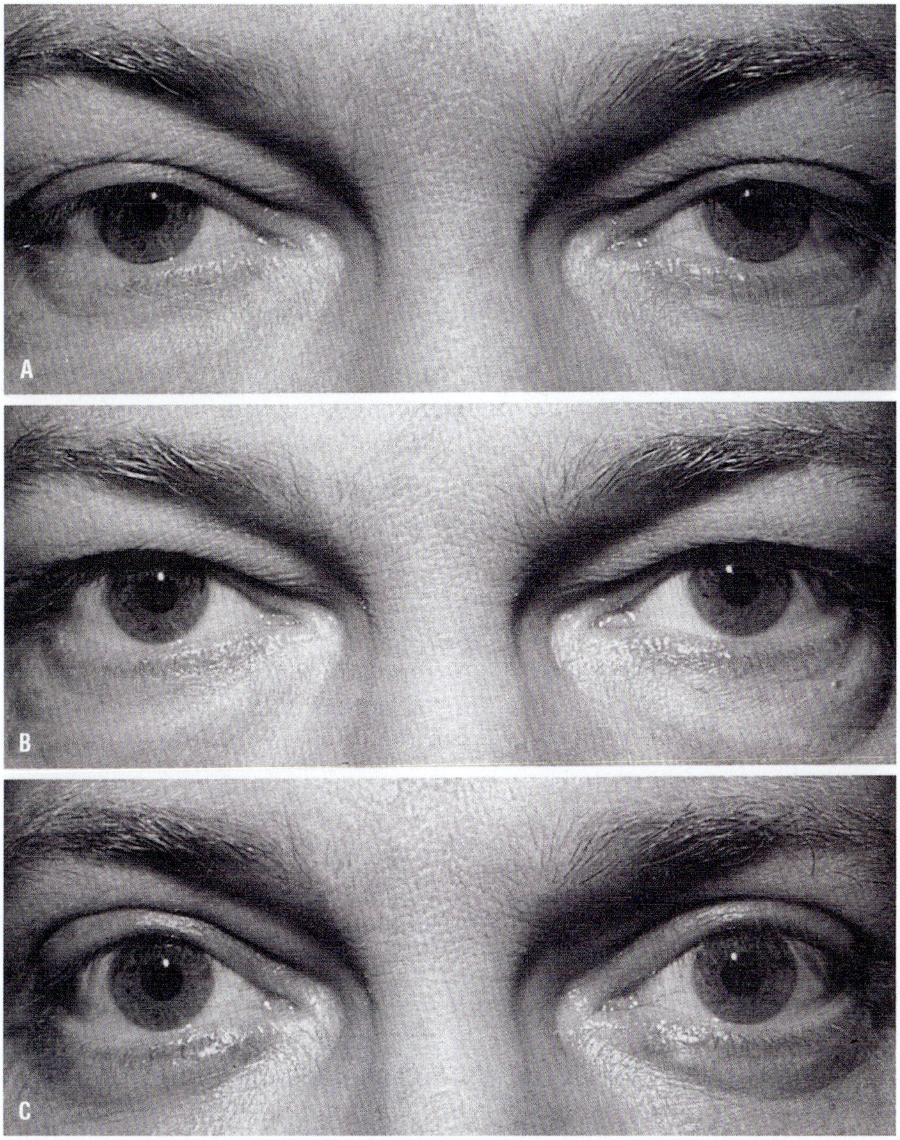

FIGURE 2.4 A: Preoperative appearance of a patient with upper eyelid ptosis associated with dermatochalasis and herniated orbital adipose tissue of all four eyelids. **B:** After instillation of phenylephrine in both upper fornices with elevation of eyelids to normal levels. **C:** After bilateral Müller's muscle–conjunctival resection–ptosis procedure with excision of skin, orbicularis oculi muscle, and orbital adipose tissue from the upper eyelids and eyelid crease reconstruction. A lower eyelid external blepharoplasty using a skin–muscle flap approach was performed simultaneously.

INSTRUMENTS TO HAVE AVAILABLE

- Putterman Müller's Muscle Conjunctival Resection Ptosis Clamp (Baush & Lomb Storz Company, Manchester, MO)
- Caliper
- Large Desmarre retractor
- Forceps with teeth
- No. 15 Bard-Parker blade and handle
- Needle holder
- Westcott scissors
- Disposable cautery

ACKNOWLEDGMENT

The material presented in this Chapter is a revision of Chapter 11 in Putterman's Cosmetic Oculoplastic Surgery 4th Edition titled "Müller's Muscle–Conjunctival Resection–Ptosis Procedure Combined with Upper Blepharoplasty" Putterman, A., Fagien, S., p. 123-133, Ed. Fagien, S., Elsevier, 2008 and is published with permission from Elsevier Publishing Co.

SUGGESTED READING

Fraunfelder FT, Scafidi A. Possible adverse effect from topical ocular 10% phenylephrine. *Am J Ophthalmol* 1978;85:447–453.

Glatt HJ, Fett DR, Putterman AM. Comparison of 2.5% and 10% phenylephrine in the elevation of upper eyelids with ptosis. *Ophthalmic Surg* 1990;21:173:447–453.

Putterman AM. Basic oculoplastic surgery. In: Peyman GA, Saunders DR, Goldberg MF, eds. *Principles and practice of ophthalmology*. Philadelphia, PA: WB Saunders Co., 1980.

Putterman AM, Fett DR. Müller's muscle in the treatment of upper eyelid ptosis: a ten-year study. *Ophthalmic Surg* 1986;17:354–356.

Putterman AM, Urist MJ. Müller's muscle–conjunctival resection: technique for treatment of blepharoptosis. *Arch Ophthalmol* 1975;93:619–623.

3 LOWER EYELID BLEPHAROPLASTY: TRANSCUTANEOUS APPROACH

E. Gaylon McCollough

INTRODUCTION

The goal of aesthetic plastic surgery is rather simple: correct the undesirable conditions for which a surgeon has been consulted and avoid the telltale signs of surgery. This objective is best accomplished by accurately identifying the combination of issues that are responsible for the appearance of aging eyelids. Moreover, the surgeon must use the correct combination of rejuvenation procedures to create more youthful appearing eyelids. In an article coauthored with Dr. James English in 1988, I described a number of safeguards that tend to preserve naturally appearing eyes following lower lid blepharoplasty. These points are crucial in ensuring success with this approach.

HISTORY

During the consultation, if the surgeon suspects or identifies pathologic conditions of the eyes, a preoperative consultation with an Ophthalmologist should be considered. Any history of dry eyes, visual changes, or tearing is important to elicit.

PHYSICAL EXAMINATION

The eye should be evaluated for symmetry and the position of the lower eyelids with respect to the limbus. Baseline visual acuity should be documented ideally by a complete examination performed by an Ophthalmologist. Schirmer's test and tear film break up times can be used as necessary when dry eye symptoms are present or suspected.

Strength of the lower lid suspensory hammock can be determined by the "distraction test," that is, gently pulling the lid away from the globe. A distraction of more than 10 mm indicates lids laxity. Another method of determining the tone of the lower lid is the "snap test" to forcefully pull the lid downward and release it. With either test, a lid with a good "hammock" will snap back into position. On the other hand, a lid that floats back or remains in an abnormal position will usually require additional surgical maneuvers. Otherwise, the possibility of a round eye and/or ectropion becomes more likely. Assessment of the degree and location of any protrusion of orbital adipose tissue should be made and documented.

INDICATIONS

Skin–muscle flap techniques are frequently recommended when there is bulging adipose tissue and skin/muscle also to remove. Bulging adipose tissue can be adequately removed and/or repositioned and minimal–moderate skin laxity can be adequately addressed. In experienced hands, a skin resurfacing procedure (laser or chemical peeling) can be performed at the same time to address fine lines but only if a layer of muscle remains attached to the under layer of eyelid skin (as is the case in skin–muscle flap or transconjunctival techniques).

Significant redundancy of lower lid skin is best corrected with a skin flap. When a skin flap technique is used in a lid with atonia of its tarso-fascial sling, downward traction on the lower lid during healing may occur as a sheet of contracting scar develops under the previously undetermined flap.

CONTRAINDICATIONS

Absolute and relative contraindications include significant ptosis of the eyebrows, systemic conditions such as excessive bleeding, active thyroid ophthalmopathy, blepharochalasis, blepharospasm, and symptoms of "dry eyes." A patient who has unrealistic expectations about the cosmetic outcome should also be excluded.

PREOPERATIVE PLANNING

During the preoperative consultation, a surgeon has an opportunity to identify conditions that may herald a potential problem postoperatively. The strength of the lower lid hammock and any preoperative scleral show should be noted and pointed out to the patient. Photographic documentation of the preoperative state is also essential.

As a rule, blepharoplasty tends to improve the sags and bulges but does not remove wrinkles in the skin around the eye. If wrinkling of the skin is noted at the time of consultation, the surgeon should advise the patient of the potential for a skin resurfacing procedure (chemical exfoliation or laser resurfacing) to provide additional improvement. In most cases, skin resurfacing is performed from 8 to 12 weeks following blepharoplasty. When transconjunctival adipose tissue removal is performed or when a skin–muscle technique is used, skin resurfacing may be performed at the time of blepharoplasty. Patients should be duly informed of the potential risks of combining these procedures.

The two principal approaches to removing excessive tissues in the lower lid are the skin flap technique and the skin–muscle flap technique. When bulging infraorbital adipose tissue needs to be addressed—without the presence of redundant skin—a transconjunctival approach may be considered. The correct diagnosis determines which technique is used in each individual patient.

Presence of an atonic or hypotonic lower lid should be noted, and this would require performing a pentagonal full-thickness wedge resection of the lower lid. For best results, the surgeon should place the center-most portion of pentagon (and resulting scar) at the lateral margin of the limbus.

SURGICAL TECHNIQUE

In the preoperative holding room, the appropriate blepharoplasty skin incisions are outlined with a skin-marking pen. Once the patient arrives in the operating room—and after conscious sedation anesthesia is instituted—lidocaine (1%) with epinephrine (1:100,000) is injected into the surgical areas, taking care not to injure underlying structures.

If performed in conjunction with lower lid blepharoplasty, the upper lid is corrected first. After excision of excessive upper lid skin and removal of any adipose tissue pads needed, a tacking suture is placed at a point that coincides with the lateral canthus to anchor the inferior edge of the upper lid defect to the upper edge. This maneuver tends to stabilize the lateral canthal region in its new position. Once the upper lid blepharoplasty is complete, the lower lid skin incision is made with a no. 15 blade. This incision should be placed with traction on the lower lid in the first lower lid skin crease (approximately 4 to 6 mm below the free border of the lash margin) (Fig. 3.1). The incision, which is carried only through skin, begins a few millimeters lateral to the punctum medially and courses laterally just past a vertical line dropped from the lateral canthus. At this point, the incision curves inferiorly and laterally 4 to 6 mm following a naturally occurring relaxed skin tension line (Fig. 3.2). Doing so, results in a more aesthetically pleasing postoperative scar.

In a skin flap procedure, undermining is carried inferiorly to the edge of the infraorbital rim. Access to the adipose tissue pads is achieved by dividing the fibers of the orbicularis oculi muscle approximately 5 to 6 mm cephalad to the rim.

In skin–muscle flap procedures, a small curved Iris Scissor is used to spread and penetrate the orbicularis oculi muscle laterally (Fig. 3.3). A blunt scissor is then used to undermine the entire skin–muscle flap to a point just cephalad to the infraorbital rim (Fig. 3.4). Once the undersurface of the orbicularis oculi muscle has been freed from the orbital septum, one blade of the scissor is placed in the previously created pocket beneath the muscle. The other blade of the scissor is placed externally along the initial skin incision. A beveled incision through the orbicularis oculi muscle and subcutaneous tissue is completed with the blades of the scissors (Fig. 3.5). Since the skin–muscle flap is selected in those patients with minimal skin redundancy, the flap is reflected allowing for visualization of the orbital septum (Fig. 3.6).

Bulging adipose tissue pads can be more accurately removed by incising the overlying orbital septum while placing gentle digital pressure on the globe (Fig. 3.7). This maneuver causes the excessive adipose tissue

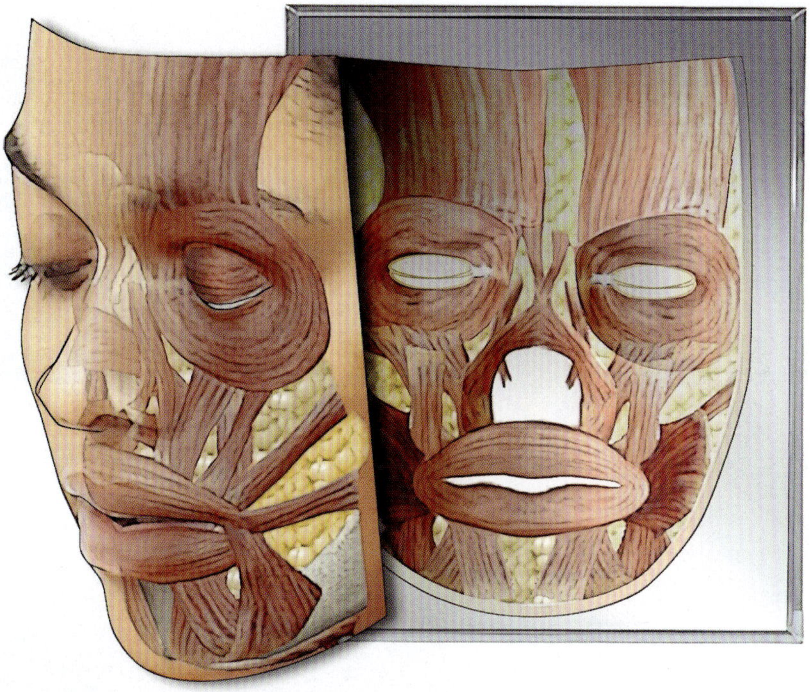

FIGURE 3.1 Note anatomic relationships of tarsal plate and pretarsal orbicularis oculi muscle. Optimal incision site is at inferior border of tarsal plate in order to preserve the pretarsal fibers of the muscle.

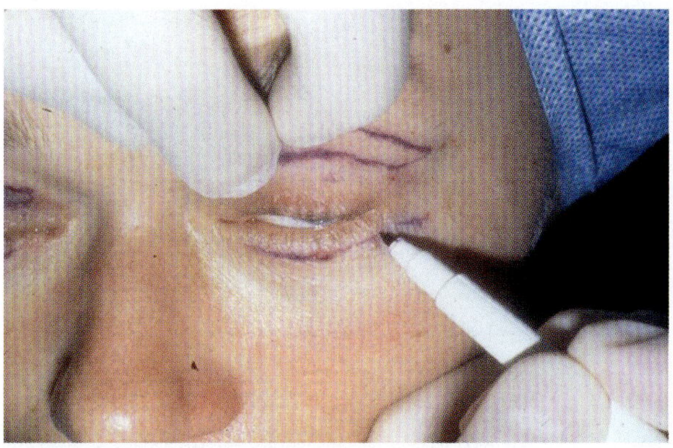

FIGURE 3.2
Marking pen outline of incision placement.

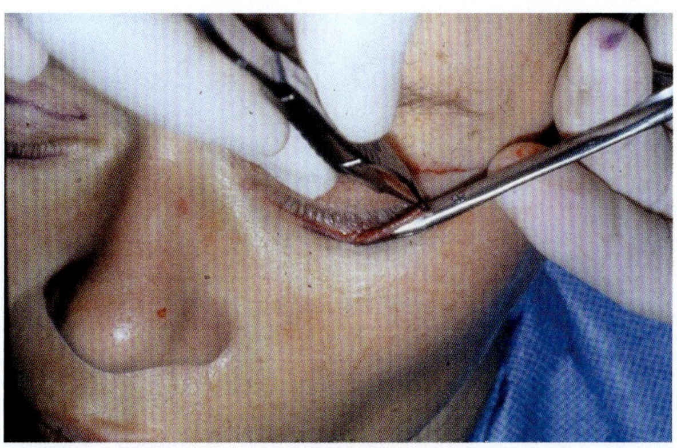

FIGURE 3.3
After the skin incision is made, submuscular dissection is begun with sharply pointed scissors.

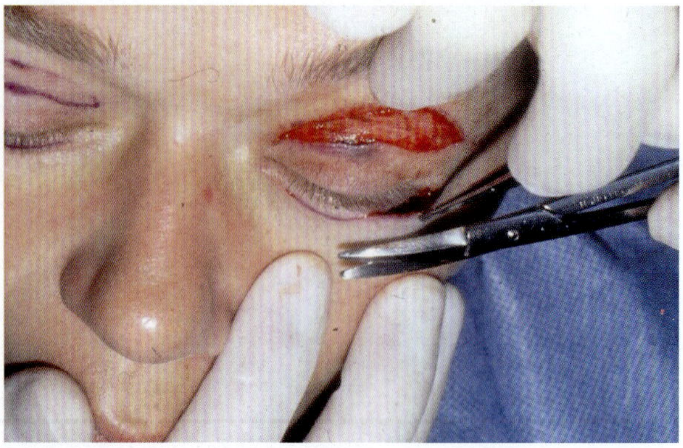

FIGURE 3.4
After a submuscular pocket is established, a blunt tip scissor is used to dissect under the muscle.

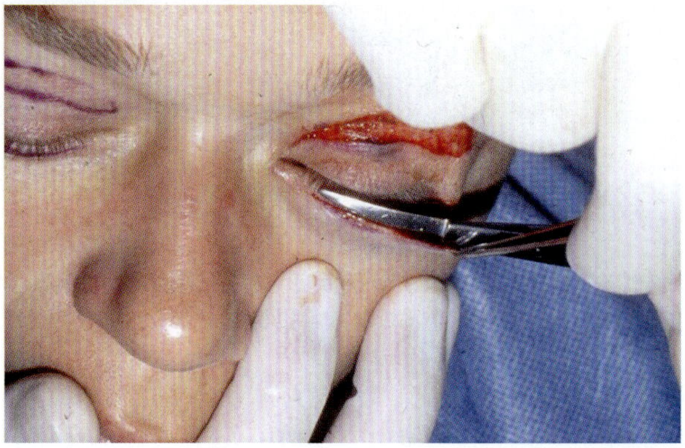

FIGURE 3.5
A beveled skin–muscle flap is created using blunt tip scissor.

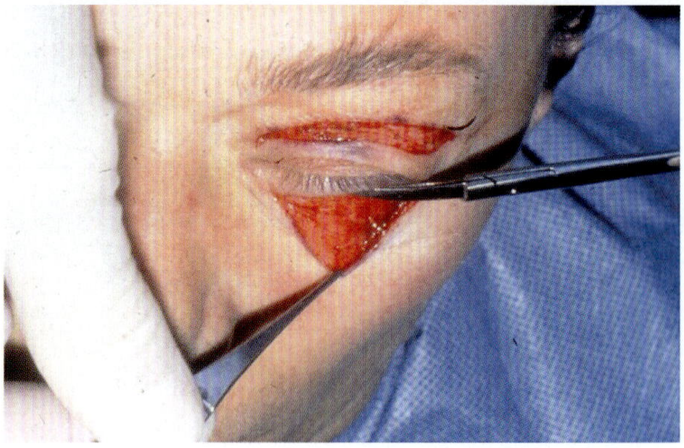

FIGURE 3.6
The skin–muscle flap is retracted exposing the orbital septum.

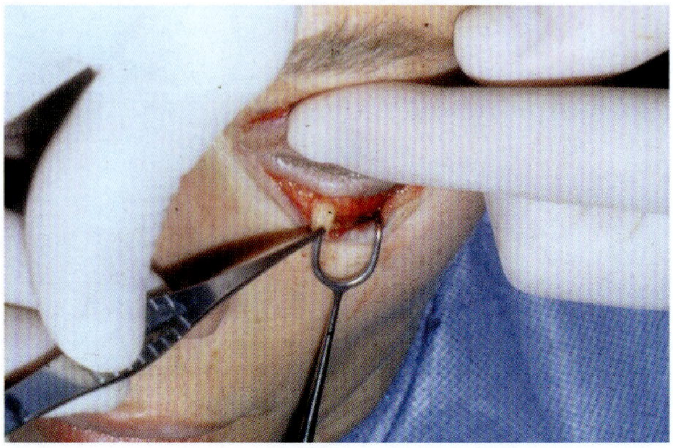

FIGURE 3.7
An incision is made into the orbital septum to expose protruding adipose tissue pads in each compartment.

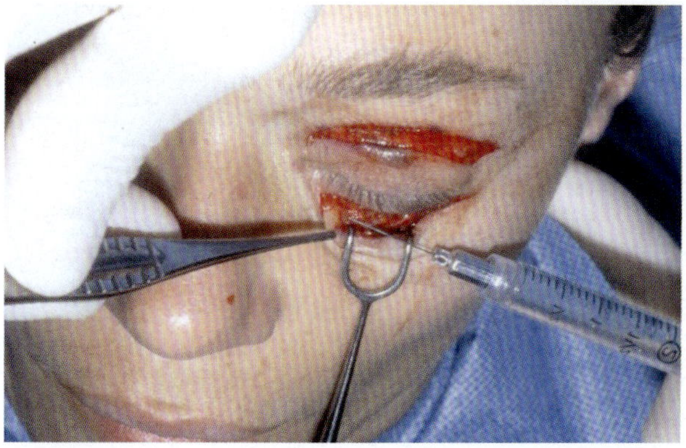

FIGURE 3.8
Injection of 1% plain lidocaine at the base of each adipose tissue pad prevents pain during cauterization.

to bulge through the orbital septum for easy amputation. Unless patients are under general anesthesia, prior to excision, the base of the adipose tissue stalk is injected with local anesthetic (without epinephrine) (Fig. 3.8). The stalk is then generously cauterized with bipolar cautery (Fig. 3.9). Only the portions of adipose tissue that exude easily through the defect in the orbital septum are removed (Fig. 3.10).

When each adipose tissue compartment has been adequately treated, redundant lid tissue is excised. If a skin flap with horizontal division of the orbicularis muscle was used, the muscle fibers are first reapproximated and secured with two to three absorbable 6-0 catgut sutures.

The flap is then advanced superiorly and laterally, draping the excess over the incision line. Small vertical incisions are now made into the overlapping portions, dividing the tissue to be removed into three or four segments. This maneuver adds a measure of safety and tends to prevent excess skin removal.

When both the skin and muscle incisions are placed at—or beyond—the inferior margin of the tarsus, it is not necessary to remove a strip of muscle from the undersurface of a skin–muscle flap. Once the overlapping skin and muscle have been removed, the wound edges are precisely closed with a 7-0 monofilament suture (Fig. 3.11). Once complete, there is often edema present at the end of the case (Fig. 3.12).

If small infraorbital festoons are present, an extended skin flap technique may be all that is needed. Conversely, if festoons are large, a direct excision of the defect may be indicated. With direct excision techniques, bulging adipose tissue that lies superior to the orbital rim can be addressed by dividing the orbicularis oculi muscle in a horizontal fashion 3 to 4 mm superior to the infraorbital rim. Once the bulging adipose tissue pads are addressed, the margins of the orbicularis oculi muscle are reapproximated with two to three interrupted 6-0 catgut sutures.

With skin–muscle flaps, the skin incision is placed 4 to 6 mm inferior to the lash line. Doing so preserves a larger number of innervated orbicularis oculi muscle fibers on the anterior aspect of the tarsal plate. Furthermore, by curving the lateral portion of the incision downward past the lateral canthus, fewer orbicularis muscle fibers are disturbed laterally. In short, the design of the skin incision, herein described, preserves more of the circumferential support mechanism of the orbicularis oculi muscle and minimizes the possibility of postoperative distortions.

The surgical scar resulting from the incision that I advocate is more than acceptable and—if sutured with care and precision—is generally imperceptible (Figs. 3.13 and 3.14). In patients who return years later for additional surgery, it is difficult—if not impossible—to find the previous incision site (Figs. 3.15 to 3.17).

In keeping with the adage: prevention is better than cure, if the safeguards herein described are embraced and carried into the operating theatre, the incidence of postoperative displacement and distortions of the lower eyelid margin can be significantly reduced and—in most cases—completely avoided (Figs. 3.18 and 3.19).

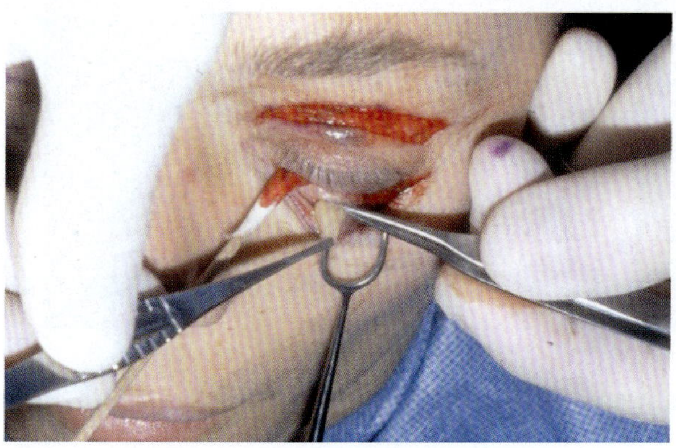

FIGURE 3.9
Bipolar cauterization of the adipose tissue pad stalk prevents bleeding.

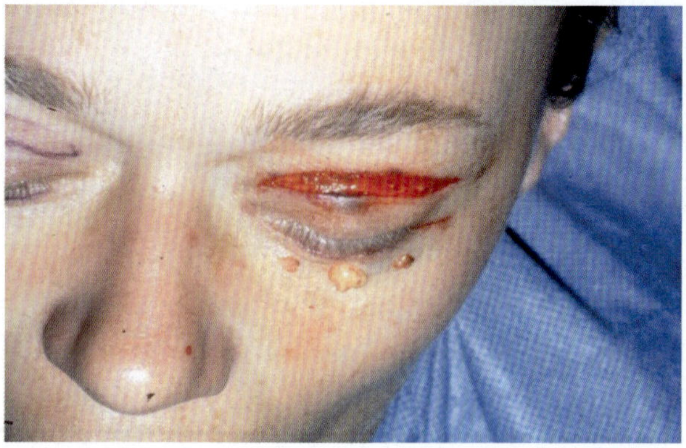

FIGURE 3.10
Adipose tissue is conservatively removed from the three compartments.

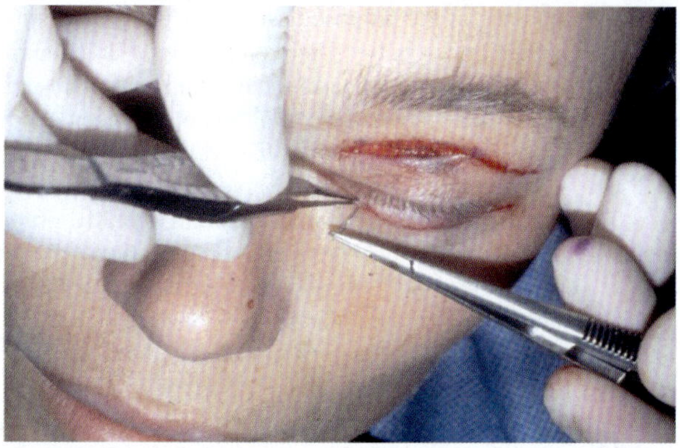

FIGURE 3.11
A 7-0 monofilament running suture is used for closing incisions.

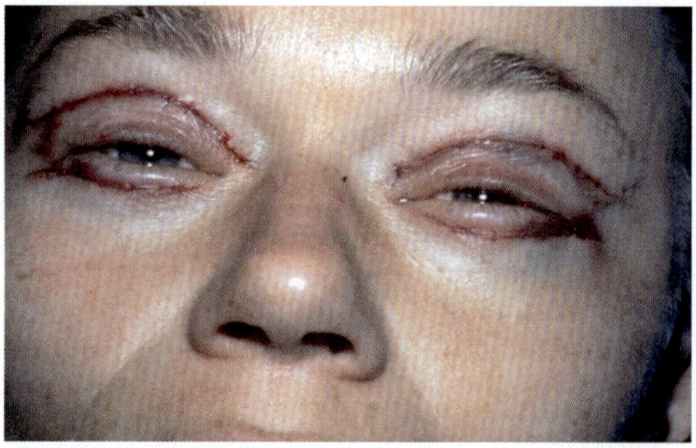

FIGURE 3.12
Immediate postoperative view of bilateral upper and lower (skin–muscle) blepharoplasties.

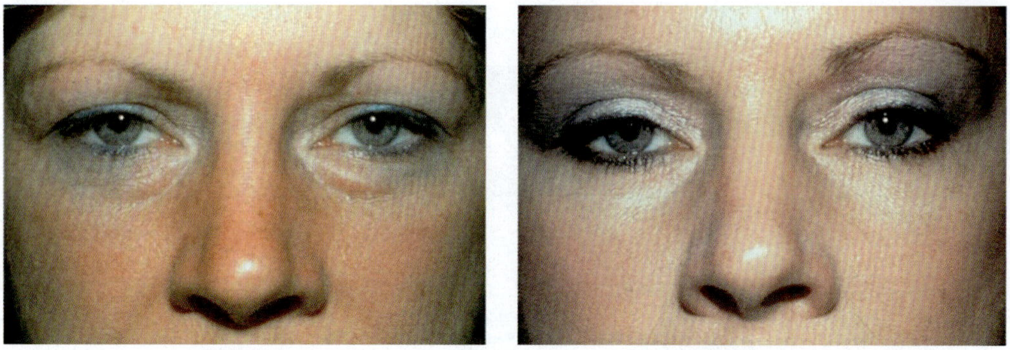

Before After

FIGURE 3.13 Patient who underwent a transcutaneous skin–muscle lower eyelid blepharoplasty with incisions placed at the lower border of the tarsus. Scars are imperceptible.

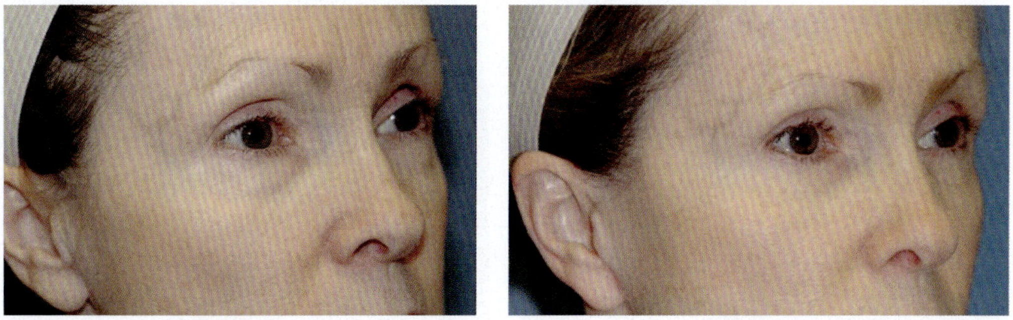

Before After

FIGURE 3.14 Patient who underwent a transcutaneous lower eyelid blepharoplasty with excision of adipose tissue.

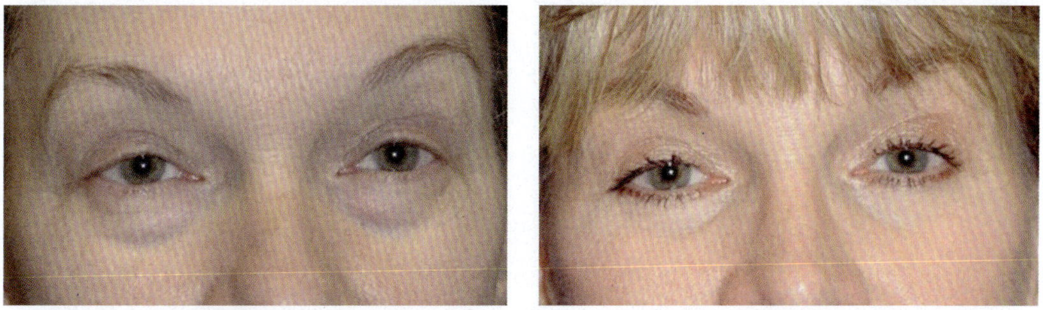

Before After

FIGURE 3.15 Patient who underwent transcutaneous skin–muscle flap blepharoplasty as herein described. Note absence of postoperative sequelae and invisible scars.

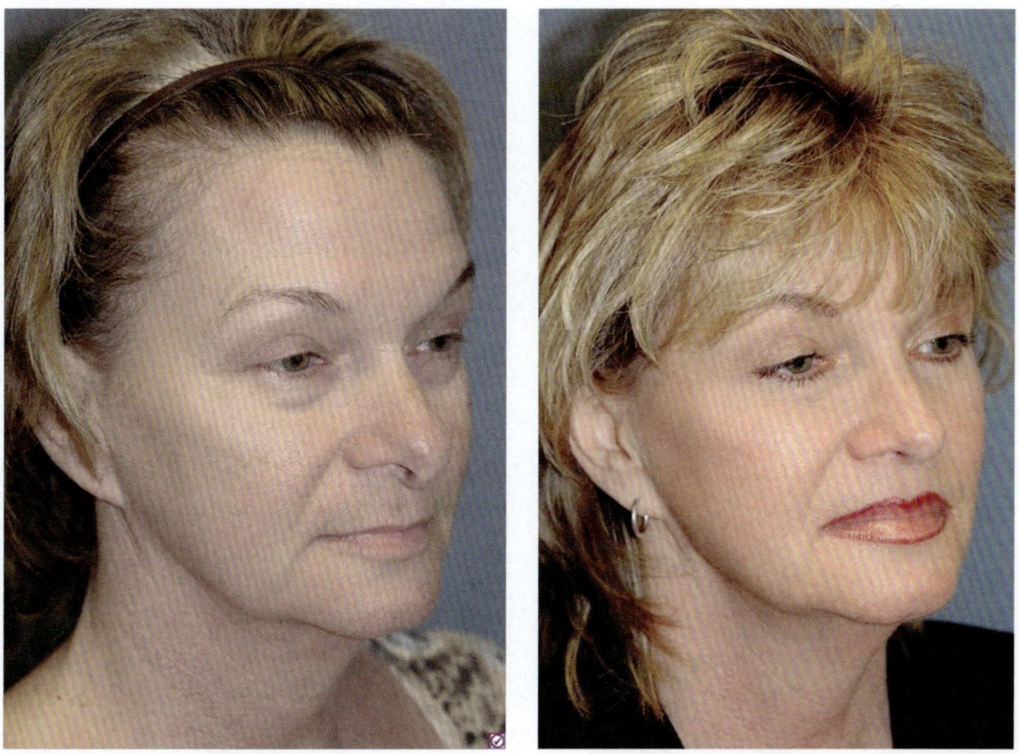

Before After

FIGURE 3.16 Another view of the same patient. Note absence of "tear trough" deformity following conservative excision of adipose tissue.

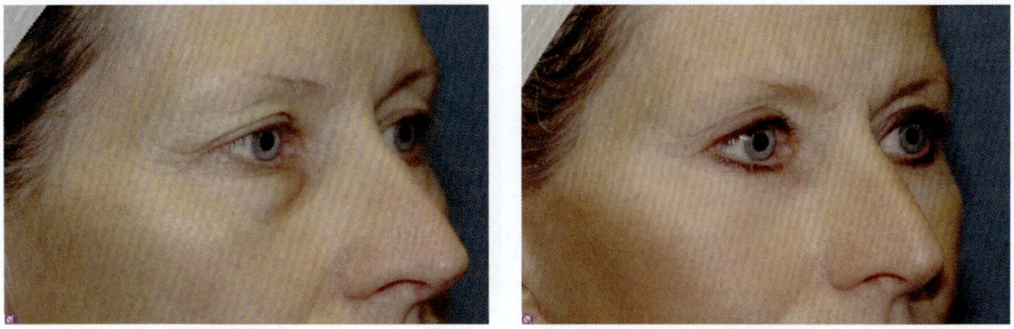

Before After

FIGURE 3.17 Transcutaneous skin–muscle flap blepharoplasty with incision at inferior border of tarsus.

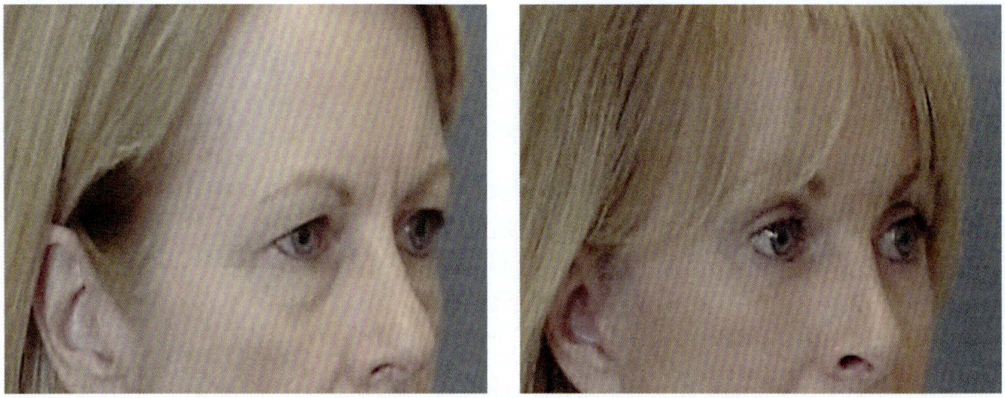

Before After

FIGURE 3.18 Skin–muscle lower lid blepharoplasty with adipose tissue excision and temporal brow/cheek lift.

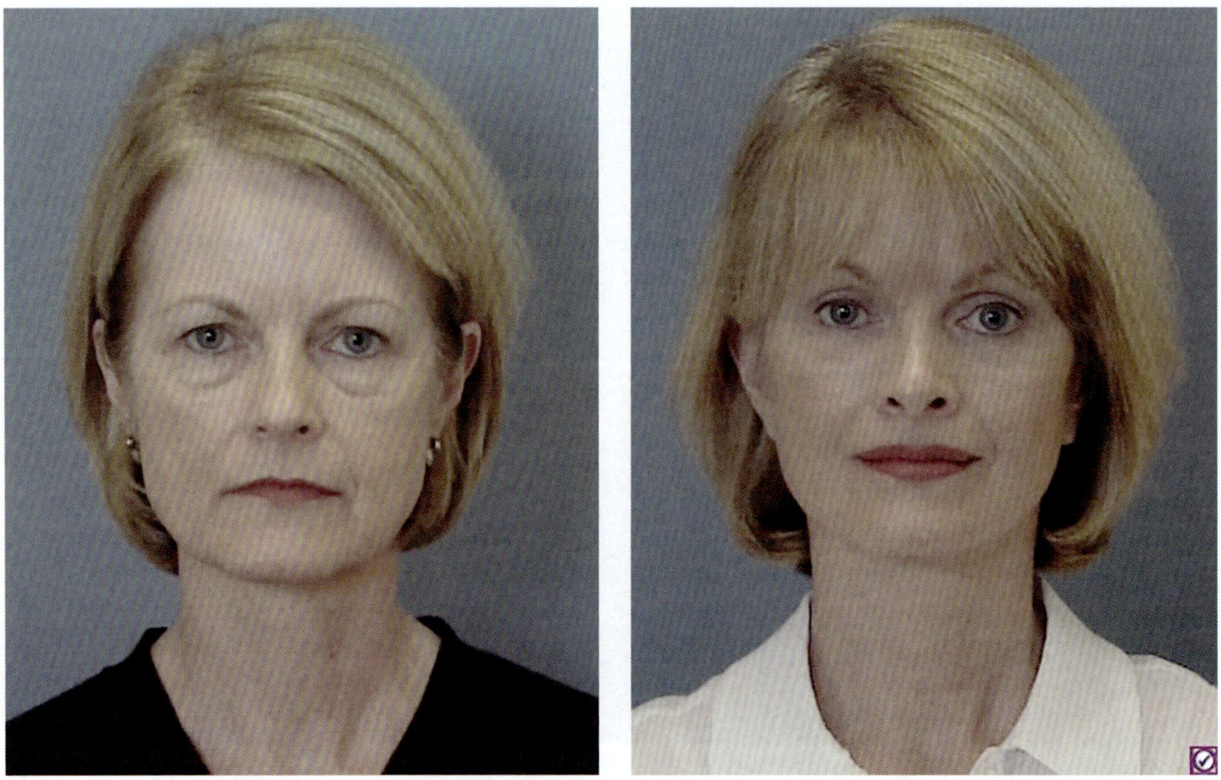

Before After

FIGURE 3.19 Another view of the same patient. Upper and lower lip augmentation performed at the same time.

COMPLICATIONS

The most common, permanent sequela following conventional lower lid blepharoplasty is inferior retraction of the lower lid, that is, scleral show and rounding of the lateral canthus (the round eye). The condition is readily identified by an increase in the amount of white-colored sclera visible between the limbus and lower lash margin with the patient gazing straight ahead.

Closer evaluation of postsurgical "round eyes" will reveal inferomedial displacement of the lateral commissure, increased slope of the lateral third of each eyelid, a flattened, unanimated, pretarsal component, and *an* unnatural infralash crease produced by the healed incisional scar. These findings are one step short of ectropion; therefore, the methods described in this chapter should help reduce the incidence of each of these unfavorable sequelae of lower eyelid blepharoplasty.

A number of factors contribute to lower eyelid malpositioning, including atonia associated with advanced aging, iatrogenic disruption of—and surgical weakening—of the lower lid tarso-fascial sling (hammock). Vertical (downward) tension on the sling, as a result of excessive skin removal and/or the forces of postoperative scarring, can also contribute to lower eyelid retraction.

Many of the aforementioned postoperative sequelae may be avoided by a simple modification in the placement of the lower eyelid incision at the time of surgery. If the skin incision is placed in the first skin crease (approximately 4 mm below the free border of the eyelid) rather than in the immediate infralash line as described by Castanares and Rees, the afore-referenced anatomic hammock is undisturbed.

POSTOPERATIVE CARE

Postoperative wound care consists of gentle application of hydrogen peroxide with a cotton swab and Tears Renewed ointment (Akorn, Inc., Buffalo Grove, IL) to the incision lines. This is repeated four to five times per day during wake hours to keep the sutures moist and aid in suture disintegration. Any remaining sutures are removed at 1 week under magnification with the aid of a Wood lamp, which allows the residual suture to glow in the dark.

RESULTS

Postoperative distortions of the eyelid are known sequelae of lower eyelid blepharoplasty. In my experience, relocating the conventional lower lid incision to a more physiologic position has proven to be an effective and safe variation of the classical technique. Avoiding injury to the pretarsal soft tissues and the anatomic tarso-fascial "hammock" at the time of surgery may reduce the occurrence of postoperative rounding and ectropion of the lower lid. The scar that results from the more inferiorly placed lower lid incision is aesthetically acceptable and, in most cases, undetectable. It can usually be camouflaged with make-up 1 week following surgery.

PEARLS

- In general, I do not advocate repositioning of adipose tissue pads. Removal of adipose tissue should not produce a hollowing of the lower eyelid if it is not excessive.
- Care must be taken not to disturb the periosteum overlying the bone, as this can allow the orbicularis muscle to heal directly to the bone during the postoperative period. This creates undue downward traction on the lower lid and might produce lid malpositions.
- In lower lids with marked excessive skin, it is wise to leave behind a millimeter or so of skin that could have been removed at the time of surgery.
- The first crease in the lower eyelid skin should be used as the incision. This usually corresponds to the inferior border of the tarsus. This allows for maintenance of the skin–orbicularis–tarsal–canthal tendon complex (hammock), which better resists the inferomedial pull of any contracting scar and/or excess skin removal.
- Canthopexy becomes unnecessary in the vast majority of cases by simply placing the skin incision farther inferiorly from the lid margin, thereby preserving the tarso-fascial sling.

PITFALLS

- Excessive cauterization of the skin and muscle at the time of surgery can result in postsurgical scarring to periorbital tissues.
- Contraction of the sheet of subcutaneous scar (which occurs in any undermined area) is absent with a skin–muscle flap technique. Still, scarring remains a factor especially in the septum that the surgeon must consider in planning the operation.

- Removal of the pretarsal orbicularis muscle can denude its support system resulting in an abnormally flattened appearance.
- Avoiding disruption of the pretarsal hammock composed of skin, orbicularis, the fibrous tarsus, and the most superior portion of the horizontal fibers of the orbital septum will tend to resist these contracting forces, providing skin (and/or muscle) removal is not excessive.

INSTRUMENTS TO HAVE AVAILABLE

- No. 15 blade
- Double prong skin hook
- 4 prong skin hook
- Desmarres lid retractor
- Castroviejo forceps
- Halsey needle driver
- Caliper
- Mosquito hemostat
- Suture scissor
- Tissue scissors
- Greene forceps
- Cotton tip applicators

SUGGESTED READING

Castenares S. Blepharoplasty for herniated intraorbital fat: anatomical basis for a new approach. *Plast Reconstr Surg* 1951;8:46–58.

Garcia RE, McCollough EG. Transcutaneous lower eyelid blepharoplasty with fat excision: a shift-resisting paradigm. *Facial Plast Surg* 2006;8:374–380.

McCollough EG, Cortez EA. Blepharoplasty in the allergic patient. In: Spencer JT, ed. *Allergy problems: current therapy*. Miami, FL: MEDED Publishers, 1981:213–218.

McCollough EG, English JL. Blepharoplasty. Avoiding plastic eyelids. *Arch Otolaryngol Head Neck Surg* 1988;114:645–648.

McCollough EG, Ha CD. The McCollough Facial Rejuvenation System: expanding the scope of a condition-specific algorithm. *Facial Plast Surg* 2012;28(1):102–115.

McCollough EG, Langsdon PR. *Dermabrasion and chemical peel: a guide for facial plastic surgeons*. New York, NY: Thieme Medical Publishers, 1988.

Webster RC. A flap suspension technique in blepharoplasty on lower lids. *J Dermatol Surg Oncol* 1978;4:159–165.

Webster RC. Suspending sutures in blepharoplasty. *Arch Otolaryngol Head Neck Surg* 1979;105:601–604.

4 LOWER EYELID BLEPHAROPLASTY TECHNIQUES

Bryan Sires

INTRODUCTION

Aging changes of the lower eyelid have been better defined over the past decade as the result of increased understanding of the anatomy. This has led to an evolving approach to rejuvenation of the lower eyelid. Two main factors are part of this evolution. These include the recognition that the lower eyelid has an anatomic relationship with the adjacent cheek region. There is a continuum from one area to the other, and what affects one will affect the other. They exist in a symbiotic relationship. One region cannot be adequately addressed unless both regions are considered in the treatment plan. The abundant suborbicularis oculi adipose tissue (SOOF) spans both structures in youth, but with age, it atrophies and descends (Fig. 4.1). The second factor is that with aging, there is not only descent, redundancy, and prolapse of tissue over time but also deflation of the facial and periorbital regions. This has led to tissue additive procedures to the lower eyelid rather than just tissue subtractive or redraping techniques. Additionally, there has been the recognition that supporting structures exist in the face (Fig. 4.2). With time, these ligaments stretch. To rehabilitate the face and eyelid, the ligaments require release in order to allow the soft tissue structure to slide over the bony hard tissue and to be anchored in an elevated and supported position, which secondarily supports the lower eyelid.

Up until the mid-1970s, lower eyelid blepharoplasty was usually performed through a skin incision in the infraciliary line. Dissection proceeded through the orbicularis oculi muscle and orbital septum if excision of adipose tissue was required. The skin and/or muscle would then be redraped and trimmed, thereby removing excess tissue. In 1950, the transconjunctival or internal approach was recognized but limited in its use. This was due to the thought that the excess skin could not be addressed via this approach. However, the combination of transconjunctival removal of adipose tissue and addressing mild to moderate excess skin with either chemical peels or laser allowed for the increased use of the transconjunctival approach. The two techniques of chemical peels and laser resurfacing that lead to skin contraction are beyond the scope of this chapter. In cases of severe amounts of excess skin, transcutaneous excision remains the procedure of choice.

Over time, there is a loss of facial volume that can create a skeletonized and aged appearance. Early efforts in facial volumization were limited by the available technologic, material, and even conceptual resources that we take for granted today. It was not until the 1980s when tumescent liposuction techniques were described that widespread use of adipose tissue and its various applications could be used. Through the continued advancement of liposuction techniques, the harvest and production of "fat pearls," which could be passed through narrow cannulas to the site of interest, became realized. These advances, along with the more complex understanding of facial volume, converged into what is considered modern facial rejuvenation.

The rationale behind using adipose tissue for volumization of the face is that you have a living autologous tissue that could potentially provide a lasting effect without repetitive injections. If the adipose tissue survives the transfer, then you have a basis for a long-lasting treatment. The adipose tissue is also readily accepted by the body as it is the patient's own autologous tissue. Typically, there is an ample supply of adipose tissue. It is unclear what cells survive and what conditions are ideal. It is known that both preadipocytes and adipocytes are transferred. Both may survive, but the transfer of preadipocytes supposes that

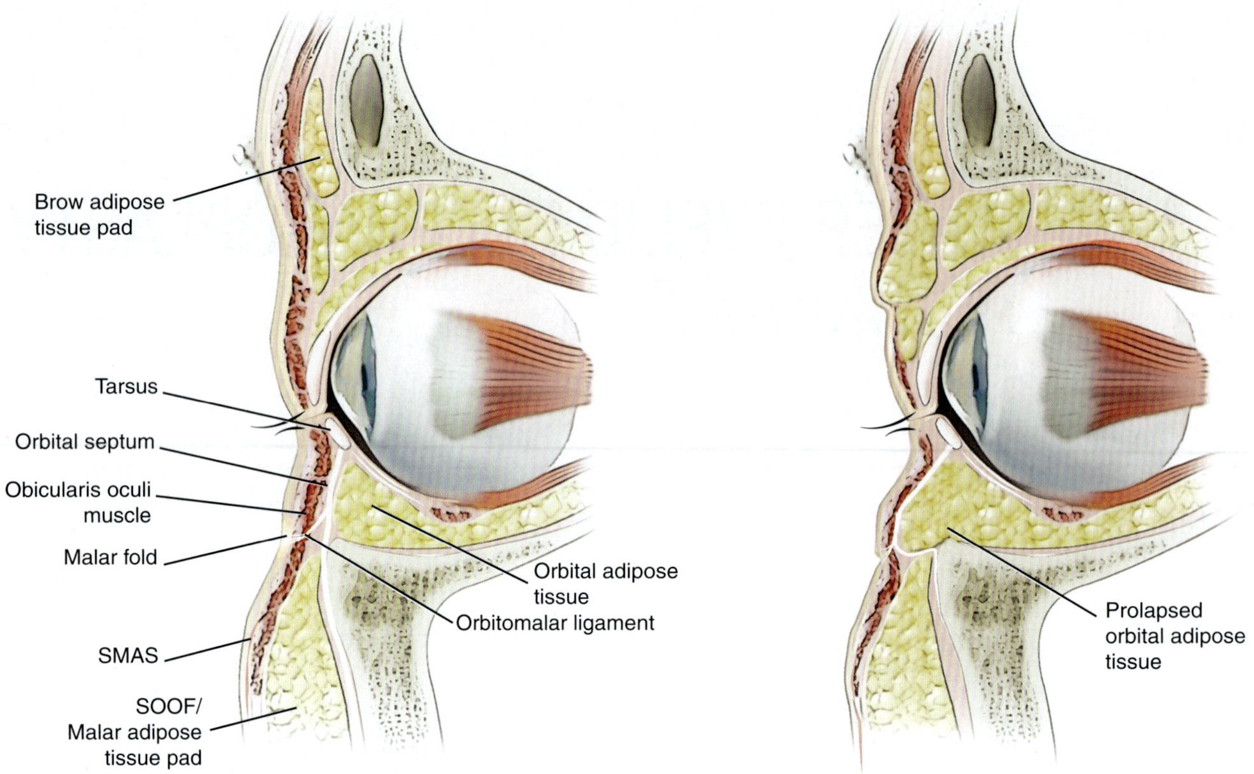

FIGURE 4.1 Anatomy of the lower eyelid–cheek junction during youth and in the aged. SOOF descent is apparent along with orbital adipose tissue prolapse and subcutaneous tissue thinning.

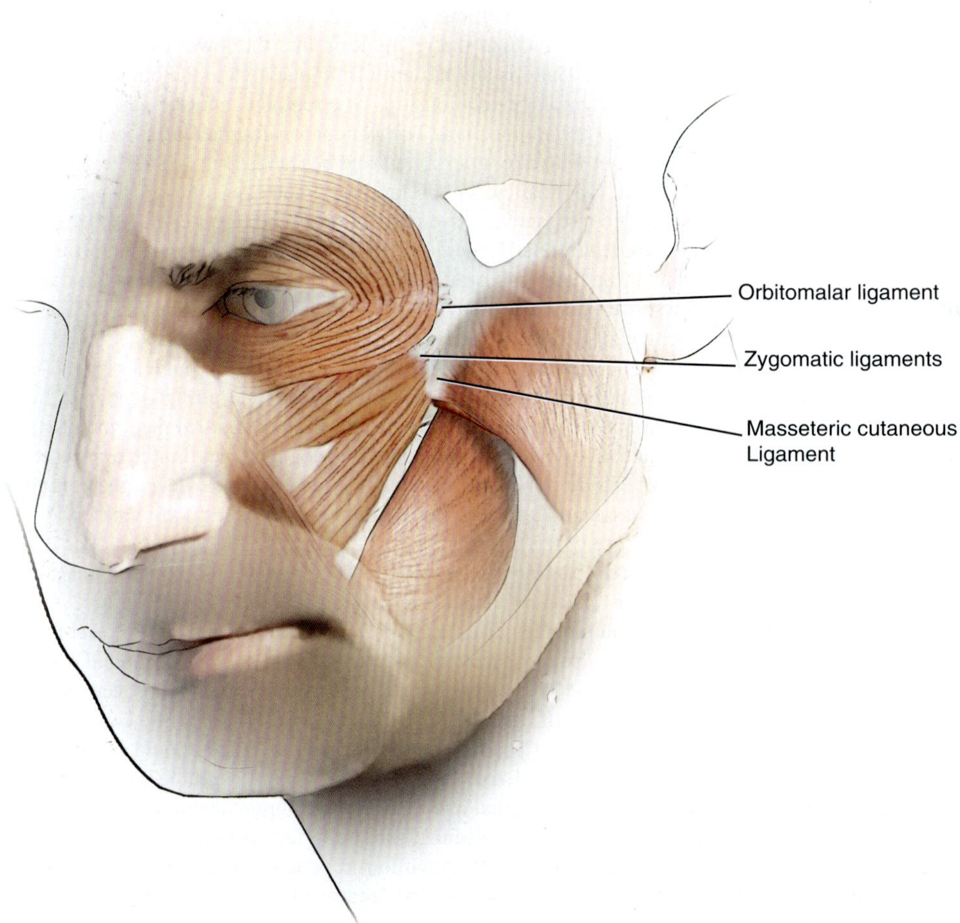

FIGURE 4.2 Location of the supporting structures of the face including the orbitomalar ligaments (OL) and zygomatic ligaments (ZL).

regeneration of new cells plays a role. It is becoming apparent that the long-term volume effect is more likely the result of regeneration of adipose tissue rather than tissue transfer. This is brought about by the transfer and differentiation of stem cells or preadipocytes. It has been shown that volume retention will often dip in the first 3 to 4 months with resolving edema and as vascularization occurs. This is followed by a rebound and improved facial volumes at 1 year or later. The delayed volumetric effect is secondary to either the uptake of fatty acids into the cytoplasm of the surviving adipocytes or the differentiation of the stem cells into adipose tissue cells that mature and grow. It is also unclear what percent of the transferred cells survive. This is important in deciding how much adipose tissue to place considering the anticipated loss. Access of the "fat pearls" to the surrounding blood supply also plays a critical role. Most surgeons are overcorrecting due to the anticipated loss. An unknown critical maximum volume exists whereby additional "fat pearl" volume will lack adequate exposure to blood supply nourishment. This will lead to cell death and atrophy due to inadequate oxygenation and nutrition. To ensure adequate blood supply, no more than a 1.5-mm layer of adipose tissue should be injected into any plane. The placement of optimal total volumes of adipose tissue rather than overfilling to get the desired effect is also crucial for adipose tissue survival. The goal is to place a total of 30 to 50 mL of adipose tissue into the facial regions compared with the 100 to 150 mL some authors advocate. Five to six mL of adipose tissue per lower eyelid/cheek interface is ideal. This helps retention and avoids contour issues as well. If further research can enhance "fat pearl" survival, then overcorrection will become less important.

Adipose tissue transfer application to the lower lid and cheek junction is important because there are patients who lose subcutaneous volume in this region. This volume loss occurs in the SOOF and malar adipose tissue pads. At the same time, some patients' orbital adipose tissue becomes more apparent leading to the impression of adipose tissue prolapse. It is unclear if the adipose tissue prolapses or it becomes manifest as the cheek adipose tissue falls and deflates. Regardless, removing this adipose tissue would lead to deepening of the area and would exacerbate the tear trough deformity. Adding adipose tissue in this region restores the volume lost due to aging with clinical effects that can last years.

HISTORY

A complete history is standard in the evaluation for any patient considering surgery. A detailed past medical history with questions about general medical, ophthalmologic, and surgical events is important. A directed history with regard to the specifics of facial surgery, trauma, congenital abnormalities, autoimmune disease, thyroid disorders, dry eyes, eyelid swelling, ease in bruising, or dermatologic conditions is essential. I ask patients to list all medications that they are taking, including herbal and over-the-counter, to assess for any risks of increased bleeding during and after surgery. I also review tobacco, caffeine, and alcohol consumption. Additionally, I inquire about any placement of neuromodulators (e.g., Botox, Dysport, Xeomin) as well as soft tissue fillers in the regions of interest.

PHYSICAL EXAMINATION

Facial and Eyelid Examination

Understanding the patients' unbiased goals and expectations of the procedure is the first step of the examination. These should align with the anatomic changes observed on the physical examination, and if so, then a customized treatment plan can be formulated. Standardized photography should be used including full face AP, oblique, and side views when relaxed as well as in positions of facial expression such as smiling and grimacing. The patient should have a good understanding of the financial commitment and the recuperation process. The latter issue may take longer than some patients are willing to tolerate due to the time for resolution of edema. This cannot be overstressed during the preoperative evaluation and discussion.

The lower eyelid should be evaluated for excess skin or dermatochalasis, prolapse of adipose tissue, eyelid laxity, and changes in the relationship between the lower eyelid and the cheek. Dermatochalasis can be determined by gently pulling the skin laterally to determine the excess amount and if skin should be excised. Fine wrinkling needs to be distinguished from tissue excess. Fine wrinkling is dealt with using retinoid, chemical peels, or laser techniques rather than actual skin excision. Prolapse of adipose tissue is determined by observing the prominence of pockets of adipose tissue. This can be accentuated by having the patient look up or by gently retropulsing the eye and noticing the forward movement of the pockets of adipose tissue. The patient is asked to lie in the supine position so that the adipose tissue falls back into the orbit. This will give the surgeon and patient an idea of the result if it is determined that adipose tissue should be removed. This will also help the surgeon determine if there is really descent and loss of SOOF and malar adipose tissue volume. If so, then an additive procedure rather than a subtractive procedure should be considered.

Eyelid laxity is determined using the snap and distraction tests. The snap test is performed while the patient is asked not to blink and the lower eyelid is pulled down and let go. The eyelid should return to its

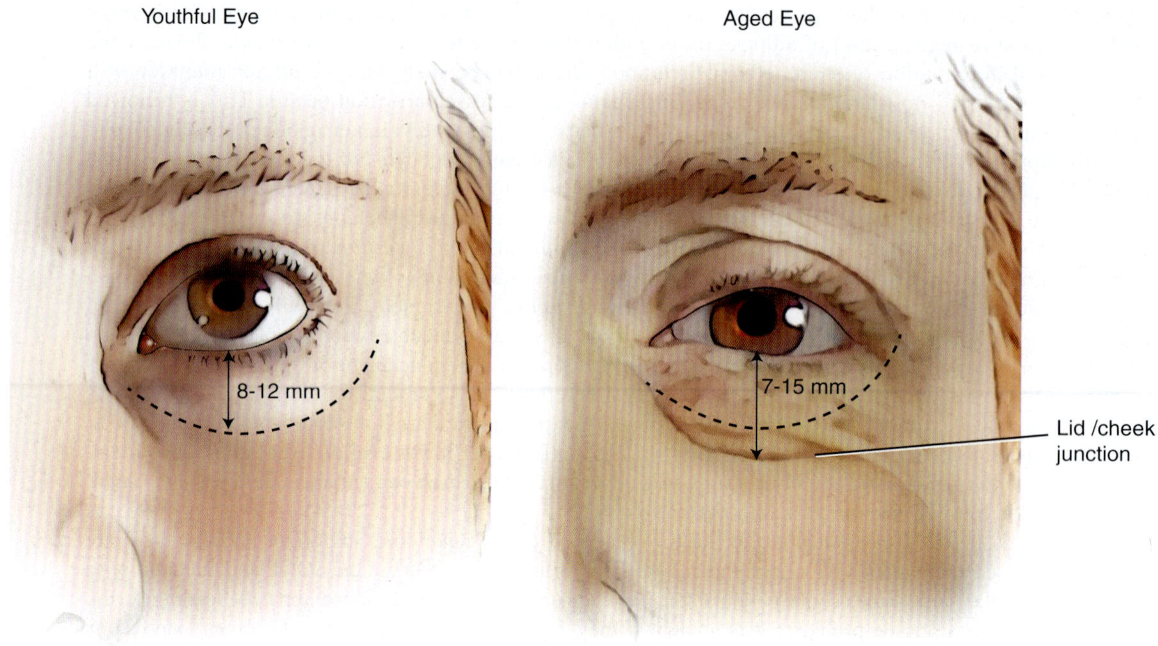

FIGURE 4.3 Demonstration of the topography of aging of the lower eyelid–cheek junction.

normal anatomic position in 2 seconds or less. The distraction test measures the distance from the eyelid to the eye when the eyelid is pulled away from the eye to its end point. This should be 7 mm or less. The snap and distraction tests help determine if the lower eyelid should be tightened to avoid postoperative ectropion or retraction.

Additional signs of aging of the lower eyelid–cheek region have been described consisting of four basic stages made up of two components. The two components of aging include the angle of the line from the lateral to medial canthal angles and the position of the lid–cheek junction. The lateral canthus is typically 2 mm higher than the medial canthus. This provides the natural gravitational slide for tears to be directed toward the nasolacrimal drain. As aging occurs, the lateral canthus can actually descend and be positioned below the medial canthal angle. Many patients will experience tearing in this setting. Along with descent of the lateral canthus, it also moves medially due to stretching leading to acquired blepharophimosis or narrowing of the horizontal palpebral fissure. The patients will describe this as loss of their "almond-shaped" eye.

The lid–cheek junction normally sits 8 to 12 mm below the lower eyelid margin in a young adult. In the aged eye, the lid–cheek junction descends to a distance of 15 to 18 mm and can give way to a tear trough deformity, a malar bag, and deepening of the nasojugal fold (Fig. 4.3). From the side, the youthful transition from the lid to the cheek is smooth, continuous, and convex. However, with aging, a biconvex deformity develops. The elevation in the eyelid is orbital adipose tissue. Inferior to this is the depression or the tear trough deformity. Finally, below this is the cheek mound/malar bag. If these findings are present, then the cheek region, as well as the eyelid, need to be addressed.

INDICATIONS

The indications for lower eyelid blepharoplasty are mostly related to the cosmetic aging changes found in this region. However, in severe cases, insurance will cover the costs of lower eyelid blepharoplasty if it interferes with the functionality of vision in the reading position. This typically occurs when the excess tissue sits on the reading segment of the glasses and obstructs the person's ability to read.

The signs of aging that would be amenable to lower lid blepharoplasty are prolapsed adipose tissue/mounds, excess skin/dermatochalasis, descent of the lid–cheek junction, deepening of the nasojugal fold/tear trough deformity, and lateral canthal dystopia.

The goal of surgery is to reposition the lateral canthus, redrape the cheek, and fill the tear trough deformity. Transfer of adipose tissue is an additive procedure that has superior longevity compared to industry-produced materials like hyaluronic acid or hydroxyapatite. It should be used in patients with deflation and deepening of their tear trough deformity. The key to planning where to inject the "fat pearls" is based on a thorough understanding of the patient's expectations along with the physical examination findings and then studying photographs for final decision-making.

An alternative to filling the tear trough with transferred "fat pearl" is to transpose the already presumed prolapsing orbital adipose tissue. This proves to be technically more challenging and invasive; so many surgeons have abandoned this technique in favor of transfer of adipose tissue.

CONTRAINDICATIONS

Patients with a significant past medical history should be eliminated from consideration for lower lid blepharoplasty. This may include patients with rheumatologic diseases or severe diabetes and those on anticoagulants for cardiovascular/vascular disease. The surgeon should decide when medical clearance is needed from the patient's primary medical doctor. Also, patients with body dysmorphic syndrome should be screened and eliminated from consideration.

PREOPERATIVE PLANNING

The main goal is to customize the decision regarding which additive, subtractive, or combination procedure should be used for each individual patient. This is decided by the severity of the findings. General guidelines have been developed and can be used as a starting point for decision-making (Table 4.1).

SURGICAL TECHNIQUE

Subtractive/Draping

The bilateral cosmetic lower lid blepharoplasty is described as follows. A transconjunctival incision is made 2 mm below the inferior tarsal border. Dissection is carried through the retractors and the septum into the lower eyelid adipose tissue. Equal amounts of adipose tissue are removed from both sides. Over the medial portion of the eyelid, dissection is carried inferiorly to the inferior orbital rim where the medial aspect of the orbitomalar ligament is released in a supraperiosteal plane. Hemostasis is obtained using a needle tip cautery device. Next, an incision over a distance of approximately 8 mm in the lateral raphe is made. A trench is then dissected down to the periosteum over the lateral orbital wall with a needle tip cautery on blend (Fig. 4.4A).

Next, the SOOF lift is performed. Starting in the trench over the lateral orbital wall, a supraperiosteal dissection is performed inferiorly and medially (Fig. 4.4B and C). This is carried along the inferior orbital rim to release the orbitomalar ligament in a sharp fashion. Special attention is given to releasing the lateral canthal component of this ligament.

TABLE 4.1 Guidelines for Using Subtractive, Additive, or Combination Procedures during Lower Lid Blepharoplasty Surgery

Findings	Procedure	
Mild prolapsed adipose tissue	Transconjunctival blepharoplasty	Subtractive (Fig. 4.9)
Mild prolapsed adipose tissue + fine wrinkles	Transconjunctival blepharoplasty + laser/peel	
Moderate adipose tissue/skin	Transconjunctival blepharoplasty (adipose tissue) + transcutaneous blepharoplasty (skin) +/– laser/peel	
Severe adipose tissue/skin	Transcutaneous blepharoplasty	
Moderate or severe adipose tissue/ skin with midface aging	Transcutaneous blepharoplasty + SOOF lift	
Mild prolapsed adipose tissue with tear trough +/– wrinkles	Adipose tissue transfer +/– laser/peel	Additive (Fig. 4.10)
Moderate adipose tissue/skin + tear trough	Transconjunctival blepharoplasty (adipose tissue) + transcutaneous blepharoplasty (skin) + adipose tissue transfer +/– SOOF lift	Combination (Fig. 4.11)
Severe adipose tissue/skin + tear trough	Transcutaneous blepharoplasty + adipose tissue transfer +/– SOOF lift	
Moderate/severe adipose tissue/ skin + tear trough + midface aging	Transcutaneous blepharoplasty +/– SOOF lift +/– adipose tissue transfer	

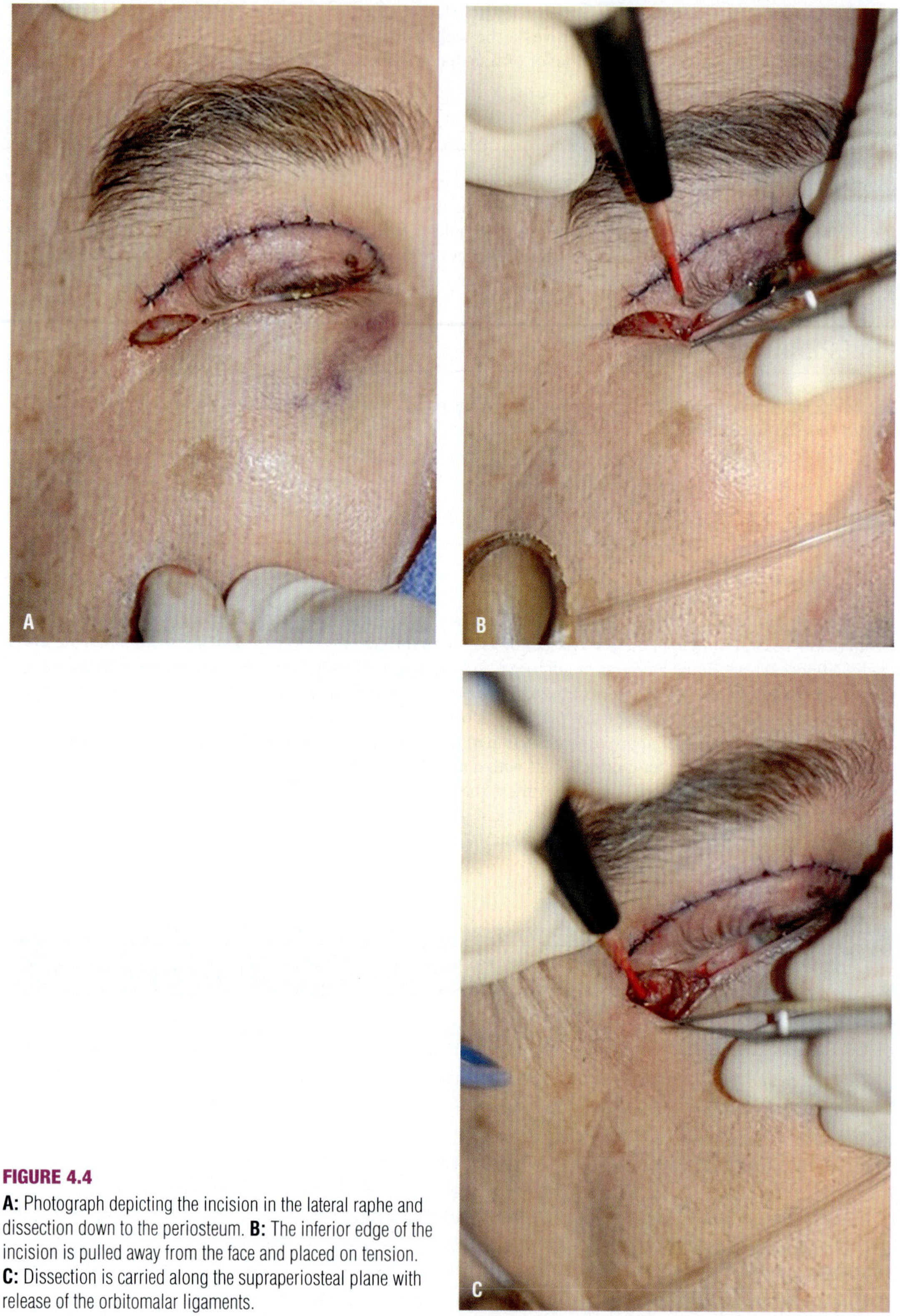

FIGURE 4.4

A: Photograph depicting the incision in the lateral raphe and dissection down to the periosteum. **B:** The inferior edge of the incision is pulled away from the face and placed on tension. **C:** Dissection is carried along the supraperiosteal plane with release of the orbitomalar ligaments.

Once the orbitomalar ligament is released, blunt dissection is carried out inferiorly to a point just superior to the buccal sulcus (Fig. 4.5A). This allows the orbicularis oculi muscle and the SOOF to slide superiorly and laterally (Fig. 4.5B and C). Special care in the region of the infraorbital nerve is taken so as not to disrupt it.

Next, using a sharp dissecting scissors, an incision is made in the infraciliary line. This is carried across approximately one-third of the lateral lower eyelid. The skin is dissected off of the overlying orbicularis muscle in this region. Using a 5-0 Vicryl suture, the angle of the lateral canthal ligament is supported to the periosteum

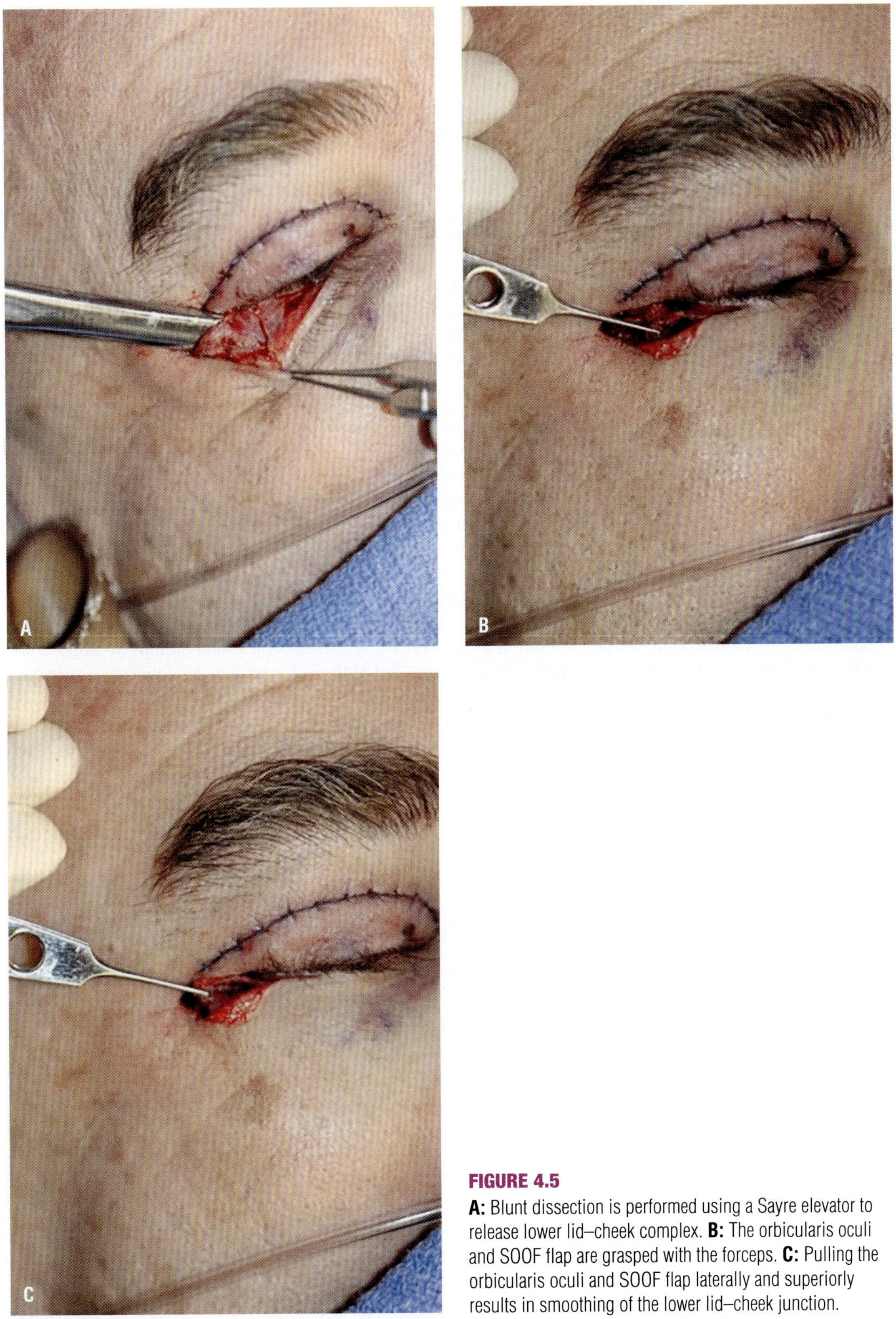

FIGURE 4.5
A: Blunt dissection is performed using a Sayre elevator to release lower lid–cheek complex. **B:** The orbicularis oculi and SOOF flap are grasped with the forceps. **C:** Pulling the orbicularis oculi and SOOF flap laterally and superiorly results in smoothing of the lower lid–cheek junction.

of the orbital tubercle. Next, the SOOF and orbicularis oculi muscle are sewn to the periosteum of the lateral orbital wall. The muscle is completely repaired with 5-0 Vicryl suture. Finally, an overlap technique is used to determine how much skin should be excised. Two triangles are excised—one triangle along the raphe and the other along the infraciliary line. The skin is then closed with multiple interrupted 6-0 plain gut suture. Alternating bites include the underlying muscle to limit dead space. The procedure is performed in a symmetric fashion on the opposite side.

Additive

The patient's face and abdomen are prepped and draped in the usual sterile fashion. The superior aspect of the umbilicus is infiltrated with local anesthetic. A stab incision with an 11 blade is made. Blunt dissection with a sharp dissecting scissors is performed. A Byron cannula and a half Monte cannula are used to infiltrate the tumescent anesthetic. This can be done either with a pump or by hand with a 60-cc syringe. This is allowed to work for 20 to 30 minutes.

Next, adipose tissue is harvested from the abdomen or saddle bags with a 14- and 16-gauge Capistrano cannula connected to a 10-cc syringe. A fine needle aspiration gun is used to provide ergonomic slow steady increases in suction 1 to 2 cc at a time. Each syringe is placed into a holder and allowed to settle over 12 minutes (Fig. 4.6). The bottom layer containing the tumescent anesthetic and blood is pushed out of the syringe. The middle layer containing the cleaned adipose tissue is then loaded into 1-cc syringes using a female–female adaptor. A top oily layer is also present but should not be injected into the face. Other alternatives for separating the adipose tissue include centrifuging or washing. Our sedimentation technique has been shown to produce more viable adipose tissue cells than do the other two methods. The setup and cleanup is also simplified.

Regional facial blocks are performed with a 1:1 mixture of 1% lidocaine with epinephrine and 0.5% Marcaine. The areas include the infraorbital, zygomaticofacial, and zygomaticotemporal nerves as well as the central transconjunctival space of the eyelid. No more than 0.5 cc is injected into each site to avoid volumetric distortion. The adipose tissue is then injected into the periocular region in a symmetric fashion. This is done in three layers (deep, intermediate, and superficial) using 1.2 and 1.4 mm Tulip cannulas. The larger cannulas are used for the deeper injections. The majority of the injections along the lower eyelid–cheek interface are done from a point corresponding to the intersection of imaginary lines oriented horizontally through ala of the nose and vertically through the lateral limbus. A smaller amount of adipose tissue is injected through a second entry point found in the lateral aspect of the lateral raphe. The entry points for these injection sites are made with a no. 18-gauge needle (Fig. 4.7). A total of 6 cc of adipose tissue is injected in a symmetric fashion on both sides. A two-handed technique is used to avoid overfilling and causing visual clumps of adipose tissue (Fig. 4.8). No more than 0.1 cc of adipose tissue is injected with each pass. Once symmetry is attained, the patient's face is cleaned and dried. Antibiotic ointment is placed on the two entry points. Crosshatched tape is placed onto the face to help support the position of the adipose tissue as well as to remind the patient not to manipulate the face. Antibiotic ointment, gauze, and a mild compression bandage are placed over the donor site(s).

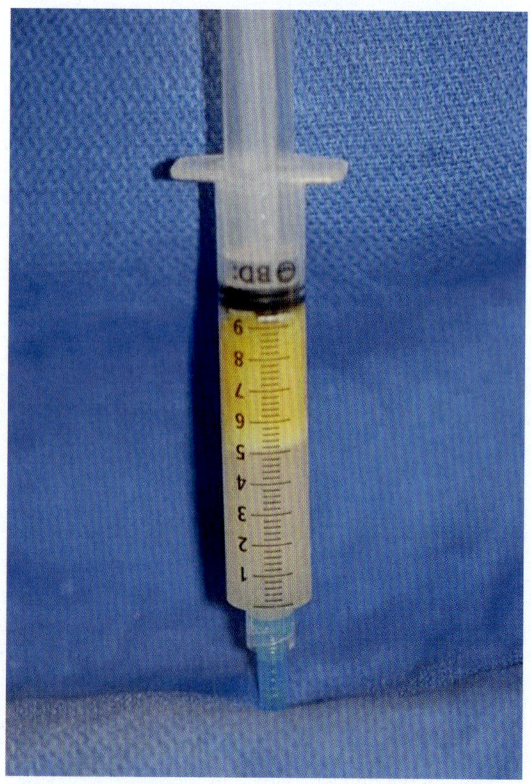

FIGURE 4.6

Photograph demonstrating the separation of the adipose tissue from the denser tumescent solution/blood mixture. A thin, oily layer rests on top of the adipose tissue, which is difficult to appreciate in this photograph.

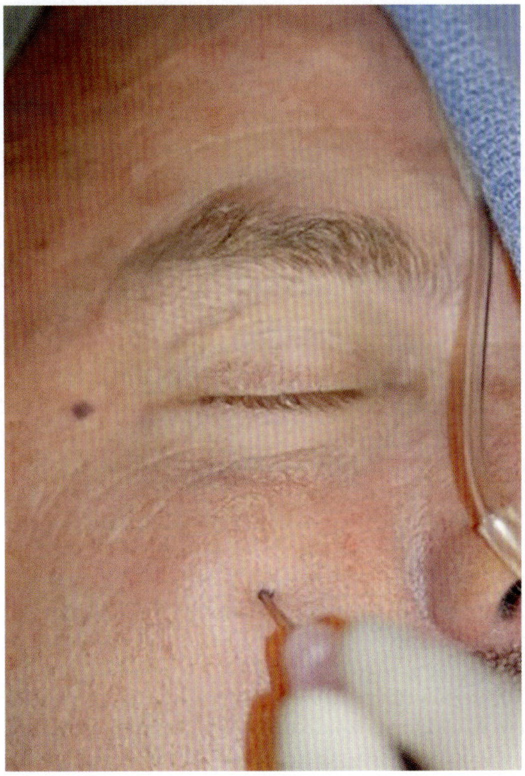

FIGURE 4.7
The two injection sites are marked with a surgical pen. An 18-gauge needle is used to create the entry points.

POSTOPERATIVE MANAGEMENT

Patients are given a series of instructions to help guide them in their postoperative recovery during their preoperative visits. Salient points include the following:

- Bruising and edema will peak at 48 to 72 hours.
- The head and shoulders elevated at 45 degrees or greater at all times by using two pillows for 10 days.
- Cold compresses can be applied to the eyelids for 20 to 30 minutes per hour for 3 days after surgery. Ice is never to be applied directly.
- Bacitracin ophthalmic ointment is applied to incisions four times daily until sutures are removed.
- Patients may shower the day after surgery, but they are not to wash their face.
- Strenuous activity is avoided for 14 days.
- Contact lenses are not worn for 1 week.
- If eyes feel dry, the patient may use artificial tears such as "Refresh Tears" as needed.
- Patients are advised to avoid the use of aspirin, ibuprofen, naproxen, vitamin E, fish oil, and herbal medications for 2 weeks after surgery.

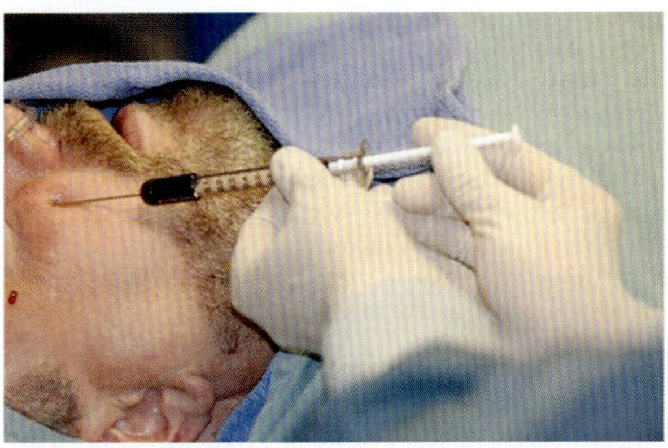

FIGURE 4.8
Two-handed technique is demonstrated and used to deliver controlled, small threads of fat pearls.

COMPLICATIONS

Complications from lower eyelid blepharoplasty usually involve either over- or undercorrection. A good guide is to aim for the amount of tissue removal wanted with error in favor of undercorrection. More tissue can be removed later when undercorrected. Attempting to put tissue back when overcorrected is more complex with less desirable outcomes. Unfortunately, a common occurrence of overcorrection in lower eyelid blepharoplasty produces lateral canthal rounding and retraction of the eyelid with scleral show. This can be managed with scar release, placement of a hard palate spacer graft, midface elevation, and a Frost suture. However, the best way to deal with these issues is to avoid them. This is done by limiting the trauma to the tissue, avoiding multiplane dissection, performing canthal tightening, and reducing manipulation of orbital adipose tissue by grafting adipose tissue to the tear trough.

Another common postoperative complication is chemosis. This occurs due to decreased lymph drainage. This comes about by shock and/or disruption to the orbicularis oculi muscle and/or the lymphatic channels. With each blink, the orbicularis oculi muscle helps massage the lymph channels and carry edema away. As the muscle recovers, the chemosis generally improves. If this does not improve, then topical or oral steroids can help. Other treatments include pressure patching with or without subbulbar conjunctival dissection. A period of 6 months is typically allowed to pass before any invasive intervention is entertained. The best preventative measure to decrease the risk of chemosis from occurring at all is to avoid the disruption of the orbicularis oculi muscle. This can be accomplished by limiting the transcutaneous incisions to no more than 50% of the entire horizontal length of the lower eyelid.

When operating in the lower eyelid, it is also important to understand the anatomy of the lower eyelid adipose tissue pads and their relationship to the inferior oblique muscle. Knowing this critical anatomy can decrease the chances of injury to the muscle, which can lead to intractable diplopia.

Complications from adipose tissue transfer range from serious loss of function to easily managed situations. Anticipation of these issues will allow the surgeon to quickly and rapidly deal with the presenting situation. The most devastating complications are death and blindness following injection. This likely occurs by the injection of adipose tissue into the vascular system akin to adipose tissue emboli. The adipose tissue likely traverses the external carotid system and occludes the cerebrovascular system leading to stroke or obstructing central retinal artery and leading to blindness. Standard treatment for central retinal artery occlusion should be attempted. These include lowering the eye pressure with drops, oral medications, and massage, along with Carbogen inhalation and anterior chamber paracentesis. Emboli of adipose tissue can also possibly lead to regional facial skin ischemia and necrosis. This has been seen with the use of industry-manufactured fillers in the glabellar furrows and nasolabial folds near the ala of the nose. Treatment of ischemia and necrosis should include aspirin, application of nitroglycerin paste, and warm compresses to the affected area. Hyperbaric oxygen may also provide a beneficial role. All of the above treatments work at reestablishing flow to the affected area and increasing oxygenation.

More easily managed complications are related to uneven, inadequate, or excess placement of the adipose tissue at the time of transfer. This would include lumps, bulges, over or undercorrection, and depressions at the injection site. Persistent edema can also be problematic. This is especially true in the area of the malar bag. Carefully check patients to determine if they may be predisposed to having this occur, and if so, have an informed discussion with them. A lump of adipose tissue usually occurs in the inferior periorbital region where the skin is thin and there is minimal subcutaneous tissue. Overapplication of adipose tissue or placement too superficial is the etiology of a lump. Treatment may consist of either local steroid injection or actual excision of the excess adipose tissue. The best way to avoid a lump that occurs along the inferior orbital rim is to inject from the malar area superiorly in a perpendicular fashion. Avoid injecting parallel to the inferior orbital rim from the lateral canthal region. A bulge is a larger area of elevation of a recipient site. The three causes include fibrosis, edema, or excess adipose tissue. Induration of the area can be determined with palpation. If indurated from fibrosis, intralesional steroids can be used. Dilute, low-dose steroid is suggested to avoid atrophy of the surrounding tissue and hypopigmentation of the overlying skin.

Excess overcorrection with adipose tissue needs to be distinguished from edema. Excess adipose tissue can be removed with liposuction after at least 6 months have passed in order to ensure that edema is no longer present. Reduction of overcorrection is performed with a fine-gauge liposuction cannula. Undercorrection is simply treated with the addition of more adipose tissue. Also, be aware that smokers and avid exercisers can have more atrophy. Some surgeons store frozen adipose tissue for this purpose, but this is not suggested according to the office-based or ambulatory surgery center accrediting or certifying agencies. Storage of adipose tissue results in the small possibility of mixing up the patient's harvested adipose tissue and placing it into the wrong individual. The best temperature and cryopreservation conditions to store it for viability have also not been determined. It is easiest to simply harvest fresh adipose tissue and refill the undercorrected areas, which is likely to give the best results.

Lifting procedures tend to have the goal of slight overcorrection in order to overcome the effects of gravity as the edema resolves. Transfer of adipose tissue on the other hand has the goal of proper correction or to err on the side of undercorrection. The addition of more adipose tissue is simpler than trying to remove adipose tissue in the complex anatomical facial region by liposuction techniques.

RESULTS

The key to accurately evaluating postoperative results is to correlate the subjective patient response with the physical examination findings, photography, and a quantitative measurement of volume or topography. To date, little work has been done in the quantification of results, but surgeons are becoming more critical of their results and are introducing objective evaluation techniques. Humans have inherent visual abilities to identify what is a good outcome and how it improves one's appearance. Fournier acuity is helpful in this regard. It is easy to see and describe with the eye, but this does not quantitatively measure the differences before and after treatment. It does not allow rigid comparison for research purposes. Until standardization of results is performed, there will be no basis to study the many remaining questions about the optimization of lower lid blepharoplasty. Fortunately, studies have been undertaken to measure the results of adipose tissue transfer over time. This includes the use of MRI and 3-dimensional imaging. Both imaging modalities show about 50% and about 33% volumetric retention at 1 and 1.5 years, respectively (Figs. 4.9 to 4.11).

PEARLS

- The surgeon must have a clear understanding of the orbitomalar ligament as well as other supporting ligaments of the face. Complete release of these structures allows for adequate resuspension of the orbicularis oculi muscle and elevation of the SOOF.
- Orbicularis oculi muscle suspension alone is like a mini-SOOF lift.
- Adipose tissue, itself, has no holding capacity but can be used to elevate the soft tissues of the cheek over the malar prominence, filling in the tear trough deformity, supporting the lower lid, and elevating the lateral canthus relative to the medial canthus.
- Elevation and tightening of the lateral canthus is a critical step in lower eyelid blepharoplasty.
- It is important to perform the snap test and distraction test to determine the severity of lower lid laxity.
- Elevation of the midface also helps to support the lateral canthus.

PITFALLS

- During subtractive procedures, it is better to err on the side of undercorrection.
- If transfer of adipose tissue is being done in conjunction with other facial surgeries, it is best to do the adipose tissue transfer first followed by the incisional surgery. If the adipose tissue transfer follows the incisional surgery, the adipose tissue during injection can overaccumulate in a dissection plane because it will follow the path of least resistance.

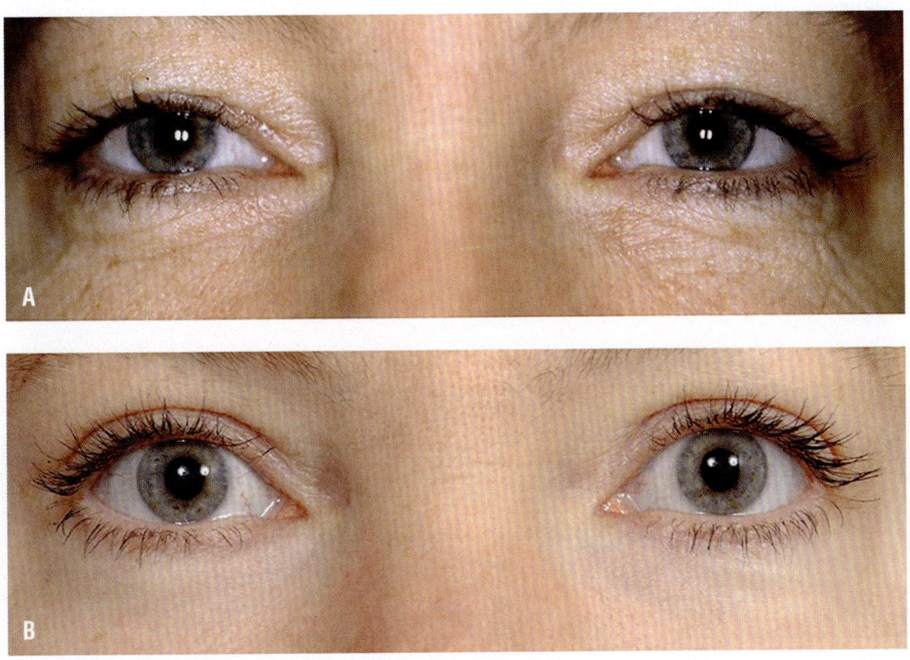

FIGURE 4.9 Before **(A)** and after **(B)** photographs showing a patient who underwent bilateral lower eyelid transconjunctival blepharoplasty with CO_2 resurfacing.

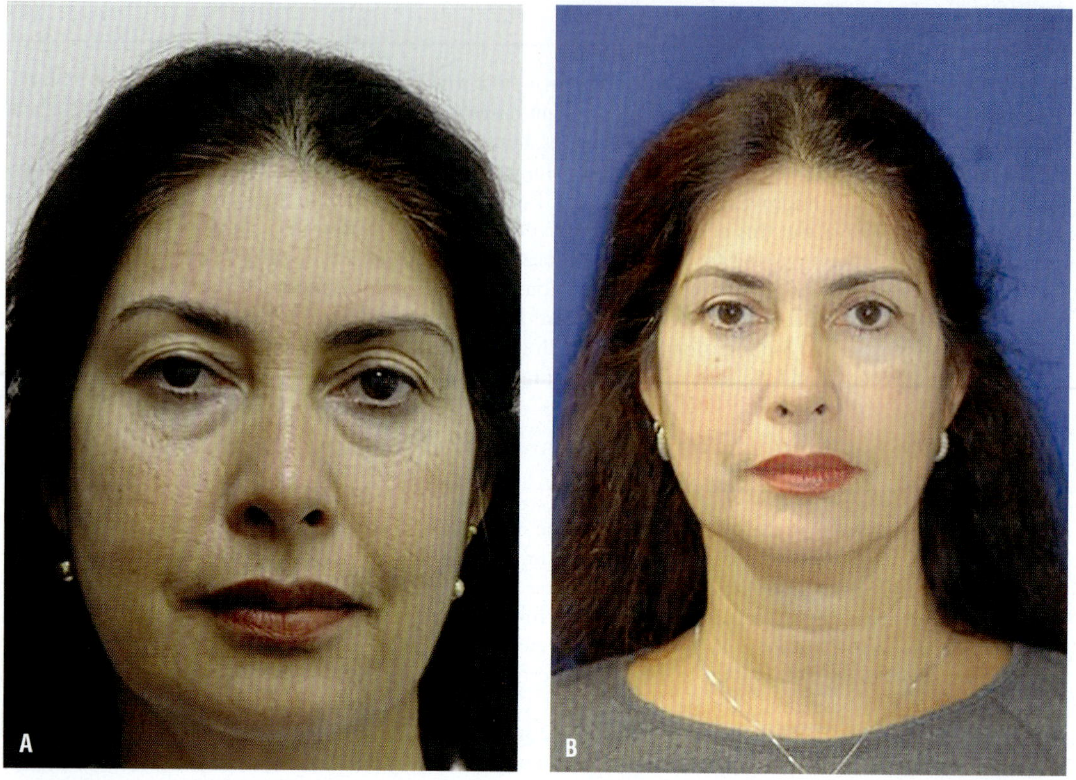

FIGURE 4.10 Before **(A)** and after **(B)** photographs of a patient who underwent bilateral lower eyelid adipose tissue transfer from her abdomen.

- Adipose tissue may also migrate out of a previously made surgical wound, which may have deleterious effects on the healing of the incisional surgery. Therefore, performing adipose tissue transfer first results in decreased risk of fat migration, increased chance of viability, and more predicable healing.

INSTRUMENTS TO HAVE AVAILABLE

- Standard plastic surgery tray
- Corneal protectors
- Caliper
- Webster needle holder
- Desmarres retractor
- Westcott scissors
- 0.5 Castroviejo forceps
- Stevens tenotomy scissors
- 14- and 16-gauge Capistrano cannulas
- Byron cannula
- Half Monte cannula

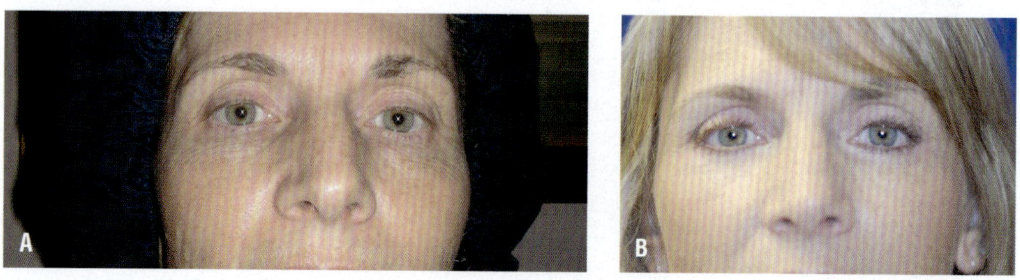

FIGURE 4.11 Before **(A)** and after **(B)** result photographs of a patient who underwent bilateral lower eyelid blepharoplasty with SOOF lift. Note improvement in the appearance of the lower lid–cheek junction.

ACKNOWLEDGMENT

I would like to acknowledge my fellow, Henry Lee, MD, for his assistance in the editing and final drafting of this chapter.

SUGGESTED READING

Donath AS, Glasgold RA, Glasgold MJ. Volume loss versus gravity: new concepts in facial aging. *Curr Opin Otolayngol Head Neck Surg* 2007;15:238–243.

Hester TR, Codner MA, McCord CD, et al. Evolution of technique of the direct transblepharoplasty approach for the correction of lower lid and midfacial aging: maximizing results and minimizing complication in a 5-year experience. *Plast Reconstr Surg* 2000;105:393–406.

Meier JD, Glasgold RA, Glasgold MJ. Autologous Fat Grafting. *Arch Facial Plast* 2009;11:24–28.

Stallworth CL, Wang TD. Fat grafting of the midface. *Facial Plast Surg* 2010;26:369–375.

Trepsat F. Periorbital rejuvenation combining fat grafting and blepharoplasties. *Aesth Plast Surg* 2003;27:243–253.

5 TARSAL STRIP CANTHOPLASTY

Richard D. Lisman

INTRODUCTION

Lower lid tarsal suspension was originally described in 1911 by Lexer and Eden, and since then, multiple modifications have been made most notably by Tenzel, Anderson, and Gordy. The alteration in the contour and position of the lower eyelid has been described by various names such as the tarsal strip procedure, the lateral canthal sling, lateral canthoplasty, canthopexy, the tarsal tongue, the periosteal strip, horizontal shortening, and tarsal suspension. The tarsal strip canthoplasty is used in the functional treatment of lower lid laxity and malpositions (i.e., ectropions and entropions) and also in aesthetic surgery of the lower eyelid.

The upper and lower eyelids serve to distribute moisturizing tears over the surface of the eye and to protect the delicate tissues of the ocular surface. Compromise of eyelid function can have significant repercussions with regard to ocular irritation and pain as well as the potential for visual loss. Abnormalities in the position of the lower eyelid can either be congenital or acquired and often relate to changes along the lateral canthus. Anatomic contributions from the lateral horn of the levator aponeurosis, Lockwood's ligament, lateral orbicularis oculi, and the check ligament from the lateral rectus muscle comprise what is collectively described as the lateral retinaculum and commonly known as the lateral canthus. Direct and effective treatment of malposition of the lower eyelid commonly entails the undertaking of a tarsal strip canthoplasty, which is the focus of this chapter.

HISTORY

It is important to obtain a general past medical and ocular history with particular attention to identifying prior eyelid, ocular, or facial plastic surgery, trauma, facial paralysis, history of rosacea, blepharitis, other cicatricial diseases, and thyroid eye disease. A review of medications and supplements that may increase bleeding is important as well.

PHYSICAL EXAMINATION

- Check visual acuity in both eyes.
- Examine the position and contour of the lower lid. Is there a malposition of the eyelid present? If there is an ectropion present, what is the etiology? Is it a result of lid laxity or does the patient have associated anterior lamellar shortening suggesting a cicatricial ectropion?
- Measure the distance of the margin of the lower lid to the center of the midpupillary light reflex (MRD2). Identify whether there is any inferior scleral show.
- Evaluate the laxity of the lower eyelid by the snap back test and the distraction test. The eyelid snap back test is performed by everting the lower lid inferiorly toward the orbital rim. Normal snap back occurs spontaneously. Abnormal lid laxity can be quantified by the number of blinks required for the lid to return to

the normal position. The eyelid distraction test is an estimation of the distance the lower lid can be pulled directly off of the globe.
- Evaluate the cornea for any keratopathy by assessing lagophthalmos during gentle closure of the eyelids. Fluorescein staining of the cornea and examination under a slit lamp microscope can identify punctate corneal changes in cases of keratopathy.

INDICATIONS

Lateral strip canthoplasty is a highly effective procedure for resuspension of the lower eyelid. This is a beneficial procedure for those:

- Who have malposition of the lower eyelid as a result of entropion or ectropion
- With lower eyelid retraction (i.e., inferior scleral show) requiring a lateral resuspension to help improve the position of the lower lid
- Who wish to change the lateral angle to a more aesthetically pleasing position
- Who are undergoing cosmetic or reconstructive lower eyelid surgery and those who require a resuspension technique to help support and reduce the incidence of postoperative retraction of the lower eyelid

CONTRAINDICATIONS

- Active infection, herpetic outbreak, or rosacea
- Stand-alone procedure in the treatment of anterior, posterior, or combined lamellar shortening
- Unrealistic patient expectations

PREOPERATIVE PLANNING

It is important to evaluate the patient preoperatively and to identify the cause of malposition of the lower eyelid. Does the patient have laxity of the lower lid with or without shortening of the anterior lamellar and lower lid retraction? In cases of isolated laxity of the lower lid, a lateral tarsal strip canthoplasty alone can be sufficient to provide an appropriate cosmetic result. When there is shortening of the anterior lamella, recruitment of anterior lamella through midface resuspension may be required. Very severe cases of shortening of the anterior lamella may require skin grafting. Patients with retraction of the lower lid may also require posterior lamellar grafting in addition to a lateral tarsal strip canthoplasty. Various substrates can be used, but the authors generally prefer autologous hard palate grafting in moderate to severe cases. Allografts such as Alloderm graft can suffice for cases of mild to moderate retraction of the lower lid.
Furthermore, it is important to assess the patient for the:

- Position of the lateral canthal angle
- Position of the lower eye lid (MRD2)
- Eyelid positional changes that have occurred with age. It is always worthwhile to evaluate the patient's premorbid photographs to avoid postoperative overcorrection of the lateral canthal angle

SURGICAL TECHNIQUE

Surgical technique: tarsal suspension technique for repairing lower lid malposition
The general steps for the lateral tarsal suspension technique including the following:

- Local anesthesia
- Lateral canthotomy
- Inferior cantholysis
- Release of the orbital septum
- Development of the strip
- Opening of a periosteal slot
- Reattachment of the strip
- Resupporting the strip
- Reformation of the lateral canthal angle
- Closure of the lateral skin incision

A number 15 blade is used to create a lateral canthal incision of approximately 1 cm in an aesthetically pleasing skin fold (Fig. 5.1). With upward traction on the lateral aspect of the lower eyelid, the inferior crus of

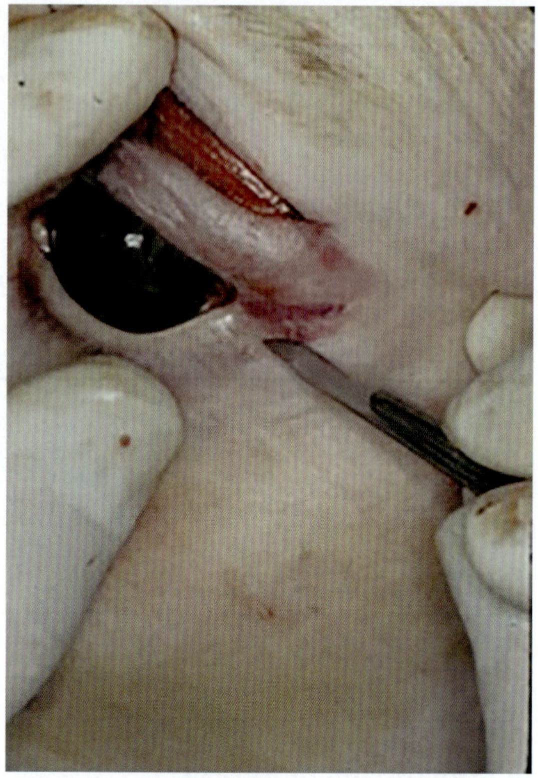

FIGURE 5.1
Lateral canthal incision.

the canthal tendon is severed with a Stevens scissors (Fig. 5.2). The scissors are directed posteromedially, and the orbital septum is released with sharp dissection (Fig. 5.3).

Next, the tarsal strip is prepared by splitting the lateral eyelid along the gray line, taking care to avoid cutting into the tarsus (Fig. 5.4). Next, a horizontal incision is made along the inferior border of the tarsal plate to detach the lower lid retractors and conjunctiva. The conjunctiva at the mucocutaneous junction is shaved off with a 15 blade (Fig. 5.5). The reasoning is that it is difficult to visualize where keratinized skin begins and ends. Conjunctiva is a nonkeratinizing epithelium and does not require removal from the posterior surface of the eyelid. The keratinizing surface at the mucocutaneous junction, if buried at the canthal angle, can produce foreign body discomfort; therefore, it is excised.

In order to determine the length of the strip, the terminal edge of the tarsal strip is grasped and pulled laterally and slightly superiorly toward Whitnall's tubercle until appropriate height, tension, and contour are achieved. Attention should be paid to confirm the correct position of the punctum. With a prominent eye, negative vector or shallow orbit the eyelid can bowstring or "hammock" under the globe if the strip is placed too low on the superior temporal orbital rim. In those circumstances, the tarsal suspension is placed higher than usual to avoid bowstringing under the globe.

A periosteal slot is indirectly opened at the inner aspect of the lateral orbital rim with a no. 15 blade (Fig. 5.6). The soft tissues are pushed with a swab to indirectly feel the lateral orbital rim. This creates a "tongue in groove" adhesion such that the strip fits into the groove within the periosteal opening.

The tarsal strip is then secured to the periosteum on the inner aspect of the lateral orbital rim with a 4-0 polydek suture on double armed, ME-2 needles. Although the surgeon may use another suture for periosteal

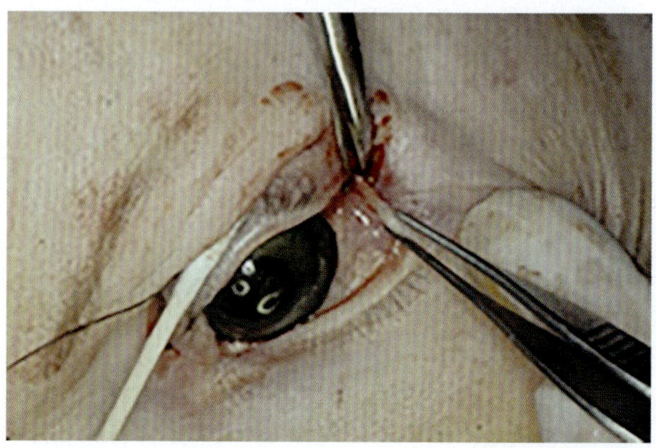

FIGURE 5.2
Inferior cantholysis.

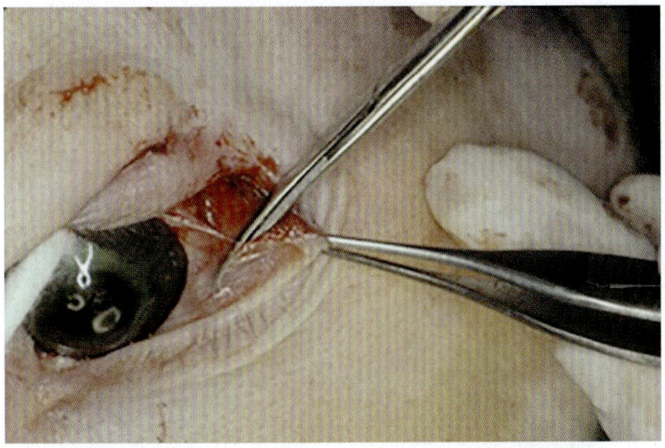

FIGURE 5.3
Orbital septal release. Note the ability to fully distract the lower lid from the globe secondary to complete release of the inferior crus of the canthal tendon and orbital septum.

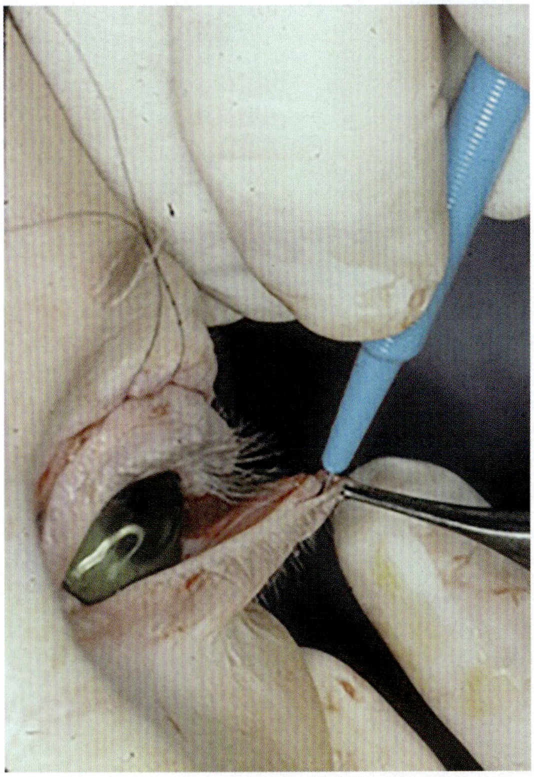

FIGURE 5.4
Splitting of the anterior and posterior lamella.

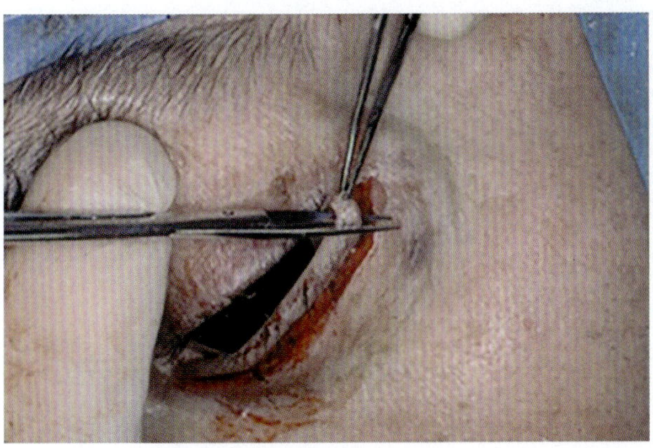

FIGURE 5.5
Completion of the lateral tarsal strip.

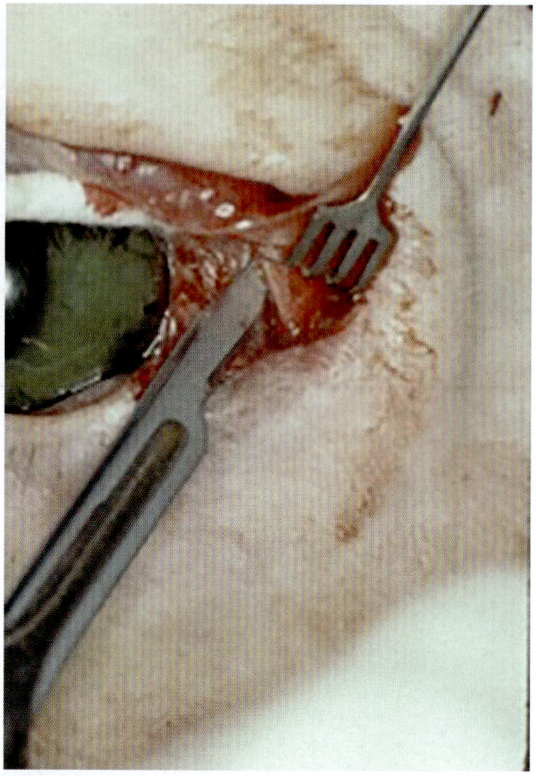

FIGURE 5.6
Opening the periosteal slot.

fixation of the tarsal strip, I recommend a suture that has a double-armed semicircular needle (i.e., ME-2 or P2) for adequate fixation of the periosteum within the orbital rim. The first needle is sutured through the superior portion of the tarsal strip while the second needle is placed through the inferior tarsus. The superior suture is first grasped and used to engage the periosteum on the inner aspect of the rim within the groove. Lid height and contour is assessed by pulling on the upper suture. If necessary, the suture can be backed out and repassed to improve the contour or height. A slight overcorrection in tautness and height is desired to allow for mild relaxation of the tissue in the early postoperative period. The inferior tarsal suture is then passed in a similar fashion approximately 2 to 3 mm inferior to the superior suture arm (Fig. 5.7).

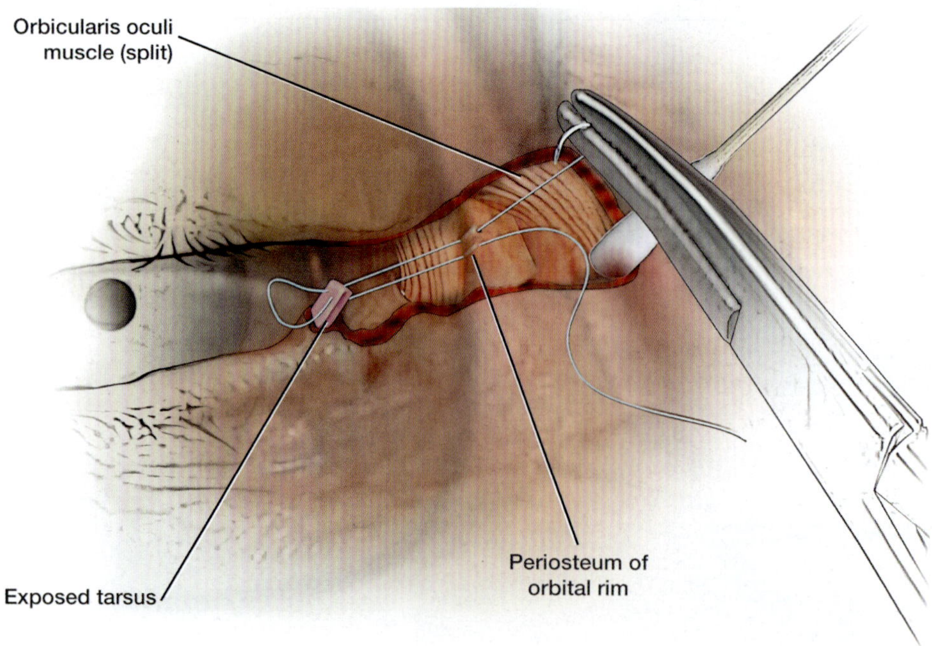

FIGURE 5.7 Attachment of the strip to the periosteum.

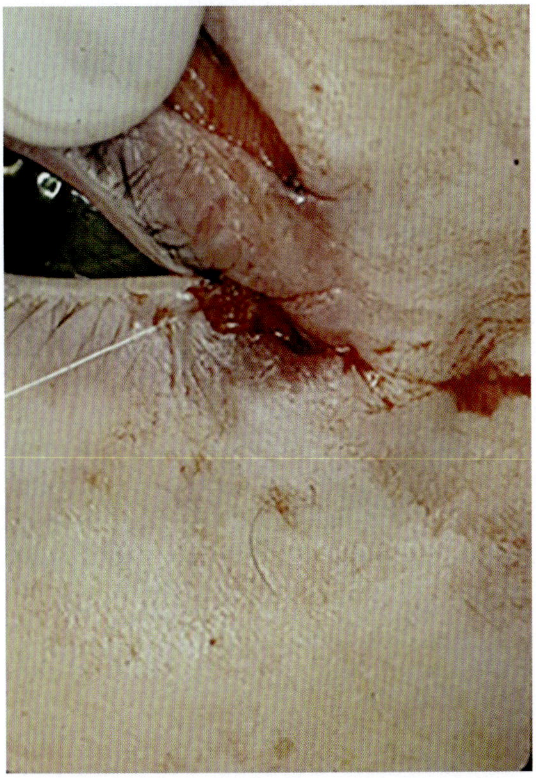

FIGURE 5.8
Resupporting the strip. Note that the polydek suture is not visible after placement of the polydioxanone suture.

The polydek suture must be cut close to the knot. Any exposed polydek is prone to externalize and create inclusion cysts or even a fistula posteriorly toward the periosteal fixation. A second suture (absorbable suture such as a 4-0 polydioxanone-PDS P3 needle) is then used to further secure the tarsal strip ("belt and suspenders" technique) and to further bury the underlying polydek suture (Fig. 5.8). This second suture further allows refining the upsweep of the lateral eyelid by moving or walking the second suture superiorly or inferiorly along the orbital rim.

Once the lateral strip is suspended properly, attention should be made at the lateral portion of the lower lid to identify any prolapsed orbital adipose tissue or pleating of the orbicularis muscle that may have been created with the retroplacement of the globe due to the tension on the newly positioned lower eyelid. The herniated orbital adipose tissue or pleated orbicularis muscle can be debulked by using a skin hook for retraction. This must be done carefully so that the lateral canthal sutures are not disrupted.

Closure begins by reforming an acute lateral canthal angle. The lateral commissure is realigned along the lid margin using 6-0 chromic suture (Fig. 5.9). The lateral skin is then closed with either a 6-0 chromic or 6-0 silk suture.

POSTOPERATIVE MANAGEMENT

Immediate postoperative care is usually minimal. Ice compresses are applied frequently for the first 48 to 72 hours. The skin sutures are removed by the seventh postoperative day. The single silk suture at the lateral canthal angle should be left for 8 to 9 days since the tarsus does not adhere until that time. Patients should avoid heavy lifting, straining, or physical activity for 2 weeks after surgery. All patients should avoid mechanically pulling their eyelid down or attempting to rub the eyelid in a downward direction when instilling eye drops or placing contact lenses.

COMPLICATIONS

Bleeding and infection are rare complications of lateral strip canthoplasty. Care is taken to obtain intraoperative hemostasis, and the well-vascularized eyelid helps to reduce the rate of postoperative infection. Careful placement of the corneal protective lenses intraoperatively prevents damage to the ocular globe and corneal abrasion during surgery. If damage to the globe is suspected, prompt evaluation by an ophthalmologist is recommended.

It is normal to have postoperative pain or discomfort in the area of the tarsal periosteal fixation; this usually resolves over weeks to months. Suture granulomas are seen infrequently, and they can either be treated with intralesional steroid injections or excision. Lower lid asymmetry or contour abnormalities can occur, and

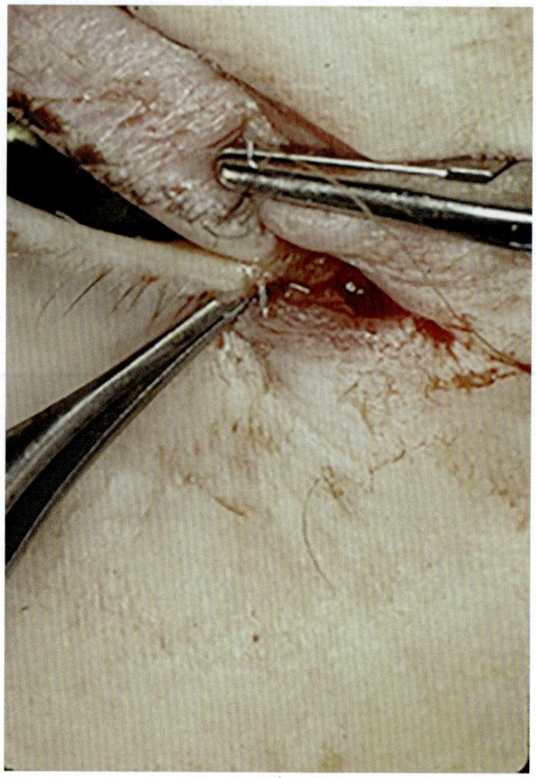

FIGURE 5.9
Reformation of the lateral canthal angle.

prevention can be optimized by careful preoperative and intraoperative evaluation. Intraoperative evaluation should assess for symmetry in lower lid contours and tension. In cases of postoperative asymmetry, the eyelid with the higher lateral canthal position can be gently massaged or stretched downward if needed.

PEARLS

- It is important to identify the cause of the malposition of the lower lids preoperatively. Cases of laxity of the lower lids respond well to the lateral tarsal strip canthoplasty; in contrast, cicatricial changes require recruitment of additional anterior lamella. Cicatricial retraction of the lower lid or ectropion, as seen in some postoperative blepharoplasty patients, often worsens with a negative vector. Patients with retraction of the lower lid or ectropion may also require a posterior lamellar graft to aid in the retraction of the lid.
- Intraoperatively, lysis of the inferior crus of the lateral canthal angle is best performed by feel. Traction is placed on the lower lid to allow the surgeon to feel the release of the inferior crus as it is "strummed" with scissors in order to identify its firm tendinous insertions to the orbital periosteum. With each cut through the inferior crus, the surgeon should feel the release of the lower lid. In cases of prior surgery, scar tissue may also need to be released around the tendon to allow for an adequate mobilization.
- Often times, a lateral strip canthoplasty technique will worsen the herniation of the lower lid adipose tissue compartments, most notably the lateral adipose tissue compartment. In order to allow for an optimal cosmetic result, the surgeon should identify such herniation and attempt to gently excise the adipose tissue pocket through the laterally based transconjunctival incision already made for the canthoplasty.
- In order to optimize postoperative healing of the incision, the lateral canthal angle should be closed first laterally in a medially directed approach toward the lateral canthal angle. Excess tissue can be "milked" toward the canthal angle, and, as a result, scarring or excess tissue can be directed toward the canthus.
- The patient should appear slightly overcorrected immediately postoperatively. Through the healing phase, the lower lid angle is expected to drop to a more "natural" position.

PITFALLS

- It is important to avoid multiple attempts at passing the suture through the tarsal strip. Multiple attempts can result in diminished integrity of the tarsal strip and "cheesewiring" of the suture.
- Appropriate fixation of the tarsal strip onto the periosteum is critical. Periosteal fixation is confirmed by having the surgeon assess the suture and its ability to not "give" with firm traction away from the orbital rim. Repassing the suture onto the periosteum is recommended if there is noted to be some "give" of the suture.

- If the tarsal strip is not fixed within the orbital rim but rather placed anteriorly (along the rim), the lateral lid may become malpositioned and result in an ectropion. The surgeon must make sure to visualize the suture fixation onto the inner aspect of the orbital rim. Note that the correct attachment of the lateral canthal tendon is deep to the rim by approximately 5 mm.
- Appropriate lateral canthal closure allows for optimal lateral canthal angle formation and prevents the upper lid from overriding in the postoperative period.

INSTRUMENTS TO HAVE AVAILABLE

- Standard oculoplastic surgical tray
- Steven's tenotomy scissors
- 0.5 Castroviejo forceps

ACKNOWLEDGMENT

The author would like to recognize Christopher I. Zoumalan, MD, for his exceptional contributions to the writing of this chapter. His work in the writing, editing, and figure creation for this chapter is greatly appreciated, without which this chapter would not have been possible.

SUGGESTED READING

Anderson RL, Gordy DD. The tarsal strip procedure. *Arch Ophthalmol* 1979;97:2192–2196.

Lisman RD, Lelli GJ Jr. Tarsal strip canthoplasty. In: Aston SJ, Steinbrech DS, Walden JL, eds. *Aesthetic plastic surgery*. London: Elsevier, 2009.

Lisman RD, Rees T, Baker D, et al. Experience with tarsal suspension as a factor in lower lid blepharoplasty. *Plast Reconstr Surg* 1987;94(6):671–681.

Ortiz-Monasterio F, Rodriquez A. Lateral canthoplasty to change the eye slant. *Plast Reconstr Surg* 1985;75(1):1–10.

Tenzel RR. Treatment of lagophthalmos of the lower lid. *Arch Ophthalmol* 1969;81:366–368.

Whitaker LA. Selective aleration of the palpebral fissure form by lateral canthopexy. *Plast Reconstr Surg* 1984;74(5):611–619.

6 ASIAN BLEPHAROPLASTY

William P. Chen

INTRODUCTION

The term double eyelid surgery has been used to describe a procedure that adds an upper eyelid crease to an eyelid that is without a crease. It is a very popular aesthetic procedure in Asian women of all ages. I first coined the term "Asian Blepharoplasty" in 1987 while attempting to define the skills and pitfalls necessary for performing primary and revision surgery in Asian patients. Along the way, various terminologies that are more precise ophthalmologically were developed. I will describe my technique, which is an external incision approach.

HISTORY

The common perception that all Asians are single lid without a crease is incorrect. There is approximately a 50% incidence of having a crease among Asians of Han origin (Chinese, Koreans, Japanese). Their crease, when present, tends to be located approximately 6.5 to 7.5 mm from the upper eyelashes. The current anatomic view of the distinguishing features of an upper eyelid with crease versus one without crease, in Asians, seems to be the presence or absence of terminal interdigitations of levator aponeurotic fibers into the pretarsal orbicularis oculi intermuscular septae and fibers, located in an area just slightly below or along the upper border of the tarsal plate (superior tarsal border).

PHYSICAL EXAMINATION

There are two main variants of the Asian crease:

- The nasally tapered crease (Fig. 6.1) is a low-set crease that runs parallel to the ciliary margin over the central and lateral portion of the upper lid, while over the medial one-third, it converges inward toward the medial canthus, and often blending into a small ethnic medial canthal fold of upper lid skin.
- The parallel crease (Fig. 6.2) runs parallel to the ciliary border over its entire extent, and at its medial section, it simply runs independent to and above any residual medial canthal fold.

Most individuals who are seen in our practice desire a *permanent* placement of a *natural*, *Asian-appearing* eyelid crease. The following are typical findings that they may present, though not necessarily having all findings listed below:

- A slight to mild excess of upper lid skin presenting as a hooded look.
- Fullness of the upper lid, especially over the preseptal portion of the lid; presumably due to a relative excess of inferior positioning of preaponeurotic adipose tissue (and to a lesser extent at times, the preseptal adipose tissue as well as pretarsal fullness).

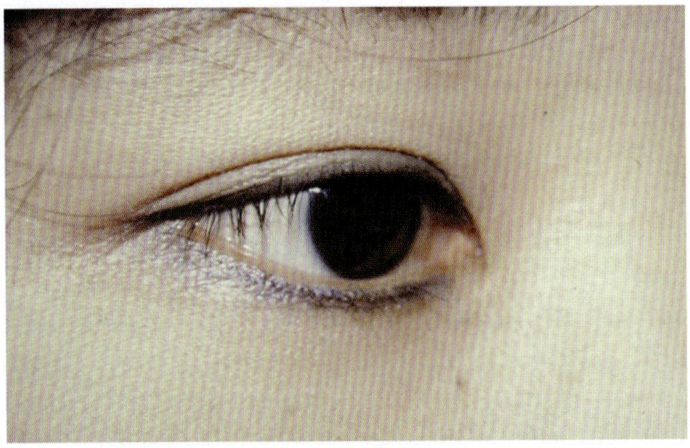

FIGURE 6.1
The nasally tapered crease.

- An absence of crease, or a mixture of incomplete or partial crease, with asymmetry between the two eyelids.
- May have a medial canthal fold of the upper lid skin.
- Secondary down-turning of the upper eyelid lashes.
- May have clinically undiagnosed latent ptosis in one or both sides.
- Pseudoesotropia (in-turning or slight crossing inward of the eyes).

INDICATIONS

A good candidate is a motivated, oriented individual who has some of the above findings and desires to have a crease added, for a valid reason. Typically, my patients have done some research as to their own needs and should be able to clearly voice what they desire. This is preferred as compared to an individual who wants the clinician to make all the decisions for them. They should understand that the individual surgical outcome may not be precise and are not completely predictable or guaranteed.

CONTRAINDICATIONS

- Patients with unrealistic expectations.
- Patients who expect instant healing.
- Patients with shifting ideas.
- Patients who do not seem to understand the preoperative discussion regarding necessary postoperative care.
- Patients who are strongly influenced in their decisions by others, including family members, no matter what their age.
- Patients with a significant history of keloid formation around the periocular areas, as well as dermatologic ailments that carry a higher incidence of unpredictability in crease formation.

PREOPERATIVE PLANNING

- Detailed in-office history and examination, noting palpebral fissure sizes, any unusual ophthalmic findings like ptosis, tear function and dry eyes, or use of contact lenses.
- Discussion of goals and expectations.

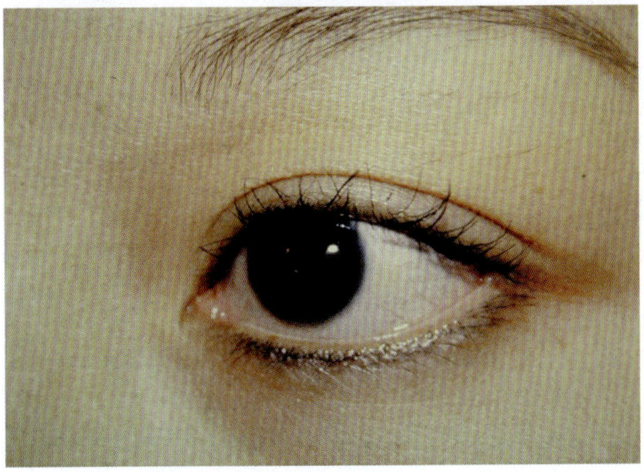

FIGURE 6.2
The parallel crease.

- Discussion of the height and shape of the crease; formulate a mutually agreed on plan. Document this in the chart.
- Signing of informed consent for primary Asian blepharoplasty or revision attempts (in revision Asian blepharoplasty, need to list exactly what is involved).
- Preoperative photos of primary findings, as well as previous eyelid scars if it is revision surgery.
- Go over it again immediately before surgery.

SURGICAL TECHNIQUE

- The appropriate oral premedications analgesic (one tablet of Vicodin and sedative; 5 to 10 mg of Valium) are given 1 hour prior to surgery. Intravenous line is started. The upper lid skin is infiltrated with 2% Xylocaine with 1:100,000 dilution of epinephrine, along the incision line. (A #30 gauge needle is used, and the volume injected is seldom over 0.5 to 0.75 mL for each eyelid.) After a 5-minute period for the anesthetic solution to disperse, the upper face and eyelids are cleansed, prepped, and draped. The patient is placed in a supine position, and cardiac monitors and a pulse oximetry sensor are applied.
- Marking—Attention is turned to the right eye. A black protective corneal eye shield is applied over the right globe. The tarsal plate of the upper lid is everted (Fig. 6.3), and a caliper is used to measure the vertical height of the central portion of the tarsal plate (it is usually between 6.5 and 8 mm). The lid is returned to its normal position, and methylene blue ink is used to mark the central point of the crease incision, usually at about 7 mm from the lashes. If the shape of the crease chosen was a nasally tapered crease, the crease marking is merged toward the medial canthus. For a parallel crease shape design, the surgeon should make a conscious effort to stay parallel to the lash line as one approaches the medial canthus.
- Skin incision—Typically, a segment of skin measuring about 2 mm centrally, 2.5 mm laterally, and 1 mm medially is included in the lines of incision. This will vary depending on clinical findings. The skin-deep incision is made using a no. 15 Bard-Parker blade (Fig. 6.4). Precise attention and repeated positioning of the lid tissue is warranted.
- Transection through the orbicularis—When the orbicularis muscle is seen, control of capillary oozing is carried out using bipolar cautery. The muscle layers are then carefully traversed using a surgical blade or cutting monopolar cautery on a low-energy setting (which is my preference). The cautery tip is intentionally beveled superiorly along the orbicularis such that the orbital septum is reached at a slightly higher level from the superior tarsal border. The cautery tip is likely to reach the preaponeurotic adipose tissue pad first rather than injure the levator aponeurosis with this maneuver, and it allows one to readily identify the preaponeurotic space (Fig. 6.5).
- Opening of the orbital septum—When the preaponeurotic adipose tissue is seen, it is typically fluctuant, and as one reaches, it easily prolapses through small rents in the orbital septum (this may not be as easily seen in the elderly). The septum is opened horizontally with a blunt scissors (Westcott's), avoiding blood vessels in the adipose tissue pads or the levator aponeurosis underneath (Fig. 6.6).
- Treatment of adipose tissue pad—The strip of skin-muscle bounded by the two skin incisions is retracted inferiorly using a Blair retractor. If preaponeurotic adipose tissue is overlying along the superior tarsal border, where the crease construction is to occur, it can be partially excised (no more than 20%) (Fig. 6.7). If the adipose tissue is not abundant, it is best to preserve it by freeing it and allowing it to reposition superiorly into the sulcus. This maneuver often seems to greatly facilitate the glide mechanism (glide plane) of the levator relative to the anterior skin lamella, allowing an eyelid crease to indent dynamically against a passively relaxed preseptal skin-muscle layer that forms the eyelid fold.

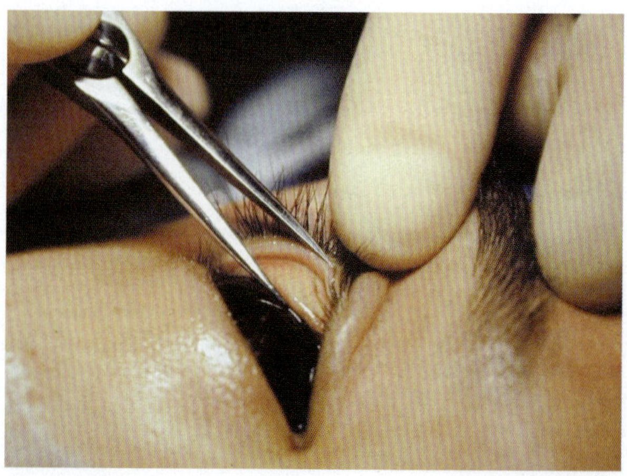

FIGURE 6.3

Eversion of the upper lid and measurement of the tarsal plate with a caliper.

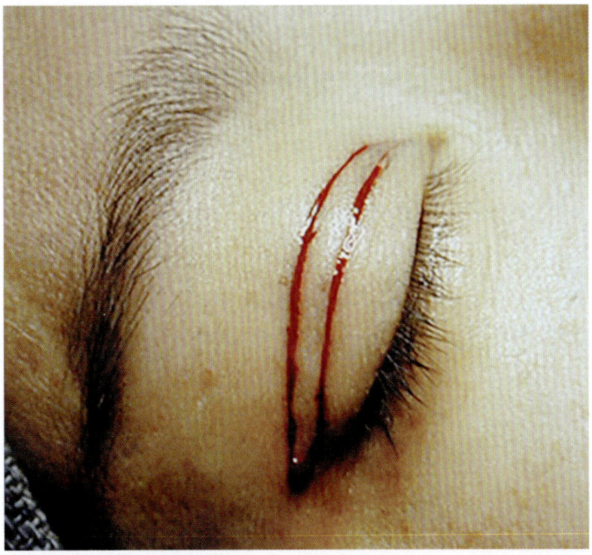

FIGURE 6.4

Incision through the skin only. Measurements increasing from 1 to 2 to 2.5 mm in a medial to lateral direction.

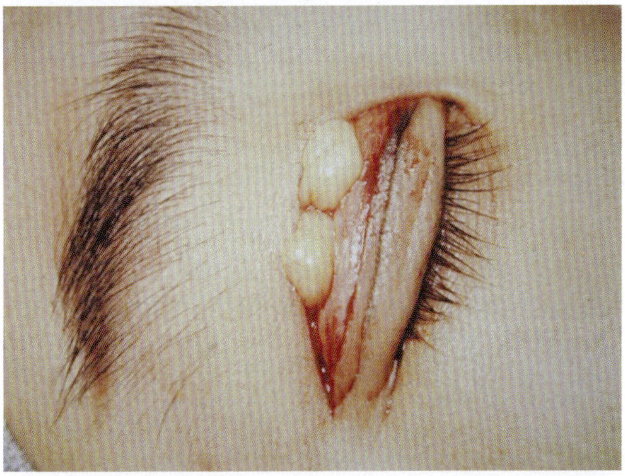

FIGURE 6.5

Transection through the orbicularis oculi and direct visualization of the preaponeurotic adipose tissue pads.

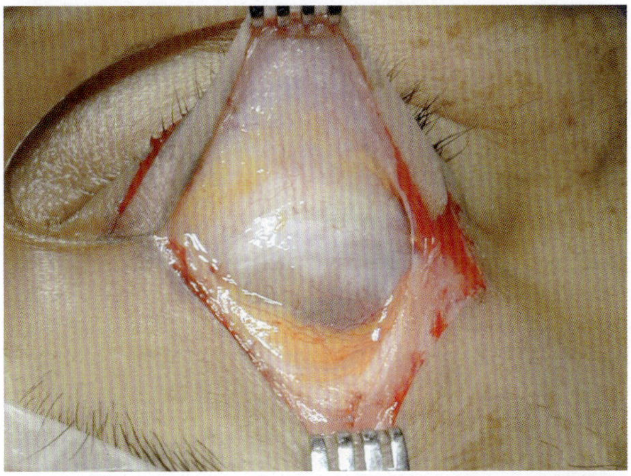

FIGURE 6.6

Horizontal opening of the orbital septum.

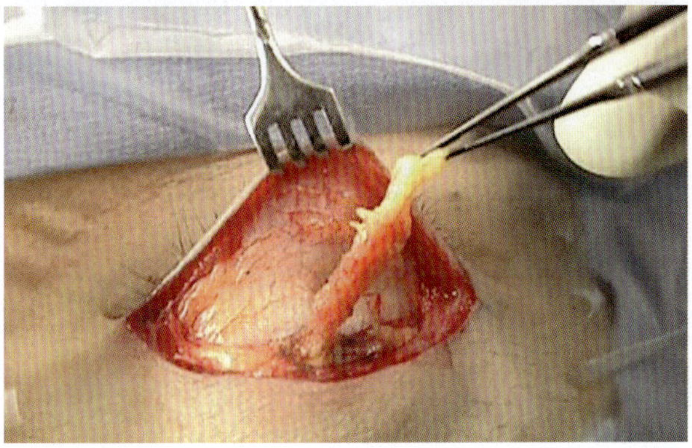

FIGURE 6.7

Partial removal of the preaponeurotic adipose tissue pad that overlies the tarsal plate and impairs the future placement of the skin–levator–skin sutures.

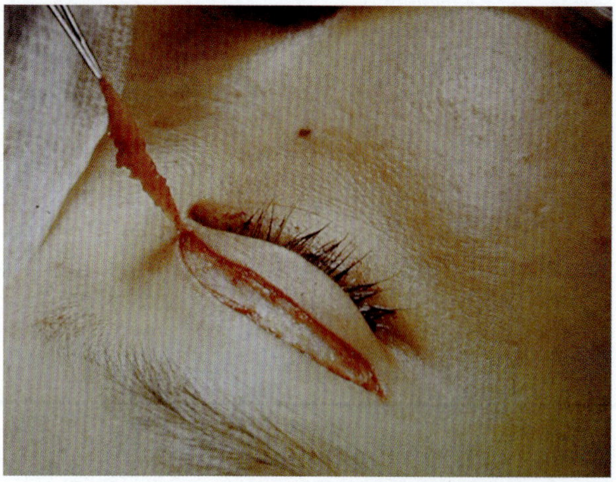

FIGURE 6.8
Excision of the skin and orbicularis oculi trapezoidal fragment and a fragment of orbital septum.

- Trimming of the skin-muscle strip—The small slip of preseptal skin and orbicularis oculi muscle (2-mm skin plus a slightly larger fragment of preseptal muscle just above the upper tarsus) is excised using cutting cautery (Fig. 6.8). This is an efficient and a precise maneuver. With the lid crease skin incision and only two additional steps (first superiorly beveled vector was through the orbicularis and septum, second vector through orbicularis along the superior tarsal border), one can complete a uniform and beveled excision of these layers: skin and orbicularis oculi as a trapezoidal fragment and fragment of orbital septum overlying the distal 4 to 5 mm of the levator aponeurosis.
- Resetting of the tissue plane—This is the most underappreciated step in upper blepharoplasty in general. After the steps above, it is essential to release the forehead drapes and reposition the anterior skin-muscle layers properly in relation to the underlying aponeurosis. It avoids setting an exaggerated crease height, induction of secondary ptosis, lagophthalmos on downgaze, and a secondary high-arched brow as a compensatory reaction. In revision cases, this resetting allows some skin recruitment and brings in additional soft tissues to partially fill in any deep sulcus from excision of adipose tissue associated with previously aggressive blepharoplasty.
- Wound closure and crease construction—I use 6-0 silk sutures which I apply from the lower skin edge, taking a very small bite of the aponeurosis along the superior tarsal border, then through the upper skin edge and then tied down. Six to seven interrupted sutures are typically used. The rest of the skin gap is closed using 7-0 Prolene, nylon, or silk (Fig. 6.9). The corneal eye shield is removed from the right eye and applied to the left eye where the procedure is repeated. Each eye is irrigated with normal saline. The surgeon checks for symmetry in the crease and makes any necessary adjustments.

POSTOPERATIVE MANAGEMENT

The patient applies ice compresses to the upper eyelids and is instructed to continue icing as well as bed rest for 1 day. The patient may bathe and sit up for their meals the first day; they are told to have restricted physical exertion the first week. Topical gentamicin–steroid ointment (Pred-G, by Allergan) is applied four times daily for 1 week. Suture removal is usually in 1 week. Figure 6.10 shows a young Asian female patient before and 2 months after the procedure.

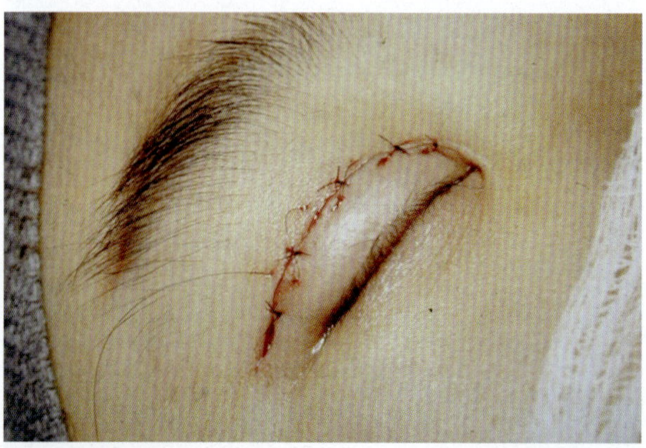

FIGURE 6.9
Placement of interrupted 6-0 silk suture in skin–levator–skin fashion. Additional closure with 7-0 nylon.

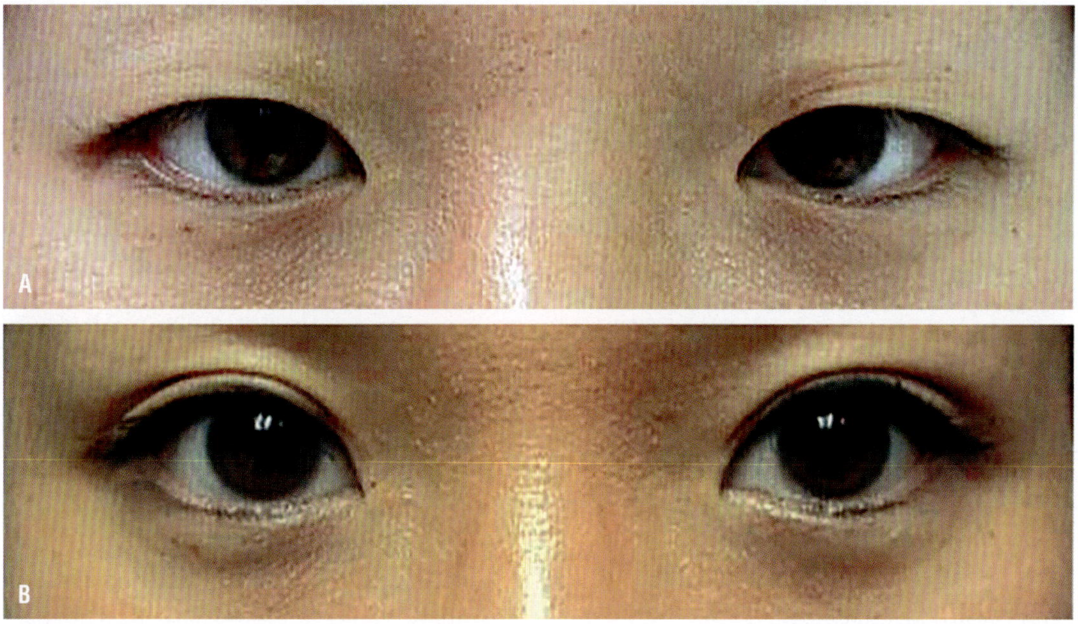

FIGURE 6.10 Pre- and postoperative images **(A and B)**.

COMPLICATIONS

There are many situations in which patients may consider their results as suboptimal, or at worst, as complications. Suboptimal results most often involve asymmetries, and this may be from insufficient formation of their crease on one or both sides, partial crease formation, and discrepancy in the height of the crease or shape. Complications involve overly aggressive removal of skin, muscle, adipose tissue, or high anchoring of crease indentation. The latter is more common among earlier practitioners of this art.

I have not covered the suture methods (suture ligation methods). Although most would agree that these variations of double eyelid surgery is simpler to perform, it has its own sets of suboptimal results including the most common complaint of disappearance of crease after several years (or months), foreign body sensation from buried permanent sutures that may be on the posterior side of lids (anterior on corneal surface) or midlamellar in nature, and static appearance on down-gaze. From an aesthetic standpoint, these are results that are unacceptable.

RESULTS

Among all practitioners, the overall consensus is that approximately 15% to 20% of primary cases with external incision methods may need touch-up revision. This is probably in line with most cosmetic procedures though the numbers may well be lower in skilled hands. I believe that when a high bench mark is set of recreating a *permanent, natural (shape and height) crease*, the current technique provides for the best control of these parameters with lessened incidence of complications.

PEARLS

- Accurate preoperative definition of the desired crease height and shape.
- A layered and selective treatment of each eyelid.
- Atraumatic dissection, precise hemostasis and prevention of tissue injury can reduce intraoperative soft tissue distortion and afford more accurate results. This establishes the proper orientation and spatial geometry of the semirigid pretarsal skin and tarsus (posterior lamella, vectored by the levator muscle) relative to the more passive preseptal skin and orbicularis (anterior lamella) when the lids are opened.
- Preservation of the preaponeurotic adipose tissue is key in preserving an Asian appearance to the upper eyelid and preventing a sunken superior sulcus.

- Resetting of the eyelid skin and forehead structures relative to the posterior lamella prevents the distortion of the skin–levator–skin closure and the resultant crease that is formed.
- Exact anastomosis of levator aponeurosis to lid crease incision along the superior tarsal border ensures a natural crease that is dynamic and disappears on downward gaze as opposed to the skin–tarsus–skin technique (static lid crease).

PITFALLS

- A high lid crease (9 to 12 mm) occurs if a surgeon empirically applies a lid crease height without regard to ethnicity.
- The semilunar (Caucasian) crease is rare in Asians and is the most common, unwanted result from surgery in the United States.

INSTRUMENTS TO HAVE AVAILABLE

- Standard oculoplasty surgical tray
- Sharp-tipped Westcott spring scissors
- Dull-tipped Westcott spring scissors
- Castroviejo needle holders (straight)
- 0.12, 0.30, and 0.50 forceps

SUGGESTED READING

Chen WPD. Concept of triangular, trapezoidal and rectangular debulking of eyelid tissues: application in Asian blepharoplasty. *Plast Reconstr Surg* 1996;97(1):212–218.

Chen WPD. The concept of a glide zone as it relates to upper lid crease, lid fold, and application in upper blepharoplasty. *Plast Reconstr Surg* 2007;119(1):379–386.

Chen WPD. Beveled approach for revisional surgery in Asian blepharoplasty. *Plast Reconstr Surg* 2007;120(2):545–552.

Chen WPD. Chapter 7 (Primary Asian blepharoplasty) and Chapter 15 (Revisional Asian blepharoplasty). In: Chen K, ed. *Color atlas of cosmetic oculofacial surgery, second edition, with DVD*. Butterworth-Heinemann/Elsevier Science, Ltd., 2010. ISBN: 07506-74229.

Chen WPD, Chen K. *The eyelid crease and double eyelid surgery*, 2013. An iBooks textbook, available through Apple's iTunes Store as a download file, readable on all Macintosh computer running the latest operating system Maverick, current iPad, iPhone and iTouch devices.

7 ENDOSCOPIC BROW LIFT

Marc H. Hohman

INTRODUCTION

The periorbital area is essential for nonverbal facial expression and communication, and critical to social engagement. With advancing age, the eyebrows descend due to gravitational forces, loss of elasticity of the scalp and forehead tissue, and repeated muscle contraction. These changes, combined with the development of vertical and horizontal rhytides of the central forehead and glabella, result in a tired, heavy, crowded, or even "angry" appearance. In patients with significant lateral hooding, visual field deficits are commonplace. Loss of volume also occurs, transforming a youthful, oval face into a more rectangular or deflated one.

To rejuvenate the upper third of the face effectively, a surgeon must place the eyebrow in an ideal position, and even restore lost volume when indicated, while maintaining harmony with the upper eyelids and minimizing surgical scarring and distortion of the hairline.

The endoscopic brow lift has become a well-established technique in upper facial rejuvenation. First described by Isse in 1992, it is preferred by patients and surgeons alike due to decreased length of the incision, less scarring, decreased risk of numbness, decreased bleeding, and a more rapid recovery when compared to traditional coronal or trichophytic approaches.

HISTORY

Prior to undertaking any cosmetic or functional procedure, the patient's motivation for surgery and expectations must be discussed. Having the patient look into a mirror, describe the specific changes he or she would like to effect, allows the surgeon to determine the patient's goals and tailor a suitable surgical plan.

Patients with brow ptosis often present with concerns of a tired, heavy, or angry appearance. They may report dissatisfaction with deep glabellar or forehead rhytides. If severe lateral hooding or eyelid ptosis is present, the patient will likely complain of visual field restriction. Frequently, patients request only upper blepharoplasty and fail to recognize the contribution of brow ptosis to the aging face.

The surgeon should inquire about previous surgical, traumatic, or minimally invasive treatments, such as neuromodulators or injectable fillers, which may affect the clinical examination. All previous orbital and periorbital surgeries should be documented, especially blepharoplasty, which may predispose the patient to postoperative lagophthalmos if aggressive brow lifting is performed.

Systemic diseases predisposing the patient to adverse outcomes should be identified during the initial consultation. Particular attention should be directed toward underlying thyroid disease, allergic symptoms, or recurrent episodes of eyelid edema suggestive of blepharochalasis. One should also make note of autoimmune diseases such as Sjögren's, rheumatoid arthritis, or myasthenia gravis. Perhaps most importantly, any history of xerophthalmia should be identified, because the surgical plan may require alteration to avoid exacerbation of the problem.

PHYSICAL EXAMINATION

In order to perform an endoscopic brow lift successfully, it is critical for the surgeon to have a precise understanding of facial anatomy and brow aesthetics as they relate to the clinical examination. The brow itself is a structure consisting of thick hair-bearing skin just superior to the thin skin of the upper eyelid. In general terms, the ideal male brow overlies the bony supraorbital ridge. The ideal female brow, as classically presented by Westmore, begins with the medial brow along the vertical plane of the alar–facial junction and ends laterally at an oblique line drawn from the lateral alar point through the lateral canthus (Fig. 7.1). The medial and lateral ends of the eyebrow are nearly level on a horizontal plane, but there is a variable degree of aesthetic arch between them. Location of the ideal brow apex has ranged from above the lateral limbus to the lateral canthus with current ideals resting somewhere in-between. There is a range of aesthetic ideals across ethnic groups, but the general differences between the ideal male and female brow positions remain fairly consistent. The brow is a naturally hair-bearing area, and variations in aesthetic taste may also affect the amount and location of the hair in this region. However, the location of the anatomical brow is determined solely by the position of the thick soft tissue and not by the presence or pattern of hair. This is important as it is the shape of the eyebrow that is a greater determinant of brow aesthetics than the elevation of the brow in relation to the orbital rim.

The patient should be examined with the head aligned in the Frankfort horizontal plane and the eyes in primary gaze. Brow ptosis appears as soft tissue overhanging the orbital rim, usually most prominent laterally. This causes the eyes to appear aged and tired. The examiner should note the skin texture, skin color, and position of the eyebrows. Many patients with dermatochalasis or brow ptosis compensate by elevating the brows. This results in prominent transverse forehead rhytides (Fig. 7.2).

Asymmetric transverse forehead rhytides may indicate asymmetric brows or ptosis. To determine the natural brow position, the patient should close his or her eyes and fully relax the forehead. The examiner should then apply gentle downward traction on the brow to simulate the effect of gravity, releasing the brow and then instructing the patient to reopen his or her eyes slowly and without raising the eyebrows. Often times, for those patients with frontalis muscle hyperactivity, the examiner may need to place his or her hand on the patient's forehead to keep the brow in a neutral position. This maneuver frequently exposes brow ptosis and upper eyelid dermatochalasis, as well as upper eyelid ptosis, if present. Palpation of the supraorbital rim is useful in determining the amount of brow ptosis present. It is important to remember that many female patients alter the quantity or pattern of brow hair, but this does not affect the position of the anatomical brow. The astute surgeon determines where the true brow is positioned during preoperative evaluation. Mobility of the forehead can be assessed with the glide test, in which the examiner manually elevates the brow to the desired position; the point of maximal elevation is then planned according to the patient's needs, generally at or lateral to the lateral limbus. Lastly, temporal hollowing should be noted in case volume augmentation needs to be performed concurrently.

The surgeon should note the position of the hairline using the Norwood's or Ludwig's classification system. The distance from the upper brow to the anterior hairline should be about 5 cm, and the distance from the midpupil to the inferior brow border should be approximately 25 mm. The distance between the medial brows

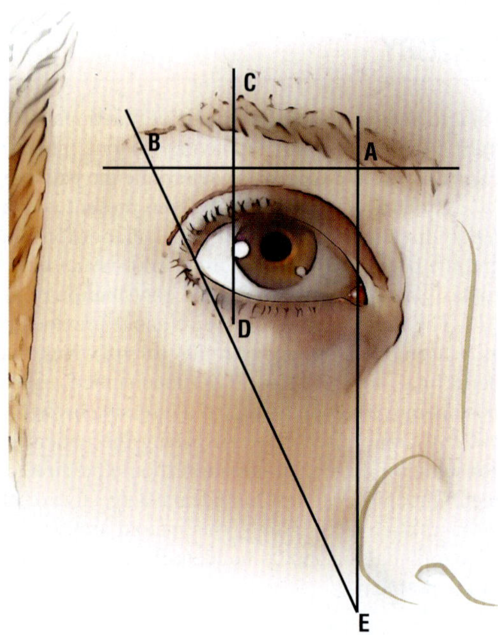

FIGURE 7.1
Key landmarks for aesthetic brow analysis include the club of the medial brow (*A*), the lateral brow tip (*B*), the peak of the brow arch (*C*), the lateral limbus of the cornea (*D*), and the alar–facial junction (*E*).

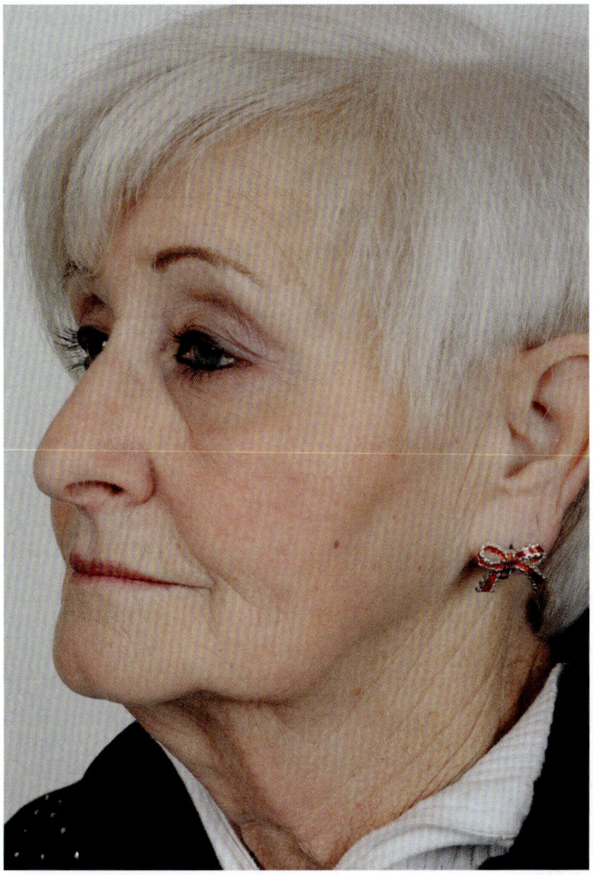

FIGURE 7.2
Hyperactive frontalis muscle resulting in prominent transverse forehead rhytides.

should approximate the distance between the medial canthi. Asymmetries should be documented and demonstrated to the patient preoperatively. Failure to recognize asymmetry prior to surgery may result in inadequate correction and patient dissatisfaction.

The texture and quality of the eyelid skin should be examined. The presence of webbing, scars, and lesions should be noted in addition to assessment of excessive skin, muscle, adipose tissue, or ptotic lacrimal glands. Accurate evaluation of the upper and lower eyelids must be completed with the brow in neutral position. The lateral canthal angle should be sharp, with the lateral canthus positioned roughly 2 mm above the medial canthus. The upper eyelid crease should be located 9 to 12 mm from the central lid margins for females and 8 to 10 mm for males. Patients with brow ptosis frequently also have excess eyelid skin, which can easily be addressed with upper lid blepharoplasties immediately following endoscopic brow lift.

Recognition of eyelid asymmetry is critical when identifying those patients with ptosis. There are many causes of eyelid ptosis, but it frequently results from dehiscence of the levator aponeurosis and presents with a decreased upper margin reflex distance 1 (MRD1). The MRD1 is the distance from the corneal light reflex to the upper eyelid margin and is usually between 3 and 4.5 mm. Disinsertion of the levator aponeurosis also results in a higher lid crease with a deepened superior sulcus. Patients typically have asymmetric brow positions with deep transverse rhytides on the affected side due to excessive frontalis activity. With an MRD1 of less than 2 mm, visual field obstruction is typically present, and ptosis repair should be considered and discussed with the patient.

The lower lid should be inspected for entropion, ectropion, and excessive laxity. The position of the globe should be assessed because a proptotic globe may cause the eyelid skin to appear retracted and predispose the patient to lagophthalmos. A retracted globe may result in pseudoptosis. Whenever malposition of the globe is noted, surgical intervention should be delayed until the appropriate etiology is identified and addressed.

Assessment of dry eyes is important in all patients undergoing brow or eyelid surgery. A simple way to screen for dry eyes is to inquire if the patient uses moisturizing eye drops. If dry eye symptoms are present, tear production should be evaluated with the Schirmer's test. If aqueous tear film deficiency is found, dry eye symptoms may require further evaluation and treatment prior to surgery. Patients with significant eye symptoms or findings should undergo a formal assessment by an ophthalmologist prior to any elective periorbital procedure.

Assessment of the cranial nerves should be performed with particular attention to the frontal and zygomatic branches of the facial nerve and the sensory status of the first branch of the trigeminal nerve. In the event that facial nerve dysfunction is identified, consideration should be given to performing either a unilateral brow lift on the affected side or an asymmetric brow lift. The goal should be to bring the paretic brow within 3 to 4 mm of the normal side's height, ideally spitting the difference between repose and elevated positions, which will minimize the appearance of asymmetry.

At the conclusion of the physical examination, preoperative photography should be performed, both for surgical planning and medicolegal documentation. Review of the photographs prior to surgery will often reveal subtle findings, such as asymmetry in brow position, thickness, or shape, that were not apparent on initial physical examination. The following views are photographed, zoomed in on the periorbital region, and zoomed out to frame the whole face: frontal view in repose, frontal view with eyes closed gently, frontal view looking upward, and frontal view with brows elevated; the same views should be documented in profile. All photographs should be taken in the Frankfort horizontal plane for the sake of consistency of perspective.

INDICATIONS

- Brow ptosis
- Lateral eyelid hooding secondary to brow ptosis
- Forehead and glabellar rhytides
- Visual field deficits

CONTRAINDICATIONS

- Those patients with uncontrolled ocular disease or systemic health problems predisposing them to anesthetic risk should not undergo surgery.
- Those patients with unrealistic expectations or who anticipate secondary gains are not good candidates for cosmetic surgery.
- Caution is advised in those patients who have a history of trauma to the forehead or prior forehead reconstruction.

PREOPERATIVE PLANNING

The preoperative plan should be clearly documented, and appropriate photography should be obtained prior to surgery. Standard preoperative photography is described above. These photos may be posted in the operating room for reference.

Preoperative counseling of the patient should include a discussion of the risks and benefits of the procedure, as well as the concerns that are anticipated to arise postoperatively. While the operation is not particularly painful, there will be mild edema and potentially some periorbital ecchymosis. Despite making all five of the incisions within the hair, the risk of infection is low. Occasionally, there can be hair loss at the incision sites, or the hairline may recede slightly. Nerve injury, both sensory and motor, temporary and permanent, has been described, but the risk is low. Many patients do, however, note persistent discomfort at the sites of implant placement, if implants are used for suspension. I advise patients to avoid palpating the implants, which usually allows tenderness to abate. Dissatisfaction with the procedure due to asymmetry or other complaints is rare.

Surgical Anatomy

The soft tissues of the forehead can be divided into five aesthetic subunits: central forehead, lateral temporal units, and eyebrows. The bony landmarks of the zygomatic arches, orbital rims, and nasal root represent the lower anatomic boundaries, while a natural hairline represents the upper limits. The temporal line divides the lateral forehead from the temporal regions, and the orbital rim serves as a consistent marker in the evaluation of brow ptosis.

An understanding of subunit interrelation is essential for conceptual planning as well as surgical outcome. The central forehead is a direct extension of the scalp and is layered, from superficial to deep, with skin, connective tissue, galea aponeurotica, loose areolar tissue, and periosteum. The first three layers of the central forehead are tightly held together, in contrast to the loosely attached skin and fascia of the temporal region. Within the soft tissues overlying the supraorbital ridges is a confluence of muscular insertions, which include the paired frontalis, orbicularis oculi, corrugator supercilii, procerus, and depressor supercilii muscles. The interplay of these muscles is responsible for the wide array of brow expressions as well as the associated observed changes with aging.

The galea aponeurotica separates along the superior origin of the frontalis muscle to form the superficial and deep galeal planes. These planes envelop the muscles along their anterior and posterior surfaces and extend to the lower forehead. Along the brow region, numerous fibrous septa from the frontalis muscles penetrate the thin superficial galea and interdigitate into the orbicularis oculi, procerus, and the overlying dermis. The frontalis muscle is the primary elevator of the brow, and contraction of this muscle produces transverse forehead rhytides.

There are numerous eyebrow depressors: the orbicularis oculi, the depressor supercilii, the procerus, and the corrugator supercilii, all of which are superficial to the frontalis. The orbicularis oculi muscle serves as a powerful lateral brow depressor due to the lack of a corresponding muscular elevator to oppose it. It is located just deep to the skin, making it a very superficial muscle, particularly the palpebral portion, which underlies the thinnest skin of the body. Repeated contraction of the orbicularis results in thin lateral rhytides, which are often referred to as "crow's feet." More medially, a smaller muscle—which some consider to be a part of the orbicularis oculi—is the depressor supercilii, a brow depressor that is frequently the target of chemodenervation in order to provide a "chemical brow lift." Deep to the orbicularis oculi at the glabella, the procerus muscle originates from the nasal bones and upper lateral cartilages and has vertically oriented fibers that insert into the dermis. The procerus causes inferior and medial displacement of the medial eyebrow with resultant horizontal rhytides in the glabella and upper nasal radix. The corrugators superciliorum are paired muscles originating from the superomedial orbital rims and lying just deep to the procerus. Their fibers are obliquely oriented and insert into the medial eyebrow dermis. They pull the brow medially and inferiorly, resulting in the vertical and oblique glabellar rhytides commonly termed "frown lines." Deep to the corrugators are the terminal fibers of the frontalis, which overly the pericranium. The periorbita and the pericranium merge to form the orbital septum, which originates from a fibrous ring around the periphery of the orbit known as the arcus marginalis. This ligamentous structure serves to anchor the periorbital soft tissues to the underlying bone, limiting their mobility when acted upon by muscles such as the frontalis.

Continuing laterally toward the temporalis muscle, the galea aponeurotica merges with the superficial temporal fascia, also known as the temporoparietal fascia (TPF), at the conjoint tendon, where this plane is adherent to the underlying pericranium and the edge of the temporalis muscle fascia. The TPF is continuous with the superficial musculoaponeurotic system (SMAS) of the lower face. Under the TPF, and directly investing the temporalis muscle, is the temporalis fascia, also known as the deep temporal fascia; this arises from the pericranium. This fascia divides into superficial and deep layers at the level of the supraorbital ridge with the superficial temporal adipose tissue pad located between these layers. The superficial and deep layers of the deep temporal fascia attach to the superior margin of the zygomatic arch at their lateral and medial locations, respectively. Medial to the deep temporal fascia is the deep temporal adipose tissue pad, which is contiguous with the buccal adipose tissue pad. Caution is taken to avoid injury of this structure as the development of temporal wasting may occur.

Motor and Sensory Nerves

The muscles of the upper face are innervated from the deep surface by the frontal branch of the facial nerve. This is the most important nerve to preserve during an endoscopic brow lift, as it is responsible for motion of the eyebrow and forehead. Though there are multiple small, variably located rami that constitute the frontal branch, a good approximation for the nerve's location is Pitanguy's line, which runs from a point 5 mm below the tragus to roughly 15 mm above the lateral aspect of the eyebrow. In the temporal area, the frontal branch of the facial nerve runs along the deep surface of, or within, the deepest layers of the TPF.

Another landmark for the frontal branch is the medial zygomaticotemporal, or "sentinel" vein, which traverses the potential space between the TPF and the temporalis fascia. The frontal branch is located superficial and superior to this vein, within a 2 to 10 mm radius (Fig. 7.3), as it courses from lateral to medial. Inferiorly, the frontal branch exits the superior border of the parotid gland and then crosses over the zygomatic arch, where it courses through the condensation of parotid fascia, SMAS, and zygomatic arch periosteum, which places it at risk for injury in this location. Because of this, the safest planes for elevating over the zygomatic arch are subperiosteal and subcutaneous.

Sensation of the brow and forehead is provided by branches of the trigeminal nerve. The supratrochlear nerve exits the orbit and pierces the medial corrugator supercilii to provide sensation to the medial forehead. The supraorbital nerve exits the orbit though a foramen along the orbital rim in nearly 90% of patients but can also exit the orbit through a foramen up to 15 mm above the orbital rim. Above the orbital rim, the supraorbital nerve branches into two divisions: superficial and deep. The superficial division travels in a supramuscular plane over the frontalis, providing sensation to the lateral forehead, scalp, and lateral upper eyelid, while the deep division travels laterally between the galea aponeurotica and pericranium to innervate the frontoparietal scalp. The supratrochlear nerve exits approximately 10 mm medial to the supraorbital nerve along the superior orbital rim and provides sensation to the glabella, medial forehead, and medial upper eyelid.

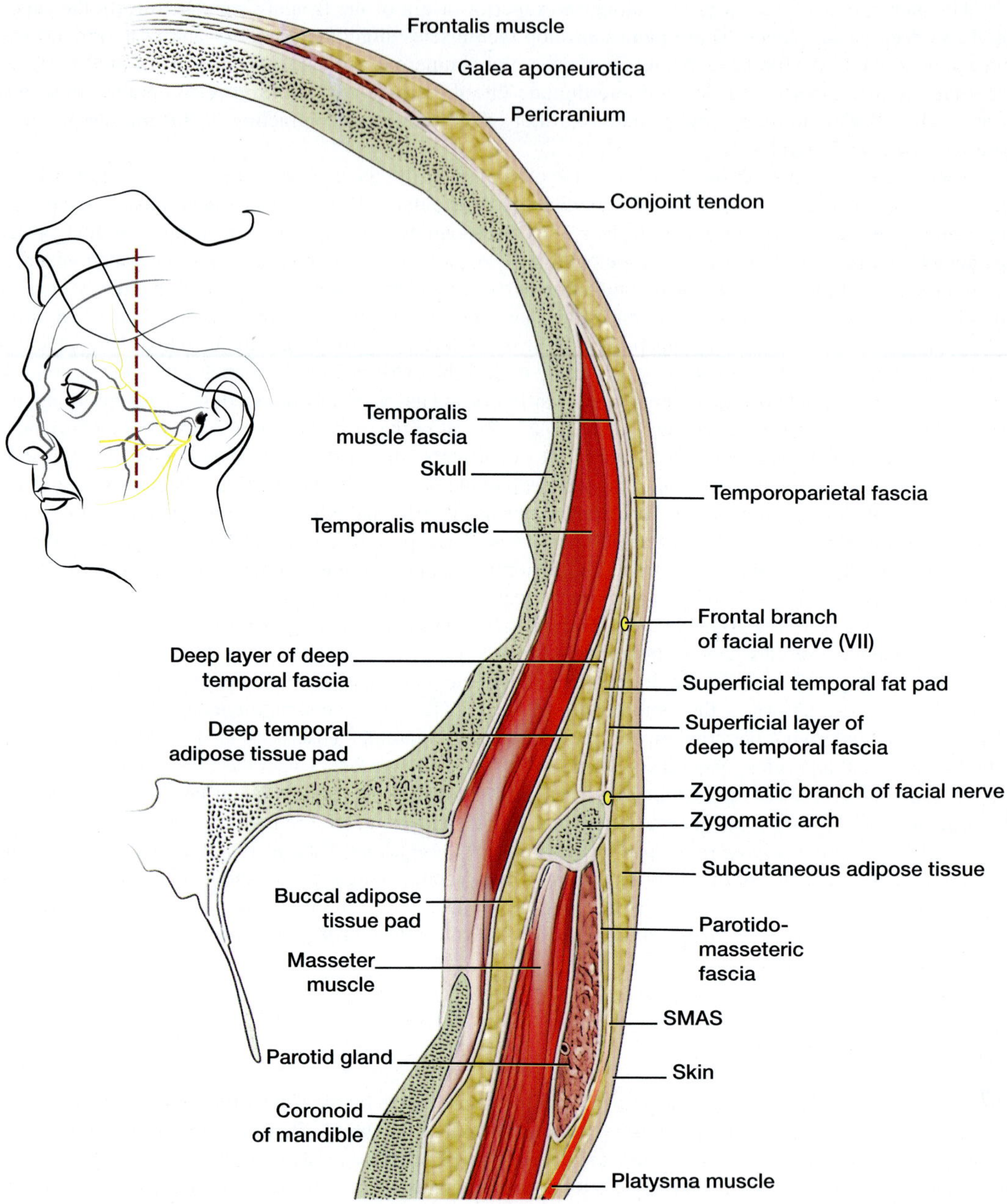

FIGURE 7.3 Anatomic layers relevant to endoscopic brow lift and the location of the temporal/frontal branch of the facial nerve.

SURGICAL TECHNIQUE

Dissection

Standard instrumentation includes a 4-mm 30-degree endoscope with a cannula, camera and video screen, a light source, multiple periosteal elevators, endoscopic graspers, insulated bipolar cautery forceps or monopolar suction cautery, and skin retractors (Fig. 7.4).

The procedure may be performed under intravenous sedation or general anesthesia. I prefer to perform the surgery under general anesthesia for superior patient comfort, especially when forehead lifting is performed in conjunction with other rejuvenation procedures. If upper blepharoplasty is to be performed concurrently, it is done after the brow lift to avoid inadvertent removal of excess skin of the upper eyelid, which would predispose the patient to postoperative lagophthalmos. Optimal patient positioning is reverse Trendelenburg with the endoscope video tower placed at the foot of the patient so it may be easily viewed by the surgeon. Marking is performed at the midline, paramedian, and temporal incision sites. The hair is

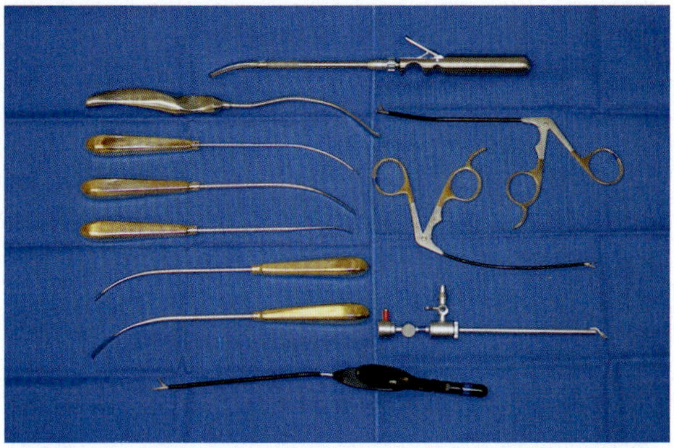

FIGURE 7.4
Standard instrumentation for endoscopic brow lift.

carefully wrapped and secured with hair ties. The surgeon sits at the patient's head, and the assistant sits beside the surgeon, opposite to the side of the video screen.

Placement of the Incision

Three sagittally oriented scalp incisions (2 cm) and two coronal temporal incisions (3.5 cm) are made. The midline scalp incision and two paramedian scalp incisions are marked 1 to 2 cm posterior to the hairline (Fig. 7.5A and B). The lateral scalp incisions are placed on a vertical line in the desired vector of maximal brow elevation. This usually corresponds to the lateral limbus in females and is more medial in males. The temporal incisions are marked 2 cm posterior and parallel to the hairline to provide for appropriate temporal lifting and redraping, typically centered on a line drawn from the lateral nasal ala through the lateral canthus or slightly above it. These temporal incisions may be incorporated into rhytidectomy incisions, if needed. After marking, the surgeon then injects the incision sites, forehead, supraorbital and supratrochlear neurovascular bundles, and arcus marginalis using 1% lidocaine with 1:100,000 epinephrine. The patient is then prepped and draped in the standard fashion.

Dissection

A no. 15 blade is used to make the incisions, avoiding excessive cautery to the skin edges to prevent damage to the hair follicles. I incise directly through skin, subcutaneous adipose tissue, and periosteum simultaneously for the central and paramedian ports; the incision is only carried down to the temporalis fascia in the lateral ports. The assistant opens the central and paramedian incisions with double-prong skin hooks, while a Freer elevator is used to open the subperiosteal plane. A quarter curved Daniel endoforehead elevator is then placed into the central incision to create a subperiosteal optical cavity. The subperiosteal plane is a relatively avascular and safe until one approaches the supraorbital rim. Blind dissection is performed centrally to within 1 to 2 cm of the supraorbital rim and several centimeters cephalically to assist with redraping following scalp advancement. A half-curved elevator may be useful closer to the brow. Laterally, dissection extends to the conjoint tendon.

After central forehead elevation, the fascia of the temporalis muscle is exposed in the lateral ports, which requires dividing TPF, which I do by spreading and snipping with long tenotomy scissors while the assistant

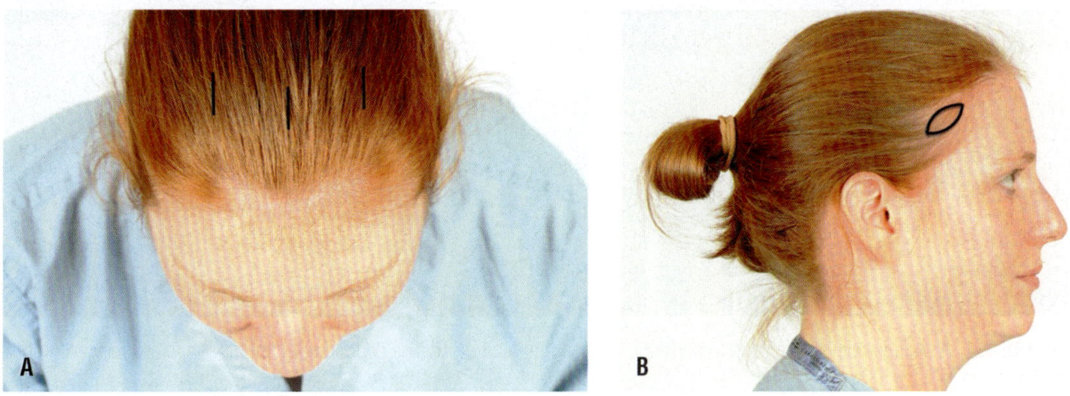

FIGURE 7.5 **A:** Median and paramedian incisions for endoscopic brow lift. **B:** Temporal incision for endoscopic brow lift.

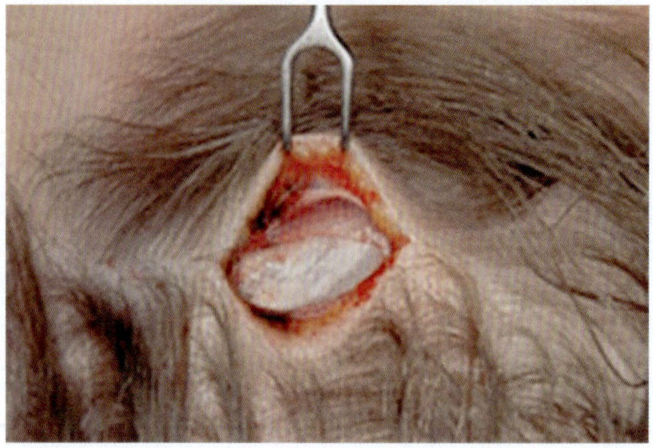

FIGURE 7.6
Surgical view of temporal incision with dissection through the TPF and exposure of the superficial layer of the deep temporal fascia (*white*) that is also known as the temporalis muscle fascia.

opens the incision with double-prong skin hooks (Fig. 7.6). A Freer elevator is used to perforate the conjoint tendon, from lateral to medial, passing into the central forehead optical cavity. A sweeping motion along the calvarium superiorly and inferiorly releases the conjoint tendon, creating continuity between the lateral and central dissection compartments and facilitating elevation of the brow as a unit (Fig. 7.7); this may be done blindly by an experienced surgeon. Under endoscopic visualization, typically through the paramedian port, dissection proceeds directly on the temporalis fascia inferiorly and along the lateral orbital rim, releasing the arcus marginalis superior to the lateral canthus (Fig. 7.8). As the dissection approaches the lateral orbital rim, the sentinel vein is encountered at approximately the level of the frontozygomatic suture (Fig. 7.9). If possible, it is left undisturbed, as reports of temporal varicosities postoperatively have been reported with sacrifice. However, when this vein or other adjacent vessels hinder dissection, bipolar cautery should be applied at the base of the vessel on the surface of the deep temporal fascia. This ensures maximum protection of the branches of the facial nerve from transmitted thermal injury. Once the sentinel vein has been located, dissection may proceed inferiorly without fear of injury to the facial nerve; this elevation may be performed blindly if the surgeon is comfortable with the technique.

After the lateral arcus marginalis release is complete, the more technical dissection at the central orbital rim is performed. The endoscope is introduced into the central scalp incision, and the supraorbital and supratrochlear neurovascular bundles are isolated with the Daniel endoforehead nerve dissector (Fig. 7.10). The remainder of the arcus marginalis is then released with the Ramirez periosteal spreader. The periosteum may be preserved medially to the supratrochlear bundle to avoid excessive medial brow elevation, which may give the patient a "surprised" or "operated" look. It is critical that the lateral orbital rim and arcus marginalis be adequately released in order for the soft tissue of the forehead and upper lid to be repositioned superiorly without tension. This may be confirmed by manually elevating the forehead for accurate assessment of mobility, although the brow will generally elevate spontaneously after forehead elevation and arcus marginalis release are complete.

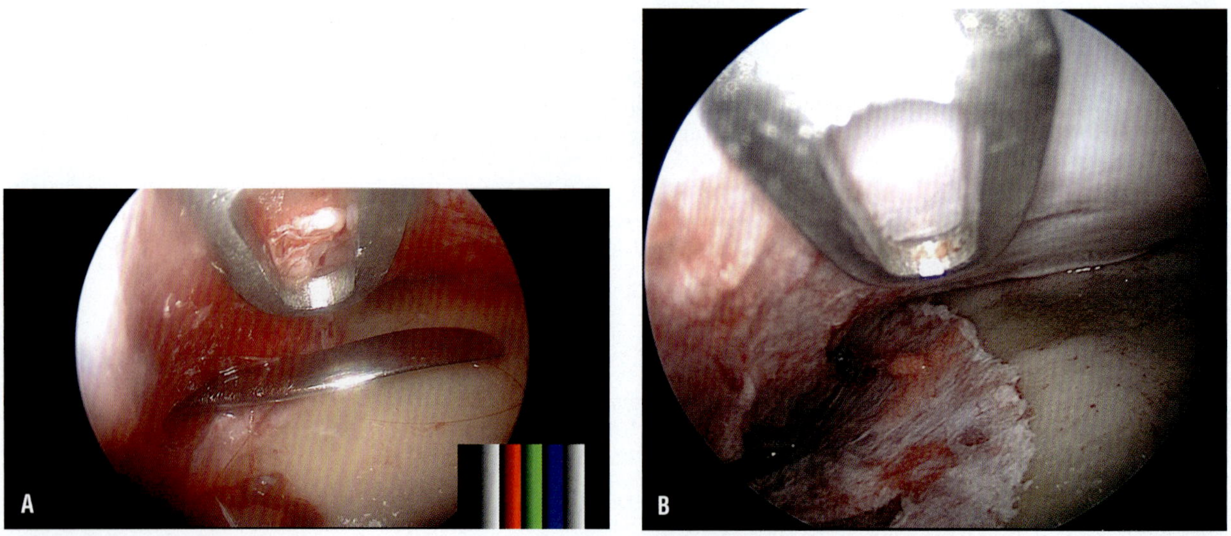

FIGURE 7.7 **A:** A Freer elevator is used to perforate the conjoint tendon. **B:** The divided conjoint tendon affords a view of the temporal line.

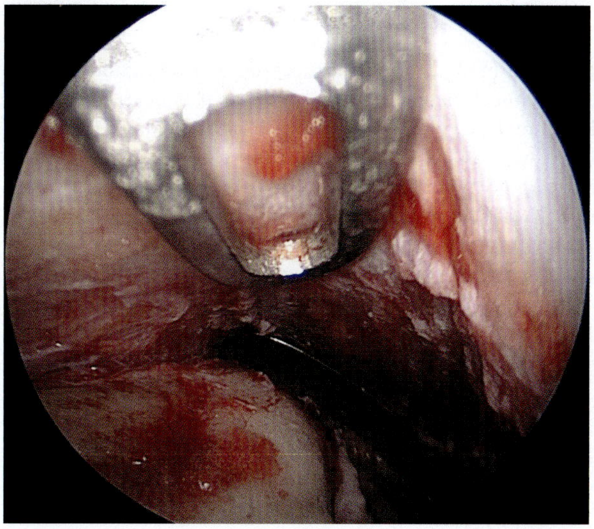

FIGURE 7.8
Release of the arcus marginalis along the lateral orbital rim permits elevation of the lateral brow.

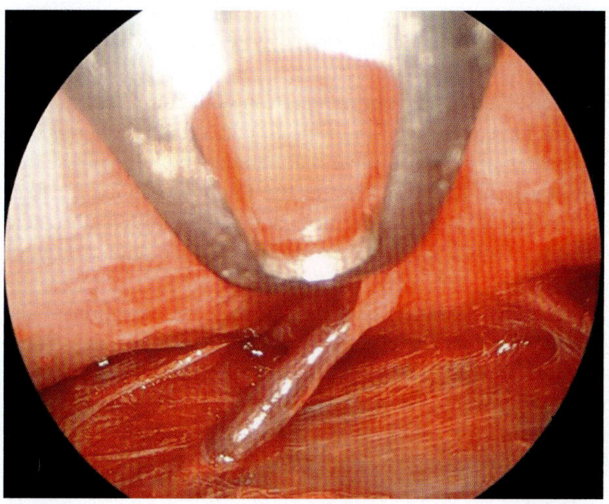

FIGURE 7.9
Endoscopic view of the sentinel vein. The temporalis fascia is deep, and the TPF is superficial. The frontal branch of the facial nerve runs in the TPF. It is found superior to and within 10 mm of the sentinel vein.

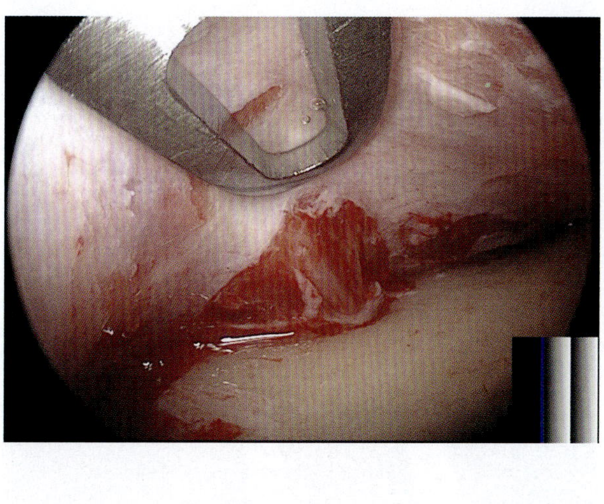

FIGURE 7.10
Identification and dissection of the supraorbital neurovascular bundle. Note the periosteal release on either side.

Muscle Release

The corrugator and procerus muscles are then identified medial to the supraorbital neurovascular bundles and exposed with careful dissection. The corrugator muscle is encountered first, as it is deep to the procerus. Corrugator fibers travel in an inferomedial direction, while the procerus muscle fibers run vertically. These muscle fibers are carefully teased apart with an elevator or nerve dissector and ablated with electrocautery. Some surgeons leave the medial corrugator muscle undisturbed to protect the supratrochlear nerve. Others suggest dissecting out the nerve prior to medial release. Symmetric corrugator muscle release is important to prevent postoperative contour irregularities. Overly aggressive muscle resection in the glabellar region may cause excessive lateralization of the medial eyebrows, potentially resulting in an operated appearance.

Temporalis fascia may be harvested through the temporal incision and placed in the glabellar region, where muscle resection was performed, to improve postoperative contour and to minimize return of muscle function. The amount harvested corresponds to the amount of corrugator and procerus muscle resected. The harvested fascia is secured with a 3-0 polydioxanone suture, which is passed transcutaneously using an endoscopic needle driver through the glabella to position it at the site of corrugator release. The suture is tied over the skin and left in place for 3 days before removal to provide adequate time to minimize fascia migration. Alternatively, one may use adipose tissue in this area if provided from a concomitant procedure.

Fixation

Long-term brow stability is dependent upon periosteal readherence at the level of fixation. A number of different techniques have been described for brow fixation with the optimal method still being debated. These include tissue sealants, suture fixation, cortical bone tunnels, permanent screws, K-wire, and resorbable screw fixation.

Regardless of the technique chosen, the surgeon must ensure appropriate fixation with complete and adequate readherence of the periosteum. Numerous studies have examined the time to periosteal readherence in rabbit models. Most report 6 to 8 weeks of fixation is necessary for complete readherence, but recent research has shown periosteal refixation may be completed as early as 12 days. I prefer the Endotine device for fixation (MicroAire Surgical Instruments, LLC, Charlottesville, VA), which are polylactic acid–polyglycolic acid polymer resorbable periosteal fixators. The recipient sites for the implants are drilled into the outer cortex of the skull (Fig. 7.11), typically centered over the lateral limbi.

No medial fixation is performed. Instead, medial brow elevation results from passive elevation of the brow complex from unopposed frontalis activity, due to release of the corrugator and procerus muscles. Some surgeons place a small round drain in the forehead, but I do not do this routinely. The skin incisions may be closed with sutures or staples. I prefer 4-0 deep dermal poliglecaprone sutures and 5-0 running plain gut along the superficial scalp. Attention is then directed to the temporal incisions.

The lateral temporal skin is fixated to the deep temporal fascia after the brow is elevated to the desired position and the temporal skin is redraped in a superolateral direction (Fig. 7.12). Excess skin is excised (typically 1 cm) with a no. 15 blade, beveling the edges to promote hair growth through the incision line, and a 3-0 polyglactin suture is used to secure the superficial temporal fascia to the deep temporal fascia using multiple buried sutures for deep fixation. A head dressing is applied at the conclusion of the case.

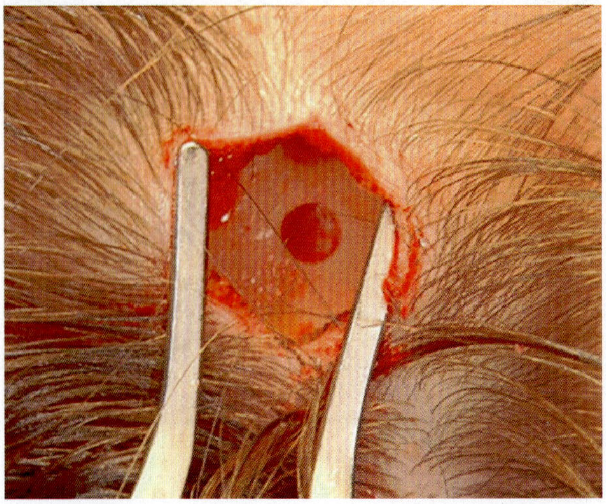

FIGURE 7.11
Intraoperative image of brow suspension recipient site after drilling of the outer cortex.

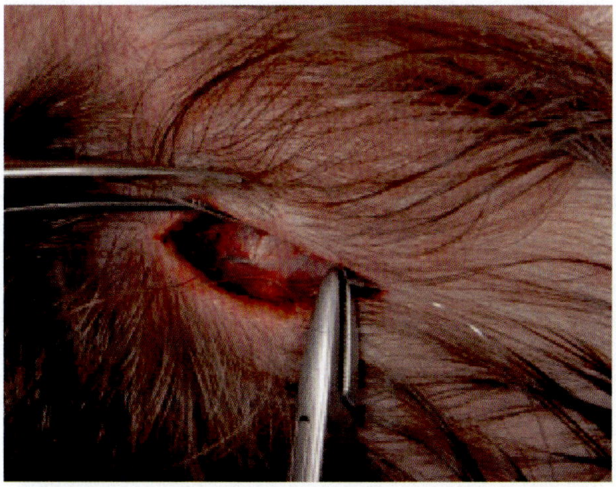

FIGURE 7.12
The lateral temporal skin is fixed to the deep temporal fascia, redraping the skin in a superolateral direction.

POSTOPERATIVE MANAGEMENT

Narcotic pain medication is prescribed for all patients in the immediate postoperative period. Drains and the head dressing are routinely removed on postoperative day 1, and washing the hair is permitted thereafter. The patient is instructed to keep the head of the bed elevated 30 to 45 degrees for the first 3 days and to avoid vigorous activity for 2 weeks after surgery. Photo documentation is performed at each patient visit for comparison and record keeping. Examples of postoperative results are shown in Figure 7.13A and B. Figure 7.14 provides a schematic of the vectors used in an endoscopic brow lift.

COMPLICATIONS

Endoscopic brow lifting remains a relatively safe procedure with a low rate of complications (Table 7.1). Even with the minimally invasive approach, up to 22% of patients report feelings of social restriction following the procedure due to pain, edema, or hematoma. These complaints are usually transient and resolve within the first 4 weeks after surgery.

- *Alopecia* occurring along the incision lines is reported as the most common complication. Careful attention to tissue handling and minimal use of electrocautery limit damage to surrounding hair follicles. All tension in closure should be at the galea, with minimal tension along the skin edges. If significant, alopecia may be treated with excision of the involved segment of the scalp or with hair grafting techniques.

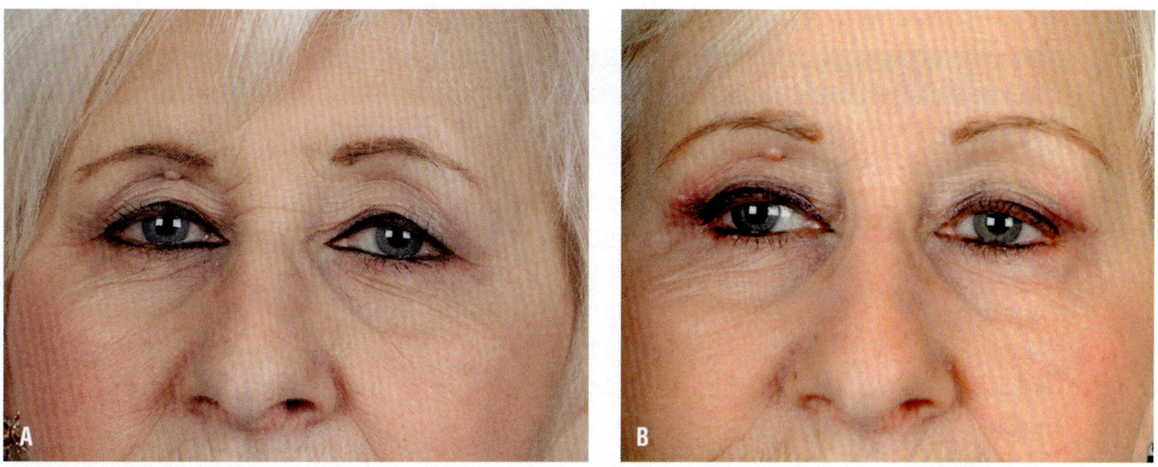

FIGURE 7.13 **A:** Preoperative photograph. Note asymmetry of brows, with both medial brows located inferior to bony supraorbital rim. The upper eyelids also have significant dermatochalasis with lateral hooding. **B:** Postoperative photograph, 9 months after endoscopic brow lift with upper blepharoplasty. Note symmetry of brows, with position just above bony supraorbital rim, and significant reduction of dermatochalasis and lateral upper lid hooding. A conservative upper blepharoplasty was performed due to a history of xerophthalmia.

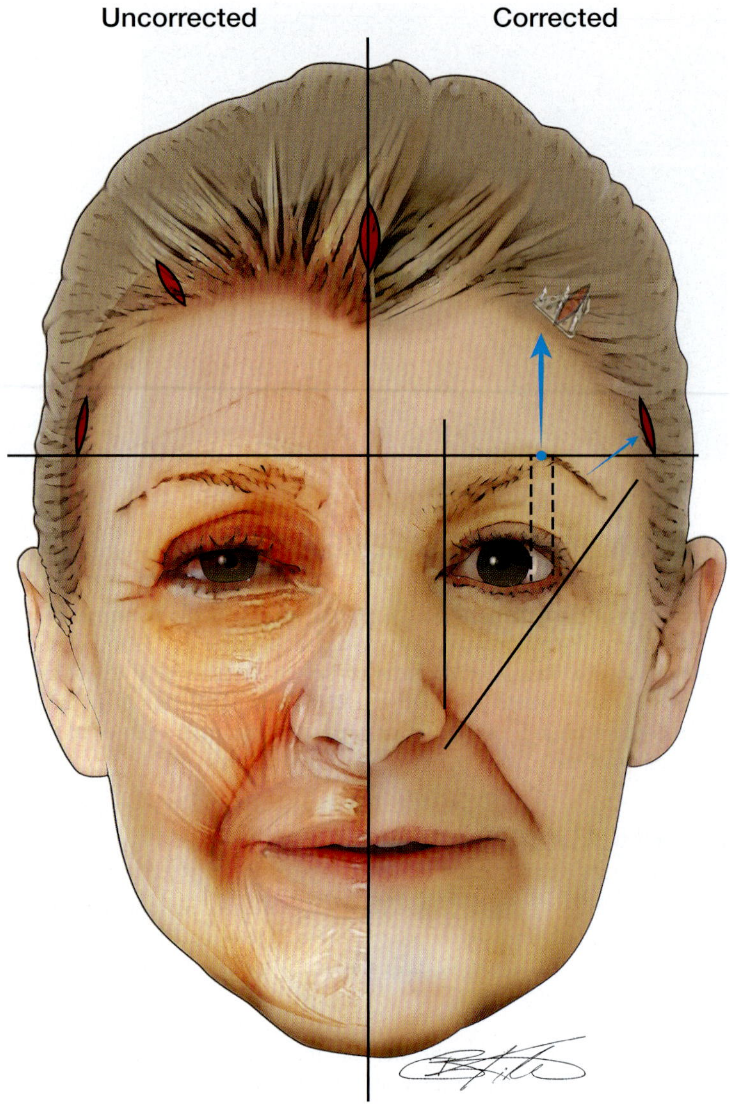

FIGURE 7.14
Composite illustration displaying brow aesthetics (line references around the left eye), surgical access points (*red lines*), brow suspension vectors (left eye), and implant (left calvarium) in preoperative and postoperative states.

TABLE 7.1 Summary of Reported Complications after Open Brow Lifts and Endoscopic Brow Lifts

Complication	Open (*n* = 3,534) (%)	Endoscopic (*n* = 3,417) (%)
Alopecia	4.0	2.9
Dissatisfaction	0.8	1.8
Scarring	0.8	<0.1
Asymmetry	0.8	1.2
Sensory loss	0.1	0.6
Infection	<0.1	<0.1
Lagophthalmus	<0.1	<0.1
Motor deficiency	<0.1	<0.1
Abnormal contour	<0.1	<0.1
Hematoma	<0.1	<0.1

From Elkwood A, Matarasso A, Rankin M, et al. National Plastic Surgery Survey: Brow Lifting Techniques and Complications. *Plast Reconstr Surg* 2001;108(7):2143–2150.

- *Asymmetry* may result from surgical error, fixation failure prior to periosteal readherence, or persistence of preoperative asymmetry. If significant, revision surgery may be required. Recurrent brow ptosis or insufficient brow elevation is frequently attributed to inadequate release of the arcus marginalis.

For minor asymmetry or ptosis, botulinum toxin injections may benefit the patient and help avoid further surgery; however, the extent of elevation with chemodenervation remains unpredictable.

- *Medial brow malposition* is an unfortunate finding after overaggressive resection of the procerus and corrugator musculature. The medial brow becomes elevated, and the distance between the medial heads is widened. A surprised appearance results when the brow is uniformly elevated with overresection, and a depressed appearance occurs when the arcus marginalis is inadequately released and the central musculature is overresected. Initial treatment is supportive, but often revision surgery is necessary for reversal of elevation. Such procedures are complex and are best avoided with conservative muscle treatment during the brow lifting procedure.
- *Numbness of the scalp* is frequently reported following brow lifting procedures due to traction on neurovascular bundles. Careful dissection of the corrugators and selective bipolar cauterization minimize avulsion and thermal injury to neurovascular bundles. It is important that the patient understand preoperatively the common but temporary nature of this complication, as the majority of this resolves in the weeks to months following surgery.
- *Contour abnormalities* have been reported in those patients with irregular corrugator and procerus release. This may be addressed intraoperatively with the placement of autologous adipose tissue or fascia, or postoperatively with autologous adipose tissue or fillers.
- *Lagophthalmos* may occur in patients with a prior history of blepharoplasty or with an aggressive brow lift combined with upper blepharoplasty. It is often preferable to perform brow lifting prior to upper blepharoplasty to avoid excessive skin resection. For those patients with prior upper eyelid surgery, conservative brow lifting is recommended to minimize the risk of lagophthalmos.
- *Injury to the facial nerve*: The most severe complication is injury of the frontalis branch of the facial nerve. Fortunately, such an event is rare and may be avoided by meticulous dissection in the appropriate surgical planes, gentle tissue handling, and attention to key anatomic landmarks (e.g., sentinel vein) as discussed. However, if neuropraxia is observed, watchful waiting is recommended with light frontalis muscle massage suggested on the side of the injury. The nerve regenerates approximately 1 mm per day, and injuries medial to the lateral canthus should recover within a 90-day time frame. If injury is persistent, contralateral chemodenervation may improve brow symmetry.

RESULTS

The endoscopic technique remains an effective method to reduce brow ptosis, improve brow symmetry, and reduce forehead and glabellar rhytides with relatively few complications. Compared to open techniques, it offers the patient shorter scar, less paresthesia, quicker recovery, and increased acceptance. Overall, the lift appears to persist well, with up to 65% of patients reporting a continued improvement in appearance 5 years following surgery.

PEARLS

- Defining the goals of each individual's procedure (ideal eyebrow position, symmetry, establishment of stable fixation, reduction of rhytides) is critical in creating natural-appearing results.
- Knowledge of aesthetic ideals of the brow and periorbital region in men and women is critical, as many aesthetic surgical procedures may feminize the face.
- Multiple techniques are available for brow fixation. Explore each option and choose the one that best suits your surgical approach. Some implants are palpable until they are resorbed.
- A single 30-degree scope will meet your surgical needs.
- The sparing use of bipolar cautery prevents loss of tissue and hair.
- Facial swelling and supine positioning can cause the brow to appear more elevated than it will after recovery.
- Aging is a panfacial process; therefore, the brow and upper eyelid must often be addressed together.

PITFALLS

- Facial asymmetries need to be reviewed with the patient preoperatively and addressed during surgery. In many circumstances, an asymmetric surgery is performed to create a symmetric result. However, this will not happen if preoperative asymmetry goes unrecognized.

- Eyebrow asymmetry and asymmetric forehead rhytides may be the result of eyelid ptosis and must be recognized preoperatively if present.
- The most common technical failure during brow lift is the failure to release the arcus marginalis completely. If the brow has not elevated after release, but before fixation, then it has not been adequately released and requires further attention.
- Aggressive muscle resection and excessive medial elevation are key partners in creating an "operated look."
- Cautery along the undersurface of the elevated flap can lead to injury of the frontal branch of the facial nerve.
- Caution is advised in patients who have undergone a previous blepharoplasty, as tension bands may become apparent after brow lifting.
- Performing upper blepharoplasty before the brow lift can result in lagophthalmos.

INSTRUMENTS TO HAVE AVAILABLE

- No. 3 Bard-Parker scalpel handle
- 10-mm two prong Joseph skin hook × 2
- Freer elevator
- Quarter curved Daniel endoforehead elevator
- Half curved Daniel endoforehead elevator
- Daniel endoforehead nerve dissector
- Daniel endoforehead cannula, single stopcock
- 10-cc syringe
- Ramirez endoforehead periosteal spreader
- Adson-Brown forceps
- Reynolds tenotomy scissors
- 5-inch Halsey or Webster needle holder
- Curved iris suture scissors
- Suction cautery
- Insulated bayonet bipolar forceps
- 30-degree rigid endoscope and camera
- TPS drill with Endotine bit
- Endotine prostheses and holder

ACKNOWLEDGMENT

The author would like to thank Patricia S. McAdams, MD, for her contributions to this chapter. Her work in writing, editing, and figure creation for this chapter is greatly appreciated.

SUGGESTED READING

Chiu ES, Baker DC. Endoscopic brow lift: a retrospective review of 628 consecutive cases over 5 years. *Plast Reconstr Surg* 2003;112(2):628–633.

Hohman MH, Kim SW, Heller ES, et al. Determining the threshold for asymmetry detection in facial expressions. *Laryngoscope* 2014;124(4):860–865.

Isse NG. Endoscopic facial rejuvenation: endoforehead, the functional lift. Case reports. *Aesthetic Plast Surg* 1994;18(1):21–29.

Ridgway JM, Larrabee WF. Anatomy for blepharoplasty and brow-lift. *Facial Plast Surg* 2010;26(3):177–185.

Terella AM, Wang TD. Technical considerations in endoscopic brow lift. *Clin Plast Surg* 2013;40(1):105–115.

8 DIRECT BROW LIFT

Tom D. Wang

INTRODUCTION

The direct brow lift is one of several effective methods to surgically reposition the brow and rejuvenate the upper face. It is one of the most straightforward surgical approaches for managing brow ptosis due to aging or facial nerve paresis. Aging results in loss of skin elasticity, decreased bulk of subcutaneous tissue, and resorption of the skull bone. Together, these factors contribute to the development of forehead and eyebrow ptosis. These changes are usually first seen in the region of the lateral eyebrow. This is due in part to the agonist/antagonist relationship between the brow elevator (frontalis muscle) and the brow depressors (corrugators, depressor supercilii, procerus, and orbicularis muscles). The attachments of the frontalis muscle do not extend laterally beyond the temporal line. Hence, the depressors have unopposed action lateral to this area, and the lateral brow descends to a greater degree than the rest of the brow.

Brow ptosis is also a common sequelae of facial paralysis and in this setting may cause significant upper eyelid hooding and impairment of the superior visual field. To an observer, these changes in brow position, regardless of cause, convey a conception of fatigue, tiredness, and lethargy, despite good rest, energy, and health. In the aging face, brow lift aims to restore a more youthful appearance, while conveying a more rested and vigorous image. In the patient with facial paresis, brow lift serves to restore brow position and symmetry; these components are important to both facial recognition and relieving possible blockage of the visual fields.

Effective rejuvenation of the upper face, or paresis, requires a thorough understanding of aesthetics of the forehead and brow. The youthful forehead of a female is generally smooth and without significant rhytids. The male forehead may have shallow glabellar furrows and soft horizontal rhytids while still appearing youthful. While the aesthetics of the ideal upper brow is debatable, no universally accepted rule exists. However, it is generally accepted that in females, the brow should arch superolaterally, with an apex in line with the lateral limbus or the lateral canthus. The medial extent of the brow should abut a line vertically tangent to the lateral nasal ala, and the lateral extent should approximate an oblique line drawn from the nasal ala through the lateral canthus. In females, the youthful brow should be arched and lie just above the supraorbital rim. In males, the youthful brow position and contour are flatter without the high arching lateral aspect and should sit at the supraorbital rim.

Advantages of the direct brow lift include the following:

- Easy to perform
- Relatively direct control of brow position
- Limited risk to supraorbital, supratrochlear, and facial nerve
- Low risk of hematoma
- A long-lasting lift from orbicularis oculi suspension

Disadvantages of the direct brow lift include the following:

- Presence of a prominent, conspicuous scar on the forehead.
- Inability to address forehead and glabellar rhytids.
- It is difficult to achieve elevation and contouring of the medial portion of the brow.
- Placement of suspension sutures to a superior position on the periosteum is difficult.

HISTORY

As with any cosmetic or functional surgical procedure, the patient's motivation and expectations for surgery must be understood. A thorough ophthalmologic history should be obtained including a history of dry eyes and previous blepharoplasty or Graves's disease. A history of hypertrophic scar formation is important. If pertinent, the cause and timing of facial paralysis should be elucidated. General medical considerations including diabetes, autoimmune disease, cardiac disease, and a history of anticoagulants are of clinical value.

PHYSICAL EXAMINATION

The assessment should proceed with an overview of the face, brow, and eyes, specifically attempting to identify facial asymmetries, brow position, natural rhytids, eyelid ptosis, lid laxity, and skin thickness. The hairline should be documented using the Norwood classification. Next, the relationship of the eyebrow to the supraorbital rim is evaluated. Brow ptosis creating hooding must be differentiated from dermatochalasis.

Predisposition to hypertrophic scarring may direct the choice of surgical approach to a less invasive technique. In the setting of facial paralysis, it is important to note and record mimetic facial tone using the House-Brackman scale. Lastly, preoperative photographs are obtained. Standardized photographic views are important for preoperative and postoperative assessments. They should include a 5-view head series, along with close-up views of the eyes closed/open/upward gaze. Other surgeons may add a photo with the eyebrows raised.

INDICATIONS

- Any degree of brow ptosis producing lateral eyelid hooding and visual field deficits
- Women who are not candidates for other approaches
- Brow ptosis or asymmetry in the setting of facial paresis

CONTRAINDICATIONS

- Tendency to form hypertrophic or unsightly scar
- Male cosmetic brow lift patients—due to loss of villus hairs bordering the superior brow giving the brow a "tweezed" or feminized appearance
- A need to address forehead and glabellar rhytids

PREOPERATIVE PLANNING

The site of skin excision is directly above the eyebrow. A lazy S-shaped incision is planned along the upper border of the eyebrow. The highest point of brow elevation is usually above the lateral limbus or lateral canthus, and the maximum width of excised skin is 8 to 10 mm, depending on the degree of elevation desired (Fig. 8.1). Some surgeons advocated marking the patient while sitting upright, where gravity is contributing to the ptosis.

SURGICAL TECHNIQUE

Direct brow lift alone is usually completed under local or monitored anesthesia care (MAC) anesthesia.

- A sterile preparation of the forehead is performed.
- Both eyes are exposed in the surgical field.
- The operative site is infiltrated with a solution of 1% lidocaine and 0.5% bupivacaine with 1:100,000 epinephrine.

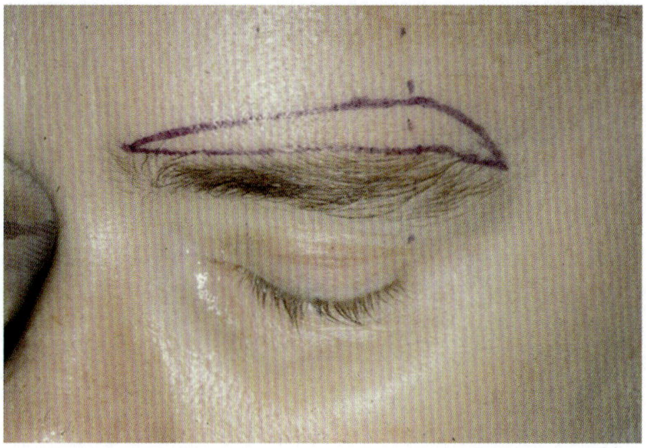

FIGURE 8.1
Skin excision is planned along the upper border of the eyebrow. The highest point of brow elevation is marked above the lateral canthus or lateral limbus.

- The skin excision is performed in the immediate subdermal plane; beveling of the incision is performed for favorable wound edge eversion.
- The subcutaneous tissue is left down on the frontalis muscle (Fig. 8.2).
- Care is taken to preserve the sensory nerves running in the supramuscular fascia.
- A small amount of undermining is carried inferiorly.
- Two buried 2-0 Vicryl sutures are used to secure the deep aspect of the orbicularis oculi (which has been split by the incision) to the pericranium at the desired level (Fig. 8.3).
- Skin is closed with a 6-0 fast-absorbing gut in a running locking fashion. Care must be taken to properly align the skin edges (Fig. 8.4).

POSTOPERATIVE MANAGEMENT

A small amount of bacitracin ointment is applied to the incision lines. A head dressing is not routinely placed.

COMPLICATIONS

One disadvantage to the direct approach is the possibility of a conspicuous scar on the face. Prominent scarring may be due to many factors but commonly is from disruption of the fine vellus hairs that border the brow superiorly. This results in an unnatural, sharply defined "tweezed" upper brow margin. Secondly, after skin excision, the skin thicknesses above and below the excision are quite different.

Other potential complications include motor nerve injury, lagophthalmos, bleeding or hematoma, and paresthesia due to supraorbital nerve injury. Ueda et al. in a review of 40 patients, who underwent direct brow lift for facial nerve palsy, reported a 27.5% incidence of postoperative paresthesia but did not state whether this was transient or permanent. There have also been rare reports of early recurrence of ptosis when absorbable suture material was used.

RESULTS

The outcome of an effectively completed brow lift is improvement in brow ptosis and visual field defects as well as a brighter, more youthful, rejuvenated appearing upper face (Fig. 8.5).

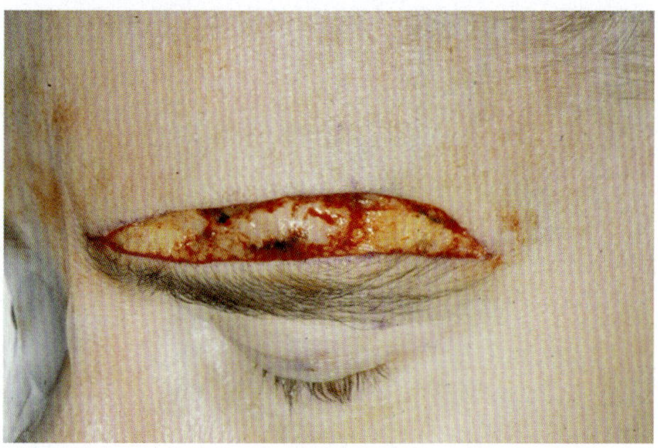

FIGURE 8.2
In order to preserve the sensory nerves running in the supramuscular fascia, the dissection is completed in a subcutaneous layer.

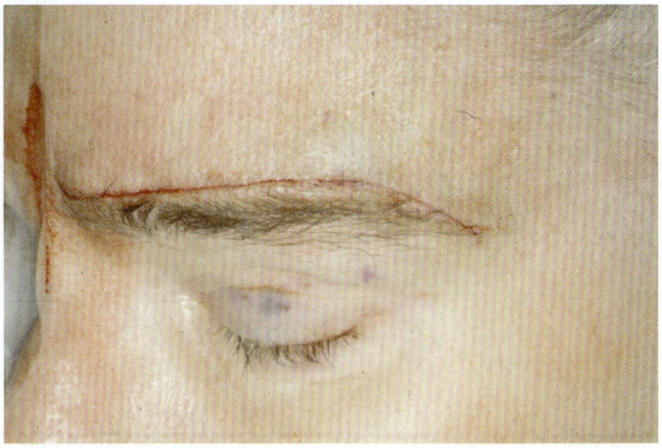

FIGURE 8.3
Two buried Vicryl sutures secure the deep aspect of the orbicularis oculi to the pericranium at the desired level.

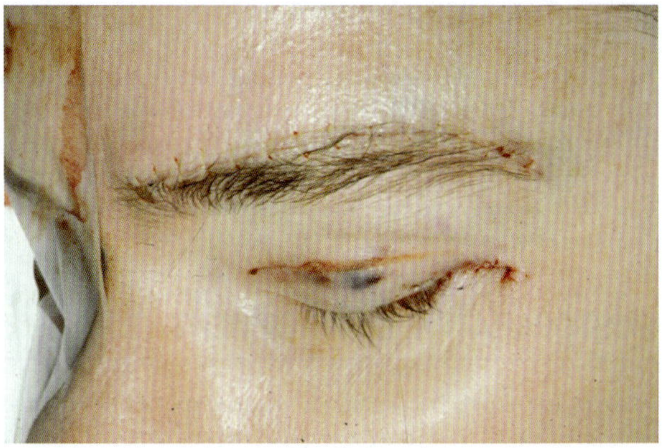

FIGURE 8.4
Skin is closed with a 6-0 fast-absorbing gut. The skin edges are carefully aligned so as to limit a conspicuous scar.

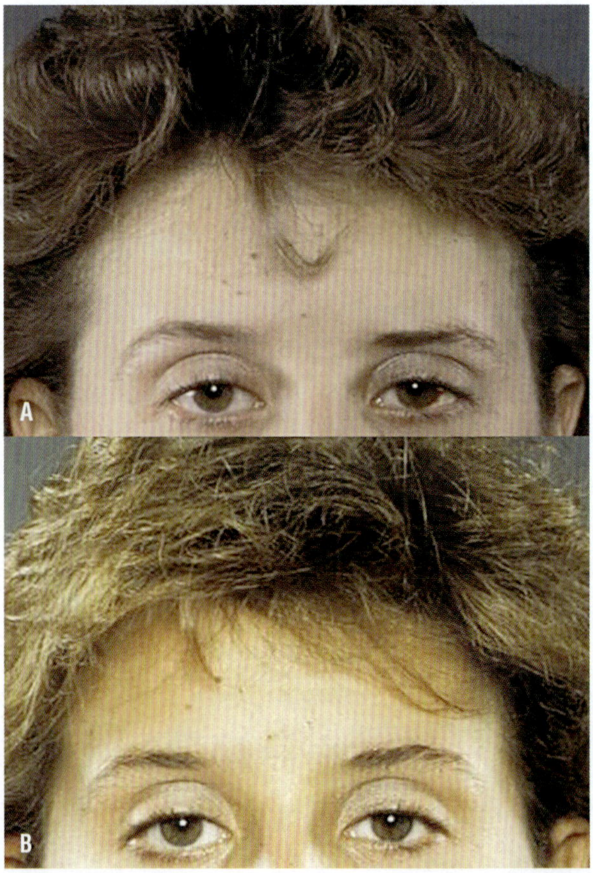

FIGURE 8.5
Left direct brow lift, pre- and postoperative images **(A, B)**.

In a postoperative evaluation of 40 patients with facial paralysis, more than 3 years after the direct brow lift, approximately 65% of patients had eyebrow symmetry.

PEARLS

- Bevel incisions parallel with hair shafts to minimize hair loss along incision line.
- The skin excision superiorly disrupts the abruptly transitioning skin thickness that occurs as the brow ascends over the supraorbital rims.
- To preserve the sensory nerves, maintain a dissection in the immediate subdermal plane, leaving subcutaneous tissue down on the frontalis muscle.

PITFALLS

- Scarring can be conspicuous and may not be an ideal technique for all patients.
- Paresthesia can occur superior to the incision.
- Soft tissue thickness mismatch after excision can potentially accentuate the frontal bar of the skull bone.

INSTRUMENTS TO HAVE AVAILABLE

- Standard plastic surgery tray
- Bishop-Harmon forceps
- 4-0 polydioxanone sutures (PDS) sutures for suspension
- 6-0 fast-absorbing gut skin sutures

ACKNOWLEDGMENT

The author would like to recognize Adam M. Terella, MD, for his exceptional contributions to the writing of this chapter. His work in the writing, editing, and figure creation for this chapter is greatly appreciated, without which this chapter would not have been possible.

SUGGESTED READING

Adamson PA, Brunner E, Pearson DC. The aging forehead, Chap. 179. In: *Bailey's head and neck surgery—otolaryngology*, 4th ed. Philadelphia, PA: Lippincott Williams & Wilkins, 2006:2663–2683.

Angelos PC, Stallworth CL, Wang TD. Forehead lifting: state of the art. *Facial Plast Surg* 2011;27(1):50–57.

Cook TA, Brownrigg PJ, Wang TD, Quatela VC. The versatile midforehead browlift. *Arch Otolaryngol Head Neck Surg* 1989;115(2):163–168.

Stallworth CL, Wang TD. Endoscopic and forehead rejuvenation. In: Massry GG, Murphy MR, Azizzadeh B, eds. *Master techniques in blepharoplasty and periorbital rejuvenation*. New York: Springer Science+Business Media, LLC, 2011.

Ueda K, Harii K, Yamada A. Long-term follow-up study of browlift for treatment of facial paralysis. *Ann Plast Surg* 1994;32(2):166–170.

9 TRICHOPHYTIC FOREHEAD LIFTING

Daniel E. Rousso

INTRODUCTION

If the eyes are considered the windows to the soul, then the eyebrow is the leading edge of the aesthetic frame in which each window resides. Each brow imparts a diversity of facial expression while directly influencing the perception of facial harmony. As a result, considerable effort has been invested in the surgical treatment of brow position and shape. In 1919, Passot initially described elliptical excisions to raise the brow complex. Hunt subsequently described coronal, anterior hairline, and direct brow lift techniques in 1926. However, it has been during the last three decades that the treatment of the brow complex has received considerable attention and focus. During this time, a constellation of techniques have been described, some more successful than others.

The importance of addressing the ptotic brow, in conjunction with or prior to excision of redundant upper eyelid tissue, has now become the operative focus. As techniques have advanced, surgeons have sought improved methods for camouflaging scars. One such improvement, the trichophytic incision technique, allows for treatment of brow and forehead ptosis while preserving hair follicles along the incision site. The resultant scar is penetrated by the patient's natural hair affording excellent camouflage and typically is very well tolerated by patients. In appropriately selected patients, the trichophytic brow lift is an effective technique for rejuvenation of the upper third of the face.

HISTORY

A complete history should be taken in conjunction with the consultation. This is usually facilitated in part by forms provided to the patient in advance of the visit. The patient's overall health status must be considered in deciding his or her candidacy for elective surgery, which includes anticoagulation status, tobacco use, autoimmune status, anesthetic risk factors, and overall wound healing capabilities. Next, the surgeon learns the patient's specific concerns and desires upon which recommendations for surgical correction are predicated. History of previous trauma, surgical interventions, facial nerve injury, and visual field deficits all contribute to the comprehensive development of an operative plan.

PHYSICAL EXAMINATION

A complete preoperative examination is performed by the surgeon during which anatomic and aesthetic principles are applied. Analysis of the forehead and brow requires consideration of multiple factors and aesthetic principles. The ideal forehead extends from the hairline to the glabella and should be in equivalent length to the midface, from glabella to the nasal base, and the inferior third of the face, from the nasal base to the menton. The typical distance from brow to hairline is 5 to 6.5 cm in women and 7 to 8 cm in men. An alternative estimate is about four fingerbreadths above the eyebrows. The ideal eyebrow should begin medially along a vertical

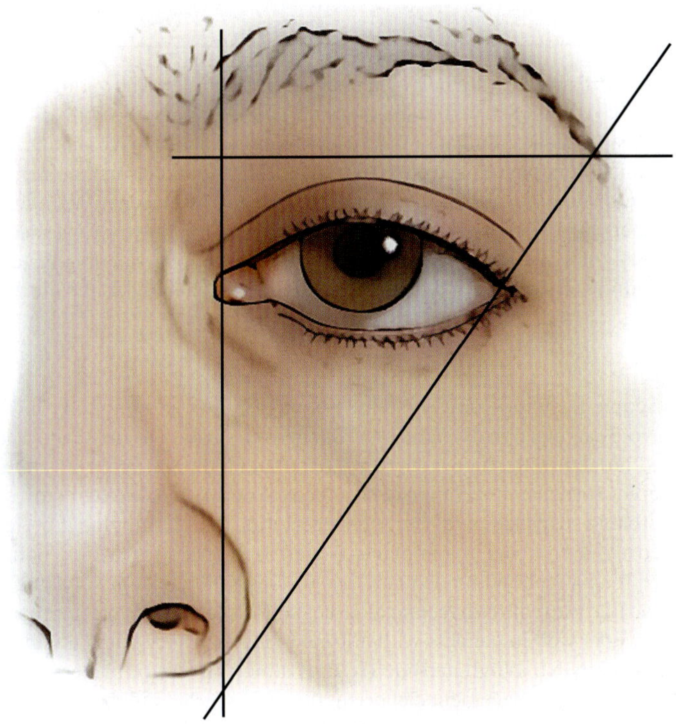

FIGURE 9.1
Ideal brow aesthetics.

line drawn from the lateral alar margin of the nose. It should extend laterally to an oblique line that begins at the lateral alar margin and extends through the lateral canthus (Fig. 9.1).

The shape and position of the eyebrows differ between men and women. In both sexes, the position of the lateral and medial ends of the eyebrows should be in close approximation. However, the lateral extent of the ideal female brow is higher. An inferior placement of the medial eyebrow confers an expression of anger or dissatisfaction, whereas a relatively inferior placement of the lateral eyebrow conveys the appearance of sadness or fatigue. Comparatively, the male eyebrow has a flat/horizontal shape and is located at or just above the orbital rim. The ideal female shape is observed as a gentle arch that peaks between the lateral limbus and lateral canthus. The medial aspect should be club shaped with a graceful taper laterally. The position is above the orbital rim, with the highest peak approaching 1 cm above the rim. The surgeon's artistic eye must be employed in order to design the most pleasing shape for each face.

Careful consideration is given with regard to which of the different brow lifting technique's is best suited for each patient. Every technique has its inherent advantages and disadvantages, and each is indicated for a specific group of findings. The height of the forehead and position of the hairline must be noted during the initial examination. This distance will play a significant role in the determination of the appropriate lifting approach. It is important to note if the patient has the natural expressive and resting tendency to spontaneously elevate the brows through inadvertent frontalis contraction. This elevation must be noted during the initial evaluation and brought to the patient's attention as it contributes to an altered position of the brow. Some authors describe a maneuver in which the patient is asked to close the eyes and relax the brows at which point the surgeon stabilizes the position of the brow. The patient then opens the eyes and sees the true position of the brow. Others simply have the patient close the eyes for 20 seconds then open. We do not routinely employ these maneuvers, but we do place emphasis on evaluating for falsely elevated brow position during each consultation. Regardless of method employed, the surgeon is well advised to evaluate the true position of the brow complex prior to surgical planning.

INDICATIONS

- Ptotic brows
- High hairline
- Adequate hair for scar camouflage

CONTRAINDICATIONS

- Low hairline
- Previous coronal brow lift
- Male gender (relative)

PREOPERATIVE PLANNING

There are several popular techniques for brow lifting, each with their own indications (Fig. 9.2). The various pros and cons of open and endoscopic techniques have been debated in the literature, but there may be little difference in the long-term outcomes between such approaches. Puig and LaFerriere found no statistically significant difference in brow position between endoscopic, trichophytic, and coronal brow lifting techniques in their series at 35- to 56-month follow-up. Guillot and Rousso demonstrated a statistically significant difference in scalp sensation in the postoperative period between open and endoscopic techniques. This difference, however, was negligible after a period of 18 months. Ultimately, there are multiple techniques that achieve long-standing results and similar long-term morbidity. The key is ultimately choosing the best technique for each individual patient.

Endoscopic Brow Lift

Described in 1992 by Vasconez, the endoscopic technique quickly gained popularity. As a "minimally invasive" approach, the endoscopic technique avoids an incision extending across the entire length of the scalp. The incisions are typically 1.5 cm in length and hidden in the hair along the frontal and temporal scalp by about 1 to 1.5 cm behind the hairline. Many different suspension techniques have been described including mattress sutures, cortical tunnels, bone screws, absorbable suspension devices, bolster fixation, and fibrin glue. I prefer a suture suspension technique that avoids costly or cumbersome implants as well as the need for drilling bone. The endoscopic technique is very effective for patients with adequate hair to cover the incision sites and a normal to low positioned hairline. A high hairline presents two technical issues. First, the endoscopic approach can tend to bring the hairline higher, which works well in patients with normal to low hairlines but is not ideal in a patient with an already broad, tall forehead. Next, a high hairline requires a more posterior placement of the incisions in order to hide them within the hair. This placement can orient the incisions behind the curvature of the frontal skull making visualization of the supraorbital structures difficult with the rigid, linear endoscope. The endoscopic approach has a clear advantage in scar camouflage and has been demonstrated to yield durable results. Many surgeons currently apply this technique as their method of choice in appropriate candidates.

Coronal Brow Lift

The coronal brow lift technique has been in use for almost a century since it was described by Hunt in 1926. The incision is designed in curvilinear fashion approximately 4 to 6 cm behind the hairline. Elevation has been described in multiple different planes, but generally, I prefer a subgaleal plane. The coronal lift will raise the hairline and therefore should be reserved for patients who begin with a lower hairline. Forehead rhytids are typically better treated with a coronal rather than endoscopic technique, especially compared to endoscopic techniques with dissection in the subperiosteal plane. The coronal approach may afford some advantage over the endoscopic approach regarding correction of asymmetry, but the direct brow lift is the best choice for reliable correction of significant brow asymmetry. Patients undergoing the coronal lift tend to complain of prolonged numbness of the scalp compared to the endoscopic technique, although the long-term difference in scalp sensation is questionable. Coronal lifts should be performed with careful consideration in men.

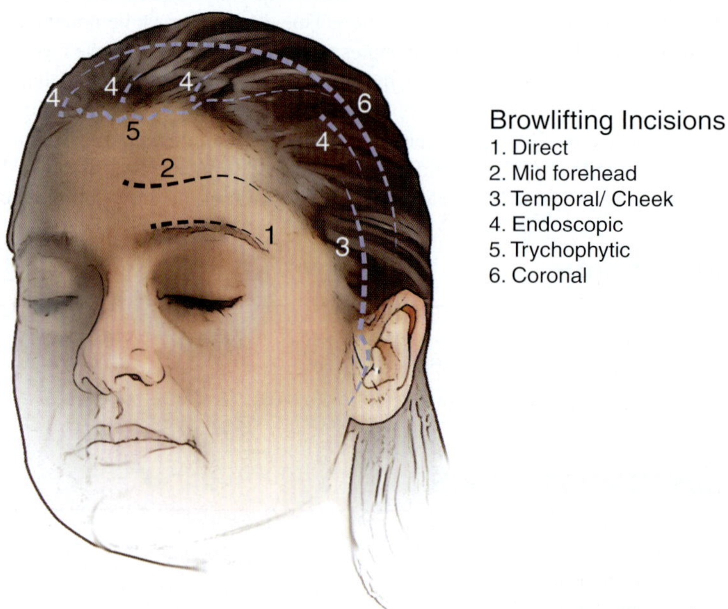

FIGURE 9.2
Placement of various brow lifting incisions.

Men prone to male pattern baldness may ultimately lose enough hair to expose the operative scar, which would be unsightly and very difficult to camouflage.

Direct Brow Lift

The direct brow lift is designed either just above the eyebrow or in a deep rhytid above the eyebrow (a midforehead lift). A subcutaneous plane is developed, and the skin excision is designed to correct the ptotic brow. The skin excision can be customized to remove more tissues laterally or medially and ultimately provide more elevation where it is needed. This is very effective approach for correction of brow asymmetry. The orbicularis is typically suspended to the periosteum, and the skin is closed meticulously in layers. The primary disadvantage of the direct and midforehead lift is the scar placement. When designed properly, both techniques can heal with acceptable results but generally are not as well camouflaged as the other approaches. Men are generally considered better candidates for midforehead incisions, which avoid a scar across the length of the scalp. The deeper rhytids in men tend to hide the incisions to a greater degree compared to women. The scar above the brow complex is equally difficult to conceal in both genders.

Trichophytic Brow Lift

The ideal patient for trichophytic forehead lift is one with either a high hairline that needs to be brought down or one with a well-placed hairline that does not need alteration. The incision is placed just within the hairline and beveled such that the hair follicles will project the hairs through the scar, thus providing camouflage (Fig. 9.3A, B).

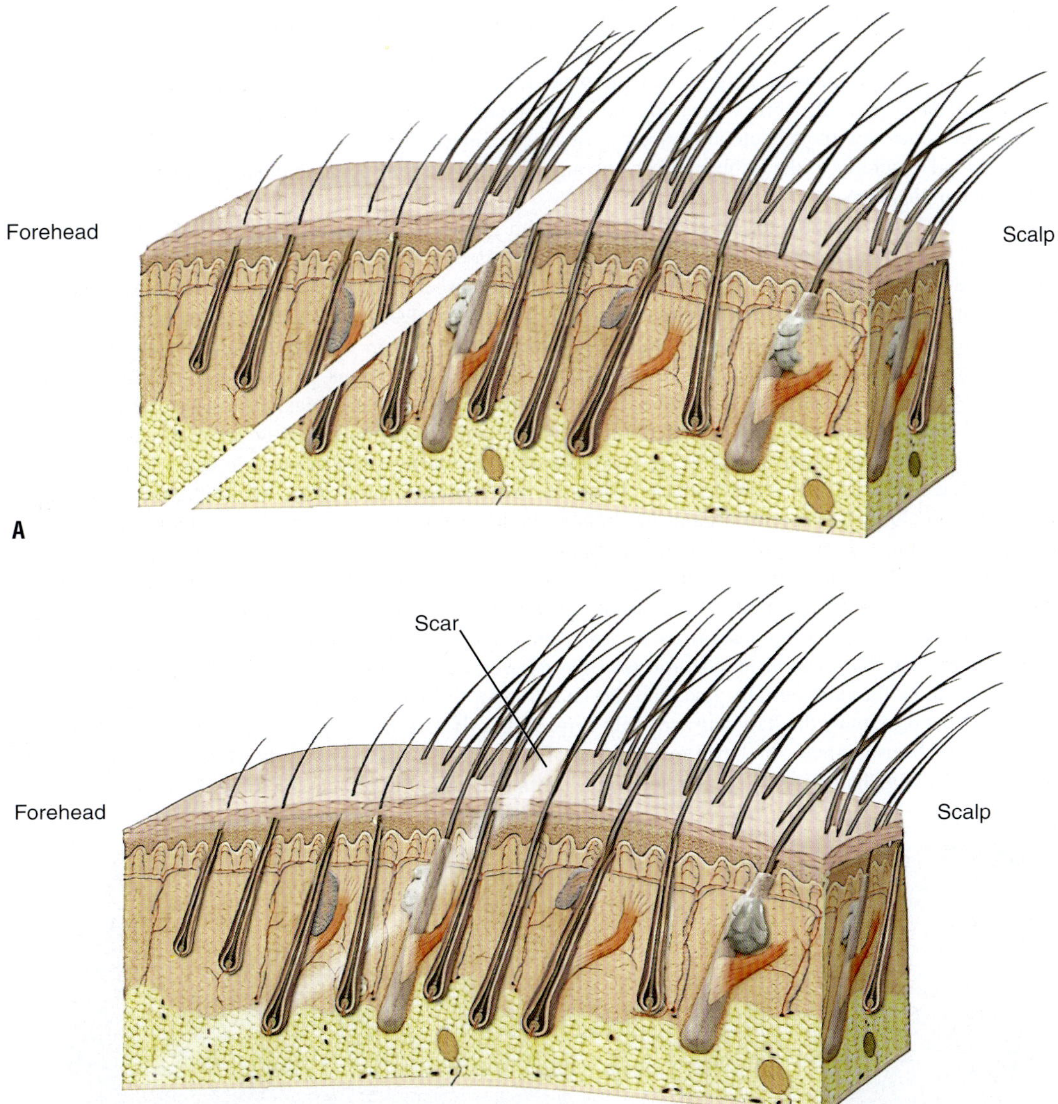

FIGURE 9.3 **A:** Trichophytic incision appropriately beveled to preserve hair follicles. **B:** Hair growth through the trichophytic incision providing scar camouflage.

While multiple planes of dissection have been described including subgaleal, subperiosteal, and subcutaneous, I prefer a subgaleal dissection plane, as mentioned. The distinct advantage of the trichophytic incision is the ability to bring a high hairline forward or maintain a hairline in the desired position. Other advantages and disadvantages are fairly similar to the coronal approach with regard to treatment of forehead rhytids, correction of brow asymmetry, and prolonged numbness. This incision is generally reserved for women due to the unpredictability of the male frontal hairline. Some surgeons believe that the trichophytic lift is more effective than the coronal lift as the incision is located closer to the brow, but there is no clear evidence to support this in the literature. When performed properly, the trichophytic incision is hidden nicely within the hairline. Given our current understanding of trichophytic incisions, the pretrichial incision is essentially never advised.

SURGICAL TECHNIQUE

Patients present to the surgery suite on the morning of surgery having taken nothing by mouth for at least 8 hours. They have been instructed to cleanse the face and hair with chlorhexidine soap the evening prior to and the morning of surgery. In the preoperative area, the incisions are marked and a final review of the case is performed. Prior to proceeding to the operating room, the patient receives a weight- and age-based dose of diazepam. It is our preference to perform this procedure under intravenous sedation (combination of midazolam and propofol) with local anesthesia (lidocaine with epinephrine).

The incision is placed in an irregular fashion mirroring the natural hairline 2 mm into the hair-bearing skin (Fig. 9.4). Meticulous attention to appropriate beveling of the incision along the hairline is absolutely crucial. It is not uncommon to require the use of more than one surgical blade for this portion of the procedure. The design of the lateral portion of the incision extending into the temporal hair depends on multiple factors. When performed in conjunction with a temple–cheek–neck lift, the lateral portion of the forehead incision continues directly into the temple incision (Fig. 9.5). Otherwise, the incision arches into the temporal hair in order to augment the lateral brow lift while concealing the incision within the temporal hair. Along the anterior hairline, the incision is created with an acute angle from posterior to anterior (or superior to inferior) (Fig. 9.6). As the incision extends laterally to the temporal hair, the angle becomes more perpendicular in order to parallel the hair follicles in this area.

The incision is carried to the level of the periosteum along the frontal region and to the deep temporal fascia, overlaying the temporalis muscle, laterally. Sharp dissection is employed to elevate the tissue away from the frontal skull in a subgaleal plane. Blunt and sharp dissection is used to elevate the tissues laterally along the surface of the deep temporal fascia (Fig. 9.7). The fascial decussation along the temporal line can be divided with either sharp or blunt dissection. It is my preference to insert my thumb behind the temporal line and lift anteriorly in order to connect the frontal and the temporal dissections. At this point, careful dissection is directed to the lower brow area (Fig. 9.8). The supraorbital and supratrochlear neurovascular bundles are identified as well as the corrugator musculature. The corrugators are debulked in order to lessen the appearance of vertical glabellar rhytids (Fig. 9.9A–D). Some of the muscle is left in place in order to preserve the integrity of the supratrochlear nerve branches. Once the neurovascular bundles are identified, the arcus marginalis is released along the superior orbital rim, bilaterally. My dissection generally halts laterally just inferior to the sentinel vein. I do not typically find it advantageous to carry dissection down to the zygomatic arch. While aggressive dissection down to the zygoma can facilitate greater mobility of the lateral brow, I find that this maneuver is not warranted in the majority of our patients. Once each forehead and brow complex is adequately mobilized, the complete soft tissue flap is laid into position and the brows are assessed. The flap is maneuvered such that ideal brow position is observed. Vertical incisions are created along the edge of the flap at the midline, the midpupillary line, and the lateral aspect of the brow at which point a staple is placed at each site to approximate the flap with the scalp (Fig. 9.10A, B). At this point, excess soft tissue is removed. In the non–hair-bearing areas, the bevel mirrors that of the initial incision so that the skin edges approximate exactly (Fig. 9.11). In hair-bearing areas, the bevel is reversed in order to protect the follicular units on the flap.

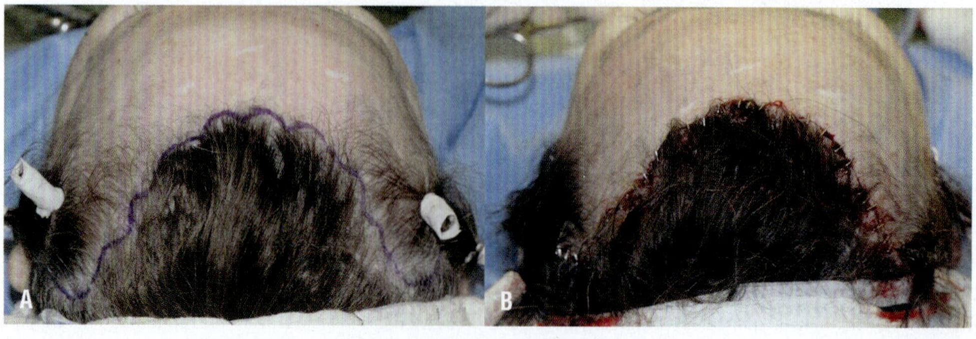

FIGURE 9.4 Design of the incision and the final closed incision.

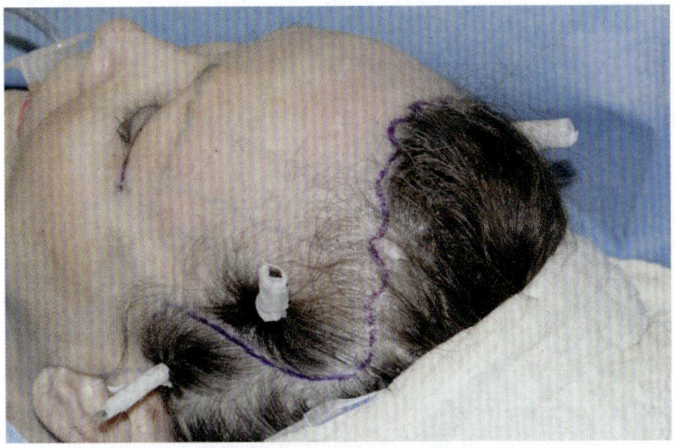

FIGURE 9.5
Extension of the incision into the temple.

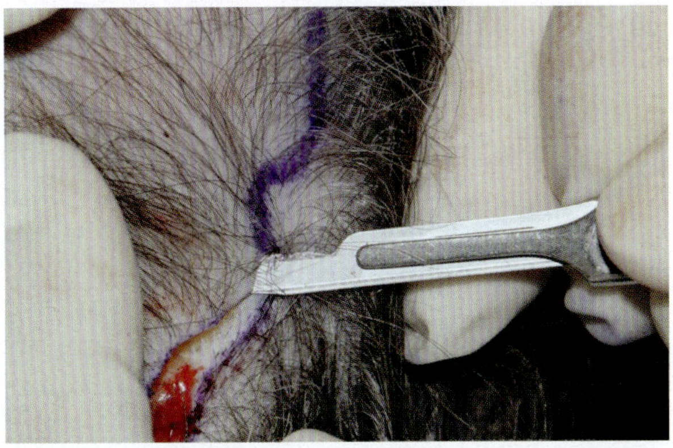

FIGURE 9.6
The blade is beveled acutely in order to preserve hair follicles on the scalp.

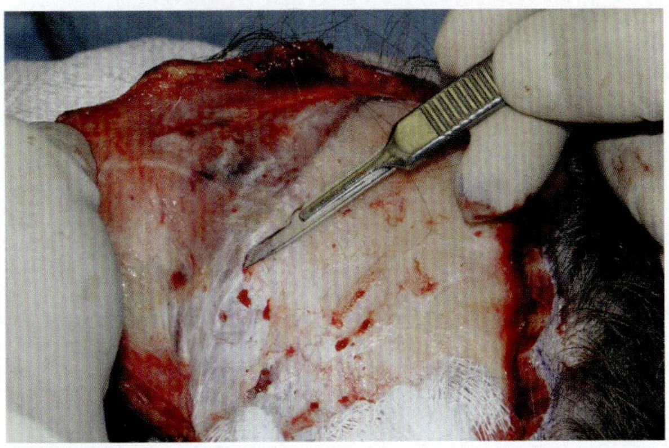

FIGURE 9.7
The flap is elevated in a subgaleal plane, superficial to the periosteum and the deep temporal fascia.

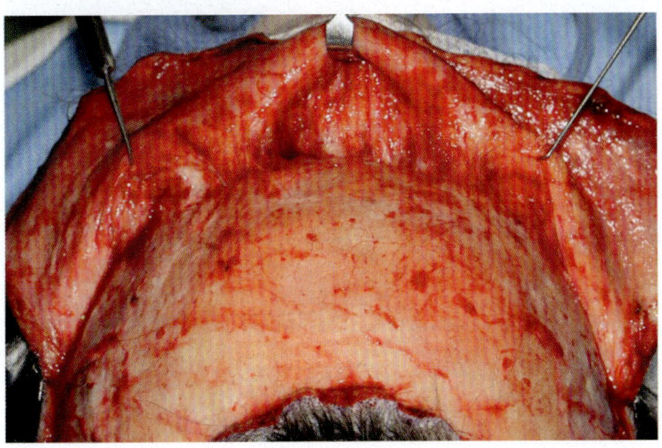

FIGURE 9.8
The flap is elevated. The corrugator muscles and the neurovascular bundles are visible.

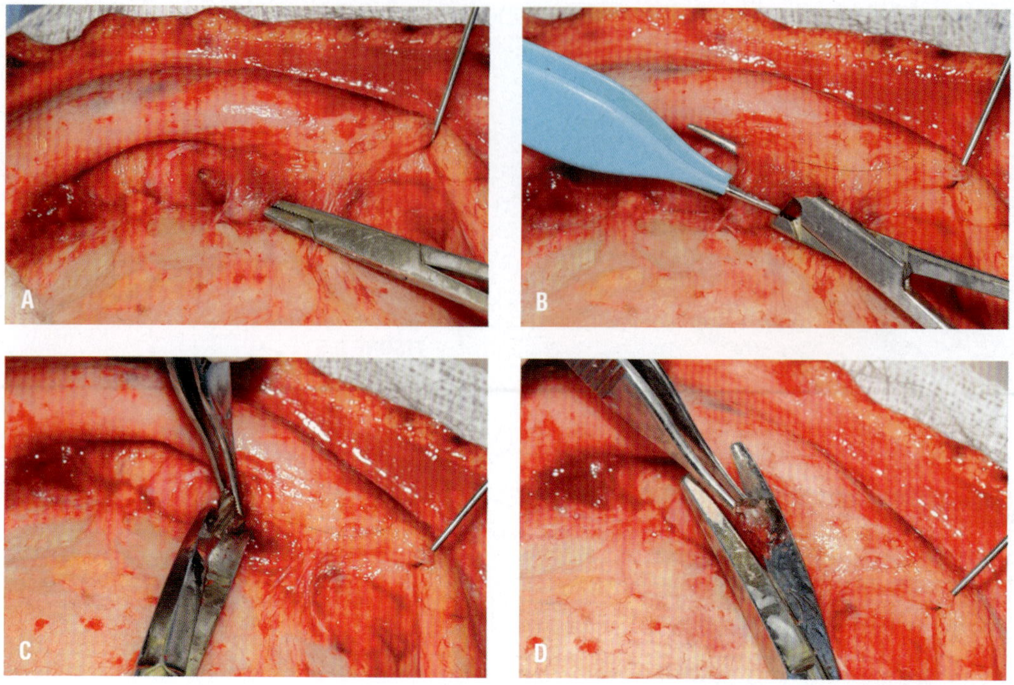

FIGURE 9.9 **A–D:** The corrugators are isolated and transected.

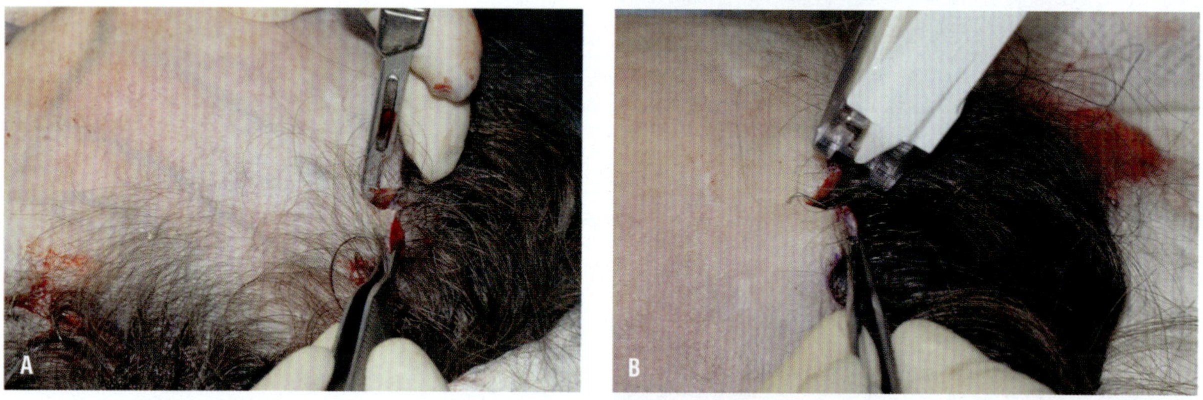

FIGURE 9.10 **A and B:** Vertical incisions are made in the flap, and key fixation points are secured with staples.

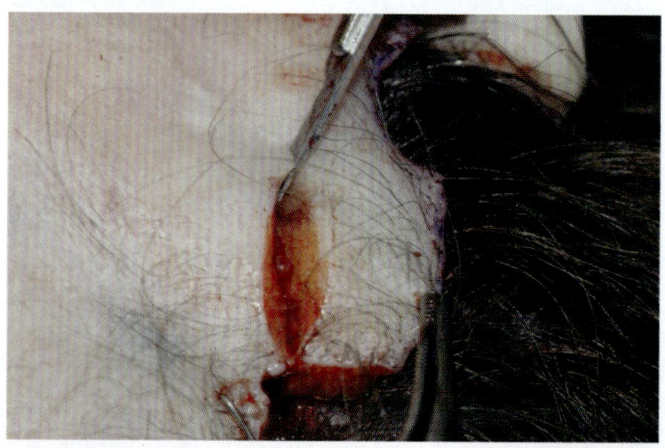

FIGURE 9.11
Excess tissue is excised from the flap.

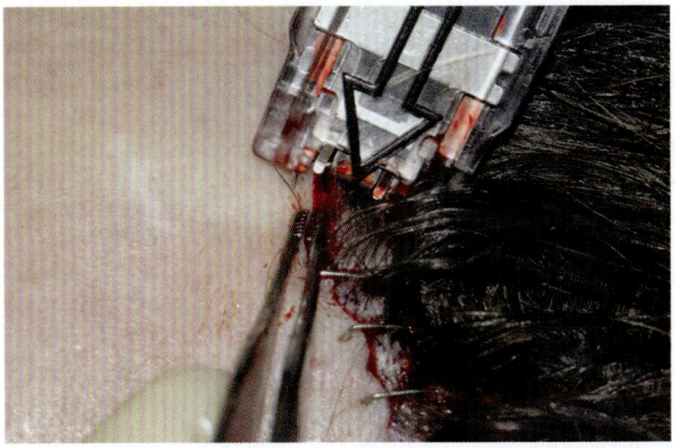

FIGURE 9.12
Staples are placed taking care to evert the skin edges.

Staples are carefully placed to approximate the skin edges with the majority of the staples placed on the scalp side of the incision and only a small amount of the staple extending across the incision onto the flap (Fig. 9.12). Meticulous tissue approximation and eversion are imperative for optimal results (Fig. 9.13).

POSTOPERATIVE MANAGEMENT

A compressive dressing consisting of Xeroform gauze, Kerlix, and Coban is carefully placed on the forehead flap. Care is taken so as to not to wrap the forehead dressing too tightly. The patient is taken to the recovery area and observed until emergence from anesthesia is complete. The patient is assisted overnight by a trained sitter and escorted back to the clinic 24 hours later for removal of the dressing, examination of the wound, and a review of postoperative instructions. The patients are permitted limited activity for 2 weeks and sleep with their head elevated. Staples are removed at 1 week. Standardized pre- and postoperative photography is imperative.

COMPLICATIONS

- Alopecia—Occasionally patients may develop some loss of hair around the incision site. This typically represents telogen effluvium and will resolve in time. If the hair loss does not resolve, it is easily remedied with hair transplants.
- Prolonged hypesthesia—Numbness lasting greater than 18 months may be permanent and is representative of injury to the supraorbital or supratrochlear nerve. In such cases, the patient must be counseled that the sensation to the scalp may never return to preoperative status. Unfortunately, there is no advisable therapy for recovery of sensation if one of the major sensory nerves is damaged.
- Hematoma—Hematoma formation is rare in my experience. In the event of a postoperative hematoma, the collection should be drained upon identification.
- Flap necrosis—Another exceedingly rare complication when dissection is confined to the subgaleal plane. If the surgeon prefers instead to elevate the flap in the subcutaneous plane, there is a slightly increased risk. Generally flap necrosis is managed conservatively with local wound care and at times can heal without significant cosmetic detriment.
- Facial nerve weakness or injury. My technique to the facial nerve exposes the nerve to very little risk. Dissection in the subgaleal plane, appropriate placement of the temporal incision, and avoidance of dissection down over the level of the zygomatic arch are all methods employed to protect the nerve. If weakness

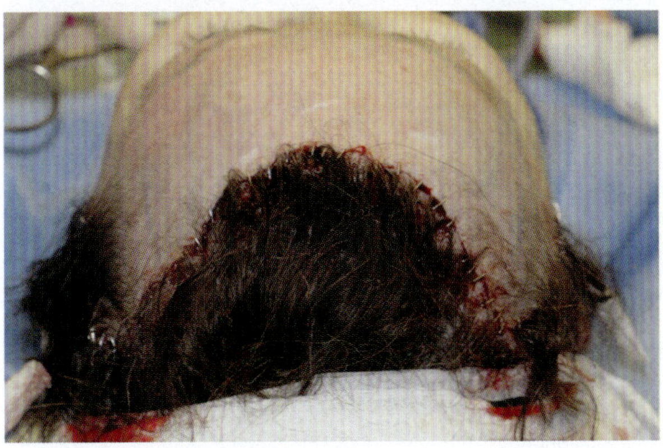

FIGURE 9.13
Final closure.

does occur, it will likely be temporary and due to traction or pressure. Symmetry can be restored to the forehead with the use of botulinum toxin along the depressors of the ipsilateral brow as well as weakening of the elevators along the contralateral brow. If function has not returned in 12 months, the nerve injury is considered permanent.

- Unacceptable scarring—A widened scar is usually an indication of excessive tension on the wound at the time of closure. The surgeon should wait at least 6 months prior to attempting scar revision. The scar can be excised and the wound closed with appropriate eversion.

RESULTS

Excellent short- and long-term results are achieved with a properly executed trichophytic brow lift. Patients should be counseled that some degree of numbness of the scalp is an expected sequelae, which typically resolves in 6 to 12 months. The healing scar is initially pink and fades over the course of 6 to 12 weeks. Illustrative photographs demonstrate easily hidden scars in the immediate postoperative period as well as durable results with long-term follow-up (Figs. 9.14 to 9.17).

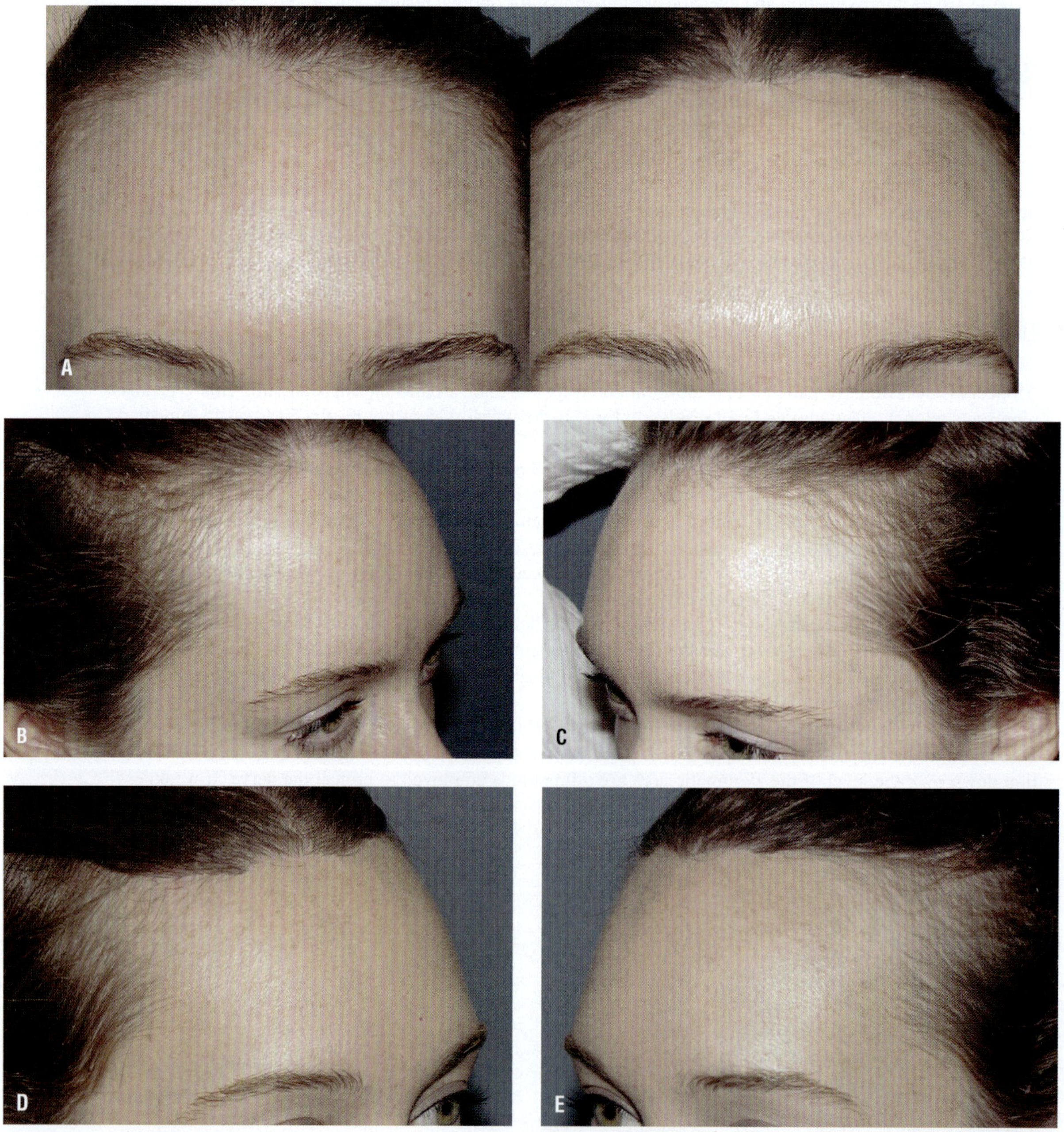

FIGURE 9.14 **A:** A 33-year-old woman who underwent trichophytic forehead lift: before and 12-month follow-up. **B:** Preoperative oblique. **C:** Preoperative oblique. **D:** Postoperative oblique, 12 months. **E:** Postoperative oblique, 12 months.

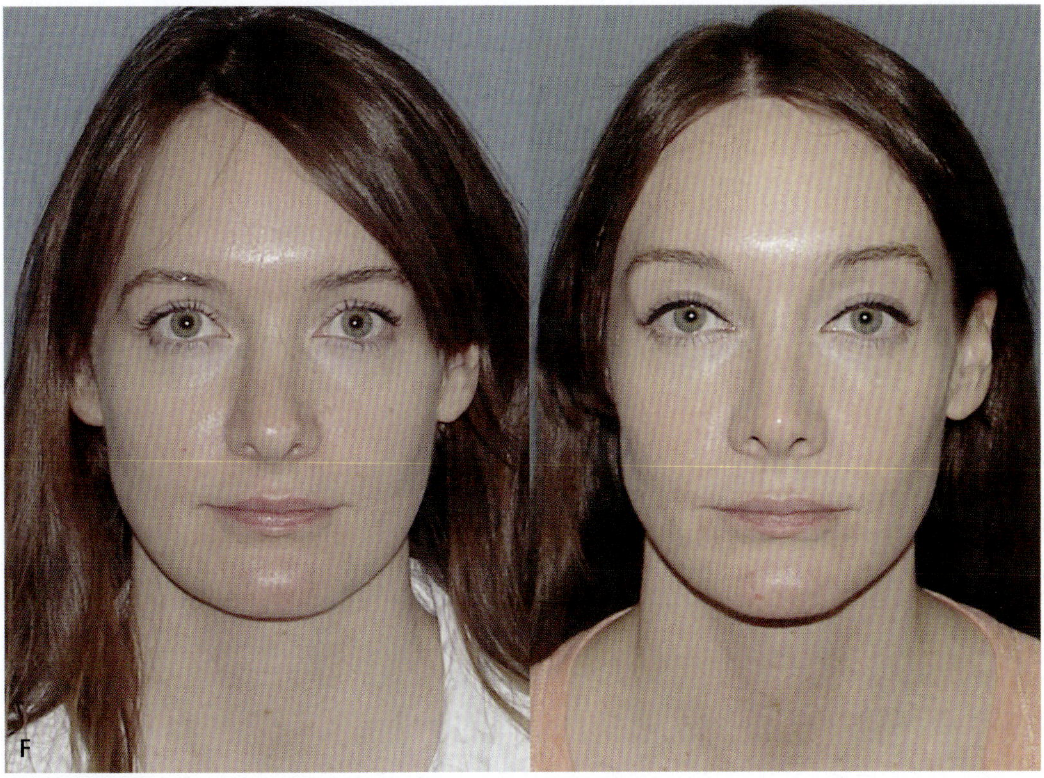

FIGURE 9.14 (*Continued*) **F:** Overall result at 12 months.

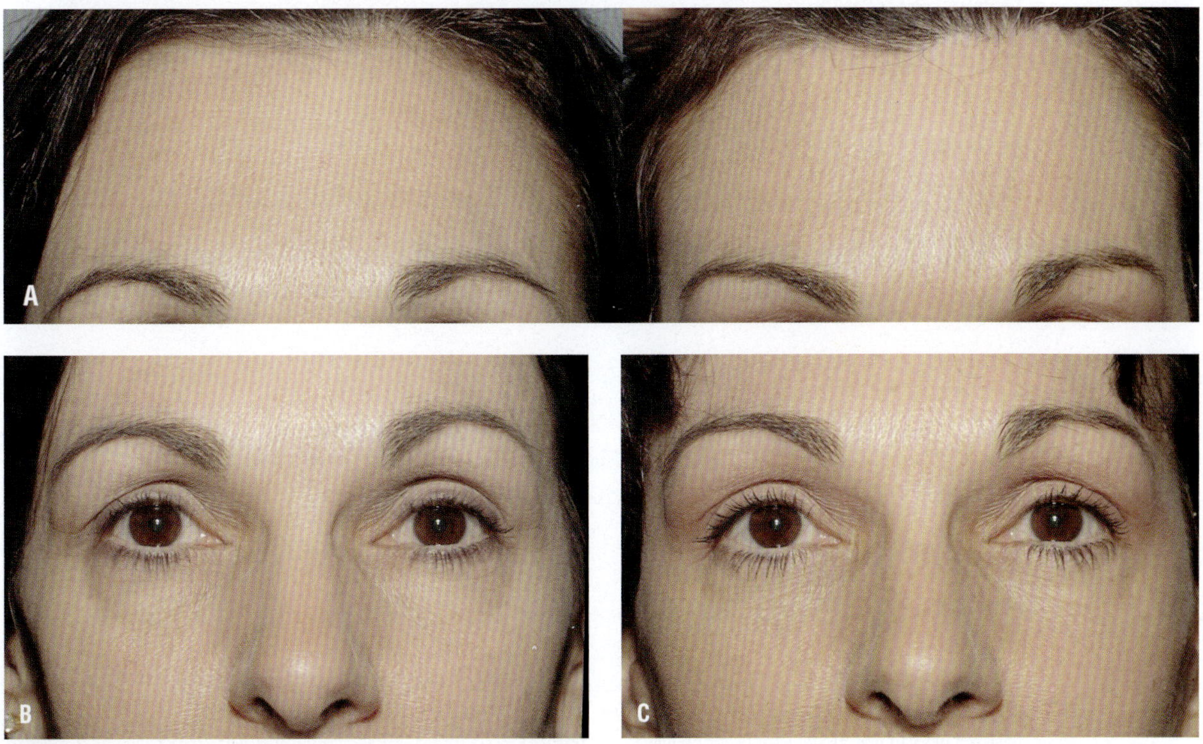

FIGURE 9.15 **A:** A 51-year-old woman who underwent trichophytic forehead lift: before and 12-month follow-up. **B:** Preoperative. **C:** 12-month follow-up.

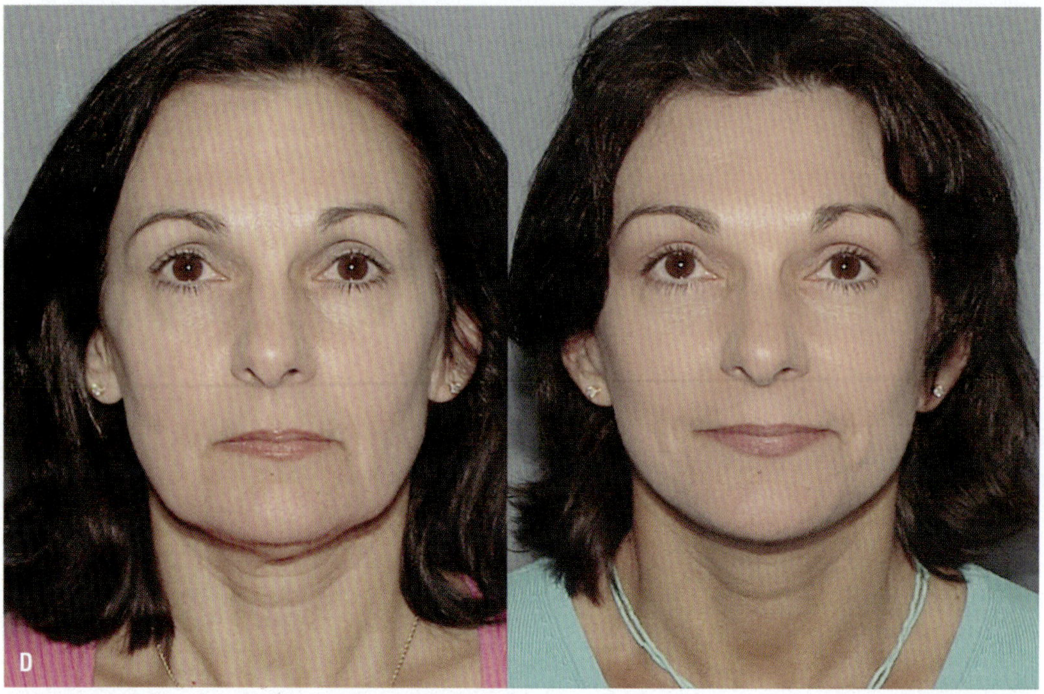

FIGURE 9.15 (*Continued*) **D:** Overall result at 12 months.

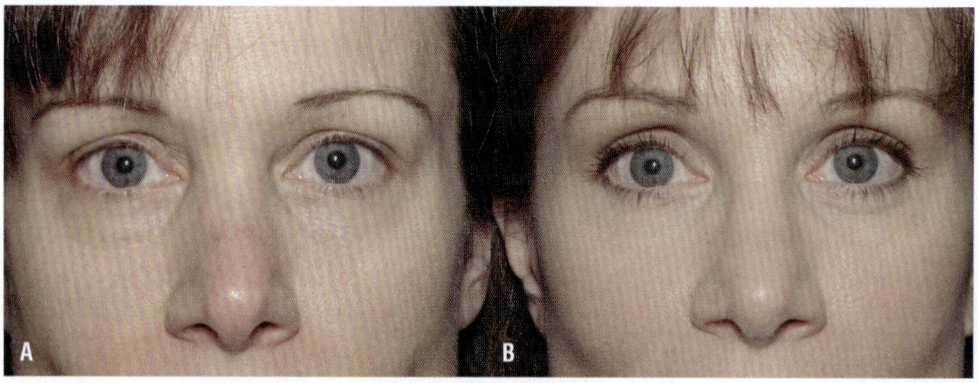

FIGURE 9.16 A 48-year-old woman who underwent trichophytic forehead lift: before and 24-month follow-up.

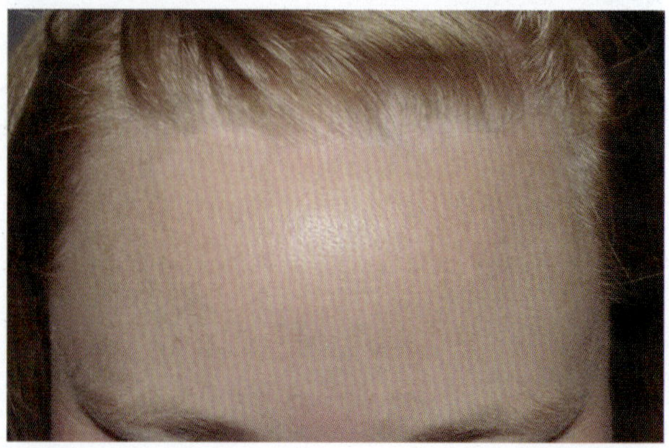

FIGURE 9.17
A 47-year-old woman who underwent trichophytic forehead lift: 48-month follow-up of well-healed incision.

PEARLS

- The trichophytic approach is ideally suited to patients with a high hairline in which case the hairline can be brought down to a more aesthetically pleasing position.
- The incision must be beveled across the hair shafts across the forehead, along the hairline, and parallel to the shaft of the temporal hair.
- Bevel during skin excision should mirror the initial incision such that the skin edges are flush upon approximation.
- Avoid overly aggressive excision of scalp so as to minimize wound closure tension.
- Eversion and approximation are essential for optimal wound healing.

PITFALLS

- Alopecia can occur if the soft tissues are not mobilized well or too much tension exists at closure.
- Compromise in scalp sensation postoperatively can lead to inadvertent trauma that goes unnoticed by the patient (e.g., curling iron burn).
- Patients who style their hair in a pulled back fashion have the potential for visible scarring.
- Soft tissues of the forehead may become fixed to the skull with injury/compromise of the periosteum.

INSTRUMENTS TO HAVE AVAILABLE

- Standard plastic surgery tray

ACKNOWLEDGMENT

I gratefully acknowledge Dr. W. Henry Barber's contributions to this chapter.

SUGGESTED READING

Freidman O. Changes associated with the aging face. *Facial Plast Surg Clin North Am* 2005;13(3):371–380.
Guillot JM, Rousso DE, Relogle W. Forehead and scalp sensation after brow lift. *Arch Facial Plast Surg* 2011;13(2):109–116.
Henderson JL, Larrabee WF. Analysis of the upper face and selection of rejuvenation techniques. *Facial Plast Surg Clin North Am* 2006;14(3):153–158.
Hunt HL. *Plastic surgery of the head, face, and neck*. Philadelphia, PA: Lea & Febiger, 1926.
Morgan JM, Farrior E. Rejuvenation of the aging forehead. *Facial Plast Surg Clin North Am* 2006;14(3):167–173.

10 SMAS FACE-LIFT

Stephen W. Perkins

INTRODUCTION

The stigmata of facial aging include, but are not limited to, facial skin ptosis, jowling, rhytids, lipoptosis, and platysmal banding. These changes can dramatically affect an individual's self-image as well as the emotional and energy states perceived by others. Often, a combination of factors leads such patients to seek facial rejuvenation. Their goal, in general, is not a drastic change in their features but simply to look as young as they feel. With realistic expectations, a face-lift can provide the desired improvement in appearance and sense of well-being. Prior to any intervention, a detailed history, focused examination, communication of expected outcomes with the assistance of preoperative digital imaging, and discussion of perioperative instructions are of utmost importance. Although many techniques have been described, the modified deep plane-extended superficial muscular aponeurotic system (SMAS) rhytidectomy with submentoplasty reliably delivers a significant improvement with lasting results.

HISTORY

A complete medical and surgical history is taken for each patient considering surgery. Attention is given to diabetic, rheumatologic, autoimmune, and psychiatric disorders. A history with regard to tobacco use is obtained as considerable soft tissue complications can arise due to circulatory compromise. Details of previous surgical interventions are discussed, and medical records are requested in all circumstances to compliment the patient's conveyed history.

Determining the patient's aesthetic concerns is an important part of the patient's history as it relates to the life experience and the sense of identity. Patients requesting a "face-lift" may specifically request correction of facial skin laxity/ptosis and jowl formation. Other patients, however, may primarily desire improvement in the appearance of their neck with reduction of submental lipoptosis, relaxation of platysmal bands, and sharpening of an oblique cervicomental angle. This latter group may also appropriately ask for a "face-lift" with different goals or request a "necklift" only. They may even say, "I don't want a face-lift, all I want is a necklift." In reality, rejuvenation of the neck and lower face are accomplished together. Conversely, a patient's focus on the cheek–lip grooves, perioral rhytids, or ptotic midfacial tissue is more appropriately managed through injectable fillers, facial resurfacing, and midface lifting techniques, respectively. After a careful discussion about appropriate treatment modalities for the anatomic problem of concern, the plan can be further refined during the clinical examination.

PHYSICAL EXAMINATION

Evaluation begins with a general assessment of the patient's overall health, facial features, and symmetry. Critical in analyzing patients presenting for rhytidectomy include those items listed in Table 10.1.

TABLE 10.1 Examination Criteria
Skin laxity, thickness, elasticity, and static rhytids
Platysma banding
Lipoptosis (submental, submandibular, and jowls)
Submandibular gland ptosis
Skeletal strength and position (mandible, maxilla, and hyoid)
Soft tissue volume (prejowl sulcus/marionette lines, nasolabial folds)

Although all factors are important, those directly related to the neck are most critical and will ultimately lead to the success of the extended sub-SMAS rhytidectomy. Together, these factors are used to grade the patient preoperatively into one of three categories: a type I face-lift patient demonstrates good skin elasticity, minimal jowling, minimal to no lipoptosis, early cheek and neck skin laxity, and minor platysmal laxity or banding (Fig. 10.1). The most common is the type II face-lift patient. This individual presents with moderate facial and neck skin ptosis, clear jowling, moderate lipoptosis, and heavier platysmal banding with an obtuse cervicomental angle (Fig. 10.2). The type III face-lift patient, including most males (Fig. 10.3), has heavy cheeks, prominent jowling with frequent prejowl grooves, loss of mandibular definition, significant platysmal bands with large amounts of lipoptosis, and absent cervicomental angle or convexity of the neck (Fig. 10.4). This grading is directly related to the expected amount of surgical work and intervention in creating a long-lasting, pleasing contour of the neck. Additionally, the underlying skeletal structure should be noted, as a low hyoid position portends difficulty creating a sharp cervicomental angle. Moreover, a chin or prejowl implant can improve the structure and overall result in select cases (Figs. 10.5 and 10.6). Lastly, the periorbital, perioral, brow, and midface should be evaluated for adjuvant procedures during rhytidectomy.

INDICATIONS

SMAS rhytidectomy in concert with a submentoplasty is warranted for motivated patients with realistic expectations. Age-related ptotic facial and neck skin, rhytids, jowl formation, platysmal banding, and lipoptosis are all indications for this surgical intervention.

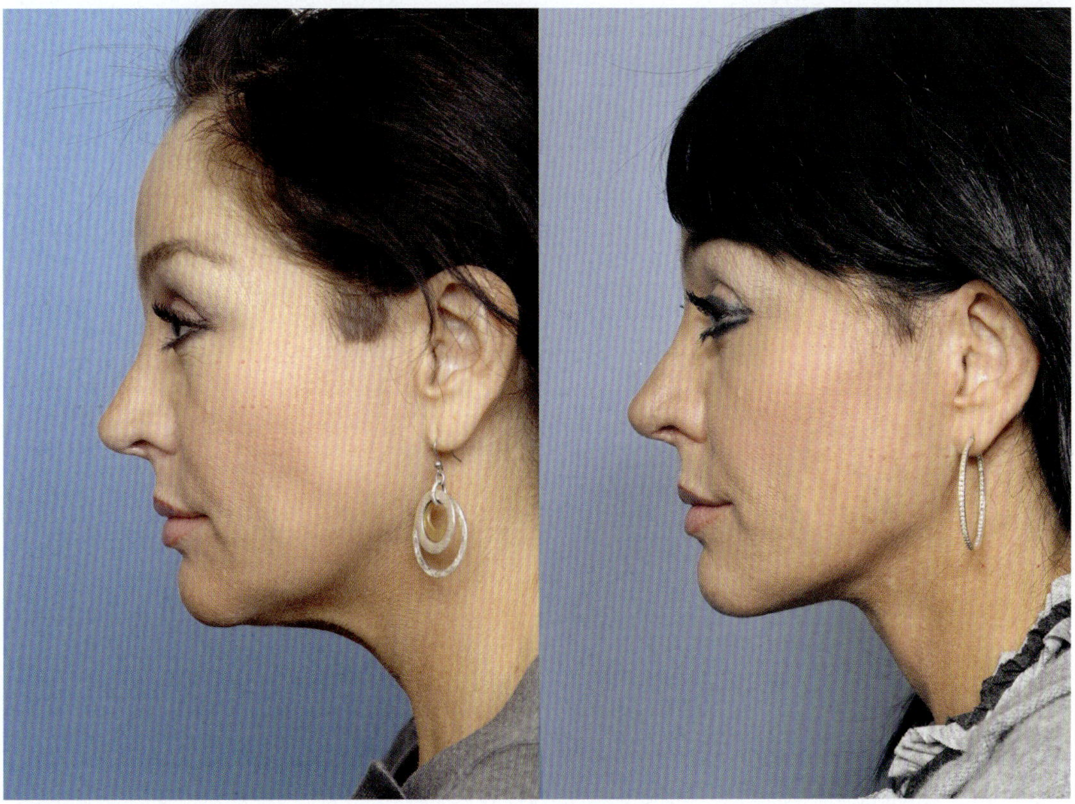

FIGURE 10.1 Type I face-lift patient (preoperative and postoperative photos).

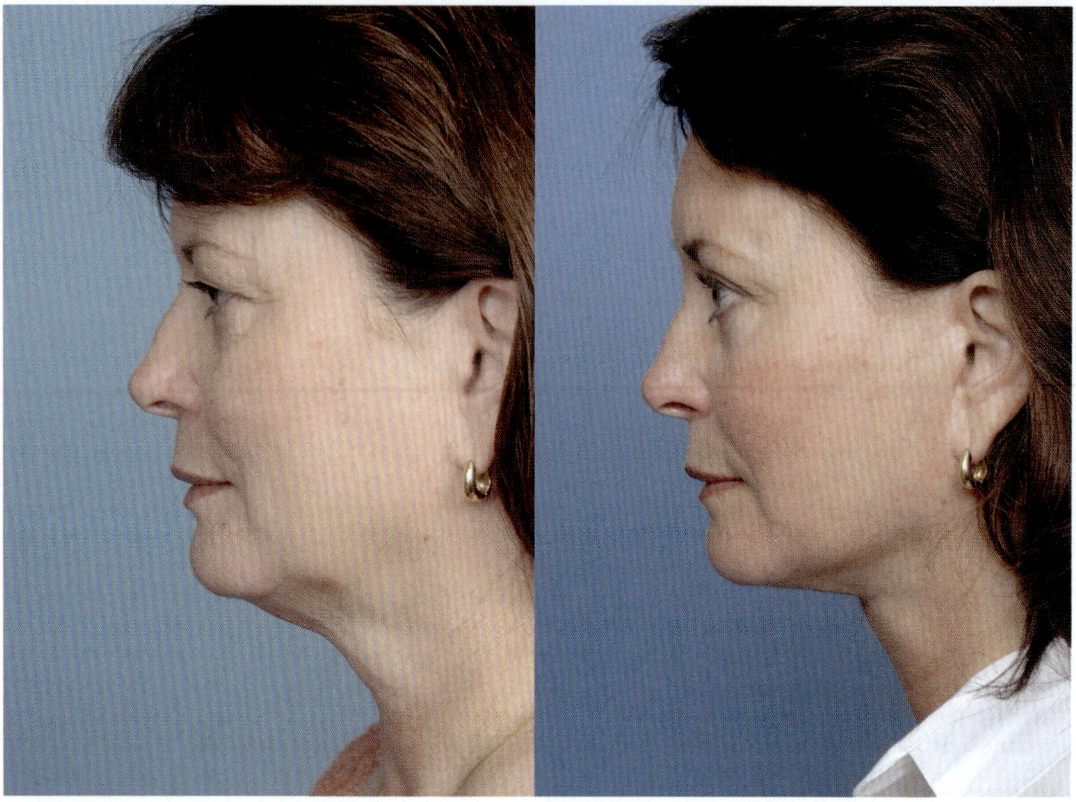

FIGURE 10.2 Type II face-lift patient (preoperative and postoperative photos).

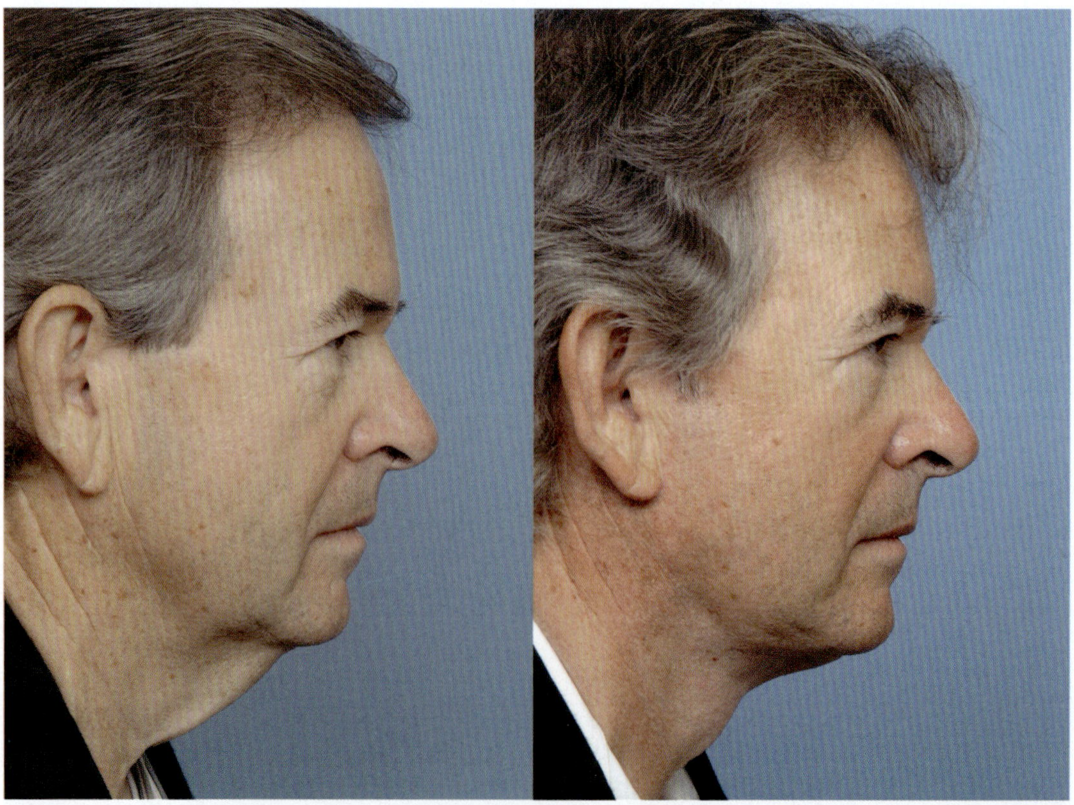

FIGURE 10.3 Type III face-lift patient (preoperative and postoperative photos).

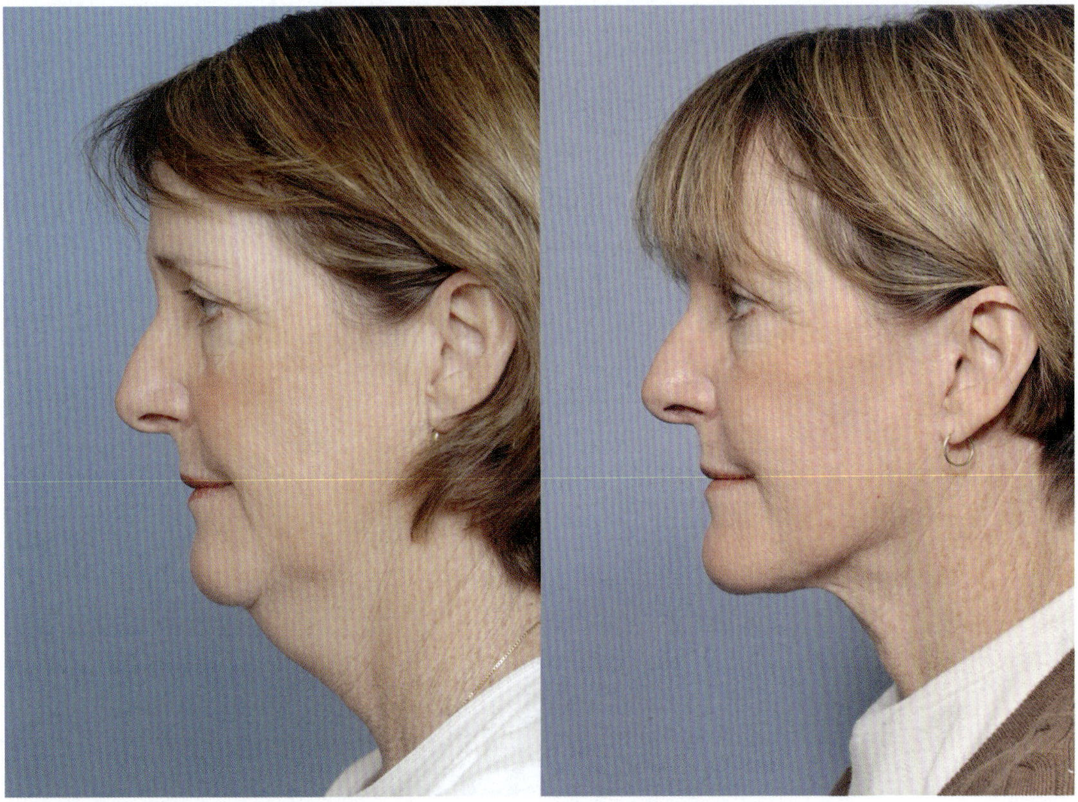

FIGURE 10.4 Type III face-lift patient (preoperative and postoperative photos).

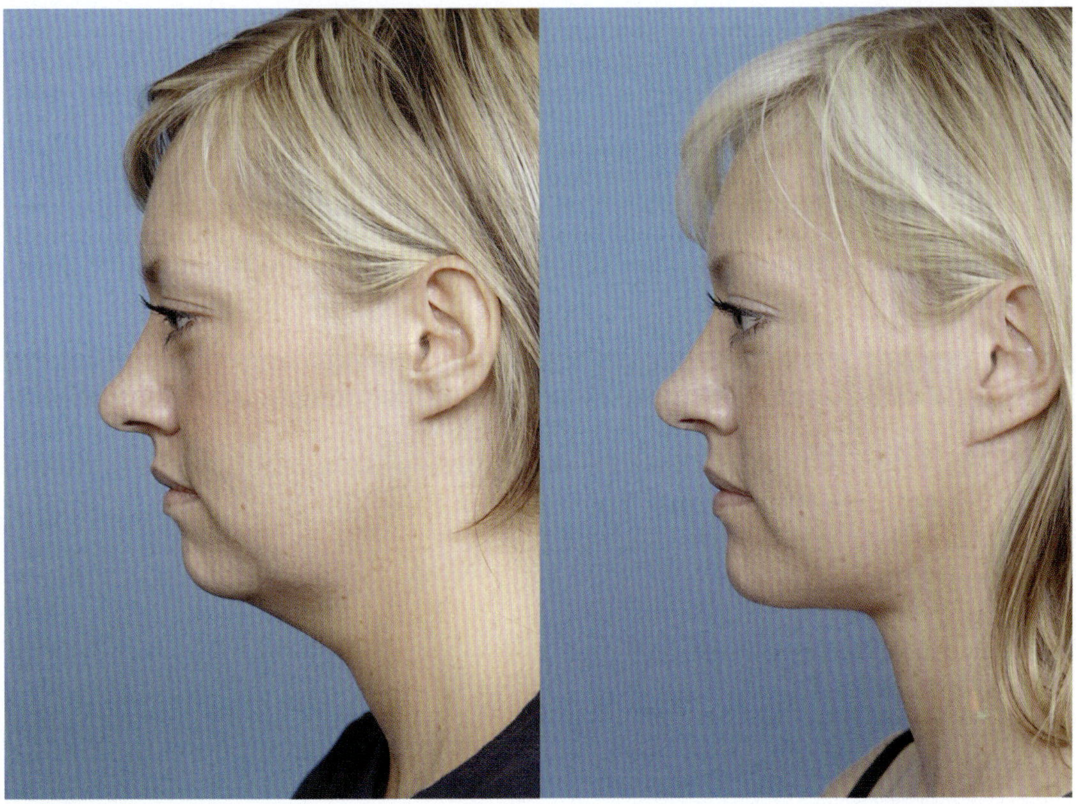

FIGURE 10.5 Type III face-lift and chin implant patient (preoperative and postoperative photos).

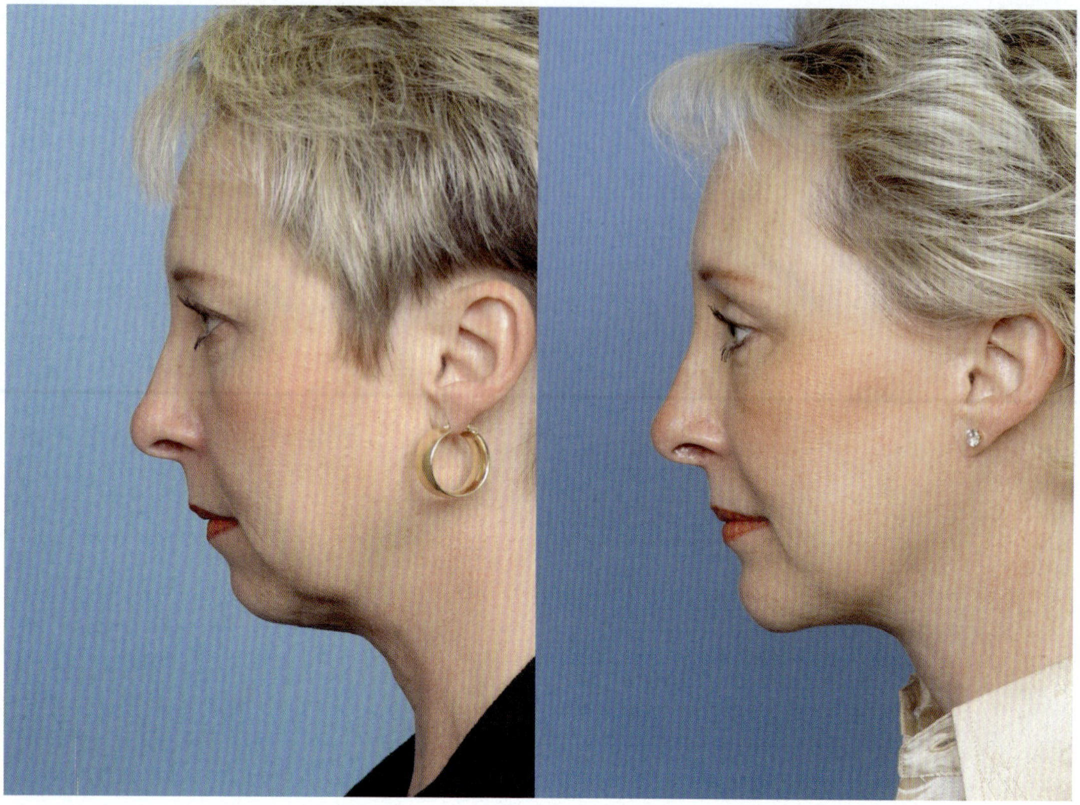

FIGURE 10.6 Type II face-lift and chin implant patient (preoperative and postoperative photos).

CONTRAINDICATIONS

The majority of absolute contraindications for rhytidectomy are factors that compromise wound healing of the large facial skin flap (Table 10.2). On the other hand, relative contraindications include characteristics that can lead to a less than satisfied patient. In particular, a low hyoid position limits the ability to recreate an acute neckline due to the underlying suprahyoid strap muscles obstructing the placement of a high, tight platysmaplasty. A weak mandible makes enhancing the transition between the face and neck a challenge even with liposuction and tightening of the heavy overlying skin. Similarly, ptotic submandibular glands can be misinterpreted as persistent lipoptosis in the neck and detract from a smooth lateral neck contour. A patient with prominent cheek mounds that deepen the nasolabial folds can expect even less than the mild correction seen in this area in a typical rhytidectomy. If present, each of these findings should be

TABLE 10.2 Absolute Contraindications to Face-lifting

Absolute Contraindications
Active autoimmune disease of facial vasculature
Active chemotherapy/immunosuppression
Active smoking
Active vasculitides
Full course facial radiation exposure
Largely fluctuating weight
Medically unfit for anesthesia
Psychologically unprepared/unfit
Uncontrolled hypertension
Unrealistic expectations

communicated to the patient so that expectations can be managed appropriately. Lastly, a patient currently experiencing a period of high stress or a major life-changing event may be prompted to surgical intervention for the wrong reasons. This may lead to an unhappy patient when facial rejuvenation does not fulfill his or her goals.

PREOPERATIVE PLANNING

With the patient's desires known and the physical examination complete, the final planning begins for the extended SMAS rhytidectomy with submentoplasty. Adjuvant procedures including neurotoxins, facial fillers, skeletal augmentation, skin resurfacing, and management of the forehead, midface, and eyes are also discussed at this time. Next, digital photographs are captured to document the patient's preoperative condition and used as a medium for digital imaging. This is routinely used as a tool to further communicate a realistic representation of the expected result. Often, this is a powerful "tool" to demonstrate to the patient the dramatic improvement that can be expected in the neckline and jowl/jawline. A patient rarely realizes and appreciates the degree of aging changes visible from the profile. This greatly helps the patient visualize and prepare for the postoperative change. If the patient is satisfied, a date is scheduled, routine laboratory tests are ordered, and the appropriate cardiac examinations and imaging are obtained. Routinely, prescriptions are given for antibiotics, analgesics, antiemetics, anxiolytics, and sleep aids at this time. Any herbals or pharmaceuticals that increase the patient's risk of hemorrhage are discontinued in a timely manner prior to surgery. Finally, verbal and written instructions for the perioperative period are given to the patient.

SURGICAL TECHNIQUE

In the preoperative holding area, the markings (Fig. 10.7) are made with a surgical pen for the rhytidectomy, as well as for any additional procedures. The preauricular marking is carefully planned so as not to distort the temporal hair tuft, as it routinely stops at the inferior extent of the tuft or no higher than the upper anterior helical insertion. It also incorporates a posttragal course, as it is continued inferiorly in all females and in some males. The marking then continues around the lobule of the ear and is placed above the postauricular sulcus on the posterior surface of the concha. As the marking reaches the level of the helical insertion, it is directed posteriorly with a gentle curve along and into the hairline. Lastly, a 3-cm marking for the submentoplasty is made in the submental crease, and the hair is twirled and taped to remove it from the operative field.

After an appropriate level of anesthesia is achieved, the incision sites of the face and neck are infiltrated with 1% lidocaine with 1:50,000 epinephrine. The areas of undermining are also infiltrated with a combination of 1% lidocaine with 1:100,000 epinephrine and 0.5% lidocaine with 1:100,000 epinephrine. If neurotoxin or filler is to be injected, it is done at this time. The patient is then prepped and draped in the usual sterile manner while vasoconstriction and analgesia from the local anesthetic take effect.

The submentoplasty is then initiated by making the submental skin incision with a no. 15 scalpel blade (Video 10.1). A short flap is then elevated with Metzenbaum scissors, and hemostasis is obtained with bipolar cautery. Through this incision, either a chin or prejowl implant can be placed without difficulty. Commonly, a 3-mm Fournier liposuction cannula is used, off suction, to make radial tunnels throughout the anterior neck within the subcutaneous plane. Once the initial tunnels are created, 1 atm of suction is applied to the same cannula, which is used to remove the excess pre-platysmal adipose tissue. The nondominant hand

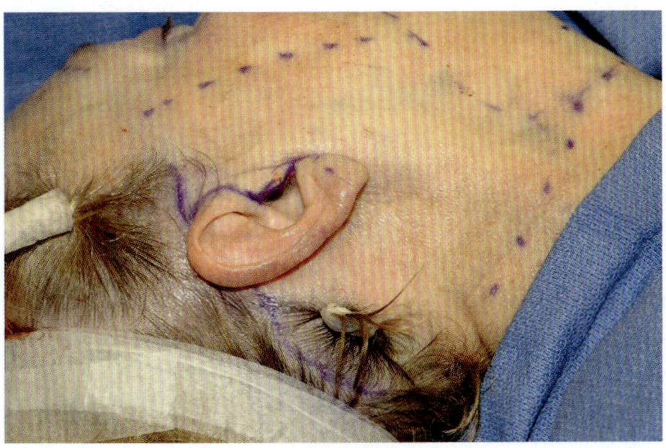

FIGURE 10.7
Rhytidectomy incision planning and surgical markings.

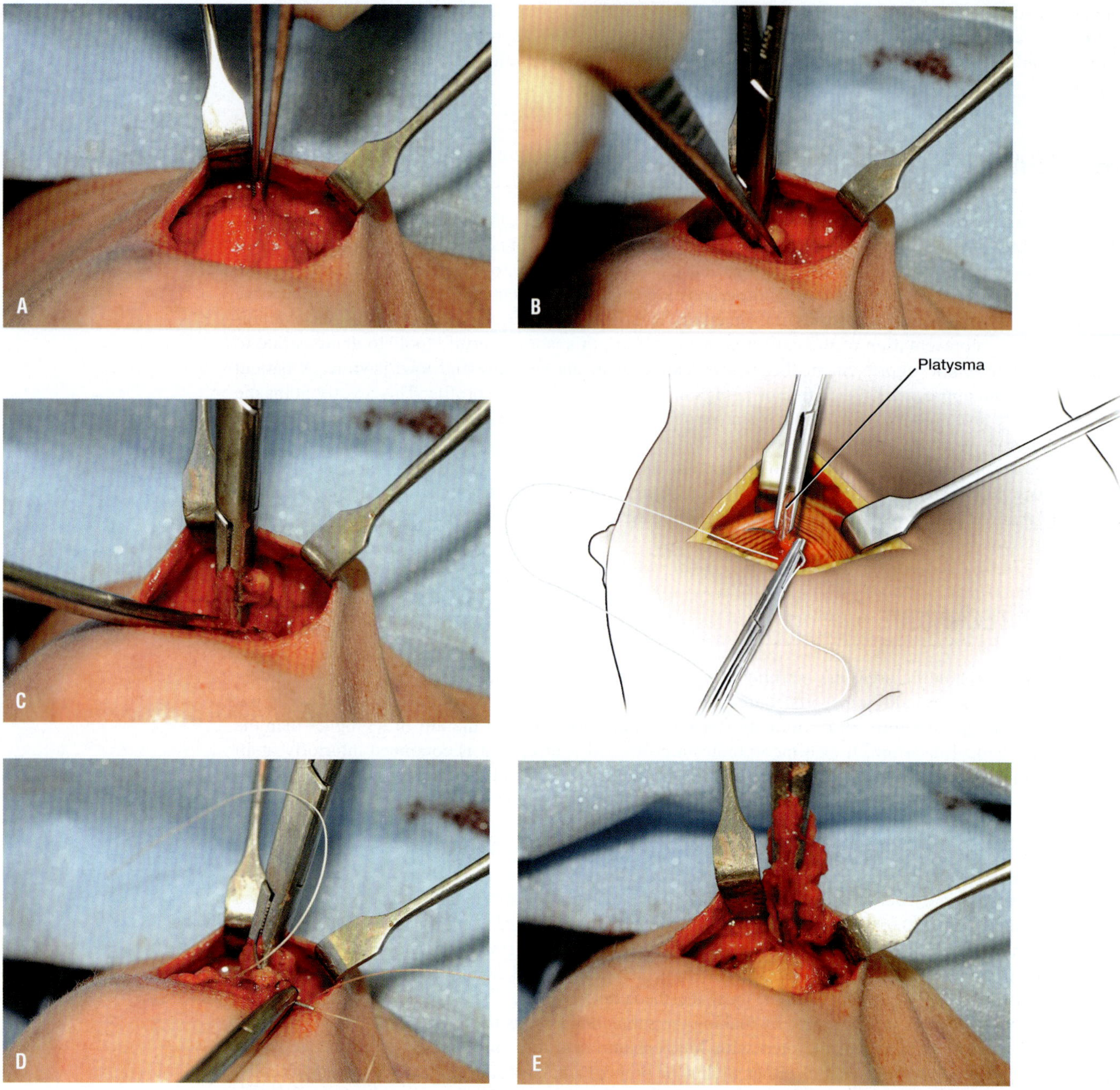

FIGURE 10.8 Kelly clamp technique for submentoplasty. **A:** Loose excess adipose tissue and platysma in submental area following liposuction prior to clamping. **B:** Cautery of clamped tissue. **C:** Division of cauterized tissue. **D:** Serial imbrication of the freed medial platysma edges. **E:** Removal of excised clamped tissue.

lifts and guides the cannula with the opening always directed away from the overlying dermis. Particular attention is given to avoid overzealous liposuctioning and subsequent dimpling in the jowl regions. In some patients, the use of a 5-mm spatula cannula is necessary to treat the submental area. Once this is complete, the entire neck flap, extending from one sternocleidomastoid (SCM) muscle border to the other, is elevated with Metzenbaum scissors. Meticulous hemostasis is then achieved with a protected bayonet-style bipolar cautery. Next, using a 6-inch long, curved, Kelly clamp (Fig. 10.8), the easily grasped redundant midline submental tissue is clamped. This may include superficial adipose tissue, loose anterior platysma bands, and subplatysmal adipose tissue extending down to the level of the hyoid bone. Once grasped, the redundancy is serially cauterized and cut, while the free margins are approximated with a 3-0 Vicryl (Ethicon, Somerville, NJ) suture. Once the clamped portion of tissue has been removed, a tightly imbricated platysma corset has been created to support the submental area. Additional back-cuts at the cervicomental junction further improve the angle and help avoid persistent postoperative banding. Once the neck has been adequately treated, attention is directed toward the face.

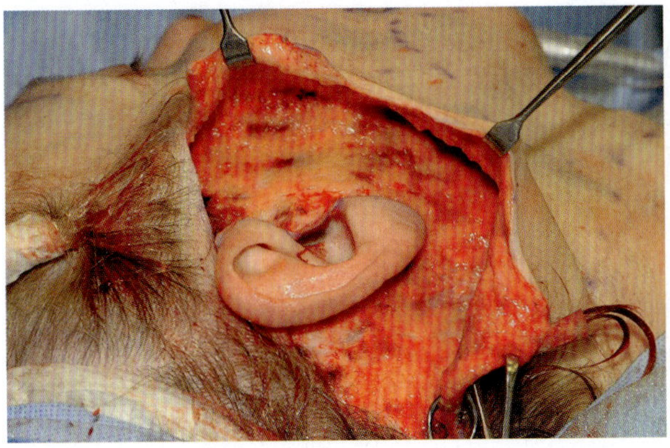

FIGURE 10.9
Complete elevation of the facial skin flap.

Rhytidectomy is initiated by incising the postauricular markings with a no. 15 scalpel blade from the lobule into the scalp (Video 10.2). In the scalp, the incision is beveled to avoid injury to adjacent hair follicles, and subsequent flap elevation remains deep to the follicles to avoid postoperative alopecia in the hair-bearing region. The flap elevation is aided by the use of nonpenetrating towel clamps for traction and performed with a scalpel dissecting just superficial to the SCM fascia. Once this short segment is elevated, complete hemostasis is again obtained with bipolar cautery. The anterior incision is made, as previously marked, and beveled appropriately when adjacent to the temporal hair tuft. Again, nonpenetrating towel clamps are placed on the temporal portion of the flap for traction and a small area is elevated in the preauricular area with the scalpel. This is followed by meticulous hemostasis with bipolar cautery.

Using modified Kahn face-lift dissecting scissors, the remaining posterior skin flap is elevated. Traction is provided by the non-dominant hand grasping the towel clamps, while counter traction is maintained on the cheek and neck with taught fingers of the assistant. The scissors, which are slightly blunted and have an outward bevel, are used in an advancing, spreading motion to achieve flap elevation. Thin, intervening bridges of adipose tissue and dermal connective tissue are then sharply released with the partially opened scissors. Once the posterior elevation is complete and is in continuity with the previously undermined neck flap, retractors are placed and hemostasis is obtained.

The anterior skin flap is then elevated in a similar manner in the subcutaneous plane. The anterior extent of this dissection is dictated by the patient's anatomy, but it does not extend medial to the nasolabial fold. Following elevation, the anterior, posterior, and neck flaps are in continuity (Fig. 10.9). Meticulous hemostasis is again obtained prior to performing the extended SMAS flap.

Using the zygomatic arch as a landmark, the SMAS is incised with a no. 15 scalpel blade in a semilunar fashion from the arch to the anterior border of the SCM. The flap is then elevated medially with a combination of sharp and blunt dissection extending anterior to the parotid gland. As the dissection continues, the masseter muscle, zygomatic major muscle, and the distal facial nerve branches are frequently visualized (Fig. 10.10). Complete hemostasis is required for safe dissection, and care must be taken to avoid injury to the facial nerve.

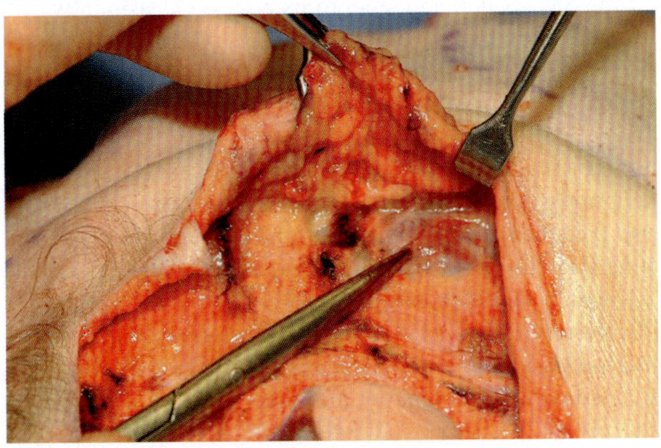

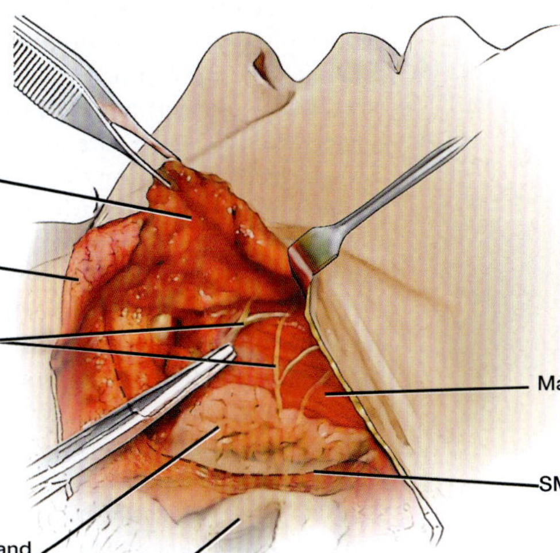

FIGURE 10.10 Complete elevation of the SMAS flap.

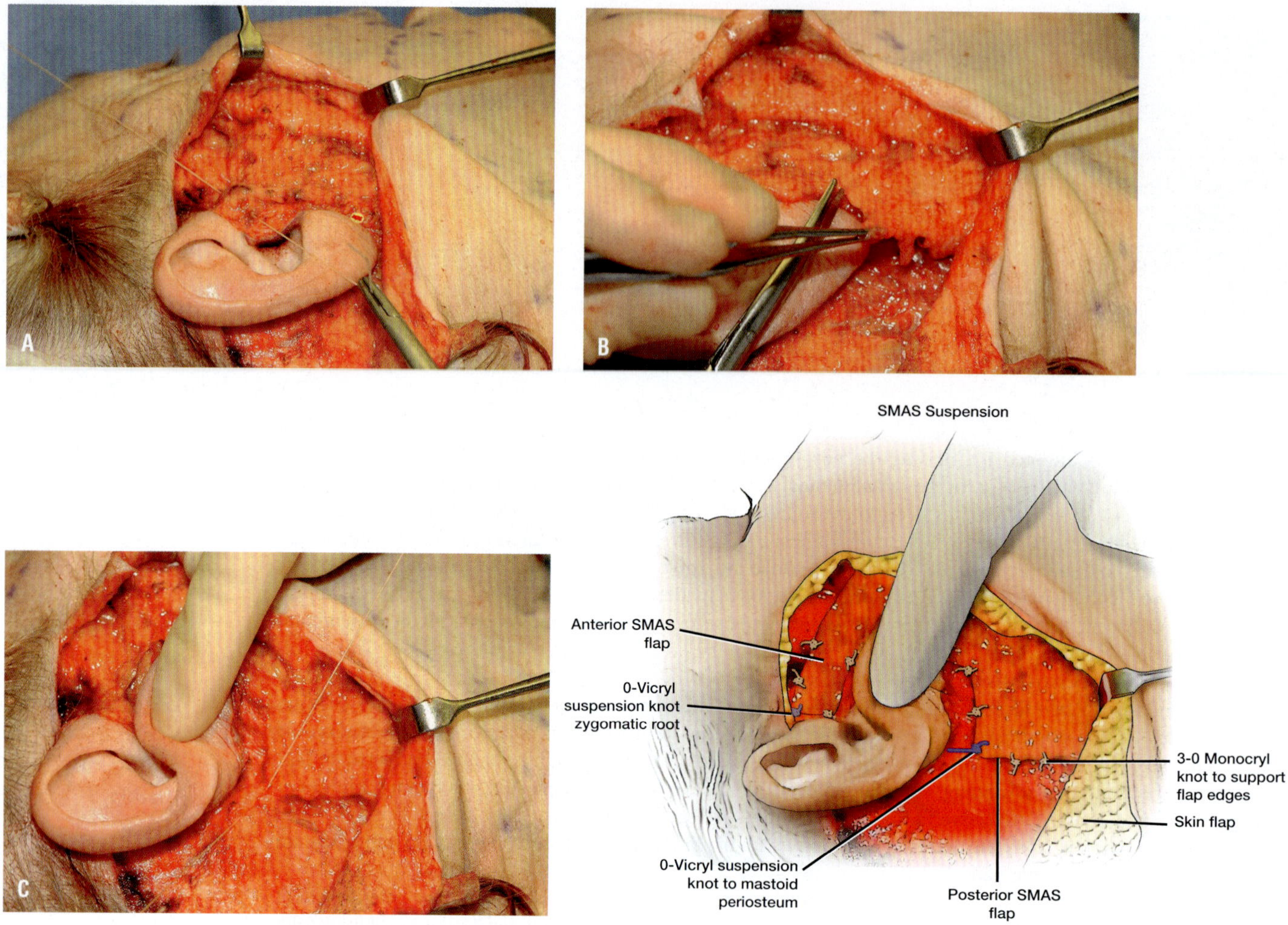

FIGURE 10.11 Two vector SMAS sling. **A:** Suspension of the anterior SMAS flap. **B:** Partial division of SMAS flap. **C:** Suspension of posterior SMAS flap.

The extent of the sub-SMAS elevation is adequate when firm traction on the SMAS flap gives the desired amount of correction. There is no absolute distance, as this varies depending upon each patient's tissues and SMAS stability. Once obtained, the SMAS is then secured to maintain this result.

SMAS imbrication begins with preauricular suspension along a posterior–superior vector (Fig. 10.11). This is then secured near the zygomatic root with a buried 0 Vicryl suture. Once placed, the SMAS is partially divided for a secondary vector of suspension. The inferior portion is then anchored posteriorly with another 0 Vicryl to the mastoid periosteum just behind the ear lobule. The SMAS is not excised but advanced over the superior and posterior fascial tissues and is used as a "sling" suspension. The only SMAS that is excised is a small portion in the immediate preauricular region. Additionally, 3-0 Monocryl (Ethicon, Somerville, NJ) sutures are used to further support the SMAS flap and smooth its edges. Occasionally, 3-0 Tevdek (Deknatel, Queens Village, NY) sutures are necessary to suspend heavier flaps. Once the SMAS is secure in its new location, all the tension of the closure rests on this deeper tissue and allows the skin to be closed without strain on the wound edges. This avoids widening of the scar and suture tract formation that would otherwise occur.

To reposition the preauricular skin flap, it is first advanced posteriorly and slightly superiorly. Next, the posterior flap is elevated posteriorly, rotated superiorly, and suspension staples are placed with particular attention to align the posterior hairline properly. It is then further secured in the preauricular area with suspension staples placed in key positions. Following this, the posterior flap redundancy is removed and the scalp is closed immediately with surgical staples. The skin flap is then tailored to cradle the ear lobule in a tension-free manner. This is a critical step to avoid a postoperative pixie or satyr ear deformity. The anterior skin flap edge is then trimmed to mirror both the anterior lobule and helical insertion. Prior to closure, a 7-mm closed suction drain is placed in a dependent position and brought out through a separate stab incision posteriorly.

After obtaining hemostasis, several 5-0 Monocryl sutures are used to reapproximate the contoured flap, and two 6-0 Ethilon (Ethicon, Somerville, NJ) sutures are placed in the lobule to maintain the tucked position. Next, the distal portion of the tragal flap is thinned of the subcutaneous tissue and left slightly redundant to help avoid blunting or anterior displacement of the underlying cartilage. The closure is then completed with removal of the suspension staples and placement of a 5-0 plain gut suture in a running, locking fashion.

The procedure is then performed on the contralateral side in an identical manner. Once both sides have been completed and closed, the submental incision is trimmed of redundant skin and similarly closed with 5-0 plain gut sutures in a running, locking fashion. Once completed, resurfacing procedures, if indicated, are performed. Although a resurfacing procedure is never performed directly over the undermined portion of the preauricular or neck skin due to the possibility of vascular compromise, the perioral area and deeper lip rhytids are frequently treated. Lastly, a light pressure dressing is applied, and the drains are attached to closed bulb suction.

POSTOPERATIVE MANAGEMENT

Overnight, the light pressure dressing and closed suction drains remain. Elevation of the head of the bed and frequent application of cool compresses is recommended. The patient should rest the first night and begin ambulation the next day. The patient's diet can be advanced as tolerated. Antibiotics, analgesics, anxiolytics, antiemetics, and sleep aids are taken as instructed to maintain comfort and minimize risk of infection. On postoperative day 1, the patient is reevaluated, and the dressing and drains are removed. Wound care is performed and demonstrated until patients have a full understanding of the postoperative instructions. A lighter, smaller dressing is applied to the neck for the next 24 hours. On the second postoperative day, the patient no longer needs the dressing and begins washing the hair daily. Light activity, continued head elevation, and frequent cool compresses are recommended. On postoperative day 7, the patient returns for removal of all but the lobule sutures and reevaluation of the results. On postoperative day 10, the lobule sutures are removed, and a makeup and skin care session is performed by my medical estheticians. At 3 weeks, normal activity can be resumed. The patient then returns for follow-up appointments at 1 week, 3 months, 6 months, and 1 year, or longer, to assess the results and confirm patient satisfaction.

COMPLICATIONS

An expanding postsurgical hematoma is a surgical emergency and requires early recognition and return to the OR under anesthesia for evacuation of the hematoma and hemostasis (Fig. 10.12). Luckily, these rarely occur, and in my experience, if treated appropriately, do not lead to adverse outcomes. More frequently, small, nonexpanding hematomas and seromas can be easily treated with needle aspiration, continued antibiotic coverage, a firm dressing, and close observation. Rarely, a small opening and insertion of a Penrose drain is required for large persistent seromas.

Infections are unlikely unless flap perfusion is compromised or a fluid collection is present. Supportive care with treatment of the underlying etiology and aggressive antibiotic management is required. Wound opening or washout is rarely required.

Skin loss from any of the above conditions, or other patient factors, such as continued smoking, can be problematic. Poor early postoperative perfusion may be improved with warm compresses, massage, and/or nitroglycerin ointment, in addition to treatment of the underlying cause, if possible. Ultimately, mild epidermolysis will usually heal quickly, while full-thickness loss may remain unsightly for many months and lead to scarring of varying significance. This almost exclusively occurs in patients who smoke in the immediate postoperative period, or who never really quit, as instructed. In full-thickness skin defects, the eschar should be allowed to slough spontaneously during wound contraction, and attempts at removal should be avoided.

Persistent edema and mild irregularities are relatively common and can be managed well with local triamcinolone injections as needed. Occasionally, mild hypervascularity is seen after rhytidectomy or following steroids injections but, given adequate time, will usually resolve spontaneously. Alternatively, asymmetries or inadequately treated areas may require a touch-up procedure if a period of watchful waiting does not resolve the problem.

Temporary sensory loss is expected, and each patient is instructed on this normal postoperative sequela. In nearly every case, complete return of sensation occurs but may take a variable length of time from several weeks to nearly 1 year. Permanent nerve injuries are also possible and should be managed as any other neural injury. This usually involves the great auricular nerve. In each of these conditions, a bit of hand-holding and reassurance is required but, with proper management and reapproximation of the injured nerve, complete return of sensation on that side can be expected. Injury to the facial nerve is reported in various series but has not occurred in my experience.

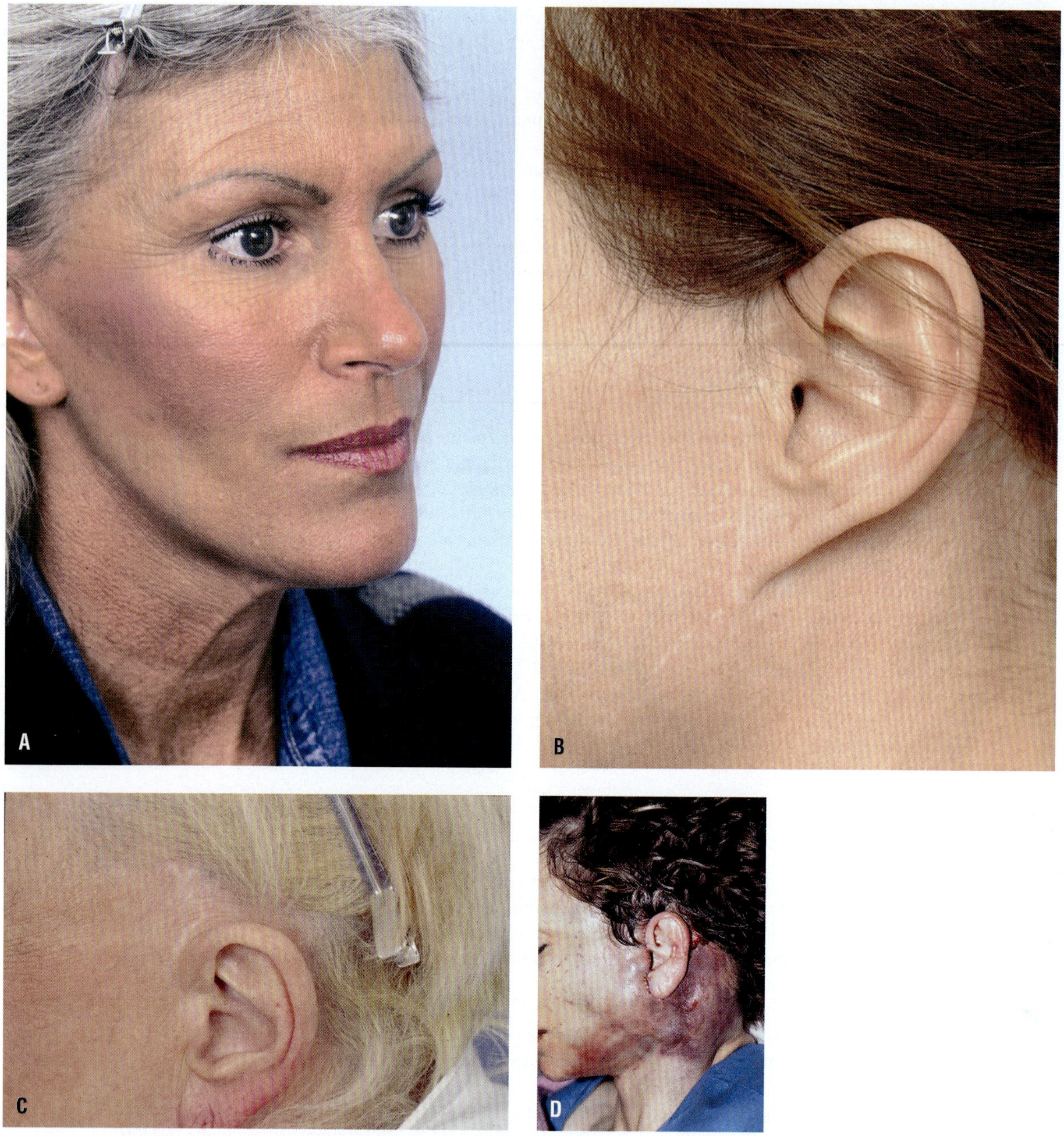

FIGURE 10.12 Complications. **A:** Persistent platysmal bands. **B:** Pretragal scarring with pixie ear and suture tracts. **C:** Loss of the temporal hair tuft. **D:** Expanding hematoma.

RESULTS

My fundamental technique has changed very little over the past 15 to 20 years. It has provided the patients with excellent, natural, lasting results, and overall satisfaction (Figs. 10.13 to 10.16). Note the use of digital imaging in planning the procedures and how close the end result comes to the planned outcome.

PEARLS

- The key to substantial, long-lasting improvement in rhytidectomy is the adequate management of the neck.
- The Kelly clamp platysmal imbrication is the foundation for an improved cervicomental angle.
- Skeletal augmentation and adjunctive procedures can further enhance the overall outcome.

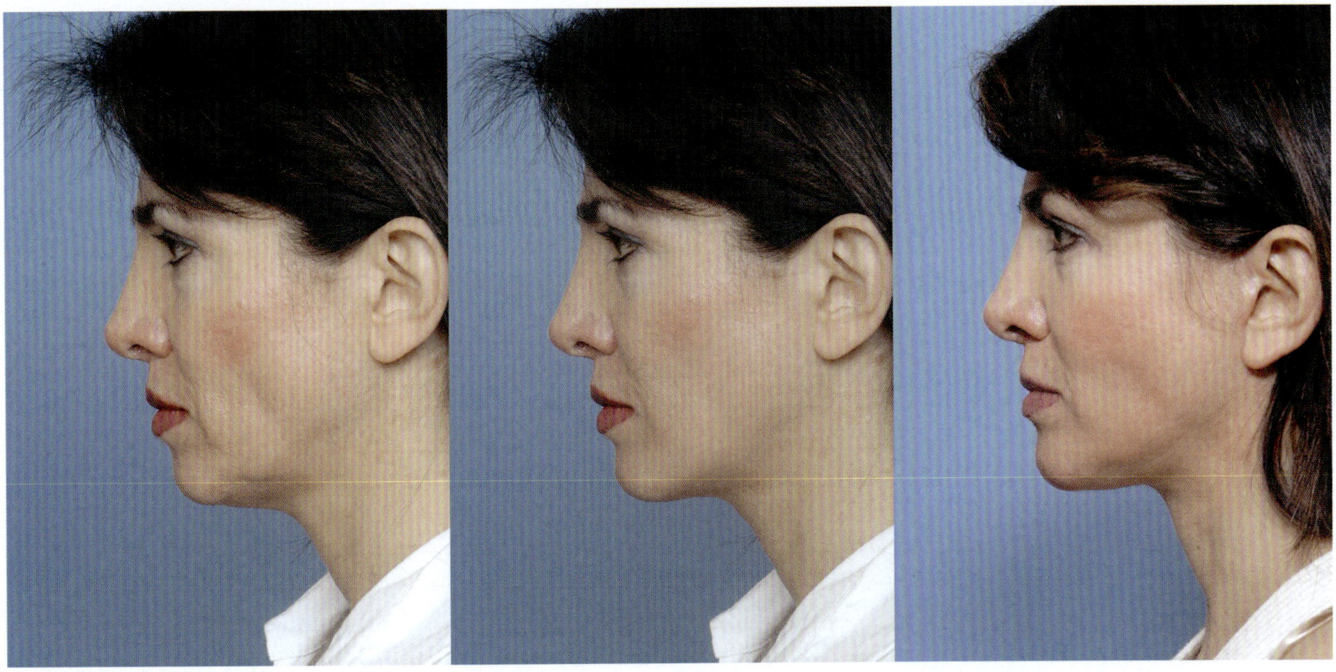

FIGURE 10.13 Type I face-lift and chin implant patient with 7-month follow-up results (preoperative photo, digital imaging, and postoperative photos).

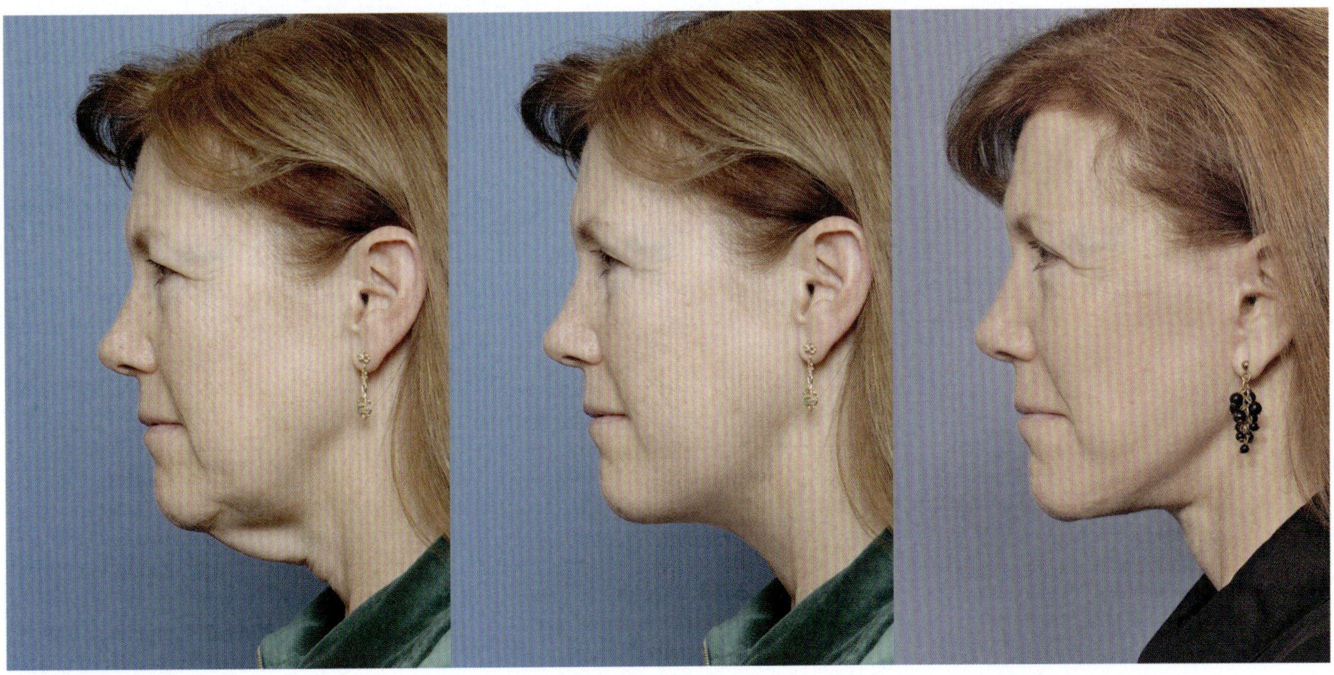

FIGURE 10.14 Type II face-lift patient with 8-month follow-up results (preoperative photo, digital imaging, and postoperative photos).

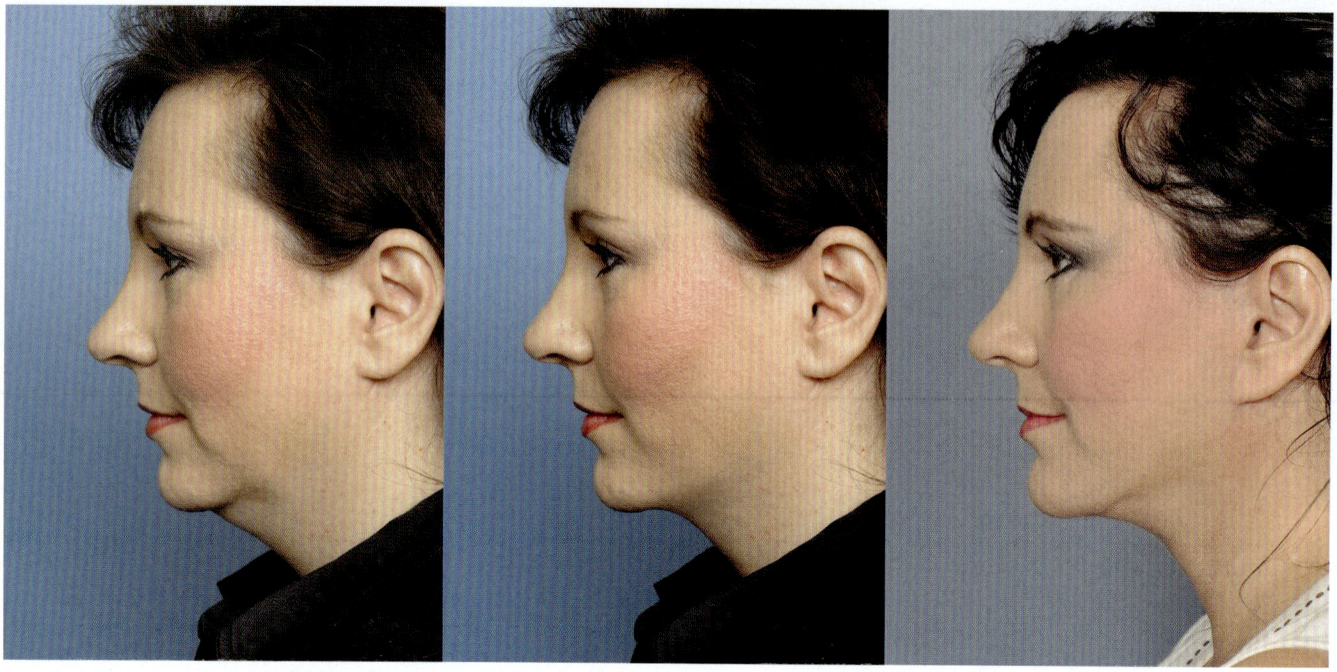

FIGURE 10.15 Type III face-lift patient with 12-month follow-up results (preoperative photo, digital imaging, and postoperative photos).

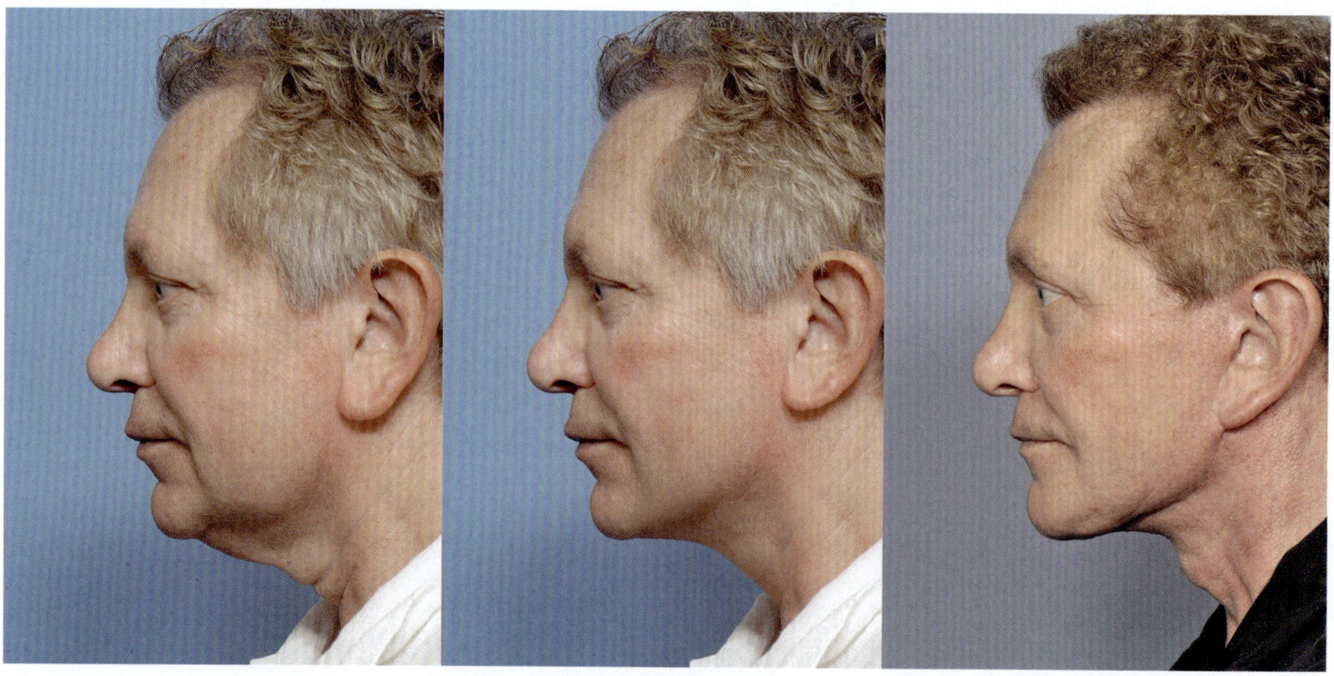

FIGURE 10.16 Type III face-lift patient with 12-month follow-up results (preoperative photo, digital imaging, and postoperative photos).

PITFALLS

- Poor incision planning with obvious scars and an altered hairline are not easily camouflaged and are a "telltale sign" of a face-lift.
- A "pulled skin" look results from excessive tension placed on the skin flap and dissection medial to the nasolabial fold.
- Overly aggressive liposuction can lead to dermal banding and visible submandibular glands.

INSTRUMENTS TO HAVE AVAILABLE

- Standard plastic surgical tray
- Fournier 3-mm liposuction cannula
- Spatulated 5/6 mm liposuction cannulas
- Lighted fiberoptic face-lift retractor
- Meyerding finger retractors
- Bumgardner needle holder
- Halsey needle holder
- Castroviejo needle holder
- Griffiths-Brown forceps
- Kelly clamp 6 inches
- Kahn face-lift scissor
- Lorna non-penetrating towel clamps

ACKNOWLEDGMENTS

The author would like to recognize Robert W. Brobst Jr, MD, for his exceptional contributions to the writing of this chapter. His work in the writing, editing, and figure creation for this chapter is greatly appreciated, without which this chapter would not have been possible.

SUGGESTED READING

Baker SR. Tri-plane rhytidectomy. *Arch Otolaryngol Head Neck Surg* 1997;123:1167–1172.

Hamra ST. The deep plane rhytidectomy. *Plast Reconstr Surg* 1990;86:53–61.

Kamer FM. One hundred consecutive deep plane face lifts. *Arch Otolaryngol Head Neck Surg* 1996;122:17–22.

Koch BB, Perkins SW. Simultaneous rhytidectomy and full-face carbon dioxide laser resurfacing: a case series and meta-analysis. *Arch Facial Plast Surg* 2002;4:227–233.

McCollough EG, Perkins SW, Langsdon PR. SMAS suspension rhytidectomy, rationale and long term experience. *Arch Otolaryngol Head Neck Surg* 1989;115:228–234.

11 EXTENDED SUPERFICIAL MUSCULOAPONEUROTIC SYSTEM (SMAS) FACE-LIFT AND CORSET PLATYSMAPLASTY

Keith A. LaFerriere

INTRODUCTION

Face-lift, or rhytidectomy, techniques have evolved in many ways over the past 50 years from being predominantly a skin operation to reliance on the deeper superficial musculoaponeurotic system (SMAS) to provide the major lifting of the sagging face and neck in facial rejuvenation. The early works of Skoog as well as Mitz and Peyronie laid much of the groundwork for the development of our current understanding of the importance of the SMAS. However, it was the seminal publication of the Deep Plane Facelift by Hamra in 1990 that has inspired over 100 articles in the plastic surgery literature and has been very influential in the approach that many facial plastic surgeons use in their face-lift techniques, including the techniques presented here.

The SMAS

The SMAS plays a role in a face-lift, regardless of the technique used. SMAS plication, derived from the Greek word *plica*, which means "to fold," consists of suturing or folding the SMAS on itself, whether a strip of SMAS is removed or not. SMAS imbrication, derived from the word *imbricate,* means "to layer, as in roofing shingles." In this instance, the SMAS is undermined as a flap and overlapped in one or more superior or superolateral directions. Many studies have been published regarding the various techniques of handling the SMAS and the preponderance of opinions would suggest that there is no clear advantage of the deep plane versus other techniques of handling the SMAS.

Hamra's classical deep plane face-lift is often misunderstood regarding the SMAS. By definition, the SMAS envelopes the mimetic muscle of the face and neck, so whenever the dissection is deep to the mimetic muscles of the face, it is considered sub-SMAS. By this anatomical definition, the original deep plane procedure is superficial to the SMAS in the neck, below the SMAS in the lower face (as it is an extended dissection below the platysma), and above the SMAS in the upper face (as the dissection is above the zygomaticus major and minor and the inferior orbicularis oculi muscles). The transition point in the face between the sub-SMAS in the lower face and the deep subcutaneous dissection in the upper face is the inferior border of the zygoma, where the nerves to the zygomaticus muscles emerge. In essence, the term "deep plane" refers to both the lower face sub-SMAS dissection and the upper face, which is really only a deep subcutaneous dissection.

In patients with a more advanced degree of aging, I do still use the extended SMAS imbrication in the lower face similar to that described by Hamra, but stop the sub-SMAS dissection at the level of the inferior border of the zygoma. I do not do the "deep plane" in the upper face, but rather undermine the skin to release the zygomatic retaining ligaments and plicate the malar adipose tissue pad in a superolateral direction (▶ Video 11.1). I do undermine the skin somewhat more anteriorly than in the classical deep plane face-lift because it allows for a different vector of the skin than the SMAS flap. The mandibular retaining ligaments are also released while the skin is being undermined. In younger patients with less aging face changes, I often elevate a shorter flap and perform SMAS excision with plication.

The Neck

For many years, I approached the neck with subcutaneous adipose tissue sculpting, removal of a small amount of platysma and subplatysma adipose tissue inferiorly to the level of the hyoid or just slightly inferior, and plication of the platysma muscle inferiorly to the level of the hyoid with many instances performing horizontal division of the anterior aspect of the platysma for several centimeters just inferior to the level of plication. This was generally my first step in the face-lift sequence. Later, when the SMAS was undermined in the face, it was continued under the posterior border of the platysma in the neck, and a posterior pull on the muscle was applied. In essence, the midline was secured with the platysma plication, and the posterior pull on the platysma tightened the neck. When I studied the results with this technique, the frequency of recurrence of platysma bands and the amount of long-term definition that was achieved were disappointing. Platysma bands recurred, in as early as a year or less, and in the difficult neck, the definition was less than desired.

The Paradigm Shift

About 5 years ago, after I analyzed my results, I radically changed my approach to the neck. Feldman had pioneered a technique that he called a "corset platysmaplasty" that at first glance did not make much sense, in that all of the work was done anteriorly without significant posterior pull on the platysma. Common sense would suggest that aging is influenced by gravity and the loss of elasticity and that a posterosuperior pull against gravity would make more sense. In spite of this, I tried this technique and was immediately impressed with the results (Video 11.1). The skin of the neck is undermined through a submental incision and the medial platysma borders are undermined laterally for several centimeters down to the level of the cricoid. This releases some of the platysma-retaining ligaments, which exposes the subplatysma adipose tissue and the anterior belly of the digastric muscles. Often, the inferior aspect of the submandibular glands can be seen. Almost always, the subplatysma adipose tissue is removed in its entirety, usually including the prelaryngeal adipose tissue as well. Occasionally, bulging anterior belly of the digastric muscles may need to be reduced. I have not reduced the submandibular glands through this approach because of potential complications, but I think that results in some patients would be better if this were performed. A complete corset platysmaplasty is performed, starting at the level of the submental incision, down to the level of the cricoid with a running suture that inverts the medial edges of the platysma muscles. Using the same continuous suture, the original suture line is inverted by suturing the platysma on itself from the cricoid back up to the submental incision, with excursions laterally as necessary on both sides of the midline to further tighten any bulging of the muscle that is identified. This creates a true corset, with lateral pleats, so the platysma completely conforms to the underlying anatomy. It is the second inverting row as one comes superiorly that really defines the neck, and this is clearly seen when one gets back up to the level of the hyoid and then to the level of the submental incision. The only posterior pull on the platysma in the neck when doing the lateral aspect of the face-lift is in the area of the angle of the mandible to increase definition.

Since I began to extend the undermining of the skin and use SMAS flaps with imbrication combined with the true corset platysmaplasty described above, the results have improved and decidedly longer lasting in the face and in the neck. This is the primary focus and purpose of this chapter. If extensive midface aging is present, the addition of a transtemporal or transblepharoplasty midface lift also improves the result and increases its longevity.

HISTORY

When evaluating a prospective patient for an aging face procedure, it is important to obtain an accurate history and clinical examination. This includes identifying and addressing the patient's concerns regarding their aging changes as well as discovering their goals and expectations with any corrective procedure. During this initial consultation, realistic goals and expectations from a face-lift procedure are discussed.

Although a face-lift is an elective procedure, a thorough medical history is obtained focusing on issues such as (cardiac, vascular, pulmonary, and endocrine) that may increase the risk of an adverse event for a 4-hour procedure under a general anesthesia. Medical clearance is acquired when indicated. A comprehensive review of medications taken is also performed to identify those that may increase the risk of bleeding or prevent optimal wound healing. The use of herbal supplements is also ascertained since many have anticoagulating properties. The overall health status of a patient is more important than the age.

PHYSICAL EXAMINATION

Along with a comprehensive physical examination, specific attention is focused on the cheek region, jawline, and neck contour. Physical examination of these three areas helps to determine whether the patient is a candidate for an extended SMAS face-lift, with or without a corset platysmaplasty, compared to a less extensive face-lift procedure. Additionally, the amount of midface aging, seen with the distance from the eyelid margin to the malar or cheek area, is noted. The extended SMAS face-lift focuses on improvement of time-related changes seen in the lower face only. The descent of the malar adipose tissue pads over time results in its redundancy and mounding against the nasolabial folds. Face-lift techniques may improve the most lateral aspect of the nasolabial folds, but complete long-term correction is elusive. These technical limitations of the face-lift procedure are discussed with the patient. Any asymmetries of the face, facial expression, skin irregularities, scars, or soft tissue prominences are noted during the examination and are pointed out to the patient. The anatomic position of the hyoid bone in the neck is also important to identify since a low and anterior placement limits the ability to contour the neck. Moreover, microgenia may prohibit achieving the maximum amount of improvement in the contour of the neck without augmentation. Ptosis of the chin, when present, needs correction for optimal contour of the neck.

INDICATIONS

Essentially, any healthy patient with realistic goals and expectations who has significant lower facial and neck aging is a candidate for an extended SMAS face-lift, with or without a corset platysmaplasty. The corset platysmaplasty is used in conjunction with the face-lift as a technique reserved to address the more difficult neck with poor contour, significant platysma bands, or both. A comprehensive approach to the aging face is important and addressing aspects outside of the lower face, such as eyelids, eyebrows, midface, volume loss, and skin changes, will maximize results and patient satisfaction.

CONTRAINDICATIONS

Absolute contraindications include the following:

- Major cardiac, pulmonary, or other systemic illnesses that would be unable to obtain medical clearance from their primary care, specialty physician, or anesthesiologist
- Patients actively undergoing chemotherapy treatments for various malignancies or other systemic diseases
- Major psychiatric conditions that will not allow clearance from their psychiatrist
- Stroke or other conditions that will not allow temporary cessation of anticoagulant medications

Relative contraindications include the following:

- Use of nicotine in any form. If the patient is not willing to discontinue nicotine use for at least 4 weeks before and after surgery, he or she is not a candidate for any type of extensive undermining face-lift. All nicotine users, regardless of whether they have agreed to abstain from nicotine use, view skin slough photos and sign a letter of acknowledgment before any face-lift procedure is performed.
- Divorce or any other major life stress. In time, these patients may be ideal candidates, but during the acute phase, it is recommended to wait and reevaluate once the patient's life has stabilized.
- Unrealistic expectations. If the main reason for undergoing a face-lift is something that most likely cannot be corrected to the patient's satisfaction, it is better to acknowledge this and move on.
- Patients who are rude to your staff. No matter how nice they are to the surgeon, if the staff identifies significant red flags, be wary of proceeding with any surgery.
- Patients with body dysmorphic syndrome often have unrealistic expectations and may be setting the surgeon up for a "patient for life." If this can be diagnosed during the preoperative phase, it may prevent future issues.
- Obese candidates who are planning to lose weight. A good rule of thumb is to have the face-lift when the patient is within 10 pounds of the weight that he or she will realistically maintain.
- Patients who "bad-mouth" other doctors. Certainly, if it is legitimate, it is reasonable to proceed, but remember that the operating surgeon could be the next doctor on the "bad-mouth" list.
- Patients who will not accept the surgeon's recommendations, but want lesser procedures that will not correct the underlying problem.
- The chronically unhappy patient who thinks that a face-lift will solve their problems. These patients can turn their unhappiness toward the surgeon in the postoperative period.
- Patients who demand exceptions to the standard rules for postoperative activity, such as caregiver or distance from the office. This can lead to unwanted complications and a substandard result.

PREOPERATIVE PLANNING

Standard preoperative photographs are obtained in the Frankfort horizontal plane including, but not limited to, frontal (smiling and nonsmiling), right and left oblique, and right and left lateral views. Medical clearance, laboratory, and imaging studies necessary for optimization before undergoing anesthesia are obtained and reviewed.

Providing postoperative care instructions in the preoperative phase is helpful in preparing the patient for the procedure and allowing them to become accustomed to the requirements during the healing phase.

SURGICAL TECHNIQUE

The bilateral face-lift incisions, and the anticipated lower face and neck limits of dissection are marked out in the preoperative area in the usual fashion for an extended SMAS face-lift with a corset platysmaplasty with the incisions running along the postauricular hairline to maximize skin removal (Fig. 11.1). The extent of the dissection in the zygomatic area down to the margin of the mandible is marked preoperatively by moving the midface tissue as far posterolaterally as possible, noting the point at which maximum movement is obtained (superior "X" in Fig. 11.1). If less skin removal is needed, the incision is placed into the postauricular hairline. The patient is then taken to the operating room for induction of sedation or general anesthesia.

Attention is then turned toward the neck and the extended SMAS imbrication lift. The submental incision is injected with a 50:50 solution of 2% lidocaine with 1:100,000 epinephrine and 0.5% bupivacaine with 1:200,000 epinephrine. The submental area is then infiltrated with tumescent injection of 1:400,000 epinephrine. Bilateral tarsorrhaphy sutures are placed if the eyelids are not completely closed under anesthesia.

An incision is made in the submental area. The anterior neck skin and adipose tissue is then dissected off the platysma muscle down to the level of the cricoid, and laterally for several centimeters, ensuring the removal of all residual adipose tissue from the surface of the platysma. The medial edges of the platysma muscles are divided in the submental midline, and the platysma is undermined bilaterally for several centimeters down to the level of the cricoid to release the retaining ligaments. In the anterior midline, the subplatysma adipose tissue is completely excised off of the anterior bellies of the digastric muscles and off of the mylohyoid muscle bilaterally with resection carried inferiorly to the level of the hyoid bone. The removal of subplatysma adipose tissue results in further sharpening the contour of the anterior cervicomental angle and allows for the infolding of the platysma muscle. A corset platysmaplasty is then completed in the usual fashion using a running 3-0 PDS suture from superior to inferior, inverting the platysma muscle edges, suturing down to approximately the level of the cricoid cartilage. The platysma muscle edges are then oversewn in a second layer as the continuous suture is passed back superiorly. Ensuring that no adipose tissue remains on the platysma muscles minimizes postoperative bulges. Prior to tying the corset suture, lateral pleating sutures are placed bilaterally to further tighten and contour the neck. The suture is then brought back superiorly and tied where placement originally began (Video 11.1).

The right-sided periauricular incision lines are injected with a 50:50 solution of 2% lidocaine with 1:100,000 epinephrine and 0.5% bupivacaine with 1:200,000 epinephrine. The right side of the face is then infiltrated with tumescent injection of 1:400,000 epinephrine. The right face-lift incisions are then made

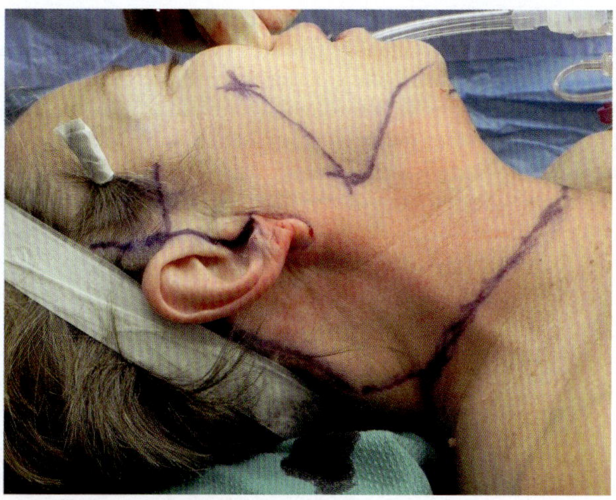

FIGURE 11.1 This figure illustrates the preoperative markings for extended SMAS face-lift with corset platysmaplasty. The incision extends superiorly into the temporal hairline. The horizontal incision along the helical root prevents the non–hair-bearing skin from raising the sideburn. The posttragal incision is outlined; note that the tragus and lobule are demarcated by a small right-angle incision improving the separation of these two structures. The postauricular incision is brought slightly onto the conchal cartilage so that the final incision will lie in the postauricular crease (postauricular incision not shown). This patient has extension of the incision along the posterior hairline. The extent of the dissection in the zygomatic area (superior "X") down to the angle of the mandible (inferior "X") is seen marked preoperatively by moving the midface tissue as far posterolaterally as possible, noting the point at which maximum movement is obtained. The inferior extent of dissection for the corset platysmaplasty is marked at the cricoid, and the inferior neck marking depicts the extent of undermining for this portion of the procedure.

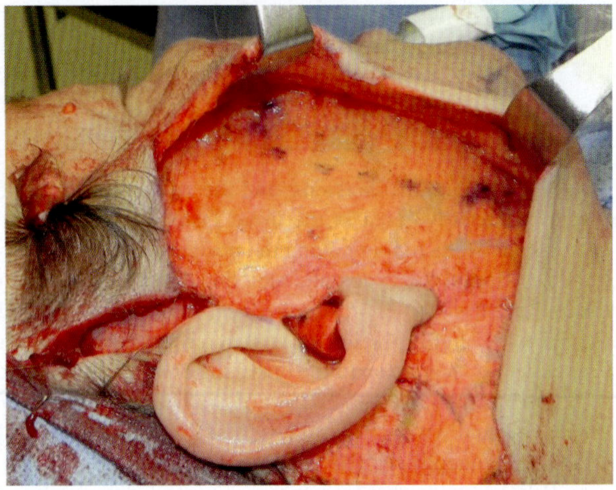

FIGURE 11.2
This figure illustrates the extended SMAS flap design. The superior mark is placed just inferior to the zygomatic arch anteriorly, and the inferior mark is placed along the angle of the mandible.

with extension of the incision superiorly into the temporal scalp. Dissection is performed anteroinferiorly on the deep temporal fascia and past the location of the frontal branch as it crosses the zygomatic arch. Next, the skin flap is elevated in the subcutaneous plane extending anteriorly to the preoperative markings in the midface and inferiorly over the platysma muscle creating a connecting tunnel to the midline submental dissection pocket. Particular attention is taken toward elevating as much adipose tissue off of the platysma as possible while preserving a thin fascial layer over the platysma muscle itself. Along the inferior rim of the mandible, dissection is carried out medially over the jowls, taking care to keep the adipose tissue pad of the jowls down on both sides and releasing the mandibular retaining ligaments. It is important to visually monitor the facial nerve during the facial and upper neck portions of the procedure for signs of facial nerve branch stimulation.

An extended SMAS imbrication lift is then performed. The SMAS flap is marked and incised along a line from the inferior border of the zygoma to the angle of the mandible (Fig. 11.2 and Video 11.1). Once incised, the platysma muscle is identified in the midportion of the flap. Dissection is then continued through the platysma muscle and on top of the parotidomasseteric fascia anteriorly to mobilize the lower facial SMAS (Figs. 11.3 to 11.5 and Video 11.1). The dissection is carried anteriorly to the level of the facial vessels. The facial nerve branches lie safely below the parotidomasseteric fascia, and it is important not to violate this fascia in order to protect the facial nerve. Once the SMAS flap is adequately created, the soft tissues overlying the preauricular area are thinned to reduce the bulk when the SMAS flap is imbricated. Prior to anchoring the SMAS flap, a 3-0 PDS suture is passed through the temporal fascia (which was previously exposed) through the malar soft tissue to create maximal movement of this area (Video 11.1). The suture is first passed from the deep temporal fascia through the malar soft tissue anterior to Pitanguy's line to protect branches of the facial nerve. It is then passed multiple times anteriorly through the midface soft tissue to the most anterior extent of the skin flap elevation, grasping the area of maximal soft tissue mobility that was marked preoperatively. The suture lines end superior to the elevated dissected SMAS flap (Video 11.1). The suture is then reversed and passed posteriorly again multiple times through the midface soft tissue and then back into the deep temporal fascia and tied, anchoring the midface soft tissue into position. Care is taken not to overtighten the suture. An additional pass is taken into the temporal fascia after the first knot is tied to provide additional strength to the anchoring suture (Video 11.1).

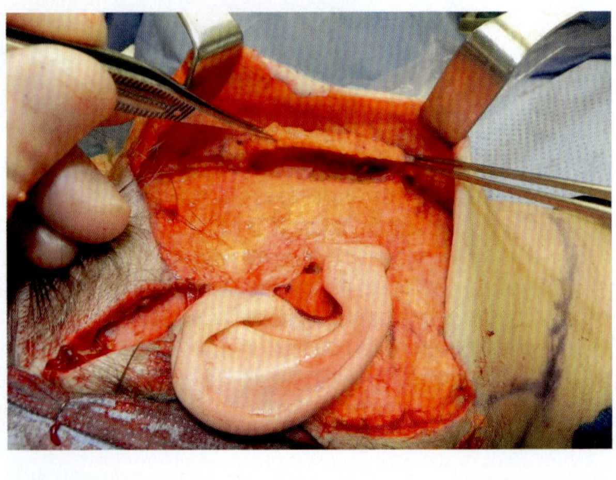

FIGURE 11.3
This figure illustrates the SMAS flap once dissected above the parotidomasseteric fascia.

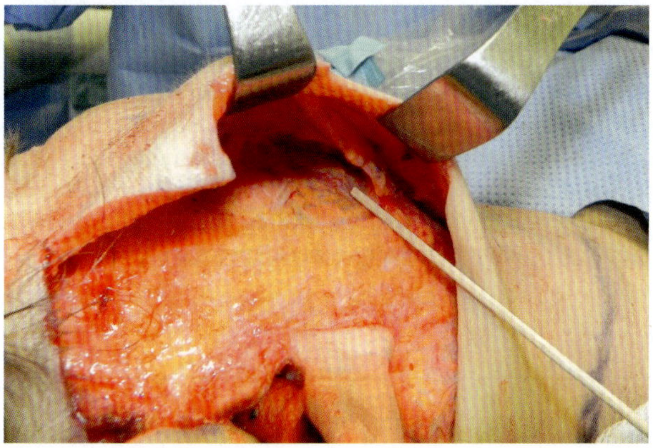

FIGURE 11.4
This figure illustrates the SMAS flap elevated and the presence of a facial nerve branch (pointer).

The SMAS flap is then imbricated in a superolateral direction with 2-0 PDS interrupted sutures. The first suture is placed in the inferior preauricular area, and a second suture is placed through the apex of the SMAS flap superiorly to the level of the zygomatic arch. A third suture is often placed in between the two for additional stabilization (Video 11.1). The earlobe is then dissected from the underlying soft tissue, which exposes the auricular ligament. A suture is then placed from the inferior aspect of the SMAS flap at the level of the angle of the mandible to the auricular ligament, underneath the earlobe, which delineates the angle of the mandible. A second suture may be placed further inferiorly, but no additional posterior pull is placed on the platysma.

Absolute hemostasis is maintained with bipolar electrocautery while carefully monitoring the facial nerve. A drain is placed through a separate stab incision in the postauricular scalp posterior to the lift incision and secured with a 2-0 silk suture. The skin is first redraped in a predominantly superior direction, bringing the postauricular earlobe cutout portion of the flap to the superior post auricular crease and anchoring it with a staple. Care is taken to ensure the postauricular hairline is realigned when the flap is anchored. A second anchor point is set at the level of the junction of the root of the helix with the face, drawing the flap in a posterosuperior direction perpendicular to the melolabial fold, and secured with a 3-0 Vicryl suture. This attaches the subcutaneous tissues both of the root of the helix and preauricular skin flap to the superficial layer of the deep temporal fascia (Video 11.1). Care is taken to tuck the flap underneath the lobule to avoid later inferior migration or "pixie" ear formation. The hair-bearing postauricular incision is trimmed and closed with a running locking 5-0 Prolene suture. The non–hair-bearing postauricular portion of the incision is closed with a running 5-0 chromic suture. The excess skin is trimmed in the preauricular area. The tragal flap is then thinned and tailored to improve its contour. Subcutaneous adipose tissue is removed from the preauricular area to allow for a slight, natural-appearing preauricular depression. This is created by suturing the tragal flap to the pretragal tissues with a single 5-0 Monocryl suture in order to achieve a natural-appearing pretragal sulcus. The hair-bearing temporal incision is closed using surgical staples, and the excess skin is tailored to maintain a natural sideburn level and closed with a running 5-0 Prolene suture. The preauricular incision is closed using a 6-0 Prolene suture. The submental incision is closed in the subcutaneous layer with 5-0 Monocryl and the skin with a running, locking 6-0 fast absorbing gut suture.

The left side of the face-lift is performed in identical fashion as the right side. The cheek and neck flaps are then checked to make sure there is no evidence of hematoma. The patient's drapes are then removed. The patient's facial and neck skin are cleaned and a face-lift dressing is then applied. The submental incision is dressed with Mastisol and taped with flesh-colored tape. The patient is awakened and taken to the recovery area.

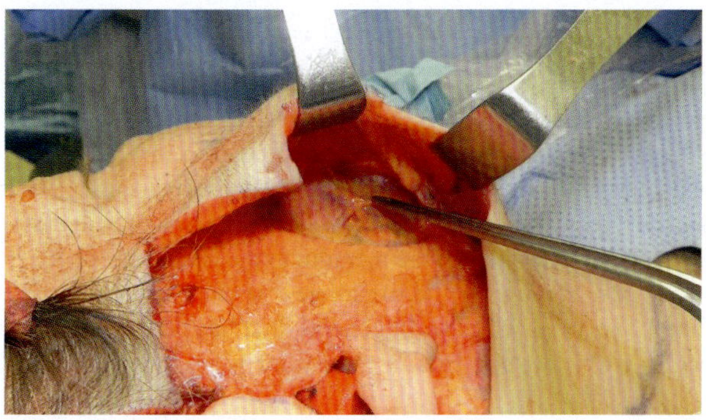

FIGURE 11.5
This figure shows the parotidomasseteric fascia layer present over the masseter muscle and facial nerve branches.

POSTOPERATIVE MANAGEMENT

Face-lift surgery is considered as outpatient surgery and may vary in recovery time, especially related to bruising and swelling. Most patients require 1 to 2 weeks for their immediate recovery period and are ready to go back out into public or work by this point. Continued healing and final results may require 6 months to 1 year. Generally, patients after surgery will go home with a standard face-lift dressing with drains, which are removed the following day. Sleeping with the head elevated is very important during the healing phase, and exercise is avoided for 4 weeks. Sutures and surgical staples are removed approximately 1 week after the procedure.

COMPLICATIONS

Complications of extended SMAS face-lift with corset platysmaplasty are similar compared to other rhytidectomy procedures. When performed carefully and with adequate preoperative evaluation and intraoperative hemostasis, these complications are rare, including the following:

- Hematoma: Postoperative hematoma is the most common complication with an incidence of 2% to 3% in females and up to 8% in males. Control of blood pressure can decrease the rate in males to 4%. Expanding hematomas generally occur within the first 24 hours and require prompt drainage. The use of closed suction drains may be helpful but rarely will prevent an expanding hematoma formation. Even though the literature states the above incidence, I have found the incidence of a significant hematoma in my patient population to be approximately 1% in females and 2% in males with this technique.
- Skin slough: Smoking is the major factor that can contribute to this complication. Other causes include overly thin flap dissection, excessive tension, hematoma, and occlusive dressings. Using correct techniques and careful dissection, this is rarely a complication in the nonsmoker.
- Infection: This is an extremely rare complication with an incidence of approximately 1%. Antibiotics that are culture directed and wound care are the mainstays of treatment.
- Facial nerve injury: May be related in the immediate postoperative period to the effects of the local anesthetic. However, true facial nerve injury may be related to traction, cautery, sutures, or (rarely) surgical division. Buccal branches are the most commonly injured branches, but due to arborization of these nerve branches, the clinical sequelae are minimal. Frontal and marginal mandibular branches are the most common motor nerves affected that create an obvious clinical impairment. In my own experience of performing this procedure for over 20 years, I have never had an injury to the facial nerve during the extended SMAS dissection portion of a lower face-lift. However, the risk of temporary paresis of the marginal mandibular branch of the facial nerve occurs less than 5% of the time when performing the corset platysmaplasty.
- Sensory nerve injury: Injury to the great auricular nerve is the most common nerve injured face-lift surgery. Sensory innervation to the skin is always disrupted, and patients should be counseled that the recovery time for this problem may be 6 to 12 months.
- Incisional issues: Complications involve widening scars, alopecia, and hypertrophic scars. Delayed scar revision may be performed for alopecia and unsightly scars. Steroid injections may be used for hypertrophic scars. Proper planning of the incision line and minimizing tension is key to preventing all of these incisional issues. If proper techniques are used, such an event is a rare occurrence.
- Earlobe deformities: "Pixie" ear deformity may be related to excess tension on the earlobe during the healing phase. Redraping the skin and tucking it up under the earlobe allows this deformity to be easily avoided or treated.
- Psychiatric illness: Following a face-lift procedure many patients may exhibit some depression as well as difficulty with sleep. This generally resolves in a short period of time. Reassurance is the key instrument in such cases.

RESULTS

Performing a careful preoperative assessment and using the techniques as described above, patients undergoing the extended SMAS face-lift with corset platysmaplasty can have very satisfying results with significant improvement of aging changes of the lower face. Typical results from performing this procedure can be seen in Figure 11.6. Additionally, the importance of recognizing microgenia during the preoperative assessment and chin augmentation as an adjunct to the procedure can help maximize results in the neck region (Fig. 11.7). The correction of chin ptosis along with the procedure allows for the smooth contour and transition from the mentum to the neck (Fig. 11.8).

I do not believe that any face-lift technique has been "proven" to be the longest lasting. It would make sense that the more extensive the procedure, the longer the result will last. In general, that has been my experience. When I did primarily short flap/SMAS excision with plication lifts in the earlier years, the number of

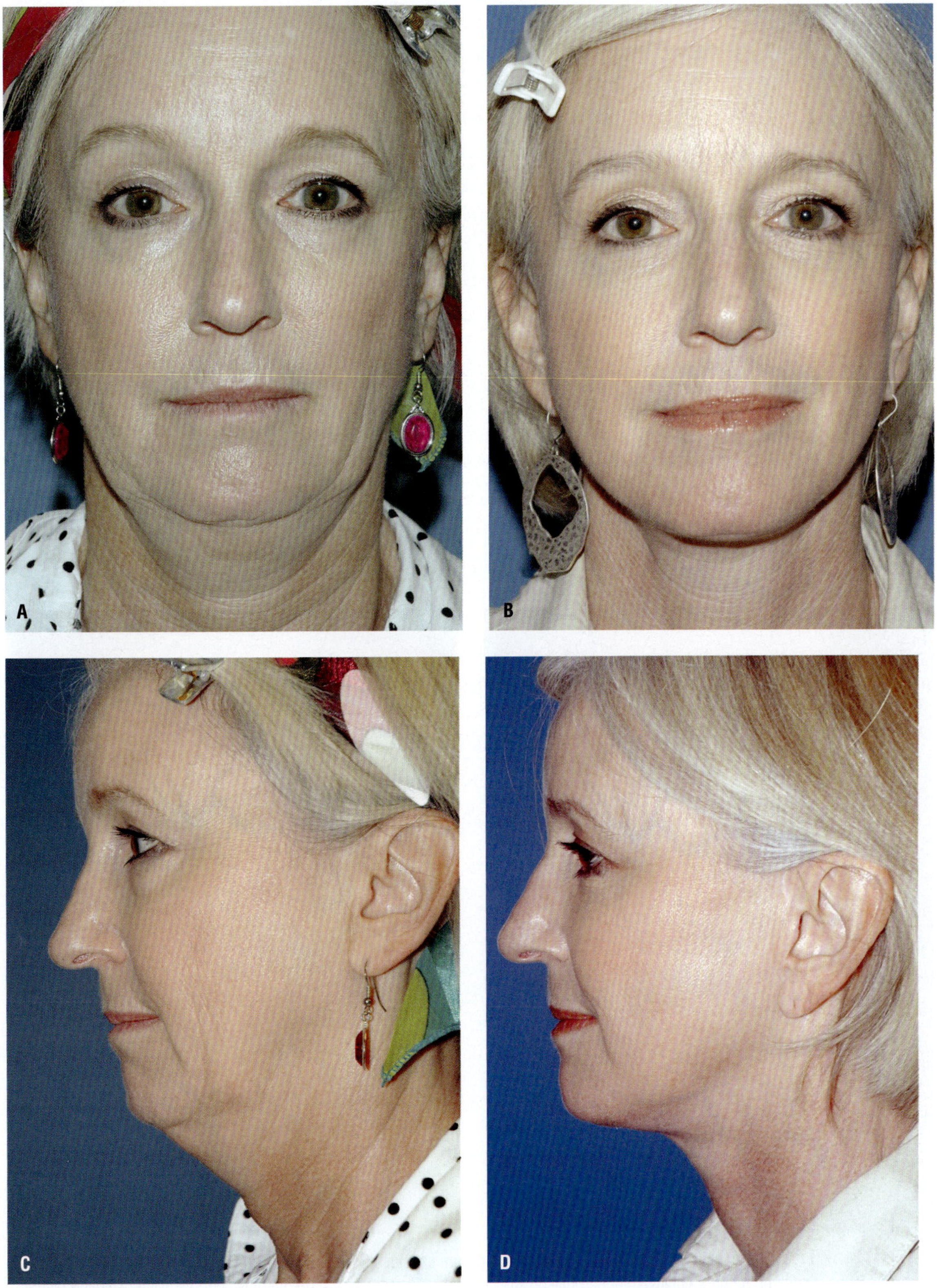

FIGURE 11.6 This is a 57-year-old female 1 year postoperative from extended SMAS rhytidectomy with corset platysmaplasty and transconjunctival lower blepharoplasty with repositioning of the adipose tissue. Preoperative photos frontal **(A)** and lateral **(C)**. Postoperative photos frontal **(B)** and lateral **(D)**.

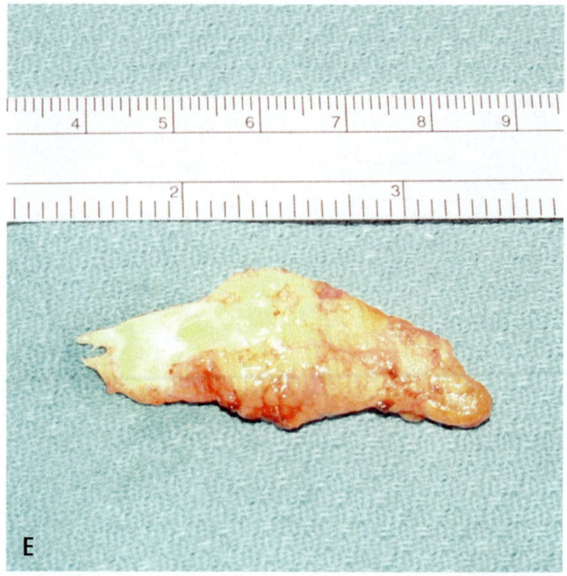

FIGURE 11.6 (*Continued*)
Subplatysma adipose tissue removed during the procedure **(E)**. Note the amount of neck definition achieved with the complete corset platysmaplasty and excision of subplatysmal adipose tissue.

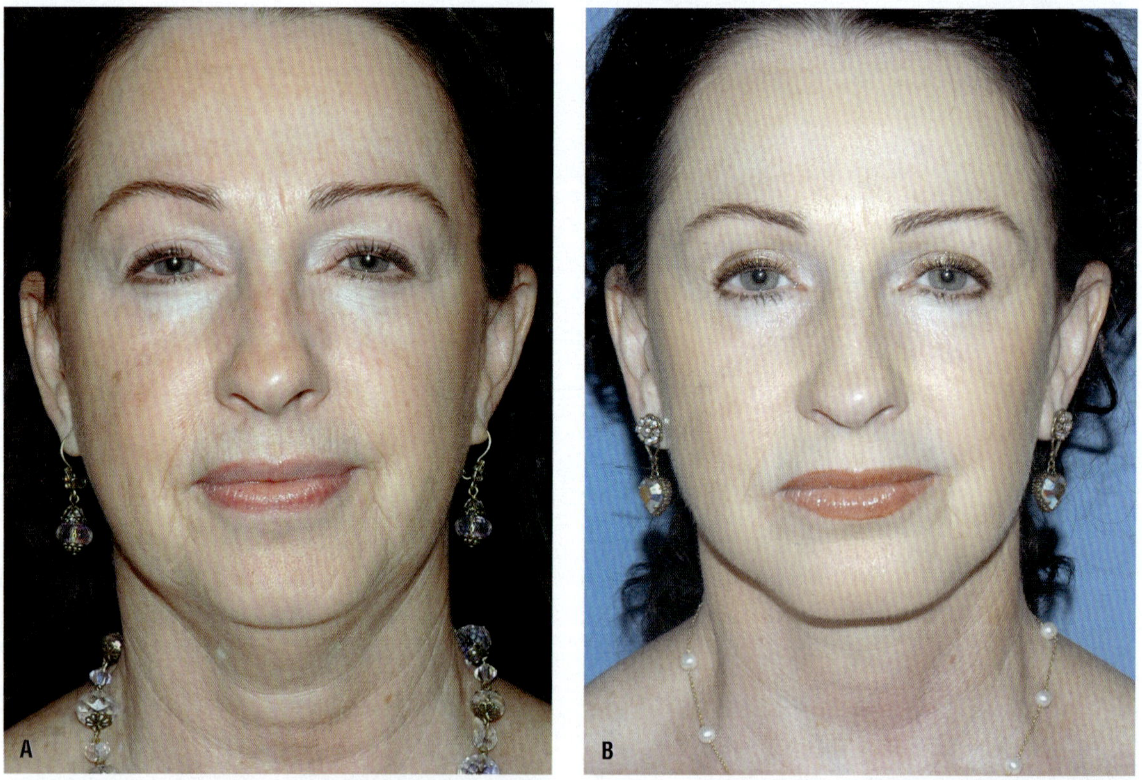

FIGURE 11.7 This is a 56-year-old female 1 year post-op from extended SMAS rhytidectomy with corset platysmaplasty, chin augmentation, upper operative blepharoplasty, and perioral laser resurfacing. Preoperative photos frontal **(A)** and lateral **(C)**. Postoperative photos frontal **(B)** and lateral **(D)**.

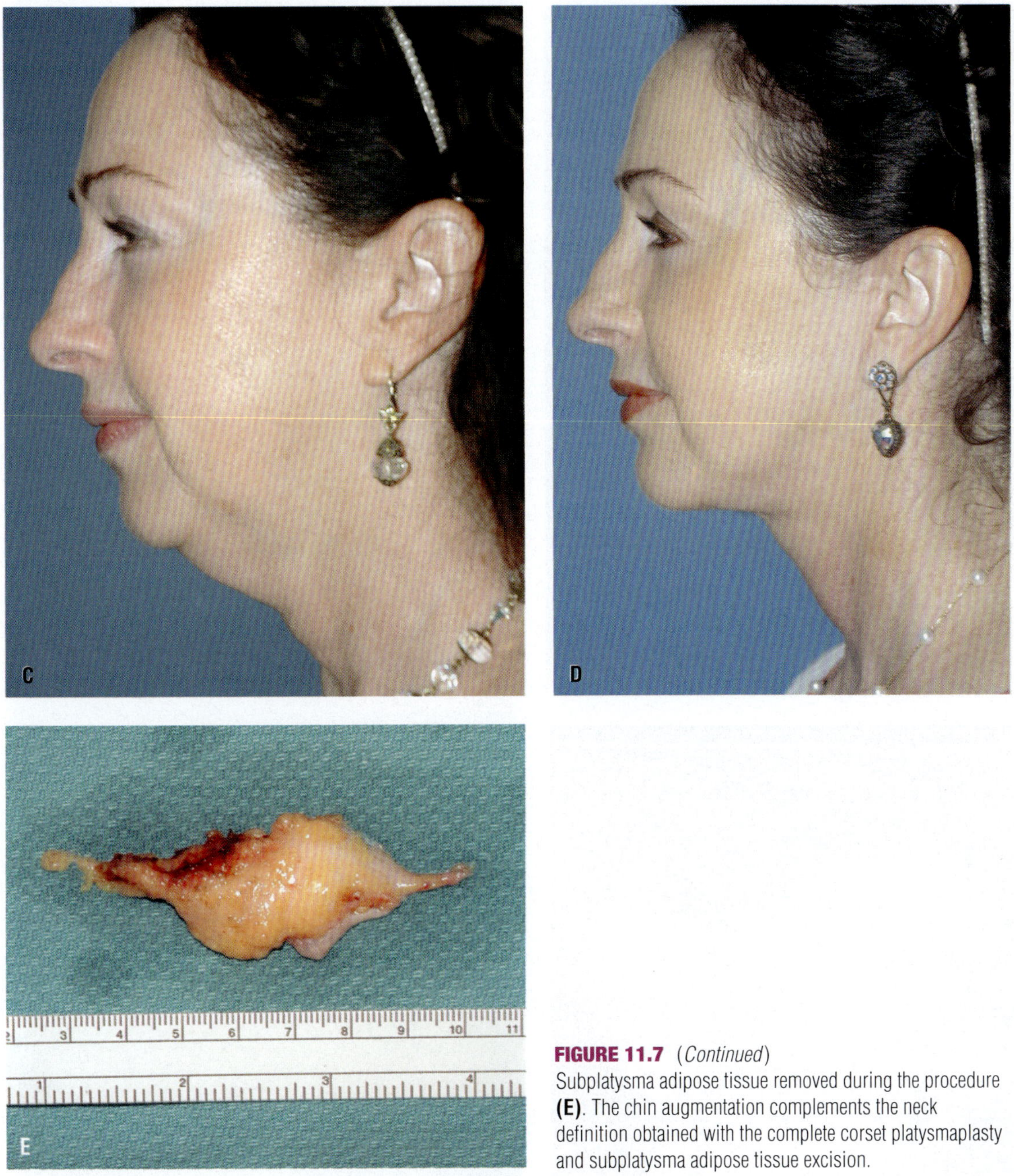

FIGURE 11.7 (*Continued*)
Subplatysma adipose tissue removed during the procedure **(E)**. The chin augmentation complements the neck definition obtained with the complete corset platysmaplasty and subplatysma adipose tissue excision.

"tuck-up" procedures necessary after the first year or two was fairly high. This revision rate was largely due to using this technique in older patients. The short flap/SMAS excision with plication is still a good procedure in younger patients with early aging changes.

As much as we all would like to say that the techniques that have evolved in our practice give us the longest lasting result in our hands, the reality is that the genetic makeup and lifestyle of the patient play a significant role in longevity. In reviewing my own patients with similar techniques at 5 years postoperative, there is a relatively wide range of findings. Some have held up quite well with only minimal signs of increased aging, and others have noticeable recurrence.

PEARLS

- The technique described is reserved for more difficult necks with poor contour and/or significant platysma bands. Less ambitious techniques are viable options for patients not needing or wanting such transformative changes.
- Defining expectations is essential in teaching the patient of what is and what is not possible.
- All patients who use tobacco products, whether they are committed to quitting or not, are required to sign a specific consent with a skin slough image on the consent.

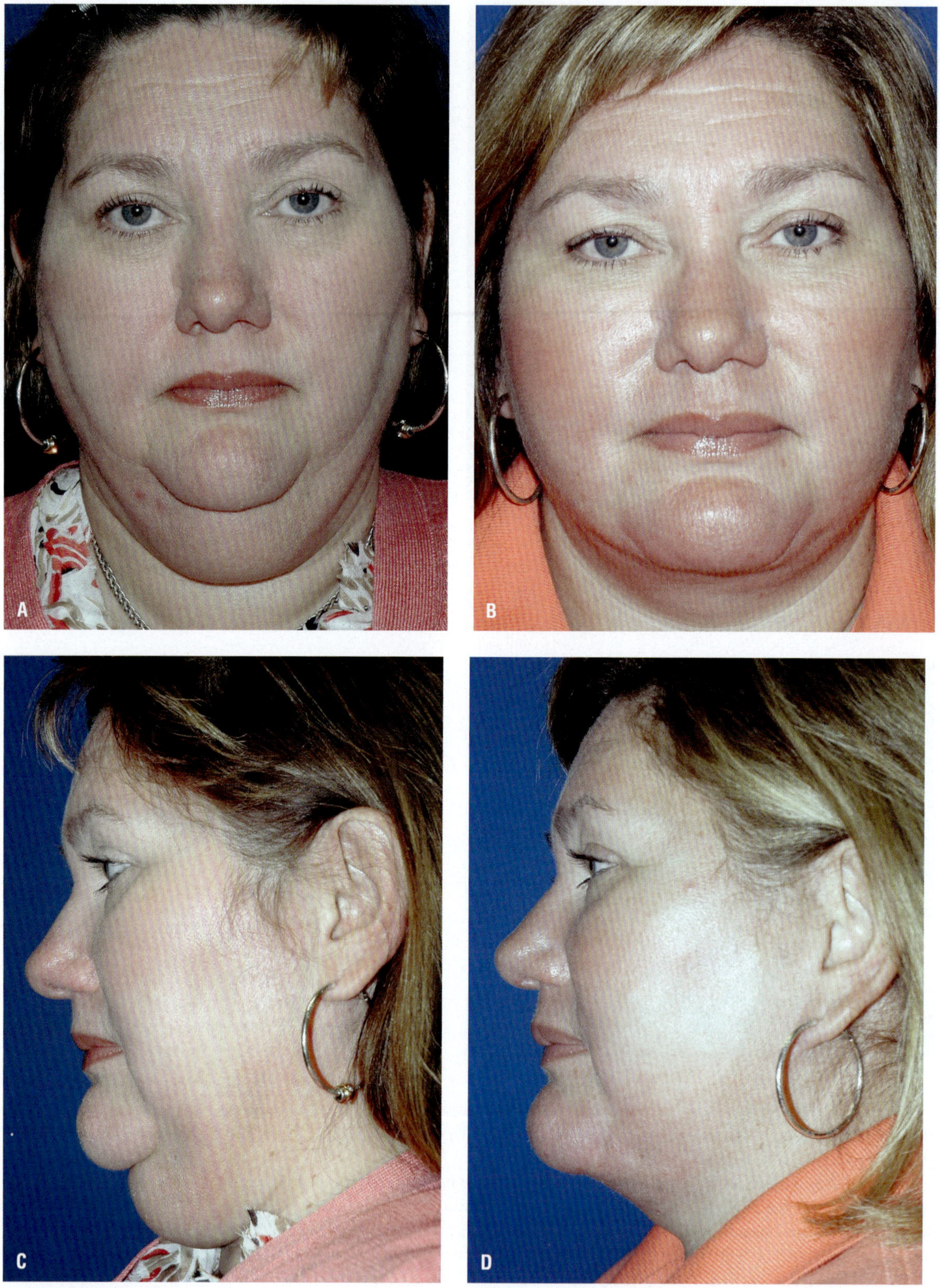

FIGURE 11.8 This is a 49-year-old female 1 year postoperative from extended SMAS rhytidectomy with corset platysmaplasty and correction of chin ptosis. Preoperative photos frontal **(A)** and lateral **(C)**. Postoperative photos frontal **(B)** and lateral **(D)**.

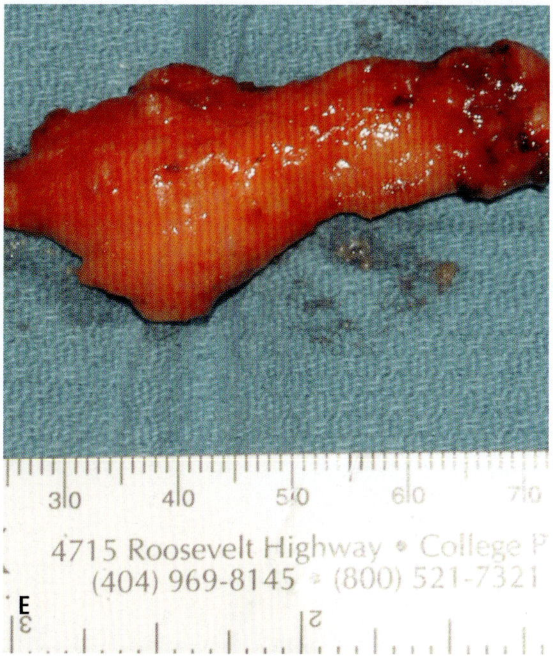

FIGURE 11.8 (*Continued*)
Subplatysma adipose tissue removed during the procedure **(E)**. Note how correction of the chin ptosis allows for a smooth transition from the mentum to the neck and how a low and anterior placed hyoid limits the depth of correction in the neck. Removal of subplatysma adipose tissue is also essential in getting the best neck definition possible.

- Take preoperative and postoperative photos of all patients.
- Meticulous hemostasis with bipolar cautery is key to preventing a hematoma.
- Tucking of the skin flap under the ear is key to concealing the scar and prevention of a pixie ear lobe deformity.
- The only posterior pull on the platysma in the neck when doing the lateral aspect of the face-lift is in the area of the angle of the mandible to increase definition.
- If you remain open and critical of your surgical outcomes, your technique will improve and your patients will be grateful.

PITFALLS

- In patients with very prominent laryngeal structures, this approach is contraindicated because it will masculinize a feminine neck and will overaccentuate the larynx in a male.
- Skin incisions should never be placed under high tension. Such techniques create "incisional issues" as described in the Complications section.
- Never operate on the patient that you do not like or the patient that does not like you.
- The chin is very important in defining the neck. Overlooking a weak or ptotic chin will markedly diminish the final surgical result.
- Complete undermining of the skin flap in the neck is essential for redraping of the skin to the underlying neck structures and a smooth soft tissue redistribution.
- It is often necessary to undermine very far inferiorly to achieve a smooth neck contour.
- There always needs to be a uniform layer of adipose tissue on the undersurface of the skin flap to avoid irregularities.
- The subplatysma adipose tissue in the submental area has to be trimmed, or there would be a residual fullness and a less than perfect result.
- The patient should never be paralyzed throughout the course of the case as nerve stimulation will not be observed and the risk of motor nerve injury will be increased.

INSTRUMENTS TO HAVE AVAILABLE

- Standard face-lift set
- Skin flap marker (Snowden-Pencer Marten flap marker)
- Castro needle driver X2
- Curved face-lift scissors (Kaye)
- Black retractor (Anodized Maliniac nasal retractor)
- Smooth Adson Forceps
- Forehead elevator (Daniel endoforehead elevator, quarter curved)

ACKNOWLEDGMENTS

I would like to acknowledge Young S. Paik, MD, and Amit Bhrany, MD. Their work in the writing, editing, and figure creation for this chapter is greatly appreciated, and without their help, this chapter would not have been possible.

SUGGESTED READING

Chang S, Pusic A, Rohrich R. A systematic review of comparison of efficacy and complication rates among face-lift techniques. *Plast Reconstr Surg* 2011;127:423–433.

Hamra ST. The deep-plane rhytidectomy. *Plast Reconstr Surg* 1990;86:53–61.

Mitz V, Peyronie M. The superficial musculoaponeurotic system (SMAS) in the parotid and cheek area. *Plast Reconstr Surg* 1976;58:80–88.

Skoog T. *Plastic surgery: new methods*. Philadelphia, PA: Saunders, 1974.

Warren R, Aston S, Mendelson B. Face lift. *Plast Reconstr Surg* 2011;128:747e–764e.

12 MIDFACE LIFT

Edwin F. Williams

INTRODUCTION

Prior to the early 1990s, the majority of surgical and nonsurgical techniques exclusively addressed the brows, eyes, neck, and jawlines. The midface region was essentially ignored until Hamra and colleagues, who first noted that the "windswept" appearance of patients whose lower face was treated while the midface was ignored, first discussed the anatomic and aesthetic importance of this area. The midface region is bordered superiorly by the inferior orbital rim, medially by the medial canthus, laterally by the lateral canthus, and inferiorly by the lateral oral commissure. Changes related to aging of this region lead to overlying ptosis of soft tissue as well as volumetric changes in the adipose and soft tissues.

During the mid to late 1990s, several techniques were developed to provide rejuvenation and lifting of the midface. Many of these procedures described the elevation of a skin–muscle flap through the lower eyelid, while additional publications described endoscopic techniques using a lateral orbital incision, a transtemporal approach, and even procedures that gained access through the gingivobuccal sulcus of the oral cavity. As time went by and experience was gained, many of the complications that arose from some of the more aggressive approaches became more apparent.

By the early 2000s, emphasis in the midfacial area had shifted to the treatment of volumetric loss in addition to the descent of the midface soft tissues. It was at this time that soft tissue fillers were developed and approved by the FDA. The reemergence and improvement in autologous adipose tissue grafting also provided a truly compatible biologic adjunct in the volumetric rejuvenation of the midface.

The midface lift has been well described by various authors. My approach of choice includes a subperiosteal midface lift that is used in conjunction with endoscopic brow lifting. For more than 15 years, this approach has proven to be safe and effective for our patient population. The following sections will attempt to describe the subtleties and nuances of my preferred approach in the rejuvenation of the midface.

HISTORY

I take a complete medical history on all surgical patients, which includes any current comorbidities, past medical history, past surgical history, medications particularly anticoagulants and alternative medicines, allergies, substance use, family history, and social history. Questions are asked concerning the use of tobacco, diabetes, connective tissue disorders, and bleeding disorders as such elements can compromise wound healing and overall surgical outcomes. Additional attention is given to the midface region regarding previous appearance, previous interventions, and current desired outcomes. Evaluation of the patient's current expectations during history taking is important as it helps to reveal appropriate or unrealistic social ramifications for and from the surgery.

PHYSICAL EXAMINATION

The physical examination requires a complete inspection of the midface region. I typically describe the midface as previously outlined, but controversy exists with regard to the superior limits of the midfacial unit. One could submit that the midface is contiguous with the lower eyelid. Better stated, the inferior boundary of the lower eyelid is typically defined by a shadow that is cast as the lower lid transitions to the midface. The dimension of this interface changes with age. The lower eyelid begins as a shorter and fuller region that subsequently elongates over time with the deflation and descent of the midface. As a result, the lower eyelid appears to lengthen while the shadowed soft tissue interface descends inferiorly into the midface region. It is important to note that the shadowing that develops along the orbital rim is created by the aforementioned soft tissue interface and the presence of the orbital retaining ligament attachment to the overlying skin. The zygomaticocutaneous ligament also extends from the orbital rim laterally and inferiorly toward the zygomatic arch to create an oblique soft tissue shadow often described in its upper limit as a malar mound or festoon. This shadow begins to show its presence in most patients by the late 1930s and becomes more prominent in the decades of the 1940s and 1950s. In addition to ptosis of the midface, I attempt to assess the degree of loss of global facial volume as well (Fig. 12.1).

INDICATIONS

My indications for the midface lift may be different from other surgeons and I will attempt to detail my rationale from this point forward. I have chosen to perform a subperiosteal midface lift in all patients who are undergoing an endoscopic-assisted brow lift. My rationale is that the brow and temporal area are contiguous with the midface. It is difficult to compartmentalize anatomy in a rejuvenation process, especially when one is elevating the brow and temple. Furthermore, I usually dissect to the zygomatic arch in an endoscopically assisted brow lift. Carrying this dissection into the midface, in a subperiosteal plane, does not present significant efforts or risks that are not counterbalanced by the favorable rejuvenation of the midface. However, I do not find the approach to the midface, through the lower eyelid, to be a favorable endeavor and so I almost never perform an isolated midface lift. It is difficult for me to justify elevation of the midface into the temporal region without addressing the soft tissue of the temple and eyebrow as there is potential for:

- Undertreating the temporal area
- Producing disharmony and bunching of soft tissues at the junction of the midface and temporal area with an effective midface lift

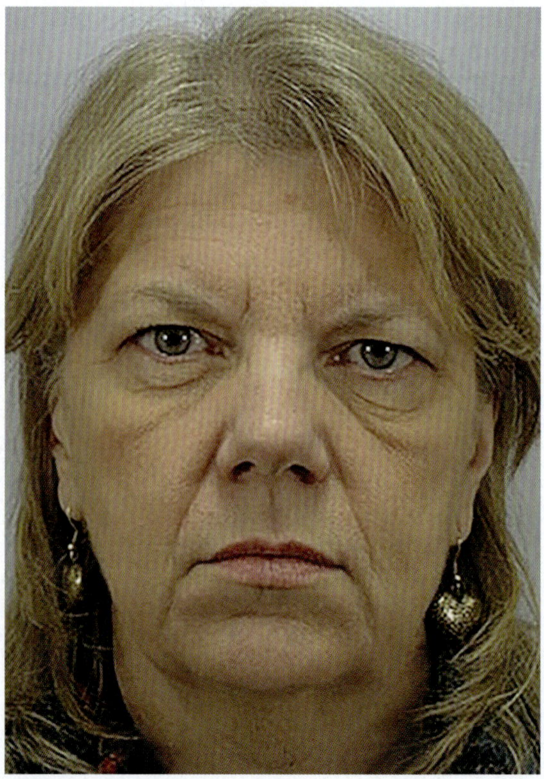

FIGURE 12.1
Aging is a panfacial process with the loss of facial volume and skeletal support in addition to the soft tissue laxity. This is well observed in the midfacial region with deflation and soft tissue ptosis.

In my hands, the indications for a subperiosteal midface lift include the following:

- Essentially all patients undergoing a subperiosteal endoscopically assisted brow lift procedure.
- The very rare situation where there is significant midfacial aging with good position and very little aging and ptosis of the brow and temporal area. In these patients, a transtemporal approach can be performed as an isolated procedure.
- I do not perform a midface lift through either a transconjunctival incision or a lower lid incision as I find the risk–benefit ratio to be unfavorable.

CONTRAINDICATIONS

Contraindications are essentially anecdotal and are based upon unfavorable or limited results. These include the following:

- *The patient who has a very round face or the patient who is obese.* Given the difficulty in achieving a rejuvenated appearance to the midface in this small population, I feel that the results are very limited and that the risk–benefit ratio is unfavorable.
- *The patient with moderate to significant isolated brow ptosis.* This is a very small patient population. Most patients who are evaluated for brow rejuvenation also display significant ptosis and settling of the midface. The additional time, effort, and marginal additional risk to rejuvenate the midface are well worth the investment. For this reason, well over 95% of patients undergoing forehead rejuvenation will receive a subperiosteal midface lift.
- *The patient who has had a previous midface lift.* This patient population has a higher incidence of neurapraxia for reasons that are currently unknown. Again, such circumstances are anecdotal, but it would be difficult to justify the additional risk in this small patient population.

PREOPERATIVE PLANNING

Preoperative planning for the subperiosteal midface lift using a transtemporal incision is essentially identical to patients undergoing an endoscopic brow lift. I prefer to use five incisions. One incision located in the midline just posterior to the hairline. There are two incisions (about 2 cm long) located in the paramedian position (approximately at the lateral canthus) just posterior to the hairline, and two additional, longer (3 cm) incisions located more temporally, camouflaged by the hairline. I believe that it is imperative to have adequate visual and functional access to the midface. Incisional lines are marked with a surgical pen and the hair is separated and tied using a one-half inch brown paper tape.

SURGICAL TECHNIQUE

I prefer to have the patient under general endotracheal anesthesia in the supine position. The table is turned 90 degrees in a counterclockwise fashion, fully elevated and placed at a 30-degree incline. This allows the surgeon to sit while operating and to visualize the dissection to the zygomatic arch with a retractor and a headlight in a stable operative field. Even a small amount of movement by the patient in an inclined setting will cause the patient to slide down the table making it more difficult for the surgeon to extend the patient's head, which allows a direct line of vision through the incision down to the zygomatic arch. I originally used the endoscopic instrumentation when performing this procedure but now reserve such techniques for teaching purposes only. I do not perform an incision in the gingivobuccal sulcus. I use local anesthetic consisting of 0.5% lidocaine, 0.5% Marcaine, and 100:100,000 epinephrine placed along the orbital rims and along the incision line. The remainder of the operative field is not anesthetized.

The five aforementioned incisions in the scalp and temporal areas are marked and infused with local anesthetic, which is allowed to set for 8 minutes. Incisions for the subperiosteal brow lift are then made down through the skin and the periosteum. Subperiosteal dissection is performed in a lateral direction to the conjoined tendon (temporal line) using a small sharp dissector and 1 tissue elevator with a fiber-optic tip or an endoscope. Dissection is carried approximately 4 to 6 cm posteriorly in the same subperiosteal plane and anteriorly to the orbital rims. A sharp, angled-down periosteal dissector is used to release attachments along the orbital rims as counter tension is provided on the soft tissue by the assistant. The most critical aspect of the browlift is the complete release of the arcus marginalis along the orbital rim to the medial region of the supratrochlear vessels. Without a complete release, the lift will be unsuccessful. The dissection is then carried to the nasion region.

At this point, I turn my attention to the transtemporal incision, first on the right and then on the left. The dissection is carried down through the soft tissue temporal–parietal fascia (TPF) and then onto the superficial

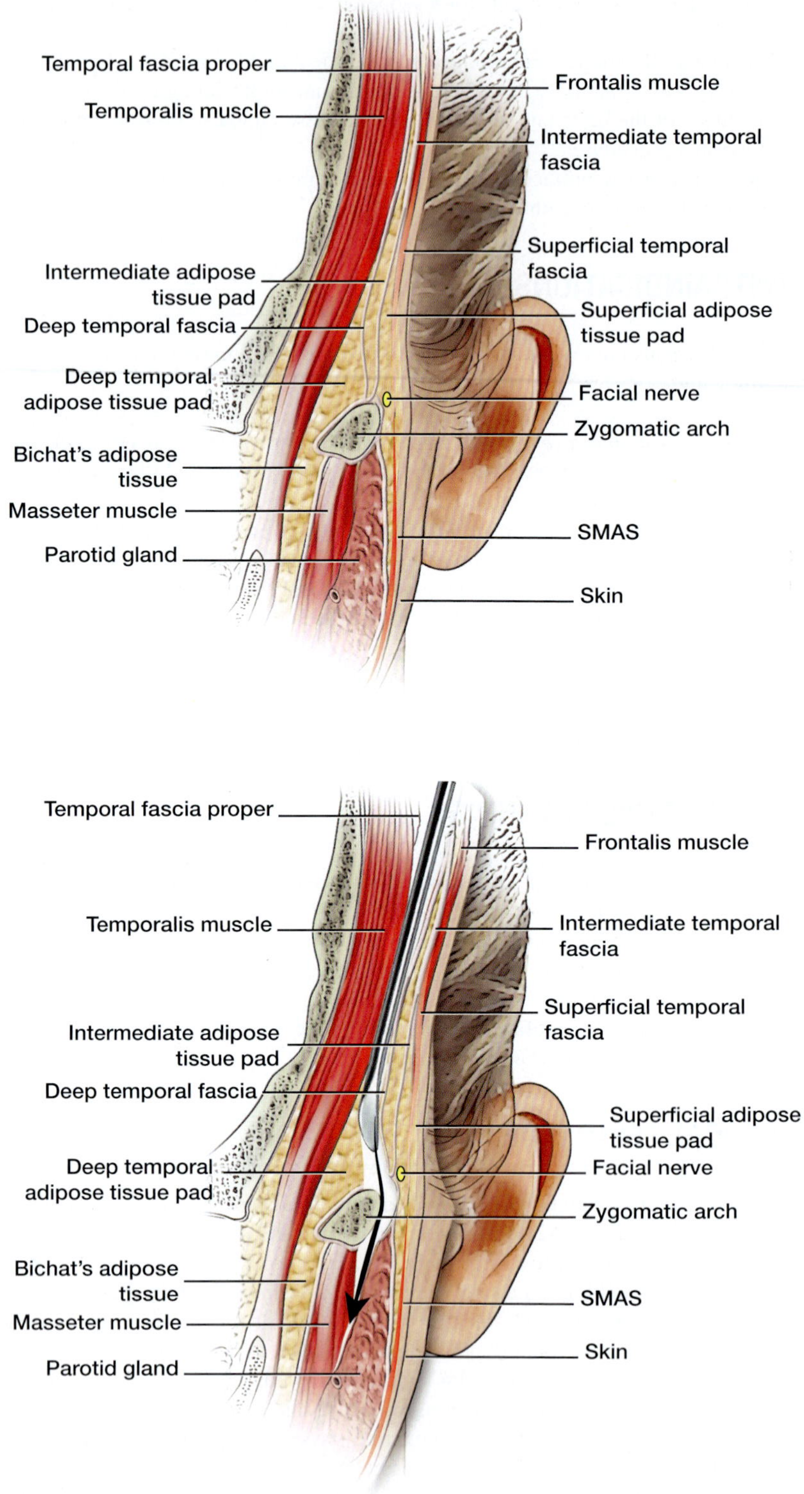

FIGURE 12.2
Tissue dissection in the temporal region is directed below the most superficial facial layer, temporal–parietal fascia (TPF), and then below the intermediate fascia layer, also known as the superficial layer of the deep temporal fascia. Dissection is then carried to the zygomatic arch, entering the subperiosteal layer, and down to the midface region.

layer of the deep temporal fascia overlying the temporalis muscle (Fig. 12.2). A dissection plane is developed below the TPF posteriorly and anteriorly. The limits of this dissection are approximately 4 to 6 cm posteriorly and to the orbital rim laterally and superiorly under direct vision. The sentinel vessels, tributaries of the superficial temporal venous system, are identified under direct or endoscopic vision. They are skeletonized and not divided unless they are in a direct path to the midface.

Dissection is now carried medially to and through the conjoint tendon using a sharp wide elevator. This is performed from lateral to medial direction so as not to place tension on the temporal branch of the facial nerve. It is critical to be certain that a release of the conjoint tendon, from its superior to its inferior orbital attachments, has been performed. Along the orbital rim, it is also critical to exclude the one centimeter of tissue

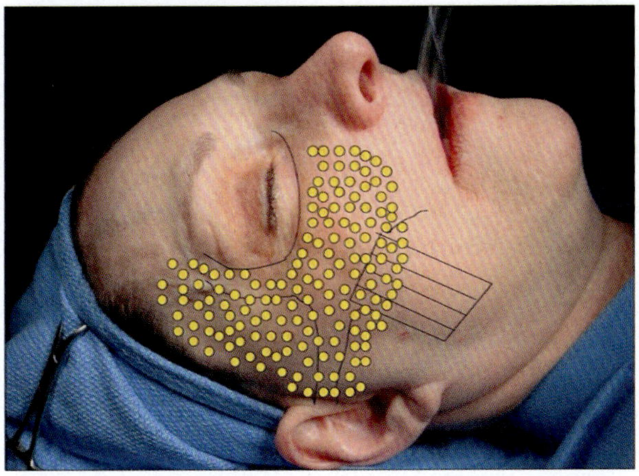

FIGURE 12.3
The yellow stippled area is overlying the malar and zygomatic bones and down over the masseter muscle (parallel black lines) showing the complete area of dissection and release prior to suture suspension.

elevation in the lateral canthal area. The assistant's finger is positioned to protect this region and the lateral canthal tendon. This tissue preservation is made to prevent anatomic distortion from the suspension that will be performed later. Dissection is then directed just below the intermediate temporal adipose tissue pad, which resides deep to the superficial layer of the deep temporal fascia (or the intermediate temporal fascia), and to the zygomatic arch (Fig. 12.3). Attention is directed along the zygomatic arch in which the periosteum is incised along the superoanterior aspect of the arch with a sharp angled-down dissector. The neurovascular bundle emanating from the zygomaticofacial foramen is preserved. Subperiosteal dissection is then carried over the arch, in a subperiosteal plane, to the midface. Endoscopes are not employed at this point, and the procedure is performed with a bimanual guided hand technique (Fig. 12.4). The continued dissection of the midface is performed using this technique, with an oblique orientation of the instrument during the subperiosteal elevation. Elevation is performed from the body of the zygoma to the piriform aperture, taking care to remain inferior to

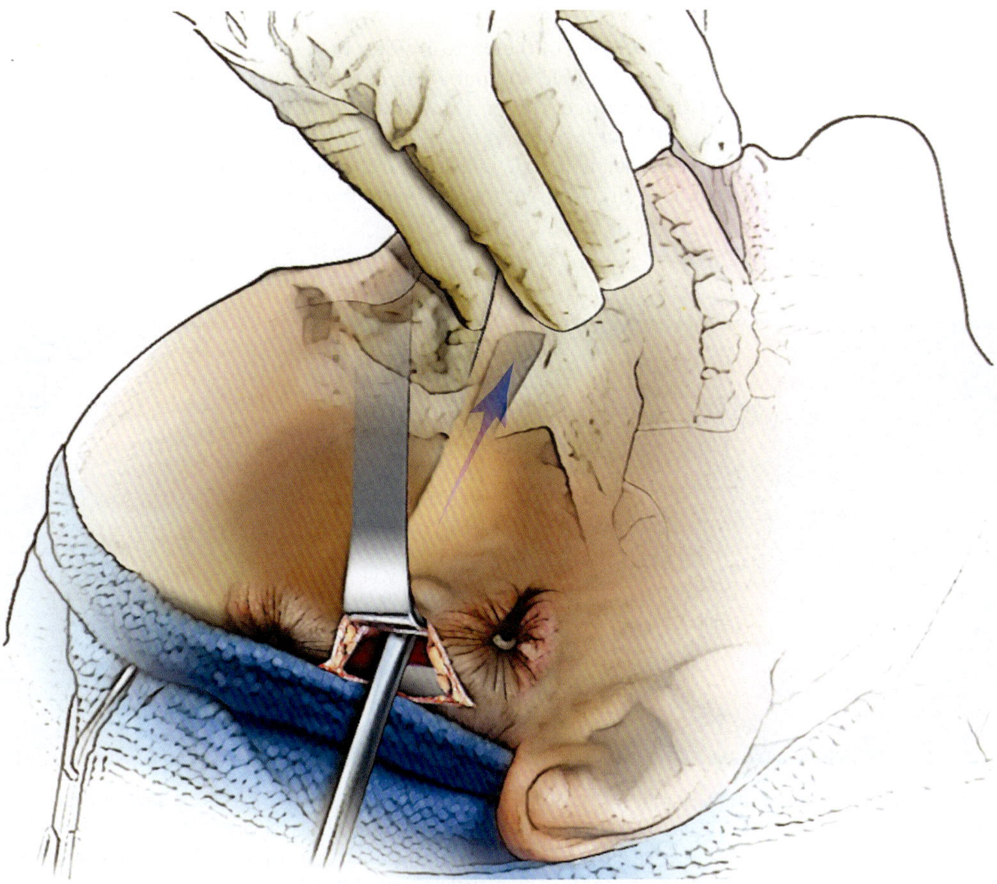

FIGURE 12.4 Subperiosteal elevation of the midface is performed with a bimanual guided hand technique with care in avoiding injury to the infraorbital nerve.

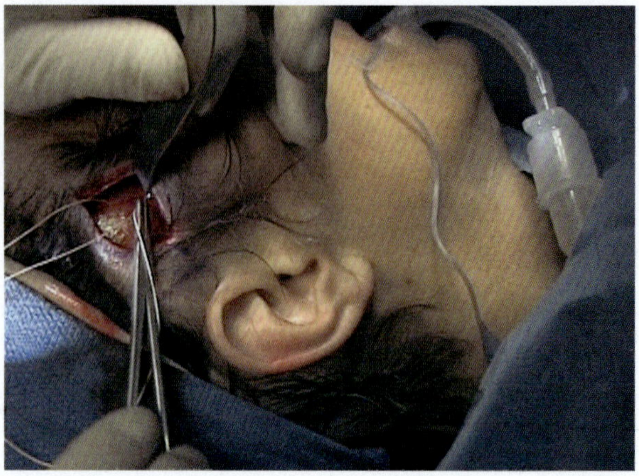

FIGURE 12.5
Under direct or endoscopic vision, through the transtemporal incision, a 2.0 Vicryl suture is placed through the released periosteum with the previously identified zygomaticofacial foramen as a central landmark.

V2 branch of the trigeminal nerve. A gentle sweeping motion is then used to dissect the soft tissues off the midface inferiorly and is carried up toward the inferior orbital rim. Direct dissection on the bone along the orbital rim is avoided so as not to injure the infraorbital nerve. Once a complete release is observed, suture suspension is then undertaken.

Through the transtemporal incision, under direct or endoscopic vision, a 2.0 Vicryl suture is placed through the released periosteum with the previously identified zygomaticofacial foramen as a central landmark (Fig. 12.5). A considerable amount of the malar adipose tissue pad, zygomatic major muscle, and periosteum is engaged at this point (Fig. 12.6A, B). Care is taken not to penetrate into the overlying dermis. The suture is then brought back through the transtemporal incision and is placed superiorly through the superficial layer of the deep temporalis fascia. The suture is oriented at a 45-degree angle extending from the soft tissue over the body of the zygoma up to the temporal region (Fig. 12.7). This is gently tied down to the appropriate adjustment height and multiple square knots are placed. Two supporting sutures are then placed anteriorly from the TPF to the deep temporal fascia to support the key suture that has been previously placed.

I then turn my attention to the suspension of the brow. I prefer the use of bone tunnels to suspend the brow as I find that patients are more comfortable without a palpable implant. The bone tunnels are developed with the use of the Browlift Bone Bridge System (Medtronic), and the brow is suspended along the desired peak of the eyebrow using 2.0 Vicryl suture (Fig. 12.8). The knot is then rotated into the channel under the bone bridge so as to not be palpable. All incisions are then closed with surgical clips and no drain is placed. A circumferential head dressing with a chin strap that consists of three cotton strips and 3- × 3-inch strips is applied.

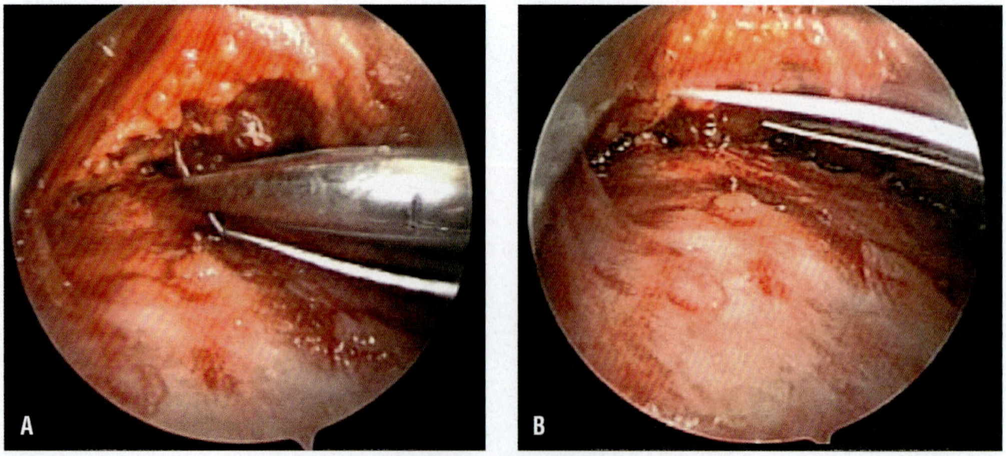

FIGURE 12.6 Visualization may be made with an endoscope or performed directly. In **(A)**, the needle driver is above the body of the zygoma and engaging the periosteum, the zygomatic major muscle and malar adipose tissue pad. The zygomatic major muscle can be seen just above the needle driver to the right of the adipose tissue pad. The 2.0 Vicryl suture is then passed through these tissues **(B)** and will be suspended in the superficial layer of the deep temporalis fascia.

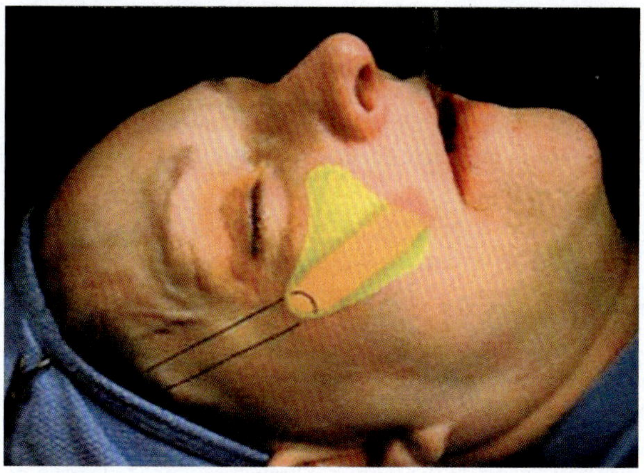

FIGURE 12.7
The artist's rendition of what occurs with suture suspension elevating the midface and moving the soft tissue of the midface back into the original anatomic position.

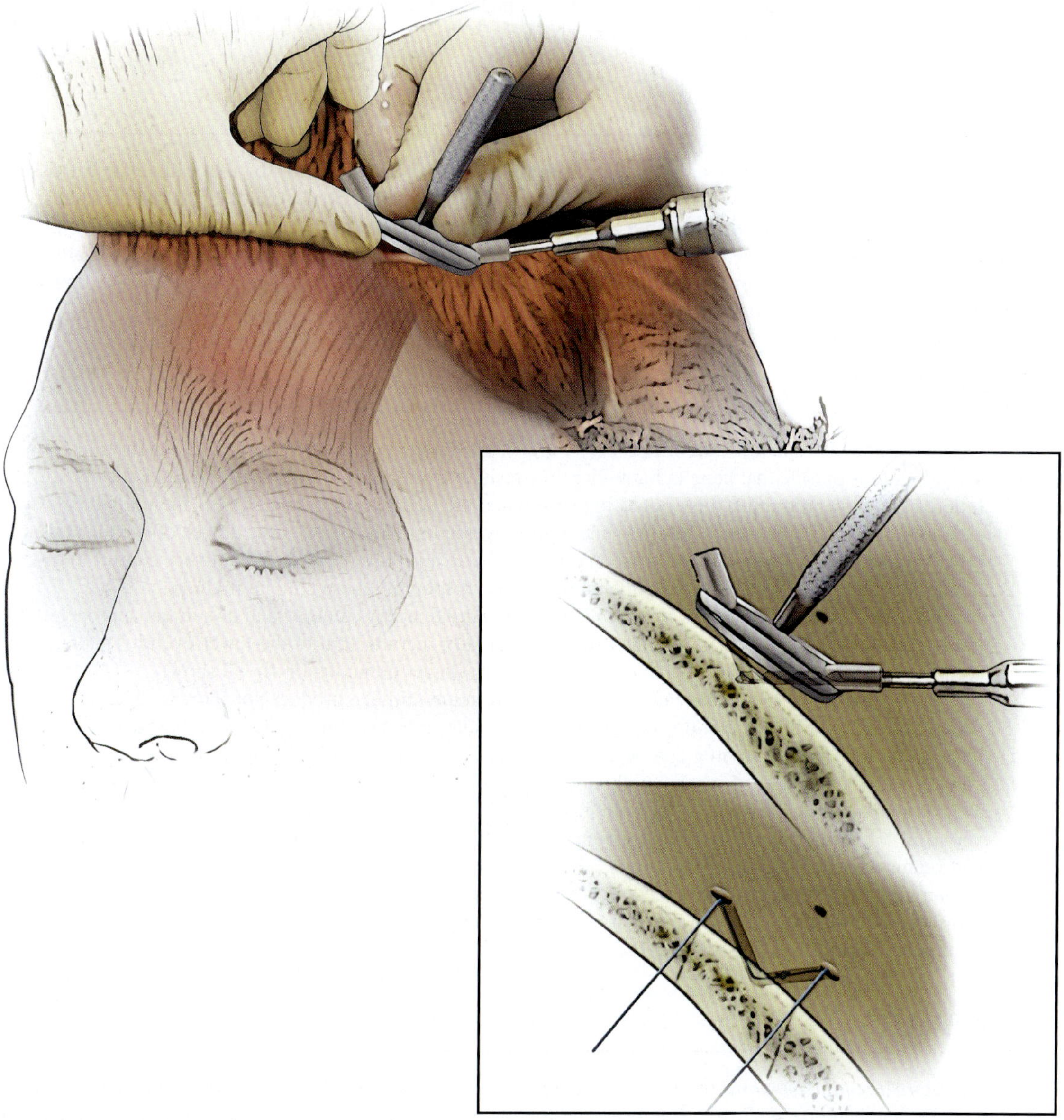

FIGURE 12.8 The bone tunnels are developed with the use of the Browlift Bone Bridge System (Medtronic), and the brow is suspended along the desired peak of the eyebrow using 2.0 Vicryl suture.

POSTOPERATIVE MANAGEMENT

On the first postoperative day, this dressing is removed and a lighter dressing is applied. This second dressing is removed in 48 hours. Surgical clips are removed on postoperative day 6. Patients are also given peri- and postoperative tapering dose of steroids for the first few days to minimize edema. Patients receive perioperative and postoperative antibiotics to prevent infections.

COMPLICATIONS

A number of potential risks are involved as with any surgery. Risks may be immediate or later. Immediate risks include bleeding, infection, corneal abrasion, neurapraxia, and paresthesia. I minimize the risks of bleeding through very meticulous hemostasis. Care must be taken to avoid injury to the cornea or any of the other important structures in the region. Neurapraxia greater than 12 hours is viewed as a complication in all circumstances, regardless of complete resolution, and is due to unwanted tension on the temporal branch of the facial nerve. In the immediate postoperative period, regional paresthesia and facial asymmetries are common due to soft tissue edema. However, in later timelines (>30 days), I view these findings as complications related to preoperative planning or surgical execution if there is no observed improvement over this timeline. The findings of hair loss and limited lifting results are commonly related to wound tension or a nontrichophytic incisions and inadequate release of all appropriate attachments, respectively.

RESULTS

Results show improvement not only in the brow temporal area but elevation of the midfacial soft tissues (Fig. 12.9). Improvement along the jawline is also apparent. The subperiosteal midface lift helps address the vertical component of the jowl, compared to the horizontal component more commonly addressed by a lower face-lift, and softens the appearance of this feature. Limitations for the midface lift include the inability to address the volumetric loss. In approximately 70% to 80% of our patients, concurrent adipose tissue transfer is performed with consistent long-term results.

PEARLS

- *Improvement of the shadow that occurs below a festoon:* Lower eyelid festoons are redundant folds of skin and orbicularis muscle that hang in hammock-like fashion from canthus to canthus when the face is upright. Intuitively, one would think this should improve when the periosteum is released off the midface elevated and suspended. In reality, there is some general improvement in this area, but the degree of such lax tissue is often best addressed with a lower lid blepharoplasty using a skin–muscle flap. I am very careful to discuss limitations of the midface lift in the patient populations displaying these clinical findings.
- *Improvement in the configuration of the lower eyelid:* Unlike a skin–muscle flap or a direct approach to the lower eyelid, the subperiosteal midface dissection actually recruits skin to the lower eyelid. This has been seen to assist the patient who has had previous rounding, lower lid laxity, or scleral show.
- *Limitation in addressing volumetric loss:* The subperiosteum midface lift does not address the aging component of excessive deflation. For this reason, we educate our patients about autologous adipose tissue transfer.
- *Overtightening:* Overtightening can occur in the area of the lateral canthus due to inexperience. This will often relax over time (2 to 6 weeks) without changing the orientation of the lateral canthal area.
- *Bunching of the skin*: This can occur from placement of the key suture too superficial or in a patient that has very thin soft tissues over the malar eminence. Care should be taken to only engage the malar fibroadipose pad versus the overlying skin and dermis.
- *Prolonged recovery:* When the procedure is executed efficiently and carefully, patients have a considerably shortened recovery period in the order of 6 to 9 days. Avoidance of a lower eyelid skin–muscle flap incision to perform the midface lift significantly reduces the recovery period.

PITFALLS

- *Neuropraxia of the temporal branch of the facial nerve* can be avoided first by placing the incision approximately 1 cm behind the hairline, but more importantly by minimizing the amount of traction with a retractor placed laterally during the dissection and visualization. Additionally, it is important to respect the potential for transmission of a current using bipolar cautery of the vessels as they have been shown to be located in close proximity to the temporal branch of the facial nerve. One should bipolar cautery down onto underlying tissues and not along the inferior aspect of the suspended (retracted) flap.

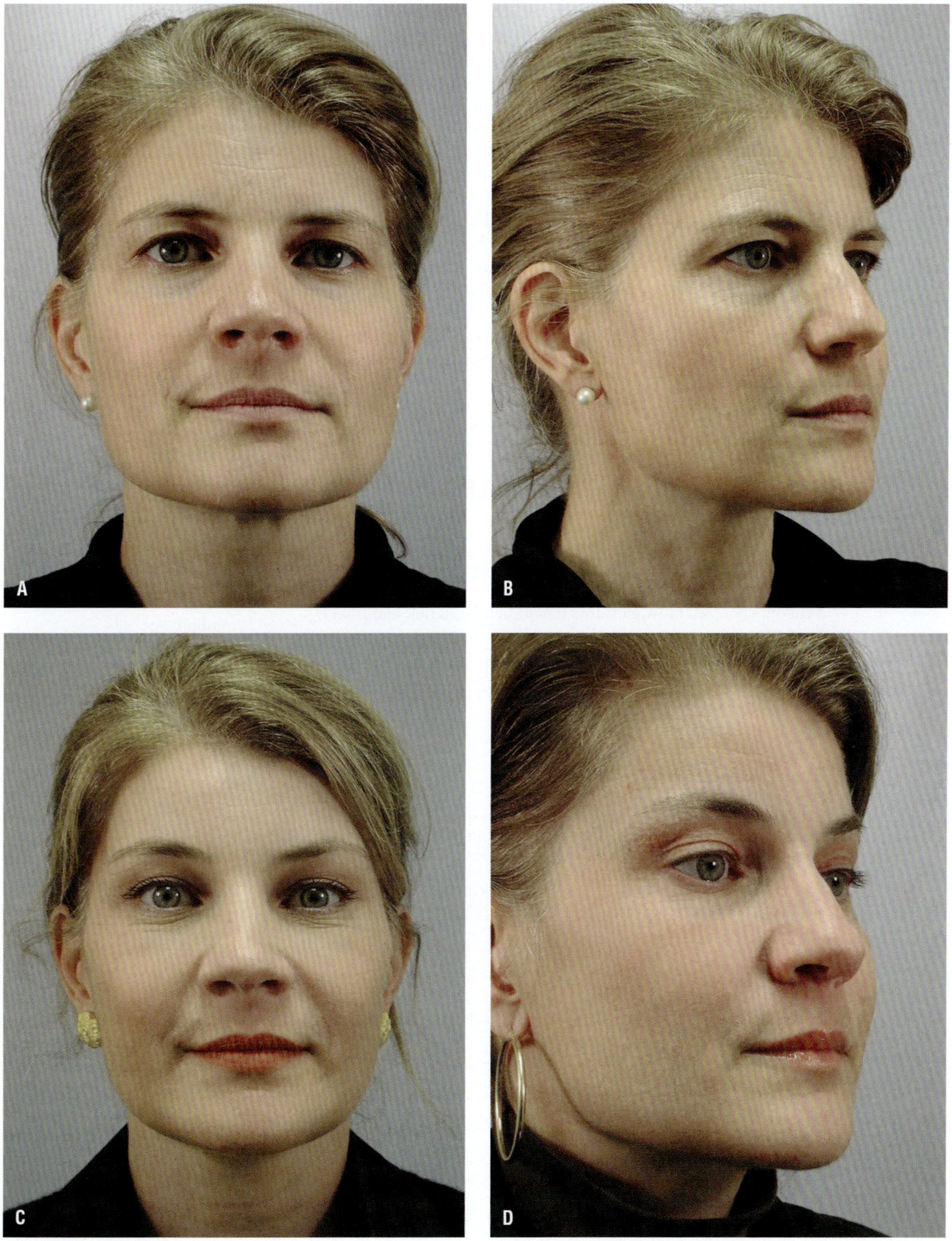

FIGURE 12.9 Preoperative and postoperative images from direct (**A and C**) and oblique (**B and D**) views after combined brow and midface lifting.

- *Paresthesia of the infraorbital nerve* can occur when the dissection is performed carelessly or with poor anatomic understanding of the region. This complication can be prevented by locating the infraorbital foramen prior to dissection and respectful treatment of tissues.
- *Increase in periorbital (temporal and superior) vascularity and varicosities* can be avoided with the meticulous preservation of transcending veins when dissecting around the periorbital area and toward the arch. If vessels are in the direct visual path of approach to the midface, they should be cauterized, but all others should be skeletonized and preserved.
- *Distortion or disruption of the lateral canthus* can occur with aggressive dissection. Preservation of a 1-cm cuff of periosteum along the lateral canthal region is sufficient to prevent from happening.
- *Ineffective or inadequate lift* can be avoided by achieving an adequate release of the periosteum and soft tissues. This concept also applies for brow-lifting procedures.
- *Paresthesia in the temporal area* is a fairly common complication that is a result of transection of the zygomaticotemporal nerve. The dimensions are approximately 2 cm and are observed above the arch, lateral to the orbit. This often resolves with time.
- *Prolonged facial edema* occurs frequently. These few patients also had concurrent autologous adipose tissue transfer to the lower lid and midface. The edema resolved between 8 and 12 months, but required a considerable amount of reassurance for the patients.
- *Alopecia along the suture line* is avoidable with careful technique and attention to detail by beveling the scalpel blade parallel to the hair follicles (trichophytic incision).

INSTRUMENTS TO HAVE AVAILABLE

- Basic soft tissue set
- Hand drill with 1.5- × 6-mm bit (for brow suspension)
- Bovie handpiece and tip
- 3 curved ebonized brow elevators (small flat, large flat, and round)
- 4 × 4 gauze
- 3″ conforming gauze bandage
- Cotton padding
- ½″ micropore tape

SUGGESTED READING

Chaiet SR, Williams EF III Understanding midfacial rejuvenation in the 21st century. *Facial Plast Surg* 2013;29(1):40–45.

Freeman MS. Rejuvenation of the midface. *Facial Plast Surg* 2003;19(2):223–236.

Pontius AT, Chaiet SR, Williams EF III. Midface injectable fillers: have they replaced midface surgery? *Facial Plast Surg Clin North Am* 2013;21(2):229–239.

Quatela VC, Azzi JP, Antunes MB. Endoscopic-assisted facelifting. *Facial Plast Surg* 2014;30(4):413–421.

Quatela VC, Olney DR. Management of the midface. *Facial Plast Surg Clin North Am* 2006;14(3):213–220.

13 REJUVENATION OF THE NECK

Gregory S. Keller

INTRODUCTION

Rejuvenation of the neck is an important aspect of the treatment of the aging face. The effects of aging are often prominently displayed in the neck. Recurrence of laxity in the neck is also a common complaint following facial rejuvenation procedures.

Common neck deformities for which surgical rejuvenation is performed include skin laxity from loss of tone of the dermal elastic fibers and loss of ligamentous support, platysma muscle banding, increased deposition of adipose tissue, prominent digastric muscles, and protrusion of the submandibular glands. Rejuvenation of the neck can be accomplished with a comprehensive cervicofacial rhytidectomy procedure or in isolation using a variety of techniques.

HISTORY

Paramount to a successful rejuvenation of the neck is to first determine what the patient wants. Often times, patients who need neck rejuvenation may not fully understand that they need a surgery of the neck. Conversely, many patients focus purely on their aging neck. Assessing patient expectations and deciding on whether expectations are achievable takes time, and a detailed history is critical. From a medical standpoint, questions pertaining to any prior surgery of the neck are important as scars will affect any neck surgery being planned. Inquiry into thyroid abnormalities is to be made as patients may expand upon either swallowing or respiratory symptoms that may be exacerbated with a tightened neck postoperatively. Patients with any history of dysphagia, globus sensation, reflux, and/or upper respiratory symptoms including obstructive sleep apnea need medical clearance for an elective neck lift. Questions should be posed to assess for any psychological concerns with the sensation of having a tighter neck postoperatively as expectations and tolerance for postoperative symptoms will be met. After a medically focused history taking, a psychological assessment focusing on the aesthetic expectations of a neck lift is important. Balancing what is achievable and what is impossible can only be done with a detailed discussion with the patient. Sometimes a repeat consultation is needed to fully inform the patient of what to expect. However, many repeat visits or unrealistic expectations by some patients may be a sign to avoid neck surgery altogether.

PHYSICAL EXAMINATION

When discussing the effects of aging on the neck, an understanding of the anatomic structures is key. Aesthetic concerns in the neck may involve one or more of these structures, and treatment of the aging or ptotic neck must be tailored to address these specific issues.

A well-defined cervicomental angle (CMA) is the hallmark of a youthful-appearing neck, and its reestablishment is often a principal goal in rejuvenation surgery of the neck. The CMA is defined by the intersection of a horizontal line drawn through the menton and an oblique line following the anterior border of the neck. The ideal angle is traditionally considered to lie within the range of 105 and 120 degrees.

The CMA has been described as being most significantly defined by the position of the hyoid bone in relation to the mentum. The hyoid typically rests at the level of the fourth cervical vertebra. Posterosuperior positioning of the hyoid contributes to a well-defined CMA, while anteroinferior displacement causes a more obtuse angle and is much more challenging to address surgically.

The platysma muscle can form undesirable, prominent bands in the aging neck. The bands correspond to pleats of the medial platysma body rather than the muscle edges themselves, as the edges are tightly adherent to the deep cervical fascia at the level of the hyoid bone.

The platysma originates in the subcutaneous tissue of the infra- and supraclavicular regions and inserts at the base of the mandible and orbicularis oris, as well as subcutaneously in the cheek and lower lip. The muscle is bilateral and obliquely oriented, joining in the midline with interdigitating fibers in the mentum. Its actions include depression of the lower lip and face, as well as forced opening of the mandible. Platysma muscle bands are thought to originate from the development of laxity in the neck skin, superficial cervical fascia, and the platysma-retaining ligaments.

Platysma bands can be categorized as static or dynamic. Static bands are the commonly bothersome variety, and lie in a paramedian vertical orientation corresponding to the medial platysma muscle. These muscle bands exist at rest and contribute to the blunting of the CMA. Dynamic muscle bands, on the other hand, present during active platysma muscle contraction and may lie along the central portions of the muscle as well as along its medial aspect. Botox has been used for dynamic bands to decrease platysma band prominence by eliminating baseline tone and causing atrophy through repeated treatments.

Excessive cervical adipose tissue can be separated into subcutaneous and subplatysmal planes. Cadaver studies have described three compartments in the subplatysmal plane: central, medial, and lateral. The central compartment is a typical yellow color, while the medial and lateral compartments are paler, similar to buccal fat.

The digastric muscle is composed of two embryologically distinct anterior and posterior bellies joined by an intermediate tendon. The anterior belly is innervated by the mylohyoid nerve from the mandibular division (V3) of the trigeminal nerve (cranial nerve V). It originates at the symphysis menti of the mandible. The posterior belly originates in the digastric groove of the mastoid bone and is innervated by the digastric branch of the facial nerve (cranial nerve VII). The intermediate tendon penetrates the stylohyoid muscle and passes through a fibrous sheath that is attached to the body and greater cornu of the hyoid bone.

The paired submandibular glands provide 70% of salivary volume and are divided into superficial and deep lobes by the mylohyoid muscle. Each gland rests within an impression on the lingual surface of the mandibular body called the submandibular fossa, just below the mylohyoid line, the site of origin of the mylohyoid muscle. Secretions are passed through Wharton's duct, which runs superior to the mylohyoid muscle and out of the sublingual caruncles located on either side of the lingual frenulum in the anterior floor of mouth. The investing layer of deep cervical fascia envelops the gland. The marginal mandibular branch of the facial nerve runs on the posterior surface of the platysma muscle, just superficial to the facial vein and submandibular gland.

Dedo described a commonly used classification to characterize the nature of neck abnormalities. Each class presents a distinct anatomic contribution to the neck deformity that must be addressed with appropriate surgical techniques.

Class I: Normal, youthful neck with a well-defined CMA, minimal adipose tissue, and good skin and platysma tone

Class II: Laxity of the cervical skin only

Class III: Abundance of subcutaneous adipose tissue

Class IV: Platysma muscle bands

Class V: Retrognathia

Class VI: Low-lying hyoid

While these classes describe different anatomical problems, many of these problems can coexist. Other problems that are not described in this classification system include prominent digastric muscles, submandibular glands, and subplatysmal fat.

INDICATIONS

Suitability for a neck lift can be determined by patients who demonstrate the following: excess subcutaneous and/or subplatysmal adipose tissue; excess, loose neck skin; platysmal banding; loss or blunting of the CMA by skin and/or fat; multilayered chin at rest and/or accentuated with head and neck flexion; loss of the mandibular border with prominent jowls; and prominent submandibular glands and/or prominent anterior belly of digastric tendons.

CONTRAINDICATIONS

The following features will not benefit from a neck lift, making these patients unsuitable for neck lift surgery: fine rhytids of the neck skin, hyperpigmentation or other textural skin changes, and/or a blunted CMA due to a low-lying hyoid. Obviously patients with substantial medical comorbidities present a contraindication to surgery.

PREOPERATIVE PLANNING

Prior to operating on the aging or ptotic neck, the surgeon must assess the various anatomic structures in order to establish the appropriate surgical plan. For many surgeons, the diagnostic process is important in the decision to perform an open neck procedure. If the soft tissues of the neck are soft and mobile, one can often manipulate the platysma and subcutaneous adipose tissue alone. If the neck is firm or other specific anatomic features are abnormally prominent, more extensive procedures may be indicated.

In order to distinguish between excessive subcutaneous and subplatysmal adipose tissue, the surgeon may grasp the superficial soft tissue of the neck between thumb and forefinger and ask the patient to swallow. Palpation of subcutaneous adipose tissue alone is soft and does not move significantly with swallowing. Abundance of subplatysmal adipose tissue and/or prominent digastric muscles manifests as firmness in the neck with more movement during swallowing. The firmer nature of the subplatysmal adipose tissue is due to the presence of fibrous bands in this plane, including the platysma-retaining ligaments. This also makes the removal of adipose tissue more difficult in the subplatysmal plane compared to the subcutaneous compartment.

A neck that is tight and resistant to manual upward pressure on physical examination is referred to as a "tension neck." This type of neck may require an open procedure to address the deep ptotic structures.

The digastric muscles demonstrate a characteristic lump in the midline submental neck. Occasionally, they can become prominent postoperatively when uncovered by a neck defatting procedure if not diagnosed early and included in the surgical plan.

Prominent submandibular glands may be seen and palpated in the lateral neck. This bulge may be due to ptosis, an enlarged gland, or an insufficient bony fossa. Occasionally, a bulge is noted following a neck lift procedure when it was not initially present. Removal of superficial adipose tissue may be the culprit, but when lipectomy has not been performed, the development of a submandibular bulge may be due to its traction into a more prominent position from adhesions of its capsule to the undersurface of the pulled platysma.

High-frequency ultrasonic images have been used to elucidate various pathologies of the aging submental neck (Fig. 13.1). The superficial cervical fascia that envelops the platysma strongly reflects sound waves, clearly delineating the boundaries of the subcutaneous and subplatysmal adipose tissue spaces. These planes can therefore be independently measured to evaluate their contributions to the full neck. The size of the underlying digastric muscles can also be assessed. When liposuction or direct excision lipectomy is performed in the fatty neck, many of the above problems can become apparent that were not identified preoperatively, and ultrasonic evaluation can aid in accurate diagnosis.

SURGICAL TECHNIQUES

Many techniques for rejuvination of the neck have been developed over the past four decades. These techniques often share the focus of correcting the obtuse CMA and platysma muscle bands. The method used is based on both the anatomic abnormality being addressed as well as the surgeon's preference.

Lipoplasty

When indicated, liposuction or direct excision can be used to address large adipose tissue deposits. Care is taken to avoid skeletonizing the underlying structures, and 4 to 5 mm of subcutaneous adipose tissue should be left on the skin flap to allow adequate coverage. Potential complications of overaggressive removal of adipose tissue in the neck include the development of irregular contour, a hollow neck appearance, skin necrosis, and unmasked prominence of underlying structures such as the submandibular gland and the larynx.

When performing liposuction, cannulas are introduced through submental and periauricular incisions. This bidirectional approach ensures thorough and even removal of adipose tissue. Subcutaneous tunnels are created through multiple repeated passes of the suction cannula resulting in both mechanical avulsion and removal of adipose tissue, as well as contraction of the subcutaneous tissues during the healing process. Suctioning aggressively on the platysma muscle is avoided to ensure that the muscle remains intact.

The elastic skin envelope then contracts over the scarring underlying tissues. It has been suggested that skin retraction may be enhanced when liposuction is performed in a superficial plane near the undersurface of the dermis.

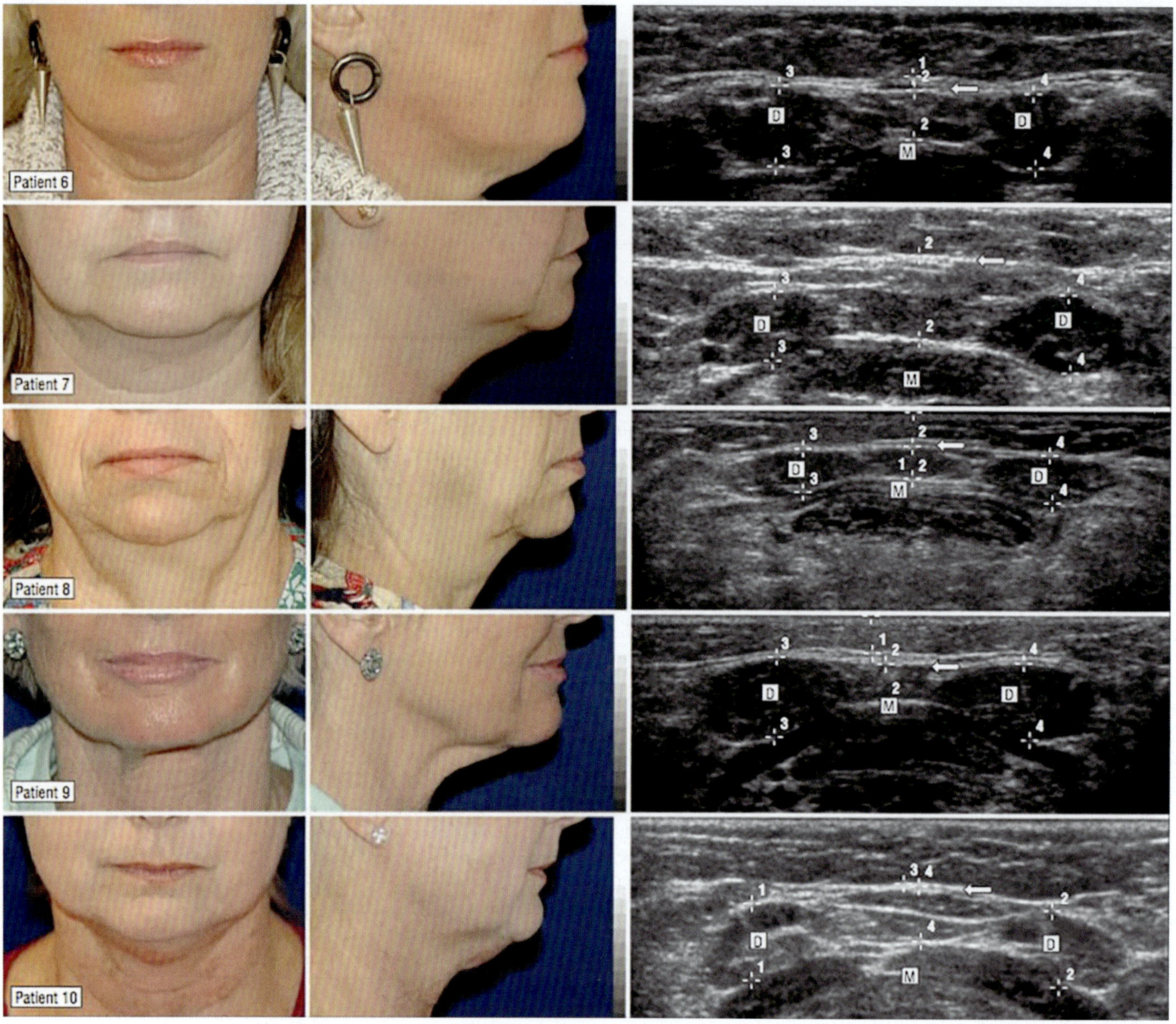

FIGURE 13.1 Ultrasound results. Frontal views, lateral views, and submental ultrasound scans of the 10 study patients. Note pseudoherniation of the subplatysmal fat in patients 1, 5, 7, 8, and 10 and the relative digastric hypertrophy in patient 3. *Arrows* indicate platysma muscle; D, digastric muscle; M, mylohyoid muscle. (Reprinted from "The Utility of Ultrasound in the Evaluation of Submental Fullness in Aging Necks," by Mashkevich G, Wang J, *JAMA Facial Plastic Surgery,* vol. 11(4), pp. 240–245. © 2009 by the American Medical Association.)

Ultrasonic energy has also been coupled to traditional suction-assisted liposuction. After tunnels are formed, the ultrasound device is introduced, causing emulsification of the adipose layer. The fibrous support system of the skin undergoes an inflammatory reaction resulting in its contraction.

The technique of laser lipolysis has developed through the supplementary use of lasers in liposuction. Laser energy is delivered transepidermally via thin laser fibers passed through cannulas. CO_2 laser use was initially described and the Nd:YAG and diode lasers have subsequently been used. Laser energy is absorbed by adipocytes triggering apoptosis and necrosis while also providing hemostasis. It also causes heating of the dermis, resulting in collagen contraction and tightening of tissue laxity. As has been reported by several authors, we feel that there is a lack of substantial clinical differences when comparing laser-assisted and traditional suction-assisted lipoplasty.

Direct excision of subcutaneous adipose tissue may also be performed. The surgeon sharply removes adipose tissue under direct vision either by first developing the subcutaneous plane of the skin flap followed by adipose tissue removal off of the platysma or by skeletonizing the platysma and then defatting the skin flap. Many surgeons feel that direct excision of adipose tissue facilitates a more precise lipoplasty.

Platysmaplasty

The treatment of platysma bands has evolved over time as each solution gave rise to new problems. These management strategies include such techniques as direct excision, z-plasty, and muscle flaps. Other techniques are discussed below.

Submentoplasty

Submentoplasty techniques address the platysma in the submental region and can be performed in isolation. An example of this type of procedure requires complete undermining of the subcutaneous plane laterally to the anterior borders of the sternocleidomastoid (SCM) muscle through a submental incision, followed by plication of the platysma in the midline down to the level of the thyroid cartilage. Direct access to the submental region also allows for removal of subplatysmal adipose tissue if indicated.

Platysmaplasty procedures often involve suturing of the medial platysmal edges in the midline from the submentum down to various levels in the neck, with resection of the more inferior medial borders and/or horizontal transection of the remaining inferior platysma muscle. Many surgeons feel that this midline conjoining of the platysma can be performed equally effectively through either running or interrupted suturing. The platysma can also be tacked posteriorly onto the mastoid fascia.

Corset Platysmaplasty

Feldman introduced the "corset platysmaplasty" in the literature in 1990. This procedure classically involves continuing the midline approximation of the medial platysmal edges inferiorly with a running suture. This so-called full-height midline plication usually extends down to at least the level of the cricoid cartilage.

Feldman describes up to three or four iterations of the running midline suture plication up and down the neck for further tightening of the platysma as necessary. Additional vertically oriented pleats of plicated platysma are created in the mid-submandibular regions to address bulging created by formation of dog-ears in the platysma muscle due to increased rotation in this area from the midline approximation. Care is taken to include only the platysma muscle so as not to damage the underlying marginal mandibular branch of the facial nerve.

The corset platysmaplasty does not involve significant skin excision but to a great degree relies on skin contraction over the manipulated underlying platysma. Feldman discusses the extent of undermining that is often necessary in the lateral neck to prevent the development of pleats or folds in the lateral neck when there is excess skin. This is performed through postauricular incisions that allow lateral undermining even to the occipital hairline, as well as removing adipose tissue from the neck.

Some advantages of the corset platysmaplasty are the elimination of platysmal bands along the entire length of the neck and avoidance of both central hollowing and skeletonization of the neck. A few potential disadvantages of this procedure include the necessity for an extensive surgery involving wide cervical subcutaneous undermining, as well as persistence of excess skin. Because excess skin is not resected, skin contraction may not be sufficient and loose skin may occasionally be observed, particularly when the patient is in the head-down position (Fig. 13.2).

Lateral Platysma Fixation

Some surgeons prefer a lateral pull of the platysma as opposed to medial approximation. Midline approaches often require extensive subcutaneous dissection and may result in a "leatherneck" appearance, while some argue that lateral approaches result in recurrent bands. In cervicofacial rhytidectomy, the platysma is commonly fixed in a superior–posterior direction to the mastoid fascia.

Fixation in a vertical direction has also been described. This is used in the S-lift and MACS-lift (minimal access cranial suspension lift). In the MACS-lift, the platysmal tacking suture is anchored to the deep temporal fascia and temporalis muscle down to the bone at a point 1 cm superior to the zygomatic arch and 1 cm anterior to the helical rim. The suture is passed in purse-string fashion through the SMAS (superficial musculoaponeurotic system) to the superior edge of the platysma.

The ligament of Lore at the base of the earlobe has also been used as a fixation point for a cephalad pull of the platysma. Labbe feels that this provides greater definition of the neck, as the ligament of Lore is a natural platysmal fixation point, providing retraction along the anatomic ligamentous suspension via the auriculoplatysmal ligament of Furnas that merges with Lore's fascia. Hamra also described platysma fixation anterior to the lobule. This avoids suture trauma to the great auricular and posterior auricular nerves that can occur with suture fixation posteriorly across these structures to the mastoid fascia.

Platysma Sectioning

Some surgeons prefer to treat platysma banding with various degrees of transverse platysma muscle sectioning. For isolated anterior bands, Connell describes medial sectioning between bilateral anterior jugular veins at the level of the cricoid cartilage. Lateral bands require extending the platysma transection laterally to include the areas of banding, while banding with lateral mandibular body or angle blunting requires complete transection in a curvilinear, superolateral direction, in continuity with the SMAS incision in the face. In all instances, the platysma is tacked superolaterally as a part of the deep-plane cervicofacial rhytidectomy.

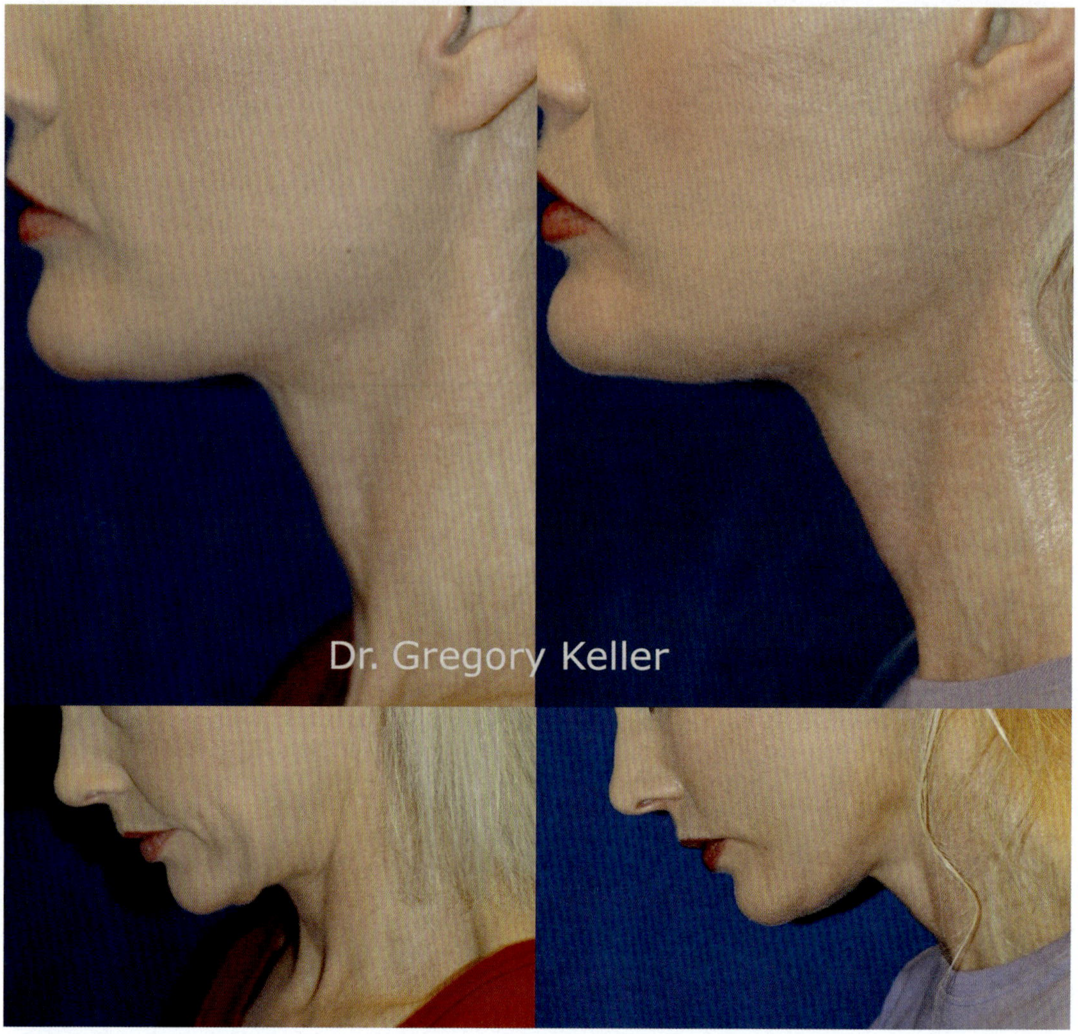

FIGURE 13.2 Loose, excess skin evident after corset platysmaplasty in the head-down position.

Suspension Platysmaplasty

The suspension type of platysmaplasty has been described in the literature in various forms. Webster described the use of a nonabsorbable suture attached anteriorly to the platysma muscle at the cervical angle and suspended back to the SCM muscle fascia. Giampapa popularized an approach using both submental and postauricular incisions with undermining of the neck in the subcutaneous plane, followed by tunneling under the edge of the mandible and plication of the medial platysma. Bilateral suspension sutures are introduced, interlocked in the midline, and anchored to the mastoid fascia on either side.

Web Lift and Posterior Platysma Pull

A closed, percutaneous procedure was recently developed for suspension of the upper neck (iGuide technique, first described by G. Mueller, marketed by Black and Black Surgical, Tucker, GA). In this procedure, liposuction tunneling is first performed, followed by percutaneous placement of an interdigitating suture in a shoelace-like configuration across the submandibular regions posteriorly, advancing anteriorly to a midline submental incision. The suture hooks the ligamentous attachments of the platysma to the dermis, tightening the skin and platysma when tied at the end of the procedure. Hence a "web" of suture is formed that acts like a hammock, suspending the submentum, accentuating the mandibular border, and redefining the CMA (Fig. 13.3).

The authors of this chapter use several techniques for correction of the aging neck. The web lift is primarily recommended and done in younger patients without significant bands as they recur in 2 to 3 years. A concomitant web lift as described above and posterior pull procedure have historically been a workhorse procedure for the senior author. The degree of tightening required and the presence of platysma bands dictate whether the posterior pull is required and how much skin is then excised, as the hammock lift alone does not, in their opinion, address banding inferior to the hyoid. A posterior pull of the platysma followed by wide running inverting platysma plication to encompass the medial neck sagging has become the more current "mainstay" procedure of choice for this group.

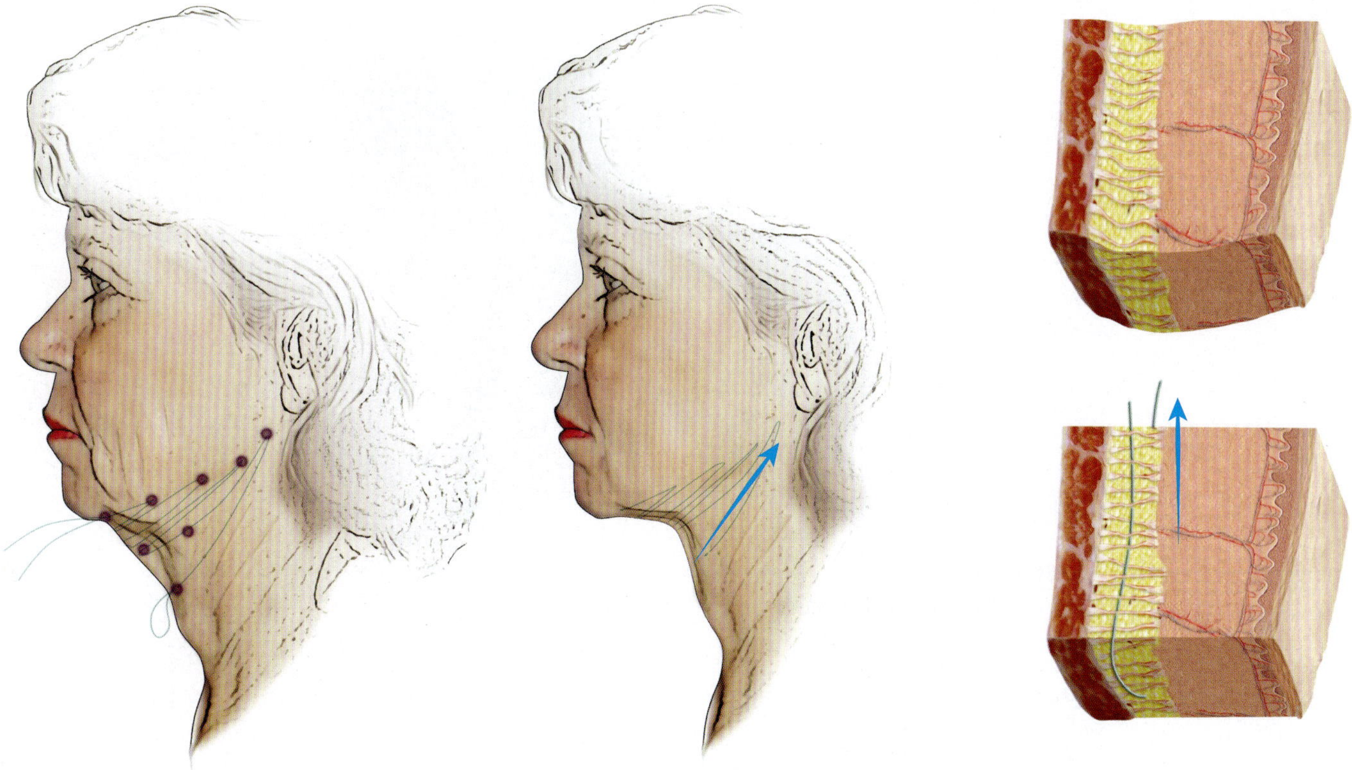

FIGURE 13.3 Placement of percutaneous sutures across the submentum (above). This suture hooks the ligamentous attachments between the dermis and platysma (below).

Operative Details

After the incision and anatomical markings are made, local anesthetic is applied throughout the surgical site. Tumescent solution (50 mL of 1% lidocaine, 12 mL of sodium bicarbonate, and 1 mL of epinephrine diluted in 1,000 mL of normal saline) is also infiltrated throughout the face and neck. Liposuction and/or tunneling of the neck and lower face are then performed. Tunneling of the lower face over the mandible is an important part of the platysmaplasty as the auriculo-cutaneous, masseteric-cutaneous, and mandibular ligaments are, to some degree, isolated by the tunnels.

A face-lift or neck lift incision (depending on the procedure desired) is made, and a skin flap is elevated over the posterior neck and SCM muscle fascia, extending only 2 cm over the edge of the posterior platysma until the level of the cricoid cartilage is reached (Fig. 13.4). If a face-lift is performed, I prefer a deep-plane rhytidectomy via an oblique SMAS excision over the parotid, and this plane is made continuous with a short, lateral subplatysmal plane in the neck.

The neck skin is undermined all the way to the midline at the level of the cricoid cartilage. The platysma is left attached to the skin in the midline, as this submental region is ultimately addressed by the web suturing. Any fat remaining on the lateral platysmal edge is removed sharply under direct visualization.

The platysma is dissected off of the anterior border of the SCM muscle, with dissection of a short, lateral 2 cm subplatysmal plane. The external and anterior jugular vein and cervical sensory nerve branches are meticulously avoided. A horizontal incision is then created across the entire platysma, and the superficial fascia (platysma and SMAS) is separate from the deep cervical fascia of the SCM muscle (Fig. 13.5).

The skin flaps are pulled in the appropriate vectors, and the free posterosuperior platysma edges are then suspended to the mastoid fascia superiorly. The remaining lateral length of the free lateral platysma edge down to the cut inferior edge is sutured in running fashion to the SCM fascia to prevent retraction of the platysma and the development of a "window shading" deformity. The inferior horizontal cut at the level of the cricoid cartilage is not reapproximated (Fig. 13.6).

Nonabsorbable braided sutures are used. Excess skin is resected appropriately, and Vicryl sutures are used to anchor the SMAS to the pretragal soft tissue, as well as to approximate the deep layer of the skin flaps. Excess skin is excised, and the superficial skin layer is closed with running 6-0 nylon suture and staples in the hair-bearing occipital scalp.

A platysmaplasty (as described by Mueller) procedure is performed last to elevate the anterior portions of the neck. Three to four "needle-size" punctures are created above the inferior border of the mandible approximately two centimeters apart. A puncture is also made at the point at which the new CMA is desired.

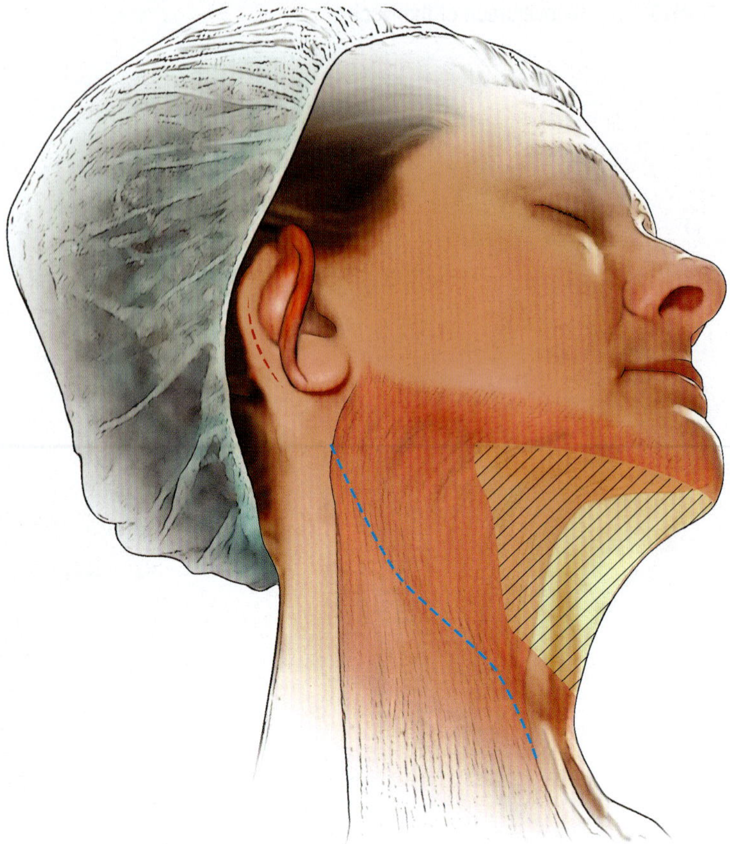

FIGURE 13.4

Neck skin flap elevation. The *dotted line* represents the incision made to elevate the platysma. The *dashed area* represents the area of the neck not undermined during the procedure as this is addressed by the percutaneous suture.

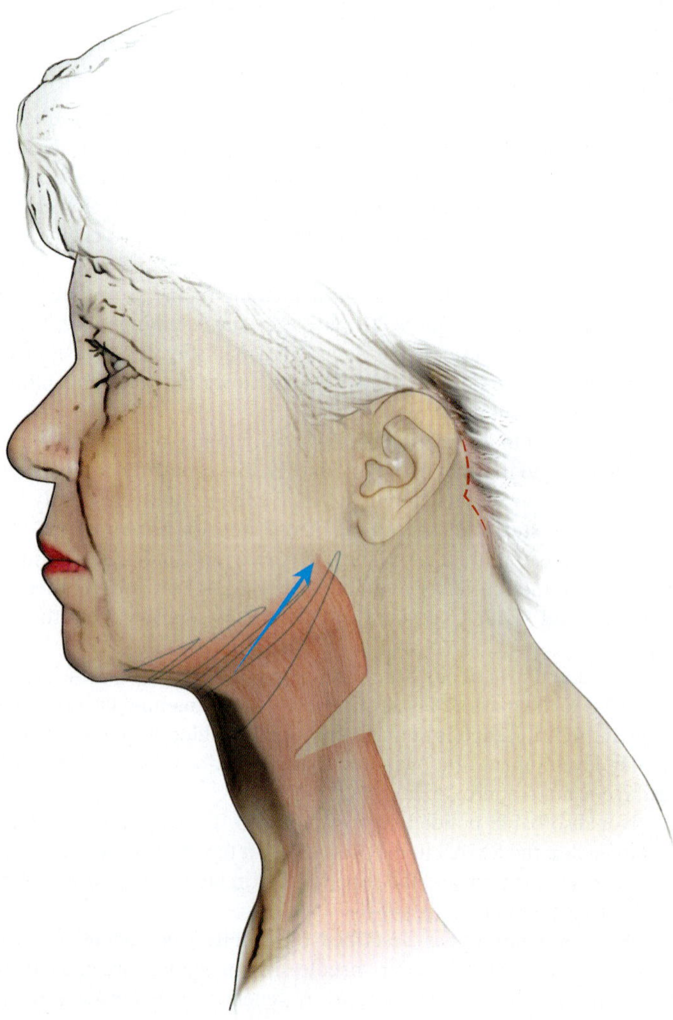

FIGURE 13.5

Platysma elevation from the deep cervical fascia overlying the SCM muscle and the horizontal incision across the entire platysma at the level of the cricoid.

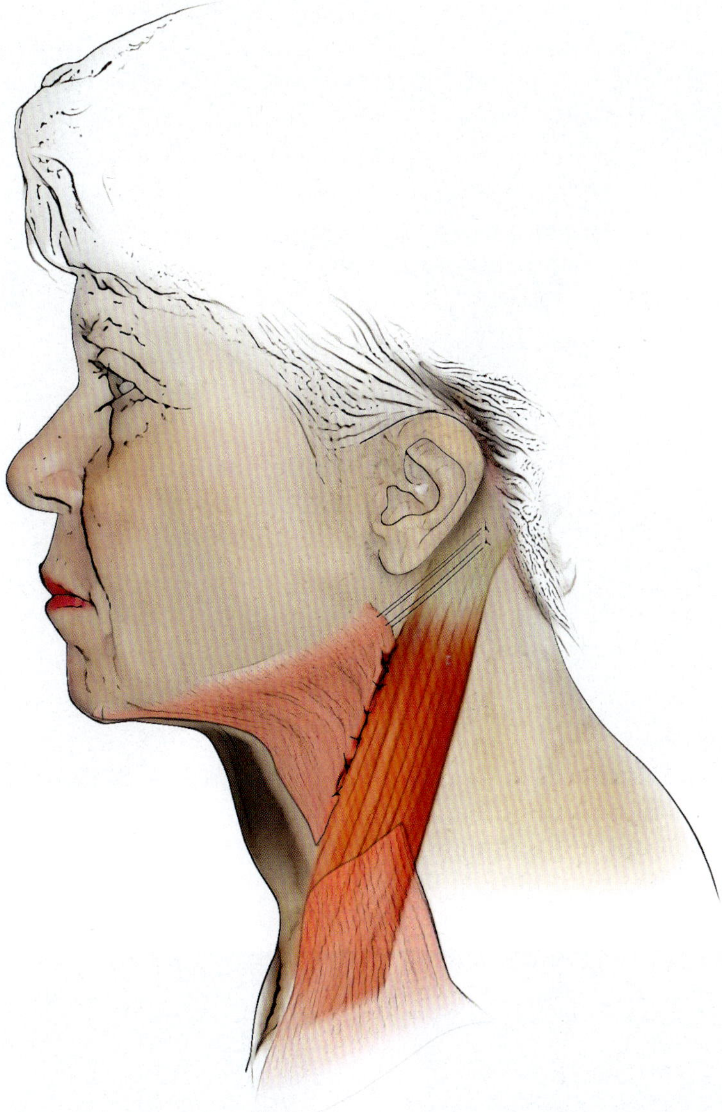

FIGURE 13.6
Final appearance of the platysma muscle with resuturing along the SCM muscle and the completely cut inferior edge.

Two punctures are then placed to either side of the midline. These punctures are then subcised to facilitate suture passage (devices for these procedures are provided in a kit).

The sutures are then woven by use of a "passer" from the inferior midline puncture to the lateral mandibular puncture, and the fibrous (preferably ligamentous) tissue is engaged. The passer with the suture is then manipulated to the second puncture on the opposite side. In the case of three punctures along the mandible on each side, the passer then engages fibrous tissue at the second puncture and is passed across the neck to the first puncture then out through the midline submental liposuction incision.

The same procedure is then repeated on the opposite side. The sutures are tightened as the procedure progresses. Too little tightening results in insufficient lifting of the neck soft tissues. Too much tightening can either break the suture or "cheese wire" the suture through the fibrous tissue. The sutures are then tied together where they exit from the submental incision (Figs. 13.7 to 13.10). An available video of this procedure provides a detailed explanation (http://www.blackandblacksurgical.com/iguide-webinar.php).

Other Techniques

Prominent submandibular glands can be addressed in many ways, such as resection, Botox injection, plication of the platysma inferior to the gland for cephalad suspension, or placement of a submental-mastoid suspension suture. Complications of submandibular gland suspension or resection always include bleeding, infection, damage to the marginal mandibular branch of the facial nerve, as well as the development of a salivary fistula. Some surgeons prefer to avoid ablative techniques due to the risk of xerostomia.

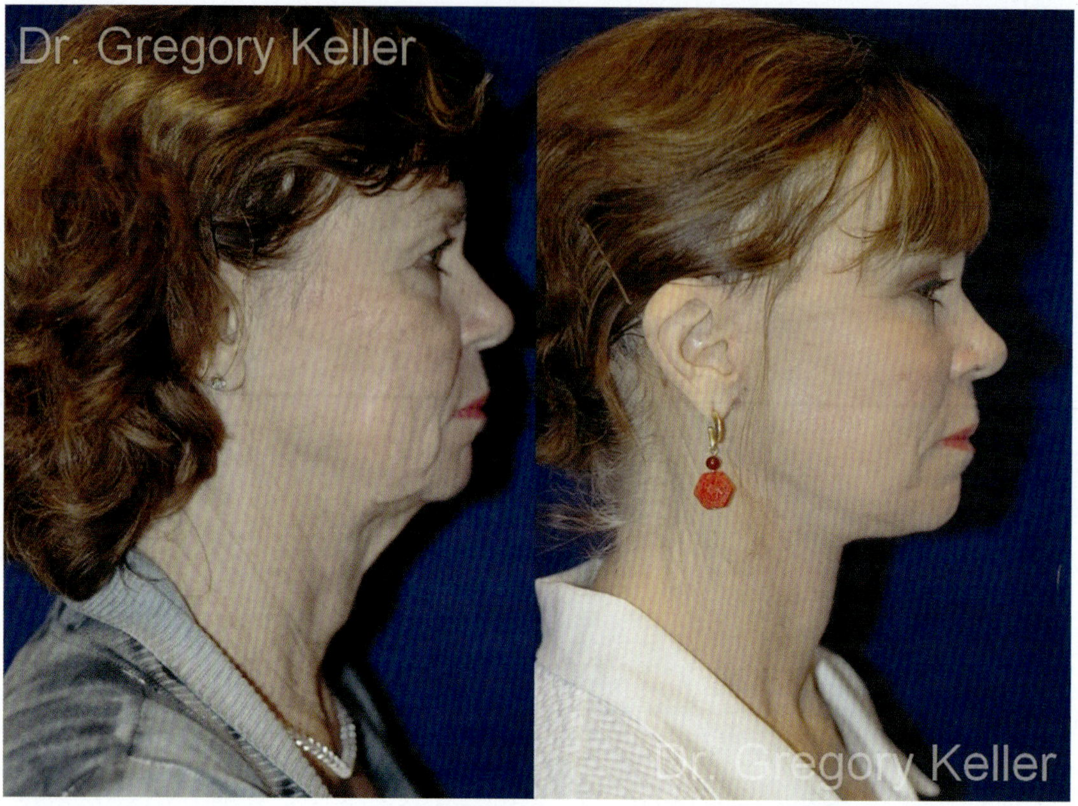

FIGURE 13.7 Web lift with posterior pull neck lift and face-lift.

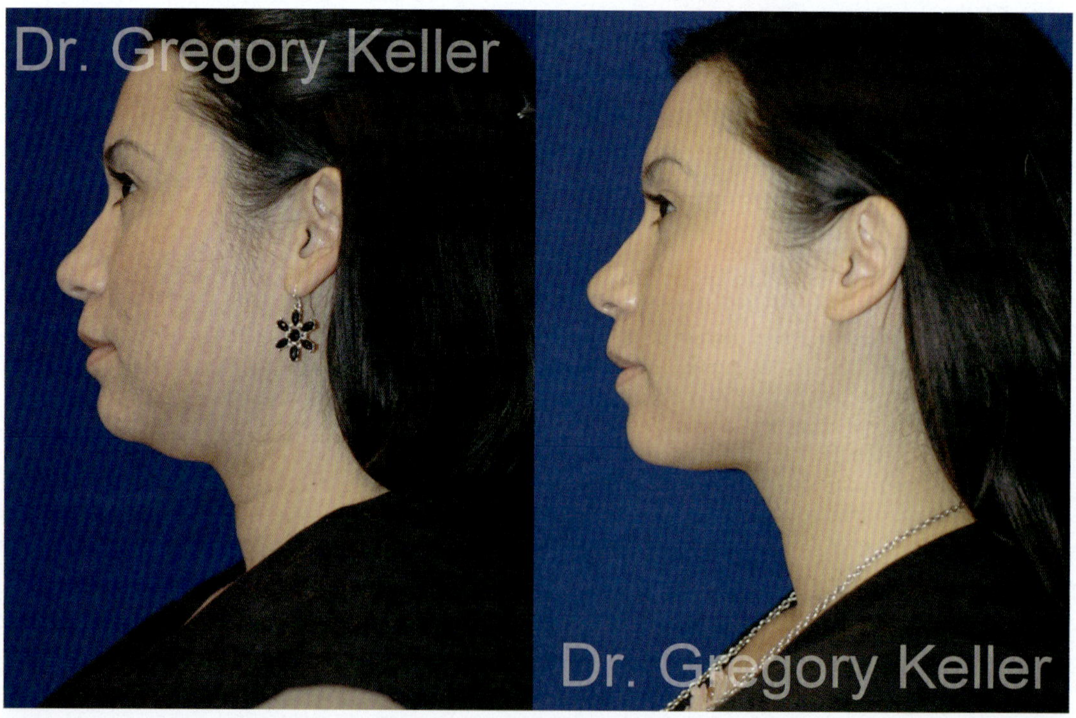

FIGURE 13.8 Web lift without posterior pull, with elevation of prominent digastric muscle. (Reprinted from "The Web Lift and Posterior Pull for the Aging Face," by Ezzat WH, Amodeo CA, and Keller GS, *Facial Plast Surg,* 2012, vol. 28(1). © Georg Thieme Verlag KG.)

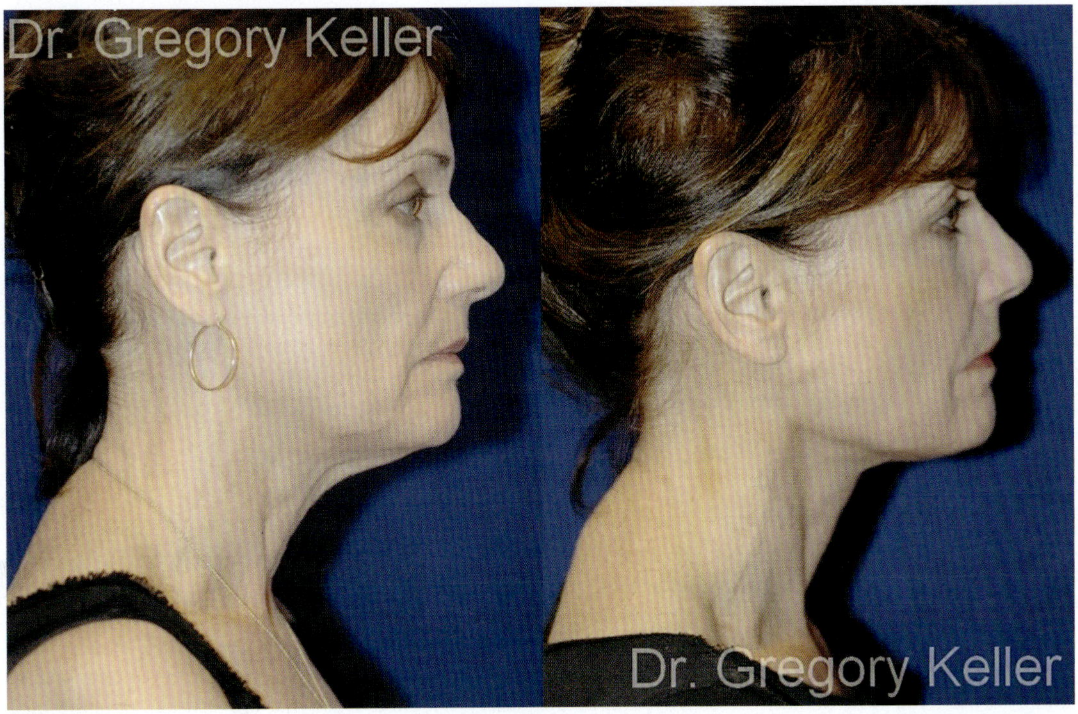

FIGURE 13.9 Web lift with posterior pull, without face-lift. (Reprinted from "The Web Lift and Posterior Pull for the Aging Face," by Ezzat WH, Amodeo CA, and Keller GS, *Facial Plast Surg,* 2012, vol. 28(1). © Georg Thieme Verlag KG.)

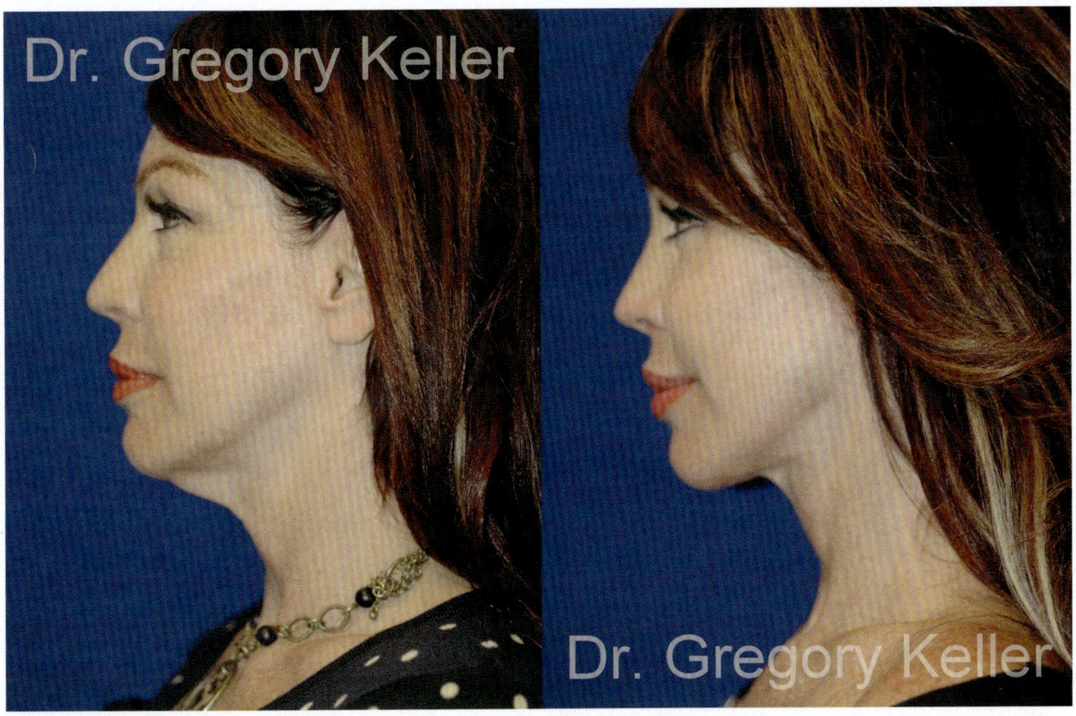

FIGURE 13.10 The web lift is often useful for neck lift revisions, particularly if lateral bands remain. (Reprinted from "The Web Lift and Posterior Pull for the Aging Face," by Ezzat WH, Amodeo CA, and Keller GS, *Facial Plast Surg,* 2012, vol. 28(1). © Georg Thieme Verlag KG.)

Digastric muscles also contribute to unwanted bulkiness in the neck. The anterior belly of the digastric muscle can be exposed through a submental incision and dissection of the subplatysmal plane through the midline. Once identified bilaterally, the inferior 70% to 90% of the muscle can be tangentially excised from its origin in the digastric fossa of the symphysis of the mandible to the intermediate tendon sling at the hyoid bone.

POSTOPERATIVE MANAGEMENT

Postoperative care includes placement of a wrapped face-lift pressure dressing that is removed on postoperative day one and replaced with a Velcro dressing. Sutures are removed on postoperative day 5, and staples on day 10. Head elevation and the ice packs are used to diminish edema in the first few postoperative days. Our patients are also encouraged to participate in hyperbaric oxygen treatments to accelerate the healing process. Antibiotics and medication for pain control and nausea are prescribed.

COMPLICATIONS

Complications with neck rejuvenation can be divided into short- and long-term sequelae. Hematomas can occur in the immediate postoperative period and are often due to inadequate hemostasis with cautery prior to closing of the neck. Meticulous inspection of the neck is needed prior to closure. Seromas can occur as well within the first postoperative week. Left untreated, fluid collections in the neck can lead to uneven rippling of the skin, asymmetry, and possibly infection and/or skin necrosis. Closing of the neck incisions under tension can lead to skin breakdown and/or ultimately widened scars that are visible. Hairline incisions that incorrectly incised opposite to the hair growth patterns can lead to visible scars due to alopecia. Moreover, step-offs of the hairline can occur after excising excess hair-bearing skin and not realigning the hairline along the skin flaps. Pleating of the skin, especially in the postauricular sulcus, can occur when either insufficient undermining was done and/or excess standing cutaneous deformities are not excised. The distorted earlobe can have many variations of complications and is usually a result of the following: excess skin tension at the lobule, incomplete reattachment of the ligament of Lore, and not insetting the lobule in a higher position to allow for natural descent over time. Finally, abnormalities of the submental skin including concavity, excess skin, asymmetric folds or dimpling, and/or excess adipose tissue or prominences can occur and present over time. These complications are often due to either excess removal of pre or subplatysmal fat, excess thinning of the skin with incomplete undermining, incomplete suturing of the platysma using a variety of methods described (e.g., corset platysmaplasty), and/or incomplete partial removal of the submandibular glands or anterior belly of the digastric tendons. Complications of a neck lift need watchful waiting for at least 6 months prior to considering revisions as skin redraping and contour changes will improve over time.

RESULTS

Rejuvenation of the aging neck requires precise diagnosis of the various contributions of the anatomic structures involved in order to design an effective surgical plan. Restoration of a well-defined CMA is the goal of any neck tightening procedure, and this can be accomplished using any of the techniques described above in isolation, or more commonly, in combination. Some surgeons prefer a comprehensive approach to neck rejuvenation, wherein select patients undergo deep-plane cervicoplasty, subplatysmal lipectomy, midline plication of the digastric muscles, short corset-type platysmaplasty, and either skin excision or suture suspension. Whatever the extent of surgery required, careful analysis, planning, precision of surgical execution, and alignment of the patient's desires and expectations together afford the best chance for a desirable outcome.

PEARLS

Surgical rejuvenation of the neck can significantly improve a patient's quality of life. Knowledge of the indications, contraindications, and balancing patient expectations with realistic operative outcomes are important in planning a neck lift. Ultimately, anatomical knowledge of the neck is a key factor to successfully be able to employ single or multiple combined techniques to improve the aesthetic appearance of the neck.

PITFALLS

Insufficient preoperative planning including history taking that misses the unrealistic expectations of the patient will lead to an unhappy patient that cannot be improved with any rejuvenating procedure of the neck. Performing neck surgery on a class VI low-lying hyoid neck will most certainly lead to failure. As mentioned above, anatomical knowledge of the neck is critical to avoid temporary or permanent damage to the skin, nerves, and contours of the neck.

INSTRUMENTS TO HAVE AVAILABLE

- 15 and 10 blade
- Baby Yankauer suction
- Short and long curved Metzenbaum scissors
- Double wide skin hooks x2
- Guarded needle tip Bovie cautery
- Bipolar cautery
- Army navy retractors
- Deaver retractor
- Headlight
- Magnifying loupes
- Adson-Brown forceps
- Liposuction cannula
- Active bulb drains

ACKNOWLEDGMENTS

The author would like to recognize Robert S. Kang, M.D., M.P.H., and Vishad Nabili, M.D., F.A.C.S., for their exceptional contributions to the writing of this chapter. Their work in the writing, editing, and figure creation for this chapter is greatly appreciated, without which this chapter would not have been possible and which merits second and third author status.

SUGGESTED READING

Feldman JJ. *Neck lift*, 1st ed. St. Louis, MO: Quality Medical Publishing, Inc., 2006.

Ramirez OM, Robertson KM. Comprehensive approach to rejuvenation of the neck. *Facial Plast Surg* 2001;17(2): 129–140.

14 NASAL VALVE DEFICIENCY: A NEW PROPOSAL TO CLASSIFY DEFORMITY AND APPLY SURGICAL REPAIR BASED ON FOUR ANATOMICAL PLANES

Charles East

INTRODUCTION

Defining the flow-limiting segments in the nose (valve) was originally proposed by Mink. The arbitrary division into internal and external nasal valves is commonly referred to in the surgical literature, and a large range of surgical innovations have been proposed to rectify deficiencies reducing nasal airflow. However, defining exactly what is meant by these areas, both in a static and dynamic form and an appropriate link with clinical correlation, has led to some confusion as to which technique(s) to apply in individual functional problems. Part of the problem rests with inconsistent anatomical diagnosis in defining the clinical area of insufficiency given the considerable variations in form, shape, strength, and dynamic stability of the nose from the nostril margin to the bony pyriform aperture. For many years, nasal function was linked directly to the septum or inferior turbinates; however, the area of interest in the airway is the region in the nose covering 2 to 3 cm from the external nares controlled by hard fixed tissue structures, mucosal changes, and a variably dynamic lateral sidewall (cartilages and musculocutaneous structures) together with clearly defined ligaments. Descriptions of the lateral wall into zones have been published previously by Tsao whose article proposes/adds a more complete method of assessment.

Recent publications point out the benefit of recreating stability in the valve region as the majority of surgical procedures weaken or destroy its various elements leading to insufficiency and a reduction in function.

This chapter does not intend to comprehensively itemize the correct treatments rather I hope to provide a more reliable method of assessment and documentation based on the principle of four planes of the valve beginning at the nostril margin and considering medial and lateral contributions to the flow-limiting segment. The proposal is based on anatomic descriptions, which have clinical relevance and encompass the entire region from medial to lateral, floor to roof of the flow-limiting segment of the nose.

Anatomy

The proposal is to consider the flow-limiting segments from the clinical viewpoint by classifying medial structures and lateral wall structures from anterior to posterior. The basis for this is to link the known fixed structures, which can be altered to increase the cross-sectional area and the variable or dynamic predominantly lateral nasal wall structure that may require augmenting or strengthening.

In addition to the medial and lateral wall of the nasal vestibule, there is also a floor composed of the sill of the vestibular/premaxilla skin and in the upper mid third, there is a vaulted roof formed by the natural Y-shaped widening of the dorsal septum as it blends with the superior aspect of each upper lateral cartilage. The forms, variations, and pathologies of the nasal septum have been exhaustively described. Its physiologic role in the support of the upper lateral cartilages and perpendicular plate form a fixed tripod of the nose. On top of this, there is the floating tripod consisting of the lower lateral cartilages, accessory cartilages, and the variable scroll cartilages, which maintains the relations between the upper and lower lateral cartilages—the intercartilaginous junction.

The lateral wall deserves more scrutiny as it is composed of variable and incomplete cartilages, mucosal spaces, ligaments, muscles, and skin that has significantly different properties between the middle and the lower third of the nose. The tough tela subcutanea cutis is the main support of the lateral alar rim/lobule after the "turn point" of the lower lateral crus. The role of the superficial muscular aponeurotic system (SMAS) extensions within the nose whereby ligamentous and muscular attachments connect the SMAS to the deeper tissues of the cartilaginous framework have a significant support role as seen by the dysfunction created from facial palsy and the laxity with aging. The transversalis nasi muscle and its extensions form the lateral scroll ligaments; the pyriform ligament attaches around the posterior margin of the lateral crus. The dilator nasi and dilator nasi anterior along with the Pitanguy ligament are the main musculoligamentous support structures, with at least three of these often being disrupted during rhinoplasty surgery.

It is often deformities relating to the lateral wall, which are responsible for the functional failure of septoplasty in functional surgery excluding, of course, the mucosal nasal respiratory diseases. In any evaluation of the dysfunctional nose, it is vital to differentiate between the structural (fixed and dynamic) elements and the mucosal diseases (rhinitis, nasal polyps) although they may often coincide but the treatment of each is separate. Clinical examination therefore should involve a combination of direct, both pre- and postdecongestion, endoscopic, and often radiologic investigation. Having a reliable systematic classification of medial, lateral, and mucosal deformities will then allow correct application of the numerous valve procedures described on a rational basis, but tailored to individual needs.

Form and function are much related. A symmetric, adequately projected, and supported lower two-thirds of the nasal skeleton is likely to produce a balanced nasal airway limited only by the resistance provided by the isthmus. Saddled, twisted, deviated noses do not work well, and the converse of abnormally large and turbulent airflow from excessive removal of intranasal structures (radical sub mucus resection (SMR), inferior turbinectomy, middle turbinectomy) produces an equally disabling "empty nose syndrome." Clinical tests such as peak nasal inspiratory flow are limited by the collapsibility of the nasal sidewall, dimensions of the pyriform aperture, and the position of the nasal septum, but are probably the best clinical correlate with the patient's perception of function.

I propose four separate planes for clinically defining areas for the flow-limiting segment beginning at the nostril (see Fig. 14.1).

Plane 1: The medial crus, nasal sill, and margin of the ala rim

Plane 2: The leading edge of the nasal septum (caudal), the nasal tip domes, the corpus of the lateral crus, and the tela of the alar

Plane 3: The upper lateral and lower lateral junctional region, the triangular part of the valve angle (the valve angle), the lateral mucosal space, pyriform ligament, lower lateral part of the pyriform aperture, and mucosa anterior to the head of the inferior turbinate

Plane 4: The chondroethmoid junction of the septum, the "spread angle" (upper middle third vault), central upper lateral cartilage, and bone of the midpyriform aperture including the bony head of the turbinate

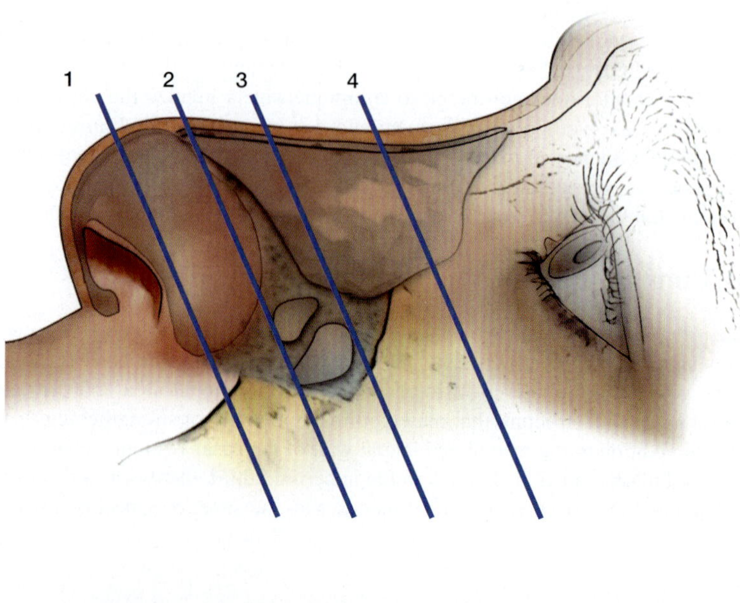

FIGURE 14.1
Profile view showing four planes clinically relevant to the valve.

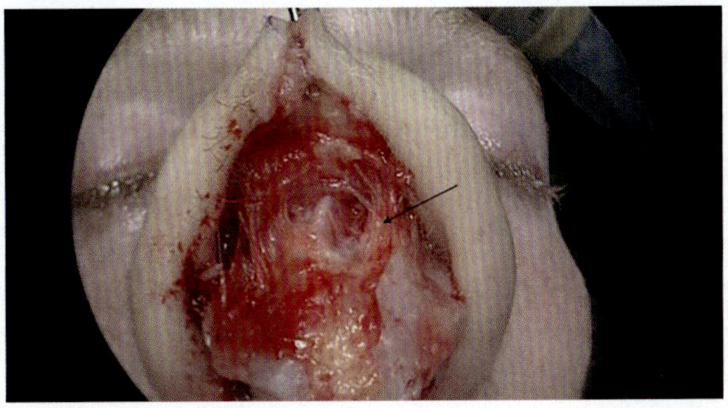

FIGURE 14.2
Lateral scroll ligaments clearly seen at the lateral Plane 3 when lifting the skin envelope.

Clinical Relevance

Based on the anatomical description, the flow-limiting segments can be classified into four basic planes detailing medial and lateral abnormalities.

Plane 1—The medial elements consist of skin and medial crus with its footplate; the floor is determined by the sill width, the alar/facial insertion point. The lateral wall is determined by the turn point of the lateral crus and the thickness of the Tela subcutanea cutis—the condensation of collagen fibers with sebaceous elements and muscle fibers that produce the form of the lateral alar lobule and give it rigidity.

Plane 2—Determined medially by the caudal end of the septum, the septal angles, membranous septum, and position of the nasal spine. Laterally, it is defined by the domes of the lower cartilages, the form and shape of the corpus of the lateral crus, the strength of the pyriform ligament, the dilator nasi muscle, and levator labii alaeque nasi muscle.

Plane 3—Medially, there is the central part of the quadrangular cartilage, the septal turbinate, and the vomer crest. Laterally, there is the upper lateral/lower lateral cartilage junction (with the accessory cartilages), the lateral mucosal space and associated pyriform bone (Webster triangle), and the transversalis nasi muscle with the lateral scroll ligament (Fig. 14.2).

Plane 4—Medially, there is the chondroethmoid junction (bifid, pneumatized), spread part (trapezoid) valve angle, the upper lateral attachment to the pyriform aperture, and the head of the inferior turbinate.

HISTORY

Deformities of the dorsum invariably reflect a displacement of the dorsal septum. Obvious sidewall asymmetry may be seen at rest particularly in the middle third of the nose. Alar pinching, abnormal curvature or position of the tip (ptosis), and caudal displacement of the cartilaginous septum are common deformities in the tip. Fixed obstructions in the nose produce a constant block. This may be reflected in the positions a patient prefers during sleep to maintain an airway, but dynamic collapse will usually be evident on increased nasal airflow.

Using this classification, with a combination of a direct, modified Cottle maneuver, endoscopic and radiologic (CBCT) investigation, deformities can be classified in the flow-limiting segment. For example, a caudal septal deformity in the left airway and a collapsed upper lateral cartilage with impingement on the septum would be area 2 medial left and area 3 right lateral. In this way, each nostril and valve can be separately categorized in a three-dimensional manner relevant to the technique required.

One must also consider patient comorbidities in the preoperative evaluation. Respiratory mucosal disease must be appropriately assessed and well controlled prior to valve surgery to optimize outcome. This includes rhinitis and nasal polyposis. Often, an extended course of medication, such as oral corticosteroids, is required pre- and postoperatively to minimize mucosal edema. Nasal steroids sprays can be used as well. Additionally, patients should be counseled to avoid nonsteroidal anti-inflammatory medications, fish oils, garlic, and any herbal remedies that have an anticoagulant effect. Prescribed anticoagulants should be held if possible from a medical standpoint and would be determined case by case.

PHYSICAL EXAMINATION

External inspection of the form and shape of the nose is crucial, with particular reference to deviations/asymmetries in the midthird and the tip, as well as the sidewalls at rest and on gentle inspiration. Evaluation of the internal aspects using nasal endoscopy using a 0- or 30-degree endoscope gives the best assessment at rest and with inspiration, noting the medial, lateral floor and roof for deviations angulations, prolapse, or lateral collapse.

Using the endoscope or lateralization using a fine looped probe for support to the areas of prolapse/instability is helpful in assessing whether that area is responsible for the airway restriction. The patient will report an improvement in airflow. It should be remembered that more than one area may be responsible for the limit (Video 14.1). Documentation of the key area is made.

Additional information can be obtained by peak nasal inspiratory flow measures or by rhinomanometry. However, in almost all cases, the valve deficiency can be diagnosed by the first two clinical examinations.

INDICATIONS

Nasal airway restriction may be due to fixed or dynamic instability in the flow-limiting segment. Indications for valve surgery should be preventative when a deficiency is seen preoperatively or if a reductive maneuver during rhinoplasty may precipitate dysfunction in an otherwise normal airway. Reconstruction of the valve should be undertaken in a symptomatic patient who undergoes rhinoplasty—aesthetic or reconstructive.

Septoplasty should be carried out to preserve as much support as possible to the lower two-thirds of the nose. To this end, the traditional L-strut leaves the septum weakest at its most vulnerable point, often leading to warping or twisting below and behind the anterior septal angle. In modern conservative rhinoplasty, a delta-shaped quadrilateral cartilage should be left in front of a line from the nasal spine to the central keystone junction with the perpendicular plate. This will help maintain an adequate height of the septum.

CONTRAINDICATIONS

None known

PREOPERATIVE PLANNING

Additional information can be obtained by cone beam CT scanning particularly where mucosal disease (e.g., allergy, nasal polyps) is suspected or coexists with structural problems. This can allow modeling of the flow-limiting step.

Valve surgery is best performed under a general anesthetic (intubation or laryngeal mask), with hypotension and careful preparation of the mucosa with vasoconstriction. There is a small margin for error so the best conditions are necessary for accuracy and grafting. Single-dose antibiotic prophylaxis and an intravenous dose of corticosteroids are given.

SURGICAL TECHNIQUE

My preferences for techniques are as follows:

General principles include that grafts must not compromise the airway by bulk when increasing the strength of the septum/lateral wall. Septal cartilage is the ideal primary source, with next best being rib cartilage. Conchal cartilage may be used if small curved grafts are required.

In the first two planes, with three-layer dissection of the nasal sidewall (outer skin, cartilage, and vestibular skin), the walls should be supported with custom soft reinforced Silastic sheets for 7 to 10 days. These are easily fashioned by cutting an oval shape, folding it, and placing a suture close to the deeper placed edge at the fold. This creates an acute angle that sits against the septum as far back as Plane 3 and then flares more caudally providing both lateral wall and medial support. A lateral onlay alar Silastic sheet can be fixed via transmural suture tied loosely (Fig. 14.3). Antibiotics are mandatory as infection is a potential disaster. Petroleum-based

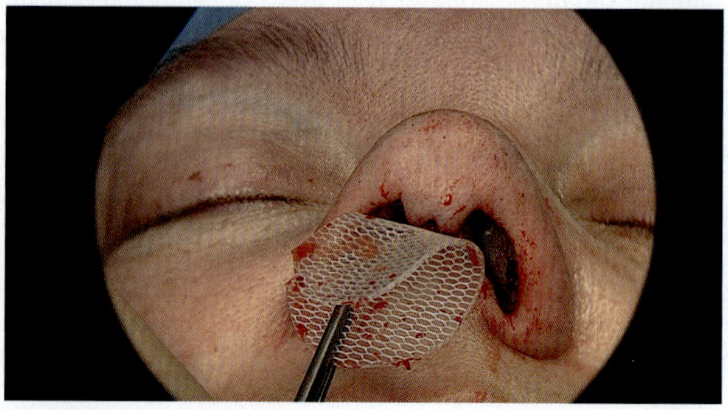

FIGURE 14.3
Custom designed reinforced Silastic internal nasal valve splint.

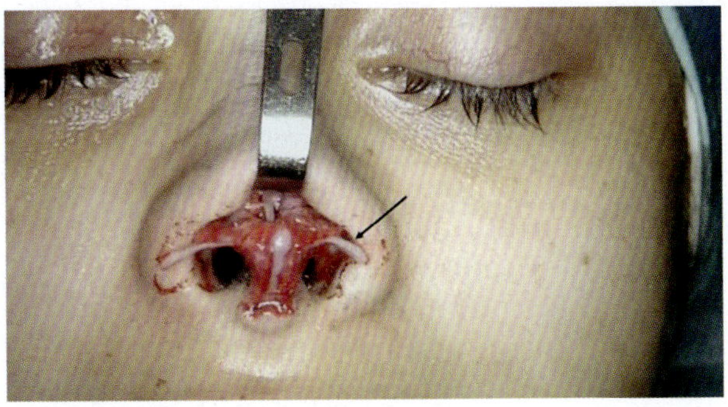

FIGURE 14.4
Articulated rim grafts fixed at the dome—axis is at right angles to the sagittal plane of the septum.

ointments applied internally in the first week, without attempt to clean the inside of the nose, reduce the risk of infection.

It is my preference not to employ any formal nasal packing. Occasional use of a hydrocolloidal dressing to the mucosa especially in Plane 4 (e.g., NasoPore), which dissolves or can be aspirated at 1 week, is well tolerated.

Plane 1

Medial: Repositioning of the medial crural footplates, narrowing of the columella base by removal of intercrural soft tissue (caudal end of the Pitanguy ligament/depressor septi nasi). Either of these can be performed endonasally via marginal incisions or by complete dissection of the crura inferiorly in external rhinoplasty

Lateral: Supporting the alar rim by eversion of the caudal edge of the lower lateral cartilage in primary rhinoplasty or a variant of a rim graft. My preference is for an articulated rim graft compared to a free floating rim graft (Fig. 14.4).

Plane 2

Medial: Caudal septoplasty with securing of the posterior septal angle to the nasal spine. Septal extension or replacement grafts may be necessary to reconstruct the anterior septal angle and provide a support for the alar lobular segment of the alar cartilages.

Lateral: Lateral crural strut graft is placed deep to the alar cartilage either caudally or cranially depending on which area needs contour/support. Careful elevation of the vestibular skin is required after hydrodissection, and the graft must not be thick and bulky. Fixation of the graft is with 6-0 PDS to the alar cartilage and the nasal sidewall supported with reinforced Silastic-flexible sheets. An alar suspension suture is placed in the lateral pyriform aperture (either to the pyriform ligament or as a guided suture brought out through the cheek skin to maintain the lateral crural graft above the bony aperture).

Plane 3

Medial: Septal curvature correction with ethmoid plate baton/resection and fixation of angulations. Spreader grafts to lateralize the caudal upper lateral cartilage edge are secured to the septum once deviated portions are excised (Fig. 14.5). M-plasty (Z-plasty) of the caudal upper lateral.

Lateral: Alar batten graft to support the scroll region. These may need to extend laterally onto the face of the maxilla to support the lateral mucosal space (bellows area). Widening of the lateral pyriform aperture at the

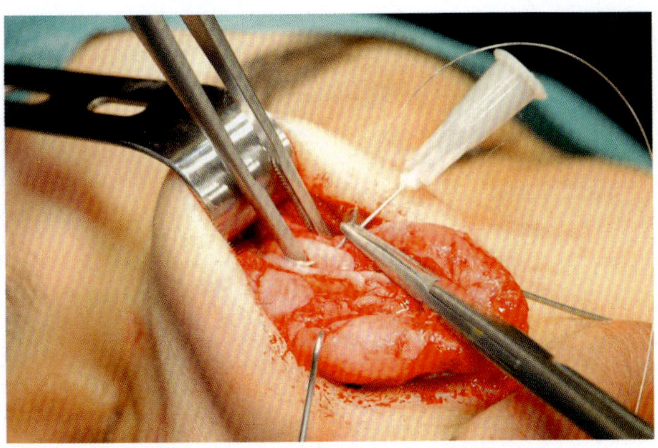

FIGURE 14.5
Fixation of a spreader flap to the septum. Each side can be tailored individually.

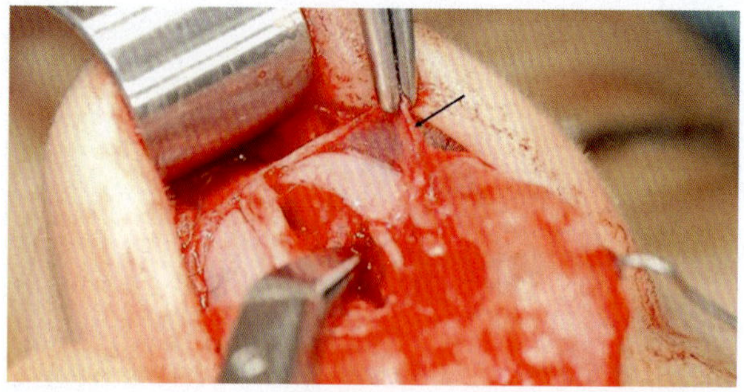

FIGURE 14.6
Release of the perichondrium to create a spreader flap. Upper lateral separated from the septum, perichondrium raised prior to turn-in flap (*arrow*).

level and below the insertion of the inferior turbinate. Titanium nasal valve prosthesis. This ultralight implant is sized and inserted above the upper lateral cartilage and beneath the cranial border of the lower lateral. Time will tell if this device replaces the butterfly graft.

Plane 4

Medial: Perpendicular plate correction and narrowing of the septal turbinate. Spreader grafts (continuous with the plane 3 medial, but slightly wider to mimic the original Y shape of the top of the septum) are also helpful.

Lateral: Autospreader flaps using the horizontal portion of the released upper lateral cartilage including the cranial extension of cartilage under the nasal bone cap turned in and sutured to the dorsal septum (Fig. 14.6). This requires release of the perichondrium to allow for appropriate placement (Fig. 14.7). This is a very effective spring mechanism to prevent inverted V deformities by creating the natural vaulted shape of the roof at this point. Spreader grafts harvested from behind the support line of the quadrilateral cartilage, either fashioned wider cranially than caudally or extended caudally, that is, to support a septal extension graft. Lateral sidewall out-fracture of the lateral bony pyriform aperture (paramedian, transverse, and lateral osteotomies) combined with a cranially placed spreader grafts is a useful technique to widen a narrow pyriform aperture as well.

Postoperatively, if the surgery is predominantly on the septum, I use a quilt suture to coapt the mucosa using a fast-absorbing running suture. This is combined with a hemostatic blanket stitch to the caudal septal incision. This negates the need for packing. If an internal dressing is needed, for example, to protect a tear, then a cellulose-type hydrogel sponge is used, for example. NasoPore. To support lateral wall surgery, a custom reinforced Silastic sheet is fashioned as per the photograph. This creates an angle to sit adjacent to the upper lateral cartilage with a flare distally that provides sidewall support in area 2 and 3 laterally.

POSTOPERATIVE MANAGEMENT

It is my preference to use sutured in place external Silastic batons when skin and vestibular lining are dissected and grafts have been used. These support the repair and minimize swelling or prolapse into the airway. In this case, oral antibiotics are continued for 5 days. In the majority of patients, the outside of the nose is covered with tapes and a three-layer plaster dressing, but without compression. The Silastic and external dressings are removed in 6 to 7 days. Chloramphenicol or similar ointment is used to cover the edges of the internal splint and internal sutures for 5 days. Irrigations are not given, and the patient is instructed not to attempt cleaning of the nose. Sniffing is permitted, but no nose blowing for 5 days. Topical steroid sprays to control rhinitis may be

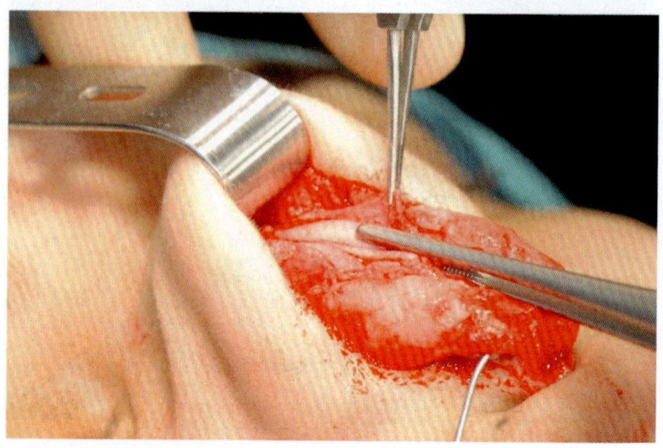

FIGURE 14.7
Turn-in spreader flaps are an effective valve support procedure often negating the use of spreader grafts.

safely resumed after 2 weeks, cover for allergies being provided by oral antihistamines preoperatively. Sesame seed sprays (Nozoil) in the first month retain moisture inside the nose and minimize crusts better than repeated saline douches.

COMPLICATIONS

The main complications are from failure to recognize the level(s) of valve deformity—usually leading to a worse functional result or technical errors, for example, malplaced endonasal incisions causing blunting of the valve angle or excessive bulk of grafts used to support the sidewall. In all valve procedures, not only must the septum be straight but the articulation to the sidewall of the midvault must be secure, so that ideally the head of the middle turbinate is visible without instrumentation in the nose. The tendency for edema in the airway during the first postoperative week can be counteracted by the customizable reinforced Silastic splints that give enough sidewall support in the lateral areas 1, 2, and 3. This is particularly important where three-layer dissections have been performed—vestibular lining, cartilage grafts, and soft tissue envelope manipulation.

RESULTS

There are few controlled studies of the outcomes of valve surgery, but recently, patient-reported outcomes indicate the value of spreader grafts and alar battens in improving the nasal airflow. It is not uncommon for the patient to recognize improvement in airflow as early as the day after surgery if the techniques have been successful. With wider adoption of patient-reported outcome measures, a firm evidence base will emerge on the benefits of valve surgery combined with either functional or aesthetic rhinoplasty.

PEARLS

- A detailed examination of the external nose at rest and during inspiration with endoscopic internal assessment is mandatory for accurate diagnosis.
- Modified Cottle test, cone beam CT, and peak nasal inspiratory flow measurements are useful tests.
- Valve compromise can occur at multiple levels in the flow-limiting segment so that more than one area may need attention.
- Preservation and reorientation of cartilage in rhinoplasty will reduce the need for extensive graft harvest.
- Don't lose in bulk what you gain in strength with alar batten or crural grafts.
- Valve surgery, the surgery of millimeters, requires high-quality fine rhinoplasty instruments.

PITFALLS

- Septoplasty and turbinectomy alone are only a small part of valve surgery.
- Valve surgery frequently requires rhinoplasty techniques and grafting.
- Mucosal disease of the nose may be reported as "nasal block."
- A knowledge of rhinitis is important in achieving an overall improvement, but structural problems require surgery.
- The multitude of techniques purported to deal with valve dysfunction need rationalizing—one technique does not fit all.
- Form and function are linked; outcomes are better when both are addressed in rhinoplasty.

INSTRUMENTS TO HAVE AVAILABLE

See Figure 14.8 for photo of all necessary instruments.

- 0- or 30-degree endoscope.
- Fine-tipped dissecting scissors (angled Walter or Converse).
- Fine dissectors.
- Multitoothed forceps.
- Round-bodied 4-0 or 5-0 PDS sutures, especially when using grafts.
- Rib graft harvesting sets.
- Sheets of reinforced Silastic, which are cut to individual shapes. See Figure 14.8 for surgical instrument layout.

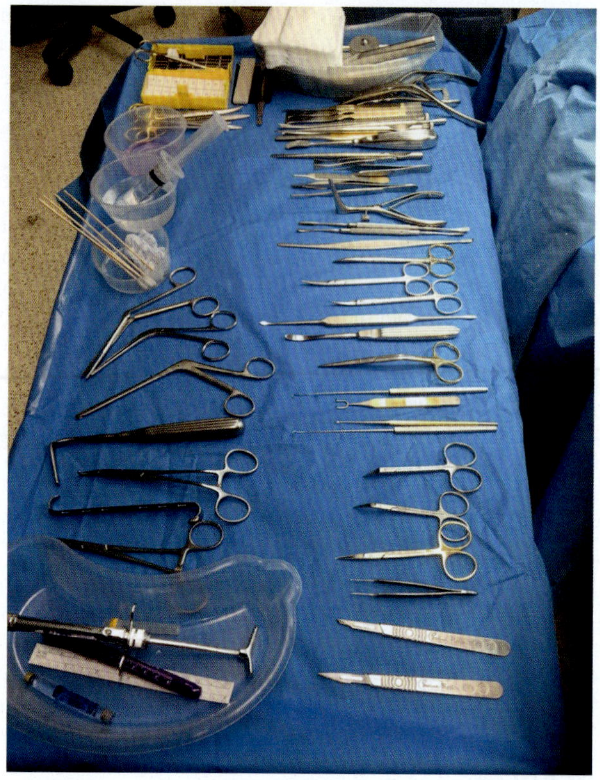

FIGURE 14.8
Surgical instruments to have available.

ACKNOWLEDGMENT

Nadeem Akhtar, FRCS (Plast) Aesthetic and Reconstructive Fellow, The London Clinic, 20 Devonshire Place, London

SUGGESTED READING

Bloching MB. Disorders of the nasal valve area. *GMS Curr Top Otorhinolaryngol Head Neck Surg* 2007;6:Doc07.
Davis RE. Rhinoplasty: contemporary innovations. *Facial Plast Surg Clin North Am* 2015;23(1):ix.
Motamedi KK, Stephan SJ, Ries WR. Innovations in nasal valve surgery. *Curr Opin Otolaryngol Head Neck Surg* 2016;24(1):31–36.
Spielmann PM, White PS, Hussain SS. Surgical techniques for the treatment of nasal valve collapse: a systematic review. *Laryngoscope* 2009;119(7):1281–1290.
Tsao GJ, Fijalkowski N, Most SP. Validation of a grading system for lateral nasal wall insufficiency, *Allergy Rhinol (Providence)* 2013;4(2):e66–e68.
Yeung A, Hassouneh B, Kim DW. Outcome of nasal valve obstruction after functional and aesthetic-functional rhinoplasty. *JAMA Facial Plast Surg* 2016;18(2):128–134.

15 RHINOPLASTY: MANAGEMENT OF THE CROOKED NOSE

Julian M. Rowe-Jones

INTRODUCTION

The crooked nose is not just one deformity, and therefore, it must not be assumed that there is a single surgical technique or set of surgical steps that can be universally applied. As a consequence, analysis is of fundamental importance to understanding the patient's anatomy and directing a surgical plan. It's critical to recognize that the crooked nose can often be associated with complex deformities involving multiple components of the nasal skeleton, skin soft tissue envelope, and mucosal lining. These anatomical elements may not just be displaced but also remodeled if there is a history of trauma. Furthermore, patient's expectations should not be assumed in advance. Functional as well as aesthetic improvement may need to be addressed.

The patient's motivation for surgery may also be complex. Special attention should be given to psychological issues not only in the patient requesting cosmetic change for congenital nasal deformity but also in those who've had nasal trauma, for example, the patient with a history of having been assaulted who hopes their nose can be returned to its premorbid appearance. The surgeon must be sensitive to patients' psychological concerns, must be capable of recognizing and understanding a wide range of anatomical deformities, and must be competent with a wide range of surgical techniques for all elements of the nasal skeleton and soft tissues.

HISTORY

A medical history should be approached in a standardized format of medical conditions, surgical interventions, current prescriptions and allergies, as well as a general examination. A rhinoplasty history should start with an open question asking the patient what they hope to achieve from the consultation and from any future surgery. It is important to establish what the patients' main hopes are. Subsequently, the patient can be guided with questions specifically addressing their aspirations and expectations with regard to both nasal function and appearance as well as their expectations as to how surgery will help them make progress generally. It is also important to ask the patients about their concerns and worries. Whether previous nasal trauma including iatrogenic has occurred should be investigated as this may warn the surgeon of increased unpredictability during any subsequent rhinoplasty. It should, however, be remembered that trauma could have occurred in childhood, and the patient may have no recollection of this event. If the patient presents after trauma, it's important to ascertain whether the patient is hoping for their preinjury nasal shape and function to be restored or whether they're looking for additional improvement. Preinjury photographs can be helpful in understanding what the patient wants. If the patients' nasal deformity was acquired through trauma, it is important to determine whether there is any pending or continuing litigation, frustration, or anger present in the patient as this could adversely affect the current doctor–patient relationship and even lead to transference of anger and disenchantment.

As with any surgery aimed at altering the shape of the nose, it's important to be sure there is no significant psychological morbidity or personality disorder. Even though at this stage the patient may not know what is possible from surgery, it's important to reflect on whether the patient's expectations are generally reasonable and whether they are embracing surgery as a positive step or not.

PHYSICAL EXAMINATION

The purpose of examination and analysis is to recognize, understand, describe, and record:

- The shape and position of each external and intranasal anatomical component
- A comparison of the symmetry of paired right and left anatomical components
- Potential anatomical pitfalls related to surgery
- Abnormal nasal function
- Pathology of the nasal mucosa
- Facial asymmetry
- Other associated deformities such as a saddle nose or dorsal hump

I like to evaluate the nose externally as upper, middle, and lower thirds and in the frontal view, half basal and full basal views, head down view, right and left oblique views, and right and left lateral views. Endoscopy can aid intranasal examination particularly when functional symptoms are present. CT scan of the face or paranasal sinuses can help to determine the nature of any bony deformity. I find that good photography with appropriate lighting and background is essential for analysis. Careful study of the photographs reinforces the initial understanding of the nose gained from the physical examination. Digital photographic processing applications that can split the frontal view and recompose the face using two right half images and two left half images may aid in assessing nasal asymmetry. General facial asymmetry is to be recognized and noted as such elements may become more noticeable after surgical correction.

INDICATIONS

The indications for surgery of the crooked nose include both aesthetic and functional aspects. Commonly, aesthetic regions of concern highlight the points of functional impairment. For example, compromise of nasal airway breathing through deviations or deflections in the bony nasal pyramid and nasal septum can reduce airflow through the internal, external, or both sets of nasal valves. Functional compromise can be either slight or near complete and must be elucidated, as previously discussed. With regard to aesthetics, a complete review of patient desires and expectations is obtained during the clinical interview and paired with desires in computer imaging. In a patient with good health, surgical treatment of the crooked nose affords an opportunity for functional improvement while optimizing nasal appearance in addition to nasal–facial harmony.

CONTRAINDICATIONS

The main contraindications to surgery are psychological. If the patient's expectations cannot be met or the patient cannot accept the risks of surgery, then these must be considered absolute contraindications. If the patient has a sense of bitterness or unfairness about considering surgery or has an excessive sense of importance and entitlement, then these may be relative contraindications to surgery. The entitled patient may feel even more embittered if they have any amount of adverse outcome. The crooked nose is often associated with complex surgical reconstruction of a nasal and septal deformity, and the surgeon's inexperience is therefore also a relative contraindication to surgery. As with any elective operation, the patient's general health must also be considered.

PREOPERATIVE PLANNING

The operative plan should take into account the foremost of the patient's aims. These must be considered alongside the surgical options and possibilities with their risks and limitations and the surgeon's level of experience. Aesthetically, special attention is given individually to the dorsum and to the lateral nasal walls. I aim to correct the position of the dorsum with regard to the midline and the shape of the dorsum, if curved. Symmetry of the dorsum is also carefully assessed, with consideration given to correction of bony and cartilaginous humps and irregularities. The length of the nasal bones is assessed. Short nasal bones increase the risk of septal disarticulation with osteotomies. The relationship of the dorsum to the lateral nasal wall—both bony and cartilaginous—is determined. The contour of the lateral walls is determined as well as their length from the dorsum to the naso-facial junction. The longer lateral wall, from dorsum to naso-facial junction, in a deviated nose may need an additional intermediate osteotomy for correction. A convex lateral wall may also need an intermediate

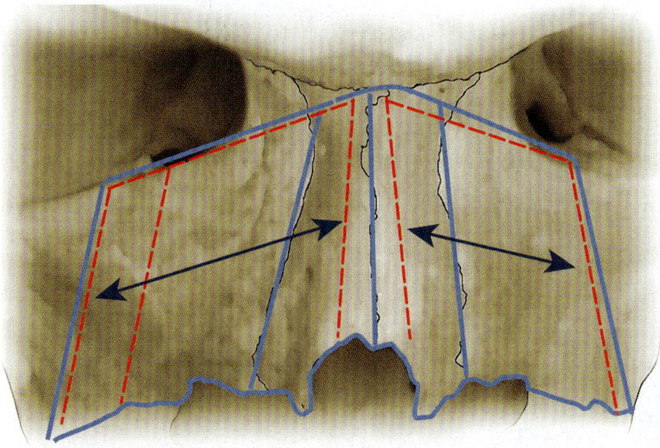

FIGURE 15.1
The right lateral nasal wall is longer from the dorsum to the naso-facial junction. Bilateral medial osteotomies, low to low lateral osteotomies flush with the face, superior transverse osteotomies, and an additional right intermediate osteotomy are shown. The right intermediate osteotomy is shown measured equidistant from the midline as the left lateral osteotomy.

osteotomy to break the curvature. The position of the lateral walls in relation to the midline is assessed when deciding on lateral, superior transverse, and medial osteotomies (Figs. 15.1 to 15.3). The half basal view is helpful in analyzing the contour and position of the lateral nasal walls, and the head down view is very helpful for assessing the position and shape of the dorsum.

Septal surgery is invariably necessary in the treatment of the crooked nose for functional and aesthetic reasons. When planning correction of the septum, particular attention is given to the position and shape of the caudal and dorsal edges of the quadrilateral cartilage. While the caudal and dorsal edges may be repositioned or reshaped, a contiguous 10-mm caudal and dorsal cartilaginous strut must be left in place. In cases of nasal blockage, particular attention must be given to the internal valves. Narrowing at this site will require high dorsal septal and upper lateral cartilage reconstruction. The position of the bony septum must be noted during planning as deviation here will influence the position of the quadrilateral cartilage. Care must be taken in planning for resection of the bony septum especially if bony hump reduction and osteotomies are required as the risk of septal disarticulation is higher. As I mentioned above, this risk is greater in the presence of short nasal bones.

The position and symmetry of the tip cartilages are also noted. Deviation of the tip may be intrinsic, thus requiring surgery to the lower lateral cartilages, or extrinsic, due to displacement secondary to septal deviation. Planning for correction of tip cartilage asymmetries must consider resection of segments of excessively long crura or grafting of short crura. Repositioning sutures may be required as may onlay grafts inserted into precise pockets to camouflage depressions.

In most cases, I use an open approach, as I feel that this is the best way to accurately diagnose anatomic deformities—particularly those of the septum. I always write each anticipated step of the surgical procedure in the notes after the initial consultation and photographic analysis are complete. This plan is reviewed at the time of informed consent for surgery and is taken to the operating room with photograph review prior to the commencement of surgery.

The surgical plan may be modified during surgery, and it's important to understand that planning is a dynamic process and continues during surgery where a better understanding of the nasal anatomy may be achieved. I find that taking intraoperative photographs from several positions and viewing them on the camera's liquid crystal display during surgery very helpful in increasing the appreciation of the patient's anatomy.

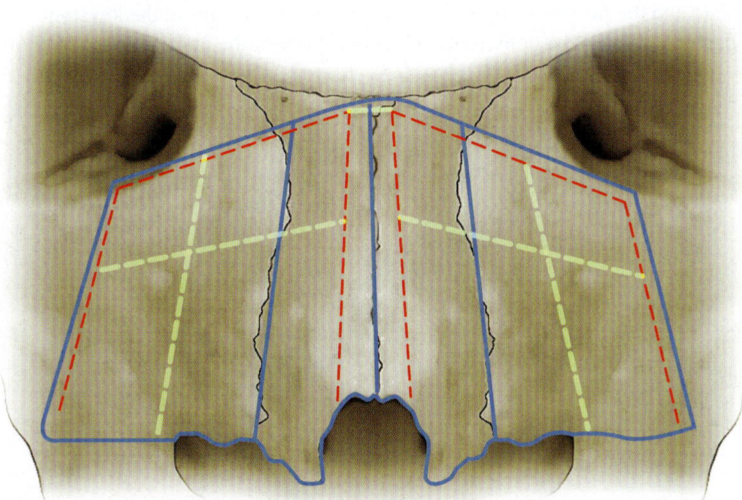

FIGURE 15.2
Bilateral lateral, superior transverse, and medial osteotomies are shown in *red.* A single midline cephalic root osteotomy and bilateral dorsal to ventral and caudal to cephalic intermediate osteotomies are shown in *green.*

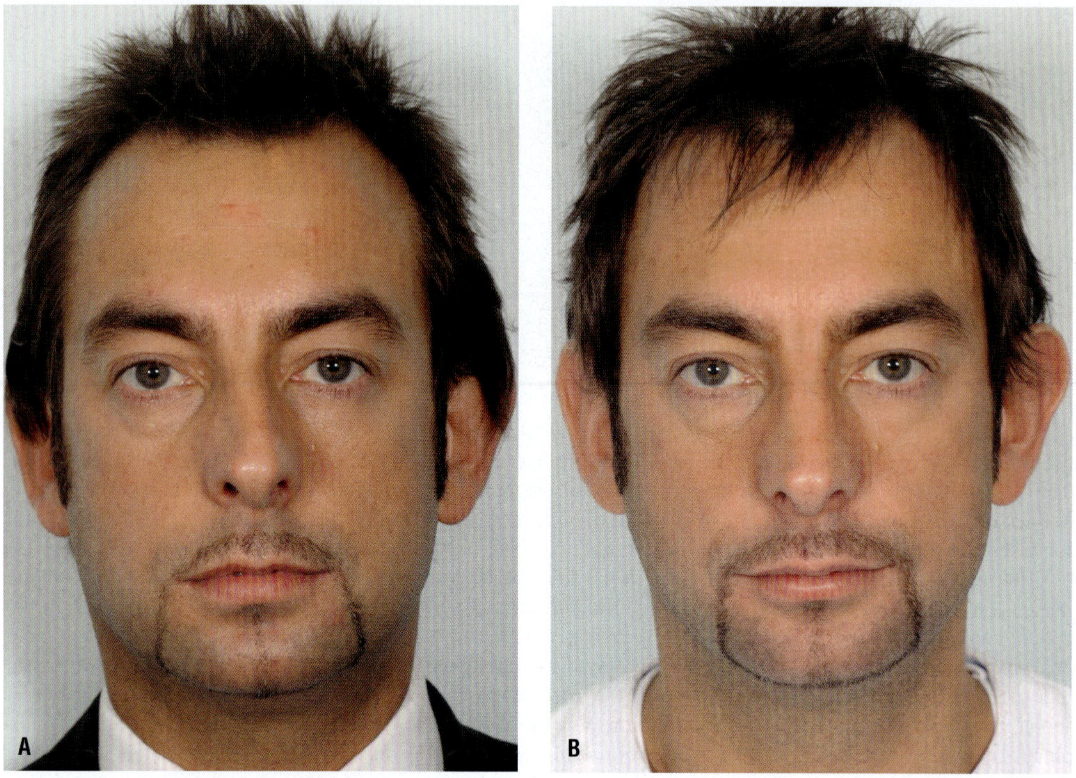

FIGURE 15.3 A swinging door septoplasty and bilateral medial, superior transverse, low to low lateral, and a right intermediate osteotomies were performed. **A:** Preoperative. **B:** Postoperative.

SURGICAL TECHNIQUES

I perform the surgery with the patient under general anesthesia with a laryngeal mask. A hypotensive technique is used and complemented by reverse Trendelenburg patient positioning. The nasal and facial skin and nasal lining are prepared with aqueous chlorhexidine and the patient is draped. The nose is marked, as necessary, to aid incisions and recognition of anatomical features, and the nose is then infiltrated with 2 to 4 mL of 1:80,000 adrenaline with 2% xylocaine. In most cases, I use an open approach, and the tip cartilages are separated to allow bilateral septal flap elevation and a full view of the entire quadrilateral cartilage. This is further enabled by release of the upper lateral cartilages flush with the quadrilateral cartilage (Fig. 15.4).

A stepwise approach is taken to septal correction. Initially, I release the ventral edge of the quadrilateral cartilage from the maxillary crest and vomer while preserving the attachment of the posterior septal angle to the anterior nasal spine if both are in the midline. This together with release of the soft tissues may allow the cartilage to be maintained straight and in the midline with no tension. It is important to maintain at least a 1-cm connection between the ethmoid plate and the posterior edge of the quadrangular cartilage at the keystone area. If the ethmoid plate is deviated, I prefer to release the bony septum from the floor of the nose with an osteotome

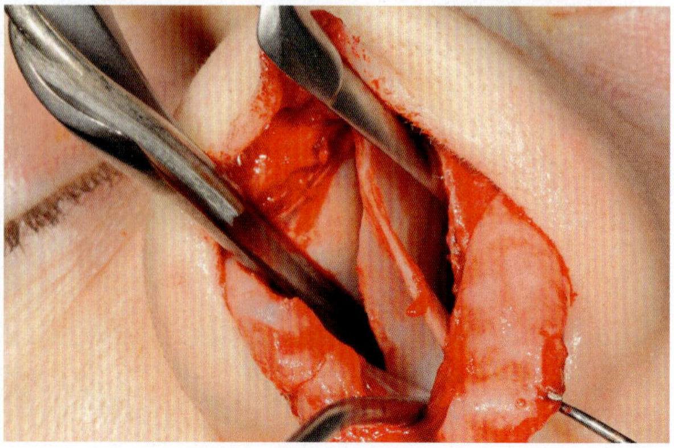

FIGURE 15.4
An open approach with separation of the lower lateral cartilages, elevation of bilateral septal mucoperichondrial flaps, and release of the upper lateral cartilage gives an excellent view of the multiple deviations in the quadrilateral cartilage.

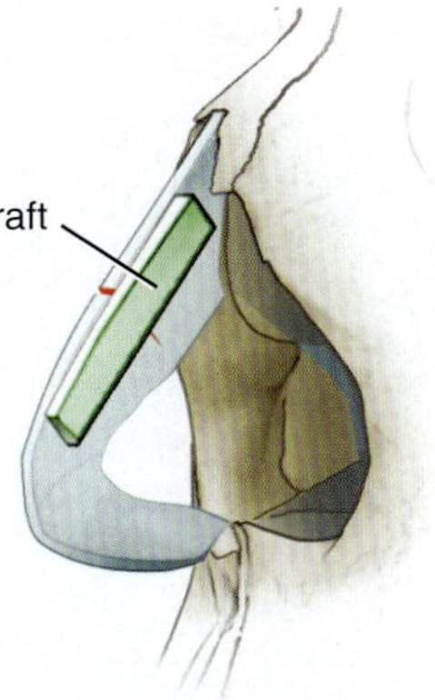

FIGURE 15.5
Incision through the dorsal strut stabilized on a left spreader graft.

or the Becker-Kaplan scissors and to fracture it to the midline, rather than resect deviated septal bone. If the quadrangular cartilage remains intrinsically deviated, I excise the deviated cartilage but ensure that at least 1 cm caudal and dorsal struts remain. Deviations in these areas are corrected by incision through the maximum points of curvature and splinting of the cartilage pieces with a batten of excised cartilage (Figs. 15.5 and 15.6) or ethmoid plate (Figs. 15.7 and 15.8). If the cartilage graft is curved, its concave surface is placed against the concave surface of the septum and sutured with 4-0 or 5-0 polydioxanone suture (Fig. 15.9). If these cartilage batten grafts (also considered spreader grafts when paradorsal in position) do not straighten a deformity, then it may be necessary to excise the deformed piece of cartilage and replace it with harvested straight cartilage or bony septum grafts (Fig. 15.10). In cases of severe deformity, an extracorporeal septoplasty may be required where the entire quadrilateral cartilage is excised, remodeled, and reconstructed on the back table and replaced. It's important that the septum is fixed well at two points—these being the anterior nasal spine and the upper lateral cartilages at the keystone area. If insufficient graft material is available for harvest from the septum, then additional cartilage can be taken from the ear or rib or the reconstructed pieces of septum can be stabilized on polydioxanone foil.

Osteotomies are required to reposition and improve symmetry in the external bony nose. If the entire bony vault is deviated but the slope of each lateral wall is symmetrical in its relationship with the dorsum, then low to low lateral and superior transverse osteotomies may be all that is necessary without necessitating medial osteotomies. The entire vault is then repositioned en bloc. If there is reluctance of the bony vault to move, then it may be necessary to use an additional midline nasal root osteotomy at the nasion. However, if one lateral wall is excessively medialized, it may be necessary to perform a medial osteotomy to enable out fracture of this bone. Intermediate osteotomies may be necessary to correct a convex nasal sidewall or excessive length (from dorsum to naso-facial junction) of one bony lateral nasal wall (Figs. 15.1 and 15.3). If an excess of length is present with a dorsal hump, asymmetric hump reduction with more hump removed from the longer side may be considered.

Bony asymmetries due to callous formation may need to be rasped and cartilage irregularities shaved. Asymmetries due to depressions may be disguised with onlay grafts inserted into precise pockets. These grafts can consist of shaved, softened, crushed cartilage or diced cartilage.

I close the incisions in the columella with 6-0 nylon and the marginal incisions with 5-0 monocryl. The septum is quilted with 4-0 vicryl rapide. Intranasal packs are not routinely used. The nose is dressed with an external splint of melolin, steri-strips, plaster of Paris, and micropore. The patient is recovered sitting up initially with the laryngeal mask still in place until fully conscious.

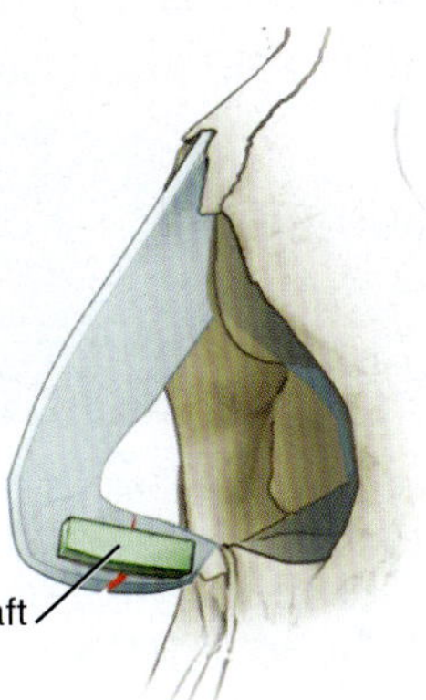

FIGURE 15.6
Incision through the caudal strut stabilized on a linear batten graft.

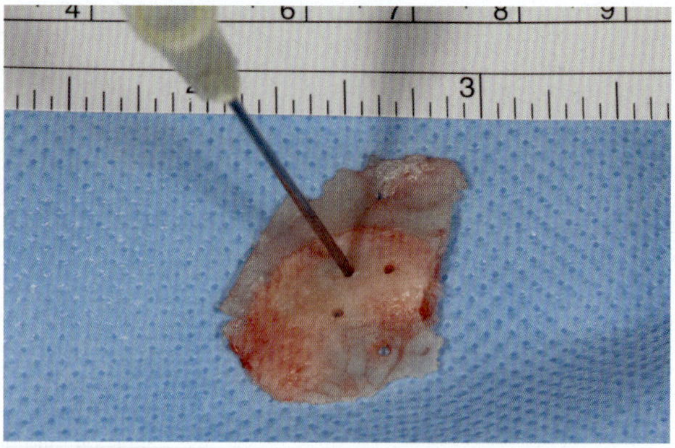

FIGURE 15.7
Holes made in ethmoid plate with a 19-gauge needle to enable suturing of this graft across curved septal cartilage. The graft stabilizes and straightens the incised septum.

POSTOPERATIVE MANAGEMENT

The patient remains in hospital for 6 hours postoperatively as this is the period during which hemorrhage is most likely. The patient is discharged with an oral broad-spectrum antibiotic such as coamoxiclav 625 mg every 8 hours for a week and instructed to perform careful cleaning of the nares and columella, nasal vestibules, and any external incisions. This is performed with 3% hydrogen peroxide solution and topical antibiotics including mupirocin ointment and ciprofloxacin two to three times daily for a week. The patient is seen in my office 1 week postoperatively for removal of external nasal dressings and nasal sutures. The patient is advised to avoid vigorous exercise for the first 2 weeks postoperatively and contact sports for 6 weeks. Strong sunlight on the nose should be avoided for 3 months.

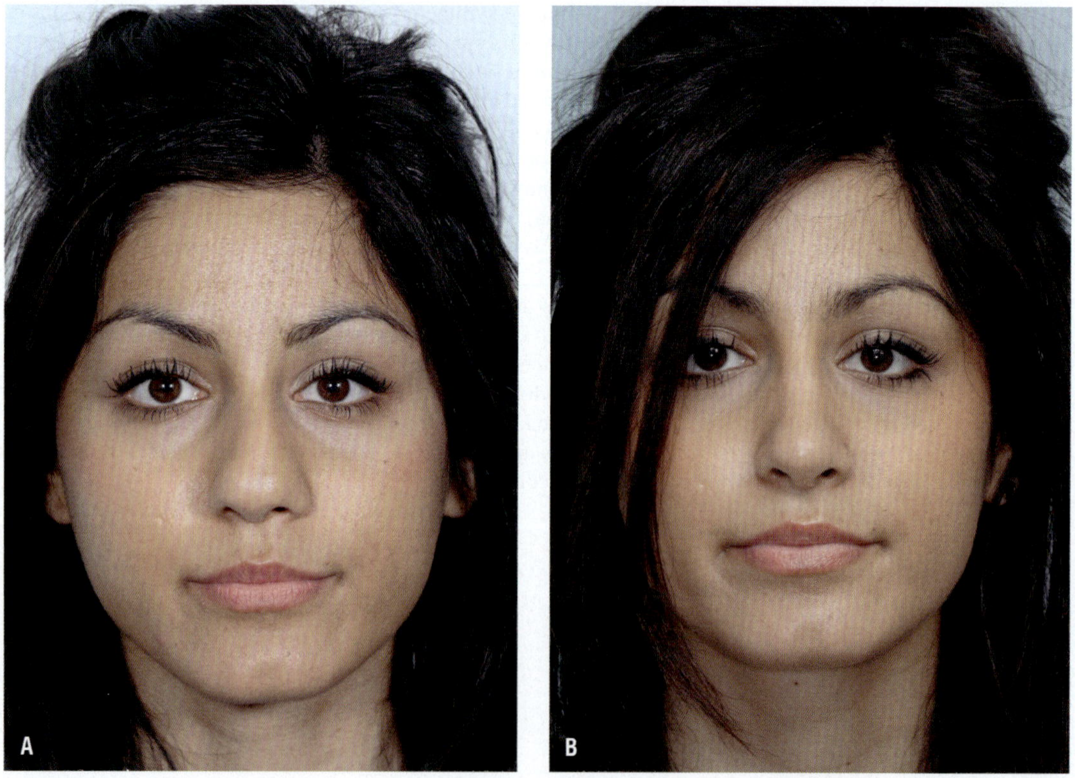

FIGURE 15.8 Bilateral medial, superior transverse, and low to low lateral osteotomies were performed. Swinging door septoplasty released the quadrilateral cartilage, and intrinsic curvature was corrected with full-thickness incisions through the axes of maximum curvature and stabilization on an ethmoid plate graft. Bilateral dome creation and a dome equalization sutures were used to correct tip asymmetry and improve definition. A right alar rim support graft was also used. **A:** Preoperative frontal view. **B:** Postoperative frontal view.

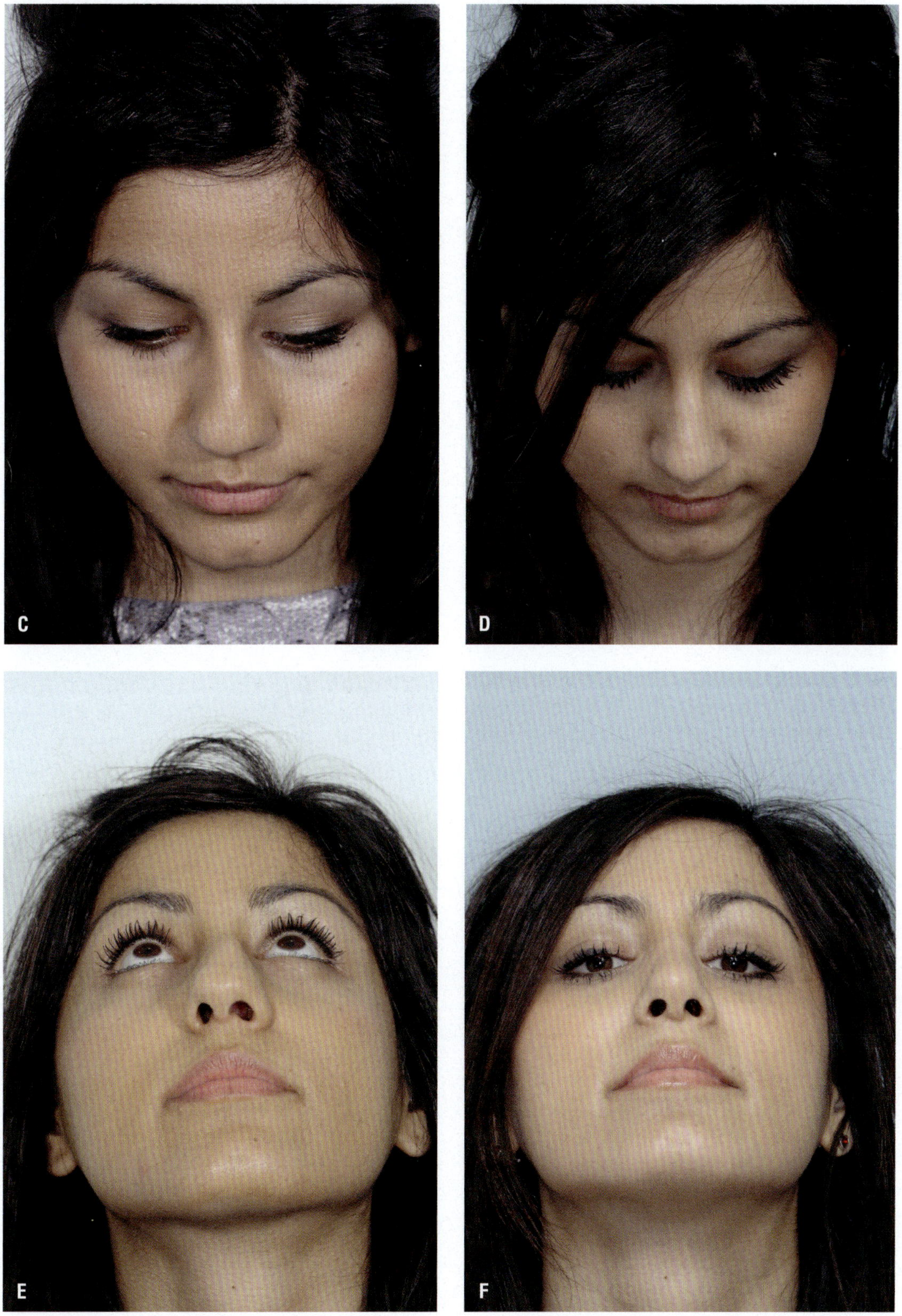

FIGURE 15.8 (*Continued*) **C:** Preoperative, head down view. **D:** Postoperative, head down view. **E:** Preoperative, basal view. **F:** Postoperative, basal view.

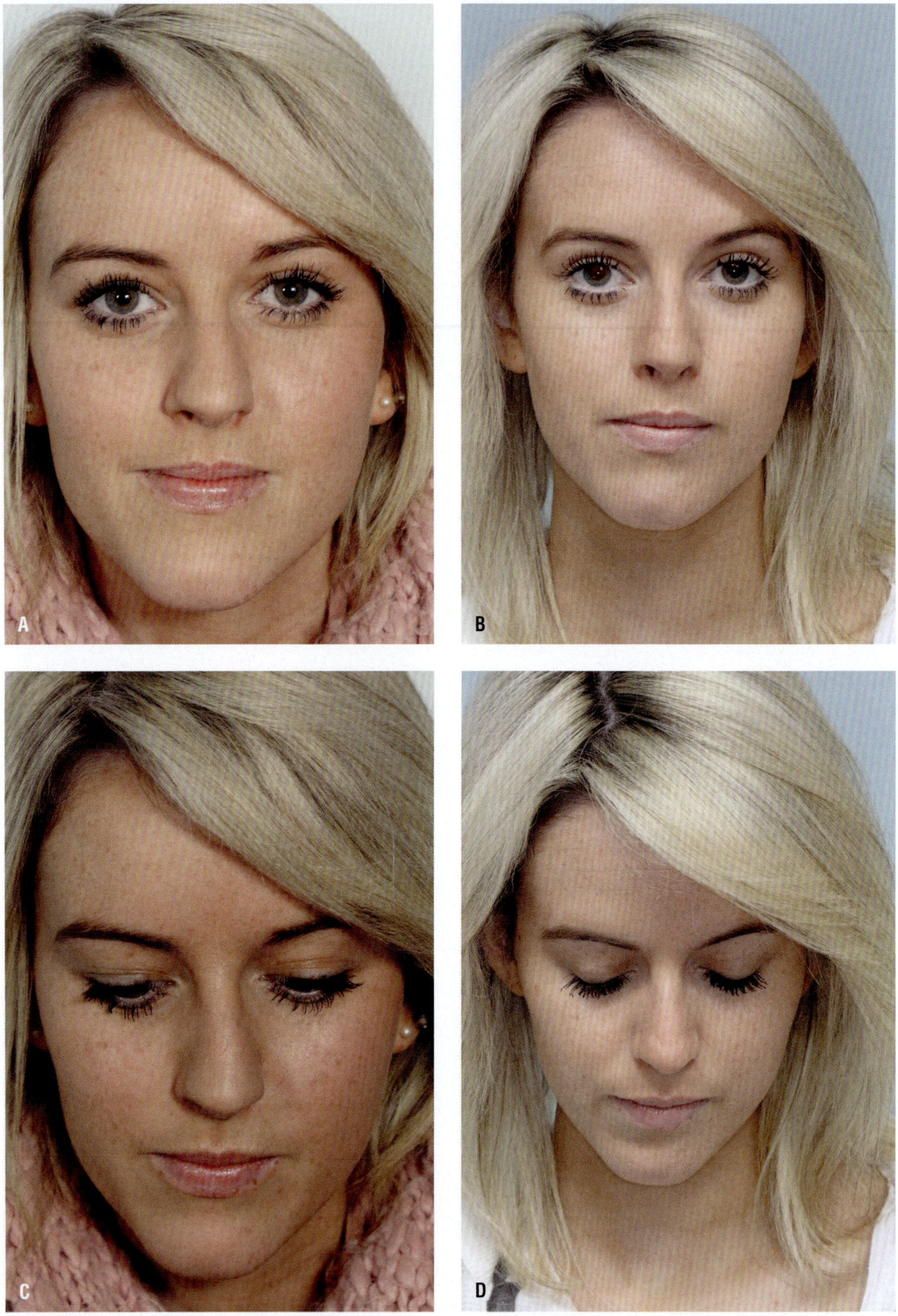

FIGURE 15.9 Bilateral medial, superior transverse, and low to low lateral osteotomies were performed; a swinging door septoplasty released the quadrilateral cartilage. A right spreader graft was inserted, and the cartilaginous junction between the left upper lateral cartilage and septum was shaved. **A:** Preoperative, frontal view. **B:** Postoperative, frontal view. **C:** Preoperative, head down view. **D:** Postoperative, head down view. **E:** Preoperative, basal view. **F:** Postoperative, basal view.

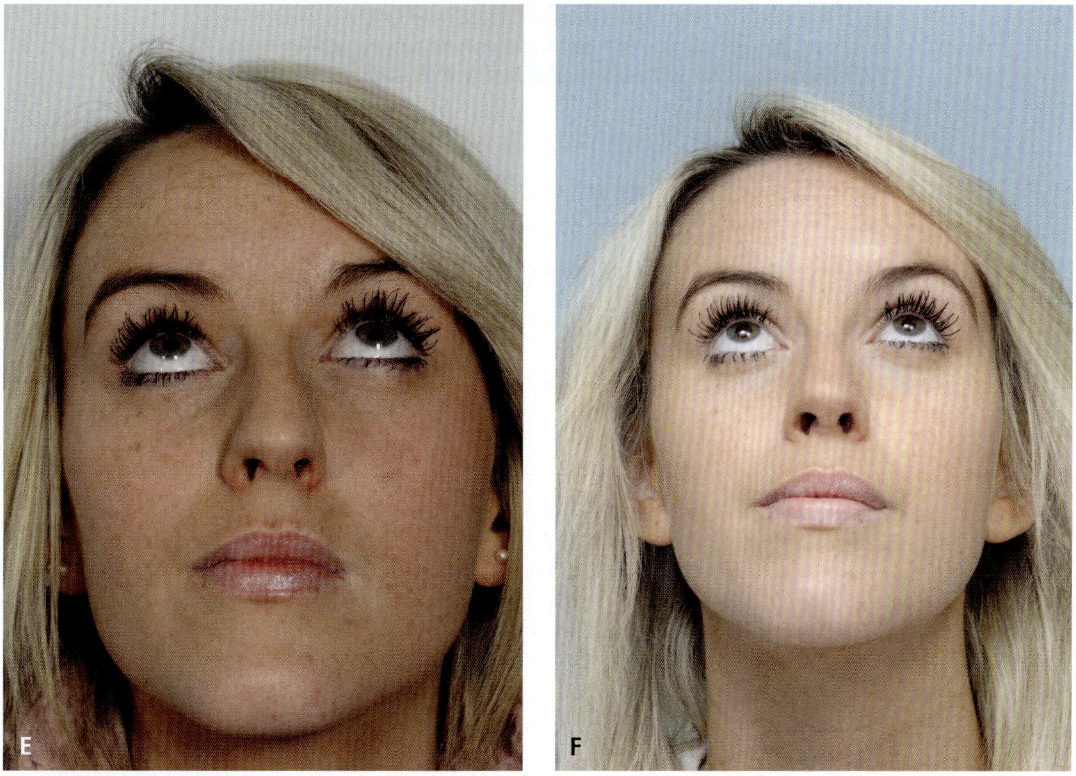

FIGURE 15.9 (*Continued*)

COMPLICATIONS

The complications are listed in Table 15.1. Complications are minimized by exacting and careful analysis and operative planning, careful patient selection, and comprehensive preoperative discussion explaining the risks limitations and unpredictability of surgery. Careful tissue handling, meticulous dissection, and good exposure aided by hypotensive anesthesia are essential. Exacting intraoperative anatomical assessment and surgical techniques that embrace reconstruction rather than resection with the maintenance of good caudal and dorsal septal struts and augmentation of tip support mechanisms with sutures and grafts are vital. Rarely does the patient with a crooked nose need any net loss of nasal skeleton tissue. Any cartilage removed that is not used for grafting or strengthening should be shaved, and divided if necessary, and replaced between the septal mucosal flaps. In my last series of rhinoplasties, the postoperative hemorrhage rate was 1.4% and the infection rate was 0.7%.

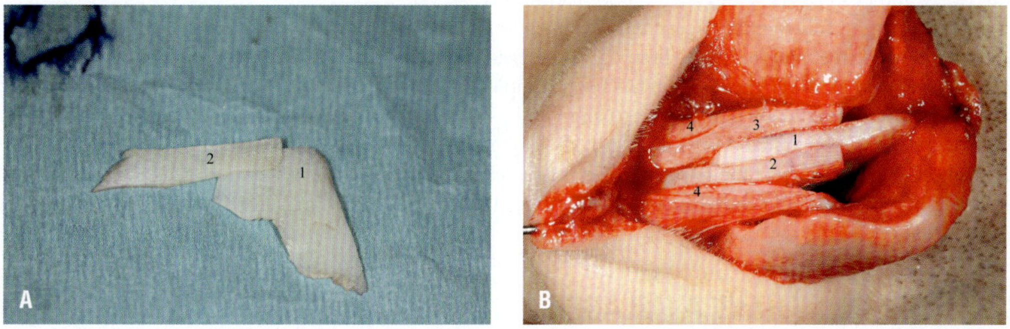

FIGURE 15.10 A: Extracorporeal construction of a new caudal septal strut with incorporated right spreader graft. *1*, New caudal septal strut; *2*, right spreader graft; *3*, remaining dorsal septal strut after caudal resection; *4*, upper lateral cartilages. **B:** The construction in situ. The new caudal strut is positioned to overlap the remaining dorsal strut on its right side. This dorsal strut was curved to the right prior to insertion of the grafts.

TABLE 15.1 Complications Associated with Septorhinoplasty for the Crooked Nose

- Primary hemorrhage
- Secondary hemorrhage which may occur up to 2 wk after surgery
- Infection
- New or residual aesthetic deformity
- New or residual functional disorder
- Visible scars
- Persistent skin—soft tissue swelling
- Skin changes
- Septal perforation
- Psychological morbidity

RESULTS

Surgical management of the crooked nose requires a meticulous review of the patient's desires, detailed facial analysis, and comprehensive photo imaging, for the development of an exacting surgical plan. Surgical aims should entail treatment of both aesthetic and functional concerns while remaining fluid enough to accommodate unforeseen anatomic findings intraoperatively. Postoperative expectations are best managed with appropriate preoperative discussions entailing surgical outcomes. Overall surgical success is contingent on proper nasal analysis and surgical expertise.

PEARLS

- Be sure you understand your patient's hopes and concerns and that you can meet their expectations.
- Recognize facial asymmetry preoperatively and explain it to the patient particularly as a limiting factor in achieving a straight nose (Fig. 15.9).
- In cases of facial asymmetry, aim to align the nose in the frontal view with the nasion, which is a fixed point and cannot be moved, rather than with the position of the columella.
- Recognize lateral wall asymmetries and concavities and disguise with onlay grafts if necessary.
- Intraoperatively pause to reassess the anatomy with the better exposure afforded, and in the light of the findings, reassess your primary operative plan.
- Recognize the crooked nose associated with tension nose deformity. These cases have higher risks of complications due to short nasal bones, narrow mid-thirds, and the excessive development of the quadrilateral cartilage.

PITFALLS

- Intrinsic curvature in the cartilaginous septum will not be corrected by releasing the quadrilateral cartilage inferiorly and posteriorly with a swing door technique.
- When performing full-thickness cartilaginous incisions for septal curvature release that extend to either the caudal or dorsal free margin, fix the bracing batten graft to the septum on one end of the incision prior to completing the incision. When the incision has been completed, the septal strut on either side of the incision is very mobile, and it is technically demanding to align and suture the graft accurately if one end has not been fixed.
- Outfracture of the medialized lateral nasal wall may not maintain a lateralized position of the bone.
- Dorsal reduction to correct the lateral profile in the crooked tension nose, when performed with osteotomies to straighten the nose and septal incisions to correct the quadrilateral cartilage, carries a high risk of septal disarticulation.

INSTRUMENTS TO HAVE AVAILABLE

- Septorhinoplasty tray

ACKNOWLEDGMENT

The author would like to thank Dr. Eugene Chu for his contributions in the writing of this chapter. His work in the writing, editing, and figure creation for this chapter is greatly appreciated, without which this chapter would not have been possible.

SUGGESTED READING

Daniel RK. Mastering rhinoplasty. In: Daniel RK, ed. *Functional factors*, 2nd ed. Berlin, Germany: Springer-Verlag, 2010:183–224.

Goldstein SA, ed. *The crooked nose facial plastic surgery*. New York, NY: Thieme Medical Publishers, 2011:27(5).

Gubisch W, Constantinescu MA. Refinements in extracorporeal septoplasty. *Plast Reconstr Surg* 1999;104:1131–1140.

Roofe SB, Murakami CS. Treatment of the posttraumatic and postrhinoplasty crooked nose. *Facial Plast Surg Clin North Am* 2006;14(4):279–290.

Tweedie D, Lo S, Rowe-Jones J. Reconstruction of the septum using perforated and non-perforated polydioxanone foil. *Arch Facial Plast Surg* 2010;12:106–113.

16

RHINOPLASTY PROFILE MANAGEMENT: THE TENSION NOSE

Edward H. Farrior

INTRODUCTION

Profile management in the tension nose encompasses almost all aspects of rhinoplasty. There is considerable work required within the bony and cartilaginous dorsum, nasal tip, caudal septum and dorsal septum, and frequently the anterior maxillary spine (Fig. 16.1). Thin skin covering the underlying skeletal abnormalities makes the care of these patients even more complex.

Reduction rhinoplasty will be necessary to correct the tension nose. This can be a disruptive procedure with interruption in the confluence of the cartilaginous dorsum (keystone), separation of the support mechanisms, and continuity of the lower lateral cartilage with division of the dome, as well as the possible resection of the anterior maxillary spine and caudal septum. All of these maneuvers create an unstable support system that must be recreated, reinforced, and redefined to achieve an ideal result.

HISTORY

Patients presenting with a high nose dorsum and tension nasal deformity must be able to identify and articulate their concerns and dislikes regarding their nose. If the patient cannot reasonably provide the surgeon with insight regarding what they perceive as unattractive, then it is unlikely that the surgeon will be able to correct their concerns. These concerns need not be expressed in an anatomically accurate description, but they do need to be able to describe their problems in layman's terms, even if vague. If they are unable to identify what makes their nose unattractive, then they will not be able to appreciate the results of a surgical intervention.

It is important to obtain an accurate head and neck history as well as general medical history. Nasal symptoms including obstruction, epistaxis, and rhinorrhea should be solicited as they may indicate an underlying pathology such as a deviation of the nasal septum, allergic rhinitis, nasal polyps, turbinate hypertrophy, or major extensive underlying pathology. A history of nasal trauma and previous nasal surgery could alter the course of surgical management and possibly require autologous grafting for structural support and reinforcement. General medical considerations such as hypertension, diabetes, bleeding disorders, or previous difficulty with anesthesia should be solicited. In the patient who has never undergone an anesthetic, a thorough family history regarding anesthesia complications is important.

Beyond the general medical history, it is imperative to assess three specific areas of the candidate for rhinoplasty: motivation, expectations, and psychological background. The patient should be self motivated and not seeking a rhinoplasty to please another individual. Expectations can be elicited by asking the patient to identify the unattractive portion of their nose and describe how they feel that it should be changed. Keeping the expectations realistic preoperatively will avoid hours of postoperative discussion. Communication throughout the entire course of patient care is important to ensure realistic expectations. The characteristics of the skin and the presence of preexisting facial asymmetries can frequently be overlooked in the preoperative discussion. If there are hints of psychological disorders, they should be pursued,

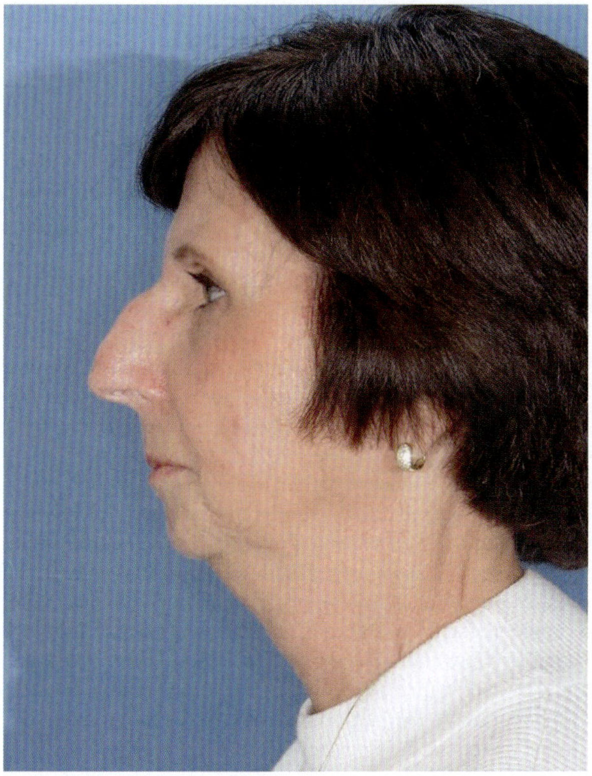

FIGURE 16.1
Clinical example of tension nose with overprojected nasal tip, a high bony and cartilaginous dorsum, an oblique nasal labial angle, and short upper lip.

not avoided. When the impression exists that a patient needs a more thorough psychological evaluation I make every effort to dissuade the patient from undergoing surgery because it becomes nearly impossible to discharge these patients from your practice postoperatively. Although rhinoplasty may help self-esteem, it will not correct true psychological disorders.

PHYSICAL EXAMINATION

Inspection of the face and nose initiates our evaluation of everyone's appearance in every encounter, in our office and on the street. This facial inspection is repeated throughout the consultation during natural animation, quiet respiration and extreme expression. Body language itself should be evaluated as it is an indication of the patient's self confidence, maturity, and understanding of the seriousness of a rhinoplasty procedure. If the patient cannot make eye contact and remains withdrawn, silly, or disinterested, they are probably not a good candidate for a rhinoplasty. Inspection provides insight to the strength, position, and length of the nasal cartilages. If the tip tripod is long in all dimensions, then some form of dome division will be necessary to accomplish shortening of all legs of the tripod, M-arch or C-ring complex.

Palpation of the nasal skeleton helps to provide an understanding of nasal structure and support. In the tension nose, there is frequently a discrepancy in the length of the nasal bones with the bony dorsum being slightly longer than the expected cephalic one third of the nose. Thickness of the nasal dorsum's cartilaginous confluence (Fig. 16.2) can be assessed on palpation and provides insight as to whether or not reconstruction of the middle vault, with either upper lateral cartilage turn-in flaps or spreader grafts, will be necessary to maintain

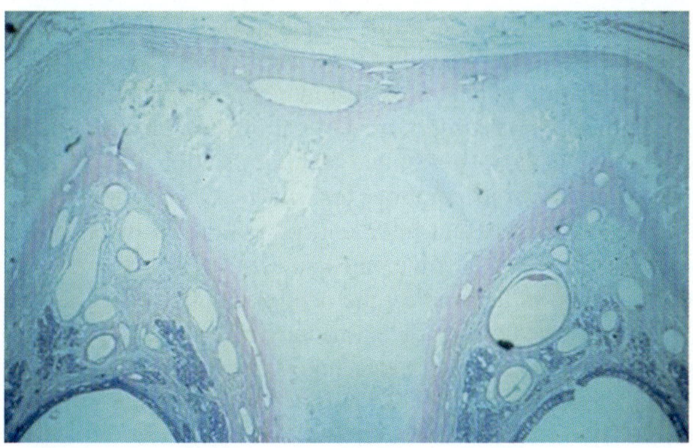

FIGURE 16.2
The nasal dorsum's cartilaginous confluence of the septum and the upper lateral cartilages.

a functional airway after reduction of the dorsum. Palpation of the nasal tip will provide information regarding the height, length, and resiliency of the lower lateral cartilages as well as the thickness of the skin of the nasal tip. The length of both the medial and lateral crus should be evaluated as well as evaluating their horizontal and vertical orientation.

Nasopharyngoscopy may be necessary in the patient with a history of recurrent sinusitis, epistaxis, or unilateral nasal obstruction that has limited anterior nasal findings. The surgeon must remain attentive to other pathologic conditions of the internal nose that may be present. In most cases, anterior rhinoscopy is sufficient and will reveal deviations of the nasal septum, high septal deflection, and abnormalities of the turbinates and nasal mucosa, which may contribute to postoperative nasal obstruction. If the nasal mucosa appears particularly atrophic, blanched, or traumatized, one must consider the possible overuse of vasoconstrictive agents or excessive digital manipulation. These behaviors will lead to an unfavorable postoperative recovery and possible complications.

There can be other abnormalities of the facial skeleton, such as microgenia and malar hypoplasia, which can exacerbate the appearance of a tension nose. These need to be demonstrated to and discussed with the patient preoperatively so the limitations they present are appreciated and they can be addressed in the final result.

Preoperative and postoperative photographs are of critical importance in patient history taking. Photographs provide an opportunity for more thorough preoperative evaluation and allow a more removed two-dimensional assessment of a three-dimensional structure. When evaluating the well-executed photographs in neutral lighting, some abnormalities will become more apparent because they are not overshadowed by facial animation. They also allow assessment of one's outcomes as well as providing physical evidence and documentation of improvement. There are six standard views and two supplemental views. The six standard views are a right and left lateral view, a right and left oblique view, and anterior view and a nasal base view (Fig. 16.3). These are supplemented, when appropriate, with smiling lateral views and a bird's eye view of the nasal dorsum. Ideally, these photographs should be taken in the absence of makeup, with the hair pulled back, and with the identical preoperative background. Photographs are taken with the patient in the Frankfort plane (Fig. 16.4).

INDICATIONS

If a patient's self-esteem and/or nasal airway can be improved with a rhinoplasty, then there is an indication to proceed with surgery. If you can achieve the defined "purpose and goal of cosmetic surgery as the enhancement of the human spirit by aesthetic considerations and technical manipulation of the physical body," then you have been successful surgically. The removal of the appearance of the nose as a distraction from other attractive features of the face, and the maintenance or creation of a patent airway, is what makes a rhinoplasty successful. However, realistic expectations of both the surgeon and the patient are essential and potentially underappreciated facets that can complicate the most elegant of undertakings.

Physical indications for hump reduction and release of the tension nose are most frequently represented by an overprojected nasal tip, with a high bony and cartilaginous dorsum, an oblique nasal labial angle, and short upper lip (Fig. 16.1). Variations in the thickness of the skin, rotation of the tip, width of the dorsum, and dimensions of the bony pyramid are common. Guidelines for nasal proportions and relationships are well described and should be applied realistically. The relative projection of the tip, as determined by Goode's method (Fig. 16.5), can be influenced by repositioning the nasion and lengthening the dorsum cephalically as well as by truly shortening the distance between the alar crease and tip. This is observed with radix augmentation to lengthen the nasal dorsum and with lowering of the radix to shorten the nasal dorsum.

CONTRAINDICATIONS

The most absolute contraindications to dorsal hump reduction and release of the tension nose are the presence of an underlying psychiatric disturbance that prevents the establishment of realistic expectations preoperatively. Psychological immaturity and an inability or unwillingness to listen would prevent me from proceeding with surgical intervention. To this date in my practice, this is the only nonmedical absolute contraindication I have encountered. Patients with medical conditions such as bleeding disorders, severe cardiovascular disease, or problems with anesthetics seldom seek rhinoplasty, although each is an absolute contraindication.

Relative contraindications usually center on socioeconomic considerations and surgical motivation. Some social issues that might influence the decision to proceed with surgical intervention include an individual's involvement in competitive sports, especially team sports that might involve physical contact such as football, soccer, and basketball. The decision to operate would also be influenced by the need for travel, especially if involving long distance or extreme changes in the climate. These contraindications may contribute to postponing surgery, but would not cause the patient to forego surgery completely. Because most rhinoplasty procedures are elective, financial considerations should also be weighed appropriately. To burden a patient financially for cosmetic concerns may result in an unhappy patient.

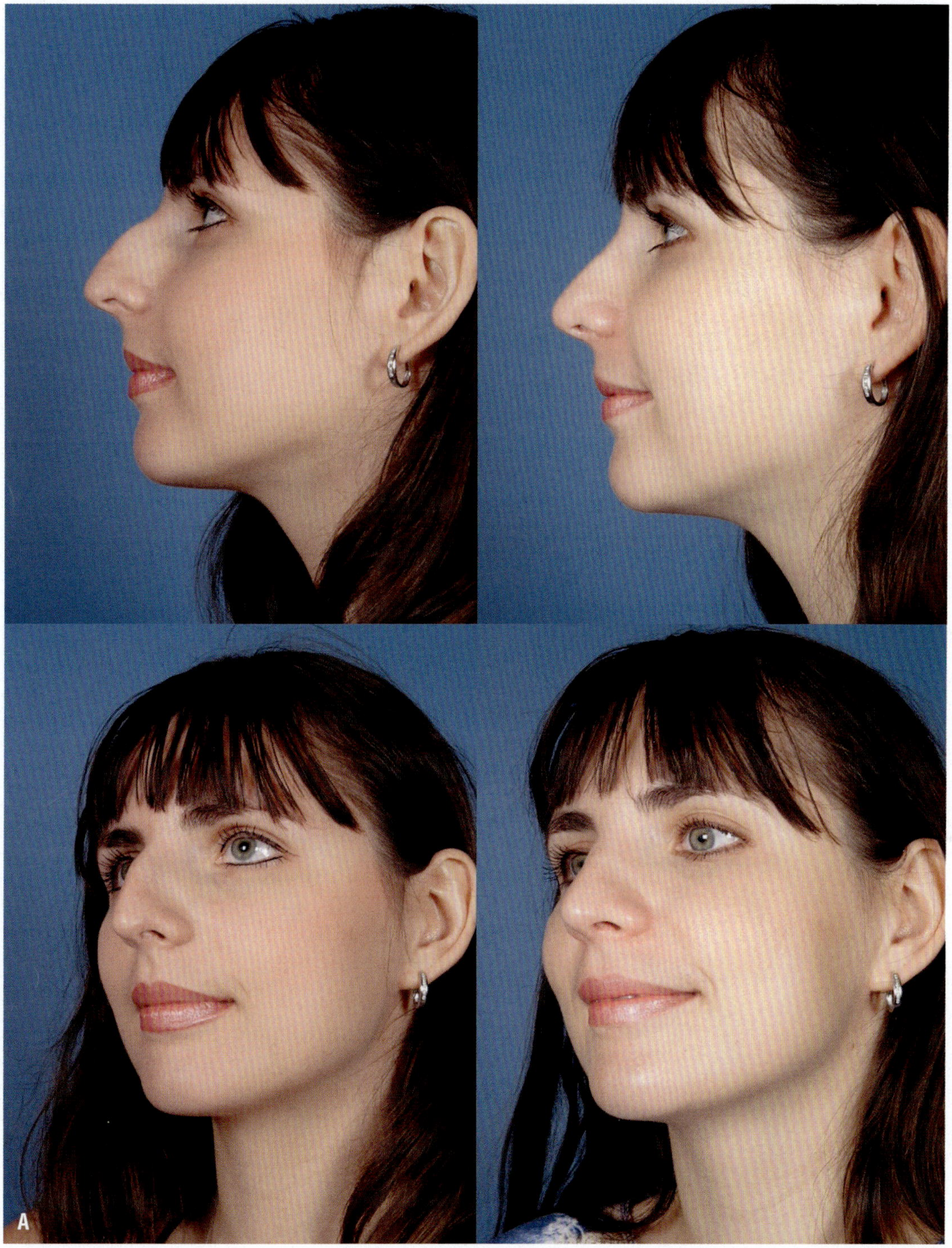

FIGURE 16.3 The six standard views for rhinoplasty imaging: right oblique and lateral views **(A)**, anterior and base views **(B)**, and left oblique and left lateral views **(C)**.

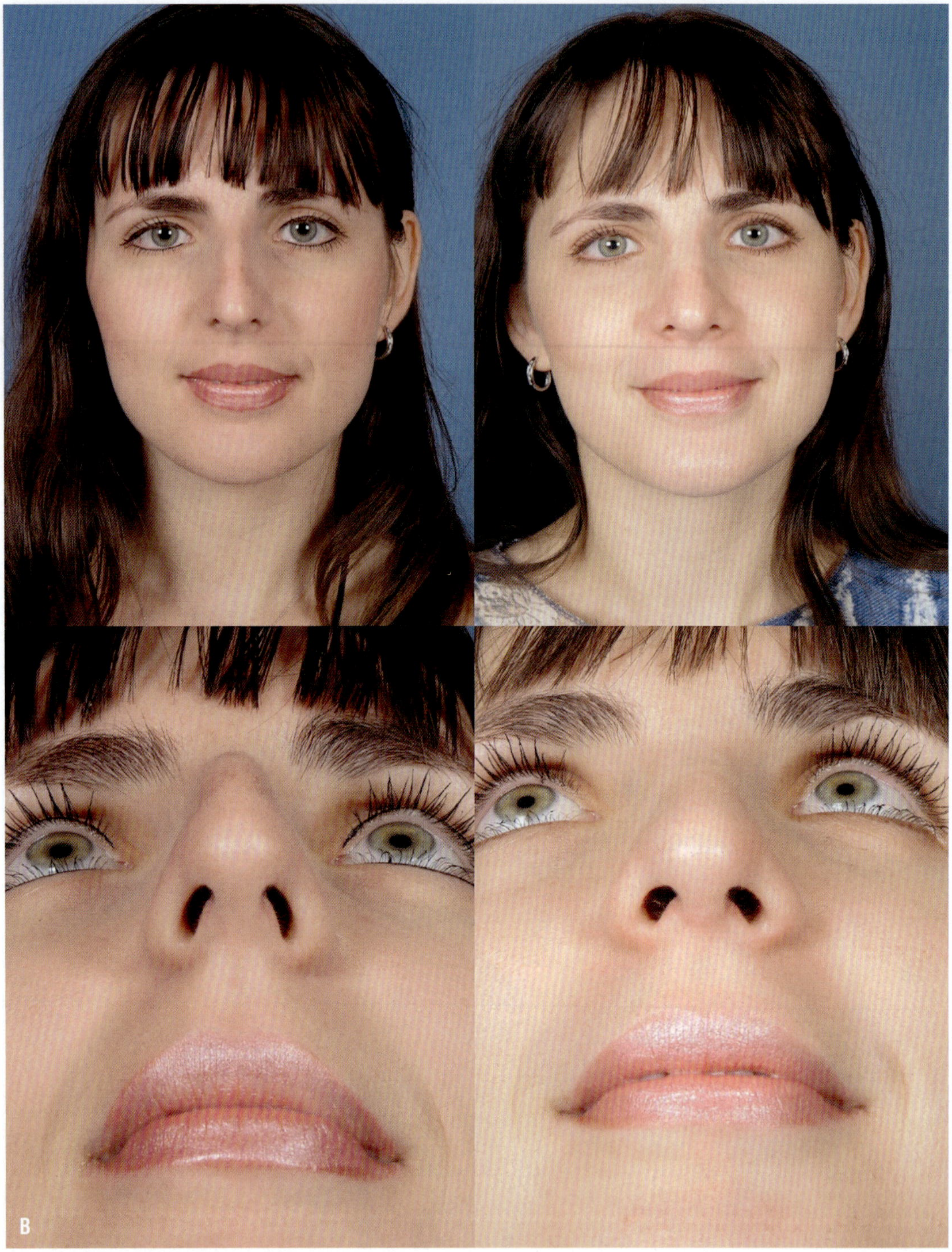

FIGURE 16.3 (*Continued*)

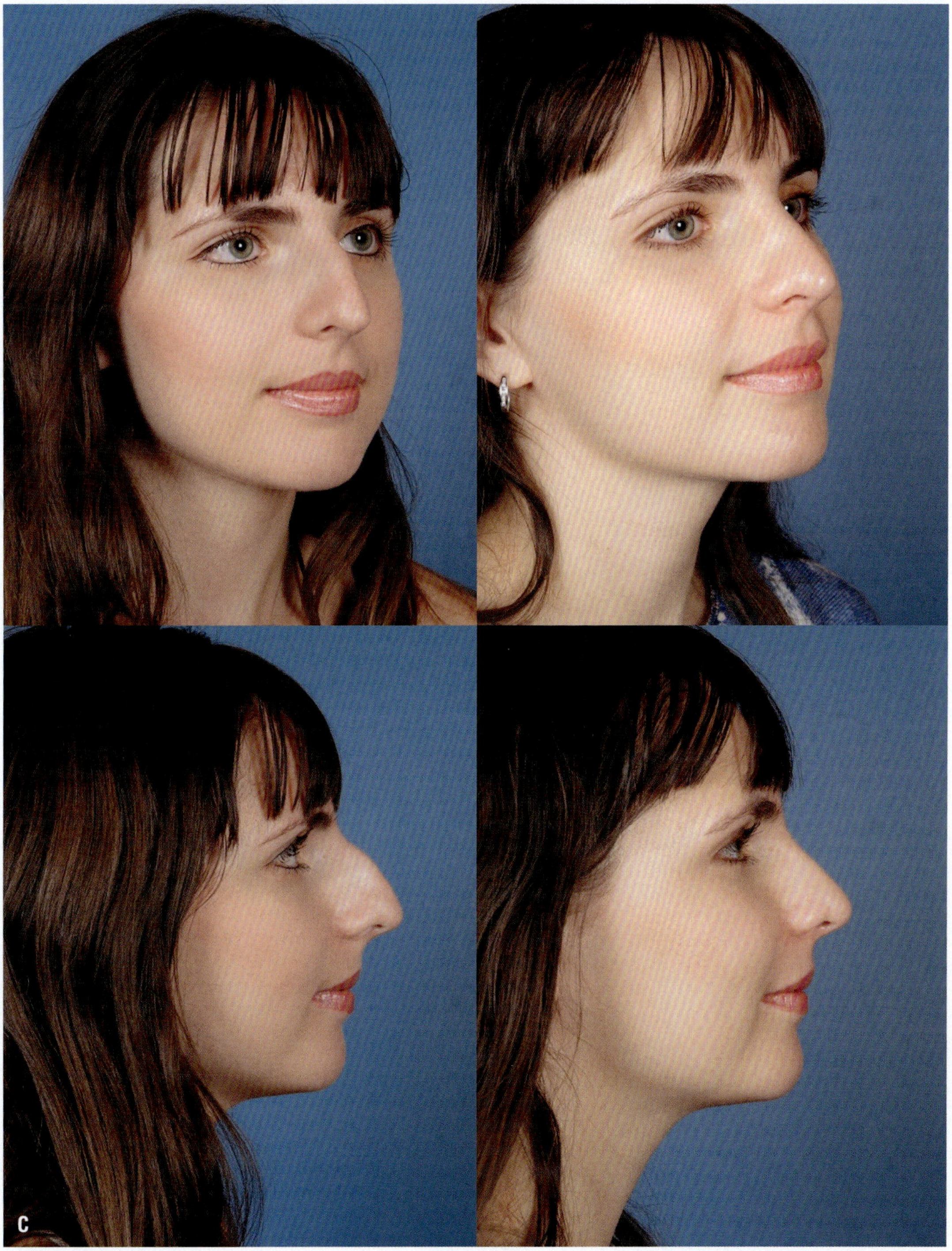

FIGURE 16.3 (*Continued*)

PREOPERATIVE PLANNING

Preoperative planning is nothing if not repetitive. This repetition occurs in private, during review of the history and physical examination as well as with the photographs. During the consultation, a plan is developed that explains the overall need to reduce the nasal dorsum and release tension on the nasal tip. The fundamental surgical principles are discussed in an effort to educate the patient regarding the seriousness and complexity of undertaking a rhinoplasty. Their photographs are reviewed with the patient in order to demonstrate the changes that will occur and the possible need for other more subtle changes to the nose that will contribute to the overall result. This is also an opportunity to point out associated facial abnormalities such microgenia, malar hypoplasia, and facial asymmetries that may or may not have been previously perceived by the patient. Digital imaging is almost always performed as part of my surgical planning exercise with the rhinoplasty patient. When altering

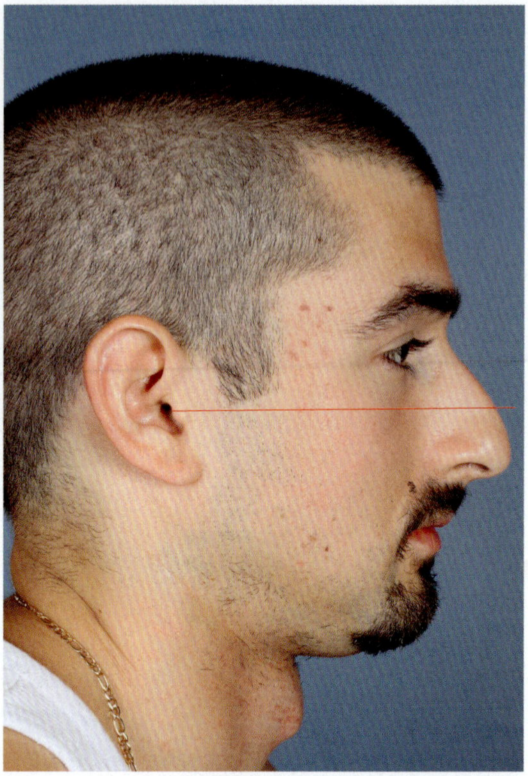

FIGURE 16.4
With the exception of base view images, all rhinoplasty images are to be taken in the Frankfort (horizontal) plane.

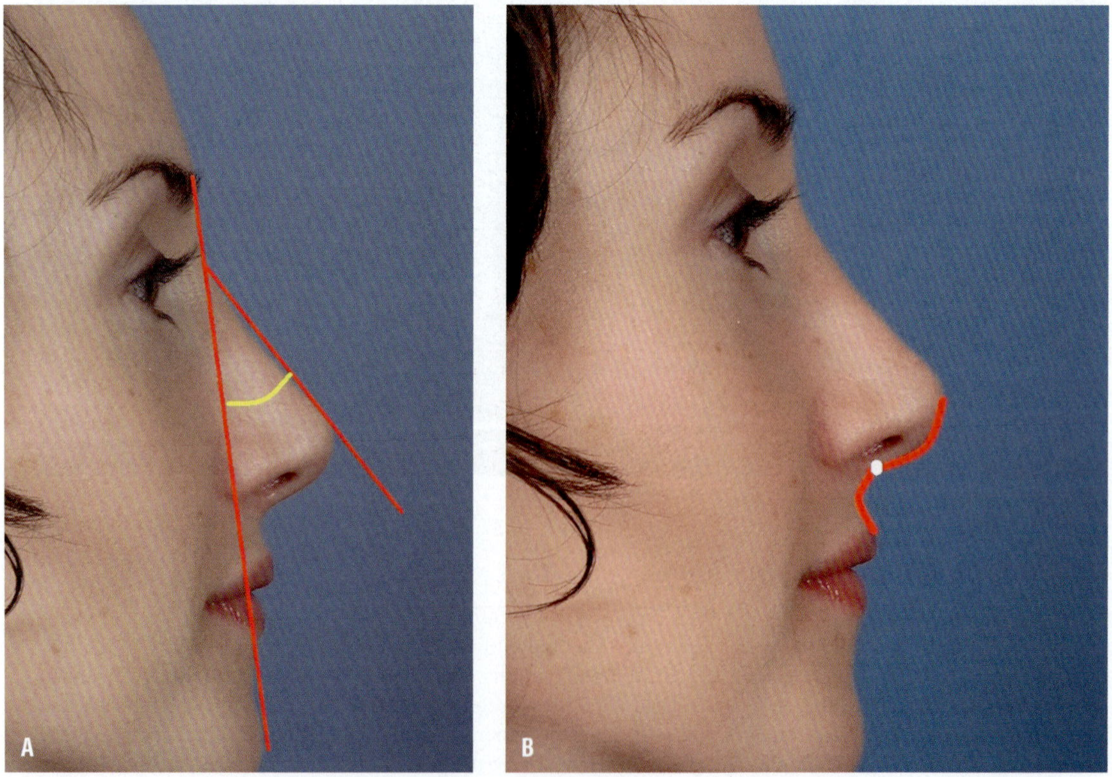

FIGURE 16.5 **A:** Daniel's analysis: line drawn from the vertical point in the ideal nasion to the ideal nasal tip and relating to the facial plane. Ideal nasofacial angles of 34 and 36 degrees in females and males, respectively. **B:** Simons ratio: nasal projection is approximately equal to the length of the upper lip with a ratio of 1:1. Although simple, the analysis has been criticized for underestimating the length of the subnasale.

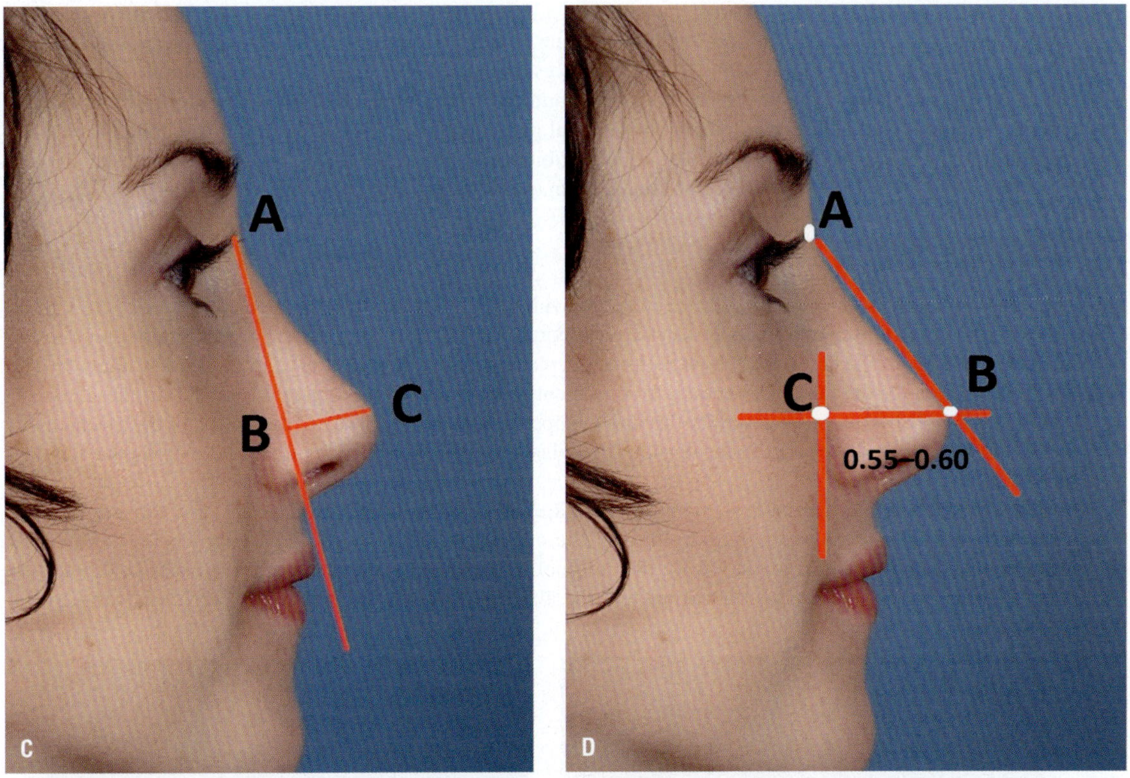

FIGURE 16.5 (*Continued*) **C:** Crumley I method: this method (and Crumley II) accounts for shortcomings that were perceived in the previously established techniques. The method is unique in that incorporates the upper lip (or chin for Crumley II) structures that affect the appearance of the nasal profile and not limiting assessment to only the nasal substructures. **D:** Goode's method: uses a triangle with the nasion and tip-defining point as landmarks that join at a 90-degree angle at the alar crease. The vertical axis is from the nasion (*A*) to the alar crease (*C*), while the horizontal axis is from the alar crease (*C*) to the nasal tip (*B*). The ratio of ala-tip: nasion-tip creating is 0.55 to 0.60.

the image with the computer, some subtleties of the existing deformity may become more evident such as alar retraction, a subtly deep radix that is camouflaged by a hump, an open nasolabial angle, broad alar base, and the more commonly observed broad bony pyramid and the nasal facial junction. The entire process of assessment and planning is repeated during the preoperative visit, in the holding area prior to surgery, and in the operating room prior to infiltration of local anesthesia.

From a more holistic standpoint, preoperative planning includes the elimination of nonsteroidal anti-inflammatory agents, nutritional supplements that may alter the coagulation pathway such as vitamin E, St. John's wort, ginger, ginkgo biloba, fish oil, and any other nonprescription medication at least 2 weeks (preferably 4 weeks) prior to surgery. Appetite suppressants, metabolic stimulants, and nasal decongestants should also be discontinued. The consumption of alcohol and the use of tobacco products must also be stopped. Excessive sun exposure is to be avoided.

Patients are counseled to arrange for postoperative care, around the clock, for 24 hours and to have someone available to assist them for 72 hours postoperatively. They are advised regarding postoperative diet, activities, and wound care and are encouraged to purchase the appropriate over-the-counter medications and supplies including food and beverages. All acute postoperative follow-up visits are scheduled at the time of scheduling the surgery.

SURGICAL TECHNIQUE

Anesthesia

My approach toward anesthesia has evolved as my appreciation for the complex nature of rhinoplasty has matured. General anesthesia with infiltration of a solution of lidocaine and epinephrine (1% lidocaine to 1:100,000 epinephrine) is now my choice in rhinoplasty procedures that require refinement of the tip and dorsum. This particularly applies to the tension nose where dome division and cartilage grafting, in addition to bone and septal work, may be required. By using a general anesthetic, there are no time constraints. The evolution of anesthetic agents, both amnestic and analgesic, to have a shorter duration of action has also helped tilt my approach toward the use of general anesthesia with a secure airway in the form of endotracheal intubation.

A minimum of 5 to 10 mL of local anesthesia is administered after the patient is anesthetized prior to the surgical prep. This includes the infiltration of the septum, which is performed in all cases even when septoplasty is not contemplated. Infiltration of the septum is necessary to achieve adequate vasoconstriction and hemostasis. Pledgets with topical epinephrine are placed onto the mucosa of the nasal cavity after infiltration, but prior to the prep. All pledgets used during the surgical procedure are moistened with topical epinephrine. The anesthesiologist is concurrently administering IV antibiotics. 1 g of cephalexin is used unless contraindicated by an allergy to penicillin then 300 mg of clindamycin or 500 mg of erythromycin is used.

Surgical Approach

The open approach is universally used for reduction rhinoplasty especially in the tension nose. There will be issues encountered with reestablishing structural support of the nasal dorsum at the bony cartilaginous junction after the resection of the keystone, which requires the placement of spreader grafts. In most cases, there will be a need to shorten the medial crus, lateral crus, or the entire tip tripod using dome division. All of these maneuvers are accomplished more successfully through the open approach. The issue of disruption of the mechanisms for tip support is one of the goals in the tension rhinoplasty as the support for the tip must be disrupted and then repositioned and secured.

The transcolumellar incision is made in the shape of a gull in flight (Fig. 16.6). This incision is made near the proximal portion in the middle third of the columella. Once the nose is deprojected, the incision will move proximally, and if made low on the columella, it could move too close to the nasolabial junction. After the transcolumellar incision is completed, the alar cartilage margin incision is performed (Fig. 16.6).

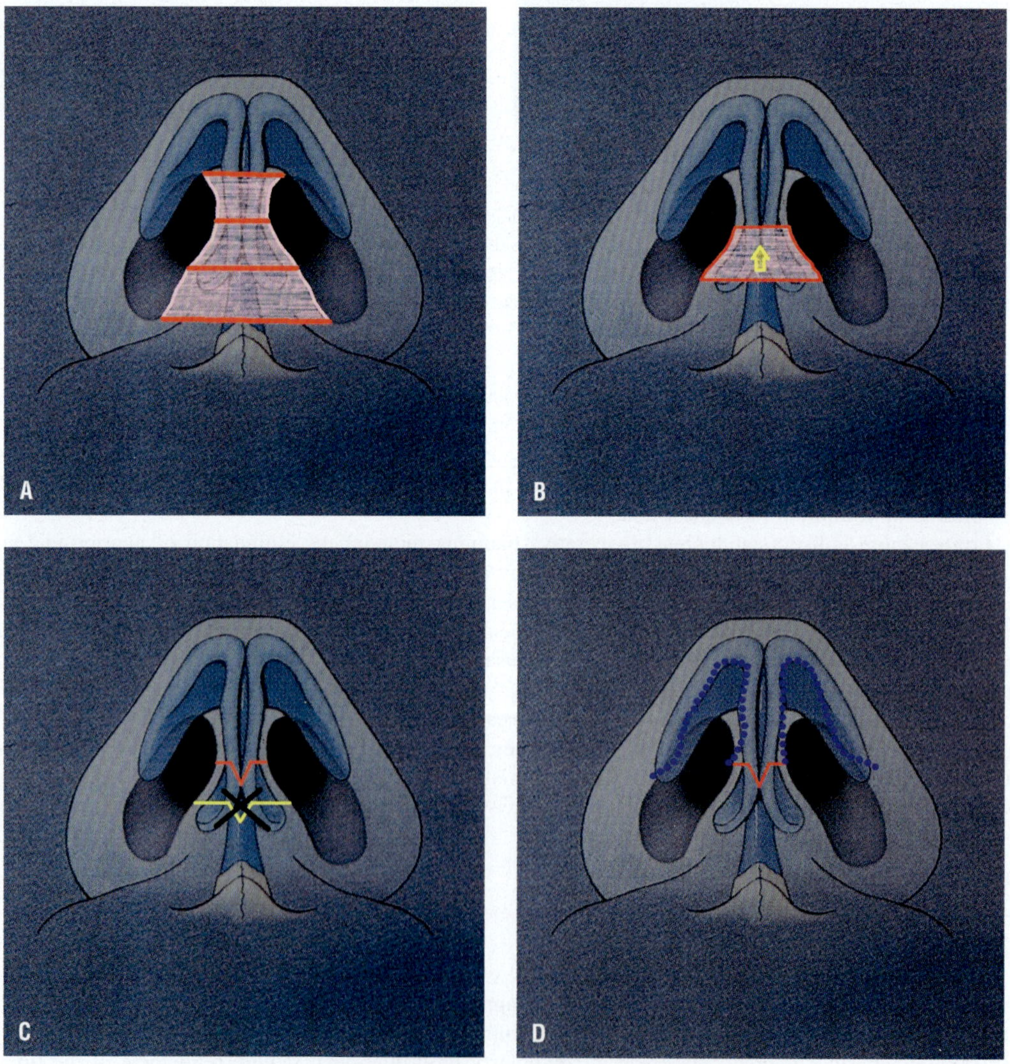

FIGURE 16.6 An analysis of where to place the transcolumellar incision. The primary goal is to shape the incision analogous to a "gull in flight." The columella is conceptually divided into equal thirds **(A)** with discarding of the upper and lower thirds **(B)**. **C:** The superior border along the middle third is chosen for the site of incision. **D:** From this point, marginal incisions along the distal border of the lower cartilages can be made.

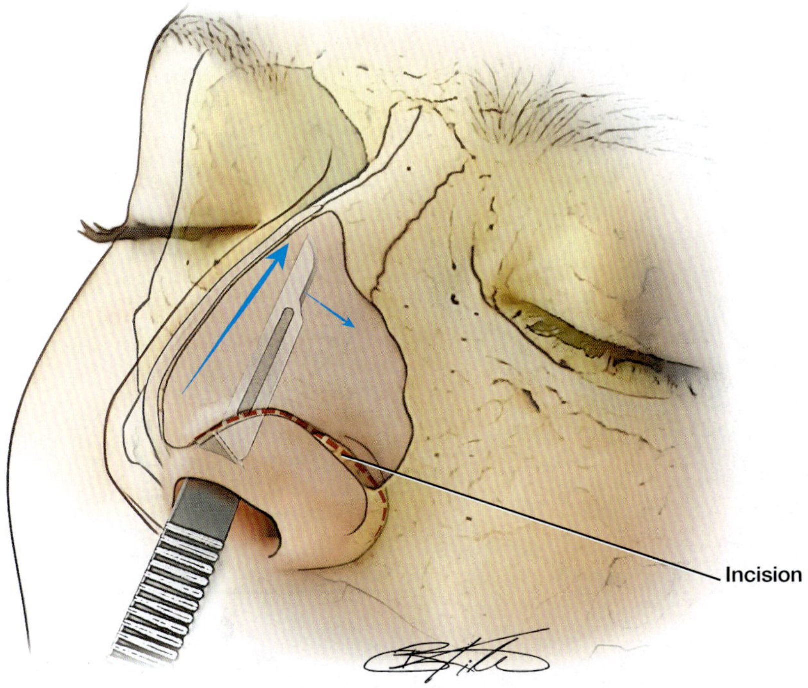

FIGURE 16.7
The perichondrium is scored at the anticipated level of the dorsal osteotomies and perichondrium elevated over the nasal dorsum only.

The lateral extent of this incision will be determined by the length and contour of the lateral crus. If excessively long, with an existing recurvature, then the lateral extent of the alar cartilage margin incision will be extended.

The soft tissue is elevated off the tip cartilages and nasal dorsum, beneath the SMAS (superficial muscular aponeurotic system) and adjacent to the perichondrium. The inferior margin of the perichondrium is scored at the anticipated level of the dorsal osteotomies and perichondrium elevated over the nasal dorsum only (Fig. 16.7). The tip cartilages are then released from the anterior septal angle using sharp dissection, which may include complete separation of the medial crura. The caudal septum is then identified, and incisions are made in the mucoperichondrium at the caudal margin of the septum bilaterally. Complete mucoperichondrial and mucoperiosteal flaps are elevated bilaterally (Fig. 16.8). This will assist in the preservation of the

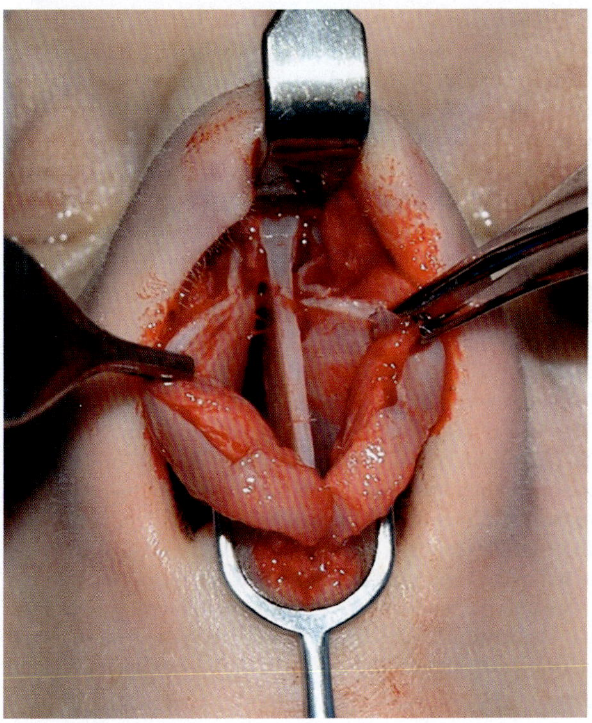

FIGURE 16.8
Complete mucoperichondrial and mucoperiosteal flaps are elevated bilaterally.

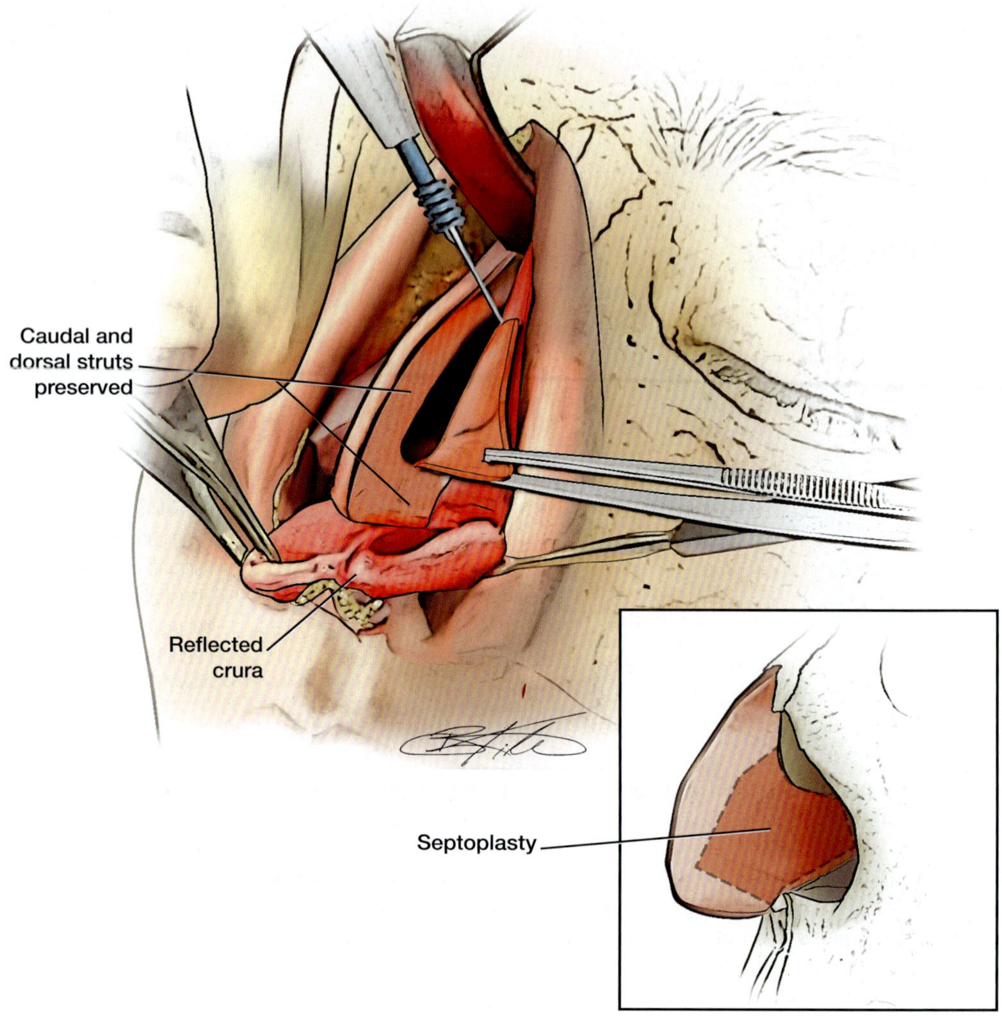

FIGURE 16.9 A septoplasty performed with the preservation of a dorsal and caudal strut.

mucoperichondrium when the cartilage is incised. It also allows the retrodisplacement and repositioning of these flaps when the nose is reduced avoiding the necessity of resecting septal mucosa after reduction. The mucoperichondrium and mucoperiosteum is also elevated beneath the nasal dorsum including the upper lateral cartilages and bony dorsum. This is done in an effort to preserve separation between the nasal cavity and nasal dorsum. It also helps to achieve stability during the repair and healing process.

The septoplasty is then performed with the preservation of a dorsal and caudal strut (Fig. 16.9). The cartilage is separated from the bony septum using a Cottle elevator. The cartilage is then incised above the deflection paralleling the nasal dorsum and 1 cm posterior to the caudal margin of the septum. These incisions intersect preserving at least 1 cm of dorsal and caudal strut. If there is tension on the caudal septum creating a caudal dislocation, the caudal strut is separated from the nasal spine, shortened appropriately, and reapproximated to the anterior maxillary spine using a 5-0 clear nylon suture.

The desired dorsal height and angulation is then determined. The upper lateral cartilages are then incised preserving the height of their distal segment. The height of the distal upper lateral cartilages is preserved, but they are released from the septal cartilage. The delayed release of the upper lateral cartilages is to preserve their stability during their proximal incision. If they are released prematurely, the accuracy of symmetric incision and reduction will be more difficult. After the upper lateral cartilages are released from the cartilaginous dorsum, reduction is extended through the dorsal quadrangular cartilage. The caudal margin of the septum will be incised in continuity with dorsal reduction if it is deemed necessary (Fig. 16.10). The Rubin osteotome is then inserted and the inferior margin of the nasal bones engaged (Fig. 16.11). The osteotome is then guided in a more superficial direction to avoid overresection of the bony dorsum. Because the nasal bones are thickest immediately beneath the nasal dorsum, the tendency is for the osteotome to dive into the thinner lateral portion of the nasal bones, predisposing to overresection. At this point, further incremental reduction of the cartilaginous dorsum will be performed to achieve the desired dorsal contour and height (Fig. 16.12).

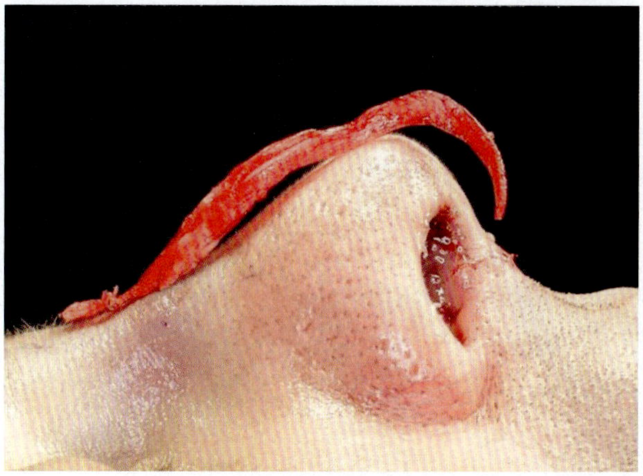

FIGURE 16.10
The caudal margin of the septum incised in continuity with dorsal reduction.

Tip refinement is now undertaken to match the nasal dorsum. The cephalic border of the lateral crus is trimmed as necessary preserving a minimum of 6 to 8 mm at the dome (Fig. 16.13). In the tension nose, with elongated medial crura, dome division with resection of a portion in the medial and lateral crura may be necessary (Fig. 16.14). This is performed in continuity with trimming of the cephalic margin. When the medial crura are not elongated, a medial crural setback and repositioning onto the caudal septum can achieve shortening of the central leg of the tripod. This technique avoids the resection of the dome cartilage. Dome division with resection of a portion of the lateral and intermediate crus may also be necessary when significant asymmetries exist in the lower lateral cartilage (Fig. 16.15). When tip contour is symmetric, the facet is aesthetically pleasing, and the medial crura are not elongated, medial crural repositioning with lateral crural

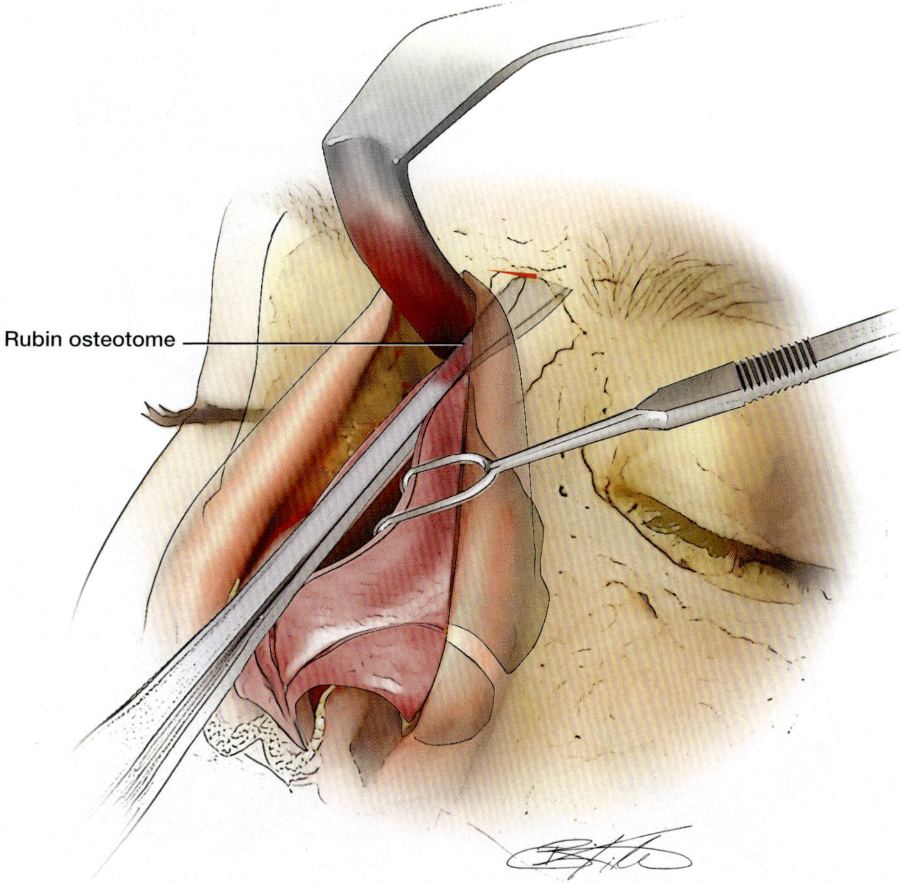

FIGURE 16.11 Engagement of the inferior margin of the nasal bones with a Rubin osteotome.

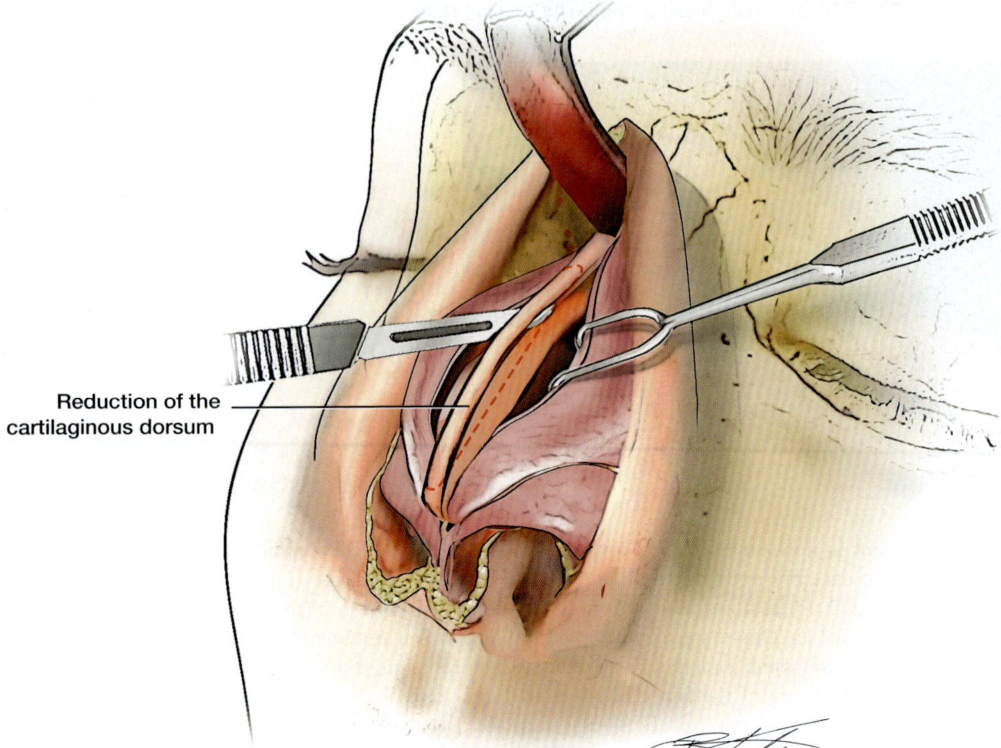

A

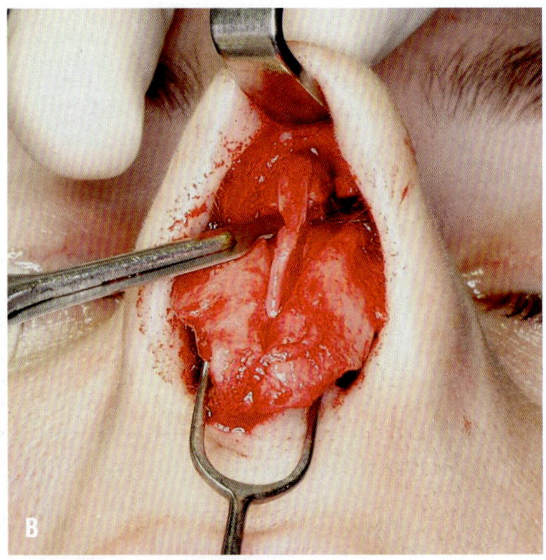

FIGURE 16.12
The incremental reduction of the cartilaginous dorsum is performed to achieve the desired dorsal contour and height. (**A**, illustration; **B**, photograph of operation.)

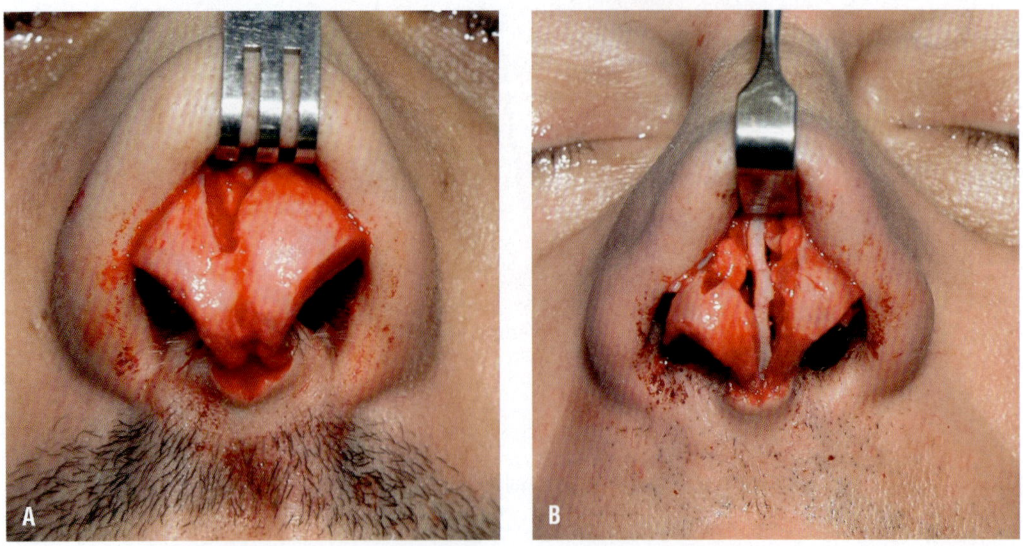

FIGURE 16.13 **A, B:** Trimming of the cephalic border along the lateral crus with preservation of a rim strip at the dome.

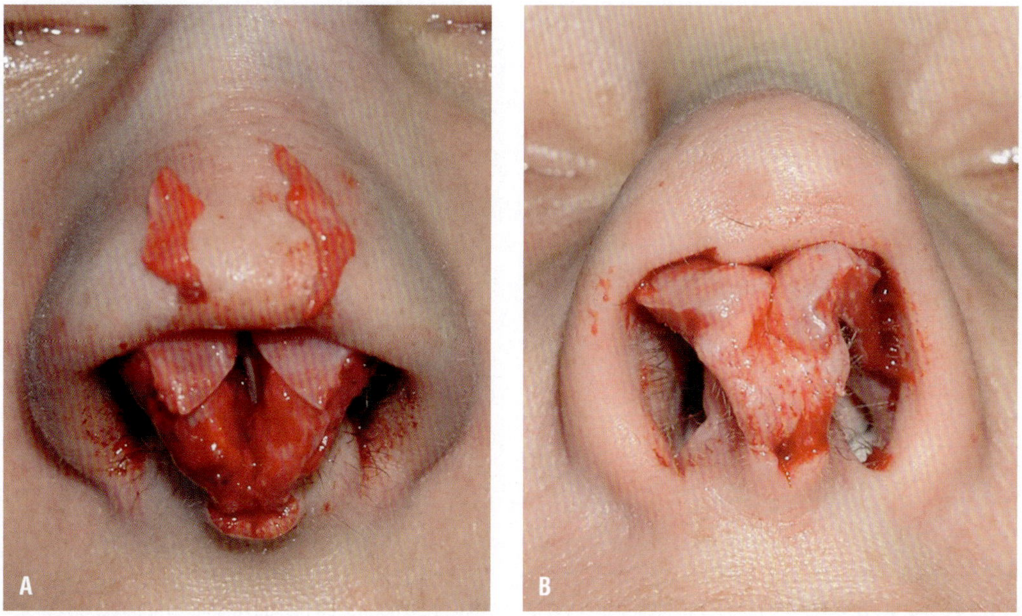

FIGURE 16.14 A, B: A tension nose with elongated medial crura where dome division, with resection of a portion of the medial and lateral crura, was necessary.

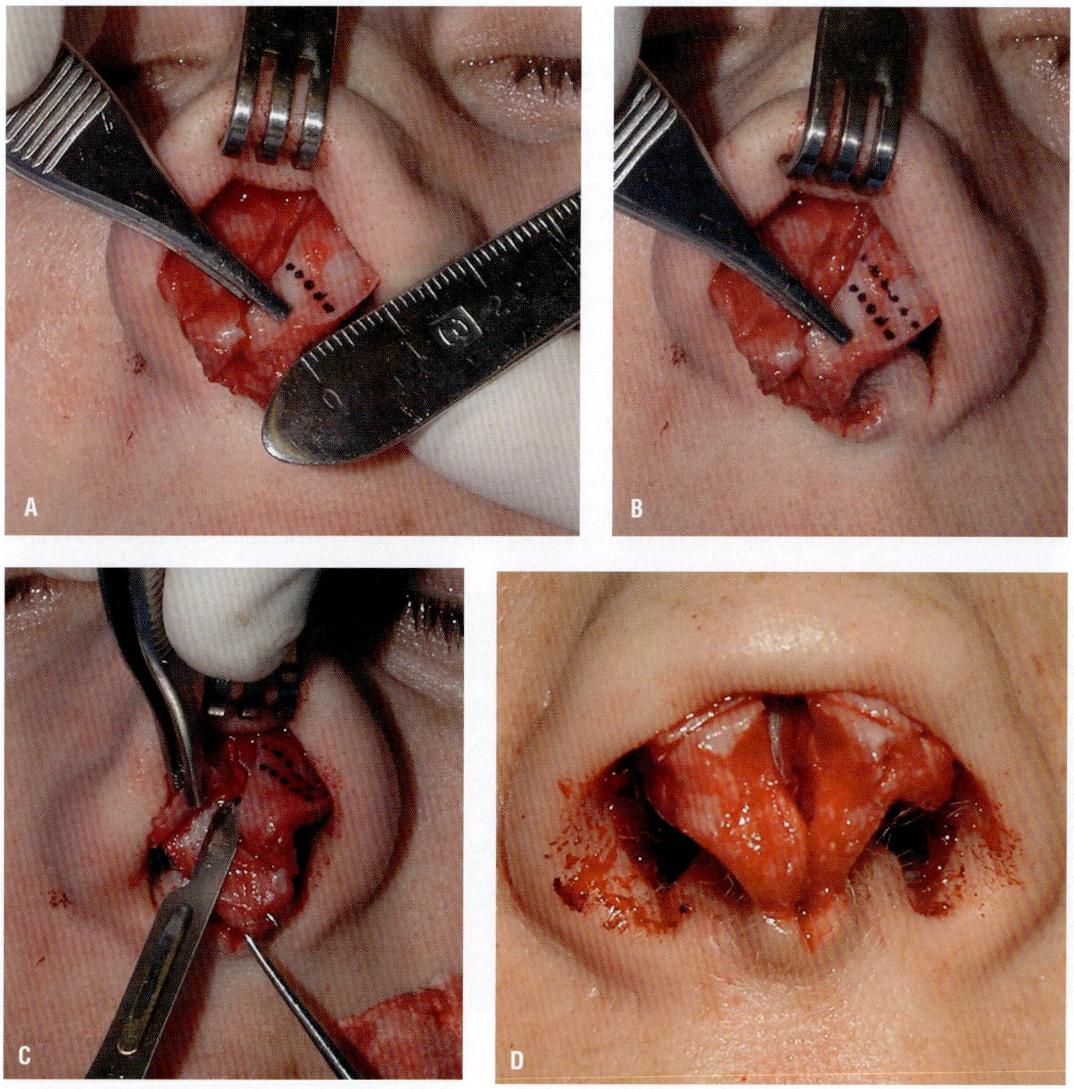

FIGURE 16.15 A–D: Dome division with resection of a portion of the lateral and intermediate crus may also be necessary when significant asymmetries exist in this portion of the lower lateral cartilage.

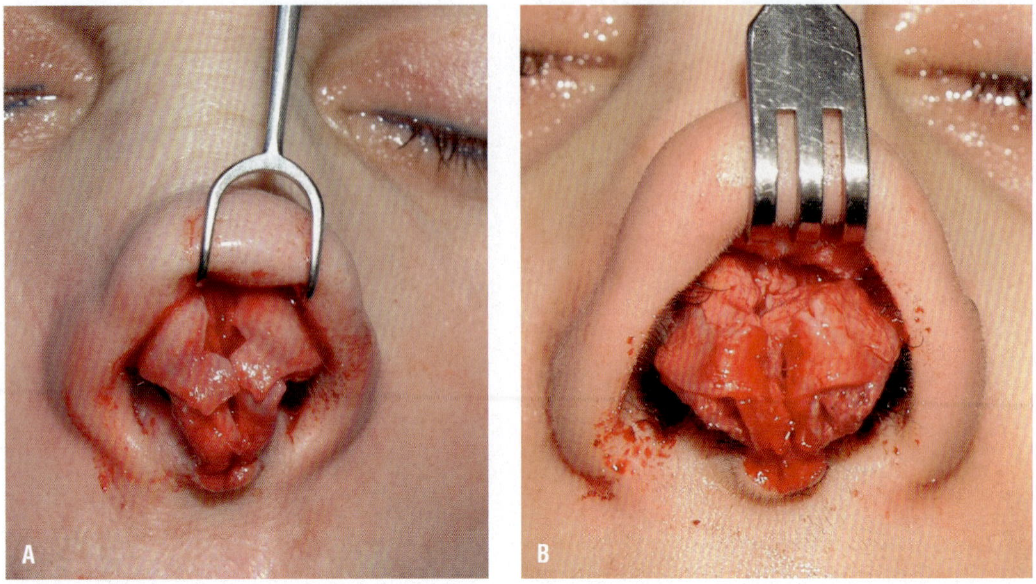

FIGURE 16.16 A, B: When tip contour is symmetric and the medial crura are not elongated, medial crural repositioning with lateral crural flap can be performed.

flap is undertaken (Fig. 16.16). This achieves shortening of all legs of the tripod while preserving the dome, in particular the caudal margin of the lower lateral cartilages of the dome. If the tip cartilages had been divided laterally, medially, or at the dome, the medial and lateral segments are reapproximated at this time with a 6-0 Maxon suture on a tapered needle. The lower lateral cartilages are not reapproximated in the midline until after the cartilaginous dorsum is reconstructed.

At this point in the rhinoplasty, spreader grafts are fashioned for the maintenance of the nasal airway as correction of the tension nose is a reductive technique. They are cut from the straightest segment of harvested septal cartilage. The spreader grafts are then divided and tapered at the superior segments, which extends under the bony cartilaginous junction of the nasal dorsum. The dorsal segment of the spreader graft is the common side of the divided cartilaginous segment. This assures that the width of the spreader grafts at the dorsum will be identical and any concavity or convexity can be used in an opposing fashion (Fig. 16.17). The spreader grafts are approximated to the quadrangular cartilage with two to three horizontal mattress sutures of 6-0 Maxon. After the spreader grafts are secured, the upper lateral cartilages are repositioned and sutured to the spreader grafts and quadrangular cartilage with the same horizontal mattress suture.

Once the dorsal architecture is secured, the cephalic margin of the intermediate crus of the lower lateral cartilages is stabilized using a dome suture and/or medial crural fixation suture (Fig. 16.18). This is performed in order to define the degree of columellar show and tip projection and equalize the domes. When appropriate, suturing the medial crura to the caudal septum is preferred to the use of a columellar strut (Fig. 16.19). This creates a more stable and reliable support mechanism for the tip cartilages. Caution is advised in this maneuver as miscalculations are unforgiving. If additional caudal septum is required, then a caudal septal extension graft

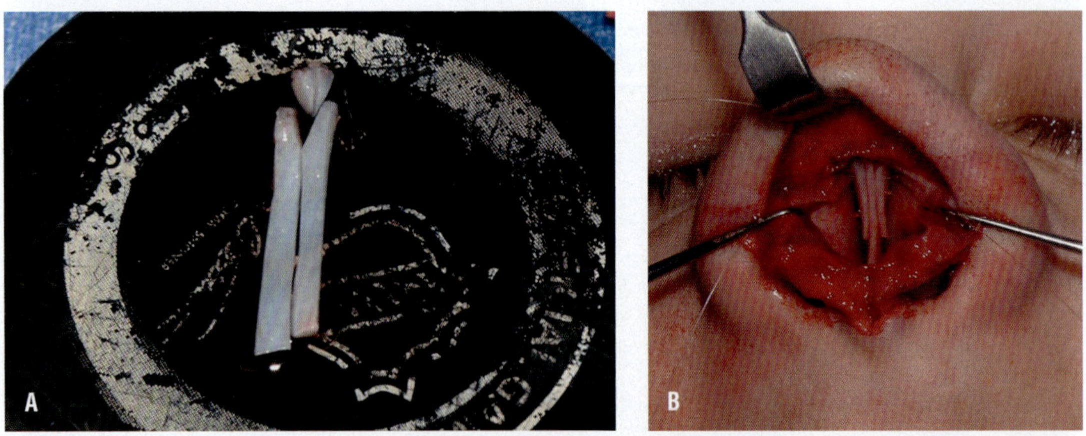

FIGURE 16.17 A: The dorsal segment of the spreader graft is the common side of the divided cartilaginous segment. This assures that the width of the spreader grafts at the dorsum will be identical and any concavity or convexity can be used in an opposing fashion **(B, C)**.

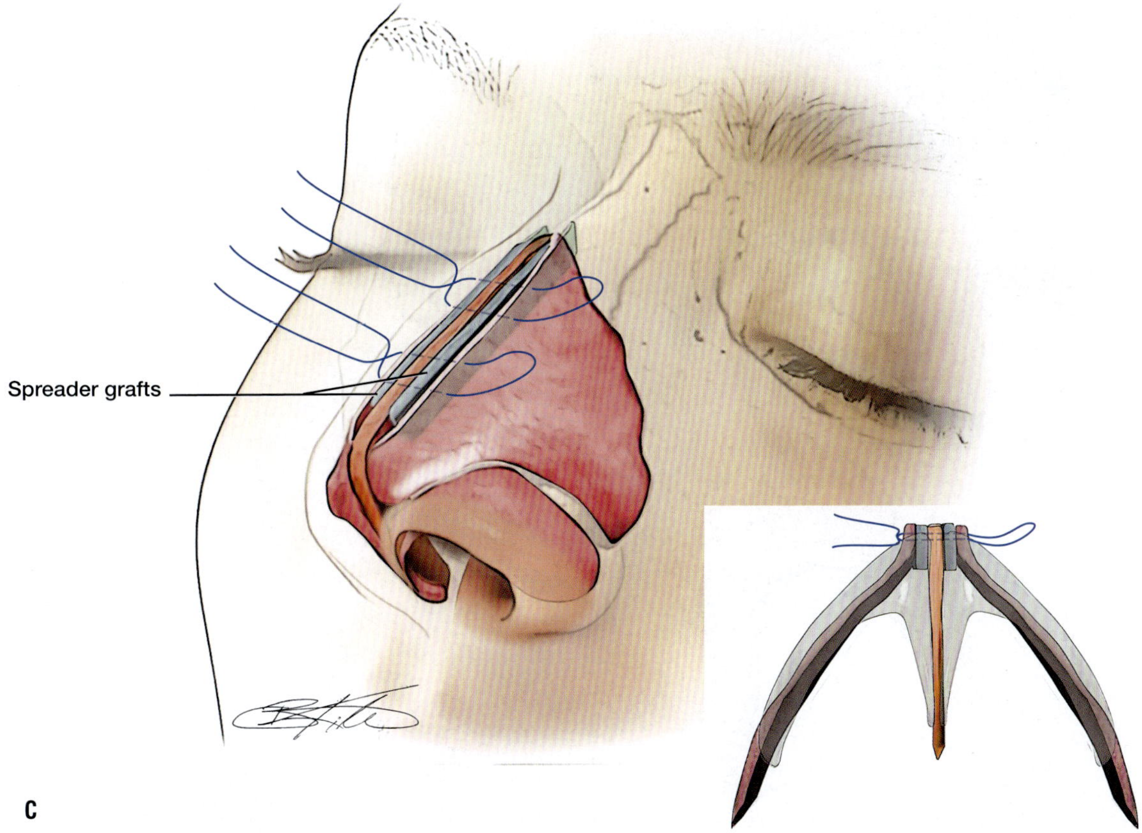

C

FIGURE 16.17 (*Continued*)

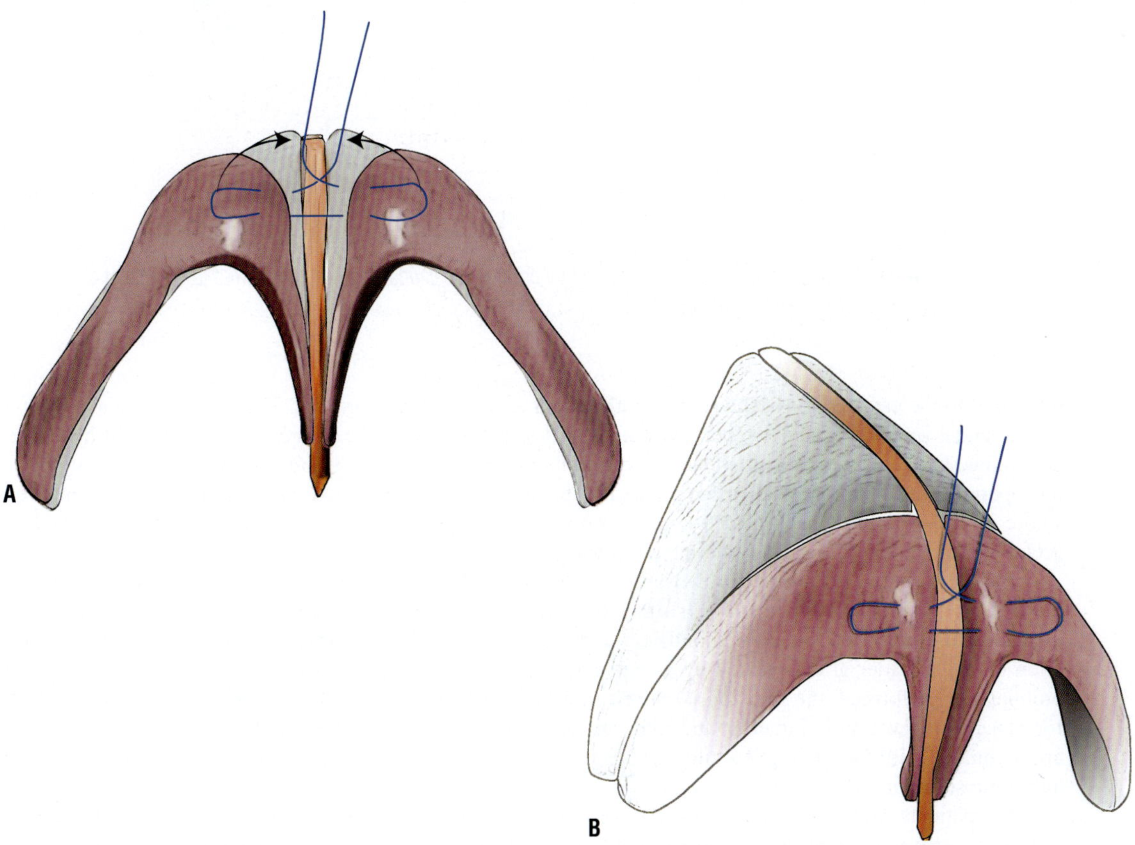

FIGURE 16.18 A, B: Suture stabilization along the cephalic margin of the intermediate crus of the lower cartilages. This helps to define the degree of columellar show, tip projection, and equalize the domes.

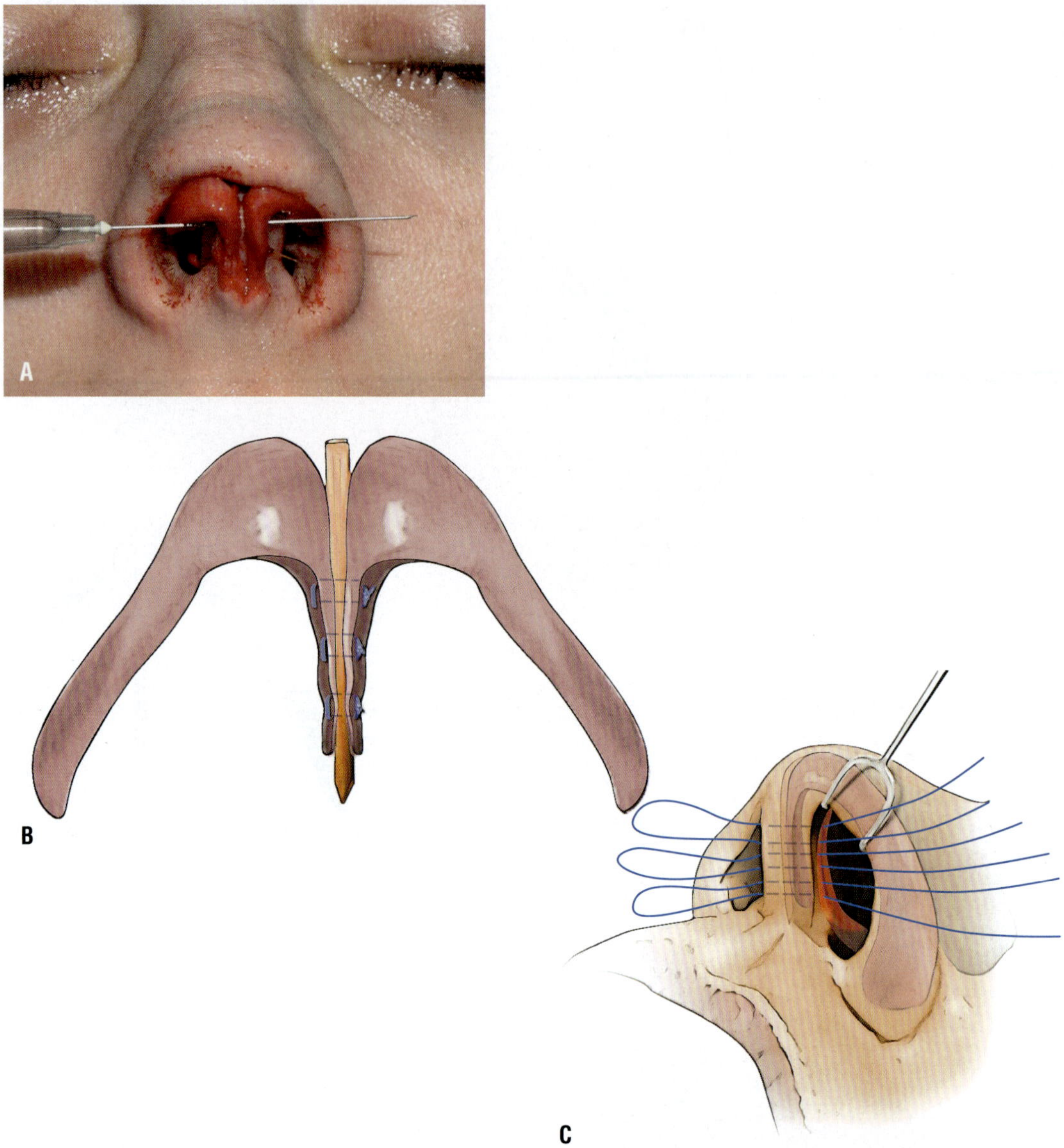

FIGURE 16.19 A–C: When appropriate, suturing the medial crura to the caudal septum is preferred to the use of a columellar strut (tongue-in-groove technique).

is sutured to the caudal strut of the septum rather than using a columellar strut. The medial crura are secured to the caudal septum or caudal septal extension graft with a 4-0 chromic suture. Tip rotation will have been determined by the degree of shortening of the lateral crus. When the tip is stabilized to the caudal septum, the mucoperichondrial flaps are then approximated to the quadrangular cartilage with a running, quilting, mattress suture of 4-0 chromic. This is placed with the retrodisplacement of the mucoperichondrial flaps to avoid the accumulation of soft tissue at the internal nasal valve.

Medial osteotomies are performed prior to closure of the transcolumellar incision. This allows placement of the osteotome from the dorsal surface of the nose. Performing the medial osteotomies in this fashion avoids disruption of the mucoperichondrium and mucoperiosteum as well as avoiding the possible subluxation of the spreader grafts created by a transnasal/transmucosal medial osteotomy. After the medial osteotomies are performed, the incision is closed in a layered fashion using subcutaneous 6-0 Maxon sutures for closure of the transcolumellar and alar cartilage margin incisions. The epidermis of the columella is approximated with 6-0 plain gut sutures. After the incisions are closed, the surgical wound is irrigated with antibiotic solution.

For patients who have had resection of the dome with shortening of the medial and lateral crus, a morselized tip graft will be fashioned and secured to the inferior margin of the lower lateral cartilages to camouflage the reconstructed rim. If there is marked recurvature of the lateral crus, an alar batten will be sutured to the lateral crus extending beyond the recurvature (Fig. 16.20).

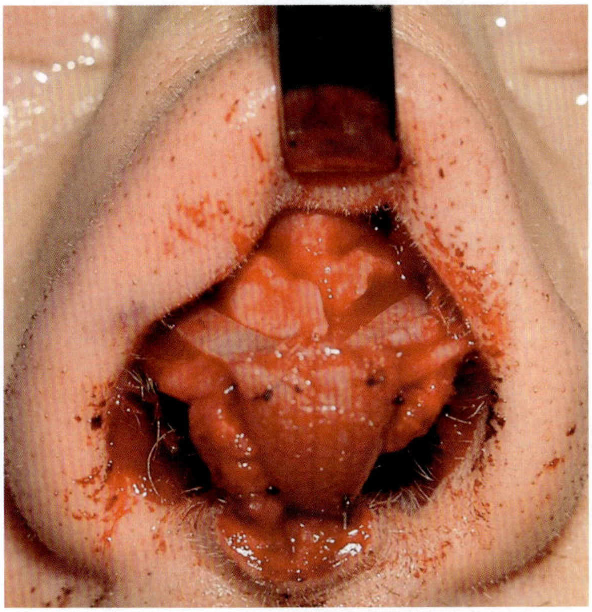

FIGURE 16.20
Correction of marked recurvature of the lateral crus with alar batten grafts that are sutured to the lateral crus extending beyond the recurvature.

Lateral osteotomies are performed after the closure of all incisions. This allows the immediate placement of the surgical dressing after the osteotomies are performed, a maneuver aimed at reducing ecchymosis and edema. The site of the lateral osteotomy is infiltrated with lidocaine and epinephrine prior to performing the medial osteotomies. A stab incision is made in the pyriform aperture at the level of the attachment of the inferior turbinate. The Joseph elevator is used to create a subperiosteal tunnel at the site of the lateral osteotomy. A freshly sharped 2-mm osteotome is used. The osteotomy is performed as a linear osteotomy inferiorly and a perforating osteotomy superiorly (Fig. 16.21). A complete back fracture is created with the intent of completely mobilizing the lateral segments of the bony pyramid. If intermediate osteotomies are performed, it is accomplished before the lateral osteotomy and at a position two-thirds of the way from the site of the lateral osteotomy to the dorsum.

Nasal Dressing

The nasal dressing cannot accomplish the desired surgical result but can splint and reinforce the subcutaneous structural components. The nasal dressing is approached in a layered fashion. After the skin is cleaned and dried, Mastisol is applied to assist in the adherence of the tape. A strip of 1-inch neurosurgical pledget is cut to extend from the supratip to the nasion. This is placed on the nasal dorsum to provide adequate compression along the dorsum as well as to assist in the ease of removal of the splint 1 week postoperatively. After taping is performed, an Aquaplast splint is applied. Getting the splint to solidify can be expedited by the use of gauze soaked in ice water. After solidification, the splint is secured to the glabella and cheeks with flesh colored 3M Micropore tape.

No internal nasal packing is used unless uncontrolled bleeding is present or nasal collapse occurs after the osteotomies. When it is necessary to pack the nose, a sleeve of a nonadhesive Telfa® dressing is created, and strips of Expandacell nasal packing® (Shippert Medical) are stacked within the sleeve. If packing is placed, it is removed on the first postoperative day and is removed as individual components (i.e., each strip of the nasal packing removed separately followed by the Telfa® sleeve).

POSTOPERATIVE MANAGEMENT

During the acute 3-week postoperative phase, the patient is instructed to avoid all physical exertion, sleep with the head elevated, not blow or digitize the nasal cavity, and only wear glasses when the splint is present. Once the splint is removed, glasses cannot be worn for 6 weeks postoperatively. The alar margin and transcolumellar incisions are to be cleaned twice a day, or more often as necessary, with hydrogen peroxide followed by the application of antibiotic ointment. I now use an antibiotic ointment, which covers methicillin-resistant *Staphylococcus aureus*. Postoperative oral antibiotics are also provided for 8 days following the surgery.

The patient is seen frequently during the first 10 postoperative days. The first postoperative visit occurs at 24 to 48 hours after surgery. Nasal packing, if present, is removed at this time. The nasal cavity is debrided. This is performed after using a topical decongestant. The nasal incisions are also cleaned and postoperative instructions are again reviewed with the patient. The next visit takes place on postoperative day 7. The nasal cavity is

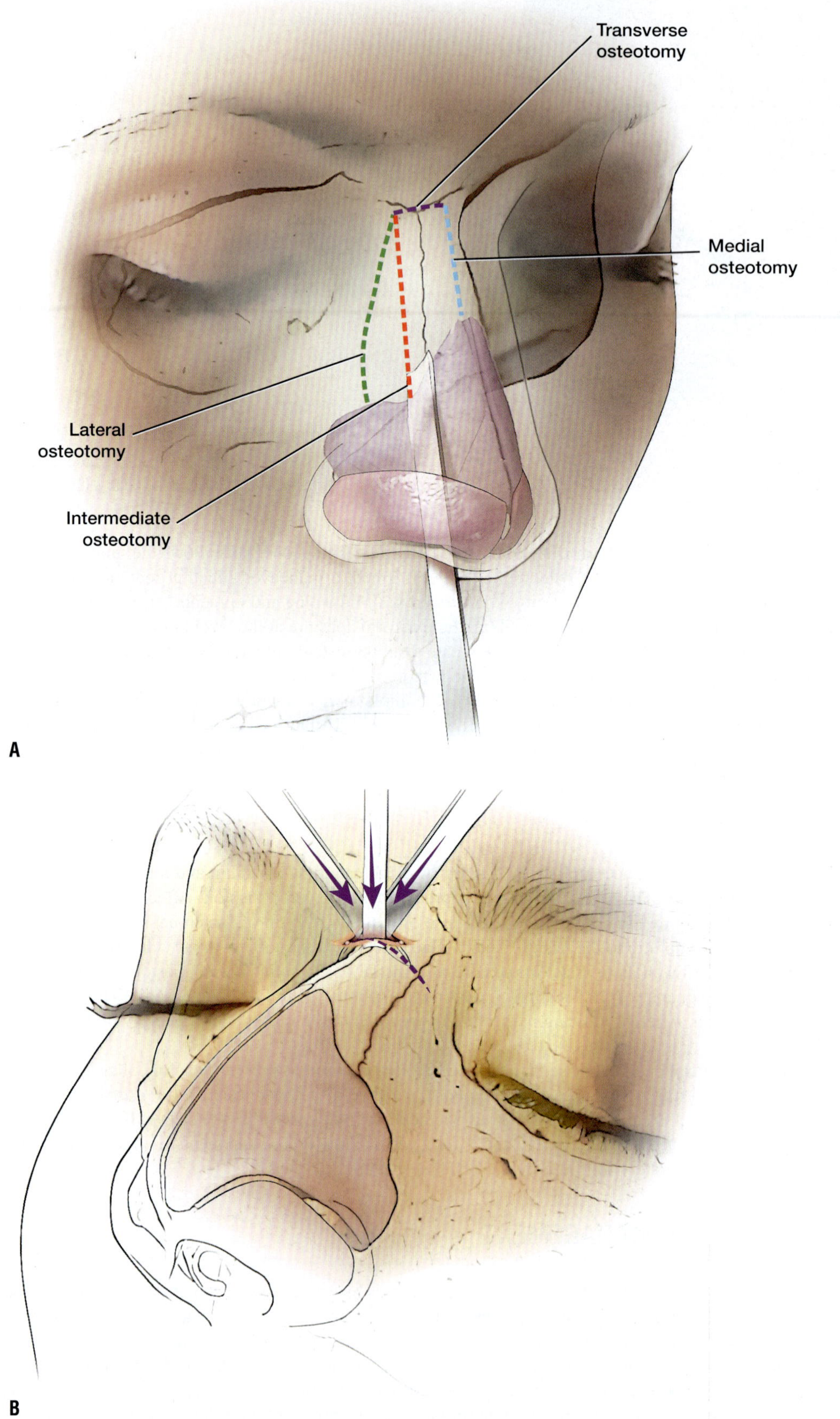

FIGURE 16.21 The osteotomy is performed as a linear osteotomy inferiorly **(A)** and a perforating osteotomy superiorly **(B)**.

again debrided and cleaned, and the nasal splint is removed. If internal nasal septal splints were placed, they are removed at this time. The nose is retaped, but not splinted. At this point, the patient is allowed to perform nasal irrigation with normal saline rinses but is not allowed to blow the nose or use topical nasal decongestants. The patient is also instructed in nasal exercises to overcome edema that might separate the nasal bones. These exercises are accomplished by placing the index fingers along the sidewall of the nasal pyramid parallel to the nasal dorsum with the application of firm pressure in a direction perpendicular to the plane of the nasal bones. This corresponds to the position of the opposite ear. These exercises are continued for 6 weeks postoperatively and are to be performed regularly at a rate of 50 to 100 times a day. The compression with the exercises is maintained for 10 to 15 seconds.

The patient returns again at postoperatively day 10 to have the tape removed and the nasal cavity debrided. Further postoperative visits will be scheduled at 3 and 6 weeks, as well as 3, 6, and 12 months. All patients are encouraged to return every 2 to 3 years for the duration of my practice.

COMPLICATIONS

Consequences must be distinguished from complications and are expected acutely but will resolve. With rhinoplasty, there will be a period of edema and the duration of which is difficult to determine. The edema will be accompanied by decreased sensation in the nasal skin and nasal tenderness. In the majority of cases, the edema has resolved by 3 weeks postoperatively; however, the hypoesthesia of the nasal tip can persist for 6 to 12 months. There will be acute postoperative nasal congestion, which should resolve in 7 to 10 days. Exquisite nasal tenderness will be present, and it may persist for 6 weeks after surgery. Some degree of nasal tenderness may persist for 6 to 12 months. The transcolumellar incision will have some degree of erythema, which should not persist beyond 3 months postoperatively. The patient is informed that their nose will feel alien for 6 weeks to 3 months and that normal sensation may not return for 12 months. During the first 24 to 48 hours after surgery, there may be mild nasal bleeding, which will resolve spontaneously. This is different from acute postoperative epistaxis, which requires intervention.

The most frequent complications of rhinoplasty are unsatisfactory results. This may be cosmetic or functional and occurs in 5% to 10% of the patients requiring revision rhinoplasty. The cosmetic complications are most often related to asymmetry of the nasal tip or dorsum and are easily managed under local anesthesia with a transnasal approach. Nasal congestion may arise from internal or external valve collapse, recurrent septal deflection, persistent or recurrent turbinate hypertrophy, and nasal synechiae. Occasionally, these problems can be managed in the clinic or medically, but often, they will require surgical intervention.

More serious complications such as epistaxis, septal hematoma, and infection are much less common. In 25 years of practice, I have had one postoperative infection that led to a compromised outcome requiring revision rhinoplasty—this event occurred in a posttraumatic rhinoplasty. During that same period of time, there have been two cases of severe epistaxis requiring emergency management with one requiring nasal packing and the other a blood transfusion. Each of these episodes occurred more than 7 days after surgery. One case was an elderly gentleman who had resumed his aspirin therapy, while the other occurred in a young woman on multiple medications for severe endometriosis. Each event involved the patient's resumption of nonsteroidal anti-inflammatory medications.

There are reported cases of CSF rhinorrhea, persistent discomfort at the osteotomy or the nasal dorsum, and numbness of the central incisors. These complications are as rare as they are difficult to manage and require a great deal of expertise, patience, and understanding. I have found it necessary to revise only one transcolumellar scar following an open rhinoplasty.

RESULTS

The patient in Figure 16.22 represents a tension tip with a relative dorsal hump secondary to a deep radix. If the tip and dorsum were reduced to match deep radix, the nose would be too small and unsatisfactory. In this case, it was necessary to reduce the tension in the cartilaginous dorsum and tip while augmenting the radix to address the relative dorsal hump.

This patient with a high radix as well as bony dorsum with a tension nose and short upper lip will require the resection of the radix and anterior maxillary spine (Fig. 16.23). Resection of the radix and creating an identifiable nasion helps to shorten the nasal dorsum as well as lowering the nasal dorsum profile. Resection of the anterior septal angle, caudal margin of the septum, and anterior maxillary spine allows the elevation of the columella without necessarily creating rotation. In spite of placement of spreader grafts and suturing of the upper lateral cartilages, there is still collapse of the left nasal sidewall.

Caudal septal deviation frequently exists in the tension nose (Fig. 16.24). This is most often addressed by shortening of the caudal strut to assist in the release of tension that is accomplished by reducing the anterior septal angle. Lateral crural flap is performed to create rotation, while projection is controlled by the positioning of the medial crura on the caudal septum (Fig. 16.25).

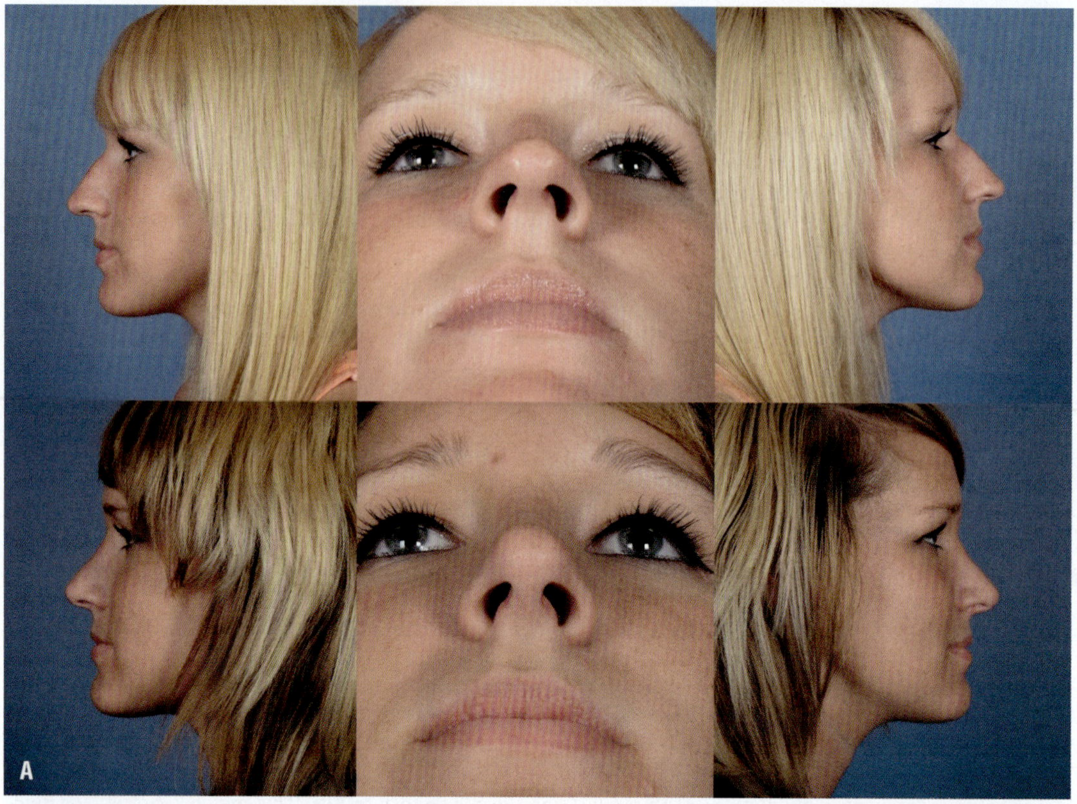

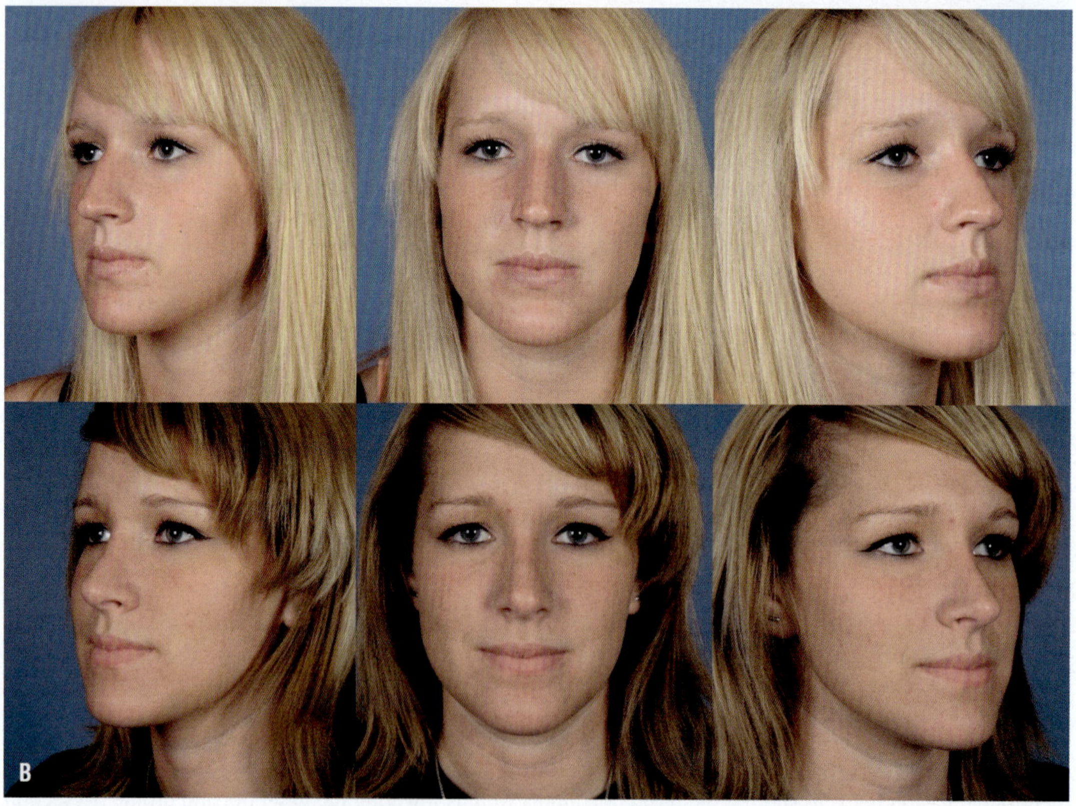

FIGURE 16.22 A–D: Reduction of the tension in the cartilaginous dorsal and tip while augmenting the radix a cartilage graft to address the relative dorsal hump. The purple in **(C)** represents lateral crural overlay technique for the reduction of the domal cartilages.

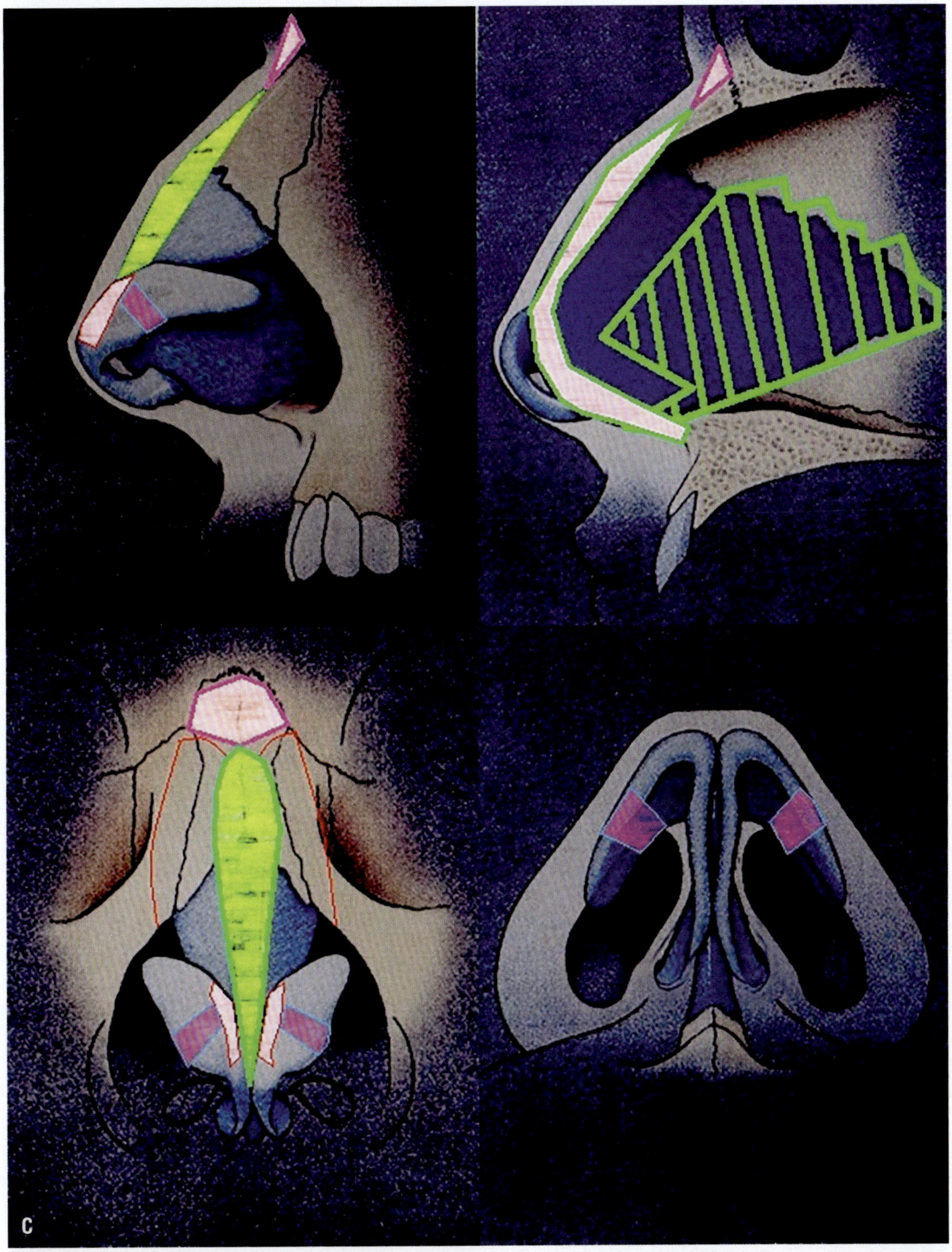

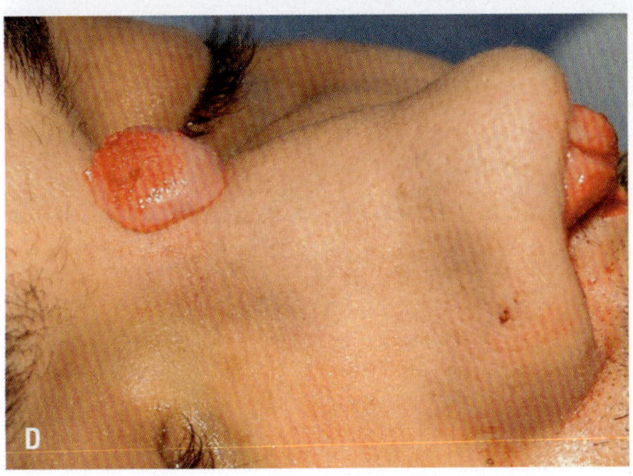

FIGURE 16.22 (*Continued*)

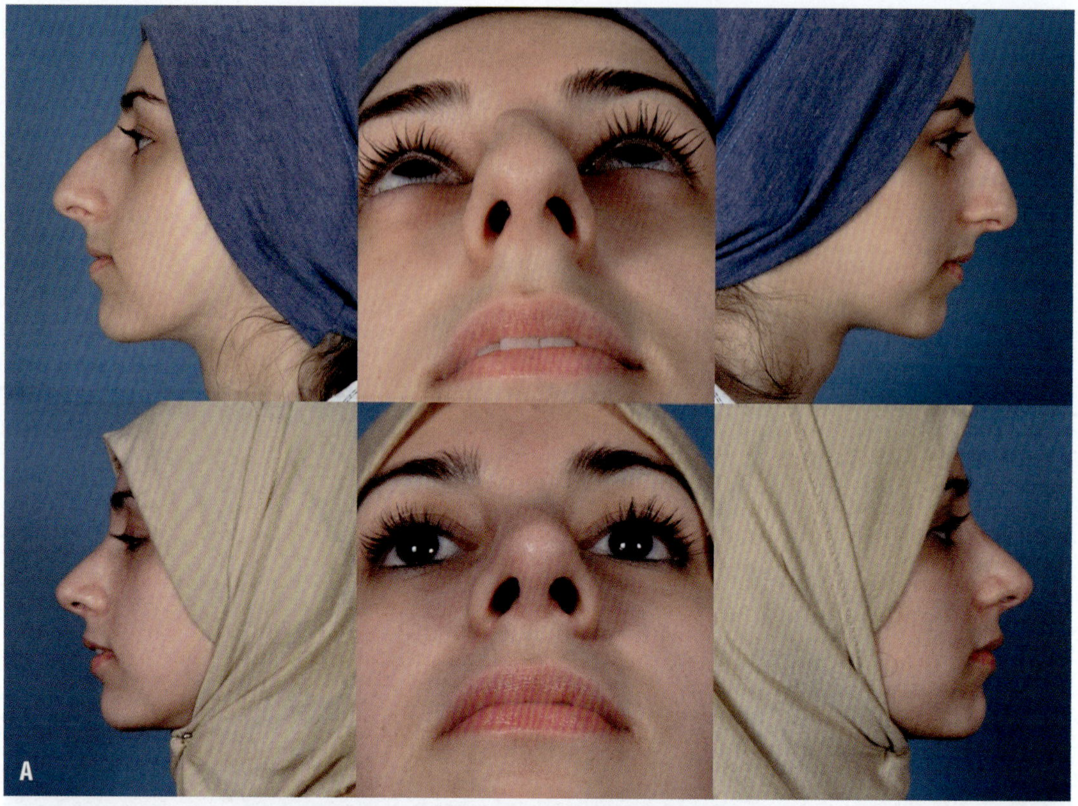

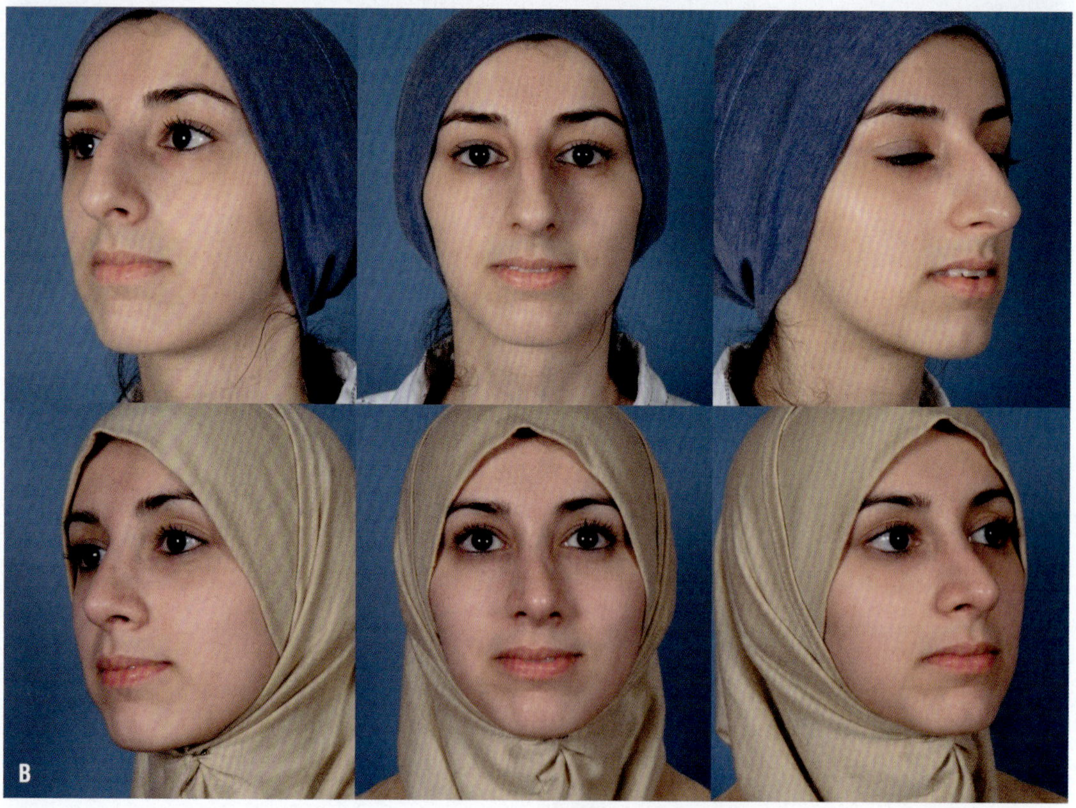

FIGURE 16.23 A–E: Resection of the radix, caudal margin of the septum, and anterior maxillary spine as well as bony dorsum to treat a high radix, a tension nose, and short upper lip.

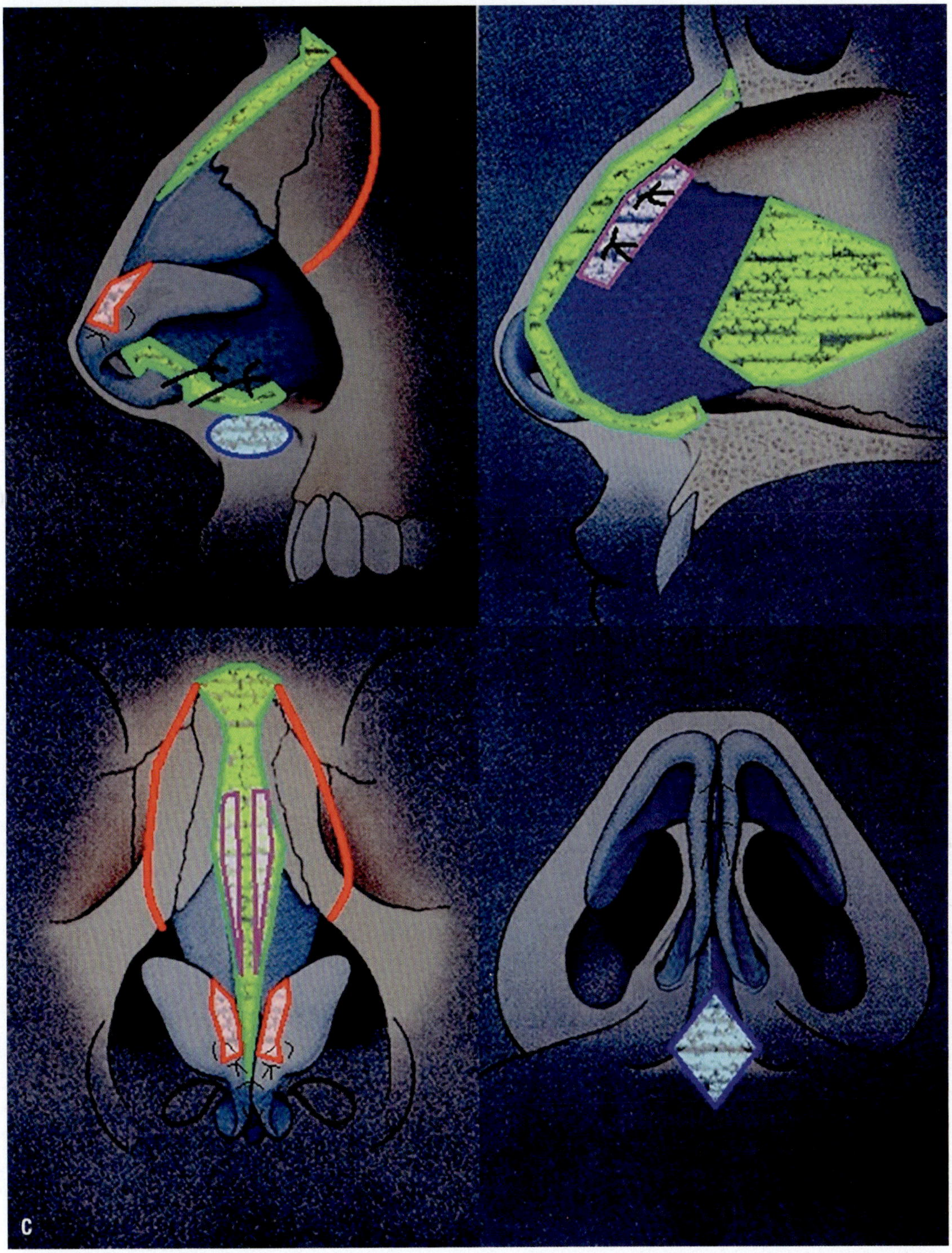

FIGURE 16.23 (*Continued*)

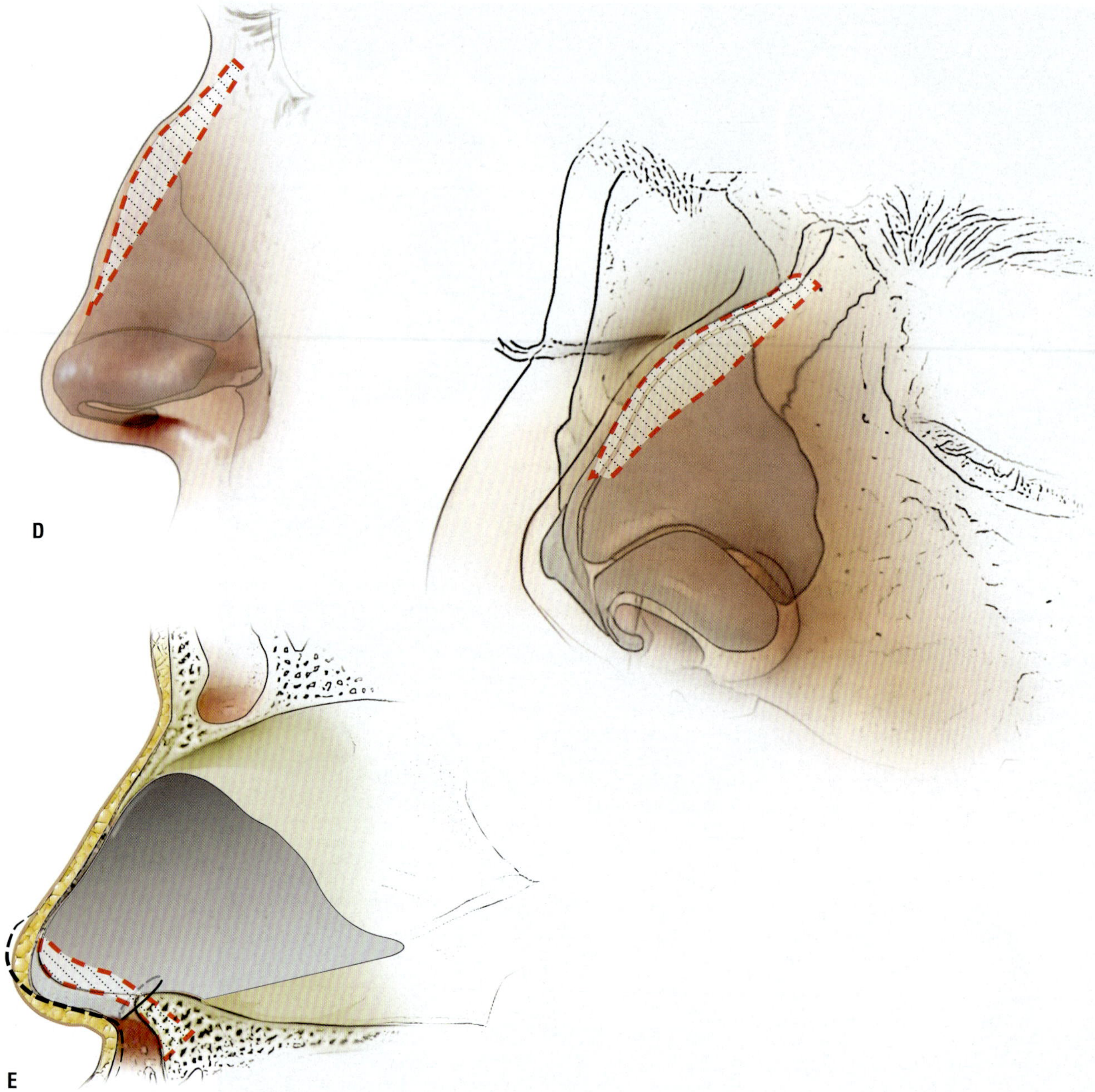

FIGURE 16.23 (*Continued*)

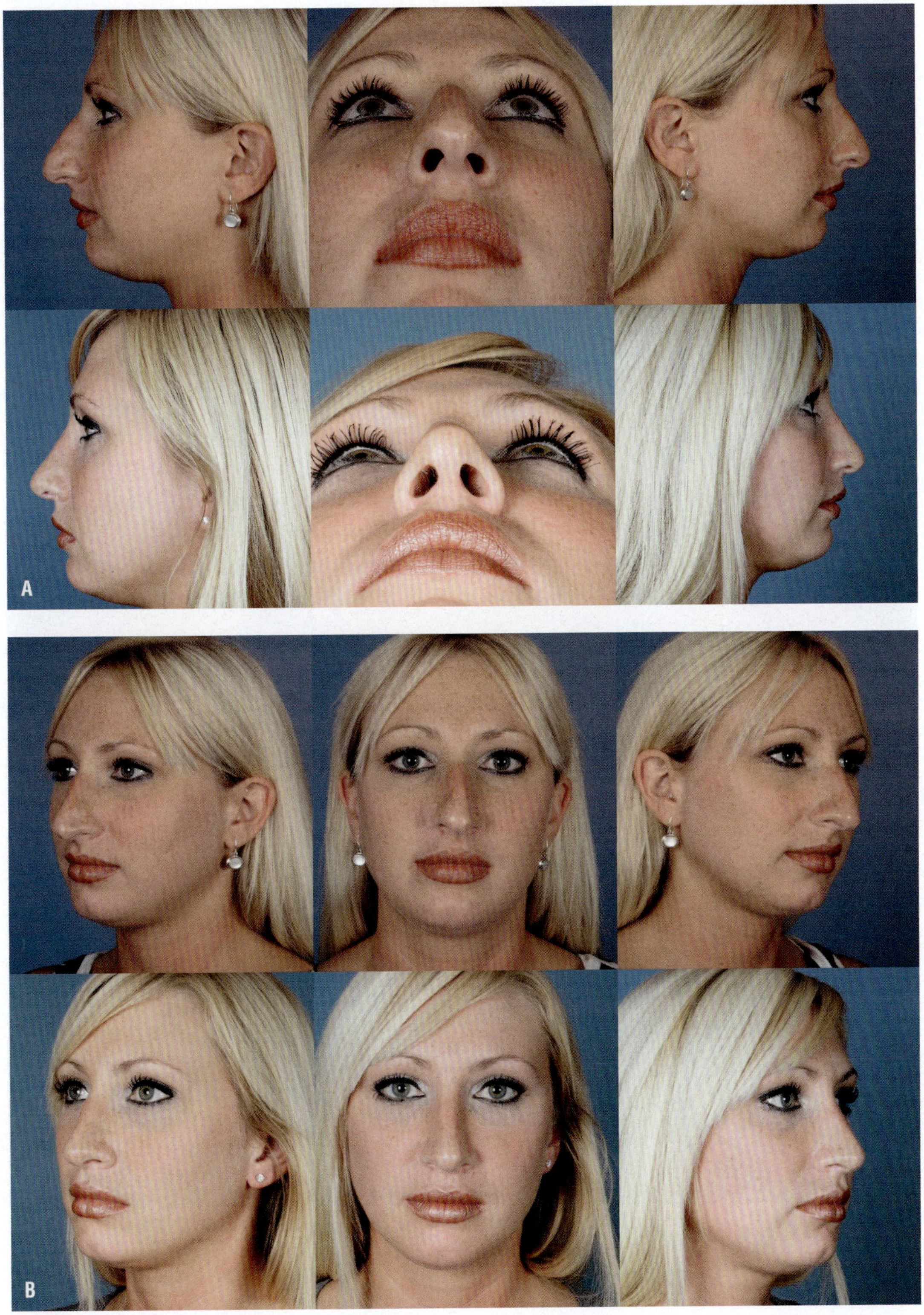

FIGURE 16.24 **A–C:** Caudal septal deviation frequently exists in the tension nose as a result of cartilage overgrowth in relation to the bony pedestal on which it rests. This is commonly addressed by release and shortening of the caudal strut. The diagram of **(C)** reveals the areas of cartilage reduction (*red*), cartilage preservation (*green*), and cartilage overlay (*purple outline*).

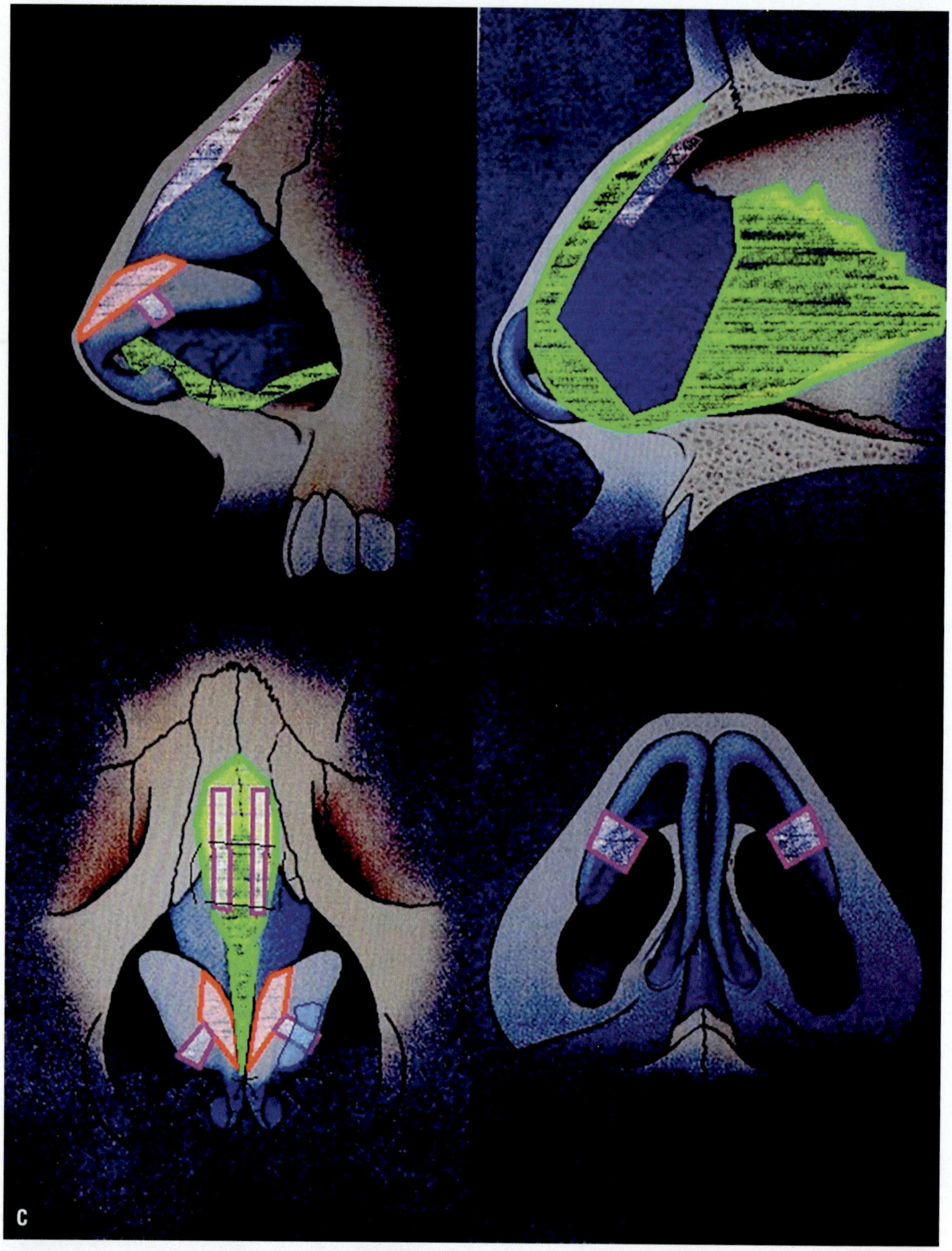

FIGURE 16.24 (*Continued*)

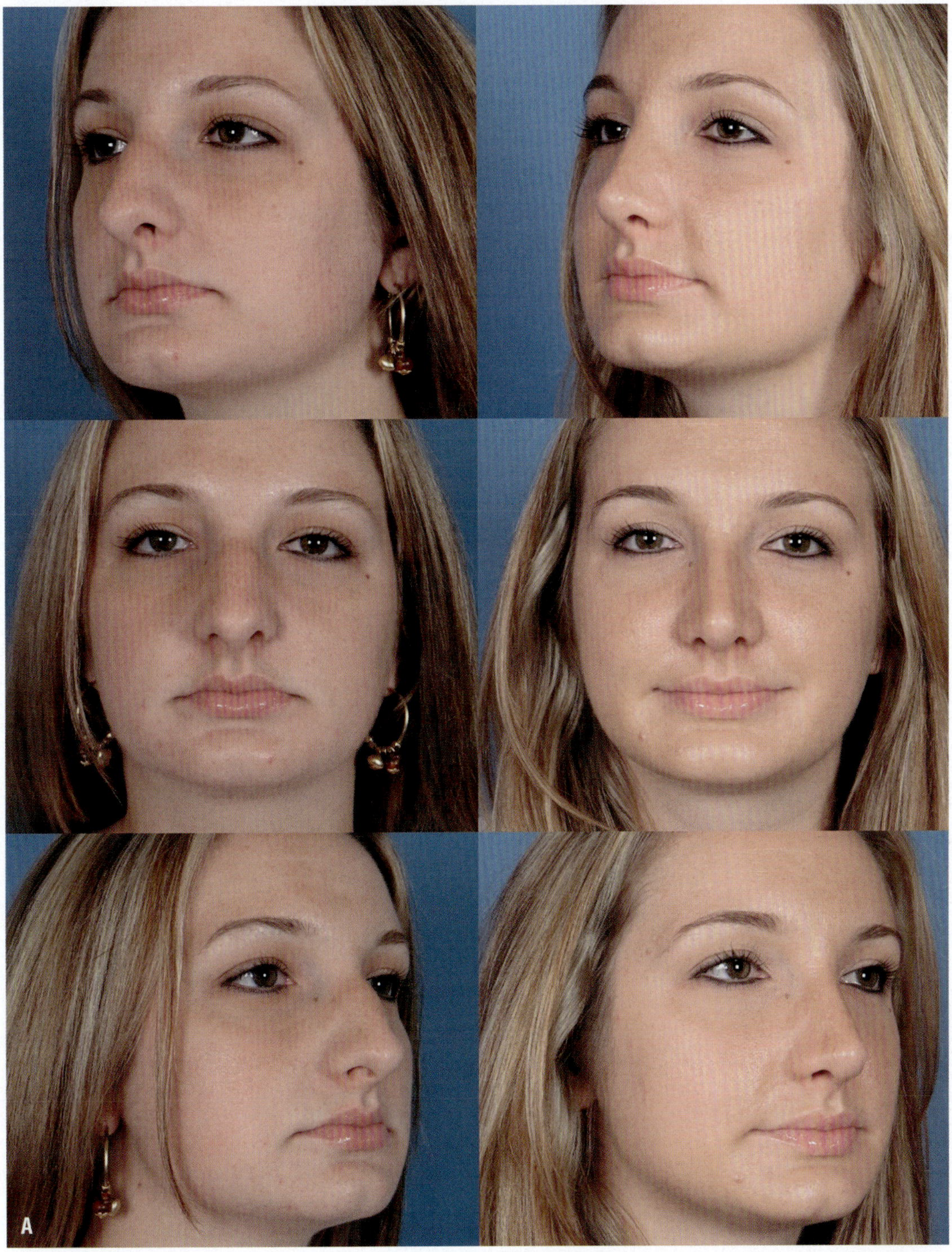

FIGURE 16.25 **A, B:** Lateral crural flaps are performed to create rotation, while projection is controlled by the positioning of the medial crura on the caudal septum.

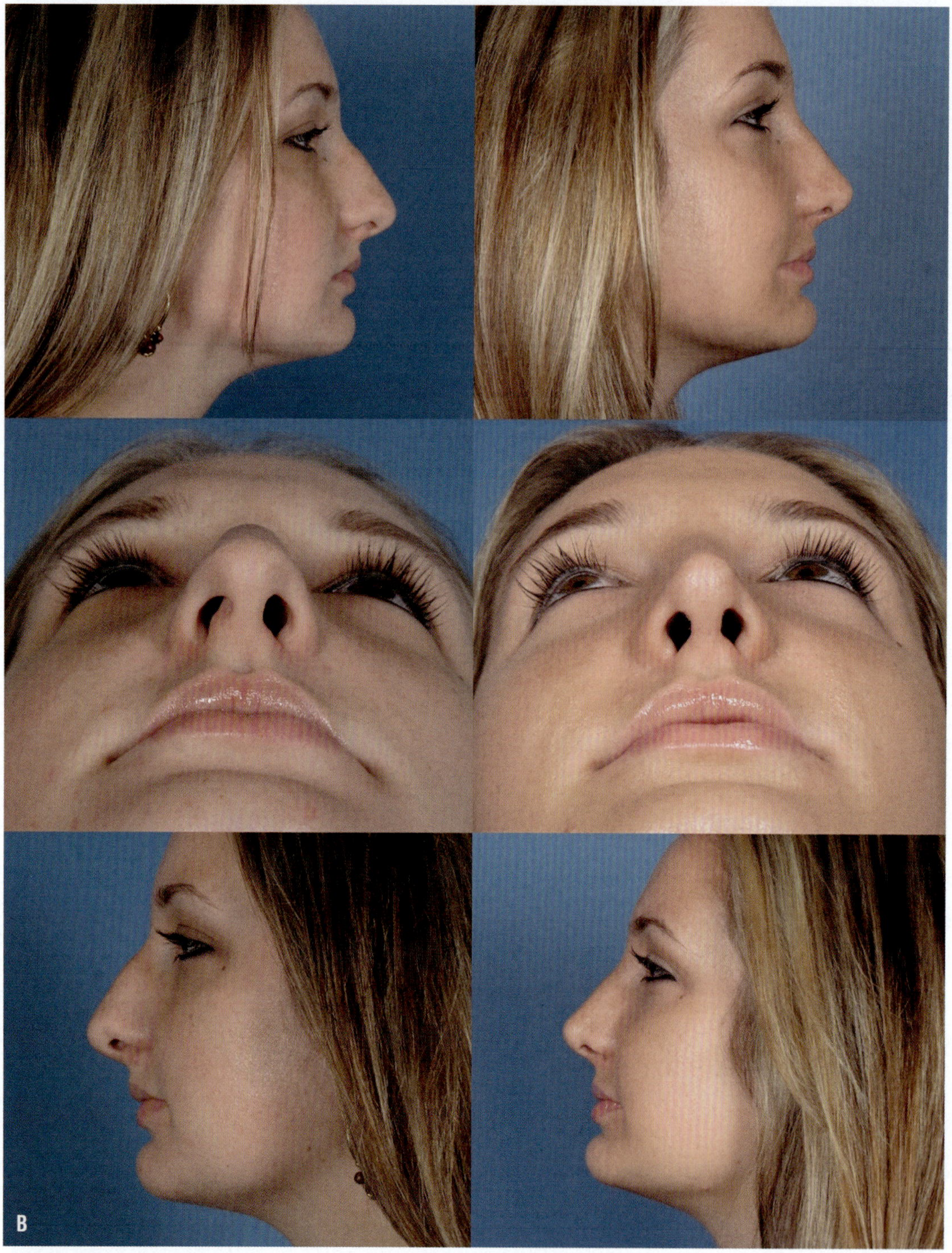

FIGURE 16.25 (*Continued*)

PEARLS

- Spreader grafts are used universally if the dorsal reduction is greater than 3 mm because this will consistently resect the confluence of the quadrangular cartilage (Fig. 16.1) and upper lateral cartilages resulting in a narrowing of the combined cartilaginous nasal dorsal width.
- Patients need to be forewarned that the nasal skin may take longer to accommodate its smaller underlying skeleton; therefore, the final results may take a longer time.
- Shortening of the alar lobule may be required in the tension nose to avoid the lateral flare of the soft tissue of the alar lobule when projection is reduced (Fig. 16.26). This also shortens the overall length of the external nares.
- Placement of the columellar incision cannot be routine when a reduction rhinoplasty is performed. The incision should be placed at the more anterior portion of the middle third of the columella.

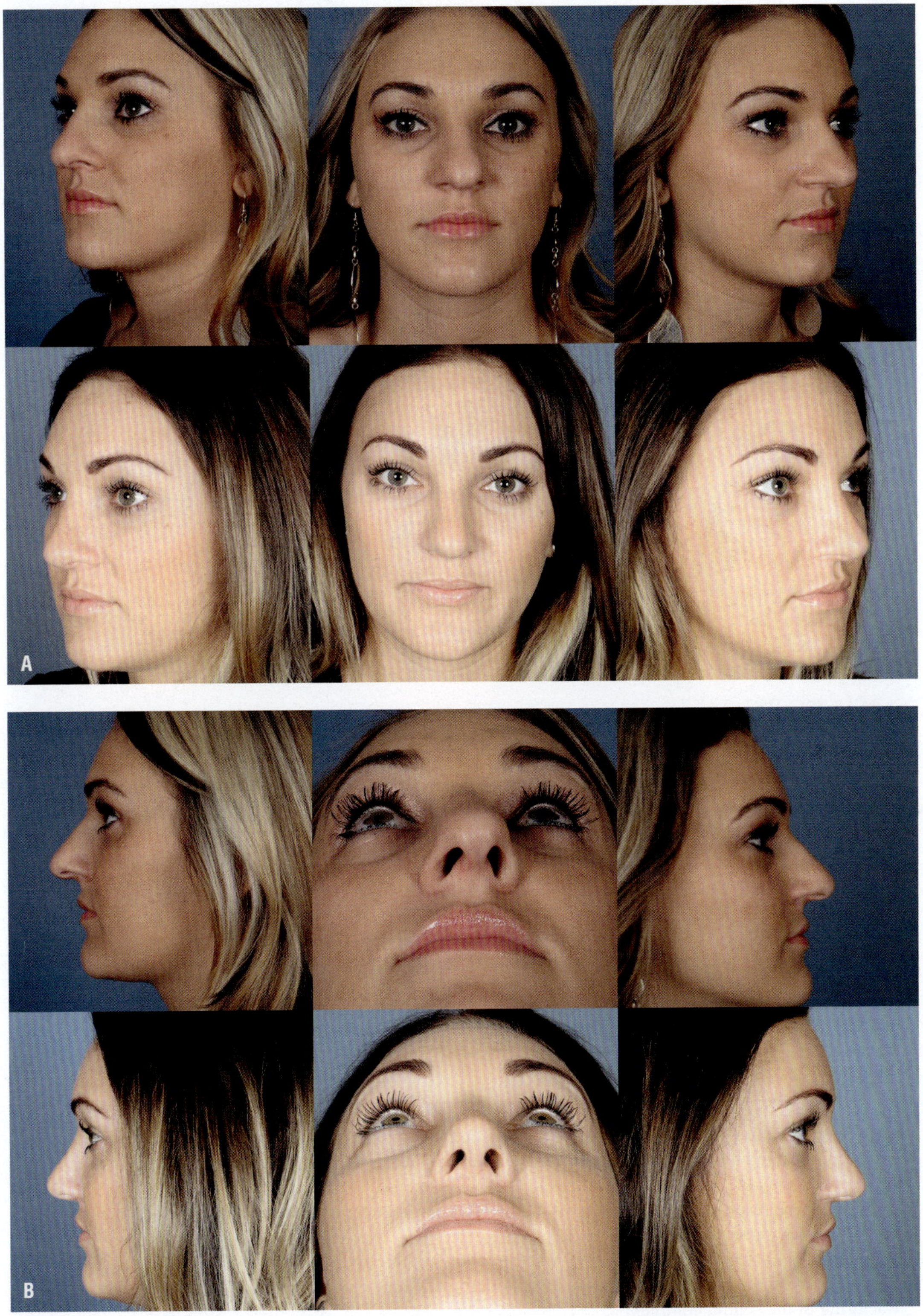

FIGURE 16.26 **A–C:** Shortening of the alar lobule was required in this tension nose to avoid the lateral flare of the soft tissue of the alar lobule when projection was reduced. Treatment of the nasal tip cartilages are seen in addition to reduction of the alar flare with intraoperative lobule shortening on the left and pretreatment observed on the right.

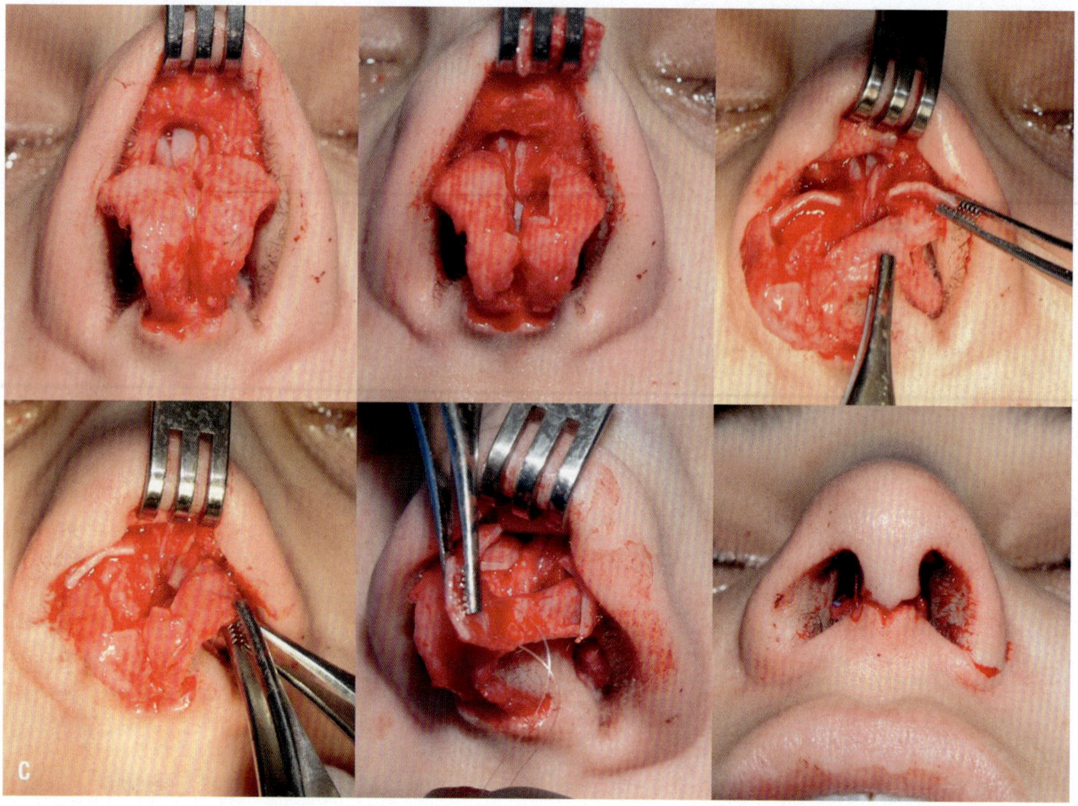

FIGURE 16.26 (*Continued*)

- The need for intermediate osteotomies may not be appreciated because of the fairly consistent narrow dorsum and the tension nose. Intermediate osteotomies are required to release the convexity of the bony pyramid when the nasal facial junction is lateral to the medial canthus.
- Preserving the alar cartilage rim in the dome is done whenever possible. This allows a consistent margin and smooth transition from the medial to lateral crus through the intermediate crus and dome.
- When the tip cartilages are symmetric, the alar cartilage rim is preserved in the dome and shortening of the medial crus may be achieved through medial crural setback for a medial crural flap.
- Temporalis fascia can help to camouflage margins of the cartilage graft that might be necessary to refine the nasal tip.

PITFALLS

Tension nose surgeries can provide some of the most remarkable results achieved in rhinoplasty, but are frequently accompanied by subtle irregularities that are unsatisfactory for the patient and the surgeon.

- Controlling the result and dorsal height as well as contour is imperative in the tension nose. Accurate planning and measurements are critical.
- If intermediate osteotomies are not performed to allow a more mobile medial segment and a flattening of the convexity of the bony pyramid, an open roof deformity may occur in spite of complete osteotomies and fracturing of the central complex.
- Failure to treat the thin skin of the tension nose will give an opportunity for any irregularity of bone, cartilage, or grafting to be seen. Temporalis fascia is the ideal soft tissue augmentation material in these cases as it is easy to harvest and place over the nasal tip and dorsum.
- Attention to the reconstruction of the structural integrity of the bony cartilaginous junction as well as the nasal dorsum is imperative for form and stability. Complete failure results in the classic "inverted V" deformity.
- Have patients refrain from the restart of medications, holistic and otherwise, until cleared by the operating surgeon.

INSTRUMENTS TO HAVE AVAILABLE

- Standard rhinoplasty set
- Freshly sharpened 2-mm osteotome
- 6-0 Maxon suture
- 4-0 chromic suture
- 6-0 plain gut sutures
- Aquaplast splint
- 3M Micropore tape

SUGGESTED READING

Christophel JJ, Hilger PA. Osseocartilaginous rib graft rhinoplasty: a stable, predictable technique for major dorsal reconstruction. *Arch Facial Plast Surg* 2011;13(2):78–83.

Dyer WK. Nasal tip support and it's surgical modification. *Facial Plast Surg Clin North Am* 2004;12:1–13.

Papel I. Secondary rhinoplasty. In: Papel I, Frodel JL, Holt GR, et al., eds. *Facial plastic and reconstructive surgery*. New York: Thieme, 2009:589–603.

Paun SH, Trenite GJN. Revision rhinoplasty: an overview of deformities and techniques. *Facial Plast Surg* 2008;24(3):271–287.

Sandel IV HD, Perkins SW. Management of the short nose deformity in revision rhinoplasty. *Facial Plast Surg* 2008;24(3):310–325.

17 RHINOPLASTY: RECONSTRUCTION OF THE SADDLE NOSE DEFORMITY USING COSTAL CARTILAGE HARVEST

Dean M. Toriumi

INTRODUCTION

The saddle nose deformity is characterized by a depression of the nasal dorsum that extends from the bony dorsum to the nasal tip. Deficiencies of the nasal septum are frequently implicated in the development of this problem. There are differing degrees of deformity, which may not be related to the severity of the septal damage. Reconstruction of the saddle nose deformity can be accomplished by using either onlay cartilage grafting or reconstruction of the damaged nasal septum using cartilage grafting. Selection of the method of reconstruction will depend upon the severity of the saddle nose deformity, the patient's expectations, and the experience of the surgeon. Materials for reconstruction include autologous cartilage, homologous cartilage, and alloplastic implants. I prefer using autologous materials including nasal septal cartilage, auricular cartilage, and costal cartilage. This chapter describes the technique of costal cartilage reconstruction of the saddle nose deformity.

HISTORY

The preoperative evaluation of the saddle nose deformity requires a thorough history. History of any nasal trauma or previous septal surgery is very important. Previous nasal trauma could have left the patient with a septal hematoma (with or without infection) that could compromise the blood supply to the septal cartilage and result in a loss of septal support. Loss of septal support of the dorsum can result in a saddle nose deformity. Immediate drainage of a septal hematoma can help prevent damage to the septal cartilage and subsequent saddling of the nasal dorsum.

Saddle nose deformity can also occur after septal surgery if there is loss of integrity of the L-shaped septal strut. Saddling of the middle nasal vault or other related deformities can occur. When performing a septoplasty, care must be taken to preserve a continuous cartilaginous support structure extending from the nasal spine to the perpendicular plate of the ethmoid bone at the keystone area (Fig. 17.1).

Patients who present with a saddle nose deformity without a history of nasal trauma or previous septal surgery must be thoroughly evaluated in order to identify the etiology. Another possible etiology for saddle nose deformity includes septal perforation. The septal perforation must extend to compromise the L-shaped septal strut. Patients who have abused vasoconstrictive agents such as cocaine may develop large septal perforations that can compromise the support of the L-shaped septal strut. Disease processes such as Wegener's granulomatosis or sarcoidosis must be ruled out if no other diagnosis can be found. Historically, syphilis was an important etiology of the saddle nose deformity, although its incidence has declined substantially in the modern antibiotic era.

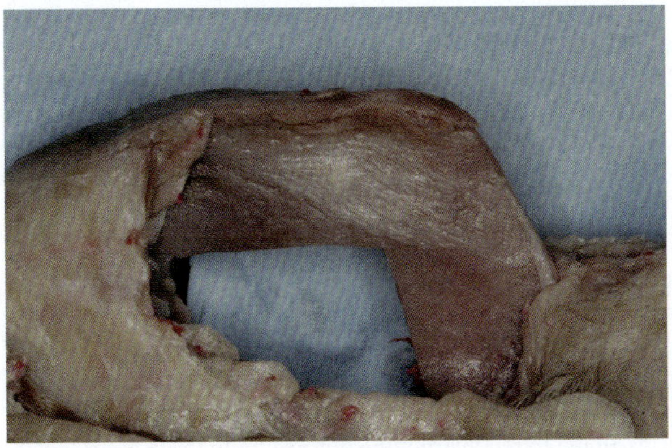

FIGURE 17.1
L-shaped septal strut showing continuous cartilage segment extending from the nasal spine to perpendicular plate of the ethmoid.

Patients are routinely assessed for the presence of nasal obstruction prior to any nasal surgery. Allergic symptoms are common and are identified at this time. In addition to obtaining a detailed symptom history, obstructive symptoms are quantified using a validated patient-reported quality of life instrument known as the Nasal Obstruction Symptom Evaluation (NOSE) scale. This is also used postoperatively as a tool to track outcomes.

Finally, a thorough medical history is obtained including any comorbid medical conditions, medication use, allergies, prior surgeries, and a social history. Medications and supplements that are known anticoagulants receive special attention. Patients are routinely advised to avoid aspirin and nonsteroidal anti-inflammatory (NSAID) medications for 3 weeks prior to surgery.

PHYSICAL EXAMINATION

A thorough examination of the head and neck is very important when evaluating patients with a saddle nose deformity. The examination should determine the degree of saddling and can be quantified by measuring the degree of concavity of the nasal dorsum. Palpation of the saddled middle nasal vault can determine the degree of support provided by the nasal septum. When pushing down on the middle nasal vault if robust resistance to compression is noted, then the dorsal strut may be partially or totally intact. If compression of the middle nasal vault reveals a weakness and little resistance to compression, this likely represents a severely damaged or absent dorsal septal strut.

The examination should include anterior rhinoscopy as well as endoscopic examination of the entire nasal cavity with particular attention to the septum. A thorough intranasal examination should reveal any septal perforations, mucosal irregularities, previous incisions, or nasal valve compromise.

INDICATIONS

Indications for reconstruction include patients with a saddle nose deformity or other similar depressed areas of the nasal dorsum. Typically, this is an aesthetic deformity of the nose and the patient may or may not present with nasal obstruction. If the patient does have nasal obstruction, reconstruction of the septal deformity will likely improve the nasal airway breathing. Patients may also have nasal valve obstruction that can be improved by stabilizing the dorsal septum and caudal margin of the upper lateral cartilages and internal nasal valve. Nasal obstruction associated with saddle nose deformity is also an indication for reconstruction. In patients with a large septal perforation that is impinging on the dorsal septal support, septal reconstruction may be indicated to avoid collapse of the middle nasal vault.

CONTRAINDICATIONS

Contraindications to repair of the saddle nose deformity include factors related to underlying pathologic problems. For example, if a patient with a saddle nose deformity has active Wegener's granulomatosis or active sarcoidosis, reconstruction should be delayed until these disease processes are stabilized or inactive. This is very important to avoid progression of the disease and worsening of the patient's condition. If the saddle nose deformity is secondary to cocaine abuse or chronic use of other vasoconstrictive agents, it is imperative that the use of these agents is discontinued. Other contraindications include medical problems prohibiting a long operation. Patients who require use of costal cartilage for repair of their deformity must have noncalcified rib cartilage. Patients older than 55 years of age will typically have some calcification of their rib cartilage, which may still be usable depending on the degree of calcification. This can be determined by transcutaneous needle palpation of the rib in the office prior to surgery. Care must be taken to avoid perforating the chest cavity during needle palpation as this can result in pneumothorax. If the patient has calcified rib cartilage, their own costal cartilage will not be usable and other sources of cartilage will need to be identified.

PREOPERATIVE PLANNING

Preoperative planning for reconstruction of the saddle nose deformity is very important. Once the etiology of the saddle nose deformity is determined, a surgical plan can be initiated. If reconstruction is planned, material for grafting must be harvested. In some cases, septal cartilage is available and can be used for the reconstruction. However, in most cases, there will be inadequate septal cartilage for complete correction of the deformity. Therefore, auricular cartilage may be needed in addition to whatever septal cartilage is available. In some cases, there may be inadequate septal and auricular cartilage to reconstruct the deformity. In these cases, costal cartilage may be needed to reconstruct the nasal septum and correct the saddle nose deformity. Alloplastic materials can be used for reconstruction but carry the risk of infection, extrusion, and deformity. I prefer not to use alloplastic materials in the nose as the risks of infection or extrusion are always present.

Decisions must be made as to whether any other cosmetic changes will be made to the nose. Patients with a saddle nose deformity may also have retraction of the columella, ptotic nasal tip and underprojected nasal tip, acute nasolabial angle (Fig. 17.2A–E). Correction of these deformities may require more extensive use of cartilage grafting.

Preoperative computer imaging is a very effective means of communicating realistic expectations to the patient and family. Care must be taken in showing the patient realistic outcomes based on the experience of the surgeon. Preoperative computer imaging does not guarantee an outcome but provides an estimation of what is a realistic proposed outcome.

Imaging

Imaging studies are not very helpful in the diagnosis and management of the saddle nose deformity. On rare occasions a CT scan of the sinuses may be helpful to rule out chronic sinus disease. Patients with Wegener's granulomatosis or other metabolic disorders should have a CT scan to evaluate the sinuses.

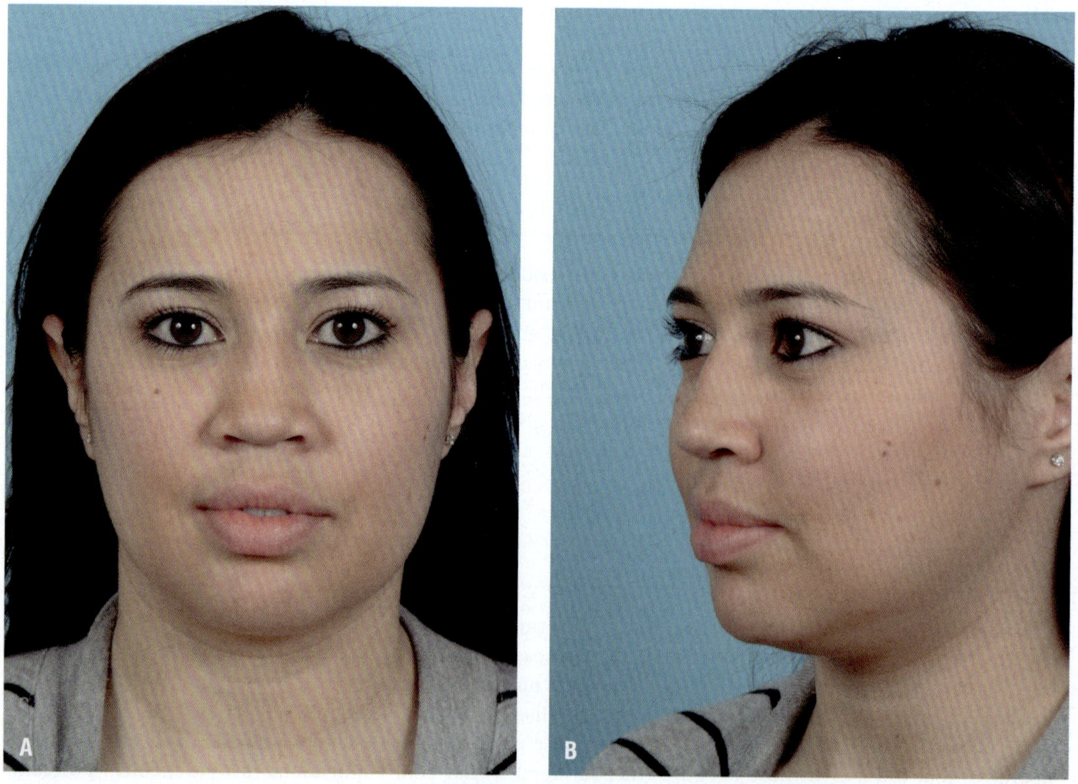

FIGURE 17.2 A–E. Patient with a saddle nose deformity demonstrating a depressed middle nasal vault, retracted columella, acute nasolabial angle, and underprojected nasal tip. This patient is the primary case used in this chapter to demonstrate the surgical technique for costal cartilage reconstruction of the nasal septum and saddle nose deformity.

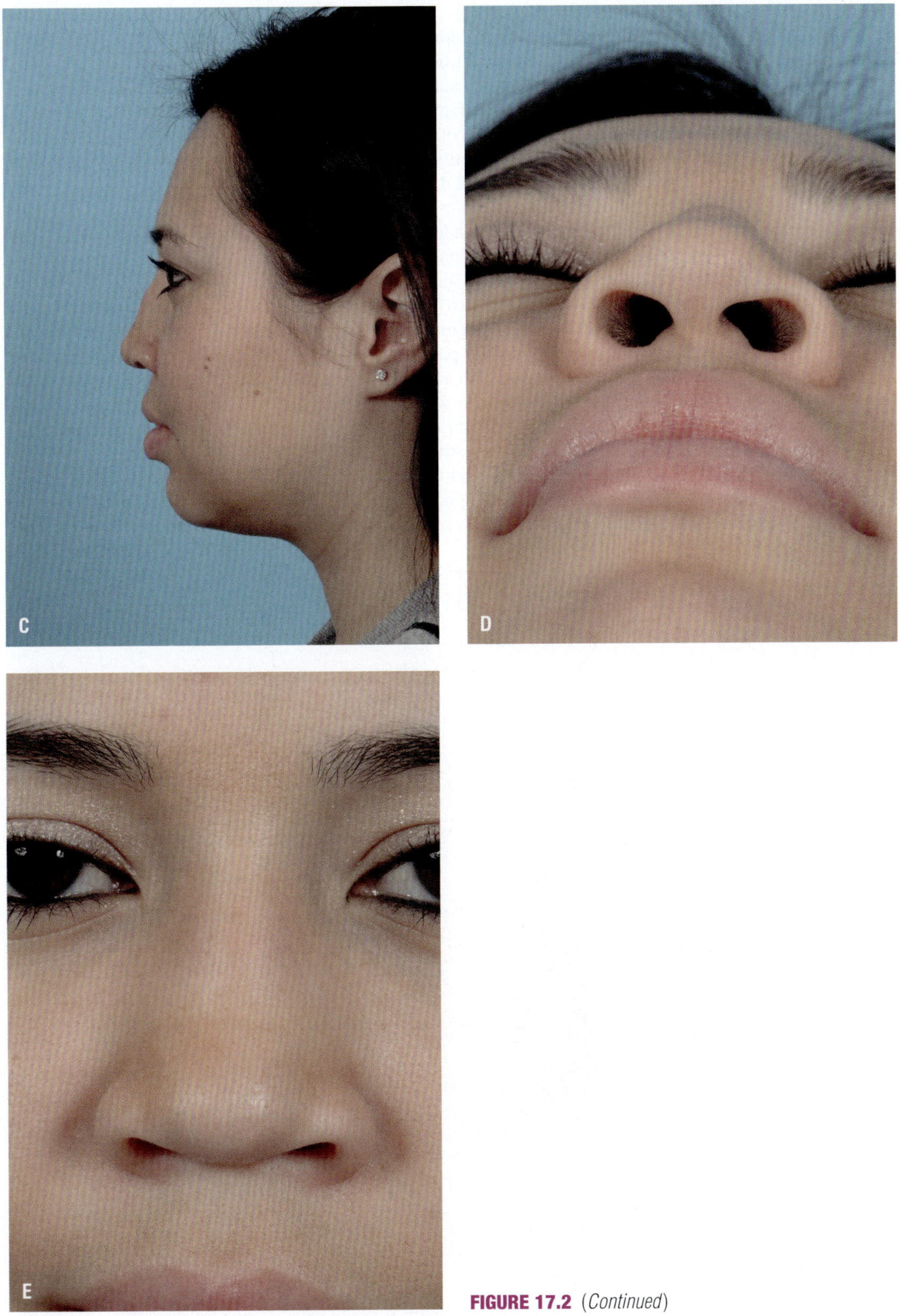

FIGURE 17.2 (*Continued*)

SURGICAL TECHNIQUE

Correction of the saddle nose deformity will usually require gaining exposure using the external rhinoplasty approach. The surgery is performed under general anesthesia, typically in an ambulatory surgery setting. The patient is placed in supine position with the head stabilized by a foam donut pillow. Perioperative antibiotics are administered prior to making incision. I typically perform a thorough endoscopic examination prior to beginning the operation. Local anesthetic (lidocaine 1% to 1:100,000 epinephrine) is injected into the nasal septum and external nose. The patient is then widely prepped with Betadine at both surgical sites and draped in sterile fashion. The clean-contaminated nasal surgical field is kept separate from the sterile chest surgical field throughout the case, including maintaining separate instruments for each site.

The external rhinoplasty approach is carried out using a midcolumellar inverted-V incision in combination with bilateral marginal incisions. Once the lower lateral cartilages are exposed, dissection between the medial crura will permit direct exposure of the caudal margin of the nasal septum. If this approach is used, it is important to reconstitute the support of the lower lateral cartilages. Many patients will benefit from placement of an end-to-end caudal septal extension graft or caudal septal replacement graft.

Saddle nose deformities with a stable dorsal septum by palpation can be treated with an onlay dorsal graft. An onlay dorsal graft can be positioned through an endonasal approach. Bilateral intercartilaginous incisions can be made and a pocket created over the nasal dorsum. The dorsal pocket should be as tight as possible and should allow the dorsal graft to fit snugly onto the dorsum of the nose.

If it is clear that costal cartilage will be required for reconstruction of the saddle nose deformity, the rib cartilage harvest can be performed prior to beginning the saddle nose repair. I typically harvest the rib cartilage from the 6th rib, which in the female patient is located at the inferior margin of the breast (Fig. 17.3). If the patient has a large pendulous breast or has breast implants, the inferior aspect of the breast may be overlapping the 7th rib. I usually harvest the rib using a 1.1- to 1.5-cm incision placed along the inframammary crease of the right breast (Fig. 17.4). This places the incision just over the 6th rib in most patients. If a smaller incision is made, the location of the correct length and shape of the rib is very important as the size of the incision will limit access to a relatively small area of the rib. Alternatively, if a large incision (over 3 cm) is made, the positioning of the incision is less critical as a large portion of the 6th rib will be exposed and easily accessible. I do not recommend using a small incision for costal cartilage

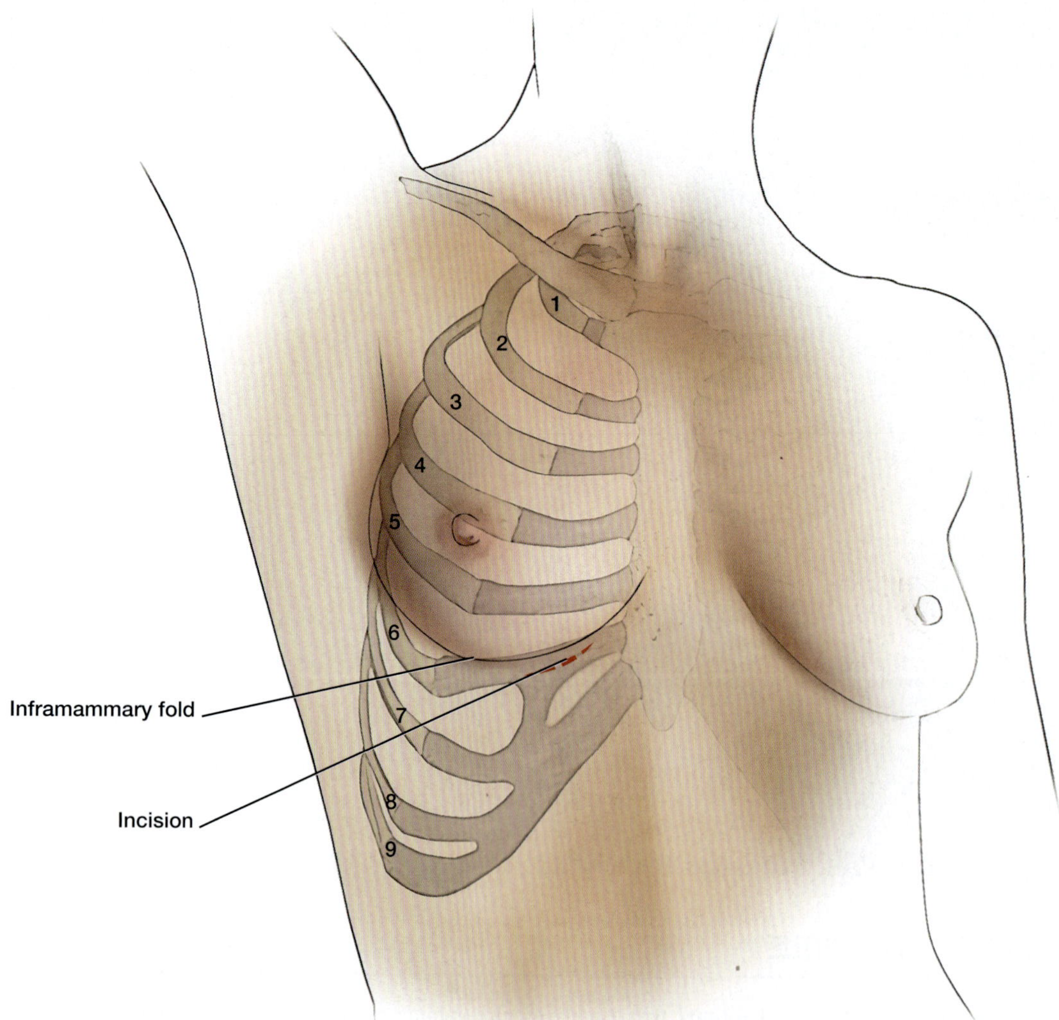

FIGURE 17.3 The 6th rib is typically located at the level of the inframammary crease allowing access to this rib through an inframammary incision.

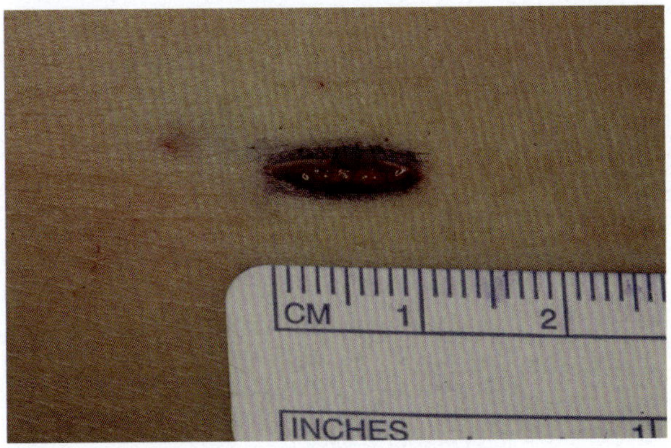

FIGURE 17.4
Inframammary crease incision over the 6th rib.

harvest unless the surgeon has extensive experience harvesting rib cartilage in order to avoid complication such as pneumothorax.

The 6th rib has a rather predictable curvature with a genu along the ribs contour. This is usually not a problem unless a long (>3 cm) straight segment of cartilage is needed for dorsal augmentation or long spreader grafts. In this case, the placement of the incision is important as the majority of the cartilage will need to be harvested either medial or lateral to the genu. Additionally, if the cartilage/bone junction is positioned more medial, this will leave less cartilage to harvest lateral to the genu. If the cartilage/bone junction is more lateral, then there will be a larger segment of cartilage available lateral to the genu. Most younger patients have a more laterally positioned cartilage/bone junction. As patients age, the cartilage/bone junction tends to advance medially. In patients with a prominent genu, I prefer to harvest the 7th rib even though the incision is not in the inframammary crease.

To know precisely where the cartilage/bone junction is located, a 1.5-inch long 27-gauge needle can be inserted through the skin and used to transcutaneously palpate the costal cartilage. The tip of the needle can be used to penetrate the outer 1 to 2 mm of the surface of the rib cartilage. The tip of the needle can be advanced along the rib cartilage until bone is encountered. The cartilage/bone junction is identified, and the bone is encountered with the tip of the 27-gauge needle. If a needle is used to palpate the rib cartilage, special care must be taken to avoid advancing the needle deep to or between the ribs as this will risk puncturing the parenchyma of the lung creating a small air leak that could develop into a pneumothorax.

Once the site of the incision is determined, local anesthetic (1% lidocaine with 1:100,000 epinephrine) is injected into the area around the incision. The incision is made using no. 15 blade initially cutting through skin and subcutaneous tissues. Dissection is then advanced down to the muscle layer. I try to avoid cutting the muscle as this will increase postoperative pain. The muscle fibers are separated to expose the underlying rib cartilage. Once the rib is exposed, the cartilaginous segment is assessed for curvature and contour. It is helpful to remove a large strip of perichondrium off of the surface of the 6th rib. Once the perichondrium is removed from the outside surface, the remaining perichondrium on the superior and inferior margins of the rib cartilage can be dissected away from the rib. To insure that dissection of the perichondrium is performed in the proper plane, I make a superficial incision into the rib cartilage using a Freer elevator and then continue the dissection around the superior and inferior equator points of the rib (Fig. 17.5). By making a superficial incision into the cartilage, it is less likely that the elevator will leave the proper plane and perforate the pleura. Once the perichondrium is elevated off of the superior and inferior surface of the 6th rib, the cartilage can be incised medially and laterally and then lifted from the chest. When making the medial and lateral incisions, a no. 15 blade is used to cut halfway through the rib, and then, a freer elevator is used to cut through the remainder of the rib. In most patients, a 3-cm-long segment of costal cartilage will be adequate for reconstruction as most cartilage grafts are 3 cm or less in length (Fig. 17.6).

After the rib cartilage is removed, saline solution is placed into the rib harvest site and a Valsalva maneuver is used to see if there is a pleura leak. If an obvious defect in the pleura is noted, the wound can be closed after placing a red rubber catheter into the defect. After closing the wound, the lungs can be expanded and the catheter can be pulled out. A postoperative chest radiograph can be performed postoperatively to assess the presence of pneumothorax.

Prior to closure, the edges of the remaining rib cartilage should be trimmed using a Takahashi forceps to prevent any sharp edges that may be palpable or can cause postoperative pain. I prefer to close the chest incision at the end of the operation so we can harvest additional cartilage or perichondrium if necessary. Initially, the muscle layer is closed tightly using 3-0 PDS sutures. Then, the subcutaneous tissue layer is closed with 4-0 PDS sutures. Care is taken to make sure that the breast moves freely over the deep layer closure so the breast tissue does not pucker when the patient stands. The skin can be closed using 5-0 nylon sutures. Typically, the scars for the rib cartilage harvest are small and not very noticeable (Fig. 17.7).

Reconstruction of the saddle nose repair begins with execution of the external rhinoplasty approach. An inverted-V incision is marked out on the columella. In most cases, the incision is made midway between the

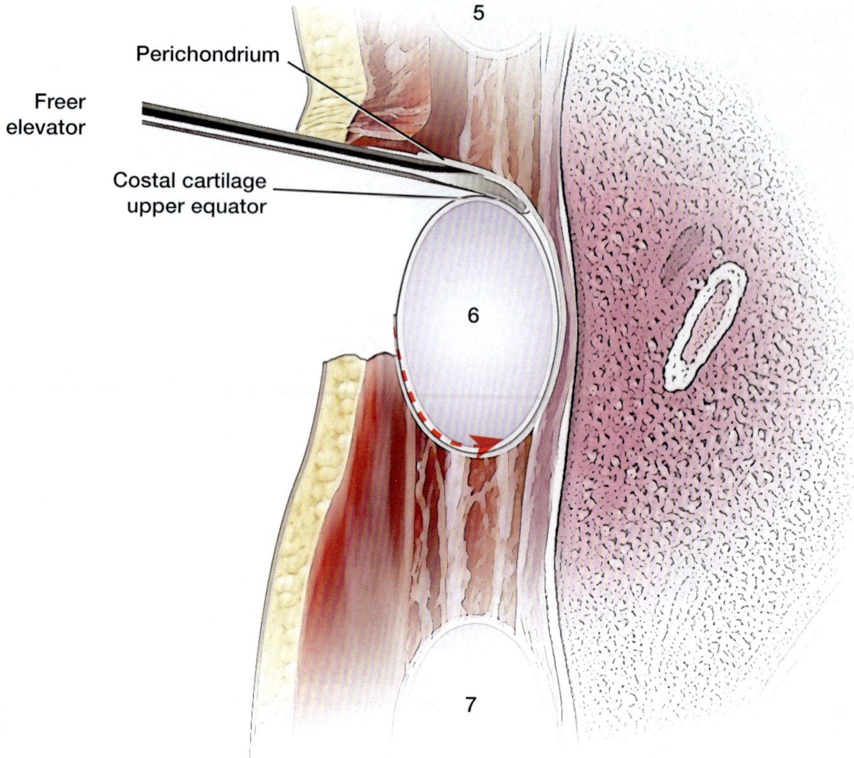

FIGURE 17.5 To ensure that the perichondrium of the rib is elevated in the proper plane, a small incision is made into the costal cartilage to start the perichondrial elevation. This helps to keep the elevator over the cartilage in order to not penetrate the perichondrium.

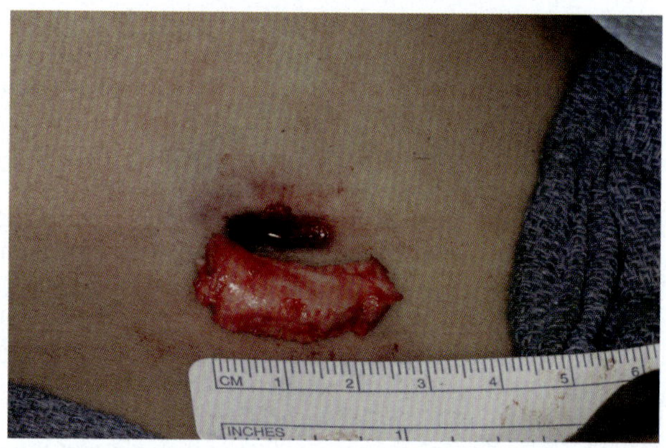

FIGURE 17.6
Costal cartilage segment measuring approximately 3 cm in length.

FIGURE 17.7
Typical healed scar following rib cartilage harvest.

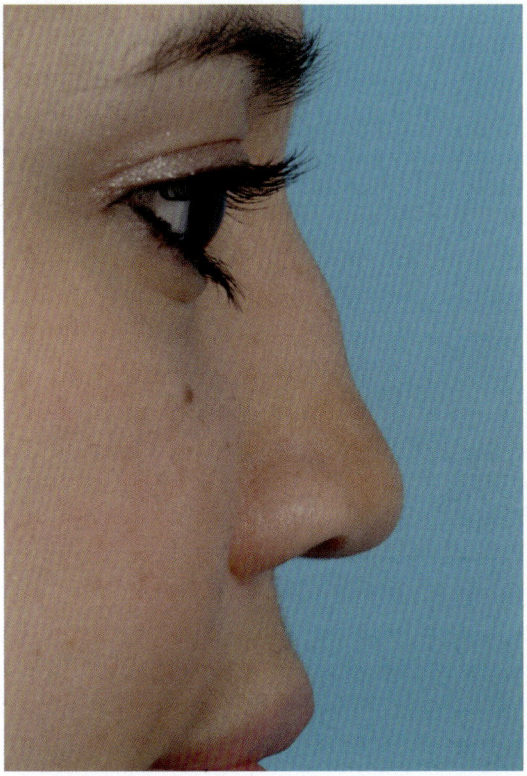

FIGURE 17.8
Patient with a dorsal hump and saddle nose deformity. Conservative dorsal hump reduction will be performed in conjunction with correcting the depressed middle nasal vault.

top of the nostril and the base of the nose. If tip projection is to be increased, the columellar incision can be placed a millimeter lower on the columella. The incision is made with a no. 11 blade using a sawing motion to allow accurate execution of the incision. The marginal extension of the columellar incision is made following the medial crura. Care is taken to avoid damaging the underlying medial crura. The columellar flap is elevated over the lower lateral cartilages, and then, dissection is extended over the nasal dorsum. A Joseph periosteal elevator is used to elevate the periosteum off of the bony nasal vault. If dorsal augmentation is planned over the nasal dorsum, a very narrow subperiosteal pocket is made over the bony dorsum. This is very important in order to create a tight fit of the dorsal graft over the nasal dorsum. If a wide dissection is performed over the nasal dorsum, the surgeon will be forced to perform a method of fixation to insure that the graft does not move.

Many patients with a saddle nose deformity have a dorsal hump with the concave saddling below the hump (Fig. 17.8). In this situation, the surgeon must make a decision as to whether to perform a dorsal hump reduction or to augment around the dorsal hump. In most cases, this will depend on the original height of the dorsum and the requests of the patient. Computer imaging is very important to help determine the proposed contour of the profile. If dorsal hump reduction is planned, a 2-mm straight osteotome can be used to create bone cut at the cephalic endpoint of the hump reduction. Then, a Rubin osteotome can be used to complete the dorsal hump reduction with the osteotomy completed at the site of the cephalic bone cut (Fig. 17.9). If the nasal bones are too wide or deviated, bilateral lateral osteotomies can be performed to narrow the bony nasal vault. In some cases, bilateral medial osteotomies may be necessary to allow symmetric alignment of the nasal bones.

Once the bony nasal vault is set, the lower two-thirds of the nose can be reconstructed. Initially, a decision must be made whether reconstruction of the saddle nose deformity will be limited to grafting the middle vault concavity or if the middle vault will be dissected and the dorsal septal deficiency reconstructed. If the reconstruction is limited to dorsal onlay grafting, the graft should be carved to fill the defect. The graft can be sutured into position under direct visualization. The nasal skin is then replaced in order to evaluate the contour. Once the concavity is filled with a cartilage graft, the nasal tip must be evaluated.

If the decision is made to reconstruct the dorsal septal deficiency, costal cartilage may be necessary to adequately replace the absent dorsal nasal strut. After performing the external rhinoplasty approach, the upper lateral cartilages are dissected free from the septum and retracted laterally to expose the dorsal septal deformity (Fig. 17.10). Patients with this degree of septal deformity usually require a more aggressive approach to septal reconstruction. The damaged septal cartilage can be removed and then reconstructed. It is helpful to leave a dorsal strut attached to the perpendicular plate of the ethmoid bone to act as a fixation point for the reconstruction. When the etiology of saddling is a large septal perforation not amenable to simultaneous repair, it is important to keep the dorsal dissection away from the perforation margin to avoid intranasal exposure of the cartilage grafts. In cases with a severe loss of caudal septal support, a caudal septal replacement

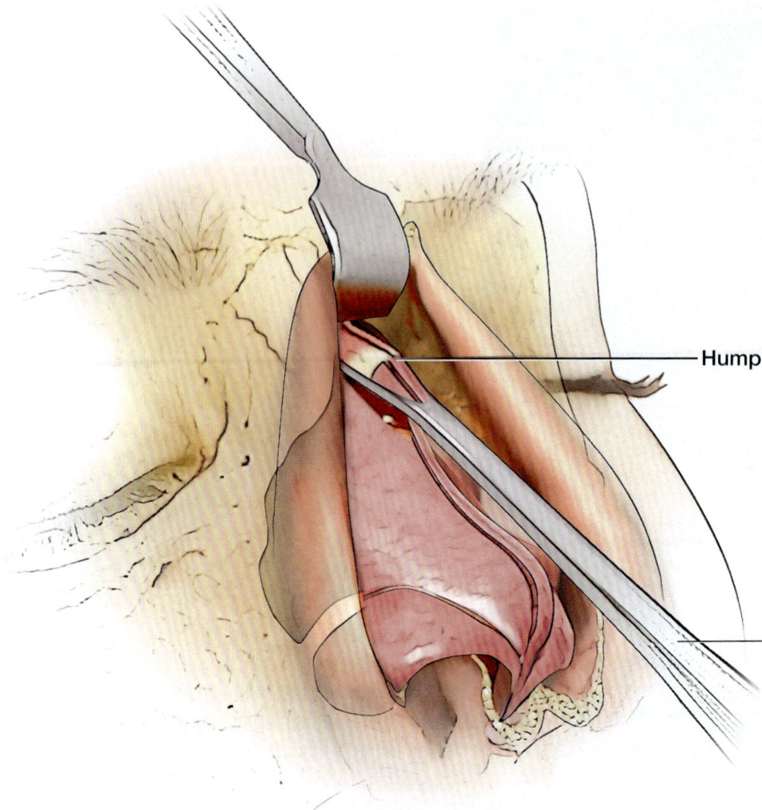

FIGURE 17.9 Dorsal hump reduction is initiated by making a 2-mm osteotome perforation at the superior aspect of the proposed dorsal hump reduction. Then, a Rubin osteotome is used to complete the reduction from below with the bony hump breaking off at the site of the perforations.

graft is fixated to the nasal spine region. A 5-mm straight osteotome is used to make a notch in the nasal spine and then a rectangular shaped cartilage graft is sutured into the notch and fixated superiorly using extended spreader grafts (Fig. 17.11). Care is taken to insure that the graft is in the precise midline as the medial crura will be sutured to the septal replacement graft. In some patients, the nasal spine is off of midline and may require an angled osteotomy to shift the notch into alignment with the dorsum of the nose. Once the notch is created and the graft is fashioned, the caudal septal replacement graft can be sutured into position using one or two 4-0 PDS sutures. These sutures are passed through soft tissue around the nasal spine. If there is no soft tissue that can be grasped, a small hole can be drilled near the base of the nasal spine using several 16-gauge needles. Then, the 4-0 PDS sutures can be passed through the holes and passed through the graft to fixate it into position. This fixation is very important as it creates a very major problem if the graft becomes displaced postoperatively. Once the caudal septal replacement graft is fixed to the nasal spine, bilateral extended spreader grafts are sutured to the remnant dorsal septum and extended inferiorly (Fig. 17.12). This is a "component reconstruction" of the L-shaped septal strut. The length of the spreader grafts and their orientation in relation to the caudal septal replacement graft will control tip projection, tip rotation, nasal length, alar–columellar

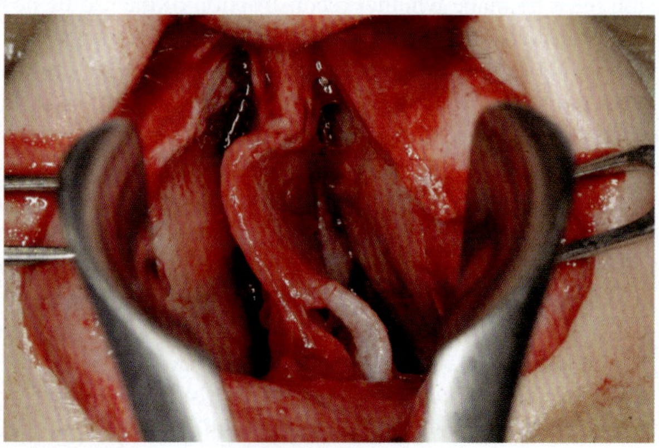

FIGURE 17.10
Septal deformity exposed after dissecting between medial crura and freeing upper lateral cartilages from the dorsal septum. Note the severity of the septal damage, which has left the patient with inadequate dorsal septal support.

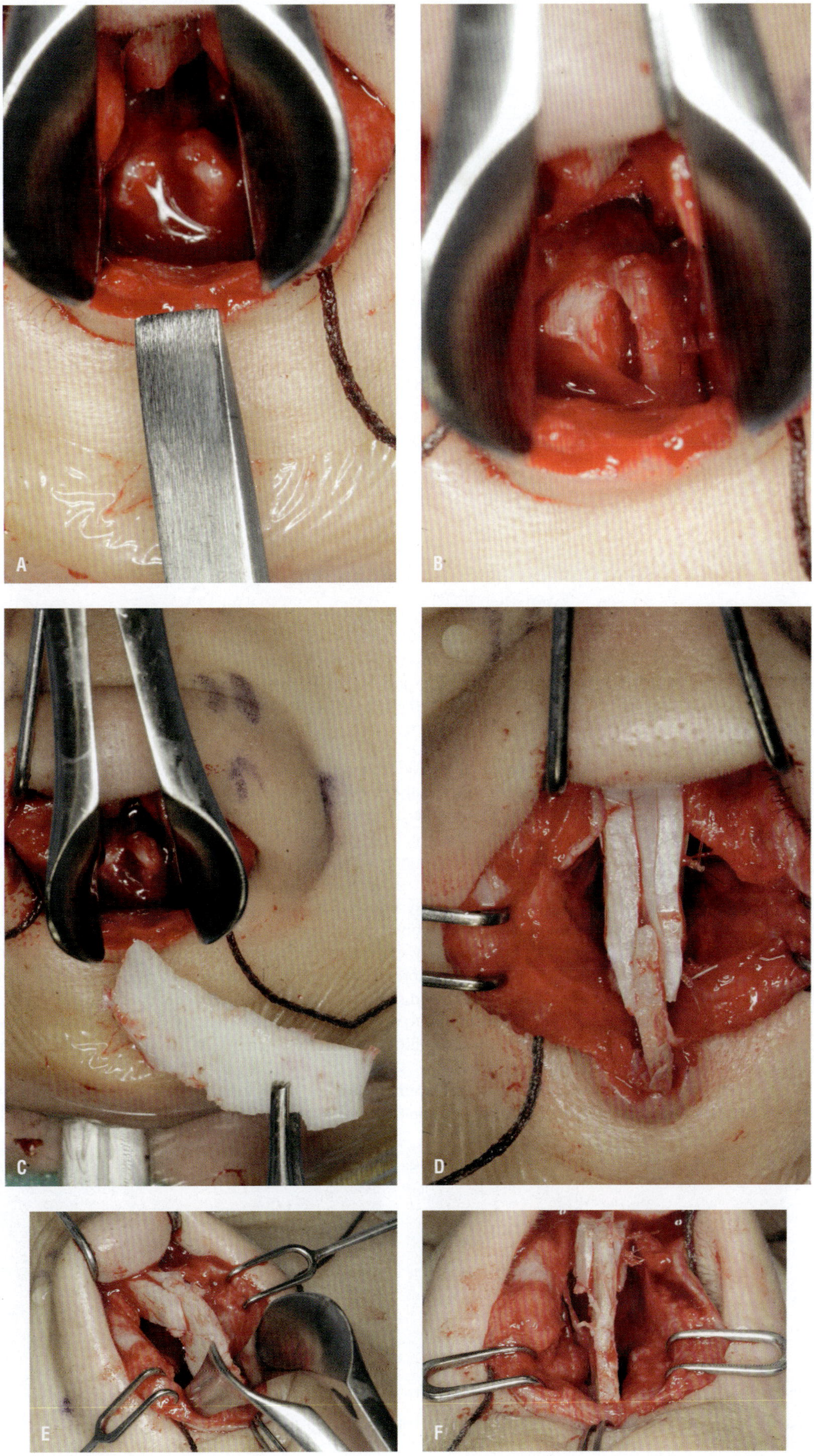

FIGURE 17.11
Reconstruction of L-shaped septal strut. **A:** A 5-mm straight osteotome is used to make a notch in the nasal spine. **B:** Note the notch in the nasal spine. **C:** Caudal septal replacement graft. **D–F:** Caudal septal replacement graft sutured into notch in nasal spine and then stabilized with bilateral extended spreader grafts.

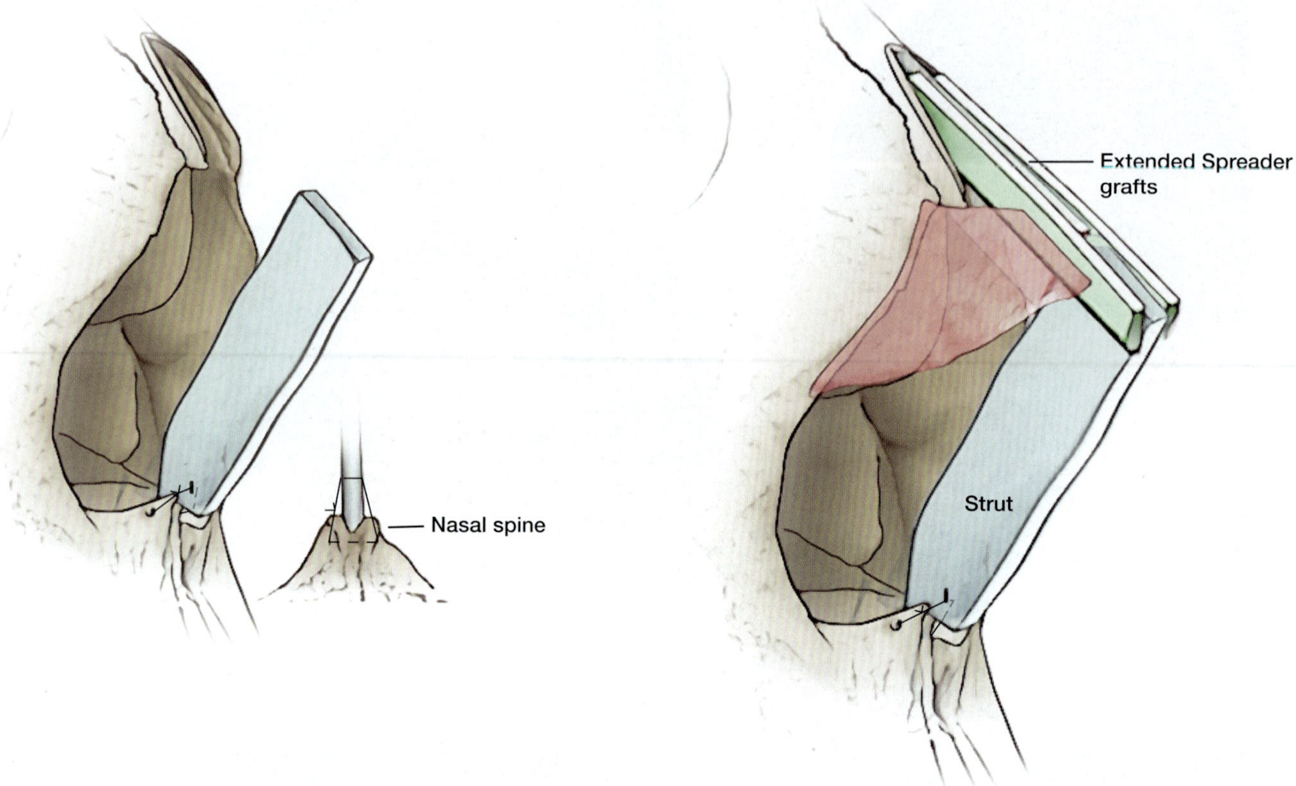

FIGURE 17.12 The caudal septal replacement graft can be positioned to move the columella inferiorly to open the nasolabial angle. The graft is fixated into the notch in the nasal spine. The notch in the strut keeps it from moving superiorly when the patient smiles.

relationship, and supratip break. The extended spreader grafts should be beveled caudally to avoid widening of the columella. Once the L-strut is reconstructed, the upper lateral cartilages can be sutured to the spreader grafts to complete the reconstruction of the middle nasal vault. The caudal septal replacement graft can be positioned to push the nasolabial angle out and down to create a more favorable nasolabial angle. Additionally, the medial crura can be advanced anteriorly on the caudal septal replacement graft to increase tip projection and open the nasolabial angle (Fig. 17.13).

Patients must be forewarned that this graft may limit the upward movement of their upper lip and they could experience a change in their smile and possibly a crease in their upper lip. Patients who have a lateral smile where the corner of the mouth moves laterally will be less likely to form a crease. Patients with a smile where the corners of the mouth move upward are more likely to form a crease in their upper lip. In the patient with this type of smile, it may be preferable to avoid rigid fixation to the nasal spine region. In these patients, the caudal septal replacement graft can be sutured to soft tissue behind the nasal spine, which will allow the graft to move upward when the patient smiles. Additionally, soft tissue can be left between the caudal margin of the septal replacement graft and the columella.

Once the extension graft or caudal septal replacement graft are in position, the medial crura can be sutured to the caudal margin of these grafts to set tip position, tip projection, rotation, columellar show, and the contour

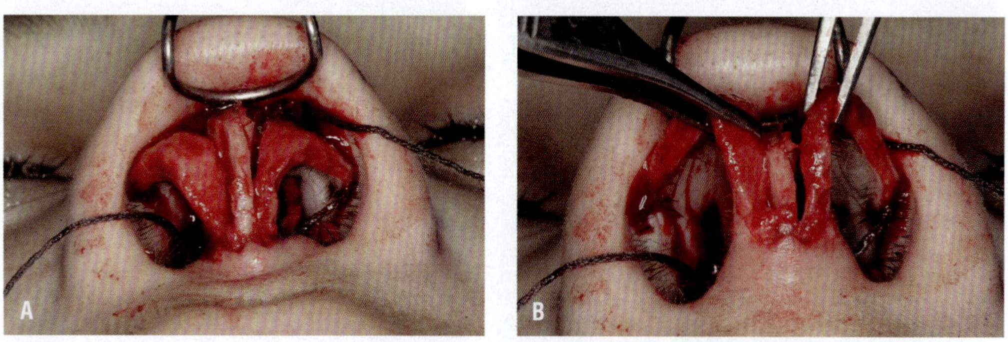

FIGURE 17.13 **A:** The caudal septal extension graft is set between the medial crura. **B:** The medial crura are advanced anteriorly to increase tip projection and open the nasolabial angle.

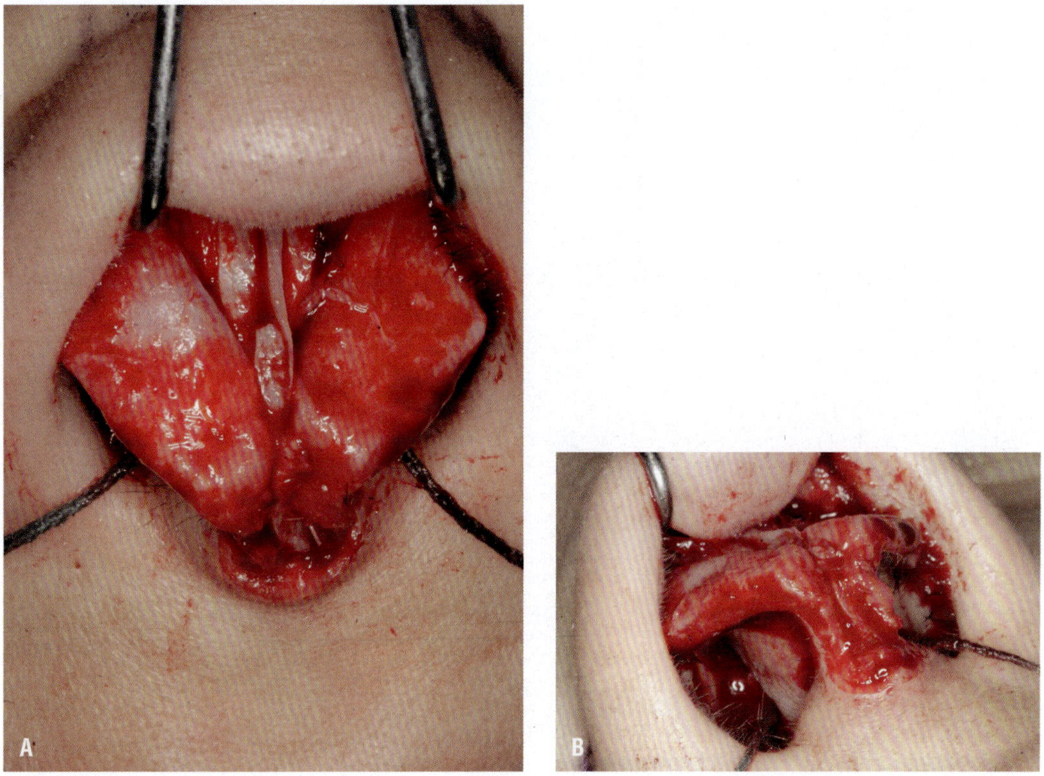

FIGURE 17.14 A: Lateral crura are flattened after placement of bilateral dome-binding sutures. **B:** Base view shows fixation of medial crura to septal extension graft.

of the nasolabial angle. This maneuver is very important as it sets many aesthetic parameters that will greatly impact the outcome. If the surgeon does not feel comfortable controlling these parameters, they may wish to limit stabilization of the nasal base and use a columellar strut.

Once the nasal base is stabilized, the tip lobule can be modified. This may involve conservative trimming of the cephalic margins of the lateral crura, dome-binding sutures, lateral crural strut grafts, or repositioning of the lateral crura to correct cephalic malpositioning (Fig. 17.14). In most patients, the projection is adequately corrected by stabilizing the nasal base and contour of the tip can be achieved using less invasive methods. Shield tip grafts are usually not necessary, but horizontally oriented onlay tip grafts are ideal for slightly increasing tip projection and providing a subtle increase in tip definition (Fig. 17.15). This method of septal reconstruction is an effective means for reconstructing the saddle nose deformity (Fig. 17.16A–J).

If the entire dorsal line needs to be reconstructed, a costal cartilage dorsal graft can be carved to accommodate the defect. This is accomplished by cutting the harvested rib cartilage into three separate segments (Fig. 17.17A, B). Then, the segments are placed into saline solution to observe for bending or warping. It is preferable to use a dorsal graft that has a distinct curvature so there is no question as to the tendency of the bending. The curve of the graft is then used in a fashion to counteract the tendency to curve by implanting the dorsal graft with the concave side of the graft facing downward against the nasal dorsum (Fig. 17.18). Costal cartilage perichondrium is sutured to the undersurface of the dorsal graft using a running 6-0 Monocryl suture (Fig. 17.19). Perichondrium can also be sutured to the lateral margins of the dorsal graft to camouflage the edges of the graft and prevent visible contour deformities postoperatively. Then, a fine-toothed rasp is used to roughen up the bone on the nasal dorsum to create a rough bone surface that will adhere to the perichondrium on the undersurface of the dorsal graft (Fig. 17.20). If rasping is not possible due to scarring, a 2-mm straight osteotome can be used to make multiple punctures into the bone that will accomplish the same effect of allowing the perichondrium to become fixed down to the bone. In order for this fixation to occur, there must be a tight pocket of periosteum over the nasal dorsum, which forces the dorsal graft to closely adhere the roughened surface of the bone. This adhesion will act to fixate the dorsal graft to the bony dorsum. By fixating the dorsal graft to the bony dorsum, it is much less likely to bend or warp and this will also create a more natural-looking stable bridge.

In some cases, there is a wide, loose pocket over the nasal dorsum that will not allow the dorsal graft to fit tightly over the roughened bone. In these cases, it may be necessary to use a Kirschner wire to fixate the cartilage dorsal graft down onto the bony dorsum. A no. 11 blade is used to make a small stab incision in the skin over the superior aspect of the graft (Fig. 17.21). Then, a 0.45-inch threaded K-wire

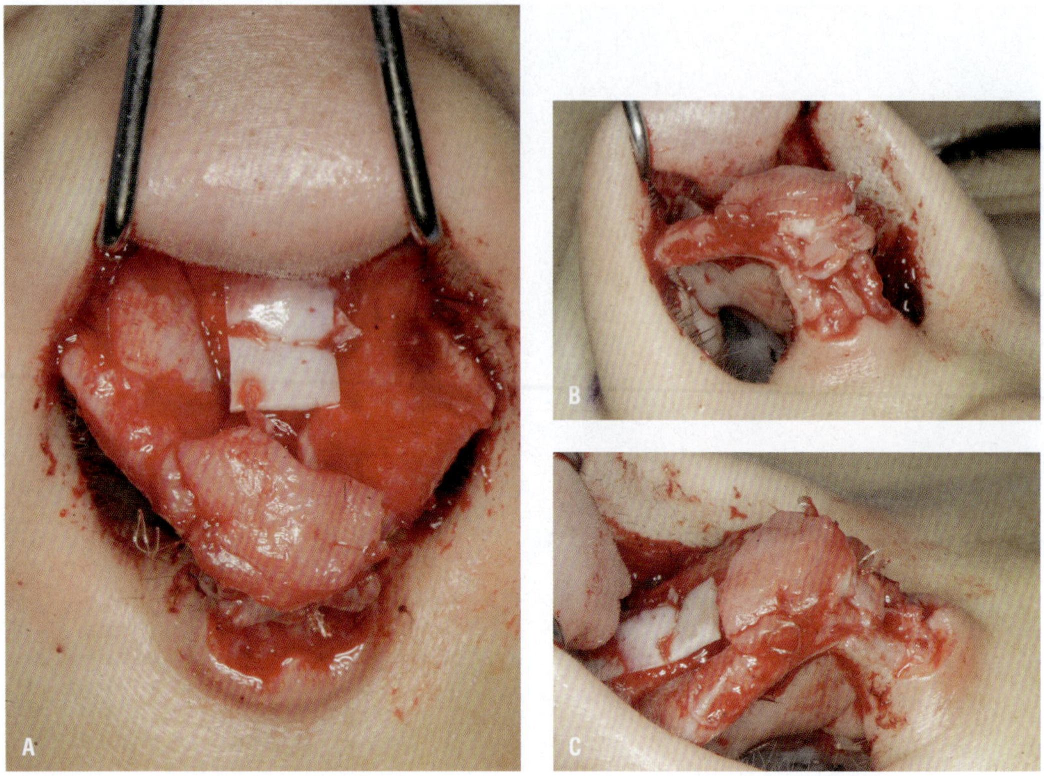

FIGURE 17.15 **A–C:** Onlay tip graft placed horizontally over the domes to increase tip projection, improve tip definition, and preserve horizontally oriented tip-defining points.

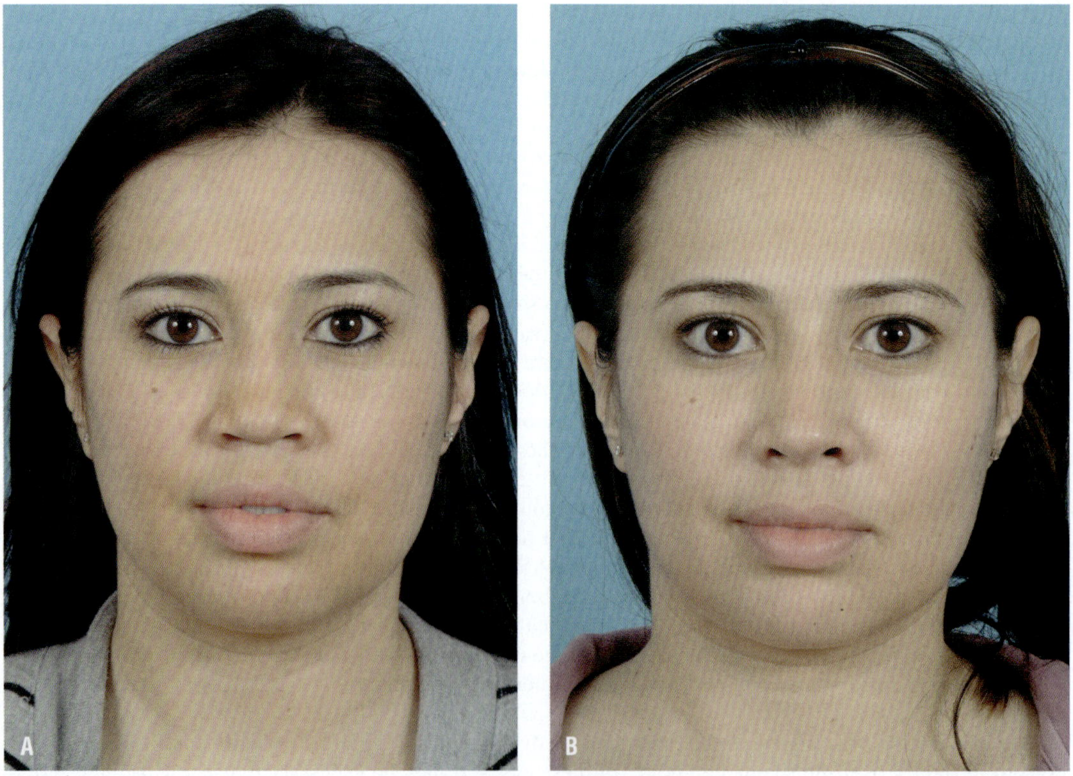

FIGURE 17.16 Saddle nose repair. **A:** Preoperative frontal view. **B:** Postoperative frontal view shows correction of depressed middle nasal vault and narrowing of nasal tip.

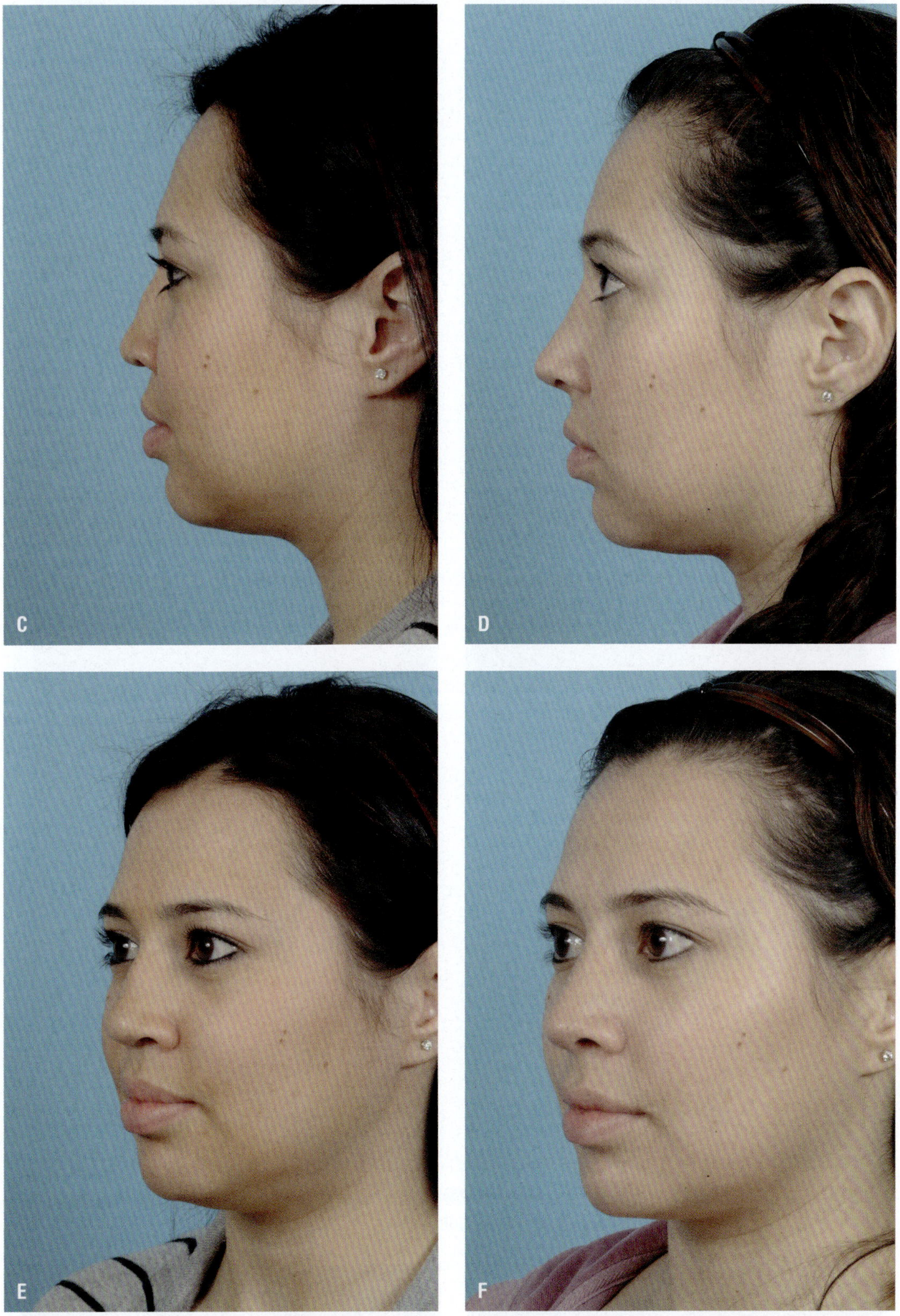

FIGURE 17.16 (*Continued*) **C:** Preoperative lateral view. **D:** Postoperative lateral view demonstrates correction of saddling of the middle nasal vault, correction of the nasolabial angle, and increase in nasal tip projection. **E:** Preoperative oblique view. **F:** Postoperative oblique view demonstrates correction of middle vault deformity.

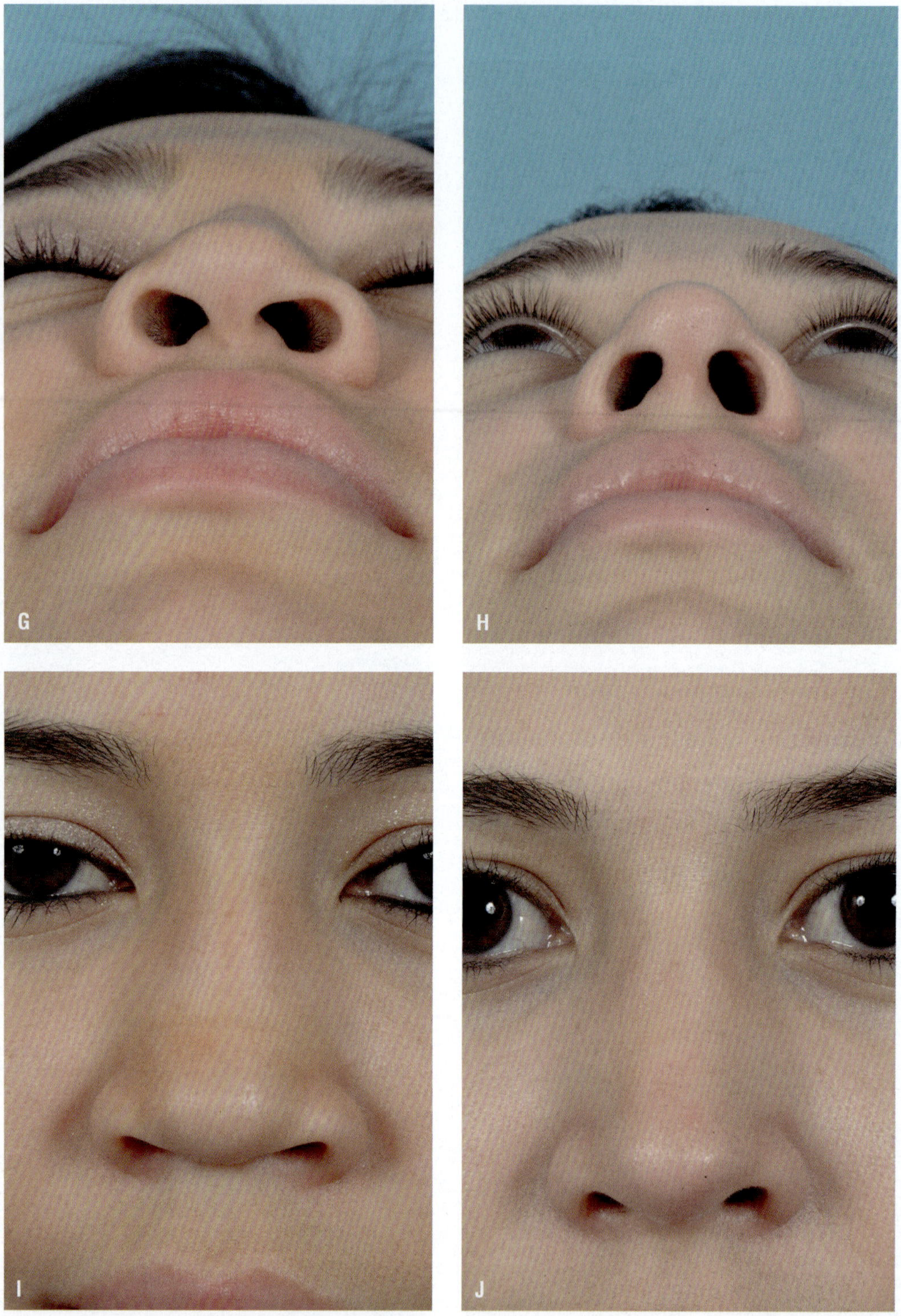

FIGURE 17.16 (*Continued*) **G:** Preoperative base view. **H:** Postoperative base view demonstrates increased tip projection and narrowing. **I.** Preoperative frontal view. **J.** Postoperative frontal view.

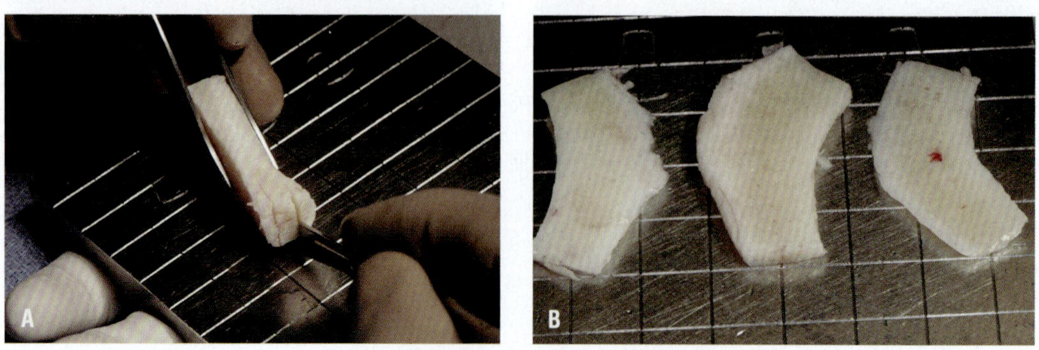

FIGURE 17.17
Carving costal cartilage. **A:** Rib is carved into three segments of cartilage. **B:** Once carved, the segments can be assessed for curvature.

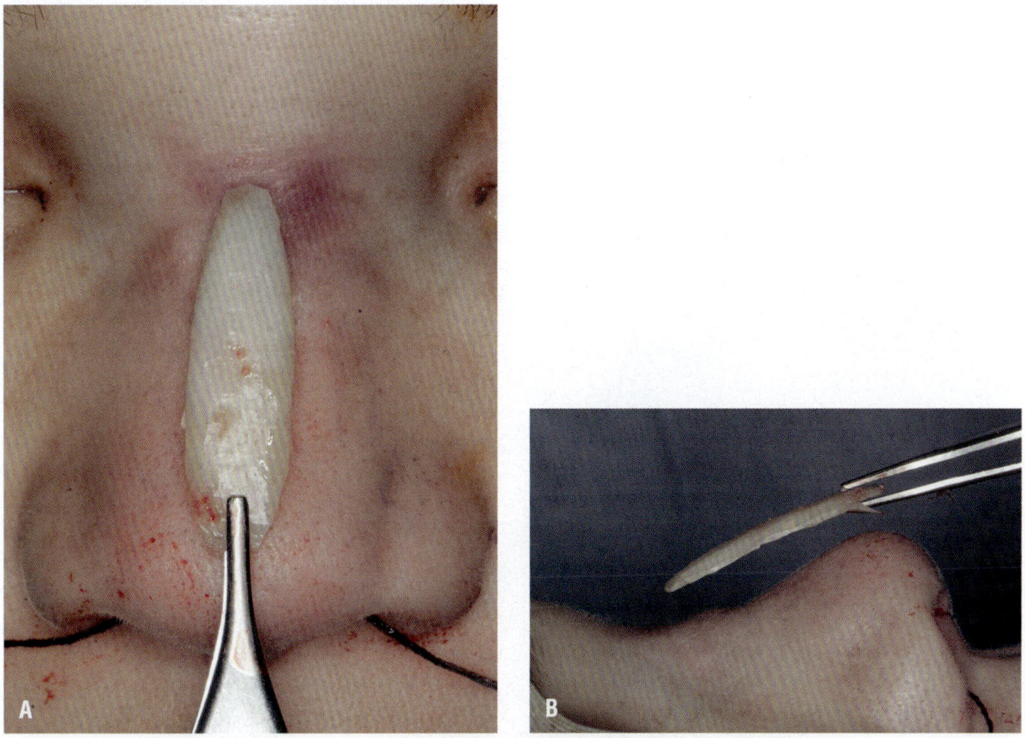

FIGURE 17.18
Dorsal graft. **A:** Dorsal graft is canoe shaped. **B:** The dorsal graft is curved so the concave surface is facing down to the dorsum.

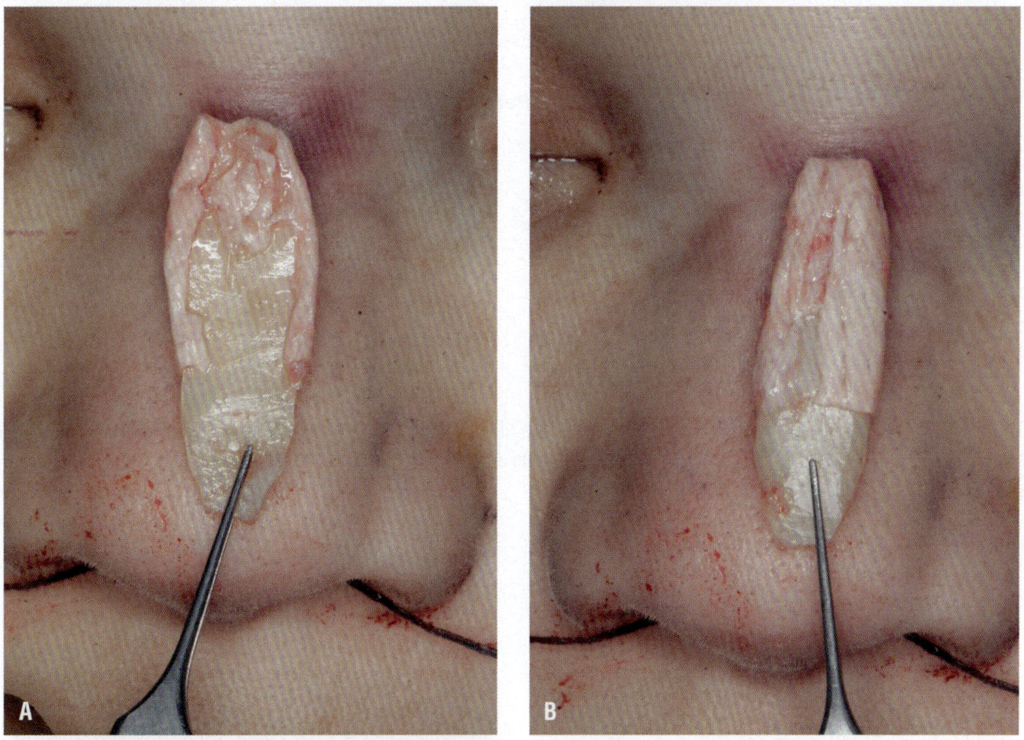

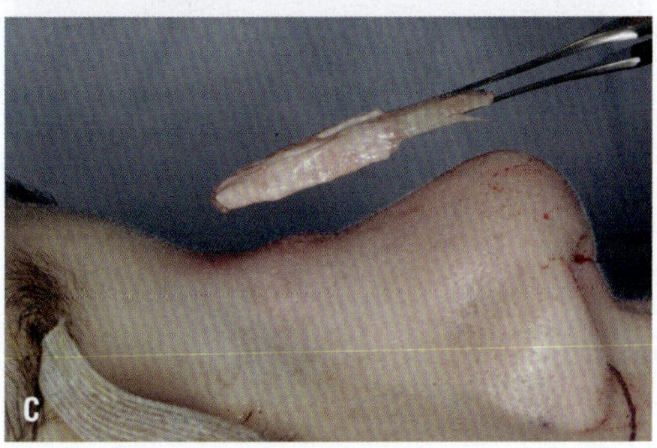

FIGURE 17.19
Perichondrium is sutured to the undersurface of the dorsal graft. This will provide a tissue fixation interface with the bony dorsum. **A:** Dorsal graft with perichondrium sutured to the undersurface of the dorsal graft to provide a fixation interface with the bony dorsum. **B:** Perichondrium sutured to the lateral margins of the dorsal graft. **C:** Perichondrium hangs over the edge of the graft.

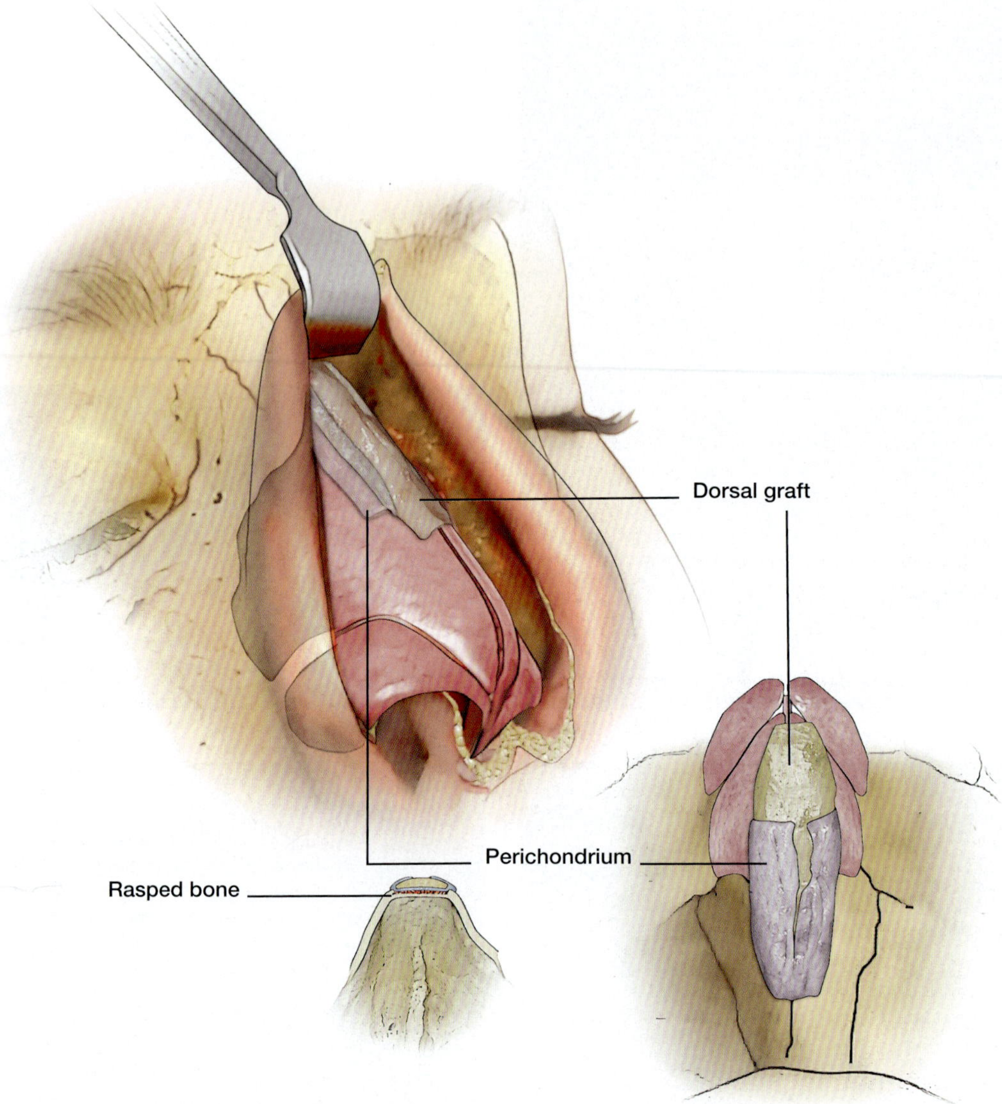

FIGURE 17.20 Perichondrium is sutured to the undersurface of the dorsal graft and then placed against a bony dorsum that has been rasped or perforated using a 2-mm straight osteotome. The perichondrium fixes to the perforated bone and allow fixation of the dorsal graft to the bony dorsum.

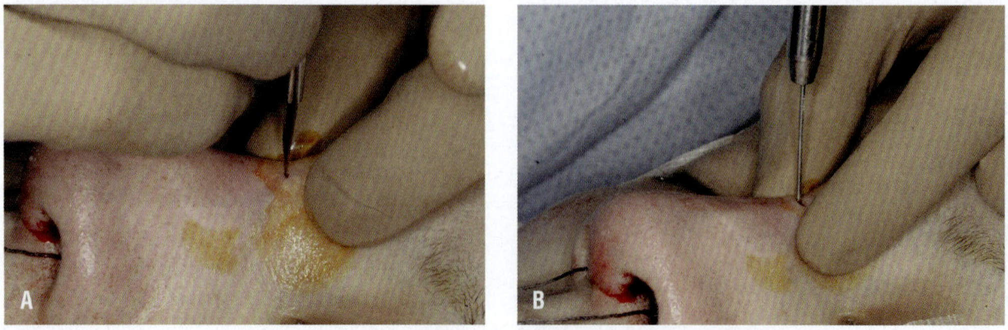

FIGURE 17.21 Placement of Kirschner wire. **A:** Stab incision made into dorsal skin over the dorsal graft. **B:** Using a Hall air-powered drill is used to advance the K-wire through the dorsal graft and into the bony dorsum.

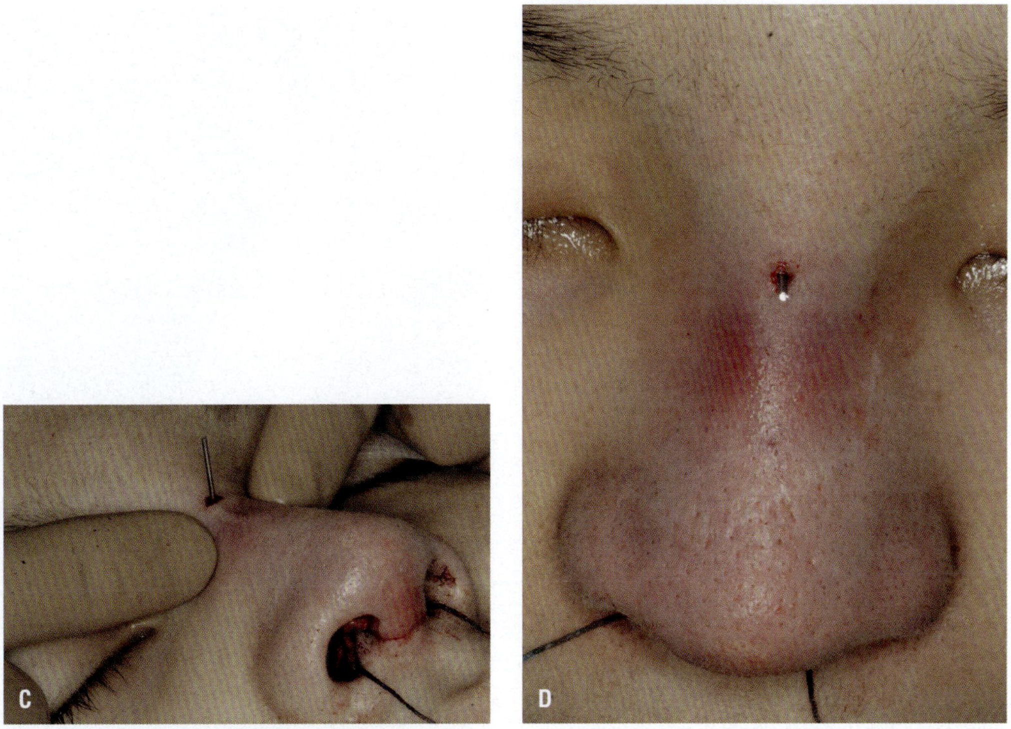

FIGURE 17.21 (*Continued*) **C:** Palpation insures that the dorsal graft is midline and closely fixed to the bone. **D:** K-wire in position with 2 to 3 cm left protruding through skin.

is advanced through the cartilage dorsal graft and on into the bone of the nasal dorsum. Care is taken to make sure that the dorsal graft stays down against the bone. The K-wire should only penetrate the bony dorsum by about 4 to 6 mm (Fig. 17.22). Special care must be taken to insure that the dorsal graft is fixated into the midline and not tilted as the graft will fixate on the dorsum in that orientation. An Aquaplast cast and Steri-Strips are applied over the dorsum allowing the K-wire to pass through the Steri-Strips and also through the holes in the Aquaplast cast (Fig. 17.23). The Aquaplast cast can be removed on the 7th postoperative day and the K-wire can be backed out using pliers. The stab incision on the nasal dorsum should heal without noticeable scarring.

As an alternative to a K-wire, holes can be drilled into the sidewalls of the bony dorsum below the graft and a 4-0 PDS suture can be passed through these holes and then over the top of the dorsal graft (Figs. 17.24 and 17.25). The holes can be drilled using a small hand drill or 16-gauge needles. Care must be taken to avoid making the holes too close to the facial plane as it may then present itself in the nasal airway. Most patients that are undergoing dorsal augmentation have a relatively low bony dorsum and the holes must be drilled horizontally across the bridge. The suture can be passed over the dorsal graft through small stab incisions in the sidewall skin of the bridge in order to allow it to be passed over the dorsal graft and then tied.

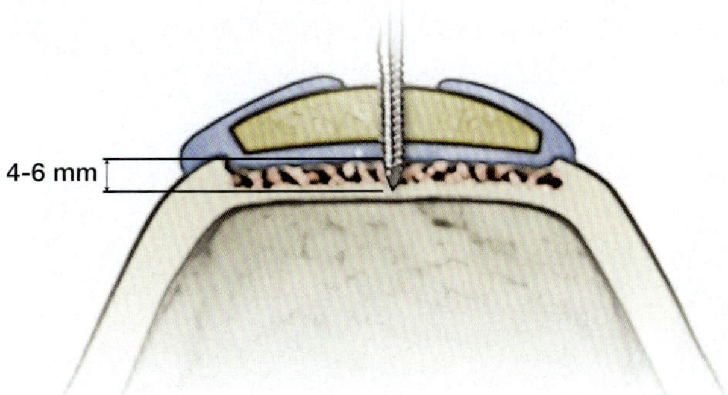

FIGURE 17.22

Kirschner wire passes through the dorsal graft and into the underlying bony dorsum penetrating the bone by about 8 to 10 mm.

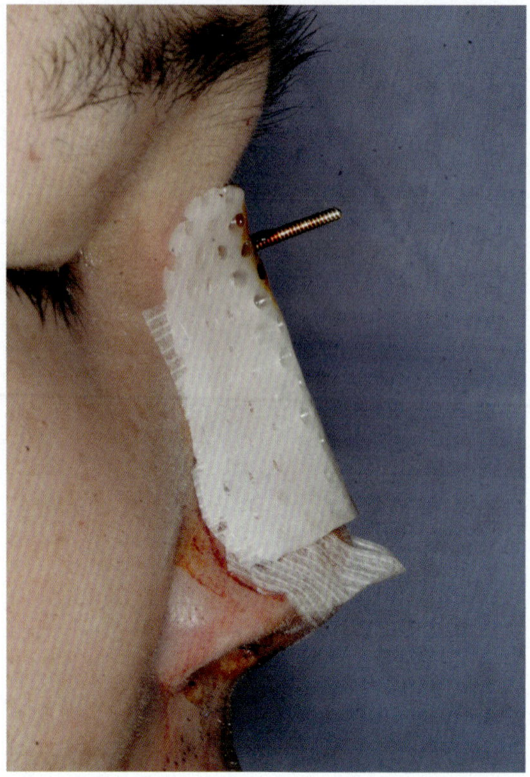

FIGURE 17.23
Aquaplast cast with holes allows the K-wire to pass through the cast.

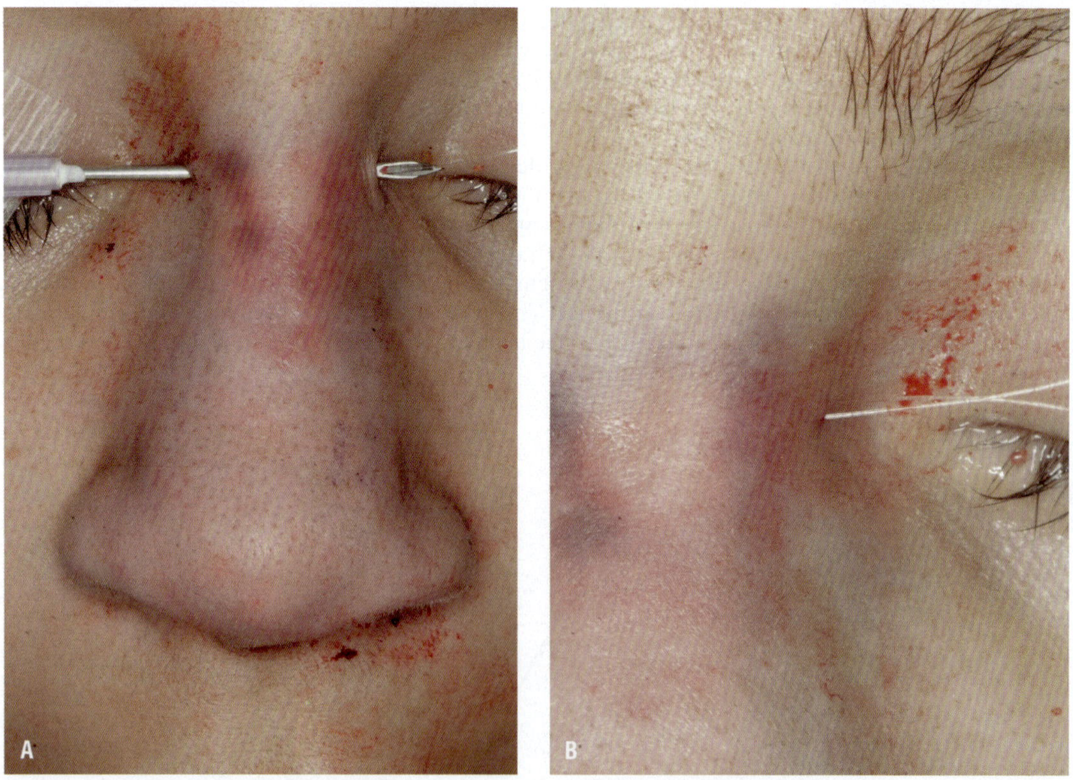

FIGURE 17.24 A: Using a 16-gauge needle, holes are drilled through the nasal dorsum using a 16-gauge needle and a 4-0 PDS suture is passed through the holes, over the dorsal graft, and then tied tightly to fixate the dorsal graft against the bony dorsum. **B:** Suture is tied to fixate dorsal graft.

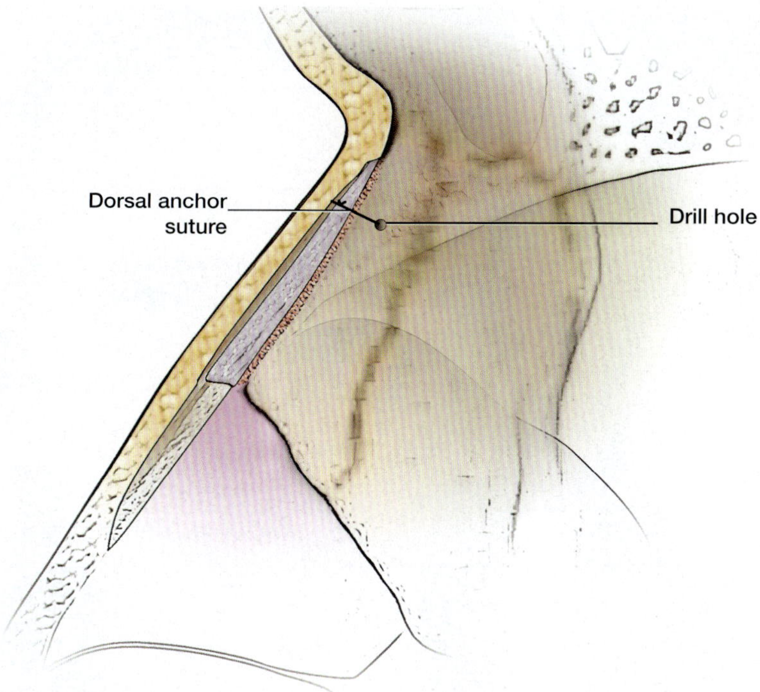

FIGURE 17.25
Suture is passed through the holes in the bony dorsum and then over the top of the dorsal graft to fixate it to the bony dorsum.

Once the dorsal graft is fixated superiorly over the bony dorsum, it should also be fixated over the middle nasal vault using two 5-0 PDS sutures placed through the upper lateral cartilages and then through the dorsal graft laterally. With the fixation over the bony dorsum and fixation of the middle nasal vault, the dorsal graft should be stable and will not move or shift postoperatively (Fig. 17.26).

In patients with thin skin, the lateral margin of the dorsal graft may be detectable with time as the thinner skin contracts over the dorsal graft. To avoid visualization of the lateral margins of the dorsal graft strips of costal cartilage, perichondrium can be placed along the sidewalls of the nose. The perichondrium can be sutured to the lateral margins of the dorsal graft and then inserted or the strips of perichondrium can be placed along the margins of the dorsal graft and fixated transcutaneously using 6-0 Monocryl sutures placed through the skin, into the perichondrium, and then tied over the skin. Betadine can be painted over the suture knots to help prevent infection. These sutures can be removed when the cast is removed.

POSTOPERATIVE MANAGEMENT

The patients are discharged the same day with antibiotics and instructions to clean their nose once a day using hydrogen peroxide on a cotton-tip applicator. More novice surgeons should consider overnight observation with a postoperative chest radiograph after any rib graft harvest. Nasal packing can be removed on the first postoperative day. The nasal cast and sutures are removed on the 7th postoperative day. If costal cartilage was harvested, the sutures are also removed on the 7th postoperative day. The patient is given Silastic sheeting to place over the chest incision beginning on the 14th postoperative day. This can be used primarily at night.

COMPLICATIONS

Complications from this type of repair can be categorized into shorter-term complications and longer-term complications. Shorter-term complications include bleeding, infection, and excessive bruising or swelling. Early complications associated with the rib cartilage harvest include pneumothorax, warping of the rib cartilage (early warping), excessive pain, and deformity. Longer-term complications include nasal deformity, deviation, warping of the rib cartilage, septal perforation, and prolonged swelling. Longer-term complications associated with the rib cartilage harvest include scarring, chest wall depression, and pain with chest wall compression. Fortunately, these problems are very rare.

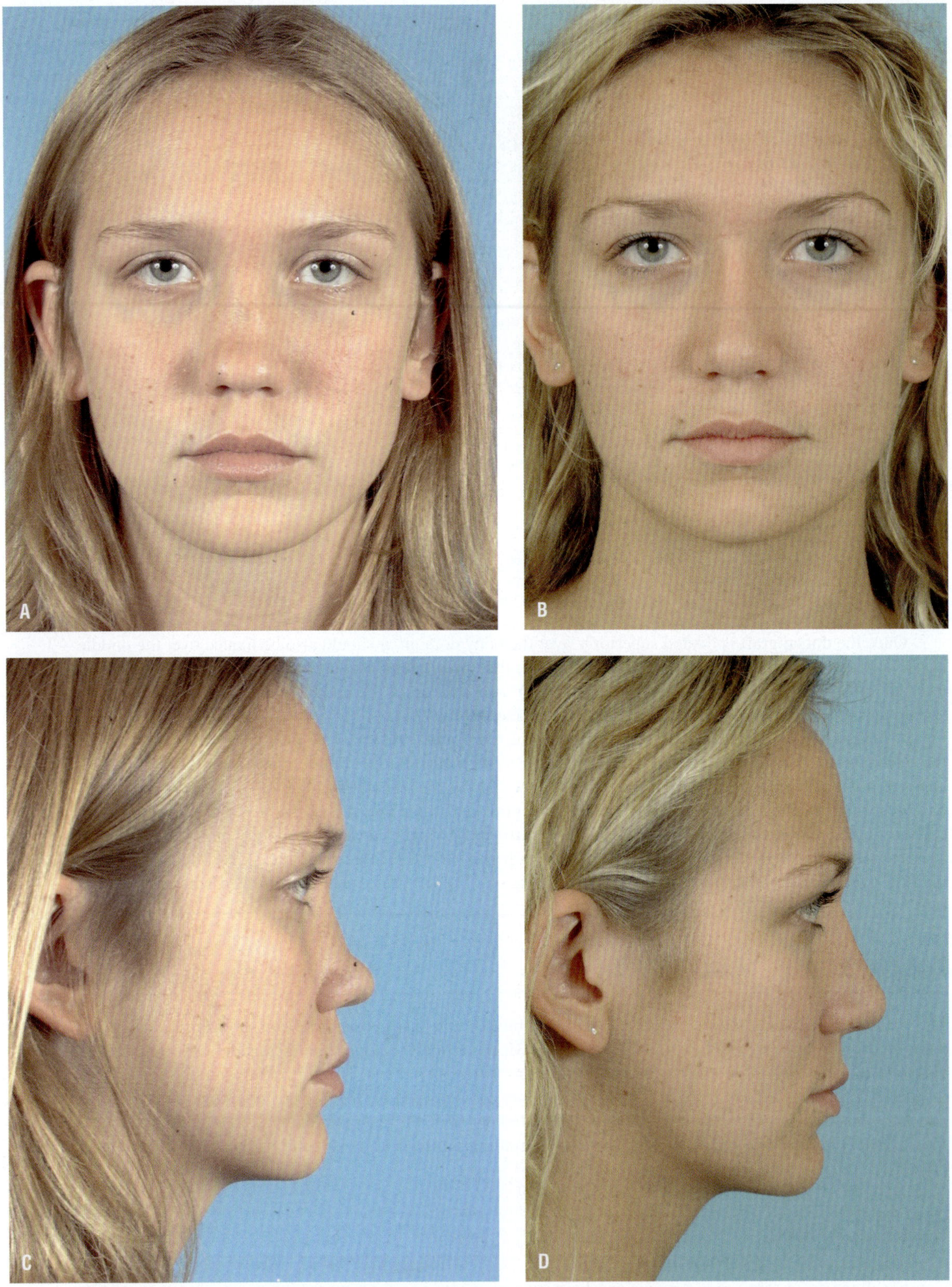

FIGURE 17.26 Patient with saddle nose deformity corrected using dorsal augmentation with costal cartilage graft. **A:** Preoperative frontal view. **B:** Postoperative frontal view showing improved dorsal lines with straight dorsal graft. The nasal tip is narrowed as well. **C:** Preoperative lateral view. **D:** Postoperative lateral view shows improved dorsal profile with improved tip projection.

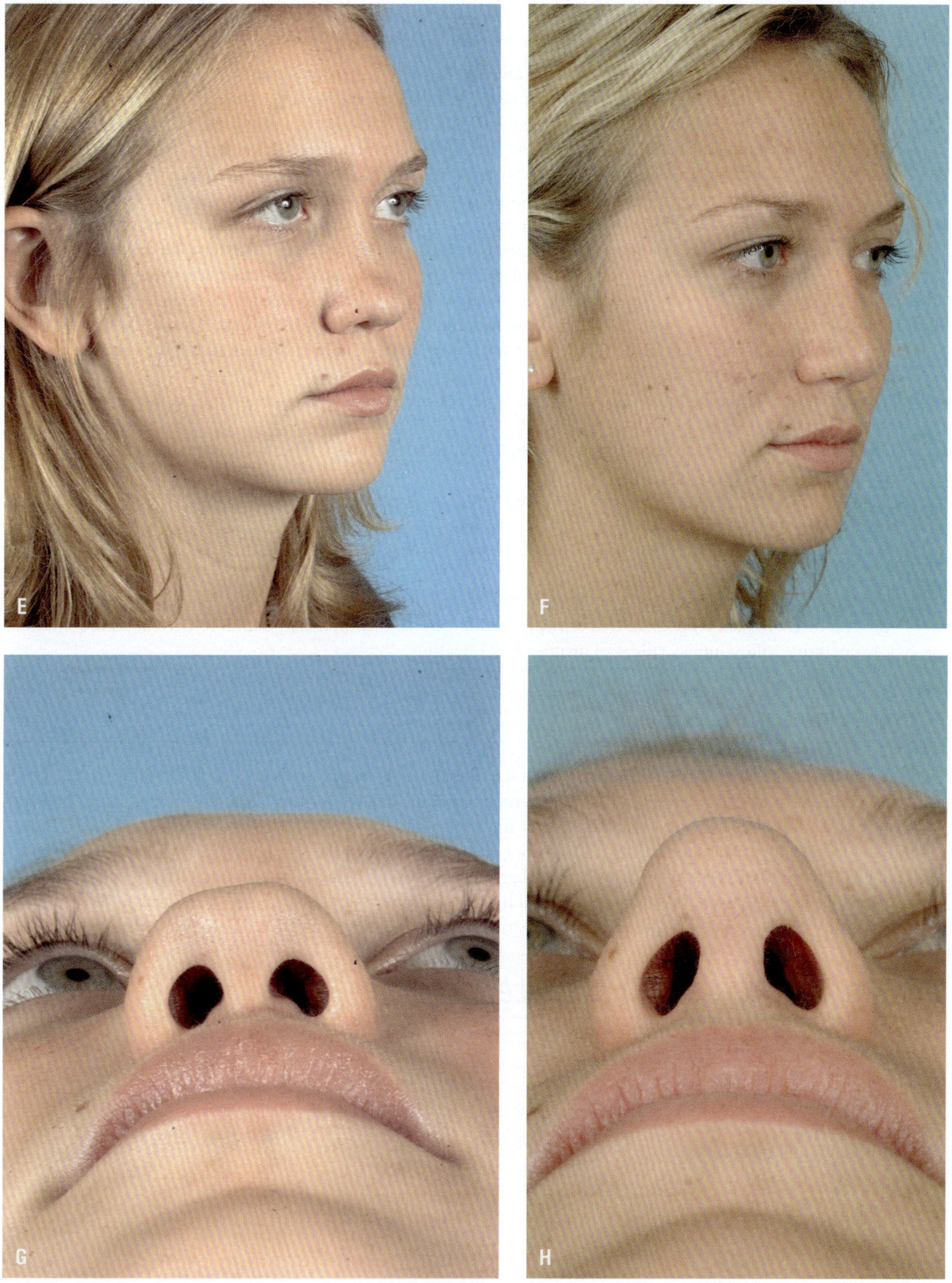

FIGURE 17.26 (*Continued*) **E:** Preoperative oblique view. **F:** Postoperative oblique view. **G:** Preoperative base view. **H:** Postoperative base view demonstrating the improved shape of the tip.

RESULTS

Reconstruction of the saddle nose deformity can be relatively simple or more complex depending on the severity of the deformity and the status of the underlying septal damage. In many patients, the saddle nose deformity can be corrected using simple onlay cartilage grafting techniques that do not correct the underlying septal deficiency. Correction of the underlying septal deficiency requires complete dissection of the nasal septum with wide exposure and reconstruction of the L-shaped septal strut using spreader grafts and possible caudal septal replacement. In the latter case, costal cartilage is frequently needed to complete the reconstruction and provide a stable nasal structure.

PEARLS

- Proper diagnosis of the underlying septal deficiency should begin with a complete examination of the head and neck and nasal endoscopy to evaluate for septal perforation and severe septal deformities.
- Palpation and compression of the nasal bridge and middle nasal vault can provide important information as to the stability of the underlying dorsal septum. If compression reveals a weakness in the middle nasal vault, that may represent a severe deficiency in dorsal septal support. This would require more than a simple onlay cartilage graft as this could result in descent of the graft over time with partial recurrence of the deformity.
- Prior to reconstructing a saddle nose deformity, the surgeon must be sure there is adequate grafting material present. If the surgeon is contemplating the use of costal cartilage for repair of the deformity, the degree of calcification of the ribs can be assessed by passing a needle into the rib transcutaneously and walking the needle along the rib to detect calcification. Care must be taken to avoid puncturing the pleura as this can lead to a pneumothorax.
- If costal cartilage is to be harvested, the 6th rib lies at the level of the inframammary crease in most women and has a genu that may not be an ideal shape for saddle nose repair. If a longer straighter segment of rib is needed, the 7th rib is the ideal option.
- Reconstruction of the L-shaped septal strut can be performed using a caudal septal replacement graft and bilateral extended spreader grafts.
- Care must be taken to be certain that appropriate tip projection, nasal length, rotation, alar–columellar relationship are set properly.
- Costal cartilage dorsal grafts should be carved with a curvature so the concave surface is oriented against the bony dorsum.
- Perichondrium is sutured to the undersurface of the dorsal graft and fixated to the rasped bony dorsum to promote osseous fixation.
- The dorsal graft must be closely adherent to the rasped nasal dorsum to allow the dorsal graft to fixate. In the case of a wide dorsal pocket, this critical fixation can be accomplished with a K-wire or suture fixation.
- Postoperative follow-up is critical to insure proper healing.

PITFALLS

- Avoid using auricular cartilage to reconstruct the dorsal nasal strut as this may destabilize over time.
- Avoid performing onlay dorsal grafting to correct the saddle nose deformity if there is inadequate septal support as the middle nasal vault may settle over time.
- Patients with an upward elevation of the corner of the mouth when they smile will be at higher risk of forming a crease in their upper lip when they smile if the septal replacement graft is fixated to the nasal spine.
- Carefully assess tip rotation, nasal length, and tip projection when reconstructing the L-strut since significant deformity can be created if these important parameters are not set properly.

INSTRUMENTS TO HAVE AVAILABLE

- Converse scissors
- Ragnell retractors
- Sharp Freer elevator
- 2-mm straight osteotome
- 5-mm straight osteotome
- Narrow fine-tooth rasp
- Hall drill if Kirschner wire needed
- 0.45-inch threaded Kirschner wire

ACKNOWLEDGMENT

The author would like to thank Gregory S. Dibelius, MD, for his contributions to this chapter. His work in the writing, editing, and figure creation for this chapter is greatly appreciated.

SUGGESTED READING

Guyuron B, Varghai V. Lengthening the nose with a tongue-and-groove technique. *Plast Reconstr Surg* 2003;111(4):1533–1539.
Toriumi DM. Subtotal reconstruction of the nasal septum. *Laryngoscope* 1994;104:906–913.
Toriumi DM. New concepts in nasal tip contouring. *Arch Facial Plast Surg* 2006;8:156–185.
Toriumi DM. Subtotal septal reconstruction: an update. *Facial Plast Surg* 2013;29:492–501.

18 RHINOPLASTY: SUTURE TECHNIQUES

Ira Papel

INTRODUCTION

The nasal tip is one of the most varied anatomic units in the human body. For that reason, multiple techniques in tip modification have been described throughout the history of rhinoplasty. Excision techniques were used primarily in the early procedures. In the more recent rhinoplasty literature, conservation techniques and the use of sutures has become the dominant theme.

Nasal tip width, contour, projection, and rotation are all elements that can be modified or enhanced by tip suture techniques. To accomplish this, narrowing sutures can be used to reduce the interdomal space which may also modify projection and rotation at the same time. The convexity of the lateral ala can be altered by the use of lateral crural convexity sutures.

The first published tip suture techniques were by Joseph who used direct interdomal sutures. This method was intended to stabilize the lower lateral cartilages after significant cephalic resection or cross-section. Goldman later used bilateral medial crural–vestibular flaps sutured to the caudal septum. This resulted in occasional extreme rotation, increased projection, and a signature appearance in which the cut ends of the domes became visible through the skin in later years. McCullough and English described the double-dome suture in 1985. This technique effectively narrows the interdomal space, but care must be taken to avoid medialization of the external valve. Kridel described a transdomal suture designed to recruit lateral crura to increase tip projection titled the "lateral crural steal." Daniel and Tebbets later described intradomal dome-shaping sutures and several variations of tip sutures. Guyuron also described tip suture techniques to alter the domes and columella. Baker and Guyuron have summarized these techniques in review articles.

HISTORY

As with any surgical procedure, it is important to gather pertinent patient history. Prior surgical procedures, cosmetic and functional, must be considered in planning further surgery. Medical conditions such as diabetes, hypertension, and sleep apnea are important to consider and advise about risk. Psychiatric conditions and medications are equally important as physical findings, especially disorders such as body dysmorphic disorder. Surgeons must identify risk factors and use their best judgment in planning rhinoplasty surgical procedures.

PHYSICAL EXAMINATION

The widened interdomal space is an esthetic finding often associated with a wide lobule, poor projection, and boxy appearance. The underlying lower lateral cartilages may have an abnormally large divergence angle between the medial or intermediate crura. The accepted angle of divergence is up to 30 degrees. The acceptable interdomal width, between tip defining points, is up to 6 mm. Patients with an interdomal width greater than

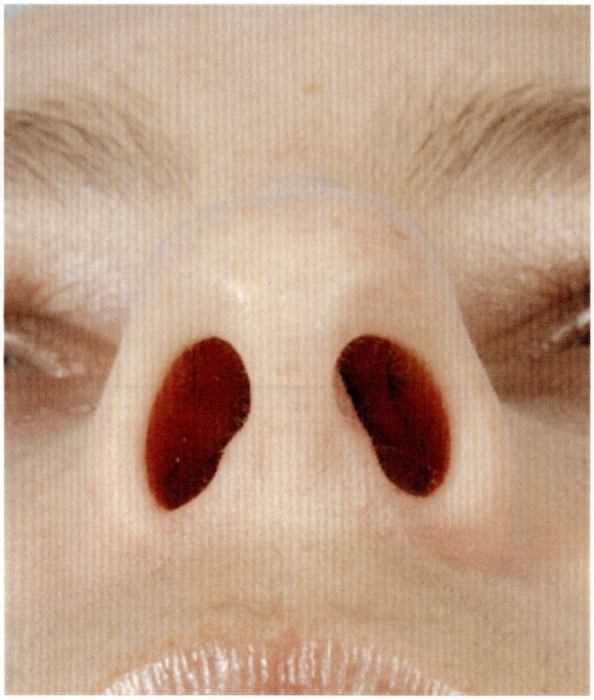

FIGURE 18.1
Base view demonstrating wide interdomal space and boxy tip.

6 mm are deemed appropriate for this technique. This chapter will illustrate a hybrid technique to accomplish tip contouring, narrowing and projection with an interlocking suture technique (Figs. 18.1 and 18.2).

INDICATIONS

Rhinoplasty tip suture techniques can be used for a myriad of nasal tip changes. The primary purpose is to narrow the interdomal space and/or contour the lower lateral cartilages. Reduction of lateral crural convexity is a common goal. Multiple suture designs have been described, but in this manuscript, I will confine myself to a description of the most common techniques of modifying the interdomal space and lateral crural convexity (Figs. 18.3 and 18.4).

CONTRAINDICATIONS

Suture techniques can be used in both intranasal and external rhinoplasty procedures. Contraindications are usually confined to known patient intolerance to suture materials. The most common suture materials are nylon, polypropylene, and polydioxanone. Suture granulomas or abscesses are rare but have been observed with essentially all suture materials.

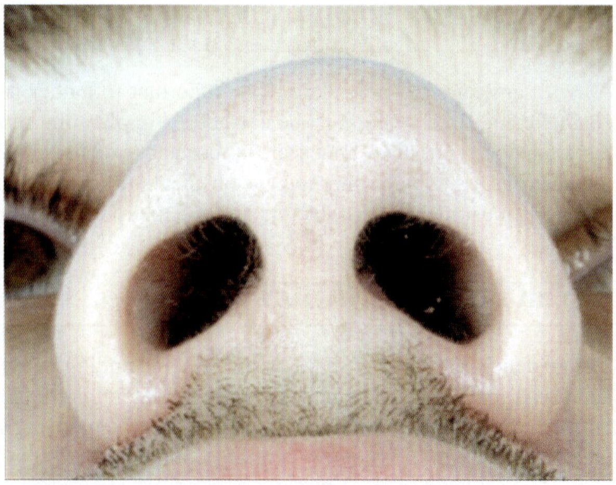

FIGURE 18.2
Base view showing wide interdomal space and convex ala.

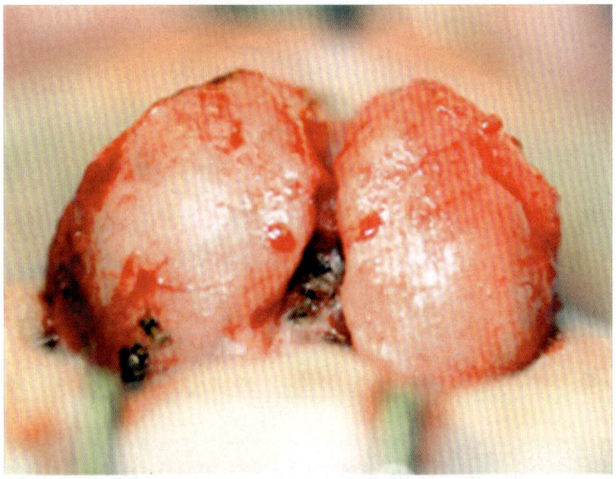

FIGURE 18.3
Operative cephalic view of lower lateral cartilages showing wide interdomal space, convex bulky, lateral crura.

PREOPERATIVE PLANNING

All patients are evaluated at a formal consultation. At this time, patient motivation, physical traits, past history, and realistic expectations are evaluated. Photographs are taken and used for further evaluation before surgery. Computer imaging is offered to selected patients, especially if the surgeon feels the patient is not visualizing the same changes as the surgeon is describing.

SURGICAL TECHNIQUE

Tip suture techniques can be performed through both intranasal and external approaches. In revision cases, the external route may be technically easier due to better visualization. Care is taken in either method to preserve the integrity of the crura and dissect as close as possible to the surface of the cartilage. The domes are each defined and marked before placement of any sutures. If the width of the lateral crura is excessive, a cephalic strip may be removed with preservation of vestibular skin. At this point, a transdomal mattress suture (5-0 polypropylene or 5-0 polydiaxanone) is placed with the knot positioned medially. In general, no scoring or morselization is necessary. The mattress suture is placed with the initial pass in the middle of the dome and the return pass more cephalic. This will help to preserve the divergence of the crura critical to maintaining a natural postoperative shape. Each transdomal suture is left with a long lead, so that the lead from the opposing domes can be tied together and narrow the space between the crura/domal complexes. As the knot is tied, the natural divergence of the medial crura is maintained. This method also avoids distortion of the lateral crura, which are often flared with traditional dome-binding sutures. Complimentary tip sculpturing sutures can be used with this procedure (Figs. 18.5 and 18.6).

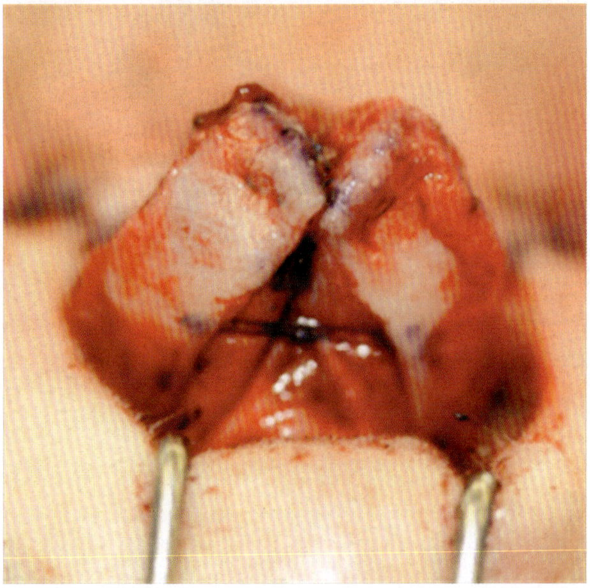

FIGURE 18.4
Intraoperative view of tip complex after cephalic strips and suture modification. Notice the narrower interdomal space and decreased convexity of the lateral crura.

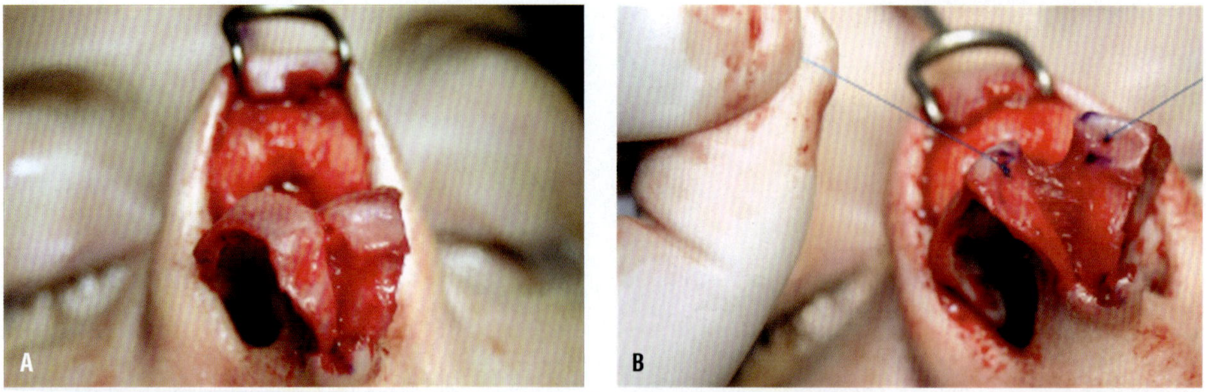

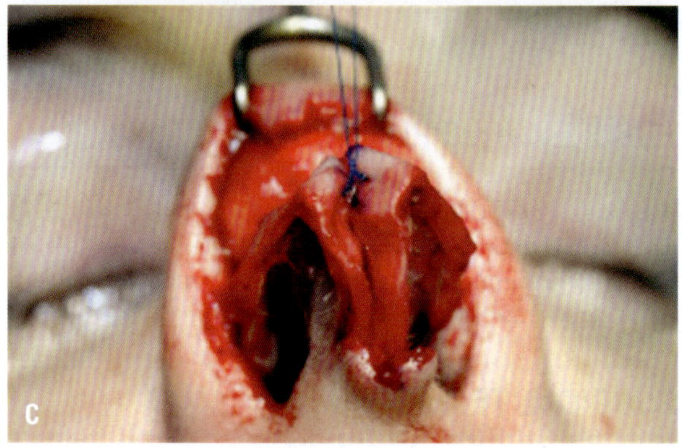

FIGURE 18.5 External approach showing the interlocked transdomal suture technique. **A:** External view of lower lateral cartilages with wide angle of domes and asymmetry. **B:** Transdomal sutures in place to approximate cephalic edge of domes. **C:** New dome formation with natural divergence and narrowed interdomal space.

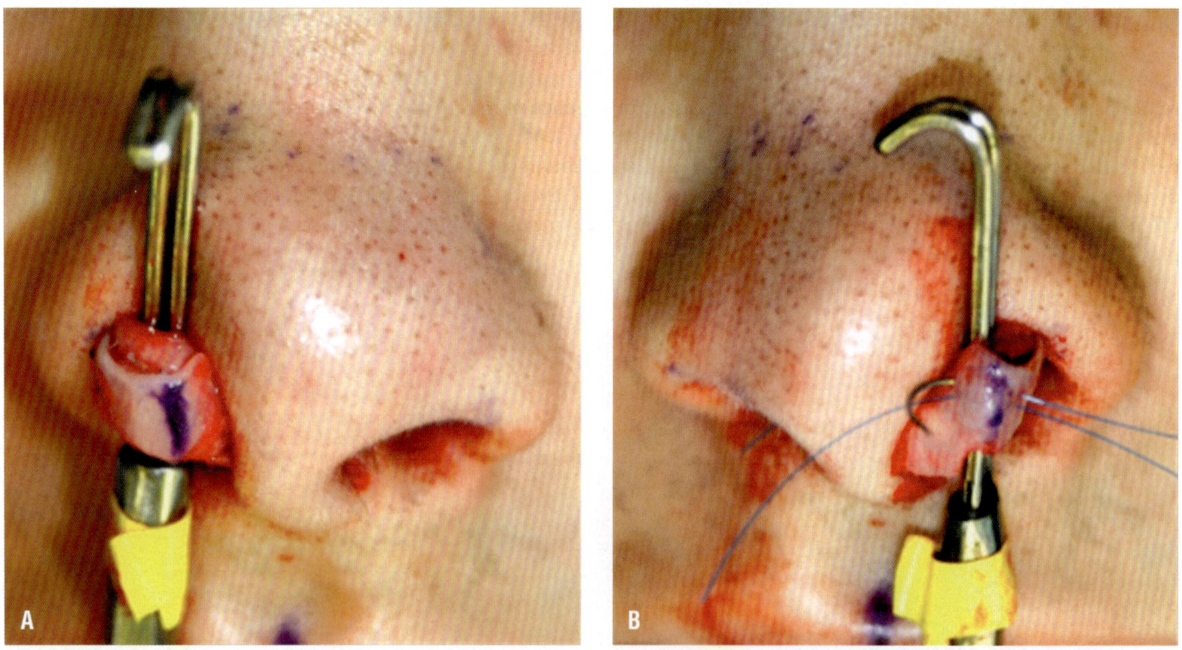

FIGURE 18.6 Endonasal approach for transdomal interlocked sutures. **A:** Delivery of lower lateral cartilage with dome marked. **B:** Mattress suture is placed with knot medial.

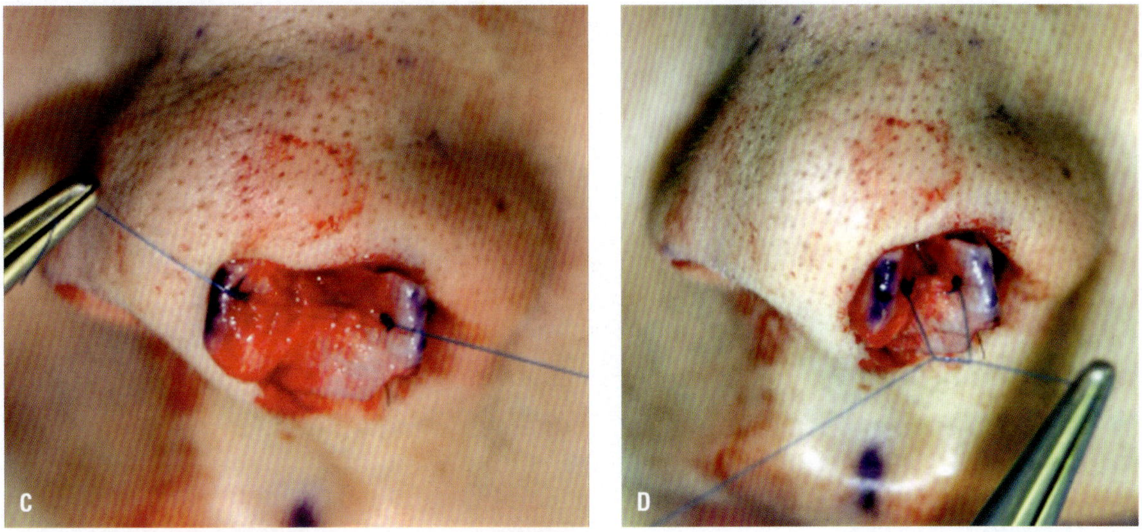

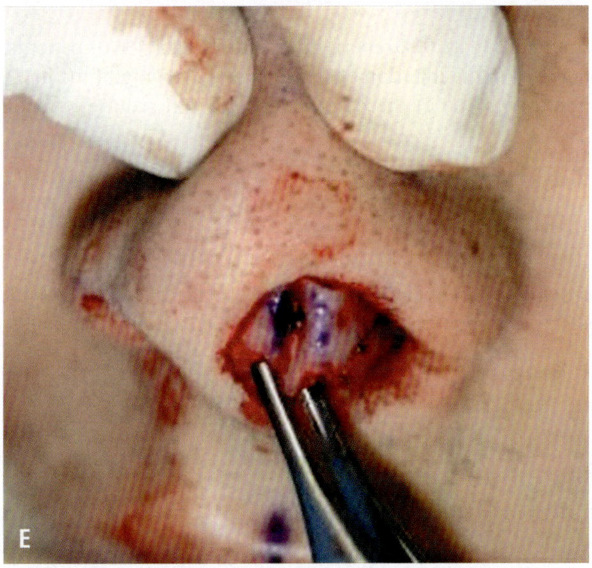

FIGURE 18.6 (*Continued*)
C: Transdomal sutures are in place bilaterally. **D:** The long ends of each transdomal suture are tied to approximate the cephalic edge of the domes. **E:** The narrowed tip complex is returned to the endonasal position.

The use of onlay tip grafts, lateral crural struts, and/or batten grafts can be incorporated into this technique. The purpose of using these grafts is to augment projection, stabilize the lateral crura, or correct contour concavities of the lateral ala (Fig. 18.7).

POSTOPERATIVE MANAGEMENT

At the conclusion of surgery, the incisions are closed with 5-0 chromic gut sutures and the nose is dressed. Mastisol or tincture of Benzoin is applied to the skin, and tape is applied in layers to help occlude potential space beneath the skin. If osteotomies have been performed, a rigid thermoplastic splint is also applied. Internal dressings are not required unless a significant septoplasty was necessary. In the recovery room, the patient's head is kept elevated and ice compresses are applied to the eyes. A drip pad is used to collect nasal drainage. After discharge, the patient is instructed to use saline irrigation frequently to clean the nostril edges with hydrogen peroxide several times per day. Bacitracin ointment is applied to the incision and internal nostril edges. The first postoperative visit is at 7 days, when all sutures and splints are removed. Care is taken to show the patient where edema is present and to reinforce that this will take several months to resolve completely. Most patients do not remember this preoperative counseling and often seem surprised by this second round of counseling. Future follow-up visits are at 1 month, 3 months, 9 months, and 1 year postsurgery. After 1 year, we ask patients to come back yearly for as long as possible, at no charge.

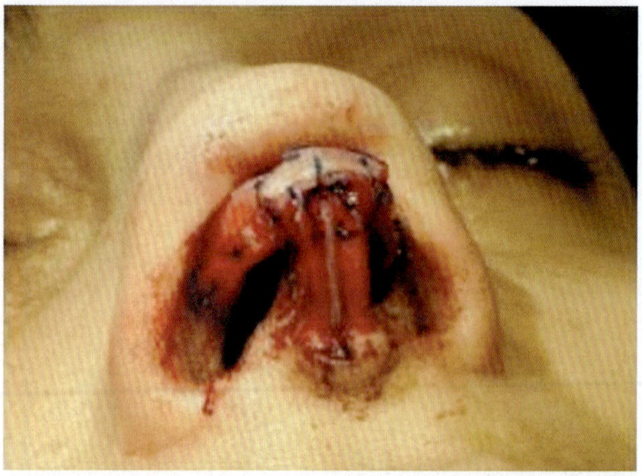

FIGURE 18.7
Tip complex with cap graft, alar batten grafts, and soft tissue graft over cap.

COMPLICATIONS

The most common complication recorded is tip asymmetry. In a 2004 report, this occurred in 4.4% of patients. Less common complications included persistent wideness of the interdomal space, over narrowing of the interdomal space, and suture extrusion. As in any rhinoplasty, some of these complications will require revision surgery (Fig. 18.8).

RESULTS

Suture techniques provide a nondestructive method of tip refinement. Sutures can be placed, and replaced if the effect is not desirable. Experimentation is possible during surgery, a major advantage over incisional or excisional methods (Figs. 18.9 and 18.10).

PEARLS

- Proper patient selection is the key to successful rhinoplasty results. Patients with appropriate anatomy and esthetic goals will benefit from the use of suture techniques.
- Careful exposure of the lower lateral cartilages by any approach, with preservation of the skin–soft tissue envelope, will lead to more consistent results.

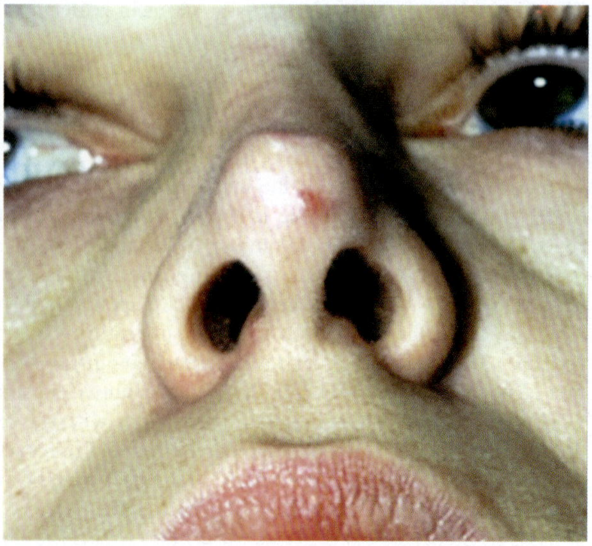

FIGURE 18.8
Suture extrusion 3 years after rhinoplasty. The suture was removed without further complications.

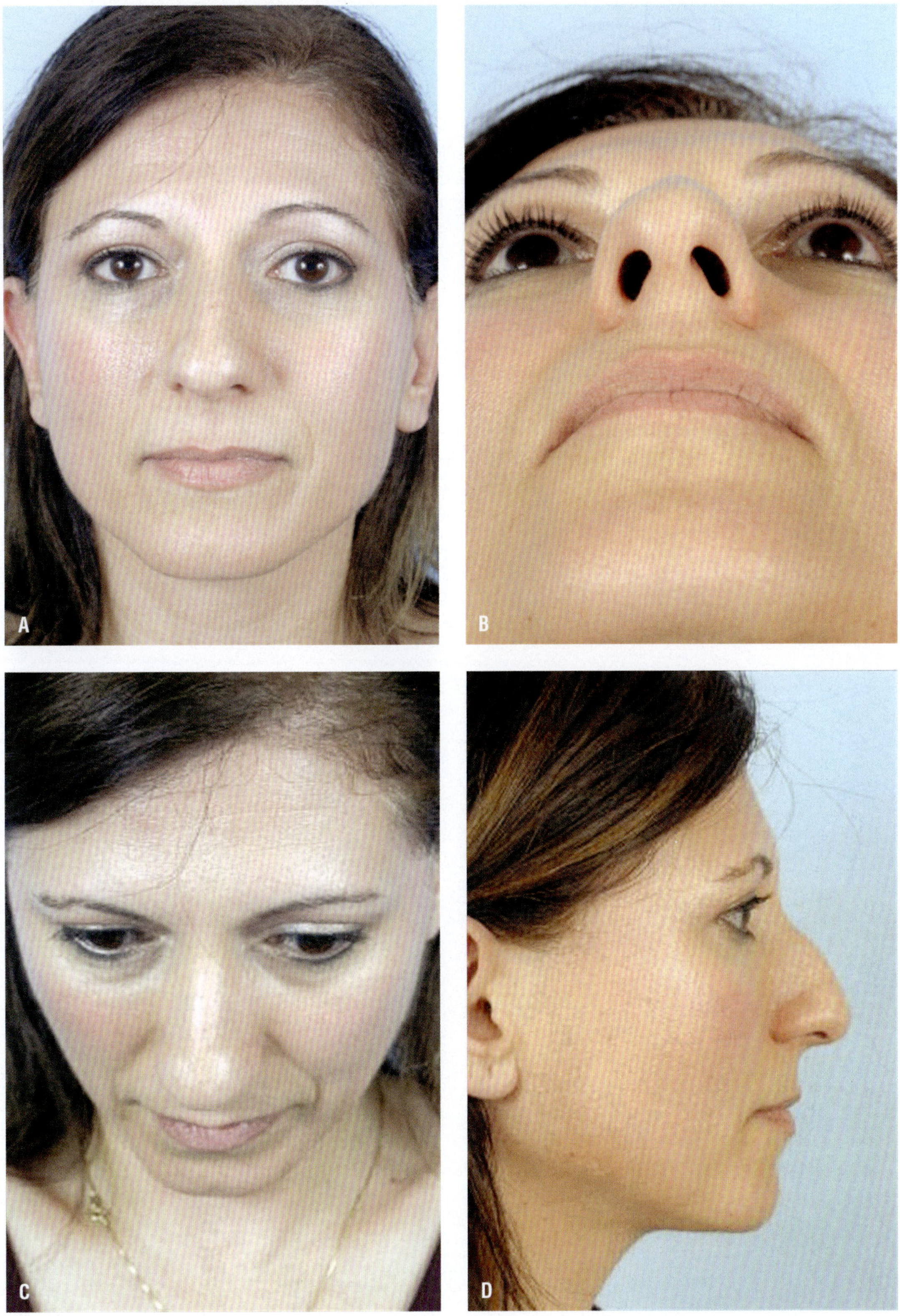

FIGURE 18.9 Patient with before **(A–D)** and 1 year after **(E–H)** rhinoplasty using interlocked transdomal sutures, cap graft, and columellar strut to define the tip.

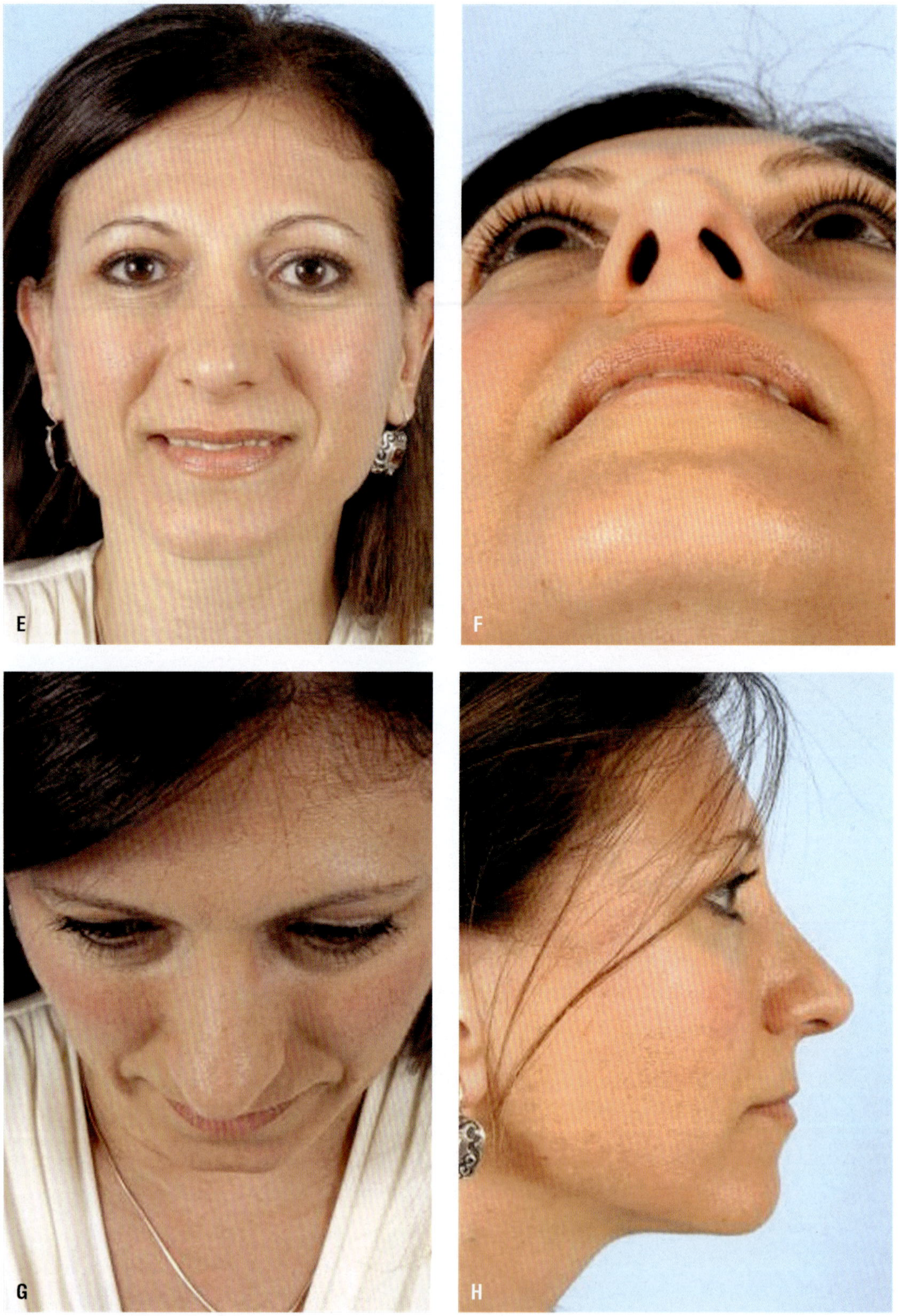

FIGURE 18.9 (*Continued*)

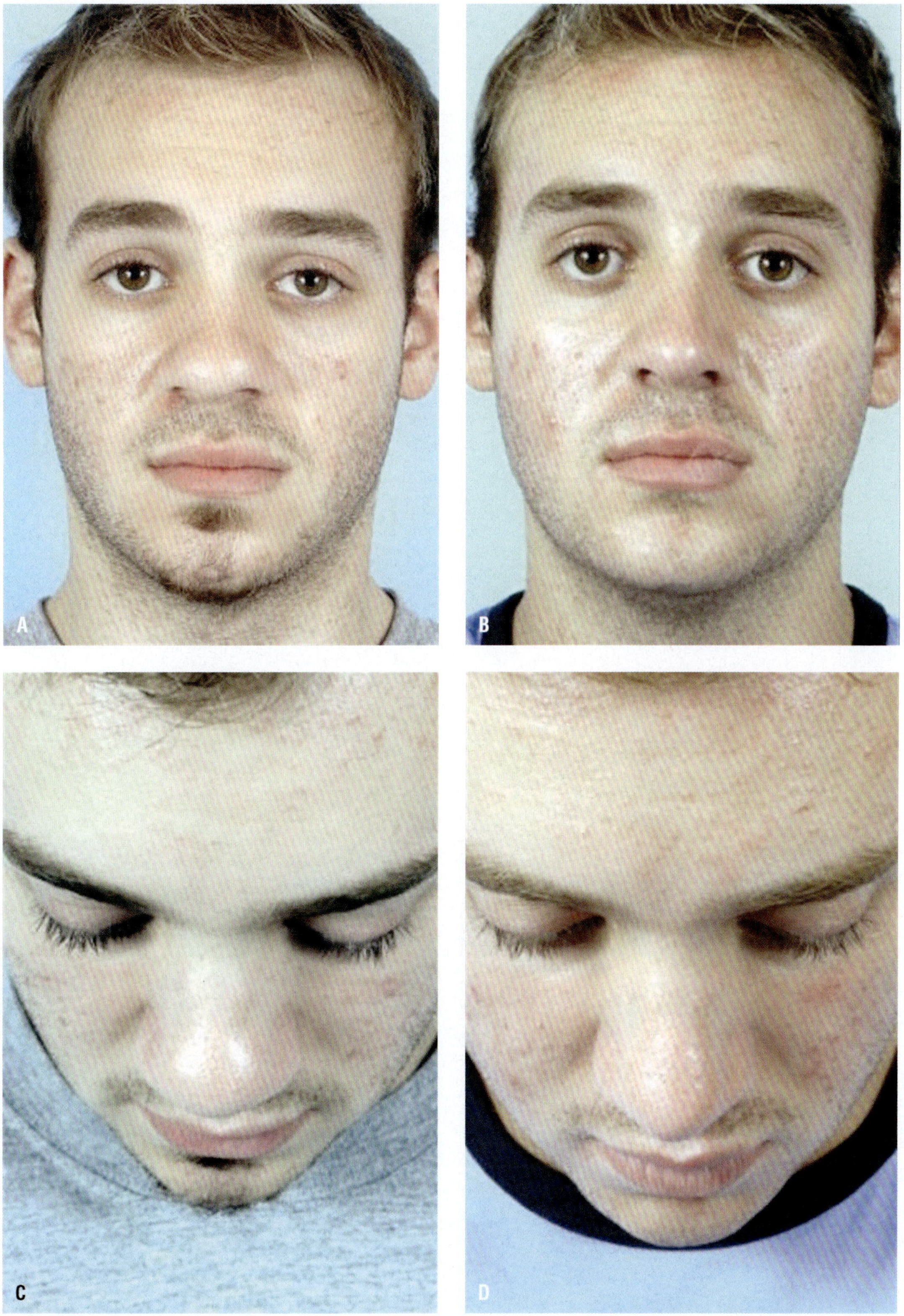

FIGURE 18.10 Patient with wide nasal tip before and 2 years after rhinoplasty using transdomal interlocked sutures, lateral spanning sutures, and columellar strut to alter the tip. (Preoperative photos in left column, postoperative photos in right column.)

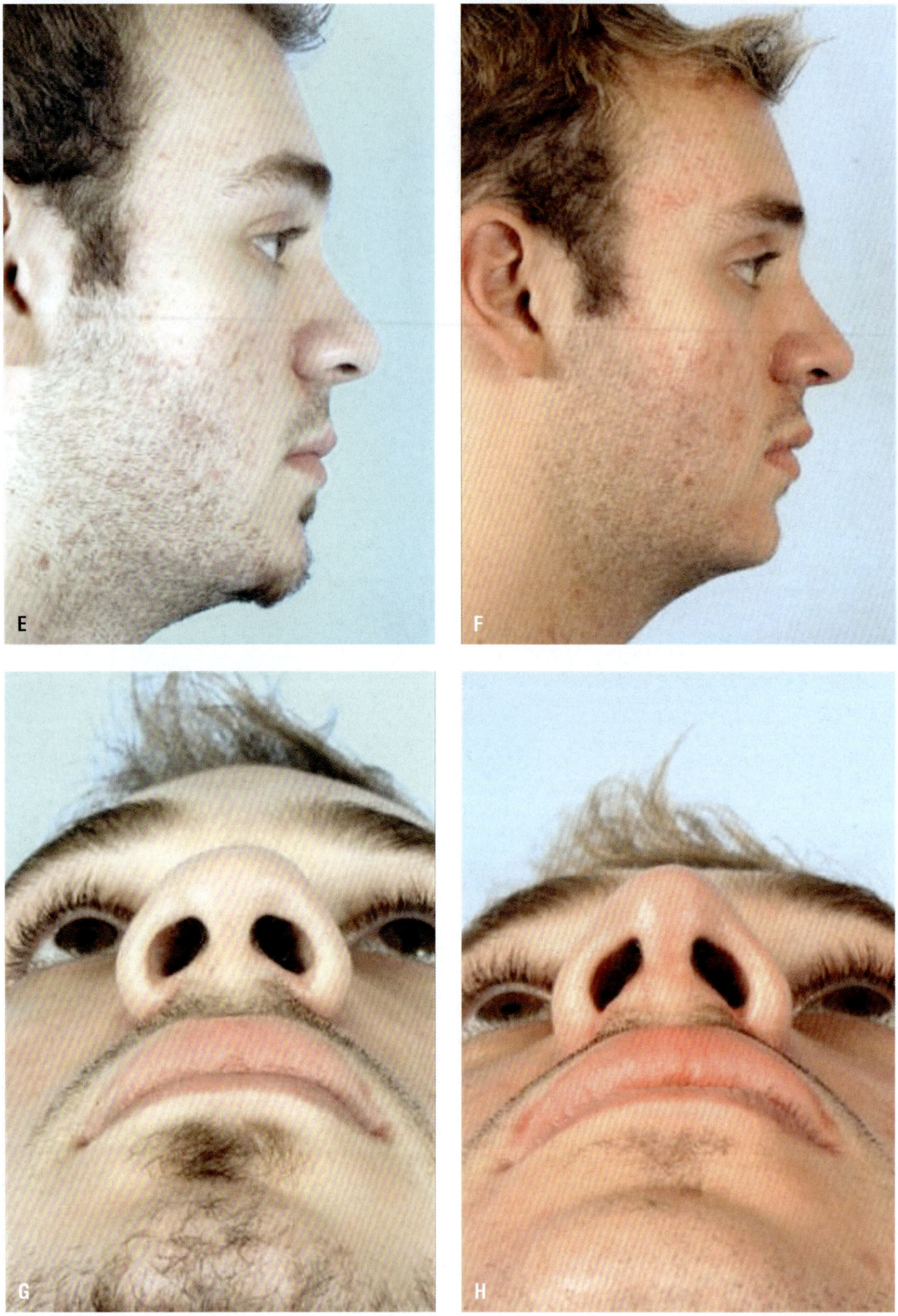

FIGURE 18.10 (*Continued*)

PITFALLS

- Preservation of a strong cartilage framework is essential to prevent the normal scar contraction of the soft tissue envelope from creating unwanted long-term results.
- Variant nasal anatomy may require modification of the basic techniques. Be flexible and original in your surgical methods.

INSTRUMENTS TO HAVE AVAILABLE

- Wide double hook retractor
- Narrow double hook retractor
- 0.5 forceps
- Adson-Brown forceps
- Converse scissors
- Blunt-tipped tenotomy scissors
- Wide double ball retractor
- Bernstein retractor
- Cottle elevator
- Webster fine needle holder
- Small suture scissors

SUGGESTED READING

Baker SR. Suture contouring of the nasal tip. *Arch Facial Plast Surg* 2000;2:34–42.

Daniel RK. Rhinoplasty: creating an aesthetic tip. A preliminary report. *Plast Reconstr Surg* 1987;4:317.

Goldman IB. The importance of the mesial crura in nasal tip reconstruction. *Arch Otolaryngol* 1957;65:143.

Guyuron B. Footplates of the medial crura. *Plast Reconstr Surg* 1998;101:1539.

Guyuron B, Behmand RA. Nasal tip sutures part II: the interplays. *Plast Reconstr Surg* 2003;112(4):1130–1145.

Joseph J. *Rhinoplasty and facial plastic surgery with a supplement on mammaplasty*. Leipzig, Germany: Verlag von Curt kabitzsch, 1931.

Kridel RW, Konior RJ, Shumrick KA, et al. Advances in nasal tip surgery: the lateral crural steal. *Arch Otolaryngol* 1989; 115:1206.

McCullough EG, English JL. A new twist in nasal tip surgery: an alternative to the Goldman tip for the wide or bulbous lobule. *Arch Otolaryngol* 1985;111:524–529.

Papel ID. Interlocked transdomal suture technique for the wide interdomal space in rhinoplasty. *Arch Facial Plast Surg* 2005;7:414–417.

Tebbets JB. Secondary tip modification: shaping and positioning the nasal tip using nondestructive techniques. In: Tebbets, JB, ed. *Primary rhinoplasty: a new approach to the logic and the techniques*. St. Louis, MO: Mosby, 1998.

19 TIP PTOSIS (THE DROOPY TIP)

Stephen S. Park

INTRODUCTION

Tip ptosis (droopy tip) is a common finding, and correcting it is a fundamental step in rhinoplasty. This maneuver is unique in that it may be applied to patients in both the young and older age group, seeking aesthetic as well as functional improvements. There are a number of different causes of tip ptosis, and it is important to distinguish between them since the precise anatomic etiology influences the choice of surgical technique, and each maneuver can be unique.

The tip may droop as a function of advanced age as the numerous support mechanisms weaken over time. The scroll between the upper and lower lateral cartilages begins to loosen and simultaneously, other structural parts loosen, such as ligaments between the medial crura and the septum and the interdomal ligament. In addition, the overlying skin and soft tissue lose its elasticity, allowing the tip to droop further. The weight of the skin of the nasal tip can pull the tip down and lengthen the nose. This is especially true for patients who have very thick and sebaceous skin, including patients with rhinophyma.

The preoperative analysis will determine if tip projection or deprojection is needed along with the cephalic tip rotation. The surgical plan then employs a series of steps designed to reposition the lower lateral cartilages and then fixate them firmly to hold against postoperative wound contracture. There are different surgical techniques that can accomplish similar changes.

HISTORY

Obtaining a history from a patient interested in a rhinoplasty who has tip ptosis is no different than with any elective procedure. The standard tenants of preoperative evaluation are undertaken and include a general review of systems. A detailed history of previous nasal trauma or nasal surgery is essential. A detailed history of past and present cardiac and pulmonary issues is recorded. A complete review of medications and allergies is performed. Attention is dedicated to any form of anticoagulant that the patient may be taking. If elective, they will be discontinued for a minimum of 2 weeks before surgery. Anticoagulation is for an underlying condition; therefore, consultation with the prescribing physician will be made to coordinate a window for a medication holiday. One must also assess such concerns as motivation, expectations, and ability to cooperate during the postoperative period. It is worthwhile to differentiate between cosmetic concerns and functional, such as nasal obstruction. Tip rotation can impart a more youthful appearance, but the magnitude of this change must be realistic.

PHYSICAL EXAMINATION

There a few key elements to the physical examination of a patient with tip ptosis. The critical step is making a careful diagnosis of the *exact anatomic etiology* of the deformity. This then leads to the most direct method

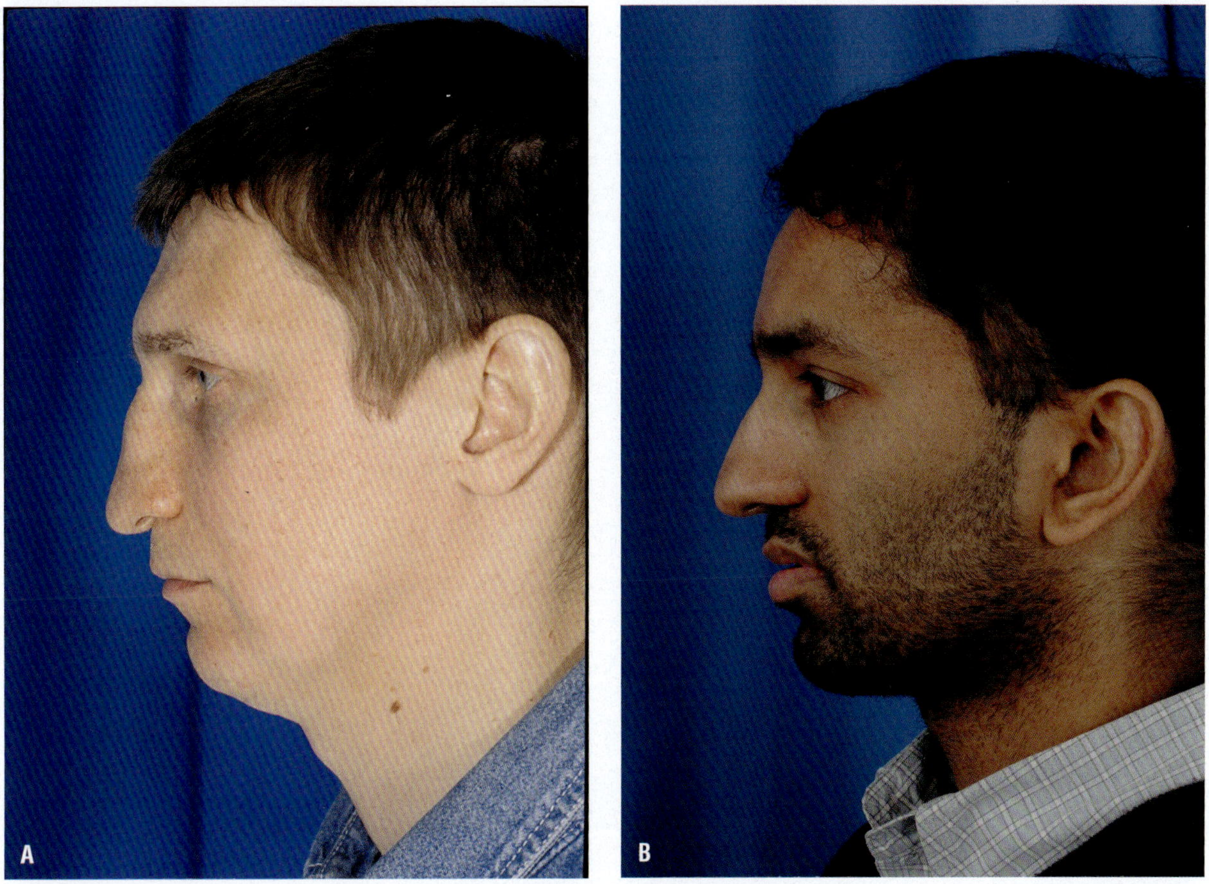

FIGURE 19.1 Tip ptosis needing cephalic rotation and *projection* **(A)** and *deprojection* **(B)**.

of repair. The first step in the examination is distinguishing between the tip that needs cephalic rotation with increased projection versus the tip that requires rotation with deprojection (Fig. 19.1A and B).

Palpation of the nose is an underemphasized aspect of the preoperative evaluation, and yet it is critical in tip ptosis. Identifying the anterior septal angle as a key anatomic landmark for tip support is accomplished best through palpation. Thickness of the skin is also an important part of the preoperative analysis also best accomplished by palpation. When extremely heavy skin is the problem, it may require a direct excision of dorsal skin since cartilage repositioning may not suffice.

INDICATIONS

Indications for repairing tip ptosis are twofold. *Aesthetically*, the ptotic tip may put the nose and face out of balance. Such a tip is often lacking in definition and tends to appear broad and wide. Moreover, tip ptosis creates several illusions to the other areas of the nose; the plunging tip and acute nasolabial angle often appear to lengthen the nose and create a "pseudohump" at the dorsum, especially the anterior septal angle. The supratip will appear *relatively* overprojected with respect to the tip. Simultaneous tip rotation and tip projection can be synergistic and reduce the amount of dorsal resection needed in order to achieve balance. Patients are rarely cognizant of a plunging tip and may request a hump or dorsal reduction rather than increased tip support; their perception is often that the nose is too large. The importance of an early diagnosis and distinction of this anatomic variant cannot be overstated (Fig. 19.2A–D).

A patients' chief complaint may be abnormal nasal *function* where the anatomic etiology for this obstruction, especially in the elderly population, is tip ptosis. Septal deviation, turbinate hypertrophy, and lateral wall collapse can all coexist within the group, but tip ptosis from lack of support can be a major contributor that should not be overlooked. Not infrequently, the patient will demonstrate a simple maneuver that alleviates the nasal obstruction—manually pushing the tip up. Once recognized, surgical correction of tip ptosis through any of the techniques discussed below will have a profound positive effect.

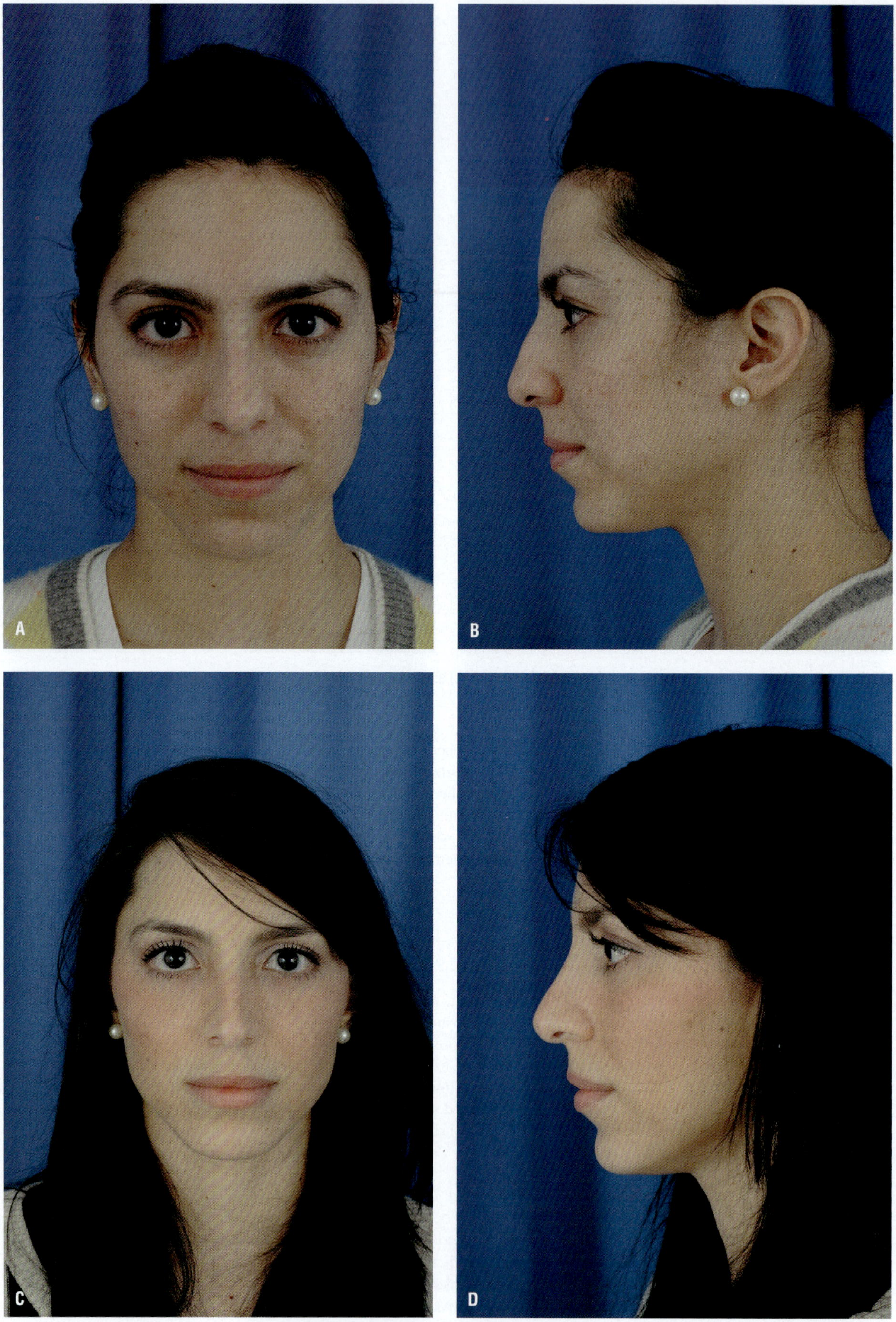

FIGURE 19.2 **A and B:** Combination of subtle dorsal hump, tip underprojection, and ptosis **C and D:** Correction with tip rotation, projection, and hump reduction. Balance is achieved by the combination of effects.

CONTRAINDICATIONS

Any surgical risk factor is amplified when considering elective procedures. In addition to this, psychological factors can be a contraindication. Fixation on one's nose is not uncommon and the surgeon must proceed with caution.

PREOPERATIVE PLANNING

Correcting tip ptosis is accomplished through a series of steps that progress in complexity and difficulty. The fundamental concept in this algorithm is the tripod model whereby the tip is supported by three well-defined "pods." The two lateral crura and the central medial crura comprise the legs that hold the tip in a 3-dimensional position. Manipulating one leg will directly impact tip position in a predictable manner. A thorough understanding of this concept allows one to design surgical maneuvers that affect the tip in terms of projection and rotation. The tripod of a camera serves as an accurate model for this concept.

Weakening or shortening the upper two limbs will lead to cephalic tip rotation and deprojection. On the other hand, lengthening them will push the tip down and out, thus increasing tip projection and causing derotation. A surgical step, which augments the central limb (i.e., the columella), will create tip projection and cephalic rotation. Conversely, weakening this central limb (e.g., full transfixion incision), overlapping medial crura, will decrease projection and create derotation.

There are a number of specific surgical maneuvers that lead to these primary and secondary effects, and the surgeon should be facile with them. A progressive algorithm allows some versatility and intraoperative decision making. There are simple steps that allow small degrees of rotation for minor deformities and more drastic techniques that afford dramatic lift. Practically speaking, a combination of techniques is usually employed.

SURGICAL TECHNIQUE

Exposure to the nasal tip can be achieved through any of the three commonly used approaches: endonasal, delivery, or external. The preferred approach is largely dictated by surgeon's preference and experience as well as the specific maneuver planned. Work on the columella, the medial crura, or caudal septum can easily be achieved through the endonasal route and a full transfixion incision. More elaborate sutures and grafts to the dorsal septum and lateral crura are for most surgeons more comfortably performed through the external approach.

Some maneuvers along the nasal tip create tip rotation and projection as a secondary effect. The *dome-binding suture* is a common suture technique used to narrow the tip and improve definition. Depending on how it is placed, it will often increase projection (Fig. 19.3A and B).

A *tip-lifting suture* is a simple technique that can be used for subtle situations requiring tip rotation and deprojection. It is a suture that passes through both domes and the dorsal septum in the region of the anterior septal angle. As the permanent suture is tightened, the domes will be pulled cephalad. It is a powerful maneuver, and one must be cautious to avoid overaggressive elevation; it is easy to create an overrotated nasal tip (Fig. 19.4A–C).

The *lateral crural overlay* has a similar result to the tip-lifting suture (i.e., tip rotation and deprojection), but is more aggressive and structurally sound. The vestibular mucosa is carefully dissected off the lateral crural cartilage along its body. One should avoid dissecting and disrupting the lateral most aspect where it is supported by fibrofatty tissue alone. The crural cartilage is then transected vertically and overlapped an appropriate

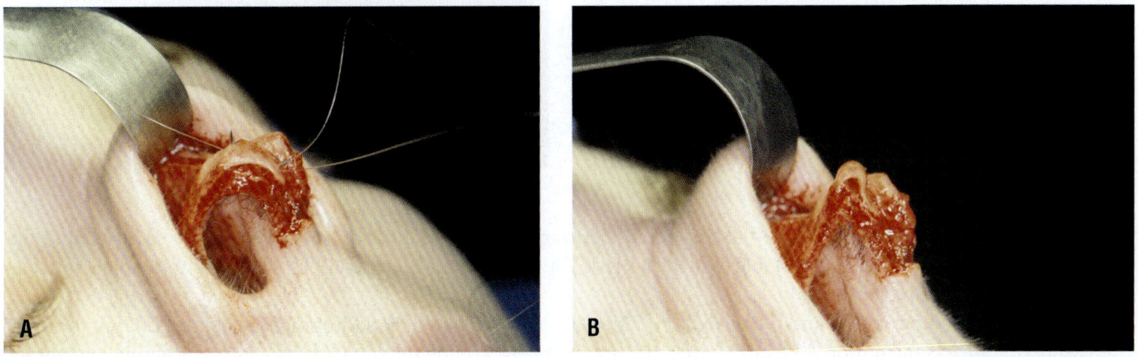

FIGURE 19.3 A and B: Dome-binding suture on the right demonstrating change in tip projection.

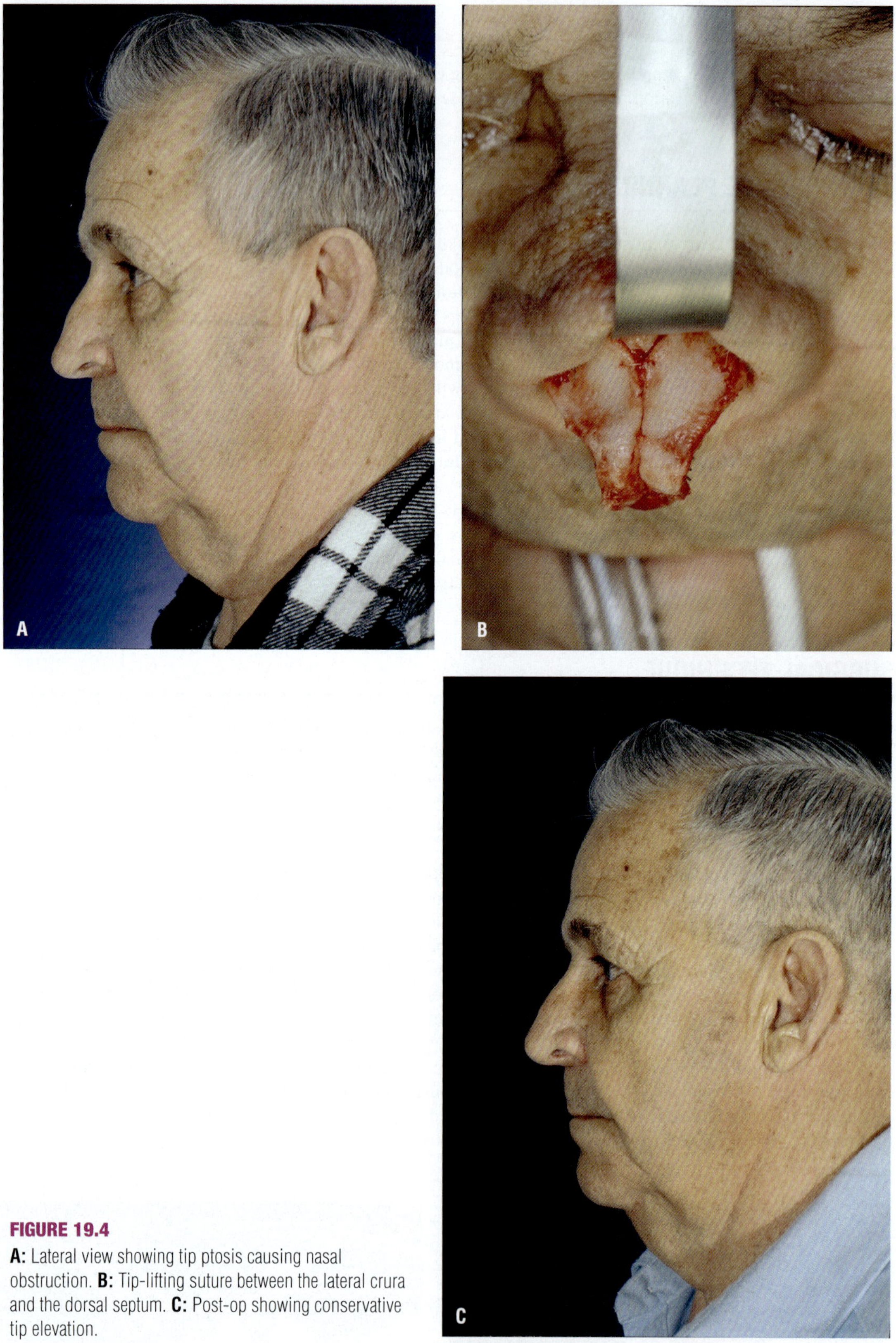

FIGURE 19.4

A: Lateral view showing tip ptosis causing nasal obstruction. **B:** Tip-lifting suture between the lateral crura and the dorsal septum. **C:** Post-op showing conservative tip elevation.

amount. There is usually no need to resect any cartilage. The overlapped portions are suture secured, and the resulting limb is once again stable with little risk for collapse or retraction. The slightly redundant mucosa intranasally contracts naturally.

Cephalic tip rotation and increased projection are accomplished by addressing the central limb in terms of support and augmentation. For mild cases, the *medial crura can be advanced up the caudal septum* and suture secured toward the anterior septal angle. Both sides of the caudal septal cartilage should be exposed for about

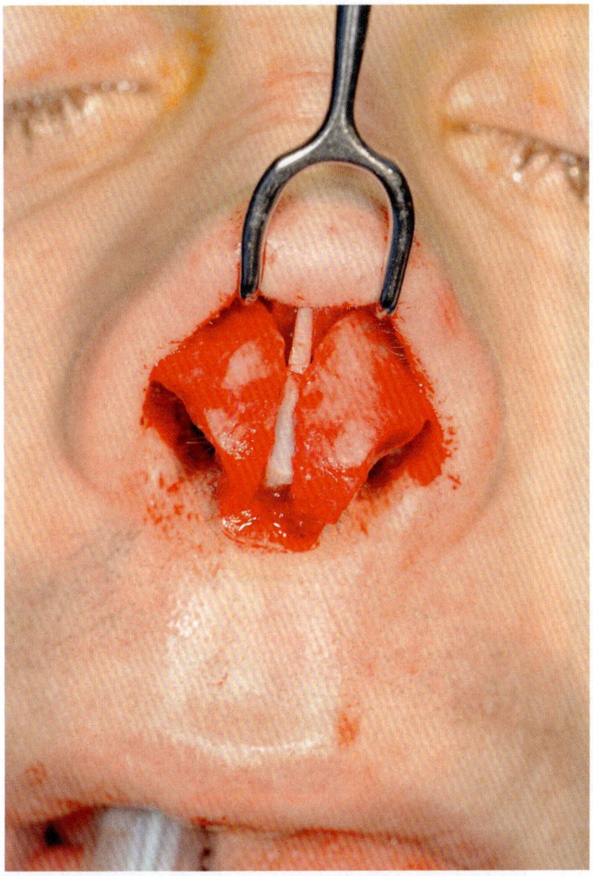

FIGURE 19.5
Caudal extension graft can serve as a pillar for repositioning and elevating the tip cartilages.

7 to 8 mm, and a small pocket created between the two medial crura. A permanent suture is used to secure the medial crura to the desired level of the caudal septum. This can create a small degree of columellar retraction as well.

A *columellar strut* lends additional support to the central limb of the tripod and can be inserted endonasally. Septal cartilage is ideal due to its rigidity and straight character. The elastic cartilage of the ear tends to be more pliable and less effective. Costal cartilage is excellent, but the donor site morbidity is excessive for this purpose. This cartilage graft is roughly 2 mm wide and 1.5 cm long. It gives rigidity to the central portion of the medial crura but should not be used to provide a structural pillar for tip projection. It should not rest on the anterior nasal spine since it will tend to slide to one side and create an asymmetry. It is suture secured to the columella.

The *Caudal Extension Graft* provides one of the more reliable methods of fixating the lower lateral cartilages in a new position, especially for projection. It works well for both cephalic rotation and derotation and lengthening the nose. A rigid cartilage graft is necessary, such as septum or rib (Fig. 19.5). The caudal septum is widely exposed bilaterally since this graft will need to be firmly fixated to this. This caudal extension graft is seated on the anterior nasal spine and the septum simultaneously. It can be placed in situ with excessive projection initially and then later trimmed to the precise dimensions. This new "anterior septal angle" serves as the platform upon which the lower lateral cartilages are based. It can be accurately fixated to any position in space, and this gives the surgeon excellent control of the tip. If tip rotation is desired, one will often separate the domes and suture them to either side of the caudal extension graft. This nonanatomic structure is a firm platform upon which the soft tissue will contract.

Tip elevation along with dorsal augmentation is a common surgical goal and is often accomplished with a strong *dorsal onlay graft (e.g., rib cartilage)*. The rib is carved to form an "L-strut" and functions to augment the dorsum and provide a platform for the tip cartilages to be secured in a more cephalic position. The cephalic border of the lateral crura can be dissected free of the vestibular mucosa to allow it to be suture secured over the dorsal rib graft, providing better camouflage (Fig. 19.6A–E).

Tip ptosis is not uncommon in elderly patients with varying degrees of rhinophyma or heavy skin. At times, a *direct skin excision* can complement the tip-lifting maneuvers performed on the framework. This can be a powerful adjunct procedure and greatly enhance postoperative results as well as longevity. Skin is directly excised from the dorsum and can be oriented in a transverse fashion at the supratip or nasion area. The incision is closed in layers. The horizontal scar often heals well in this group and is not a major concern, especially when associated with functional improvement.

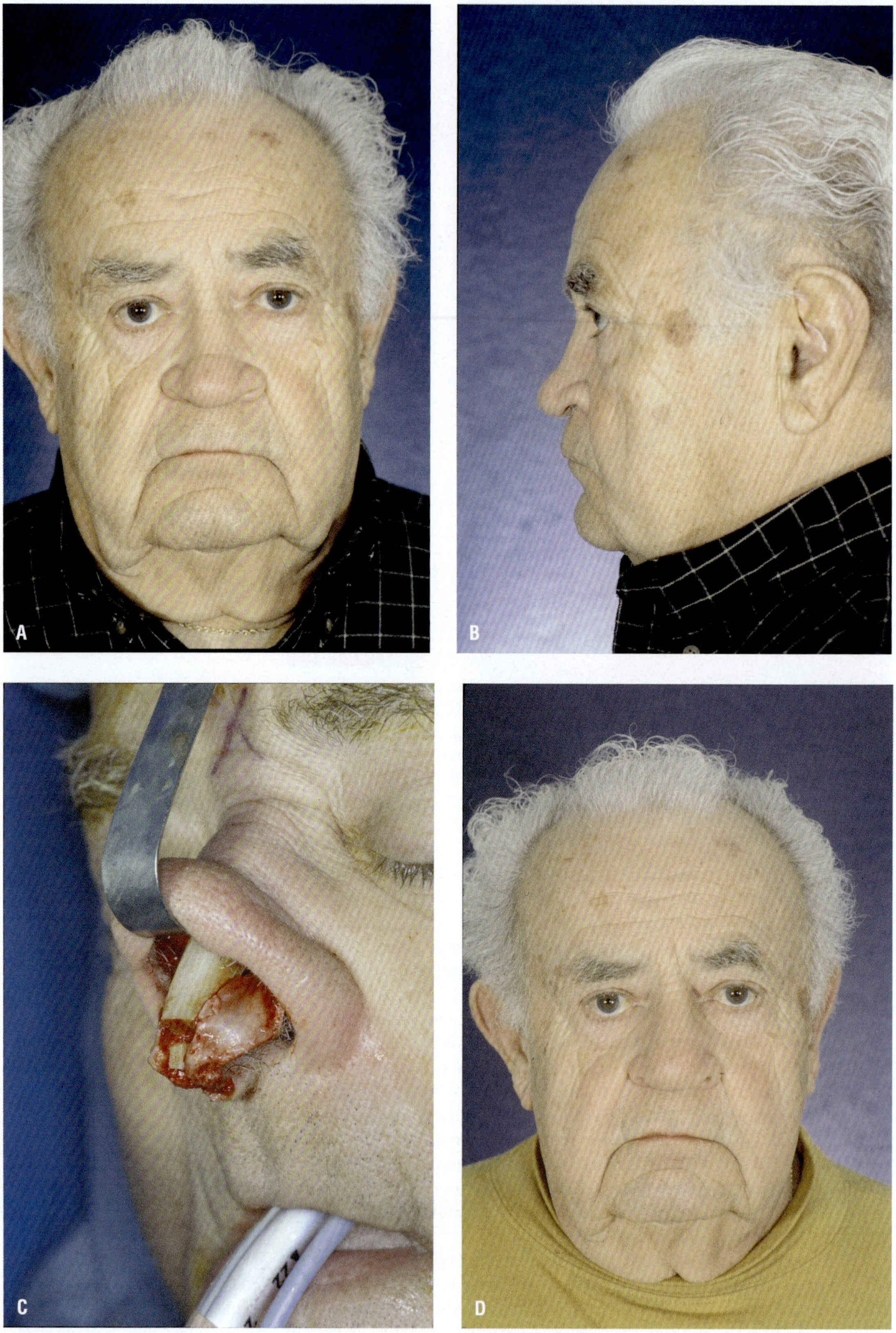

FIGURE 19.6 Tip ptosis with dorsal collapse. Preoperative photos. Anterior **(A)** and lateral views **(B)**. Rib graft in an "L-strut" to provide dorsal augmentation along with tip rotation **(C)**. 1 year postoperative views. Anterior **(D)** and lateral **(E)**.

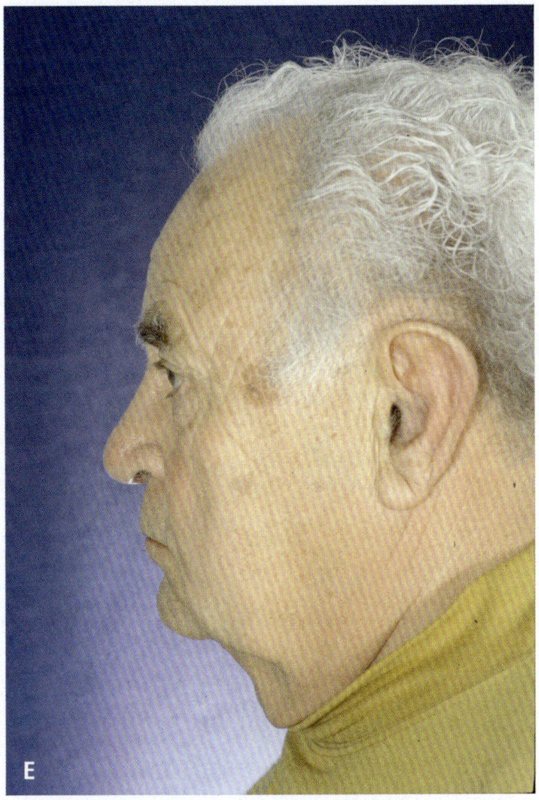

FIGURE 19.6 (*Continued*)

POSTOPERATIVE MANAGEMENT

All rhinoplasty patients are given standard instructions, which include rest, ice, bacitracin ointment in both vestibules, and head elevation. Intermittent bleeding is not uncommon. Strenuous exercise is avoided for at least 1 week. Contact sports are avoided for 4 to 6 weeks. Brief courses of a topical decongestant can help with the postoperative edema and nasal obstruction.

COMPLICATIONS

Complications of correcting tip ptosis include overcorrection and recurrence. It is easy to overrotate the nose when the patient is in the supine position and it can be dramatic, especially in the older male. Lifting the tip cartilages will easily create simultaneous alar retraction and excessive columellar show. This occurs because the lateral crura are lifted along with the domes and, in the more cephalic position, the alar rims are retracted passively. This will lead to excessive columellar show. To avoid this, concomitant caudal repositioning of the crura may be necessary with extended batten grafts, alar rim grafts, or even a vertical dome division. Shortening of the lateral crura with direct incision and overlap technique will not create this cephalic repositioning of the alar rims.

RESULTS

Surgical correction of the droopy nasal tip is a powerful maneuver that can have a dramatic effect on the balance of the nose. There are a number of different steps that are employed for this, and careful preoperative planning is essential. A tip lift can be indicated for both aesthetic and functional purposes. It is imperative to distinguish between the need for simultaneous tip projection versus deprojection. With careful planning and execution, tip repositioning can be an effective part of rhinoplasty.

PEARLS

- Patients will often overlook their droopy tip and be fixated on their dorsal hump, and this can be misleading to the surgeon. Each portion of the nose must be analyzed separately, and often, a tip repositioning is performed in conjunction with a reduction of the dorsal hump.

- Tip ptosis can be a major contributor to nasal obstruction, especially in the older age group. Rotation and projection of the tip lead to a direct improvement in the cross-sectional anatomy at the nasal valve.
- Distinguish between the need for tip projection versus deprojection. Tip rotation can be accompanied by either projection or deprojection and must be carefully mapped with distinct technical maneuvers as they are mutually exclusive. Tip rotation is not always associated with the need for increased projection.
- The "tripod concept" is the cornerstone for surgical planning of tip rotation. Shortening the lateral crura is balanced against increasing length of the medial crura.

PITFALLS

- Over tightening a tip-lifting suture can easily create an overrotated nasal tip.
- Advancement of the medial crura up and onto the caudal septum can cause columellar retrusion and widening.
- A columellar strut should not rest on the anterior nasal spine since it will tend to slide to one side and create an asymmetry.
- It is easy to overrotate the nose when the patient is in the supine position.
- The result of securing the medial crura to the caudal septum, or to a caudal extension graft, is very unforgiving if performed inaccurately.

INSTRUMENTS TO HAVE AVAILABLE

- Standard rhinoplasty set

SUGGESTED READING

Kabaker SS. An adjunctive technique to rhinoplasty of the aging nose. *Head Neck Surg* 1980;2(4):276–281.

Kridel RW, Konior RJ. Controlled nasal tip rotation via the lateral crural overlay technique. *Arch Otolaryngol Head Neck Surg* 1991;117(4):411–415.

Schlosser RJ, Park SS. Functional nasal surgery. *Otolaryngol Clin North Am* 1999;32(1):37–51.

Tardy ME Jr. Rhinoplasty tip ptosis: etiology and prevention. *Laryngoscope* 1973;83(6):923–929.

20 MEDIAL AND LATERAL CRURAL OVERLAY TECHNIQUES

Hossam M.T. Foda

INTRODUCTION

Adjusting the projection and rotation of the nasal tip is considered one of the most challenging maneuvers in rhinoplasty. The nasal tip projection refers to the posterior–anterior extension of the tip from the vertical facial plane. Tip rotation is defined as movement of the tip along an arc, with its radius maintained from the facial plane. Techniques modifying the alar cartilage can result in predictable changes in the degree of projection and rotation; these changes can be maintained only in the presence of an adequate amount of tip support.

Important mechanisms that provide support and maintain the degree of projection and rotation include the ligamentous attachment of the medial crural footplates to the caudal septal cartilage, the fibrous attachment between the upper and lower lateral cartilages, and the interdomal ligament that spans over the anterior septal angle. However, the major support of the nasal tip is derived from the alar cartilages themselves, namely, from the length and strength of the medial and lateral crura.

Techniques for repositioning the nasal tip can be divided into two categories: those that modify the existing alar cartilages and those that augment the nasal lobule with grafts or implants.

In cases where the alar cartilages are overdeveloped with long medial and lateral crura, adequate tip repositioning is practically impossible without decreasing the size of the alar cartilages.

In the 1930s, Joseph and Safian first described shortening of the medial and lateral crura to deproject the nasal tip. Since then, many refinements of shortening the lateral crura were described to preserve vestibular skin and to suture or overlap the divided segments. Later, Lipsett pioneered medial crural shortening in 1959; since then, many refinements of the procedure have been described. In the current chapter, I will present my experience in shortening the medial and lateral crura using the medial crural overlay (MCO) and lateral crural overlay (LCO) techniques.

Both the tripod concept described by Anderson in 1969 and its recent modernization into the M-arch model by Adamson are very helpful in comprehending the effects that alar cartilage-modifying techniques have on the degree of tip projection and rotation. The tripod concept depicts the alar cartilages as a tripod, with two upper legs formed by the lateral crura on each side and one lower leg formed by the conjoined medial crura. Applying the tripod analogy, the LCO, carried out alone (Fig. 20.1, top), will shorten the upper legs of the tripod which will move the tip backward and upward, thus decreasing projection, increasing rotation, and shortening the nose. MCO, carried out alone (Fig. 20.1, bottom), will shorten the lower leg of the tripod that will move the tip backward and downward, resulting in a decrease in projection, inferior rotation, and increase nasal length. Combining LCO with MCO (Fig. 20.1, center) will result in additional deprojection without altering the degree of rotation.

Furthermore, an equal amount of shortening of the M-arch may produce variable yet predictable changes in projection and rotation, depending on where the arch is shortened. For example, shortening the medial crura causes deprojection and counterrotation, whereas shortening the lateral crus causes deprojection and rotation. Shortening the intermediate crus can cause a variable degree of deprojection and rotation depending on where

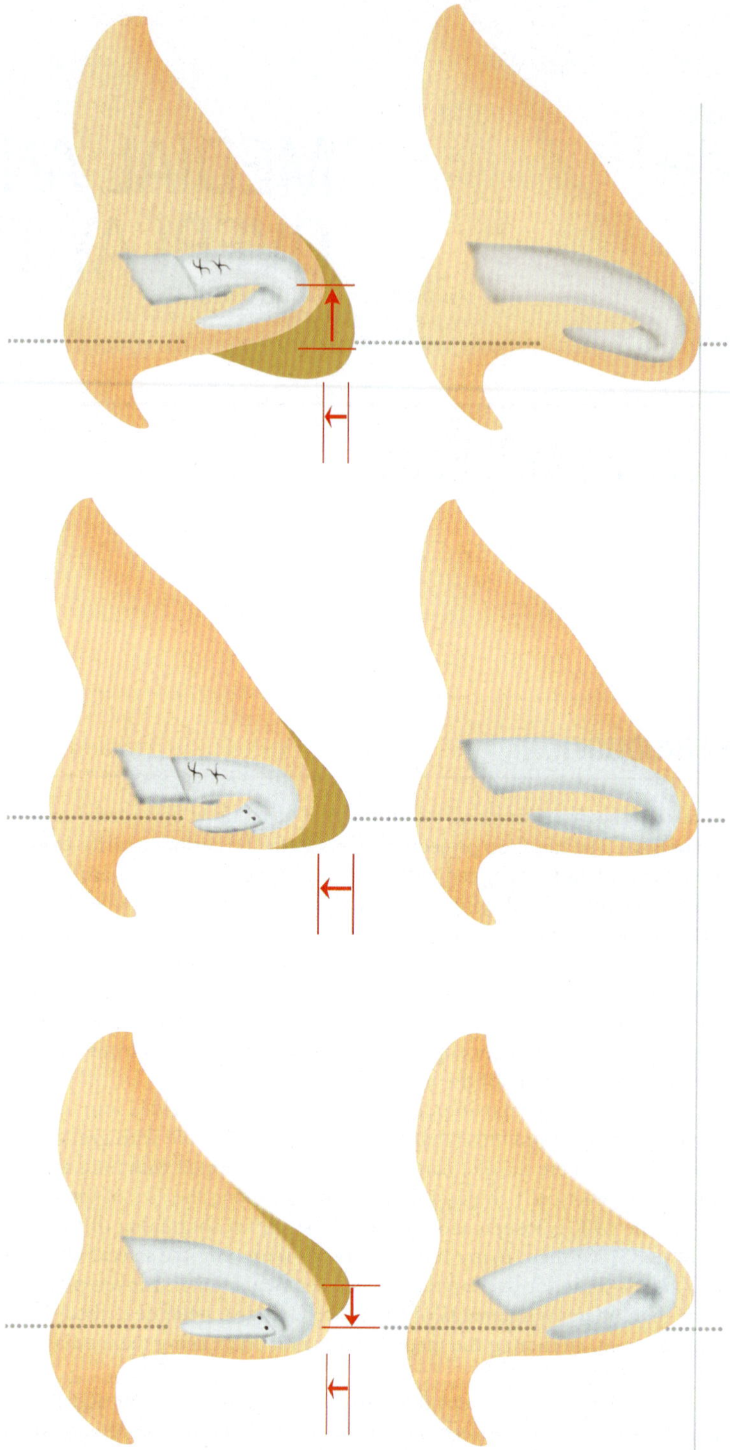

FIGURE 20.1
Schematic illustration of the effects of shortening lateral and medial crura on the degree of tip projection and rotation. **Top:** LCO decreased projection and resulted in superior rotation. **Bottom:** MCO decreased projection and resulted in inferior rotation. **Center:** The combination of LCO and MCO resulted in deprojection with no change in rotation.

the vertical division and overlap is performed. If done near the angle, at the junction of the medial and intermediate crus, there is more deprojection and less rotation. If done closer to the apex of the alar arch, there is more rotation and less deprojection.

HISTORY

A general review of the medical history is performed in relation to neurologic, cardiovascular, pulmonary, autoimmune, and overall physical fitness. Review of medications, anticoagulation therapy, tobacco and substance abuse is discussed as well. Prior to any rhinoplasty, one should exclude patients with a history of emotional problems or nervous breakdowns. A good history of nasal problems is mandatory stressing previous nasal trauma or nasal surgery and the detailed nature of these surgeries by reviewing all available operative data and analyzing the patient's photos before and after each of the previous surgeries. Finally, a complete detailed history of the patient's nasal complaint, both aesthetic and functional, is performed.

PHYSICAL EXAMINATION

It is necessary to fully examine the nose both externally and internally. The first element to evaluate is the thickness of the nasal skin and the degree of tip support available, by examining the alar cartilage size, strength, and orientation as well as the condition of the caudal septum and the anterior nasal spine. Other areas that need careful evaluation include the tip, ala, and columella. The tip is evaluated for its degree of projection and rotation and any broadness, bifidity, or deflection, while the ala is examined for its thickness and any degree of retraction or collapse. Finally, the columella is evaluated and termed short, long, hanging, retracted, deflected, wide, or bifid.

INDICATIONS

The LCO and MCO are used to shorten the lateral and medial crura and are indicated in patients with overdeveloped alar cartilages with long lateral, medial, or intermediate crura.

- Long lateral crura leading to an overprojected droopy (inferiorly rotated) tip
- Long medial crura leading to a long columella with overprojected superiorly rotated tip
- Long intermediate crura leading to a disproportionately long infratip lobule
- Malpositioned cephalically oriented lateral crura leading to a droopy tip
- Abnormal concavities or convexities of medial and lateral crura
- Asymmetry of lower lateral cartilages

CONTRAINDICATIONS

- Underdeveloped alar cartilages with short medial and lateral crura
- Absence of any degree of tip overprojection as both LCO and MCO will inevitably result in a decrease in tip projection
- Previously transected alar cartilages with loss of continuity as in cases of vertical dome division
- Revision cases with overresected alar cartilages

PREOPERATIVE PLANNING

The vital part in planning for a rhinoplasty is to fully understand the patient's desires and objectives; this is greatly helped by performing computer imaging as the surgeon can monitor the patient's reaction to the modifications in the degree of tip projection and rotation. On evaluating the degree of tip projection, it is important to exclude factors that may cause an illusion of overprojection, such as a deep nasofrontal angle, marked dorsal saddling, receding chin, or short upper lip. Once true overprojection is determined, the next step is to detect if its overprojection is due to overdeveloped alar cartilages (primary), septal cartilage (secondary), or a combination of both. When the septal cartilage is the main cause for the overprojection, the deformity is referred to as "tension nose" (Fig. 20.2) and is characterized by a high anterior septal angle and overdeveloped caudal septum and/or anterior nasal spine. Correction of the "tension nose" requires elimination of the pedestal effect of the overdeveloped septum on the normal alar cartilages which can now fall backward to a less projected position. This can be achieved through volume reduction of septal cartilage and rarely the anterior nasal spine. In cases of primary overprojection, where the main cause of overprojection is the overdeveloped alar cartilages with long medial and lateral crura (Fig. 20.3), adequate deprojection is only possible through shortening the crural length by MCO, LCO, or both. The choice depends largely upon whether rotation is adequate or will need to be increased or decreased. The droopy, inferiorly rotated tip which occurs in approximately 75% of my rhinoplasty patients is a much more common finding than the superiorly rotated tip. The pathogenesis of the droopy tip may be divided into two groups. The first group has "*abnormal*" alar cartilages with excessively long lateral crura, vertically malpositioned lateral crura with high abutment to the pyriform aperture, or short, weak medial crura. The second group has "*normal*" alar cartilages which are displaced inferiorly by the effect of extrinsic forces. These forces may be pushing from above, as in cases with long upper lateral cartilages, high anterior septal angle, and overdeveloped caudal septum, or forces pulling from below, as in cases with thick heavy nasal skin, overactive depressor septi nasi muscle, or by the effect of gravity on cases with weakened tip support as a result of aging or previous operations. The first step in the management of the droopy tip is to eliminate any

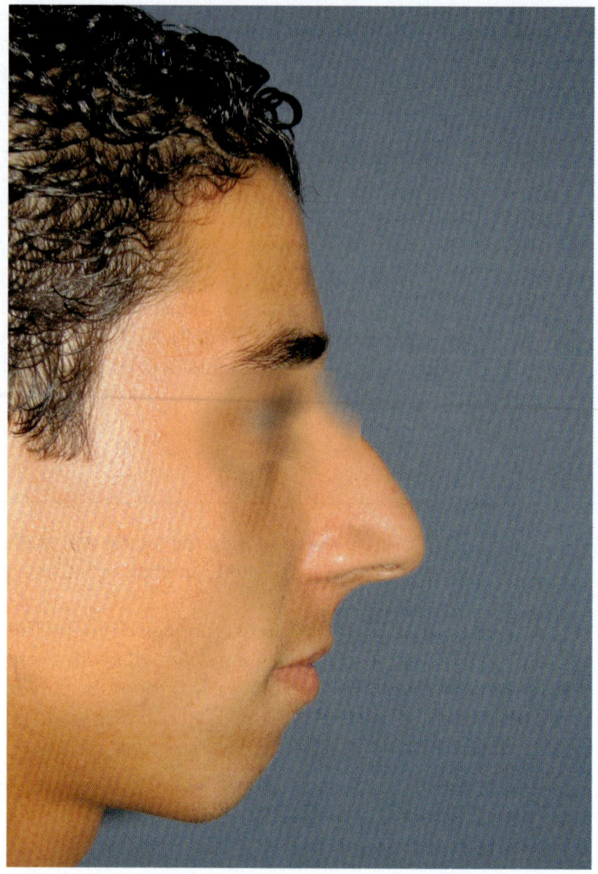

FIGURE 20.2
A case of secondary overprojection or tension nose where the septum is the main cause of overprojection.

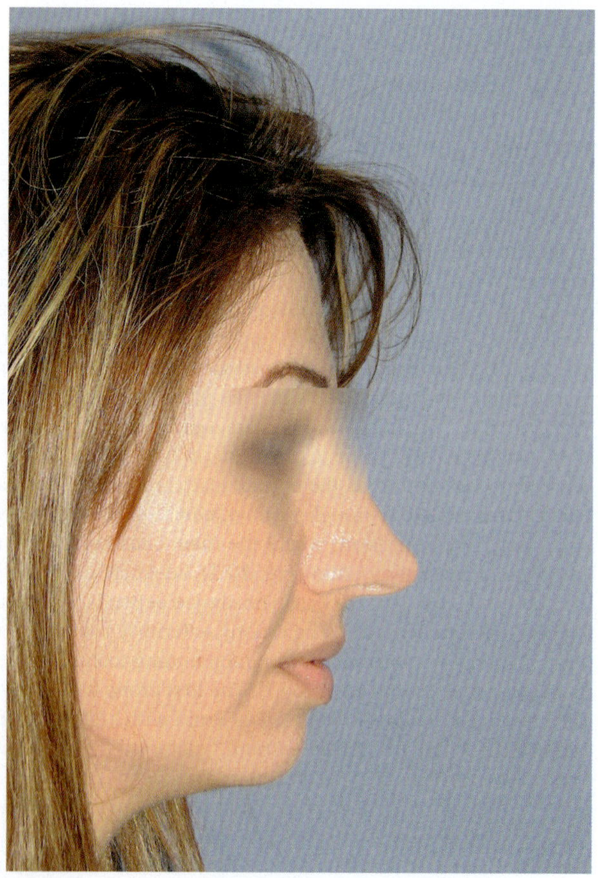

FIGURE 20.3
A case of primary overprojection where the overdeveloped alar cartilages are the main cause of the overprojection.

extrinsic forces pushing the tip downwards, thus allowing the alar cartilages the freedom to move upward, during the healing phase, and to rest in a more cephalic orientation. This is possible through such maneuvers as excision of overdeveloped scrolls of upper lateral cartilages, cephalic trim of lateral crura, lowering the anterior septal angle, or weakening of the depressor septi muscle. These maneuvers may be sufficient in cases with mild degrees of droopy tip. However, cases with more advanced degrees of droopy tip can only be corrected by alar cartilage-modifying techniques aiming at shortening the lateral crura as in LCO.

SURGICAL TECHNIQUE

The surgical procedure is performed through an external rhinoplasty approach as the exposure provided with this approach allows an accurate and direct appraisal of the tip cartilages in their natural, undistorted position. The approach also permits alar cartilage modifications to be performed in a precise manner and under direct vision. Bilateral marginal incisions are connected via an inverted V-shaped midcolumellar incision. The columellar skin flap is carefully elevated off the medial crura, and dissection is continued in the supraperichondrial plane to fully expose the alar cartilages. Elevation of the dorsal skin flap proceeds upward over the bony cartilaginous framework making sure to stay in the avascular sub-SMAS plane, until reaching the nasofrontal angle. Wide undermining is necessary to allow for better redraping of the skin–soft tissue envelope after deprojecting the nose. Any subcutaneous adipose tissue found between the domes or medial crura is carefully removed. Alar cartilage modification starts by performing a conservative cephalic trim of lateral crura; the width of the remaining lateral crus should not be less than 6 mm to maintain adequate tip support; this may go up to 8 mm in cases with thick heavy nasal skin. Any required dorsal modifications are made before modifying the tip cartilages to avoid inadvertent disruption of the delicate reconstructed alar cartilages.

Lateral Crural Overlay

In cases where the lateral crura are overly long leading to an overprojected, inferiorly rotated tip, an incision is planned in the lateral crus at the junction of its lateral third with the medial two thirds (Fig. 20.4A). The alar skin is relatively thicker in this area and can easily camouflage the cut and overlapped edges of the lateral crus. Before the cartilage cut is made, the vestibular skin is elevated off the undersurface of lateral crus for about 5 mm on each side of the planned cartilaginous incision (Fig. 20.4B) to release the tethering forces that may prevent the free overlap of the cut edges. The incision in the cartilage is made with a no. 15 blade extending in a straight line from the cephalic to the caudal margin of the lateral crus. The free medial segment of the lateral crus is advanced and rotated over the lateral segment in order to shorten the lateral crus to achieve the desired degree of deprojection and rotation. The integrity of the lateral crus is then reestablished by fixing the overlapped segments with a 6-0 Prolene suture in a horizontal mattress fashion (Fig. 20.4C). This maneuver will move the domes upward and backward resulting in an increase in tip rotation and decrease in tip projection (Fig. 20.5).

Medial Crural Overlay

This is performed to shorten the medial crura in cases where the overly long medial crura result in an overprojected or overrotated nasal tip. The level of the columella–lobular junction, which usually corresponds to the apex of the nostrils, is identified and marked on the medial crura using a surgical pen. The level of transection of the medial crura (Fig. 20.6A, C, E) is planned according to the preexisting relative length of the lobule to the columella. If the columella was found to be disproportionately longer than the lobule, then the transection is performed within the columellar segment of the medial crura. However, in cases where the lobule is relatively

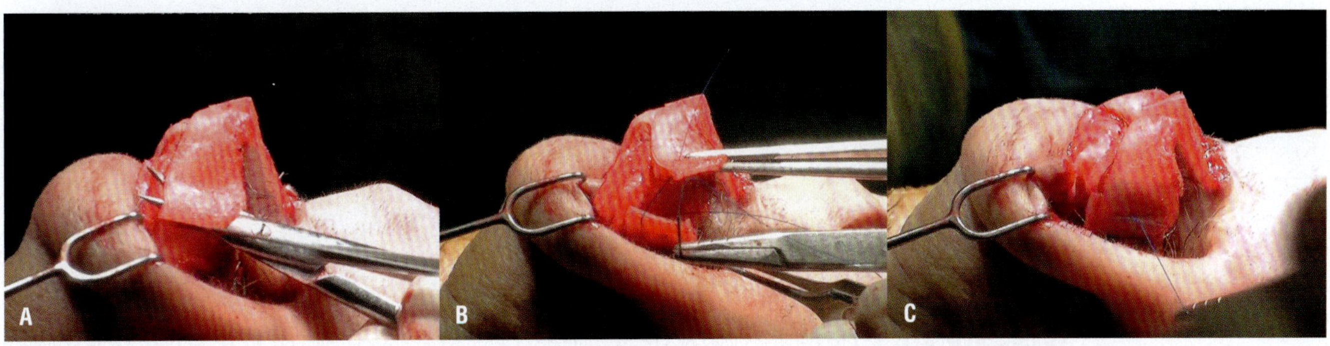

FIGURE 20.4 Intraoperative photos of the steps of LCO technique. **A:** Lateral crural transection. **B:** Overlap of cut segments. **C:** Suture fixation of overlapped cartilage.

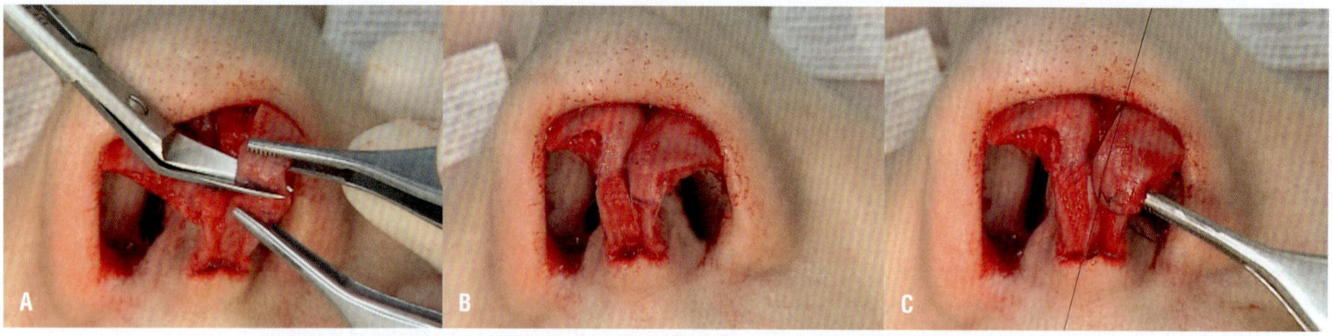

FIGURE 20.5 Intraoperative photos of the steps of MCO technique. **A:** Medial crural transection. **B:** Overlap of cut segments moved the dome posteriorly and inferiorly. **C:** Suture fixation of overlapped cartilage.

long as compared to the columella, the transection is completed in the lobular segment of the medial crura in order to shorten the lobule and correct the preexisting disproportion between the lobule and the columella.

After determining the desired level of transection, the vestibular skin is elevated from the overlying medial crus for a few millimeters on each side; the integrity of the medial crus is reestablished by overlapping and fixing the cut edges together with 6-0 Prolene sutures in a horizontal mattress fashion (Fig. 20.6B, D, F). At the completion of MCO, the domes move posteriorly and inferiorly resulting in deprojection and inferior rotation of nasal tip (Fig. 20.7). To avoid excessive widening of the columella in cases where a columellar strut is used in combination with MCO, the overlapped segments of medial crura are excised and the cut ends are directly approximated and splinted to the columellar strut using 5-0 PDS in a horizontal mattress fashion as described in the alar setback technique.

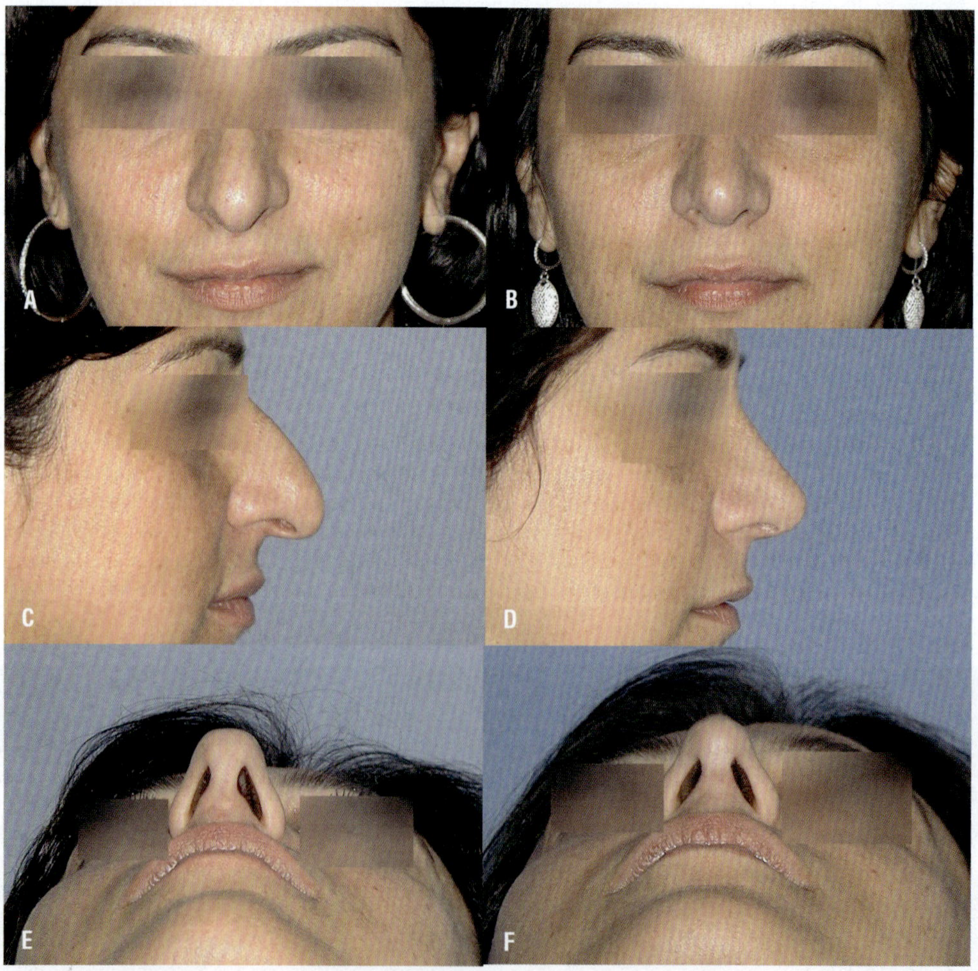

FIGURE 20.6 **A, C, E:** Preoperative views of a patient with an overprojected droopy nasal tip. **B, D, F:** Postoperative views of the patient 2 years after using the LCO technique to deproject and superiorly rotate the nasal tip. Additional maneuvers included conservative hump reduction and osteotomies.

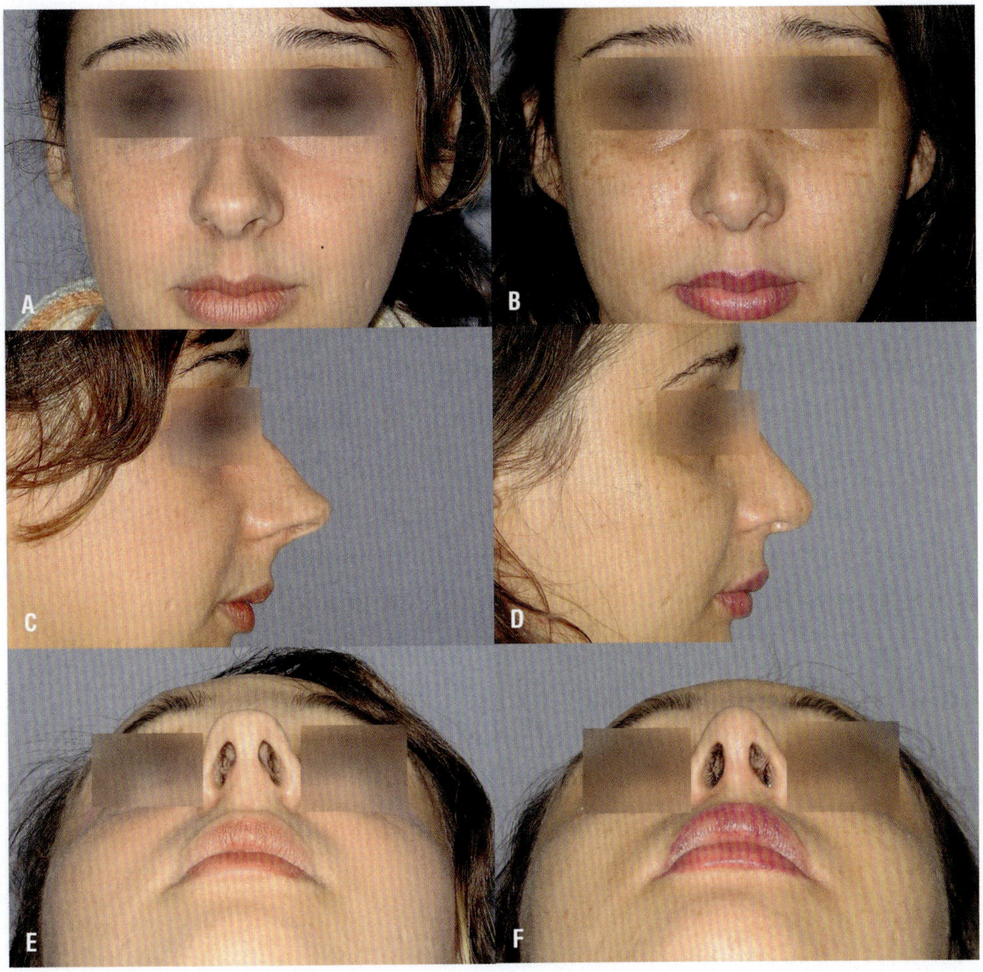

FIGURE 20.7 **A, C, E:** Preoperative views of a patient with an overprojected superiorly rotated tip. **B, D, F:** Postoperative views of the patient 3 years after using MCO technique to deproject and inferiorly rotate the nasal tip. A conservative alar base excision was performed.

Combining LCO and MCO

In cases with severe overprojection that could not be corrected by LCO or MCO alone, a combination of both techniques can be used to provide maximum deprojection without significantly changing the degree of rotation (Fig. 20.8). In these cases, I usually start with the LCO. After LCO completion, one can precisely determine any need for further deprojection or alteration in the degree of tip rotation.

At the completion of the procedure, the nasal skin is redraped to its normal anatomic position and the external rhinoplasty incisions are closed starting with the columellar incision which is closed using a 6-0 PDS deep subcutaneous suture in a horizontal mattress fashion followed by 6-0 Prolene interrupted sutures on the skin surface. The marginal incisions are closed using 5-0 Vicryl rapid sutures. Meticulous taping is necessary to maintain the proper positioning of the reconstructed tip cartilages; this is performed using 0.5-inch brown Micropore tape after applying Mastisol to the skin surface, and then a metal splint is positioned over the dorsum and secured by a second layer of tape.

POSTOPERATIVE CARE

The patient is advised to sleep in the supine position with the back of the bed raised for 3 days to minimize postoperative facial edema. Oral antibiotics are given for 5 days, and the patient uses antibiotic ointment intranasally until all the sutures in the nasal cavity fall off, which may take 4 to 6 weeks. Saline nasal irrigations can be used before ointment application to decrease the stuffy nose sensation. The splint is removed after 1 week along with the columellar sutures, and the nose is retaped for another week to help support the tip during the early healing phase where new fibrous attachments are being developed between the bony and cartilaginous nasal framework and the overlying skin. Sunscreen is used on the columellar incision as well as any external alar incisions prior to sun exposure for the first 2 months.

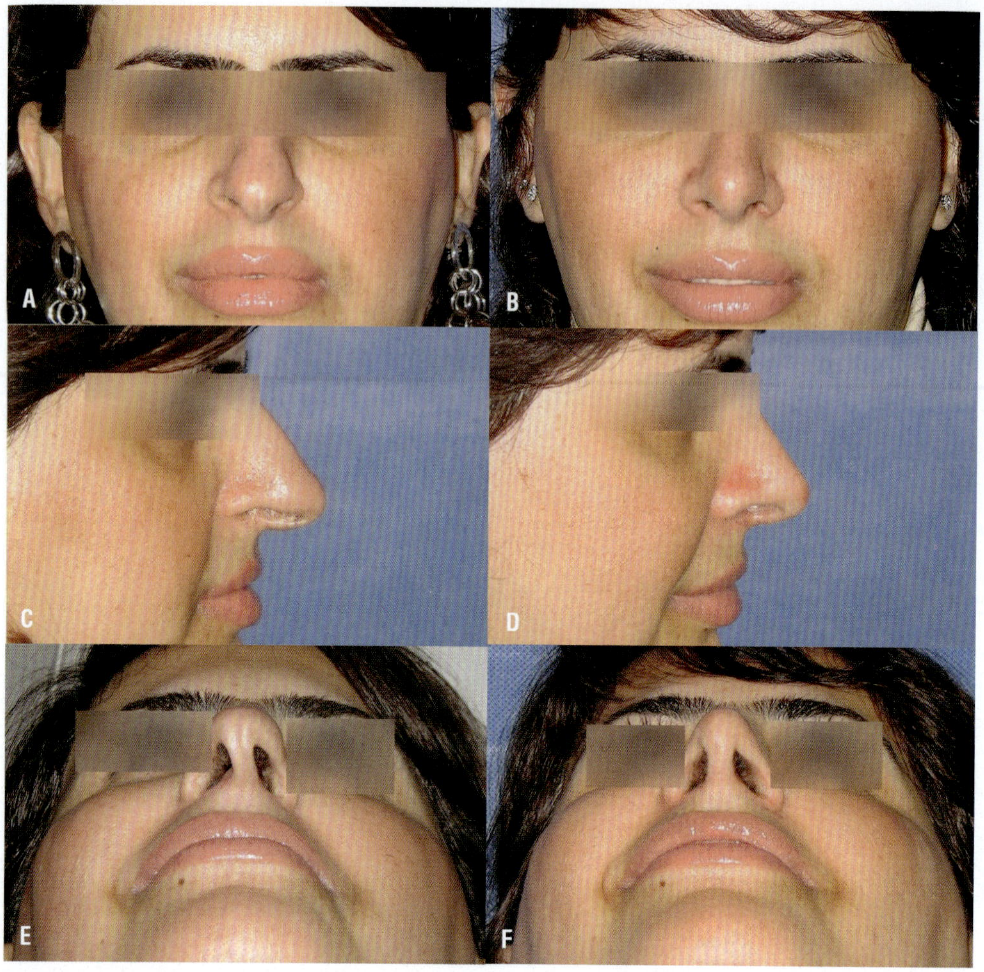

FIGURE 20.8 **A, C, E:** Preoperative views of a patient with a severely overprojected tip due to overdeveloped alar cartilages with long medial and lateral crura. **B, D, F:** Postoperative views of the patient after using both LCO and MCO to achieve deprojection without altering tip rotation. Additional maneuvers included hump reduction, osteotomies to centralize the deviated nasal bones, and septoplasty to correct a caudal septum deflection.

COMPLICATIONS

- Excessive loss of projection may result from an error in judgment on the part of the surgeon regarding the amount of overlap needed to achieve the desired degree of deprojection. This may also be due to failure to provide adequate support to the nasal tip which results in postoperative tip drop.
- Increase in the width of the nasal base due to increased alar flaring, which occurs more with MCO than with LCO. This can be avoided by performing a simultaneous nasal base narrowing procedure in all cases where major deprojection was achieved.
- Tip asymmetries due to failure to achieve equal amounts of overlap of both alar cartilages.
- Widening of the columella especially if MCO was combined with a columellar strut.
- Alar contour surface irregularity may occur if the LCO is taken too medially in patients with thin nasal skin.

PEARLS

- The LCO and MCO results in controlled predictable changes in the degree of tip projection and rotation depending on to the level of cartilage transection and degree of overlap of the cut segments.
- The MCO and LCO allow incremental shortening of medial and lateral crura to be conducted without any cartilage excision thus eliminating the risk of cartilage weakening or buckling.
- The use of sutures to fix and stabilize the overlapped cartilage helps maintain the achieved degree of projection and rotation and avoids any migration or displacement of the transected cartilages that may cause lobular contour irregularities.

PITFALLS

- LCO and MCO are powerful maneuvers that are unforgiving.
- With the patient in a spine position, overrotation is a natural tendency for the novice surgeon.

INSTRUMENTS TO HAVE AVAILABLE

- Standard rhinoplasty set

SUGGESTED READING

Adamson PA, Litner JA, Dahiya R. The M-arch model: a new concept of nasal tip dynamics. *Arch Facial Plast Surg* 2006;8:16–25.

Anderson JR. The dynamics of rhinoplasty. In: Bustamant GA, ed. *Proceedings of the Ninth International Congress of Otolaryngology*, Mexico City, August 10–14, 1969. Amsterdam, the Netherlands: Excerpta Medica, 1970.

Foda HMT. Alar setback technique: a controlled method of nasal tip deprojection. *Arch Otolaryngol Head Neck Surg* 2001;127:1341–1346.

Foda HMT, Kridel RWH. Lateral crural steal and lateral crural overlay: an objective evaluation. *Arch Otolaryngol Head Neck Surg* 1999;125:1365–1370.

Kridel WHK, Konior RJ. Controlled nasal tip rotation via the lateral crural overlay technique. *Arch Otolaryngol Head Neck Surg* 1991;117:411–415.

21 MANAGEMENT OF THE ALAR BASE

Minas Constantinides

INTRODUCTION

The alar base serves as the esthetic foundation for the inferior third of the nose. In the pantheon of rhinoplasty techniques, treatment of the alar base can be among the more challenging maneuvers. It is in addressing the disharmonies of this region that the rhinoplasty surgeon can maximize the esthetic outcome.

Weir first described resection of the alar base in 1892 when the patient developed alar flare following a deprojecting rhinoplasty. Weir excised a wedge of tissue, hiding the incision in the alar-facial groove. Subsequently, in 1931, Joseph modified the Weir technique by removing an internal wedge of tissue from the vestibular side of the ala. In 1943, Aufricht expounded on the technique further by developing over 20 geometric excisions of tissue from the alar rim to the nasal sill. Many variations of Weir's original technique have been investigated since his original description. However, the fundamental concepts necessary to manage the alar base can be distilled down to a stepwise approach that will lead to surgical success.

HISTORY

Overall evaluation focuses on the patient's cosmetic concerns as alar base modification typically does not impact nasal airflow. The patient's motivations for surgery and cosmetic goals are discussed, with the guiding principle directed toward achieving nasal and facial harmony. Previous surgeries of the nose or face are documented as these could contribute to the current structure of the alar base. A detailed list of medications, including anticoagulants, corticosteroids, herbal medications, and isotretinoin is imperative since some herbal medications can increase the risk of bleeding. Isotretinoin should be stopped for a minimum of 6 months due to its negative effect on wound healing. One may also take the opportunity to inquire about keloid formation from previous surgical interventions. The history taking is also the surgeon's opportunity to determine if the patient is psychologically fit to undergo rhinoplasty surgery.

PHYSICAL EXAMINATION

Physical examination includes an appropriate global facial analysis as well as focused internal and external nasal examination. Obviously, the most important component of the assessment is evaluation of the alar base.

Alar Base Anatomy

The topography of the region is highlighted by the shadows and curvatures that make this area a visual landmark. These relationships are critical to the appearance of the alar base: the curved insertion of the ala into the face, the shadows of the alar-facial groove and the alar crease, the convex reflection of the ala, and the smooth transitions between the ala, nasal tip, and nasal sidewall. These subtle intricacies make modification of the alar base a surgery of millimeters (Fig. 21.1).

The alar base occupies the caudal third of the nose. The boundaries of the alar base include (1) the alar crease, which separates the ala from the nasal sidewall superiorly; (2) the alar-facial groove, which separates it from the cheek and apical triangle of the upper lip laterally; and (3) the crease across the nasal sills and subnasale, which divides the upper lip from the nose and delineates the inferior border of the alar base.

The external structure of the alar base is comprised primarily of the ala and alar lobule, which is comprised of skin, muscle, and fibroadipose tissue. There is no cartilage in this region, and the soft tissue support arises from the tight attachments of the skin to underlying fibroadipose ligaments. The columella is the skin and soft tissue overlying the paired medial crura of the lower lateral cartilages. This structure commonly makes a smooth transition from the infratip and soft triangle regions, over the medial crural footplates, and then curves laterally to join the nasal sills. Internally, the nasal vestibule is bounded by the membranous septum medially, the medial aspect of the ala laterally, and the nasal sill inferiorly. The nasal sill is the soft tissue area between the medial crural footplate and the alar-facial groove. Functionally, the external nasal valve is framed by the ala, the membranous septum, and the nasal sill/nostril floor.

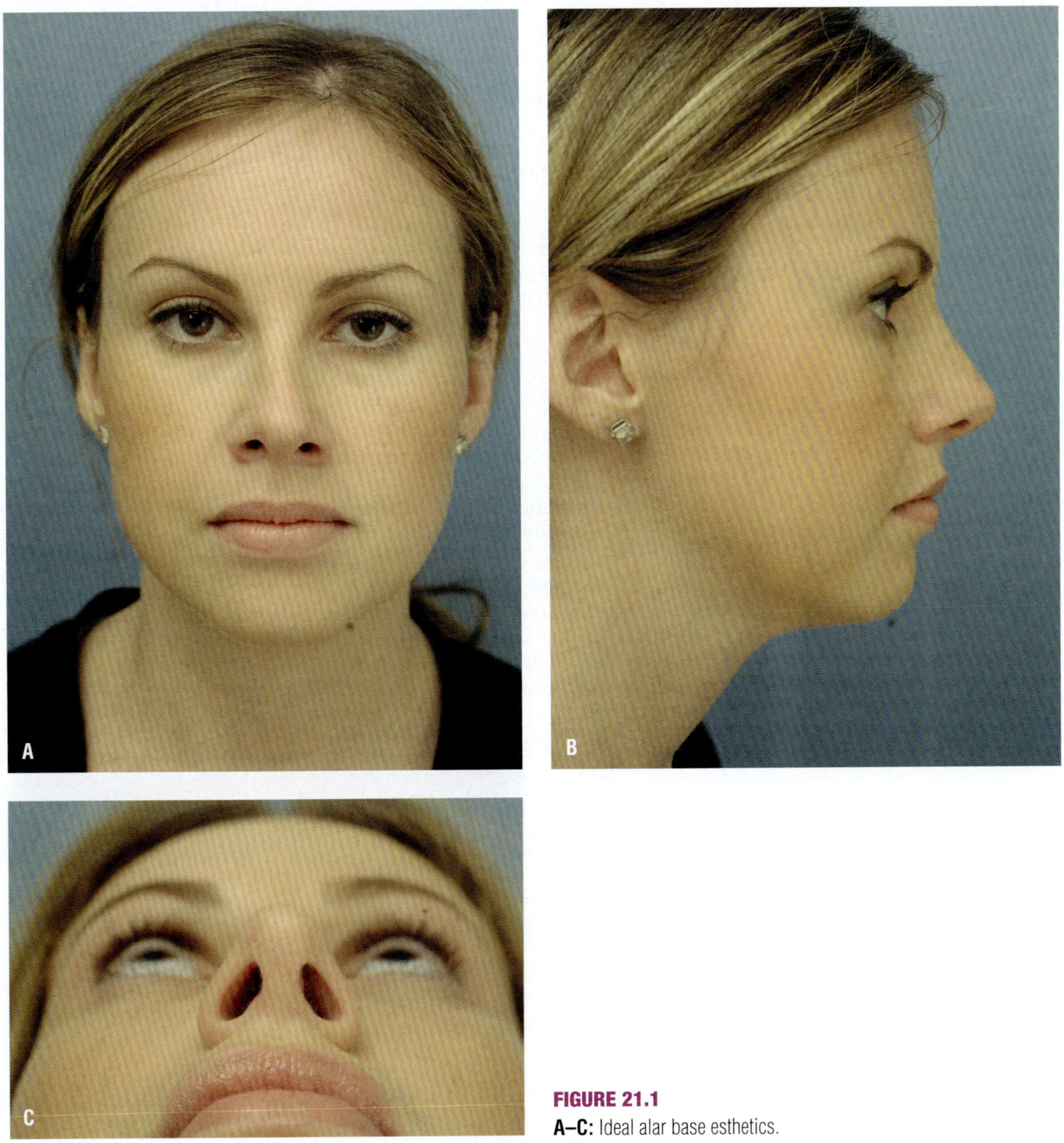

FIGURE 21.1
A–C: Ideal alar base esthetics.

TABLE 21.1 Anatomic Components of the Alar Base

Components	Photographic Views: Frontal	Photographic Views: Lateral	Photographic Views: Base
Alar base	Width	Facial insertion point	Width Curvature at insertion point
Nostril	Nostril show ("gull in flight")	Nostril show (alar rim contour; hanging columella)	Shape Width Orientation
Nasal sill	Width (face tilted slightly inferiorly)		Shape Nostril symmetry
Columella	Infratip lobule show; excessive columellar show when overrotated	Alar–columellar relationship	Width Height Medial crural footplate flare
Ala	Alar rim contour	Alar rim contour Alar lobule width Alar–columellar relationship (e.g., hooding)	Alar lobule width Alar wall thickness Flare

Physical examination of the alar base requires a structured approach. The following five components should be evaluated (see Table 21.1):

- Alar base (insertion point position and curvature, width)
- Nostril (shape, width, orientation)
- Nostril floor/sill (width, shape)
- Columella (height, relationship to tip lobule height, width, medial crural footplate flare)
- Ala (lobule width, thickness, alar–columellar relationship, alar rim contour, alar flare)

Anatomical Esthetic Ideals

The ideal Caucasian *alar base width*, measured as the transverse distance between the two insertions of the alae into the face, is typically equal to or slightly more than the intercanthal distance (Fig. 21.2). Alternatively, desirable alar base width can be measured as approximately 70% of the nasal length, defined by the distance from the nasal tip to the nasion. This value is variable, dependent on ethnicity as well as patient and surgeon preferences. For example, in African American men, the ratio of inter-alar to intercanthal distance is approximately 1.3:1, whereas the female ratio is 1.25:1. In southern Chinese women, it is also more common to have a nasal width greater than the intercanthal distance in addition to the alae having increased flare and the nostrils having a greater horizontal orientation. At the facial insertion point, the alar base should typically assume a medially directed curvature, rather than a straight insertion. The position of insertion of the ala into the face can dramatically impact esthetics, producing excessive columellar exposure or a snarl-like appearance.

In Caucasians, the *nostrils* should be pear shaped, approximately equal in width to the columella, and their long axis should be oriented at a 30 to 45 degrees angle to the vertical axis of the columella. Farkas and colleagues have developed an objective assessment system for different nostril types.

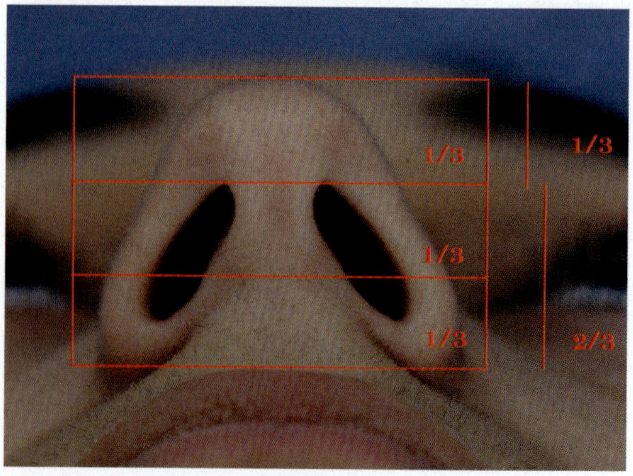

FIGURE 21.2
Ideal anatomic proportions of the alar base.

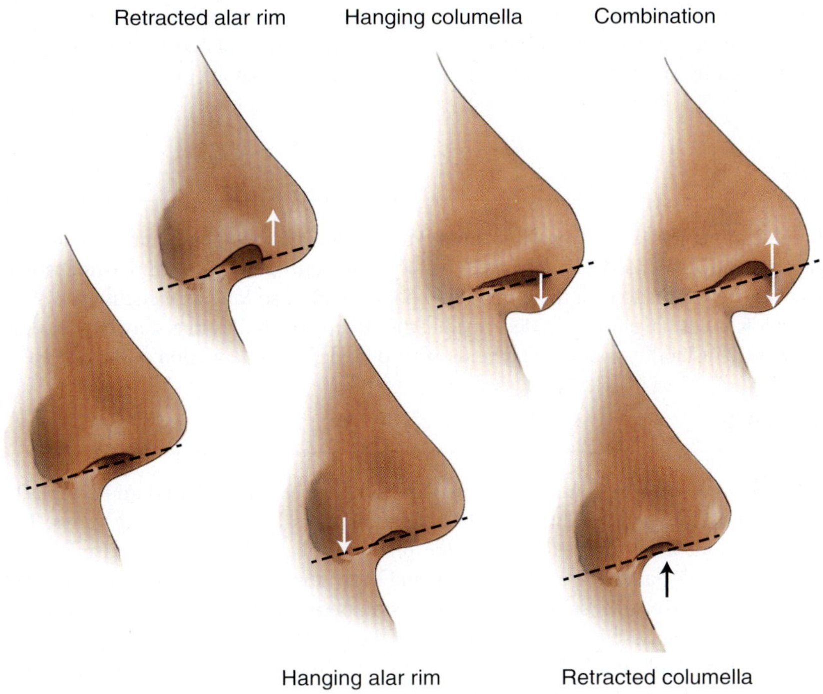

FIGURE 21.3 Depiction of various alar–columellar relationships indicated by arrows.

The *nostril sill* region may be normally notched or smooth, depending on its transition with the alar-facial groove. In some patients, the sill is flat, while in others, it is a slightly elevated roll of skin. Regardless, it is commonly recognized as the anterior base of the nasal aperture (nostril) and is commonly, but often overlooked, nasal landmark.

The *columella* width is largely a function of the medial crurae and should appear symmetric without significant medial crural footplate flare. The Caucasian nasal base is ideally shaped like an equilateral triangle, with a 2:1 ratio of columellar height to tip lobule height.

On frontal view, the *alar* margins should take on the appearance of a "gull in flight." On lateral view, the alar contour should describe a gentle curve. Crumley noted an ideal 1:2:3 relationship between the length of the alar base, the nasal tip lobule, and the length of the nostril in the profile view. On base view, the alar lobule width should be less than one-fifth of the total transverse width of the nasal base. Alar flare is best appreciated on base view and is defined as the portion of the ala extending laterally past the alar-facial insertion point. Silver has suggested that lateral excursion of the alar rim greater than 2 mm beyond the alar-facial insertion point should be considered significant.

The alar–columellar relationship is best described by drawing a meridian line between the anterior and posterior terminal points of the nostril. If the alar rim is greater than 2 mm above this line, there is alar retraction. If the alar rim is less than 1 mm above this line, then alar "hooding" is present. Alar hooding can be due to excessive alar bulk or from a distal caudal insertion point of the ala, thereby obscuring the columella on lateral view. If the columella is greater than 2 mm below this line, there is a hanging columella. If the columella is less than 1 mm below this line, the columella is considered retracted (Fig. 21.3).

INDICATIONS

In broad terms, alar base modification is indicated when the patient desires it and the surgeon deems it appropriate and achievable. The goal is to create balance between the anatomic proportions of the alar base. Specifically, four abnormalities can be addressed surgically:

- Large, asymmetric or horizontally oriented nostril
- Wide alar base
- Excessive alar flare
- Alar hooding

In Caucasian patients, the generally accepted criterion for nasal base reduction is when the width of the alar base is greater than the intercanthal distance. This standard may be modified based on ethnicity and patient preference.

Excessive alar flare, such as that caused by retrodisplacement of the nasal tip during rhinoplasty, can be reduced with alar base modification techniques. A nostril that is wide, asymmetric, or has a horizontal axis (without alar flare) can be improved by sill reduction alone. Finally, intranasal excisions can be employed to help reduce alar hooding.

CONTRAINDICATIONS

There are no absolute contraindications for alar base modification. Patients who are medically unfit for surgery could potentially undergo the procedure under local anesthesia. A history of hypertrophic or keloid scarring would raise some concern, but I have not found this to be a region prone to poor scarring, so long as meticulous wound closure techniques are employed. Keloids have not been described in this area, though fibromas may be mistaken for keloids. Patients with psychiatric instability may also be better served by deferring reduction of the alar base.

PREOPERATIVE PLANNING

Preoperative planning begins with a careful assessment of the patient as described above. Standard rhinoplasty photographs should be taken: frontal, right and left lateral, right and left oblique, base, and smiling views. The patient consultation should include a detailed discussion about the proposed changes to the alar base. Digital morphing software can help the patient visualize the eventual result and show nuances of change that may guide the surgeon's decision making intraoperatively. Most human faces are asymmetric, and the preoperative consultation is an excellent opportunity to point out these irregularities as part of the management of patient expectations.

Modification of the alar base is typically performed at the conclusion of the rhinoplasty. At this point, any changes to the alar base resulting from the preceding rhinoplasty maneuvers can be identified and addressed. If there is any doubt as to the need for alar base reduction, the procedure can be deferred for 6 to 8 weeks to allow for postoperative healing to dictate the final decision.

The goals of alar base modification are to preserve the natural curvature of the ala, to avoid overstraightening of the ala, and to prevent visible scar formation. Of course, it is important to review all relevant changes proposed in a chosen rhinoplasty as deprojection can cause increased alar flare and nostril widening (Fig. 21.4). Conversely, increasing tip projection can decrease alar flare (Fig. 21.5).

SURGICAL TECHNIQUE

Reviewing the anatomy of the alar base allows conceptualization of the surgical techniques. The alar base has an inner circumference comprised by the vestibular mucosa of the nostrils and an outer circumference consisting of alar skin. Considering these two circumferences separately can allow one to preferentially manipulate excessive nostril size and shape, alar base width, and alar flare.

Reduction of the inner circumference is accomplished via a nostril sill excision. An "internal alar base reduction" is a V-shaped excision of the sill that narrows the nostril. An "external alar base reduction" is an inverted V-shaped excision of the nostril sill, which decreases the columellar–alar base distance and narrows the alar base width. Nostril sill excisions do not address alar flare. A wedge resection from the external surface of the ala at the alar lobule reduces the outer circumference of the ala and is termed "Alar Flare Reduction." The surgeon can manipulate these three techniques to tailor the amount of nostril narrowing, decrease of alar base width, and alar flare reduction to the individual patient needs.

Effective scar camouflage at the alar-facial junction can be challenging due to the abundance of sebaceous glands, which can compromise precise healing. However, with careful planning and meticulous technique, such scars can be made virtually imperceptible. Wound closure must achieve good tissue eversion without tension. Importantly, incisions into the lateral ala should be made one half to one millimeter *above* the alar-facial groove so that the natural sulcus is not violated. This scar typically heals beautifully, while the normal groove is preserved. The 0.5 to 1 mm cuff of remaining skin facilitates exact closure of the cut edges. Regarding nostril sill incisions, these should be placed within the normal crease lines of the sill, such that there is no notching and the natural alar curves are maintained.

Structured Approach

The simplified approach to alar base modification attempts to address the following four factors:

- Wide alar base
- Large, asymmetric or horizontally oriented nostril
- Alar hooding
- Excessive alar flare

Figure 21.6 provides a detailed, stepwise treatment algorithm.

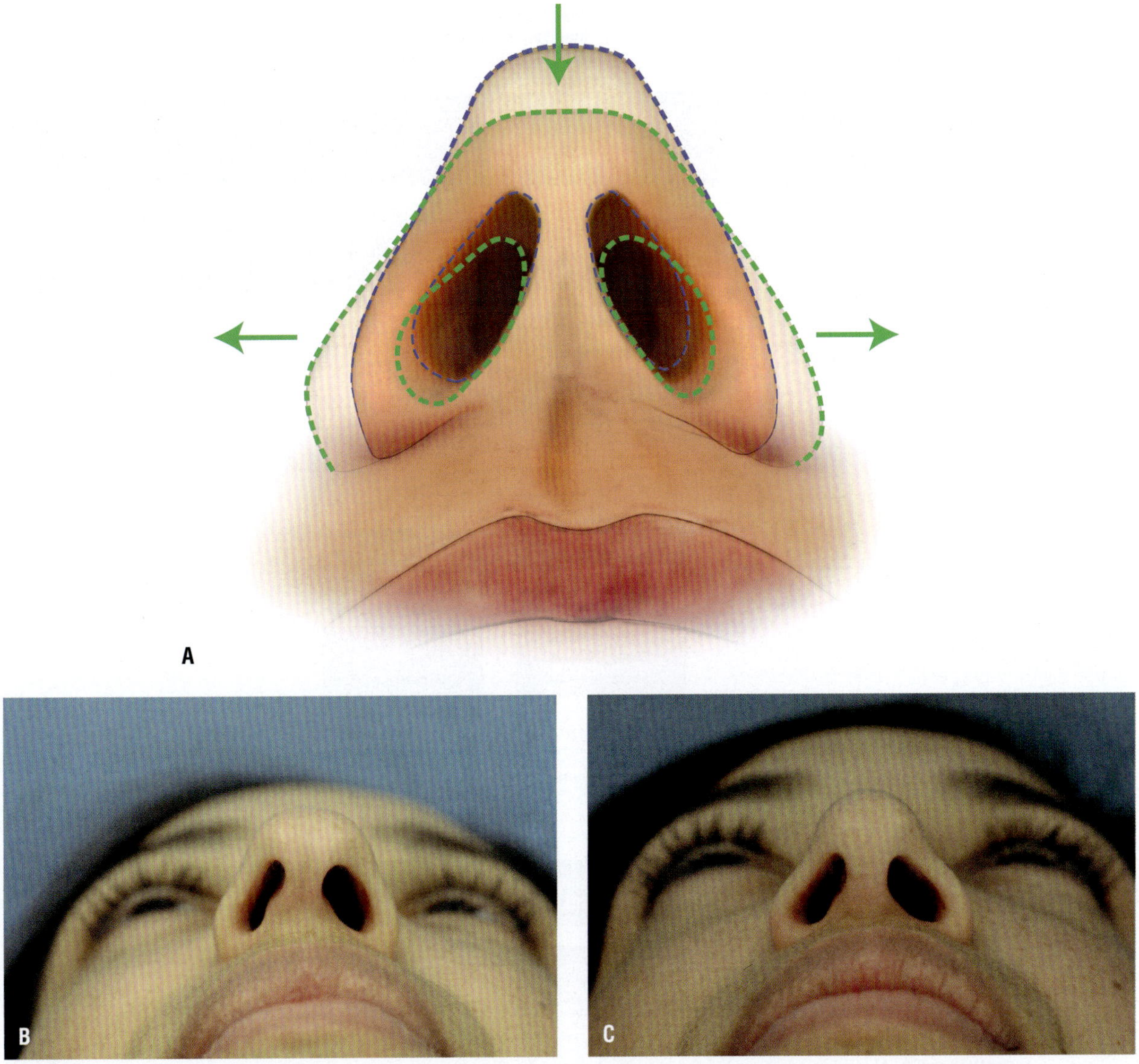

FIGURE 21.4 **A:** Significant deprojection can cause alar flare to compensate for decreased tip support. Preoperative **(B)** and 1-year postoperative **(C)** base views showing increased alar flare following deprojection rhinoplasty.

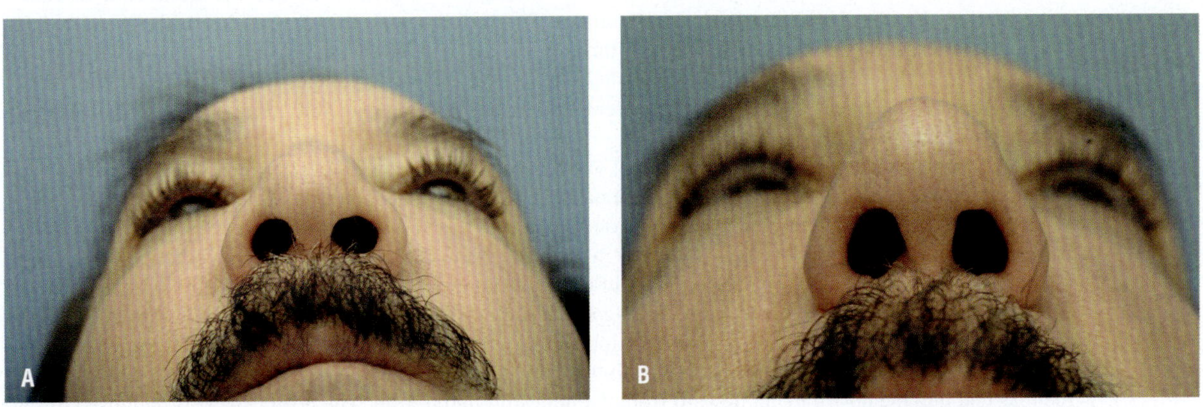

FIGURE 21.5 Preoperative **(A)** and 18-month postoperative **(B)** base views showing decreased alar flare following rhinoplasty to increase tip projection.

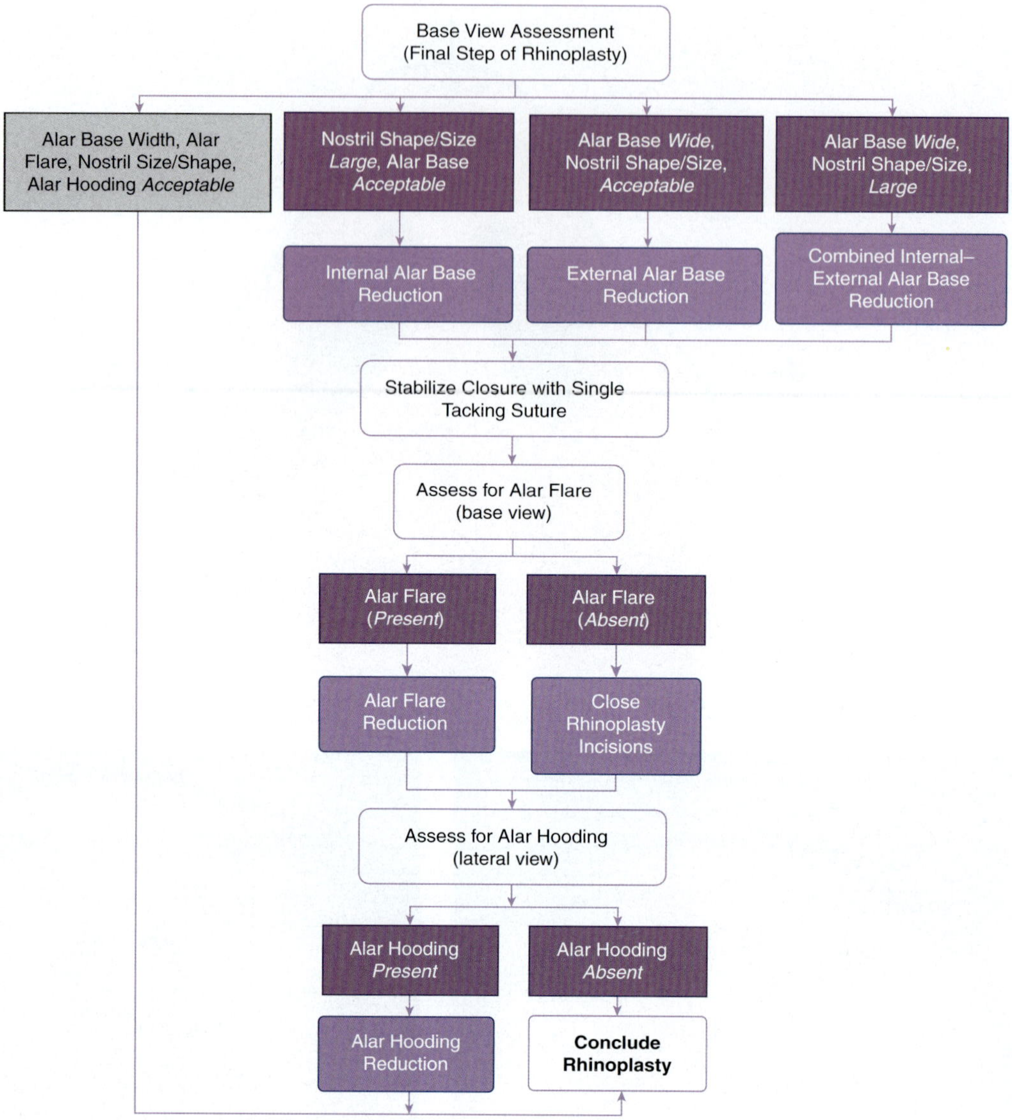

FIGURE 21.6 Algorithmic approach to management of the alar base.

I. Wide Alar Base (External Alar Base Reduction)

At the conclusion of the rhinoplasty, the columellar incision is closed if an open approach was used, and the alar base is evaluated. If the width of the alar base is deemed excessive, an external alar base reduction may be employed. Similar to the internal alar base reduction (see below), an internal nostril sill resection is performed. However, the two critical differences which distinguish this approach are the "inverted V" shape of the resection and the lateral incision through the ala. The effect is twofold: the alar-facial junction is medialized without changing nostril shape, and the through-and-through alar incision allows the ala to act as a rotation-advancement flap (hereinafter referred to as the "sliding alar flap") that can be mobilized with minimal tension.

A surgical pen is used to mark the midpoint of the base of the columella and the lateral border of the nostril sill. A third mark is placed halfway between the nasal alar base and the top of the alar-facial groove that delineates the superior extent of the alar crease incision. Calipers are used to measure the precise amount of tissue to be resected, and a fourth mark is made medially in the nasal sill to define the width of the resection (this will be the base of the "inverted V"). The region is infiltrated with 1% lidocaine with 1:100,000 epinephrine, buffered 9:1 with 8.4% sodium bicarbonate, using a 27-gauge needle. After allowing 10 minutes for vasoconstriction, the sharp calipers are kept at the desired excision setting and pierce into the sill to mark the exact excision. Then the tip of the no. 11 blade is inserted, with the cutting surface facing upward, into the pierced holes. It is then pushed into the nostril to cut upward from the holes through the sill. The no. 11 blade is then used to saw out the triangular wedge of tissue. Mobilizing the ala as a rotation-advancement flap allows for a more natural curvature while reducing wound closure tension and avoiding notching with healing (Figs. 21.7 to 21.11).

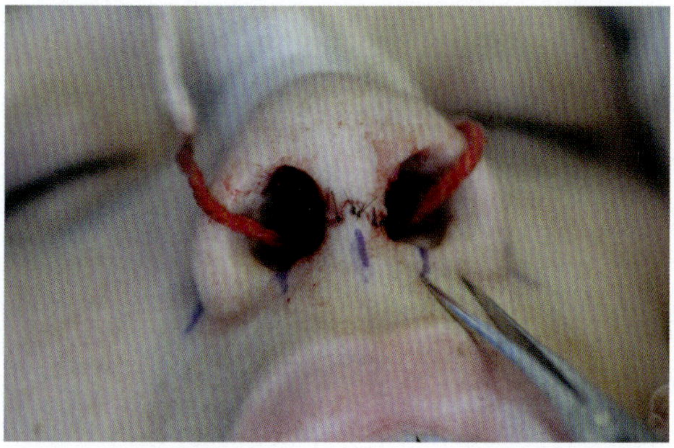

FIGURE 21.7
Markings are placed in the columellar midline, in the lateral-most points of the alar-facial grooves, and in the creases equidistant from the midline. The desired narrowing of the outer diameter of the ala is determined and marked with calipers.

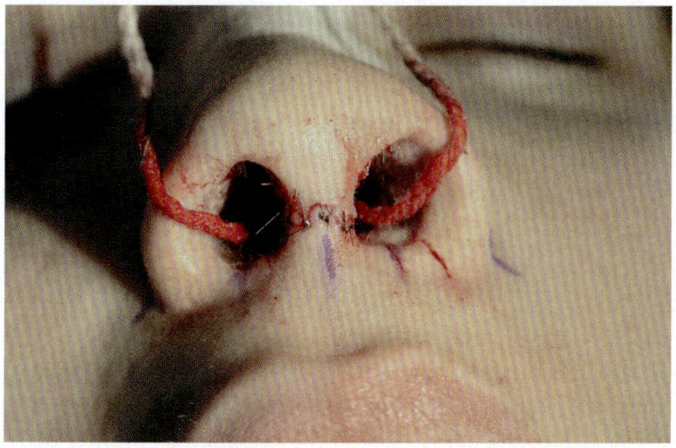

FIGURE 21.8
Sill incisions are performed with a no. 11 blade cutting upward from the stab. The starting point of the lateral incision will determine the outside nostril diameter, while the end point in the nasal vestibule determines the ultimate diameter of the inner nostril.

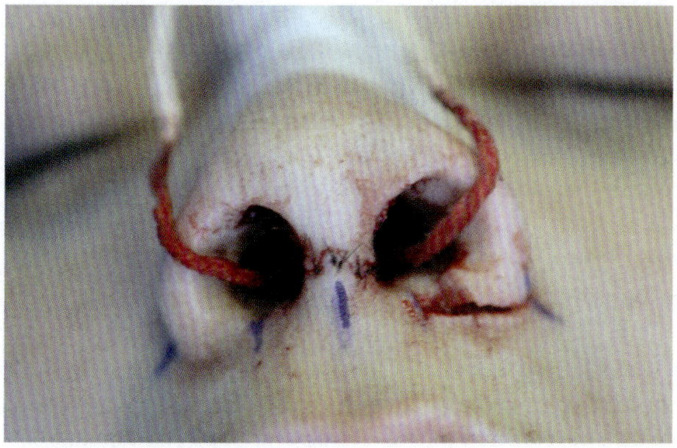

FIGURE 21.9
The caudal extent of both incisions is connected with a no. 11 blade along a line that begins medially parallel to the sill and travels to the lateral alar-facial mark.

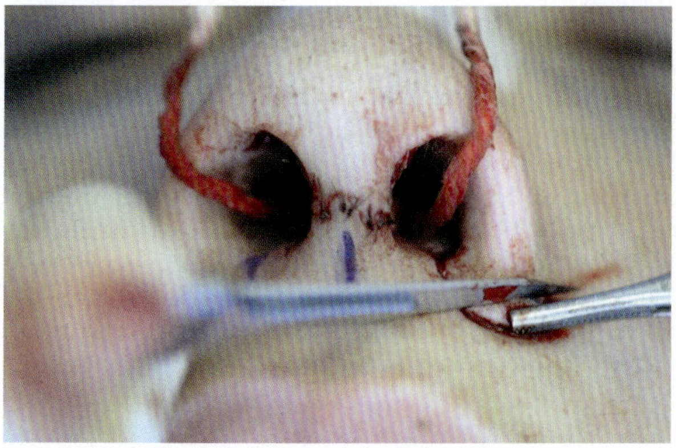

FIGURE 21.10
After the sill is tacked medially, the alar lobule edge is grasped with a Brown-Adson forceps and pulled inferiorly to estimate the amount of alar flare reduction. A no. 11 blade is used to excise this wedge of tissue.

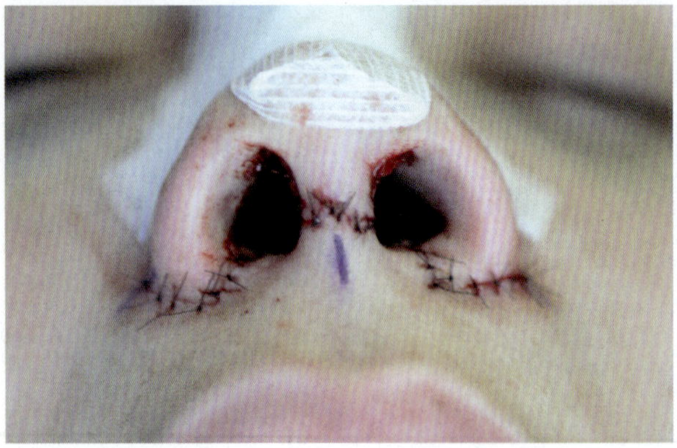

FIGURE 21.11
Alar sill and wedge resection is completed on the opposite side, and the wound is meticulously closed with simple interrupted 5-0 nylon sutures, which are removed on postoperative day 5.

Meticulous closure is critical to achieve satisfactory scarring postoperatively. If needed, a 5-0 Monocryl (Ethicon Inc.; Somerville, NJ) deep dermal suture can be used to reduce wound closure tension. A single 5-0 nylon tacking suture is placed at the medial, most intranasal aspect of the wound edges. The alar base is again evaluated for alar flare and addressed accordingly (see below). If there is no flare, the incisions are closed with interrupted 5-0 nylon sutures. Wound closure should achieve appropriate tissue eversion, no tension, and no step-offs. The nasal base is cleaned with wet gauze and antibiotic ointment is applied liberally to the incisions.

II. Large Horizontal Axis or Asymmetric Nostrils (Internal Alar Base Reduction)

If the patient has large, horizontally oriented or asymmetric nostrils, in the absence of excessive alar base width, then an internal alar base reduction is employed via excision of the nostril sill. This particular situation is extremely rare, since large nostrils are almost always accompanied by a wide alar base.

A surgical pen is used to mark the midpoint of the columella at the base of the columella. Another mark is made at the lateral border of the nostril sill, at its junction with the ala. Excisions should not extend laterally along the natural curve of the ala, as this can lead to unnatural curves, notches, or abnormal insertions of the alae postoperatively. Calipers are used to measure the appropriate width of vestibular surface of the ala to be excised. The area to be resected is then marked out in a V shape. In so doing, the resection affects the nostril size only, without causing any medialization of the alar-facial junction. The region is infiltrated with a local anesthetic, which is allowed to set for 10 minutes, as previously described. A no. 11 blade is used to make a stab incision into each of the limbs of the V-shaped markings. The wedge is grasped with a toothed Brown-Adson forceps and resected with the scalpel. Cautery is avoided to prevent excessive thermal damage to the tissues. Wound closure is carried out in the same manner as described for external alar base reduction.

III. Wide Alar Base and Excessive Nostril Size/Shape (Combined Internal–External Alar Base Reduction)

Commonly, such a patient will have both excessive alar base width and excessive nostril size/shape. In these circumstances, a combined internal–external alar base reduction can be employed. The two excision patterns are merely combined, resulting in a trapezoidal nostril sill resection plus a sliding alar flap. The top and bottom of this trapezoid may be made shorter or longer to modulate the relative amount of nostril reduction and alar base narrowing that is achieved. The remainder of the surgical steps are then identical to those described above.

IV. Excessive Alar Flare (Alar Flare Reduction)

Alar flare is addressed after the nostril and alar base widths have been set into their final positions. When the ala is excessively flared, a crescentic wedge of skin and soft tissue from the lateral aspect of the ala just above the alar-facial groove is excised (Fig. 21.12). The amount of excision is best judged by simply grasping the cut end of the ala and pulling it caudally. The amount of excision that corresponds to the improvement of alar flare is then noted and excised with the no. 11 blade. If too large a wedge is removed, the ala may become overly straight and unnatural in appearance. If a sliding alar flap had been performed in a previous step, it is prudent to close the medial nostril sill incision prior to excising the crescentic alar wedge. The crescentic wedge resection can also be carried out independently, in the absence of an alar base reduction procedure, for isolated alar flare. Meticulous wound closure is carried out with interrupted 5-0 nylon sutures, as described above.

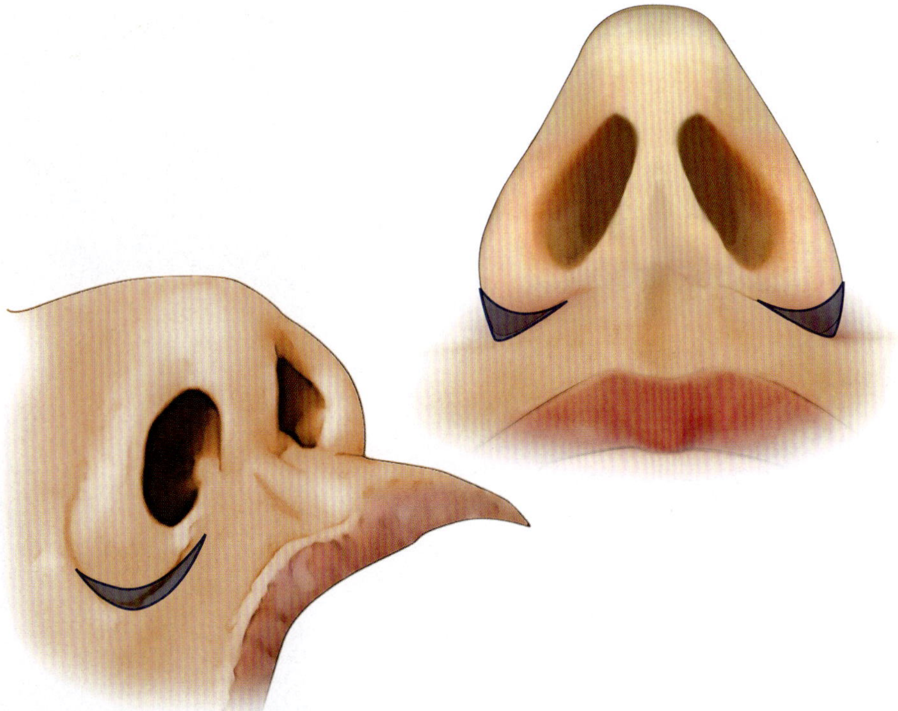

FIGURE 21.12 Alar flare reduction with wedge excision.

V. Alar Hooding (Alar Hooding Reduction)

Nostril size, alar base width, and alar flare are dependent variables, meaning that manipulating one factor may have an impact on the other. Alar hooding on the other hand is independent of these entities, so its assessment is left to the final step. As described above, excessive alar hooding occurs when the alar rim is less than 1 mm above the nostril meridian, with resultant obscuring of the columella on lateral view (Fig. 21.13). This is often of insufficient cosmetic impact to warrant correction, and the surgeon should weigh the possibility of a visible scar on the alar rim against the relative improvement that may be achieved through surgical excision. If excision is decided upon, the visual border of the ideal alar curve is marked. A corresponding ellipse is then defined on the inner portion of the ala that curves gently to avoid distortion of the alar border. Following excision, the wound is closed with interrupted 6-0 nylon suture along the most caudal aspect of the ala. The suture line falls along the visual border with this technique and scarring has been satisfactory.

POSTOPERATIVE MANAGEMENT

The patient is instructed to apply antibiotic ointment to the wound three times daily, starting immediately after the procedure. Patients are given hydrogen peroxide solution and instructed to clean any crusts forming around the sutures. Patients are seen on postoperative day no. 1 and incisions are inspected, crusts gently debrided and antibiotic ointment reapplied. Typically, sutures are removed on postoperative day seven. During suture removal, any epidermal debris in the suture holes is gently teased away with a fine forceps to avoid suture marks.

COMPLICATIONS

Broadly speaking, the complications specific to alar base surgery can be categorized as notching, scarring, asymmetry, and deformity. In general, notching of the alar rim or nostril is the most common complication in Weir-style excision techniques. However, with excisions confined to the sill, as in the sliding alar flap technique, notching is not seen along the alar rim or nostril. Notching at the sill incision may occur. Fortunately, since the sill incision is planned at the natural shadow where the sill meets the nostril, even a significant notch is of little cosmetic consequence. When it is visible, it is usually a result of poor incision placement or excessive wound tension. If excess wound tension is suspected upon closure, consider mobilization of the wound edges

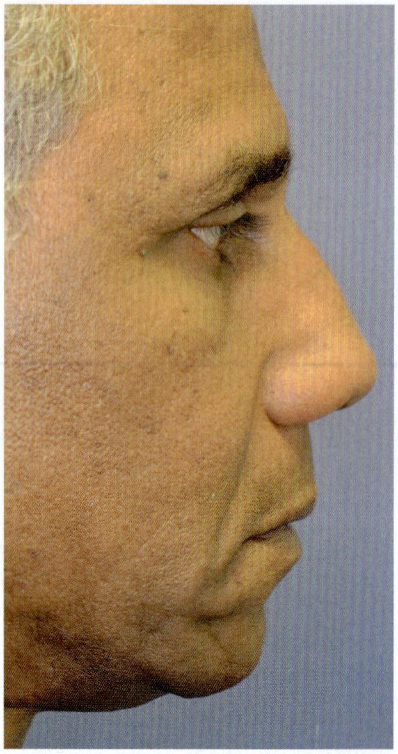

FIGURE 21.13
Patient with alar hooding.

and placement of a deep absorbable suture. Repair of this complication may require resection of the notched area with remobilization of the sliding alar flap and a more meticulous closure.

Abnormal scarring, including prominent, wide, or uneven scars, can be a significant esthetic problem. Usually, this is due to poor intraoperative eversion of skin edges or very sebaceous skin that holds sutures poorly. For irregular, conspicuous scars, dermabrasion may be considered 3 to 6 weeks postoperatively in the appropriate patient. Hyperpigmentation is a particularly challenging problem. Fortunately, when the incisions are placed in natural shadows of the alar creases, this problem may not become esthetically important. If it is, then topical lightening creams such as hydroquinone 4% can be beneficial.

A variety of deformities of the nasal base can occur as a consequence of surgery: Q deformity, tent pole deformity, and bowling pin deformity. The "Q deformity" (also known as a "teardrop deformity") occurs when a through-and-through resection of a segment of the lateral alar wall is performed at the alar-facial junction. The resultant deformity, where the scar is the "tail" of the Q-shape, is a telltale sign of alar base surgery, which can be obvious to others and is exceedingly difficult to correct (Fig. 21.14). Prevention is key, giving rise to the phrase "preserve the curve," as described above. "Tent pole deformity" can be a result of excessive alar flare reduction or overprojection of the tip, resulting in abnormally straight alae, with loss of the natural curvature of the alar-facial junction. Again, conservative resection in this area is preventative. Deprojection can be attempted to help reduce the tent pole effect. Finally, the "bowling pin deformity" refers to a postoperative alar axis that is directed inferiorly and medially. This tends to occur in patients with a preoperative vertical nostril axis who undergo nasal base narrowing, resulting in a pinched alar base appearance. Accurate preoperative evaluation is

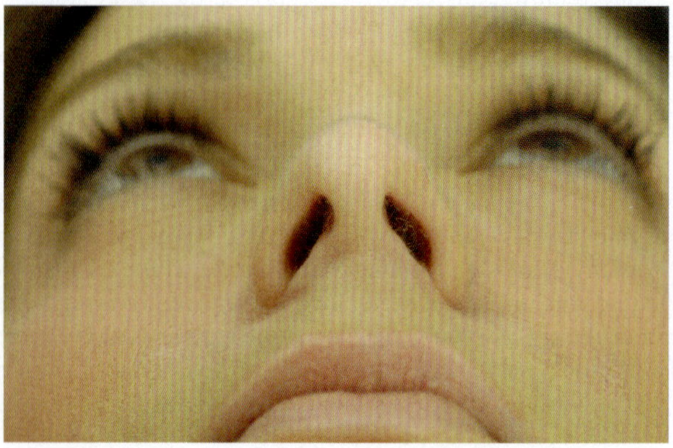

FIGURE 21.14
Postoperative base view following alar base reduction by another surgeon. Obvious stigmata of full-thickness lateral alar wall resection with resultant "Q" deformity and straightened lateral ala.

TABLE 21.2 Complications in Alar Base Modification

Complication	Etiology	Management
Alar rim/nostril notching	Poor incision placement Excessive wound closure tension Resection of deep muscle layer	"Preserve the curve" (e.g., alar incision above alar-facial groove) Tension-free wound closure with edge eversion Resect skin and subcutaneous tissue only
Abnormal scarring	Poor incision placement Excessive wound closure tension Imprecise wound edge approximation	"Preserve the curve" Tension-free wound closure with edge eversion Dermabrasion Scar excision and reapproximation
Asymmetry	Congenital asymmetry Unequal resection	Careful measurement with calipers
Nostril stenosis	Excessive sill reduction or alar base narrowing	Conservative resection Nostril stenosis repair
Q-deformity (aka teardrop deformity)	Through-and-through resection of ala at alar-facial junction	"Preserve the curve" Precise wound closure
Tent pole deformity	Excess alar flare reduction Overprojection of tip	Conservative alar flare reduction Deprojection of tip
Bowling pin deformity	Nasal base narrowing on a vertically oriented nostril axis	Careful preoperative planning Alar base widening procedure

important to anticipate this unfavorable outcome. Repair of this deformity would require widening of the alar base, possibly with the aid of a composite graft to the nostril sill.

In summary, as with any surgical complication, prevention is the best approach to management (see Table 21.2). Deformity in the nasal base region is exceedingly difficult to repair. Alar base modification is a surgery of millimeters where planning and precision are pivotal to achieving success.

RESULTS

In 2005, Kridel and Castellano published their 20-year experience of alar base reduction in 124 patients. They found their techniques to be effective, though 25% of patients did require dermabrasion for improvement of their scars. Adamson and colleagues examined their outcomes in 100 patients who underwent alar base reduction and they also found that excellent scar outcomes could be achieved.

Bennett and Constantinides evaluated the long-term effects of alar base reduction and found that vertical flare and nostril height were the only significant long-term differences seen in patients who required alar reduction. No significant changes were seen in alar base width, flare width, or base height. Proposed explanations for this unpredictability included (i) that the preceding deprojection rhinoplasty diminished the effect of the alar base modification, and without reduction, postoperative flare would have been excessive; (ii) that the alar base surgery was overly conservative; and (iii) that the flare was initially reduced but stretched back to a more flared position during wound healing.

PEARLS

- Four issues can be addressed with alar base modifications: wide, asymmetric, or horizontally oriented nostrils; wide alar base; alar flare; excessive alar hooding.
- Alar base modification should be performed as the final step of rhinoplasty.
- Meticulous, tension-free wound closure is paramount.
- "Preserve the curve."
- Incisions into the lateral ala should be placed 0.5 to 1 mm above the alar-facial groove.
- Incisions in the nostril sill should be placed at the sill margin.
- If there is any doubt, defer alar base modification to a later date to allow for postoperative healing.

PITFALLS

- Be mindful that deprojection rhinoplasty may lead to alar flare.
- Avoid through-and-through resections of the ala, which distort the natural alar curvature.
- Be conservative with tissue resection.

INSTRUMENTS TO HAVE AVAILABLE

- Standard rhinoplasty set

ACKNOWLEDGMENT

The author would like to recognize Ashlin J. Alexander, MD, for his exceptional contributions to this chapter. His work in the writing, editing, and figure creation for this chapter is greatly appreciated, without which this chapter would not have been possible.

SUGGESTED READING

Adamson PA, Oakley S, Tropper GJ, et al. Analysis of alar base narrowing. *Am J Cosmet Surg* 1990;(7):239–243.

Bennett GH, Lessow A, Song P, et al. The long-term effects of alar base reduction. *Arch Facial Plast Surg* 2005;7(2):94–97.

Crumley RL. Aesthetics and surgery of the nasal base. *Facial Plast Surg* 1988;5(2):135–142.

Kridel RW, Castellano RD. A simplified approach to alar base reduction: a review of 124 patients over 20 years. *Arch Facial Plast Surg* 2005;7(2):81–93.

Warner JP, Chauhan N, Adamson PA. Alar soft-tissue techniques in rhinoplasty: algorithmic approach, quantifiable guidelines, and scar outcomes from a single surgeon experience. *Arch Facial Plast Surg* 2010;12(3):149–158.

22 PEDIATRIC RHINOPLASTY

Dirk Jan Menger

INTRODUCTION

Pediatric rhinoplasty remains a topic of controversy as the cartilaginous nasal septum is a dominant growth center of the nose. This concern arises from surgical interventions impairing the outgrowth of the nasal skeleton, leading to facial underdevelopment and progressive malformations. Specifically, resection or detachment of specific cartilaginous structures of the nasal skeleton carries the risk of growth disturbances of both the nose and maxilla. Therefore, rhinoplasty in children is fundamentally different from rhinoplasty in adults.

During the last decade, recommended techniques have become more conservative, with emphasis in tissue reorientation and augmentation rather than resection and reduction. In children, both external and endonasal approaches can be used to reallocate or reconstruct the nasal skeleton after trauma, infection, or in congenital deformities. Alternatively, these approaches can be used as a route to remove malignant or benign pathology.

Anatomy and Development of the Growing Nose

The nose of a baby is much smaller compared to an adult as it has a short nasal dorsum, less projection of the nasal tip and columella, rounder nostrils, and a large nasolabial angle. The overlying soft tissue envelope has a thick layer of subcutaneous adipose tissue, and the nasal skeleton of a newborn is mainly cartilaginous. The nasal septum initially develops due to the formation of new cartilage, but within the first postnatal year, an endochondral ossification process starts in the region of the anterior skull base. This is the beginning of the formation of the perpendicular plate. At a later stage, the perpendicular plate extends due to progressive ossification of nasal septal cartilage. Due to this ossification, most of the cartilaginous part of the nasal septum loses contact with the sphenoid. In adults, only a small remnant of septal cartilage, the so-called "sphenoid tail," can be found between the cartilaginous nasal septum and the sphenoid. It separates the perpendicular plate from the vomer. The formation of the vomer is the result of extracartilaginous ossification.

In females, nasal growth is completed earlier (16 to 18 years) than in males (18 to 20 years). There are two significant periods of nasal growth: during the first 2 years of life and puberty. The typical "baby face" disappears due to the more rapid and longer-lasting development of the nose, maxilla, and mandible in relation to the neurocranium. The cartilaginous nasal septum plays a crucial role in both nasal and midfacial growth. The nasal septum has two thicker areas with different mitotic activity and histologic maturation. These growth zones have a transverse diameter of approximately 3 mm, whereas the surrounding thinner cartilage is 0.4-mm thick. Both zones extend from the sphenoid. The "sphenodorsal" zone is located between the sphenoid and the nasal dorsum and appears to be primarily responsible for the normal increase in length and height of the nasal dorsum. The "sphenospinal" zone is located between the sphenoid and the anterior nasal spine and is the driving force in forward outgrowth of the premaxilla region. Experimental studies and clinical observations have shown that destruction of these zones during childhood result in underdevelopment of both the nose and the maxilla. The effect of destruction is age related with younger children developing more severe malformation compared to their older counterparts. A young child with complete destruction of the nasal septum will clinically appear with an underdeveloped nose displaying a saddle deformity, columellar retraction, overrotation of the nasal tip, and a retroposition of the midface. Destruction of these zones can be the result of trauma, nasal septal hematoma, or abscess. However, it is the dedicated interventions of the well-meaning surgeon that remain the primary concern. The goal of this chapter is to review the indications and goals for pediatric rhinoplasty and surgical guidelines to avoid growth disturbances and postoperative sequelae.

HISTORY

Rhinoplasty in children may be indicated due to trauma, infections, congenital features, or psychological or functional problems. Therefore, history and examination should be focused on the specific clinical picture. An accurate history and physical examination are mandatory for correct diagnosis and treatment; therefore, a good relationship with parents and child is essential. Esthetics and function should be evaluated separately. How does the nose look like on the outside? Does it cause problems, distress, or anxiety at school or in relation with other children or adults? Does the child breath well? How is the right side compared with the left side? Is it blocked continuously or intermittently? Does the impairment of nasal breathing interfere with the child's daily activities? Specifically in children, the age and length of the child are important and the question whether further outgrowth of the nose is to be expected. The medical history should also include the use of medication and any medication that can influence blood coagulation should be stopped prior to surgery.

PHYSICAL EXAMINATION

A standardized rhinoplasty protocol is essential for a successful outcome. This includes standardized preoperative documentation using an assessment and surgical rhinoplasty sheet. In most children, evaluation of the nasal airway can be performed using a headlight and a small nasal speculum. What is the condition of the nasal septum: is it in the midline or deviated? Does the septum provide sufficient support to the upper lateral cartilages and nasal tip? Is the external and internal nasal valve region open or blocked? Does the lateral side wall collapse during forced inspiration? What is the condition of the mucosa? Inhalation allergies should be tested in selected cases and when required treated with antihistamine and nasal corticosteroids. Is there evidence of nasal polyps or other mucosal abnormalities? Does the child have hypertrophy of the adenoids? Inspection of the nasal cavity and nasopharynx using an endoscope is essential in selected cases. Examination under general anesthesia might be required in some cases of recent trauma, hematoma, or abscess of the nasal septum or dorsum (Fig. 22.1). Standardized preoperative rhinoplasty photographs (frontal, oblique, lateral, basal and bird view) should always be performed and documented. Sometimes 3-D imaging or computer-simulated imaging might be helpful in the communication with the patient. Imaging, like magnetic resonance imaging (MRI) of the anterior skull base, is essential in the preoperative assessment of dermoid cysts. In all cases, a written informed consent with all possible side effects of the surgery and postoperative period should be given and signed by the patient's parents.

INDICATIONS

The goal of rhinoplasty in children is to restore the anatomy and function or to promote normal development and outgrowth of the nose. For every indication, the expected benefits of intervention should be weighed against the possible adverse outcomes on nasal and midfacial growth. Ideally, surgery should be postponed until after the pubertal growth spurt. However, there are distinct indications for immediate intervention. Apart from tumors like malignancies, these indications include destruction of the nasal skeleton due to nasal septal abscess or severe nasal trauma. In these cases, the skeleton should be reconstructed in order to avoid inhibition of growth due to

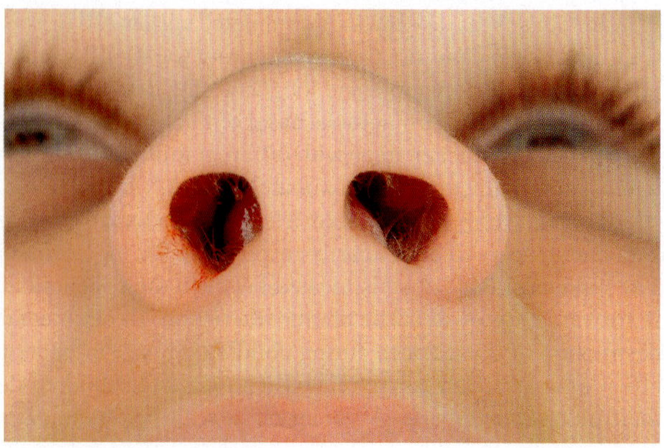

FIGURE 22.1
Nasal septal hematoma. Note the swollen septum in the right and left nasal vestibule, 1 week after nasal trauma.

destruction of the nasal septal growth centers. Other indications for immediate surgical intervention are severely impaired nasal breathing and nasal deformity causing psychological problems. A nasal deformity presents a serious psychosocial challenge to children; they have to cope with an appearance that is different that cannot be concealed and is subject to social stigma. The increasing use of facial plastic surgery in a culture that is focused on appearance heightens the pressure on those who look different. Patients with facial disfigurement or severe nasal deformities often report increased social anxiety, feelings of low self-esteem and self-worth, and depression. The degree of deformity, however, does not show a linear correlation with the degree of experienced distress. From a psychological point of view, similar to, for example, otoplasty, the ideal timing of surgery is at preschool ages in which children do not note the deformity. The decision to perform rhinoplasty, however, depends on the degree of the deformity, the psychological effect on the child, and the impact on nasal growth and development.

CONTRAINDICATIONS

In general, rhinoplasty for esthetic features without functional or psychological complaints should be avoided in children. There are two reasons for this. First, as mentioned before, surgery can induce disturbances of the normal development and outgrowth of the nasal skeleton. For example, resection of a basal strip (sphenospinal zone) from the nasal septum will disturb the development of the anterior nasal spine and the maxilla. For example, separating the upper lateral cartilages from the nasal septum before the puberty growth spurt can induce a hump-like deformity as the septum will grow anterior the upper lateral cartilage. Secondly, children are not yet able to decide emotionally whether a certain physical condition, for example, a minor hump deformation, should be corrected surgically or not. Special attention should be focused on parents who try to advocate and persuade the surgeon to perform surgery on their child. These parents believe that they support their child by exaggerating functional and psychological complaints accompanying the esthetic deformation. In those cases, it is important to educate and explain to the parents and the child how the nose develops and grows and what sequels can occur postoperatively when rhinoplasty is carried out before full maturation of the nose and midface. Sometimes, it is to be advocated to evaluate the condition at certain regular intervals like 12 months. If the functional, esthetic, or psychological situation changes, surgical intervention might be reconsidered.

PREOPERATIVE PLANNING

Patients and parents should be informed that long-term results cannot be predicted and the need for revision surgery at a later stage should be discussed. For this reason, both patient and parents should also be informed about continuing follow-up until after the adolescent growth spurt. Similar to rhinoplasty in adults, standardized preoperative and postoperative photography should be performed. A standardized assessment and operation form are recommended for meticulous assessment and documentation of the preoperative anatomical condition and the clinical findings during surgery. The risk of inhibition of nasal growth and development is lower when surgical technique conforms to the following guidelines for rhinoplasty in the pediatric age group.

SURGICAL TECHNIQUE

The child is brought into slight reverse Trendelenburg position as this position reduces bleeding. Surgery is usually performed under general anesthesia in combination with a local infiltration anesthetic and topical application of cocaine in order to promote vasoconstriction and to prevent bleeding. The local anesthetic should be given at least 10 minutes before starting surgery.

Guidelines for Pediatric Rhinoplasty

Based on clinical observations, experimental data of surgical procedures, and knowledge of the anatomical development of the nose, "conservative" guidelines can be given in order to avoid disturbances of the normal outgrowth and development of the nose.

Elevation of the mucoperichondrium of the nasal septum or elevation of the soft tissue envelope from the rest of the nasal skeleton can be performed safely if the skeleton is left intact. Several approaches, including endonasal approaches and the open approach through a transcolumellar incision, can be used, though cartilage-splitting techniques should be avoided. Due to the small dimensions of the nose and nostril size of children, the open approach often provides optimal visualization of the deformities and excellent exposure for reconstruction. Elevation and tunneling of the mucosa on one or both sides do not interfere with normal development of the nose. Be aware, however, when elevating the mucosa from the nasal floor not to damage the incisive nerves. After the septal mucosa is elevated and the cartilaginous and bony septum is exposed, be conservative with incisions, scoring, and chondrotomies of the cartilaginous septum and with disruption of the bony septum. Avoid incisions or excisions of the growth zones. For the sphenodorsal zone, this will result in growth inhibition of the nasal dorsum, causing a low and broad middle nasal vault. Incisions or excisions of the sphenospinal zone will result in underdevelopment of the nasal spine and the maxilla. Incisions or scoring of deviated areas of cartilage do not achieve predictable results and thus should be avoided as well. Incisions or excisions of the thinner, central part of the cartilaginous nasal septum do not inhibit growth of the septum. Chondrotomies, such as a posterior chondrotomy, in which the cartilaginous septum is separated from the perpendicular plate, should also be avoided because this will inhibit further growth of the nasal septum. The connection between the cartilaginous septum to the premaxilla, the septospinal ligament, should not be transected as it anchors the septum in the midline and plays a role in the forward outgrowth of the maxilla. Deviations of the premaxilla and vomer can be mobilized and realigned or removed without disturbing the normal outgrowth of the nose.

In the case of nasal trauma, defects and fractures of the septum should be identified. Mobilize deviated or overlapping fragments of cartilage and adjust form and size of the fragments in order to reconstruct a straight septum in the midline. Polydioxanone (PDS) plate (0.15 mm) may be used as a temporary resorbable carrier to support and stabilize the fragments or where the septum needs support. For defects that cannot be reconstructed with septal cartilage, autologous cartilage from the auricle or rib should be used. Homologous or other biomaterials are not capable of growth and may induce growth inhibition when implanted in the growing septum. Leftover cartilage should be crushed gently and placed back into cartilaginous septal defects to allow restrengthening and to avoid a septal perforation. The formation of a hematoma between the septum and the mucoperichondrium should be avoided by using mattress sutures to ensure good tissue approximation to avoid a potential space.

Osteotomies of the bony pyramid can be performed without inhibition of growth. Alar base wedge resections, repositioning and augmentation as used in the cleft lip patient, will not interfere with nasal growth and development. Avoid separating the upper lateral cartilages from the nasal septum; this bears the risk of outgrowth of the septum anterior to the upper laterals resulting in irregularities of the nasal dorsum. Disturbing the T-bar structure of the cartilaginous vault, as in hump reduction and the use of spreader grafts, should therefore be postponed until after the pubertal growth spurt. The use of nasal grafts, other than in the reconstruction of the growing nasal septum, may lead to unpredictable results.

Dermoid Cyst

Dermoid cysts are slow-growing masses that may contain skin, hair follicles, or sweat or sebaceous glands. Dermoid cysts may become infected or drain through a sinus opening. The origin of nasal dermoid cysts may be the result of faulty closure of the fonticulus frontalis, which permits dermal elements to invaginate between the developing nasal bones and cartilage. Alternatively, they may be the result of dura that remains in the prenasal space instead of being retracted through the foramen cecum. The lesions can be localized on the nasal dorsum anywhere along the midline from the nasal tip to the glabella, in the nasal septum or intracranial. In all cases, they can be attached to the central nervous system (CNS) by a fibrous stalk. Therefore, imaging with computed tomography (CT) and/or MRI should be performed prior to surgery to rule out defects of the anterior skull base or CNS connections (Fig. 22.2). An external approach rhinoplasty provides a wide exposure for excision of the

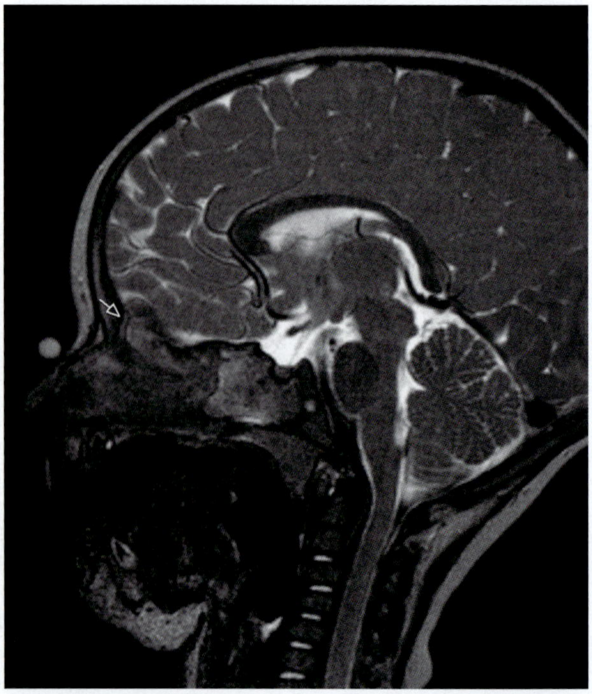

FIGURE 22.2
MRI scan, T2 sagittal plane. Opening of sinus tract at the nasal dorsum (*marker*) with extension intracranial through the foramen cecum (*arrow*).

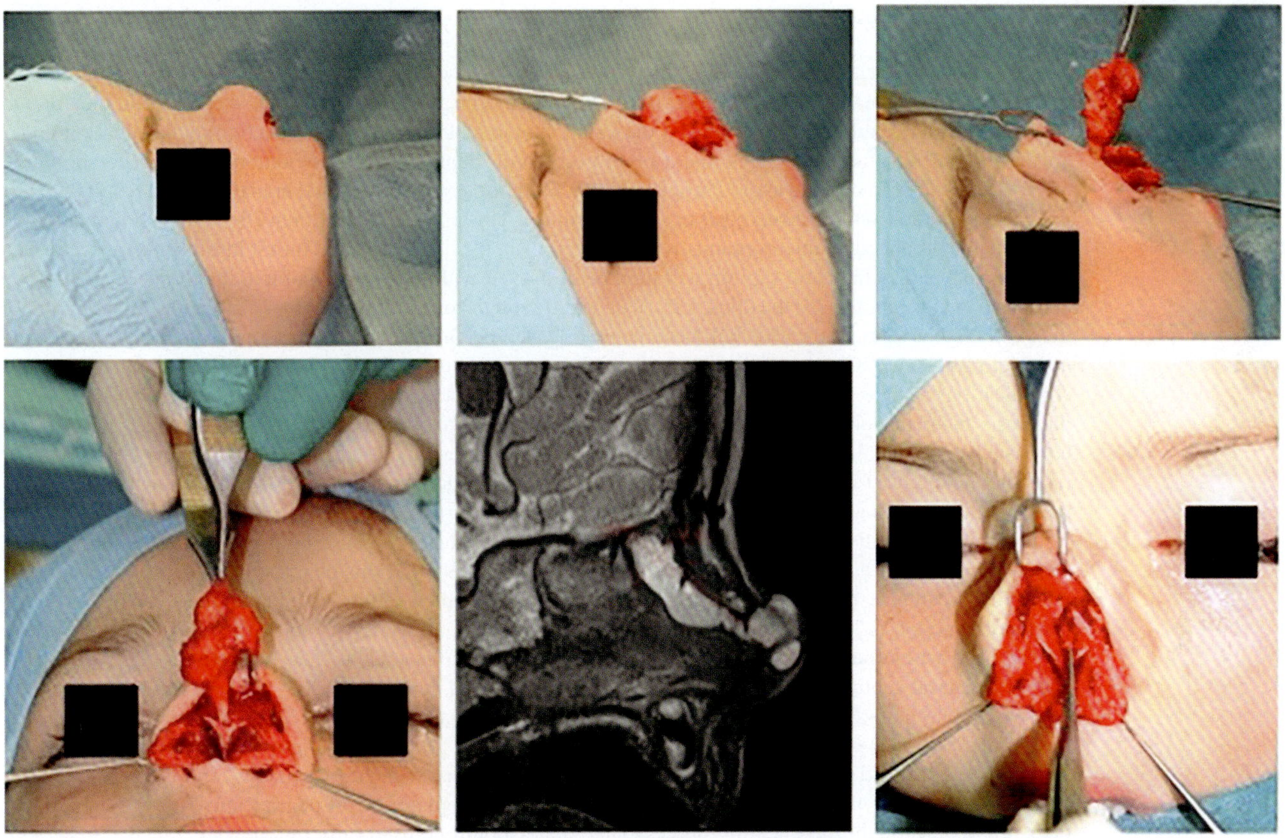

FIGURE 22.3 Intraoperative views of an external approach rhinoplasty. The nasal tip is bulbous due to a large dermoid cyst. The cyst is attached to the anterior skull base through a tunnel in the cartilaginous nasal septum but has no connections to the CNS.

tract, which may be required as far as the anterior skull base (Fig. 22.3). Open approach rhinoplasty through a broken transcolumellar incision gives a superior cosmetic result compared with skin incisions such as paracanthal incisions over the dorsum of the nose, without compromising the recurrence rate (Fig. 22.4). Surgical excision prevents expansion, infection, and destruction of adjacent tissues. In order to avoid recurrence, it is important to leave no remnants; the use of methylene blue might be helpful to follow the tract. The nasal skeleton should be left intact so that no growth disturbance is to be expected.

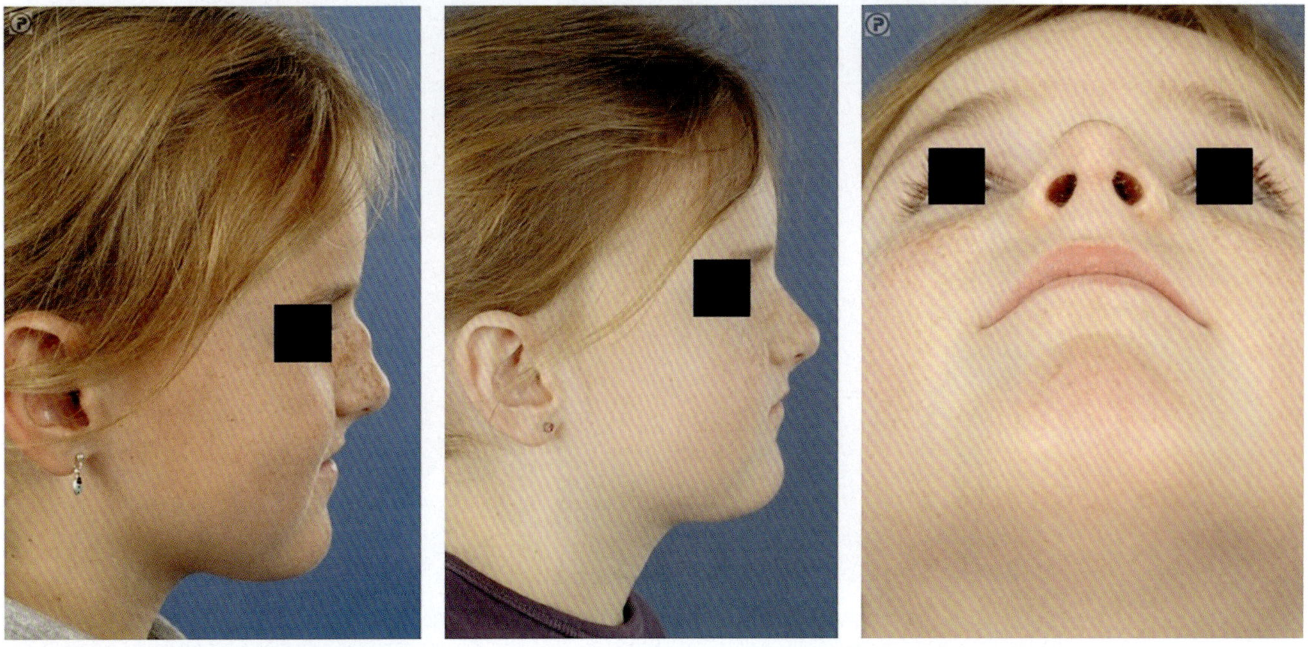

FIGURE 22.4 Pre- and postoperative lateral view of a girl with a dermoid cyst of the nasal dorsum. On the *right* side, the postoperative basal view shows the broken columellar incision, which is hardly visible.

Nasal Trauma, Hematoma, and Abscess

Trauma of the nose can result in dislocation or fractures of the cartilaginous and bony skeleton or in the formation of a hematoma or abscess (Fig. 22.1). In small children, an accurate diagnosis can be complex due to edema of the surrounding soft tissues and the small anatomical dimensions. Inspection and evaluation under general anesthesia after a few days might be more helpful. Septal or dorsal hematomas, however, should be ruled out promptly in order to avoid iatrogenic delay. Without treatment, a septal hematoma will result in insufficient oxygenation and sterile necrosis of septal cartilage. This process can be intensified due to liquefaction by collagenases produced by microorganisms that contaminate the hematoma and turn it into a septal abscess. The cartilaginous part of the nasal septum will then be destroyed within a few days. First, the thinner parts will be destroyed but eventually also the thicker areas or septal growth zones. Without proper surgical reconstruction of the cartilaginous septum, the nose will become underdeveloped including overrotation of the nasal tip, a saddle nose deformity and retraction of the columella with a retroposition of the midface (Fig. 22.5). Life-threatening complications such as cavernous sinus thrombosis or brain abscess are rare and often associated with delayed diagnosis and management. A dorsal hematoma can be diagnosed as a swollen bluish hue at the site of the internal nasal valve, cephalic to the lower lateral cartilages. Both a dorsal and septal hematoma should be evacuated (aspirated or drained) as soon as possible. It is recommended to do this under general anesthesia and to evaluate the condition of the nasal septum carefully.

After opening the submucosal space, cultures should be taken for microbiologic examination, and the abscess should be drained and cleaned using soaks of saline 0.9%. At this phase, the diameter of absent septal cartilage can be estimated to ensure total reconstruction of the septum. If the amount of cartilage needed for reconstruction is large, costal cartilage can be harvested on the right side. Auricular conchal cartilage can be used when the quantity needed is less than one auricular concha. The next step is the reconstruction of the nasal septum. The cartilage grafts can be stabilized and fixed (using polyglactin 4-0 sutures) on polydioxanone plate (0.15 × 50 × 40 mm; Ethicon, Norderstedt, Germany). This thin but strong material ensures good tissue to tissue approximation of the cartilage grafts in a single large implant (Fig. 22.6). This implant is positioned precisely between the vomer, the upper lateral cartilages, and the perpendicular plate or remnants of the cartilaginous septum. Polydioxanone plate or foil degrades in 10 to 25 weeks and does not disturb the normal healing process. The plate should be used only on one side, since if placed on both sides, it may lead to insufficient oxygenation of the cartilage grafts. Furthermore, the mucosal lining should be intact; PDS should not be exposed to the nasal cavity. Studies have shown that this material has a positive effect on the regeneration of septal cartilage in a rabbit model and in the regeneration of bone in the reconstruction of orbital defects. The next step is to fixate the implant with the use of soluble mattress sutures. An internal nose dressing should be applied for 1 or 2 days. Systemic broad-spectrum antibiotics

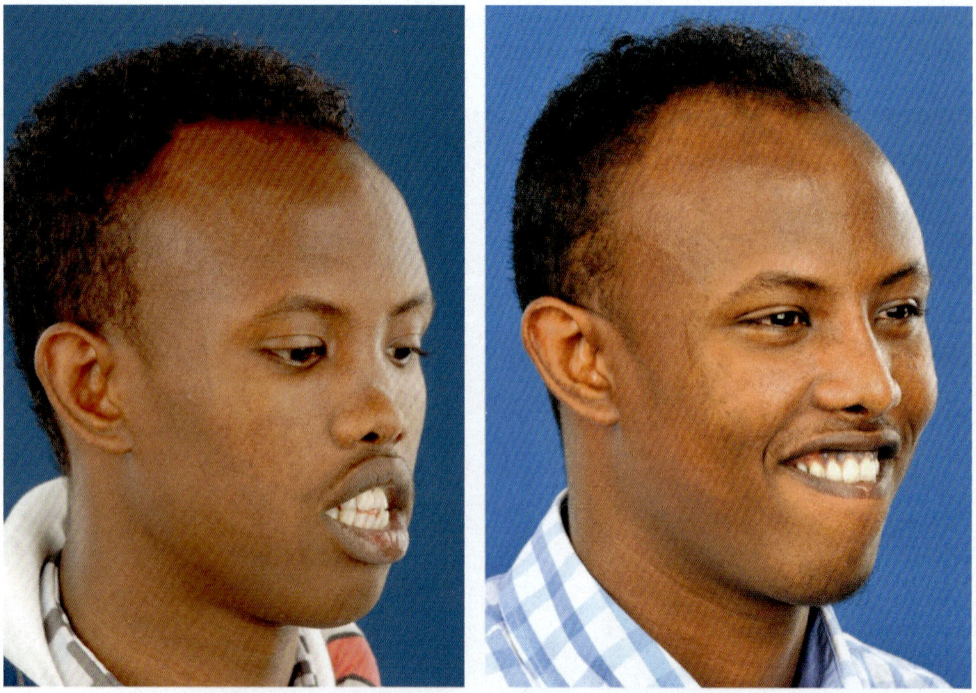

FIGURE 22.5 Pre- and postoperative photos of a male patient. Severe underdevelopment of the nose due to destruction of the nasal septum at childhood after a nasal septal abscess. The nose was reconstructed with the use of rib grafts, a dorsal onlay attached to a columellar strut graft and reconstruction of the nasal septum.

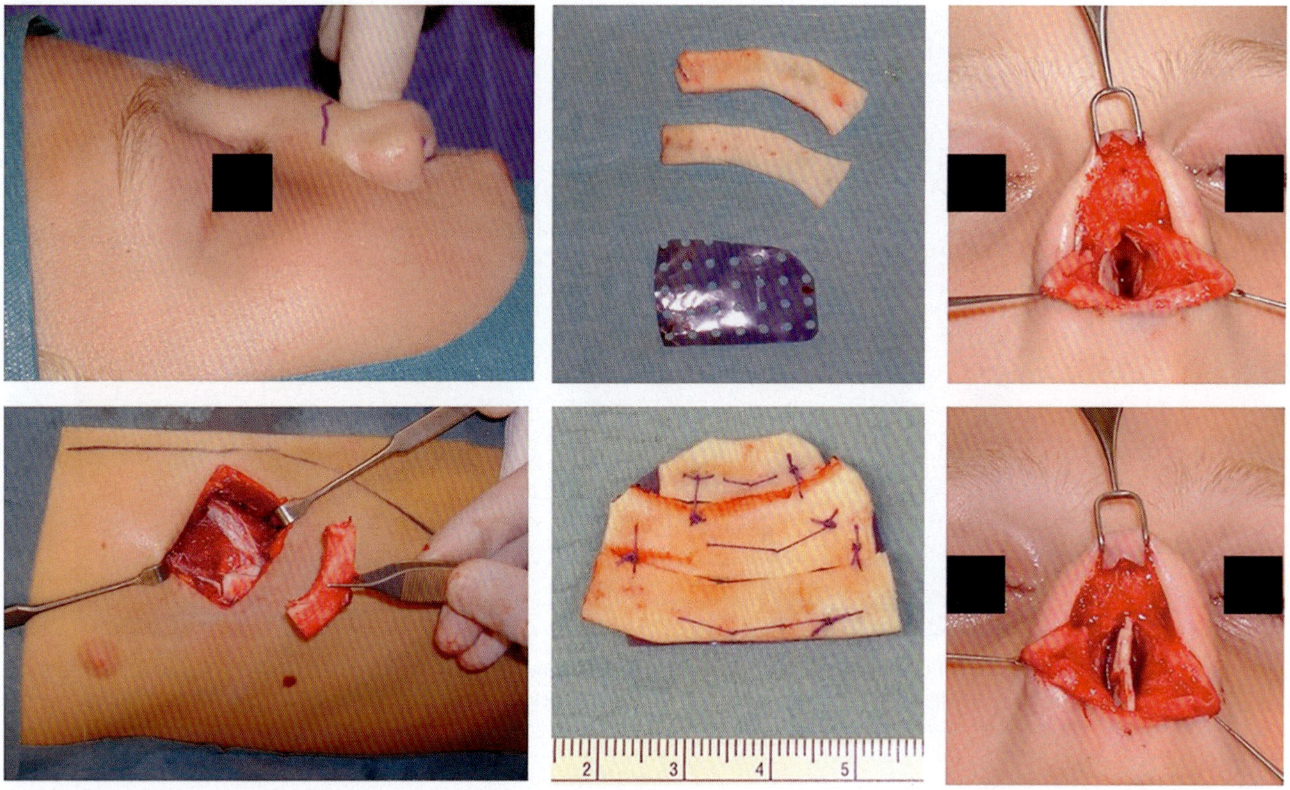

FIGURE 22.6 Perioperative view of an 11-year-old boy with complete destruction of the cartilaginous nasal septum. Costal cartilage of the seventh rib was harvested to reconstruct the cartilaginous septum, which was absent. Two-millimeter sections of rib cartilage affixed to polydioxanone foil with polyglactin 4-0 soluble sutures. The polydioxanone plate was exactly the same shape as the absent septum. To avoid warping the graft, only the central part of the rib was used after removal of the outer layers, which have a greater tendency to warp. The rib implant on polydioxanone plate was positioned between the perpendicular plate, the vomer, and the upper lateral cartilages and was fixated between the mucoperichondrium layers with polyglactin 4-0 mattress sutures.

(a combination of amoxicillin [50 mg/kg] and clavulanic acid [5 mg/kg], every 6 hours) are administered during 7 days. Depending on culture results, the antibiotic regimen is changed if necessary. Clinical observations have shown that this technique showed normal nasal development during follow-up, without expected esthetic problems (Fig. 22.7).

In a case in which the nasal skeleton is fractured or dislocated, examination and surgical intervention should take place under general anesthesia (Fig. 22.8). Mild fractures, with minimal or no dislocation of the nasal framework and without breathing disorders, can be treated conservative. As mentioned in the guidelines for pediatric rhinoplasty, repositioning and reallocation of fractures of the nasal bones can be carried out without disturbing the normal development of the nose. In the acute phase, this can be achieved by mobilizing the bones manually. In older fractures, osteotomies should be carried out, as is done in adult patients. Fractures of the cartilaginous nasal septum, however, should be realigned to improve nasal breathing and in order to prevent progression of deviation when the nose grows and develops. However, this can be difficult especially in older or healed fracture lines. In those cases, the fracture lines can be incised fully to release the stresses and strains; realignment can then be carried out with PDS plate. The foil is placed on one side of the septum, and the cartilage fragments are sutured to the plate in a straight fashion. As mentioned throughout the chapter, resection of cartilage should not be performed as the growth zones should not be interrupted in order to avoid underdevelopment of the nose. Sometimes, a cartilaginous deviation can be mobilized by moving the nasal dorsum upward thereby elevating the nasal septum in the midline.

Impaired Nasal Breathing

Impaired nasal breathing in childhood may be the result of severe septal deviations. Other causes must be ruled out before surgical intervention of the nasal septum is considered, for example, choanal atresia, benign or malignant tumors of the nose or nasopharynx, juvenile nasal polyposis, allergy, or hypertrophy of the adenoid. Decongestion of the nasal mucosa, nasal endoscopy, and imaging might be mandatory for correct assessment and diagnosis. Severe septal deviations are likely to worsen with growth and may cause progressive distortion

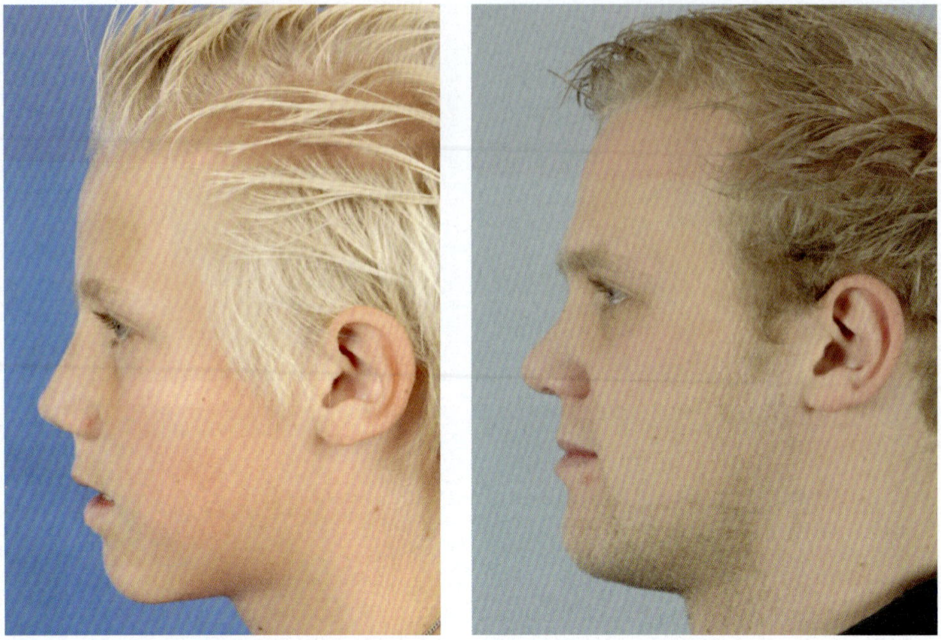

FIGURE 22.7 Pre- and postoperative photos of the patient shown in Figure 22.6. Before surgery, the patient was 11 years old; the postoperative picture shows the patient at the age of 19 years, after his puberty growth spurt. The nose shows a normal development; there are no signs of a saddle nose deformity.

and inhibition of growth of the nose and midface. Septoplasty restores the anatomy and function and may promote normal development and outgrowth of the nose. However, septoplasty may also cause growth inhibition. This dilemma should be weighed and discussed with the patient and parents. In case of less evident deformities, close monitoring might be a good alternative. Follow-up will give the opportunity to evaluate the development of the nose and the functional complaints of the child. If the decision for surgical intervention is made, it should be conservative according to the guidelines in this chapter. Particularly, in younger children, the external approach might be helpful since the small nostrils may diminish the visualization of the operative field in endonasal approaches.

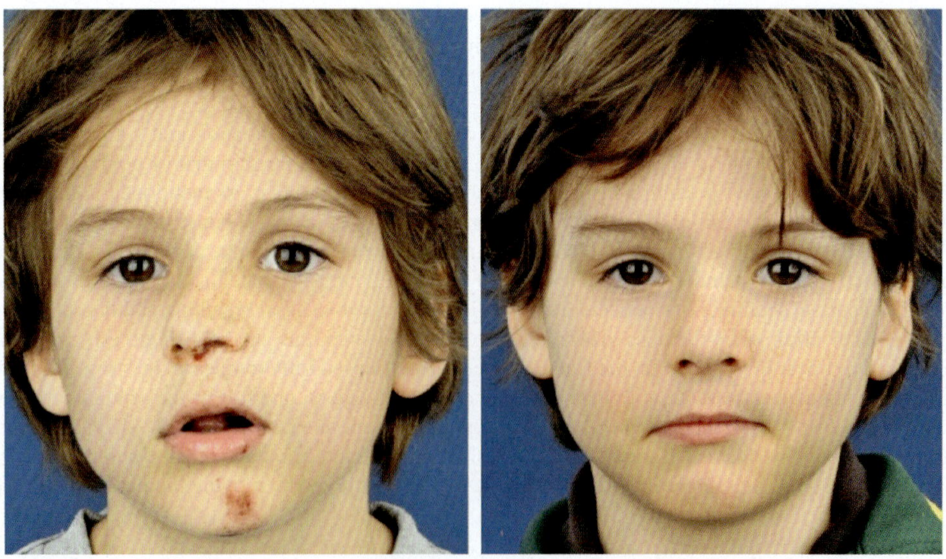

FIGURE 22.8 Pre- and postoperative view of severe nasal trauma. The nose was realigned under a general anesthesia without resections or incisions in the cartilaginous framework but with the use of PDS plate, in order to promote a normal development of the nose.

POSTOPERATIVE MANAGEMENT

Newborns and young children are habitual nose breathers; packing of the nose should therefore be avoided. Instead of packing, mattress sutures through the nasal septum can be used as they prevent potential space and the formation of a hematoma. In the postoperative management of nasal trauma of the bony pyramid, a small nasal splint may be applied for 1 week. In open approach rhinoplasty, the columellar incision can be closed using thin absorbable sutures (e.g., 7-0 Vicryl) so they don't have to be removed. Systemic broad-spectrum antibiotics for 7 days (e.g., amoxicillin/clavulanic acid: 50/5 mg/kg, every 6 hours) are recommended in children with a septal or dorsal hematoma or abscess. Depending on the culture results, the antibiotic regimen should be changed if necessary. Follow-up should be prolonged until after the pubertal growth spurt. A routine examination, including photography, should be performed at least annually to evaluate the development of the nose. A calibrated scale should be held in position on the lateral view to make accurate measurements of nasal growth.

COMPLICATIONS

Complications of pediatric rhinoplasty should be avoided. Epistaxis and hematoma formation of the nasal septum in particular can induce destruction of septal cartilage and should be prevented with the use of mattress sutures and adequate nasal packing. The use of soluble packing is to be recommended since non-soluble packings need to be removed under a general anesthesia in most pediatric patients. Postoperative infection too can cause serious complications of the cartilaginous nasal septum. Therefore, the use of antibiotics in the peri- and postoperative phase is advocated, especially after reconstruction of the nasal septum in children with a septal hematoma or abscess. Despite adequate surgical intervention and following the guidelines for rhinoplasty in pediatric patients, long-term follow-up until after the puberty growth spurt is essential to evaluate the development of the nose. In some cases, it might be needed to perform (minor) revision surgery.

RESULTS

With the described surgical techniques for pediatric rhinoplasty in this chapter, results are predictable and stable for a satisfying long-term postoperative result. When the septal growth zones are destroyed or resected in childhood, underdevelopment and disfigurement of the nose is to be expected. Studies and clinical observations of children who underwent reconstruction of the nasal septum with autogenous cartilage grafts have shown a normal outgrowth and development of the nose.

PEARLS

- The cartilaginous nasal septum is the driving force of nasal and midfacial growth.
- Educate the patient and parents regarding nasal growth and development and the goals of surgery.
- In pediatric rhinoplasty, follow-up is necessary until after the pubertal growth spurt.
- Follow the guidelines for pediatric rhinoplasty in this chapter to avoid growth inhibition and postoperative sequels.

PITFALLS

- Surgical techniques that are considered to be safe in adults might have a negative effect on the outgrowth and development of the nasal skeleton and midface in children.
- Resection and incisions in the cartilaginous septum in childhood will result in underdevelopment and disfiguration of the nose.

INSTRUMENTS TO HAVE AVAILABLE

For meticulous dissection and reconstruction of the nose in children, the use of special rhinoplasty instruments is to be recommended (Karl Storz rhinoplasty instruments designed by Prof. Gilbert Nolst Trenité).

SUGGESTED READING

Bradbury E. Meeting the psychological needs of patients with facial disfigurement. *Br J Oral Maxillofac Surg* 2012;50(3):193–196. doi:10.1016/j.bjoms.2010.11.022.

Dennis SCR, den Herder C, Shandilya M, et al. Open rhinoplasty in children. *Facial Plast Surg* 2007;23(4):259–266.

Menger DJ, Tabink I, Nolst Trenite GJ. Nasal septal abscess in children, reconstruction with autologous cartilage grafts on polydioxanone plate. *Arch Otolaryngol Head Neck Surg* 2008;134(8):1–6.

Menger DJ, Tabink I, Nolst Trenite GJ. Treatment of septal hematomas and abscesses in children. *Facial Plast Surg* 2007;23:239–243.

Nolst Trenite GJ. Cleft lip rhinoplasty. In: Nolst Trenite GJ, ed. *Rhinoplasty*, 3rd ed. The Hague, The Netherlands: Kugler Publications, 2005:31–37, Chapter XX.

Nolst Trenite GJ. Postoperative care and complications. In: Nolst Trenite GJ, ed. *Rhinoplasty*, 3rd ed. The Hague, The Netherlands: Kugler Publications, 2005:31–37, Chapter 5.

Shandilya M, Den Herder C, Dennis SCR, et al. Pediatric rhinoplasty in an academic setting. *Facial Plast Surg* 2007;23(4):245–257.

Sykes JM, Jang YJ. Cleft lip rhinoplasty. *Facial Plast Surg Clin North Am* 2009;17:133–144.

Verwoerd CDA, Verwoerd-Verhoef HL. Rhinosurgery in children: basic concepts. *Facial Plast Surg* 2007;23:219–230.

Verwoerd CDA, Verwoerd-Verhoef HL. Rhinosurgery in children, developmental and surgical aspects. In: Nolst Trenite GJ, ed. *Rhinoplasty*, 3rd ed. The Hague, The Netherlands: Kluger Publications, 2005.

23 RHINOPLASTY: ENDONASAL STRATEGIES

Pietro Palma

INTRODUCTION

Rhinoplasty occupies a central and privileged position in contemporary facial plastic surgery. Alongside the desire for physical self-improvement, the demand for rhinoplasty in particular has grown over the past few decades to such an extent that it may now be considered the most important facial plastic operation. However, concomitant with its development and expansion, rhinoplasty has also faced major hurdles. The public is now better informed about the possible risks and pitfalls of surgery, and armed with information from the Internet, they are ready to challenge the rhinoplasty surgeon at every step with incremental levels of expectation. Rhinoplasty has now become a minefield for the novice surgeon due to increasing malpractice premiums and risks of legal action against the surgeon. This makes it absolutely critical for surgeons to be sufficiently trained in rhinoplasty before embarking on a career marked by frequent technical limitations and negative encounters with patients.

This chapter aims to lay the foundation for surgeons who seek to master the endonasal approach for dealing with both "standard" and challenging rhinoplasty patients. As the older and more rigid classification of rhinoplasty into external and endonasal has lost its luster, the reader is encouraged to think of rhinoplasty in terms of endonasal hybrid rhinoplasty, where the term "hybrid" implies the incorporation of anatomical concepts and sophisticated suturing–grafting techniques developed by "openers" into the theoretical and technical corpus of endonasal rhinoplasty. The end-result is a higher technical flexibility allowing a tailor-made procedure for each patient, while minimizing tissue trauma, unnecessary scarring, and tissue plane distortion. Technical evolution has made endonasal hybrid rhinoplasty a technical option even for the most challenging patients in both the primary and revision surgery.

HISTORY

The first encounter with the patient is the most important step in a journey that may take several months or years to reach its conclusion. The astute surgeon will have read the letter of referral and familiarized him- or herself with the important features before the patient enters the examination room. Always allow patients adequate time to express their concerns and ultimate goals. A full rhinologic history, including airflow, rhinorrhea, post-nasal drip, sense of smell, facial pain, previous trauma or nasal surgery, allergy, asthma, and other allergies should be sought. The patient's past medical history may reveal significant factors such as past experiences with aesthetic surgery, an active or previous psychiatric limitation, and the use of anticoagulants, nonsteroidal anti-inflammatory agents, or herbal products. Patients may have a combination of aesthetic and functional problems, so the surgeon must make provision for medical therapy of nasal symptoms and be prepared for a combination of hybrid rhinoplasty and endoscopic sinus surgery. Additionally, with this in mind, a complete medical and surgical history are required for surgical clearance with considerations for anesthesia, such as cardiopulmonary clearance, as well as standard laboratory, pregnancy, and coagulation testing.

PHYSICAL EXAMINATION

A detailed physical examination provides the rhinoplasty surgeon with a wealth of information about the patient's anatomy, pathology, and coincidental findings. These should be summarized and form an integral part of the ultimate surgical strategy. Start with a general assessment of the patient's height, demeanor, and facial symmetry, both static and dynamic. Having made a general examination of the face, the surgeon inspects the nose while the patient sits quietly. The head is slightly flexed, and light is shone on the patient's face.

The general appearance of the external nose is evaluated regarding its size and shape, gross deformities such as scoliosis or deviations, deficiencies, condition of the skin, and the presence of scars. From this frontal view, observe the brow–dome lines. These lines not only constitute the critical landmark for symmetry of the bony–cartilaginous framework of the external pyramid but also may act as a preliminary guide to the presence of septal pathology.

Without moving the patient, observe the secondary landmarks for the assessment of symmetry. These include (a) the nose–cheek transition areas, (b) width of the dorsum, (c) scroll areas, (d) alar–columellar relationship, and (e) width of the alar base.

After the general inspection, it is advisable to examine the external nose in detail with respect for its unique anatomical components: the bony pyramid and cartilaginous pyramids, and the inferior third. The main goal consists of determining the extent and location of nasal asymmetries. Although varying degrees of asymmetry are the rule, their extent and distribution can detract from the beauty of the individual patient. From the frontal view, observe the patient's quiet respiration and specifically look for mouth-breathing, collapse or flaring of the ala, the "allergic salute," a supratip crease that sometimes accompanies it, and surgical scars on the face that may provide information about previous surgery.

While this observation of the static nose from different angles is informative, further insight can be gained during the dynamic phase of the examination. The patient is asked to show his/her teeth in the frontal view. This will accentuate asymmetrical movements of the musculature facial and nasal muscles. Asymmetry of the nasal tip can become more obvious with these movements. In the profile view, first ask the patient to show his/her teeth. An overactive *depressor septi nas*i muscle will pull the nasal tip down and decrease the columellar–labial angle. Further movement of the nasal tip may also be observed if the patient is asked to move the upper lip down towards the lower lip.

More information about the nose can be gained by lifting the columella with the left thumb. This maneuver will allow the surgeon to determine the length, shape, and position of the caudal septum as well as its relationship with the nasal spine. As a nasal speculum can mask valuable anatomical detail, a two-prong retractor can be used instead to display a wealth of anatomical detail characteristic of this area. All prominences, recesses, and grooves, in addition to the relationship of the vestibular floor to the pyriform fossa, must be noted.

The second phase of examination, palpation of the nose, will provide vital information about the nose with practical implications for surgical planning. Special attention should be given to the following:

- Thickness and elasticity of the skin and its adherence to underlying structures.
- The shape, size, and angulation of nasal bones.
- The septal dorsum and tip cartilages can be assessed by gentle digital pressure.
- The "tip recoil test," that is, pushing the tip down and then immediately releasing it, reveals the amount of tip support.
- By placing the tip of the thumb in one vestibule and the tip of the index finger into the other, the surgeon can assess the position, thickness, shape, and mobility of the caudal septum. This technique will also allow the surgeon to feel the characteristics of the membranous septum by pulling on it.
- Palpate the nasal spine and estimate its shape, symmetry and protrusion.
- Firmness and resilience of the lateral crura should be assessed during quiet breathing and forced inspiration. Areas of collapse are identified by gently supporting the various regions of the alae from the vestibular side using a blunt instrument. If the patient reports significant improvement of the airflow, weakness of the external valve is diagnosed and the area(s) of the epicenter of the collapse is(are) precisely marked on the outer skin for possible supportive grafts. A similar maneuver is executed at the level of both upper lateral cartilages in order to diagnose incompetence of the internal nasal valve.

The third and final phase of nasal examination involves nasal endoscopy. A systematic technique ensures that no areas are overlooked. A 0 degree, 2.7-mm-diameter rigid telescope is inserted parallel to the floor of the nose. The surgeon assesses the following:

- The patency and morphology of the valve area along its whole contour
- The anterior portion of the nasal cavity
- The inferior meatus, the head and body of the inferior turbinate, and the septum in its inferior portion
- The floor of the nose, posterior aspect of the inferior turbinate, and the entire contour of the choana

- The posterior wall and the roof of the nasopharynx, fossa of Rosenmuller with the Eustachian tube orifice, and, by rotating the telescope on its longitudinal axis, the corresponding contralateral anatomical structures

The second step consists of retracting the telescope to the anterior nasal valve and adjusting its position to form a 45-degree angle above the horizontal plane in order to thoroughly inspect the middle meatus and identify polyps or purulent exudate, which would require a CT scan. When the patient presents with rhinosinusitis symptoms, computed tomography imaging (three-plane reconstruction) is mandatory in order to evaluate the nature and location of the anatomical blockage and plan for concomitant endoscopic sinus surgery.

Clinical Photography

The next step involves systematic photography of the patient's face. Ideally, the patient should sit in front of a dark screen. Two light sources are aimed at 45 degrees to the subject, while a third light source illuminates the background. The simultaneous illumination of the patient from these sources ensures adequate lighting and loss of shadows. While a detailed discussion of photographic techniques is beyond the scope of this chapter, adequate photography with standardized views is the cornerstone of facial analysis. Basic views include one frontal, two profiles, four three-quarters views (two per each side), one base, one helicopter, two "base–radix" views, two dynamic profile views, and one dynamic frontal view. Two "selfie" views, right and left, complement the standard set of preoperative pictures. In addition, two further frontal views are reconstructed: the two right halves and two left halves are each spliced together.

Aesthetic surface analysis is paramount. It consists mainly of "chiaroscuro" (lights and shadow) analysis that emphasizes the visual contrast of the different nasal areas. On the frontal view, there are 4 "chiaroscuro" border lines (2 brow–tip lines and 2 nose–cheek lines), which demarcate 3 distinct areas: a central "bridge light," and 2 bilateral sidewall shadows.

From the surface analysis point of view, the nasal tip consists of four aesthetic subunits: central (domal) light, lateral (alar) light, supra-alar shade, and scroll shade.

Consequently, aesthetic rhinoplasty can be considered a "surface-contour" operation.

Summary of the First Clinical Encounter

- History: Evaluate the patient's wishes; discover any potential pitfalls that may preclude rhinoplasty ± endoscopic sinus surgery.
- Examination: Define specific anatomical features in both the static and dynamic phases that need special attention for the operative plan. Perform a full endonasal examination to evaluate the intranasal structures and to diagnose concurrent rhinologic disease and plan intervention.
- Clinical photography: A sequence of well-defined views in static and dynamic phases that will be analyzed after the first meeting and create the foundation for a personalized strategy.
- Patient communication: Provide the patient with your understanding of their expectations, and agree to meet again at a later date to plan surgery to discuss any concern and plan realistic changes for the nose.

INDICATIONS

By the end of the history-taking and examination process, the surgeon should have a clear idea of the answer to four questions that may be conveniently remembered as the "Four Ws":

1. What specifically would the patient like the doctor to do for him or her?
2. Why does the patient want this particular change?
3. Why does the patient want the operation at this particular time?
4. Why has the patient chosen this particular surgeon?

Careful analysis of the answers to these questions can lead the surgeon to determine if the patient is a candidate for rhinoplasty. Indications for rhinoplasty include anatomic nasal deformity resulting in a functional deficit (nasal obstruction refractory to medical management being the most frequent functional issue) or cosmetic issues with a dorsal hump and tip malposition being the most common subjective complaints.

CONTRAINDICATIONS

There are relatively few contraindications for rhinoplasty. Two important contraindications are a patient with unrealistic expectations or a poor understanding of the risks of surgery. From a medical standpoint, patients who cannot tolerate a general anesthetic are obviously not candidates for a complex rhinoplasty. Patients with bleeding disorders should be treated with caution, as should revision surgery within 1 year of their primary rhinoplasty.

PREOPERATIVE PLANNING

While photography marks the end of the first consultation, both the surgeon and the patient make constructive use of their time before their next obligatory meeting. The patients are encouraged to read the literature supplied to them and to ponder the impact of surgery on their personal and working life, the possible risks of surgery, and a potential for future revision. The surgeon uses the time between the two meetings for the most important step in rhinoplasty: facial and nasal analysis. The results of facial/nasal analysis based on the clinical photographs provide a list of aesthetic defects of the face in general, and of the nose in particular. Then, a strategy is tailor-made for that particular patient based on their specific anatomical and pathologic findings and desires for change. This unique plan is meticulously drafted, such that every step of the future surgical operation has already been thoroughly analyzed. The surgeon then produces computer simulations of proposed changes. Patients are told that these simulations are by no means a guarantee of the end result, but provide the patient and the surgeon points of discussion during their second meeting.

As both the patient and the surgeon have had time to think about the patient's particular expectation in the intervening period, the second consultation is aimed at conveying the findings of the facial analysis, discussing the various options that may be possible based on the computer simulations, and allaying the patient's fears and concerns about surgery. Practical advice regarding the do's and don'ts of the postoperative period are of great importance to the patient as they often entail limitations in work and social engagement for a limited period of time. It is of utmost importance that the patient realizes that not every desire for change can be achieved, and that the possibility of revision surgery of about 10% is a real one even in the best of hands.

Summary of the Rhinoplasty Plan at the end of the Second Consultation

- Facial analysis has produced a list of aesthetic defects of the face in general and the nose in particular. Pay particular attention to anatomical and pathologic findings that can have an impact on surgery.
- Compare the patient's list of subjective complaints with that generated by facial analysis.
- Compare the patient's list of desired changes with simulations.
- Plan for the technical aspects of surgery. This provides the surgeon with a valuable and sequential list of steps in the operating room that serves as a guide from the first to the last step of the procedure.
- The patient makes final plans for the practical matters, such as arranging time off from work and social support for the postoperative period.

SURGICAL TECHNIQUE

Case Study

Once the plan has been formulated, the surgeon follows a critical sequence of maneuvers that recreate surface aesthetic lines and contours. The surgeon identifies modifiable surgical landmarks and alters them in a reversible and conservative manner. These landmarks include the following:

- Frontal: radix configuration, dorsal lines, nose–cheek junctions, bridge width, scroll areas.
- Profile: radix height and depth, nasofrontal angle, point of maximal dorsal projection, rhinion, anterior septal angle, pronasale, alar margin, infratip break, subnasale. Profileplasty does not simply mean a humpectomy. By itself, removal of a dorsal hump can be inappropriate and lead to a disastrous result. The entire profile needs to be considered for careful evaluation and recontouring.

Hybrid rhinoplasty techniques can be used to create a wide variety of effects ranging from "finesse or just-one-thing rhinoplasty" to major structural changes, both primary and revision cases. This large variety of endonasal techniques include tip modification procedures such as structural grafting, "contour" grafting through gently crushed cartilage placed in tight pockets, suturing, conservative excisions, reorientation of tip cartilages, and soft tissue peeling of SMAS adipose tissue. In the Mediterranean nose, the alae are not usually limited in their width to the intercanthal line. For most of our Mediterranean patients, the caruncle seems to be a more relevant landmark. As such, reduction of the alar base, which can lead to visible scars, is rarely necessary. Instead, alar reduction sutures that gently medialize the base of the ala without compromising the airway are more effective in this population. The astute rhinoplasty surgeon also realizes that osteotomies, far from being symmetrical and equal on both sides, need to be asymmetric in the vast majority of cases as most bony pyramids are also asymmetrical. Once the nose–cheek lines and brow–dome lines have been reestablished through osteotomies, final refinements can be gained by contour grafting. This penultimate step requires careful closure of previous incisions in order to prevent movement or displacement of the contour grafts with time. All of these techniques are reported in the patient's worksheet.

For this specific case, the endonasal hybrid approach is suitable to allow profound rearrangements of the anatomical framework of the tip, such as inversion of the curvature of the lateral crus, malposition of the tip, gross asymmetry of the tip, and derangements of the contour of the nostril. These gross deformities are readily appreciated on the preoperative photographs noted in Figures 23.1A–I. These photographs show several views of an asymmetric and malpositioned tip, among other deformities.

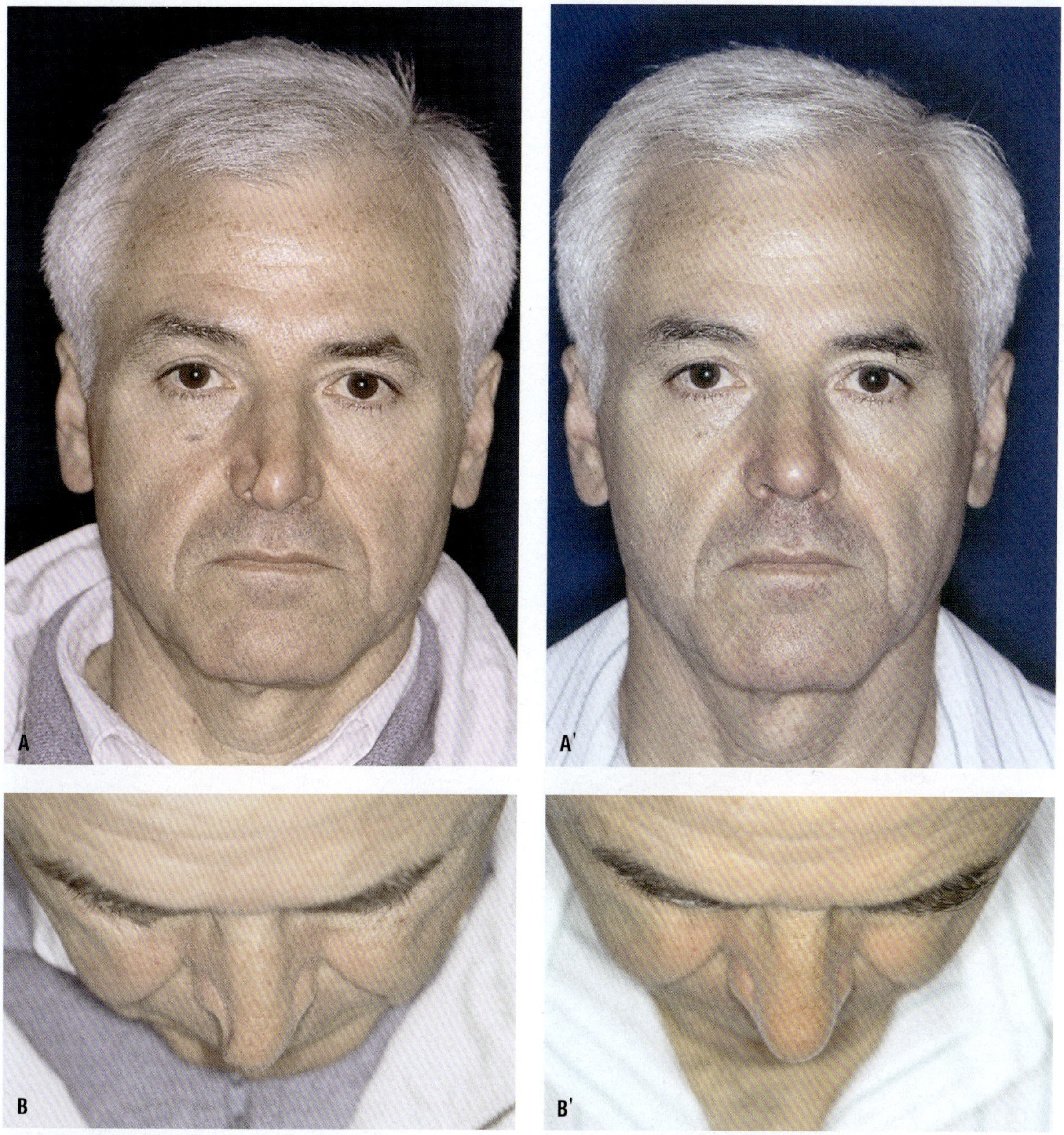

FIGURE 23.1 Preoperative views of markedly deviated tip in an adult male presenting inversion of the curvature of the right lateral crus. [**A**—frontal, **B**—helicopter, **C**—"base-radix" view, **D**—right lateral, **E and F**—right ¾ views, **G**—dynamic "tip down" right lateral view, **H**—dynamic "forced smiling" right lateral view, **I**—left lateral]. Postoperative views. Operation summary: Septoplasty and septal cartilage harvesting, "flip-flop" technique, caudal septum shortening, columellar strut, subdomal (intermediate crura) suture, dorsal lowering, bilateral basal osteotomies, right intermediate osteotomy, "tongue-in-groove" suture, and onlay cartilaginous graft over right dome. [**A′**—frontal, **B′**—helicopter, **C′**—"base–radix" view, **D′**—right lateral, **E′ and F′**—right ¾ views, **G′**—dynamic "tip down" right lateral view, **H′**—dynamic "forced smiling" right lateral view, **I′**—left lateral].

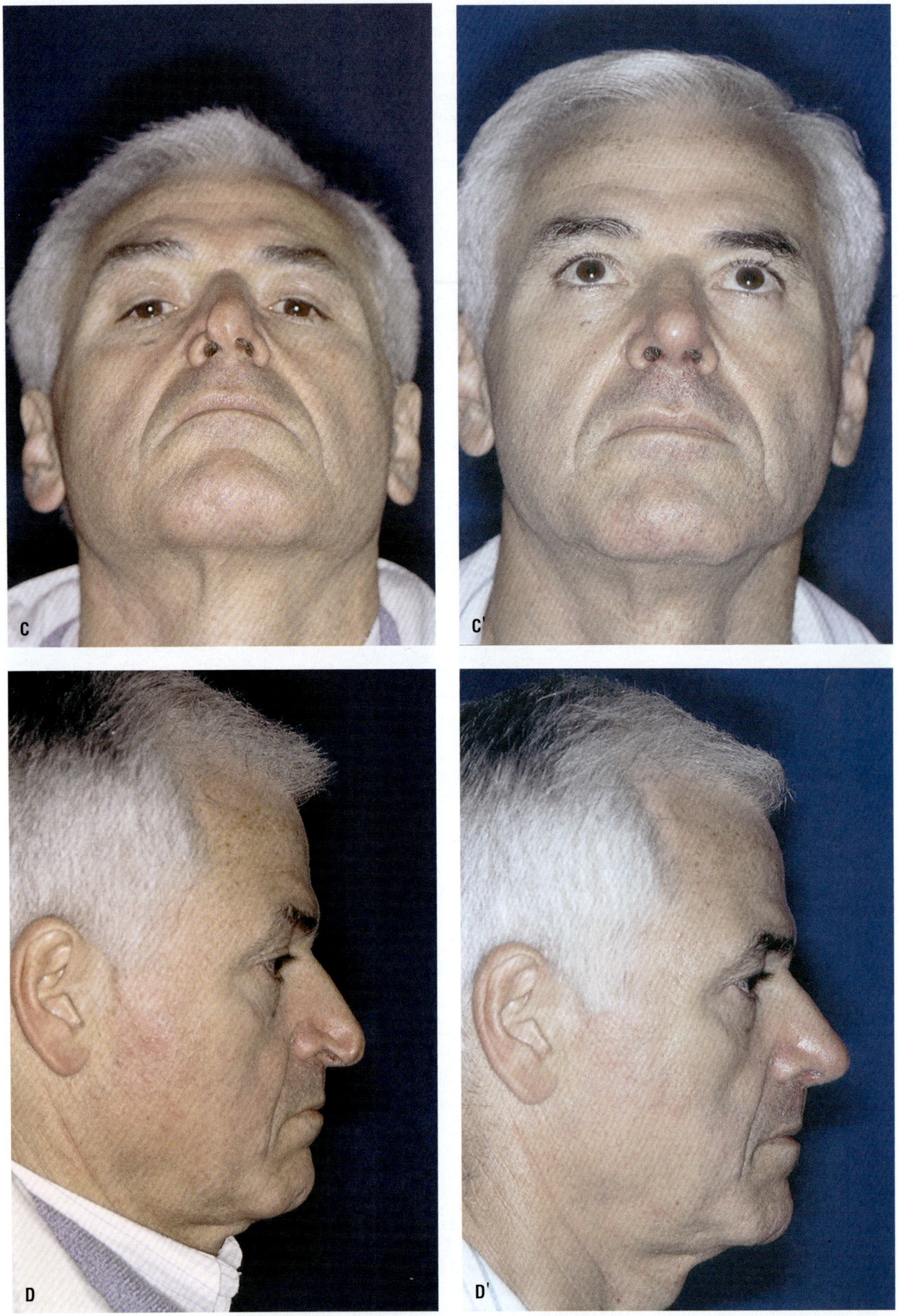

FIGURE 23.1 (*Continued*)

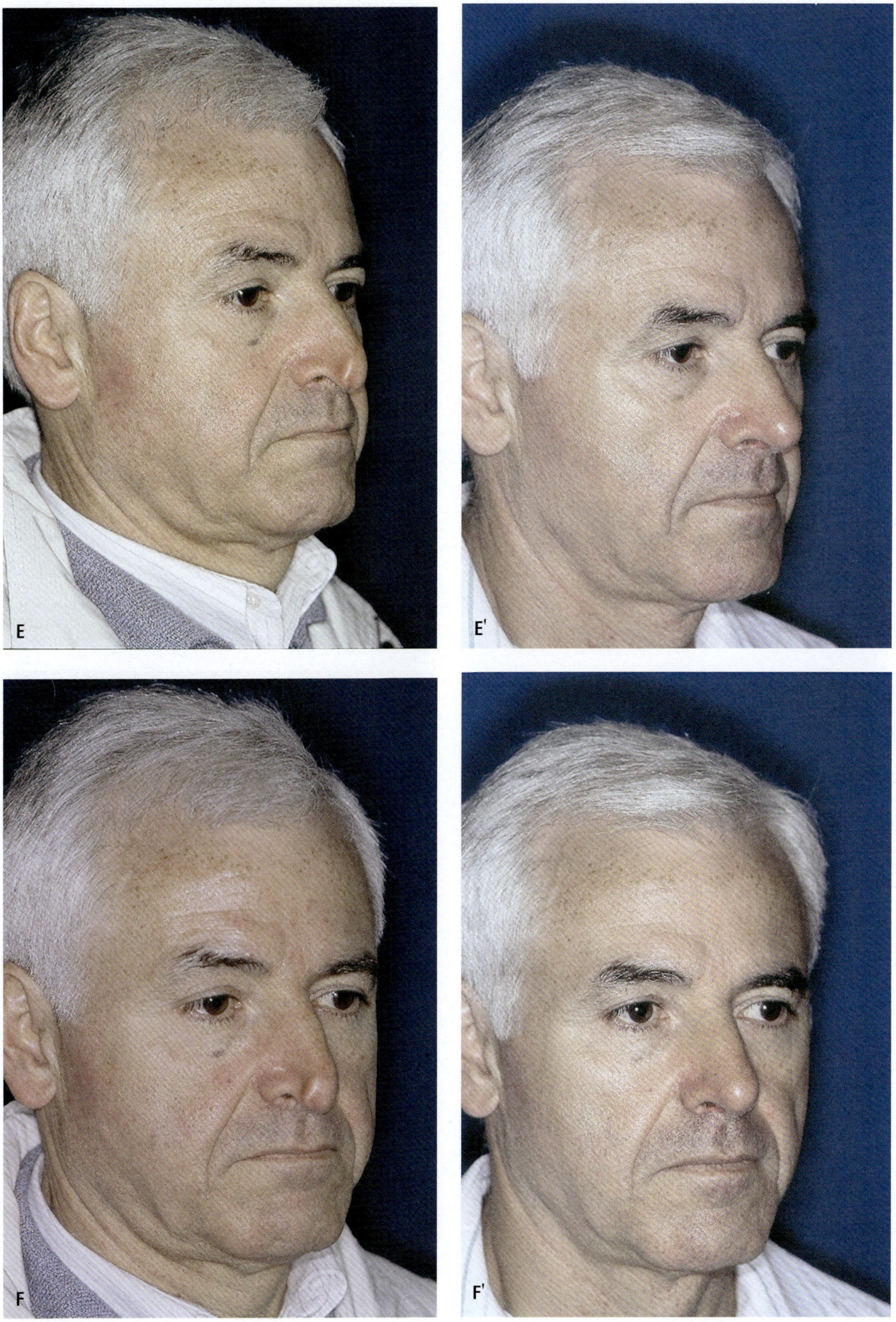

FIGURE 23.1 (*Continued*)

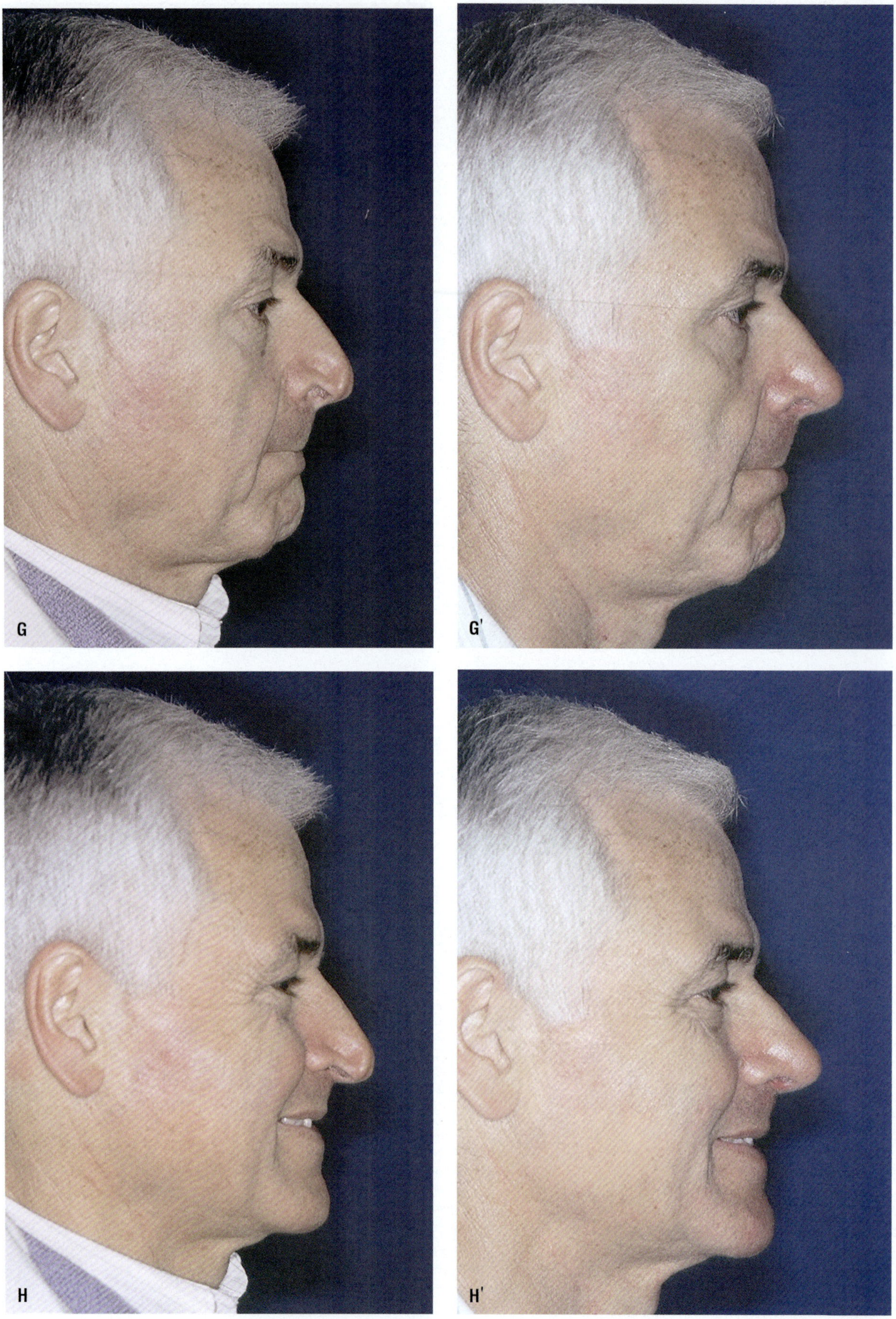

FIGURE 23.1 (*Continued*)

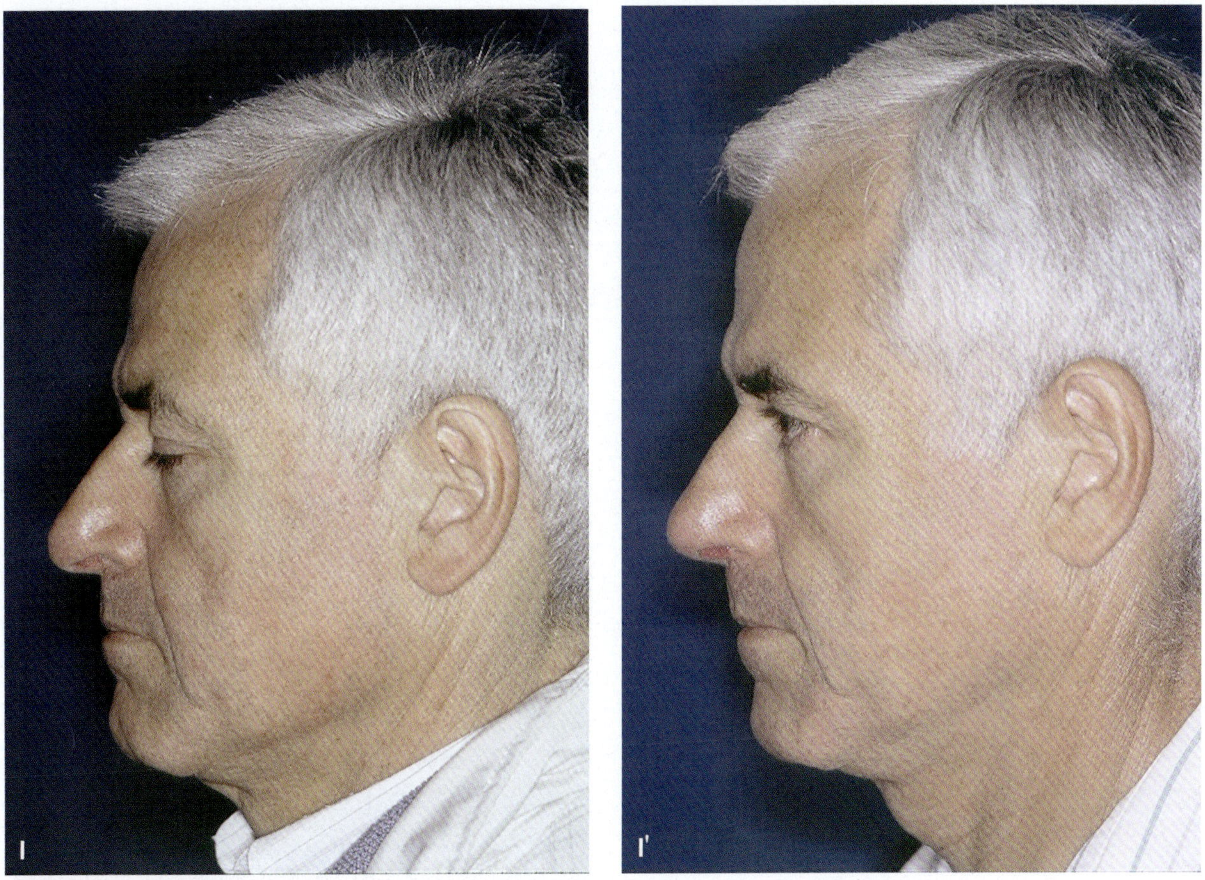

FIGURE 23.1 (*Continued*)

The procedure starts with moderate injection of local anesthetics (mepivacaine 2% + epinephrine 1:100.000) at the incision sites. The nasal dorsum is never infiltrated as we prefer to keep the constant tactile feedback of the dorsal modification. Pledgets soaked with oxymetazoline were placed inside both nasal fossae.

The septum was approached via a transfixion incision, and the caudal septum was realigned and stabilized over the inferior nasal spine. The septal deviation was corrected through the "swinging-door" technique. The inferior nasal spine was markedly asymmetrical and was reshaped by fine chiseling. Part of the central part of the septal cartilage was harvested for grafting purposes. The caudal septum is then fixed between the medial crura via a modified tongue-in-groove technique. The technique is the following: through the hemitransfixion incision, a columellar pocket is created in between the medial crura in order to create a space for the placement of the caudal septum. The shape and length of the caudal septum are adjusted so as to reach the desired columellar length/shape. The vestibular lining is trimmed bilaterally according to the new shape/length of the caudal septum. At the end of the procedure (before placing the columellar strut), the septum will be fixed into the columellar pocket through three or four septocolumellar mattress sutures using an absorbable monofilament. This "modified tongue-in-groove" technique can be used to reduce the length of the nose, treat excess of columellar show, and to finely reshape the aperture of the columellar–labial angle.

After the septoplasty, the dorsum was approached using intercartilaginous incisions. The profile was conservatively lowered, and bilateral double osteotomies (basal and intermediate) were performed in order to both moderately narrow the bony base and to create more symmetric sidewalls.

Tip refinement was the last phase of surgery. An "extended" delivery approach was performed (see Figs. 23.2 to 23.23 for a stepwise approach to the endonasal flip-flop technique)—extended because the infracartilaginous incisions were made more posterolaterally than usual. The lower lateral cartilages were skeletonized from both the overlying soft tissue envelope and the underlying vestibular skin in order to fully expose the tip framework. A conservative trim of the cephalic margin was performed on the left lower lateral cartilage. The right lower lateral cartilage was incised medially, just lateral to the dome, and laterally, at the most posterolateral aspect, close to the "hinge" area. The continuity of the right lower lateral cartilage was reconstructed by the "flip-flop technique": the free graft constituted by the excised central part of the right lower lateral was shaped in order to get it as symmetrical as possible with the lower lateral cartilage, then rotated along its major axis, and resutured to the right dome medially. The lateral aspect of the graft was inserted into an alar pocket and then bolstered. A long, curved (so to create a natural infratip break) columellar strut precisely harvested from the septum was inserted into a second columellar pocket, created through a stab incision at the columellar

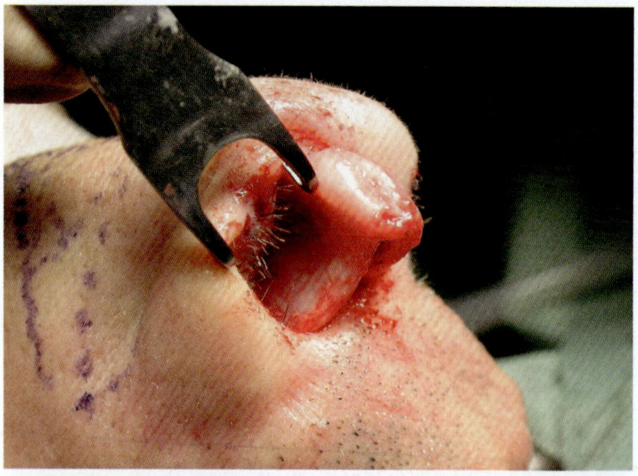

FIGURE 23.2
Delivery of the right lower lateral cartilage. The "double dome" configuration of the right nasal dome is clearly visible.

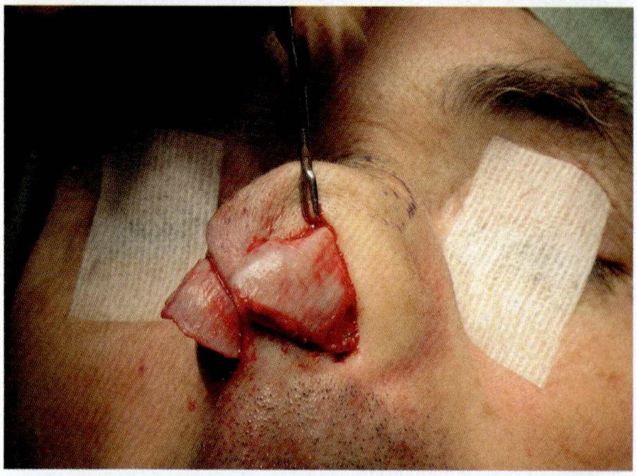

FIGURE 23.3
Delivery of the right lower lateral cartilage. Visible is the inversion of the curvature of the right lateral crus.

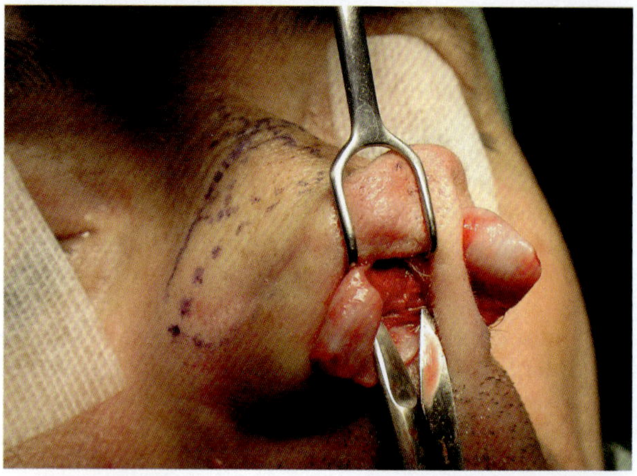

FIGURE 23.4
Delivery of the left lower lateral cartilage. The convex curvature of the left lateral crus is clearly visible.

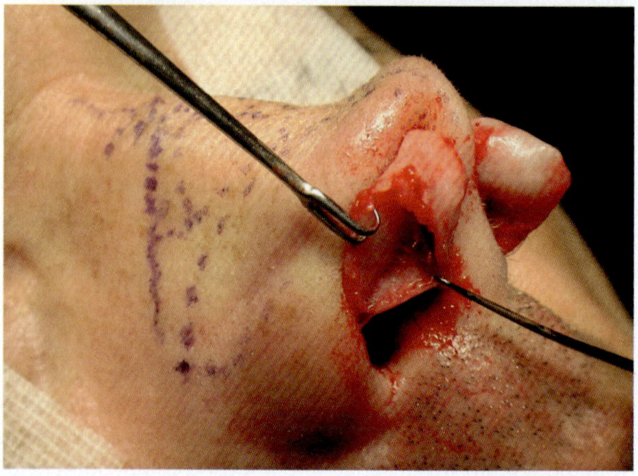

FIGURE 23.5
Dissection of the interdomal and intercrural spaces.

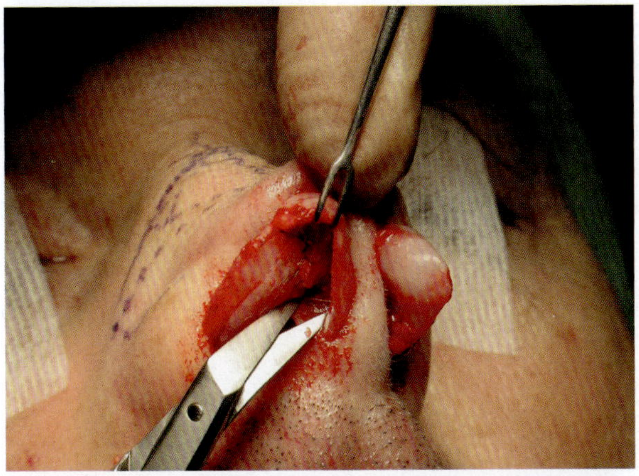

FIGURE 23.6
Dissection of the right lateral crus from the underlying vestibular skin.

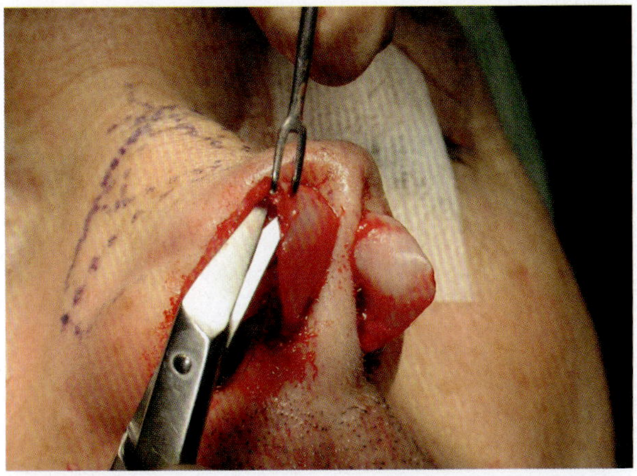

FIGURE 23.7
Dissection of the right medial crus from the underlying vestibular skin.

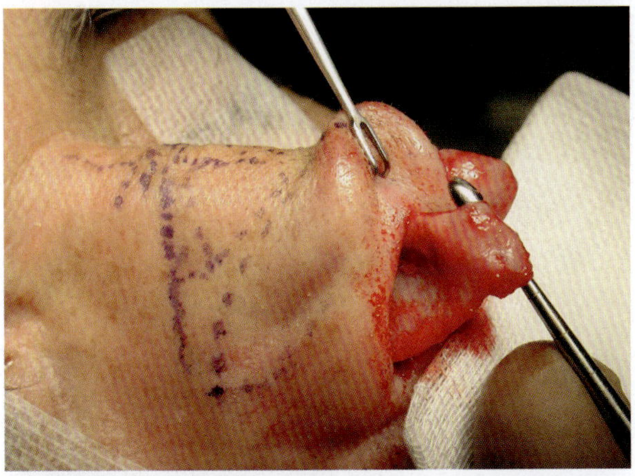

FIGURE 23.8
Delivery of the right lower lateral cartilage. Visible the "double dome" configuration of the right nasal dome.

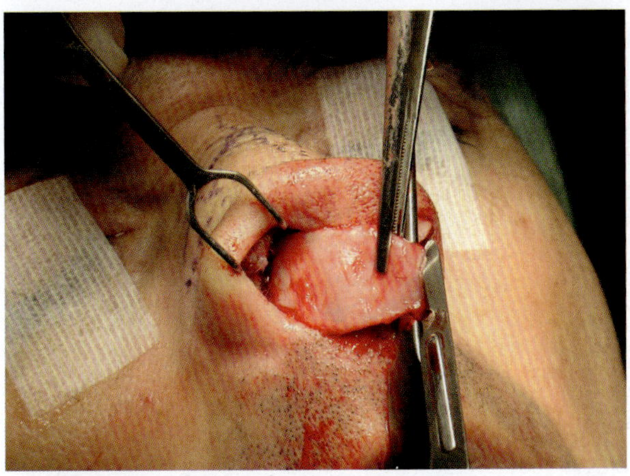

FIGURE 23.9
Full-thickness splitting of the right dome preserving the integrity of the underlying vestibular skin.

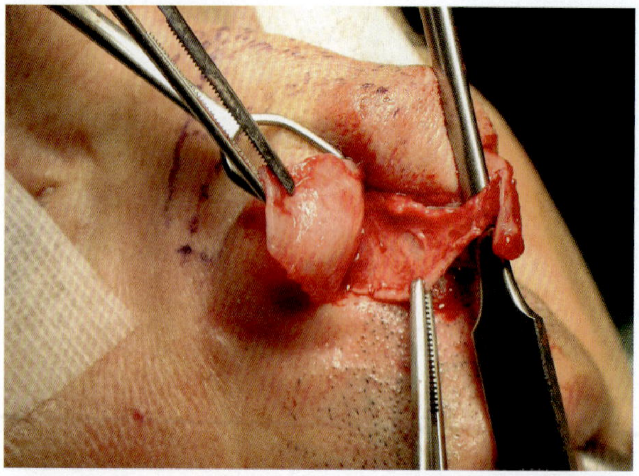

FIGURE 23.10
Full-thickness splitting of the right dome preserving the integrity of the underlying vestibular skin.

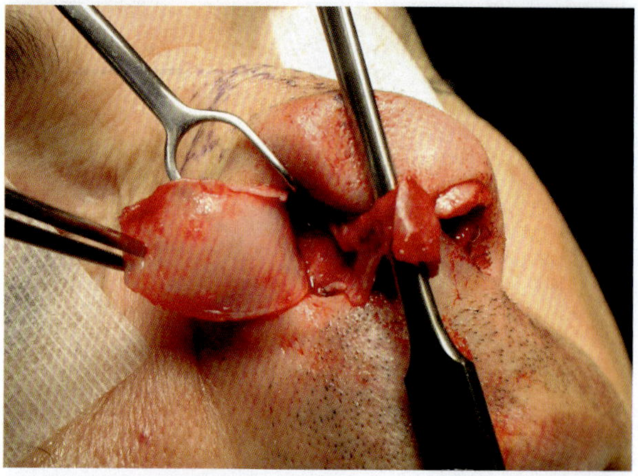

FIGURE 23.11
"Open book" dissection of the right lateral crus extended to hinge area.

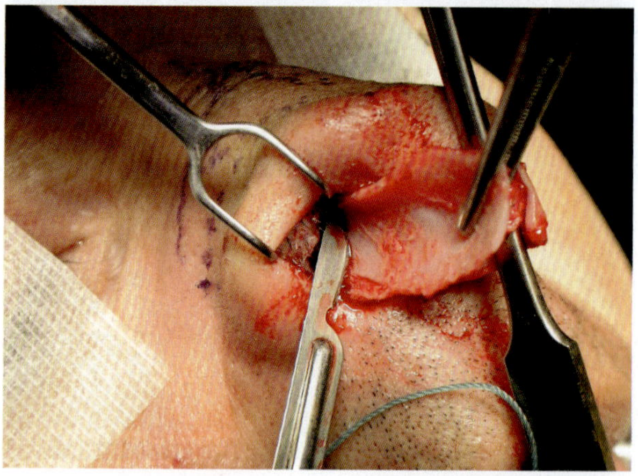

FIGURE 23.12
"Open book" dissection of the right lateral crus extended to hinge area.

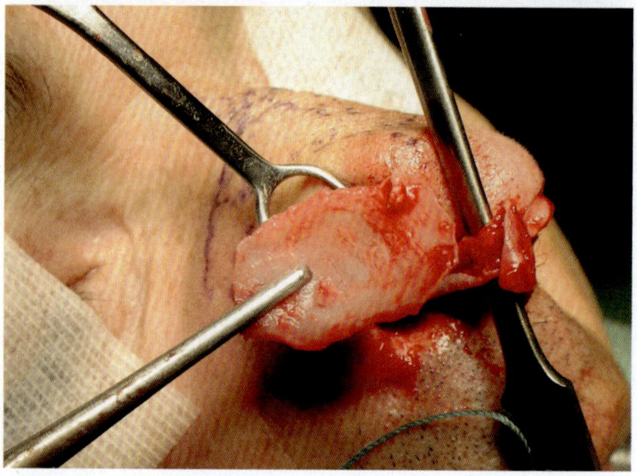

FIGURE 23.13
Section of the posterolateral aspect of the right lateral crus.

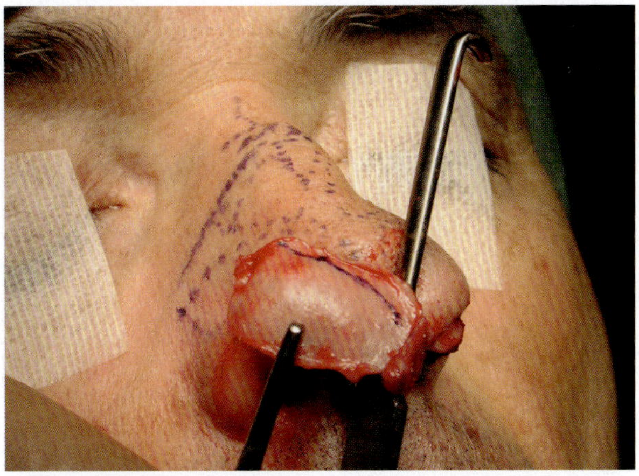

FIGURE 23.14
Inverted shape of the right lateral crus.

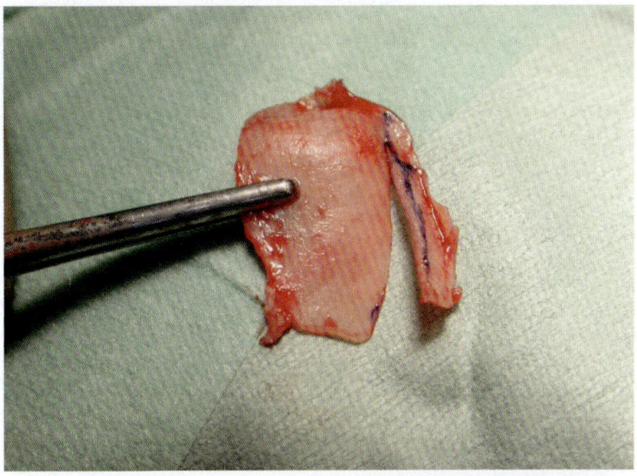

FIGURE 23.15
"Flip" of the right lateral crus. The amount of cephalic excision is marked.

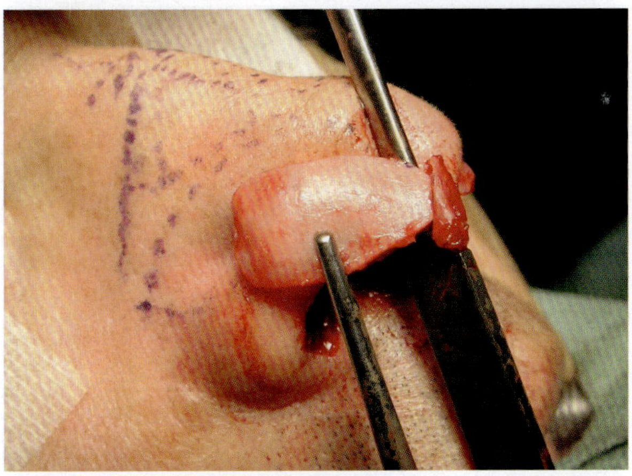

FIGURE 23.16
Sculpting of the "new" right lateral crus.

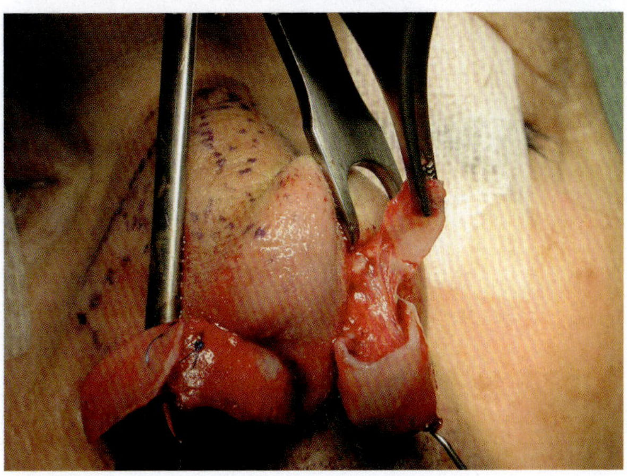

FIGURE 23.17
"Flop" of the right lateral crus.

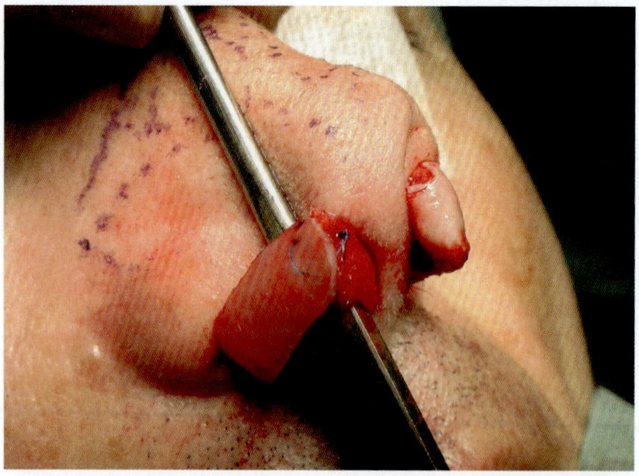

FIGURE 23.18
Reconstruction of the continuity of the domal and lateral segments of the right lower lateral cartilage. Cephalic excision of the left lower lateral cartilage.

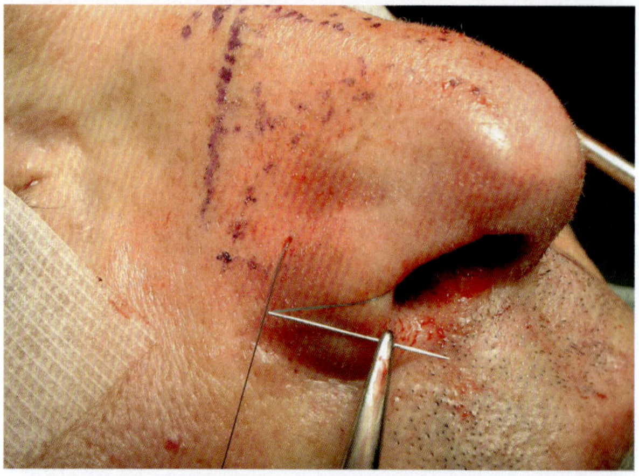

FIGURE 23.19
View of the reconstructed right lower lateral cartilage with a normal curvature of the lateral crus.

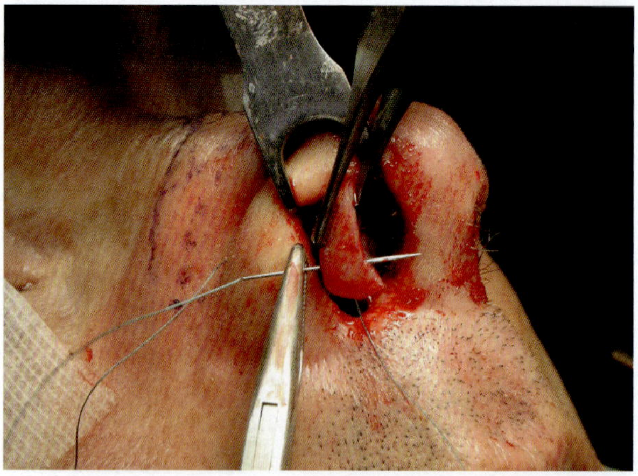

FIGURE 23.20
Fixation of the posterolateral aspect of the new lower lateral cartilages. Out–in suspension suture.

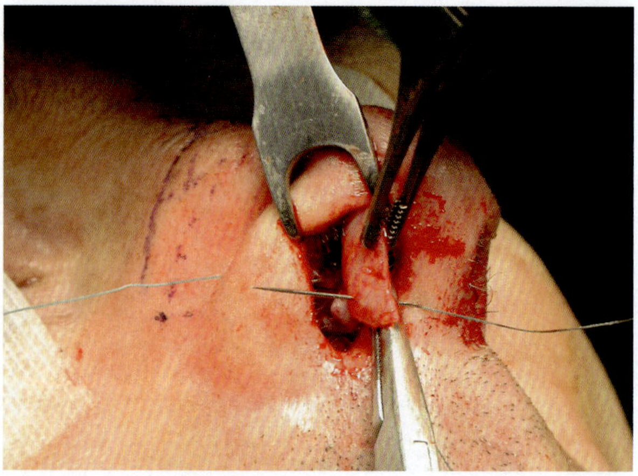

FIGURE 23.21
Fixation of the posterolateral aspect of the new lower lateral cartilages. In–out suspension suture.

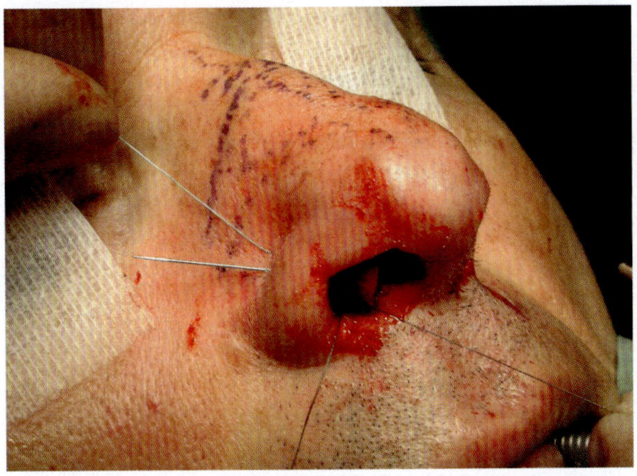

FIGURE 23.22
Fixation of the posterolateral aspect of the new lower lateral cartilages. Percutaneous fixation.

base, and positioned just caudal to the paired medial crura complex (so-called postcrural columellar strut). The stab incision was closed by a mattress suture securing the strut into the columellar pocket. "Contour" grafts are commonly positioned at the end of surgery, after closing all the vestibular incisions. "Contour" grafts are cartilage flakes obtained from the remaining septal cartilage and used as onlay in order to hide irregularities and adjust tip projection and symmetry.

POSTOPERATIVE MANAGEMENT

- Adequate analgesia and antiemetics administered by the anesthetist ensure that pain and nausea are kept to a minimum.
- Temporary, lubricated packs that have been inserted intraoperatively are removed by the surgeon usually after 24 hours. When septoplasty has not been extended, septal quilting sutures represent a valid and safe alternative to packing.
- Gentle ambulation is encouraged starting on postoperative day one.
- Elevation of the head of the bed and cool compresses may help to reduce the swelling during the immediate postoperative period.
- Removal of the splint(s) provides the patient and the doctor a "moment of truth" as they examine the result of surgery together.
- The patient is encouraged to reserve judgment for the next few months as the edema subsides. See Figure 23.1A′–I′ for postoperative photos of the case study patient.

COMPLICATIONS

Rhinoplasty is notoriously difficult for many reasons. Patients' demands have become more sophisticated and specific with time and the Internet. These requests stretch the bounds of surgical possibility, and are exacerbated by a ubiquitous culture of litigation. The long learning curve of rhinoplasty and the technical challenges of the operation also contribute to an already complicated scenario. The junior surgeon embarking on this road

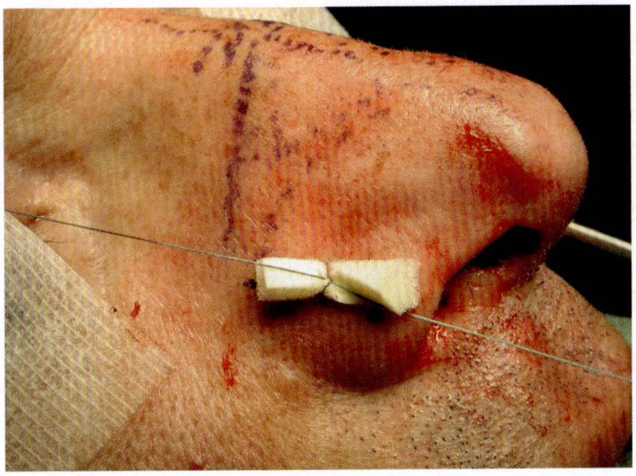

FIGURE 23.23
Bolstering.

should take every opportunity to fully understand the patient's desires for change, document and analyze the preoperative photographs, and create a detailed, tailor-made plan of management for each patient. Not operating can be much wiser than creating an unhappy patient with a grievance against that individual surgeon and the medical profession.

As a detailed description of complications goes well beyond the limitations of this chapter, it may be instructive to think of the problems of rhinoplasty in terms of the following:

- *Errors of omission.* The surgeon has failed to fully grasp the patient's list of desired changes and did not deliver the anticipated results. This shortfall may be due to poor communication with the patient, inadequate preoperative facial analysis, and/or too conservative surgery.
- *Errors of commission.* The surgeon performed an overaggressive surgery or altered the nose beyond the wishes of the patient.

RESULTS

Rhinoplasty should not be considered in the more classic terms of external or endonasal approaches, but as a hybrid of the most advanced techniques that provide reliable and long-standing results. The techniques used in surface hybrid endonasal rhinoplasty are marked by their precision, reversibility, conservative tissue handling.

Essential to the success of rhinoplasty surgery is identification of clinical and anatomic findings that directly relate to the concerns of the patient. If correctly identified, the best of external and endonasal approaches are available for the facial plastic surgeons to achieve their goal. These approaches to success are then to be shared with the patient prior to surgery. Ultimately, it affords the patient an understanding of how and what surgery can achieve and what limiting factors may exist.

PEARLS

- Know what your patients wants in great detail.
- Train your eyes to see what you should be looking for.
- The nose is not simply an organ to be operated on. Familiarize yourself with the diseases of the nose and sinuses, and be prepared to operate for more than one reason. The endoscope should never be far away from the hands of a rhinoplasty surgeon.
- Develop a personal concept and continue lifelong learning from the masters.
- Seek to improve your septoplasty and osteotomy techniques at all levels of practice.
- Never operate before meticulous and detailed facial analysis based on excellent photography. The main analytical concern consists of determining the extent and location of nasal asymmetries. Compare the two right halves and two left halves. Observe brow–dome lines, nose–cheek junctions, and alar–columella relationships. Every nasal aesthetic subunit should be evaluated in terms of symmetry and light/shadow relationship. The aim of aesthetic rhinoplasty is to create attractive surface aesthetics.
- Beauty is a matter of millimeters. Be meticulous in your handling of tissues. The nose is a complex and unforgiving organ.
- Use safe and reversible techniques.
- The nasal septum is the best source of grafts. Therefore, conservative removal of septal cartilage is the key for assuring quality graft material that the surgeon might need for fixing his/her own untoward results.

PITFALLS

- While a dorsal hump is the most common complaint and changing the dorsum, the most common request, it also forms the most common source of failure in rhinoplasty.
- Not every "hump" is a hump. Beware of pseudohumps. Don't forget radix and chin when planning/executing removal of a dorsal hump.
- Tip sutures are not a benign, low-risk procedure.
- Tip structural grafts should be used judiciously.
- Systematic, prophylactic use of spreader grafts makes surgery unnecessarily difficult.
- Most patients do not want major changes to their nose. Rhinoplasty surgeons should think in terms of surface reshaping rather than structural rebuilding.
- Thick-skinned tips often require substantial tip grafting to get a proper cartilage: SMAS thickness ratio, as well as angularity of tip contour.
- Straightening a twisted nose is a humbling experience.

- Even in the best of hands, a small number of patients require a minor touch-up operation: this is the hard reality of rhinoplasty that the patient needs to accept before coming into the operating room.
- Not every patient is suitable for an open approach.
- Failing to understand surface anatomy.
- Routinely creating a separation between the septum and upper lateral cartilages.
- Doing standard osteotomies as opposed to patient-centered ones.
- Lack of operative versatility in managing tip problems.
- Overlooking stable repositioning of the tip.
- Being surgically aggressive when not necessary.
- Telling patients that his/her surgery will be simple and 100% successful.
- "Selling" the operation.

INSTRUMENTS TO HAVE AVAILABLE

- Standard rhinoplasty set
- Ferris-Smith forceps
- Aiach clamp
- Aiach forceps
- Jost cartilage crusher
- Columellar forceps
- Grafts slider
- Rubin morselizer
- Glabellar rasp
- Double-edged Cottle elevator
- Blunt-tipped Knapp scissors

ACKNOWLEDGMENT

The author would like to thank Prabhat Bhama, MD for his contributions to the writing of this chapter. His work in the writing, editing, and figure creation for this chapter is greatly appreciated.

SUGGESTED READING

Daniel RK. *Mastering rhinoplasty*. Berlin, Heidelberg, Germany: Springer-Verlag, 2010.

Nolst Trenité GJ. *Rhinoplasty; A practical guide to functional and aesthetic surgery of the nose*. The Hague, Netherlands: Kugler Publications, 2005.

Palma P, Khodaei I. Hybrid rhinoplasty: the 21th century approach to remodeling the nose. *Arch Facial Plast Surg* 2010;12(6):412–414.

Pastorek N, Ham J. The underprojecting nasal tip: an endonasal approach. *Facial Plast Surg Clin North Am* 2004;12(1):93–106.

Perkins S, Patel A. Endonasal suture techniques in tip rhinoplasty. *Facial Plast Surg Clin North Am* 2009;17:41–54.

24 CLOSURE OF SEPTAL PERFORATION

Russell W.H. Kridel

INTRODUCTION

The presence of a nasal septal perforation, regardless of etiology, can cause significant functional, structural, and emotional consequences to the patient. Fortunately, the majority of these perforations can be closed surgically, providing that the evaluating physician does not delay surgical repair and allow the perforation to enlarge beyond the possibility of closure. It is important to emphasize that if a surgeon does not repair perforations on a routine basis, a referral to an experienced surgeon is essential as the success of the surgery is directly related to the experience of the surgeon. The success of the repair of the perforation is also related to the size of the defect and its orientation, amount of septal mucoperichondrium remaining, degree of scarring, and whether there is metaplasia or inflammation of the mucosa.

From a technical standpoint, the surgical repair is complex and tedious. The perforation represents a partial absence of three distinct layers of tissue, each of which requires closure and/or grafting. Further, the majority of suturing is performed within the narrow confines of the nasal cavity, and inadvertent enlargement of the perforation can occur easily, especially when the remaining septal flaps are thin, adherent, and friable (Fig. 24.1). Many techniques have been described in the repair of septal perforations; in my experience, the absolute best results are achieved through bilateral mucosal flap development and advancement with the interposition and anchoring of a connective tissue graft between the flaps.

HISTORY

A comprehensive past medical history of all organ systems is performed in all patients who are evaluated for surgery. Such measures are taken to optimize the general health of the patient and surgical safety. Involvement of the patient's primary care physician is important in the consolidation of the medical history and current medical conditions. Medical specialists are consulted when necessary for evaluation and management of comorbidities and clearance for anesthesia.

The etiology of a nasal septal perforation can often be determined by taking a comprehensive history. This should include eliciting a history of nasal and/or sinus problems as well as other respiratory and autoimmune medical conditions and the use of over-the-counter and prescription nasal medications. One should also consider work-related, environmental, and social factors as well. Most perforations are either iatrogenic or secondary to recreational use of cocaine. If no direct cause can be determined, a full evaluation, sometimes including a soft tissue biopsy, is needed to rule out the rare occurrence of Wegener's granulomatosis or the even rarer event of nasal-type extranodal NK-/T-cell lymphoma (NKTCL).

With regard to iatrogenic injury, the most commonly relayed history describes an antecedent septoplasty in which contiguous areas of the septal mucosa were torn on both sides, regardless of the presence or absence of intervening septal cartilage. Another common cause is the use of cautery for epistaxis in similar areas on

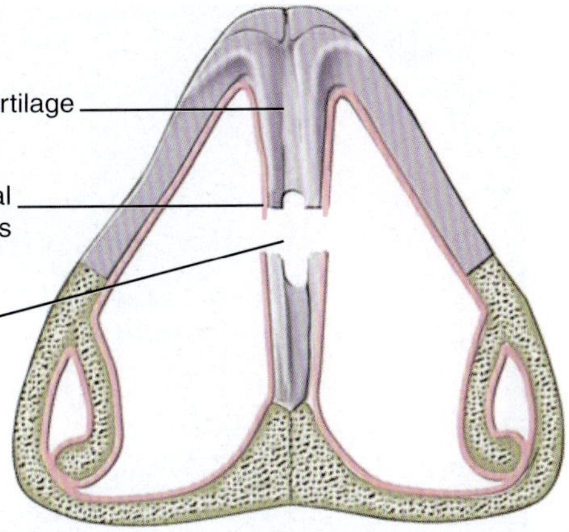

FIGURE 24.1 A septal perforation is a localized absence of the three layers, the right and left layer of mucoperichondrium septal flaps and the intervening septal cartilage.

opposing sides of the septum. Bilateral balloon nasal packing is also well known for its ability to compromise the blood supply of the mucoperichondrium and lead to a large perforation.

Additional etiologies include facial trauma resulting in substantial nasal fractures or septal hematomas, self-induced trauma from nose picking as well as placement of a foreign body (e.g., button battery) in the nose. The chronic use of nasal spray, both vasoconstrictive and anti-inflammatory, has been implicated as a causative factor. The use of cocaine has increased significantly as a major cause of septal perforation due to the intense vasoconstriction caused by the drug combined with the adulterated chemical irritants used as fillers. Chronic use of cocaine can totally destroy the mucosa of the nasal cavity creating intranasal stenosis and irreparable scarring.

PHYSICAL EXAMINATION

A comprehensive examination of the head and neck is performed on all patients as incidental and significant medical conditions not related to the consultation may be discovered. With regard to the analysis of a nasal septal perforation, a complete diagnosis cannot be made until all crusts have been removed and decongestion of the turbinates has taken place so that the entire nasal septum can be visualized. Examination of a patient with a deviation of the septum and enlarged turbinates is difficult, and a posterior septal perforation may be missed. When a septal perforation is noted, its circumference and relative position should be documented. An ominous sign exists when there is crusting not only around the edge of the perforation but all over the mucosa of the nasal septum and turbinates. Such a finding is seen more often in patients with causes suggestive of a granulomatous process or vasculitis. Findings of overall crusting in a cocaine user or in a patient with a granulomatous process make the prognosis for long-term operative success guarded and usually reflect a metaplasia of the normal respiratory epithelium to a fibrotic nonfunctioning epithelium.

The septum should be palpated with a cotton-tip applicator to identify the presence of cartilage between the mucosal flaps and to determine whether cartilage extends close to the edges of the perforation (Fig. 24.2). There is usually very little cartilage left in perforations that have occurred following septoplasty, which makes dissection of the flaps more difficult. If I find extensive inflammation and/or swelling of the membrane or see synechiae or collapse of the nasal cavity, I definitely consider an ongoing disease process or the active use of cocaine. Previous cocaine use may result in a clean-edged perforation with cartilage present almost all the way to the edges of the perforation. The more inflamed mucosa and crusting there is around a perforation, the more I am suspicious of a generalized process such as continued abuse,

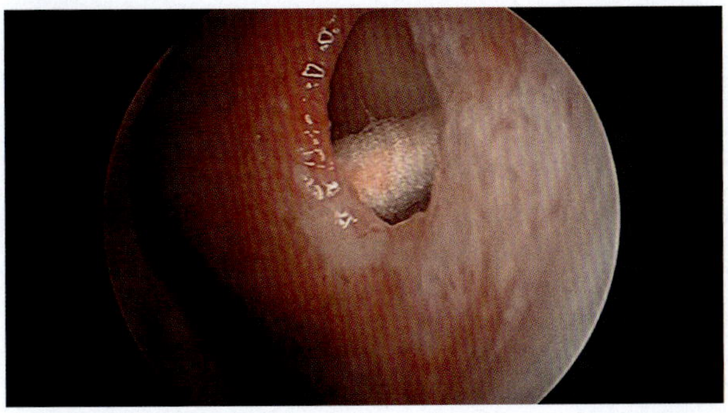

FIGURE 24.2
A cotton-tipped applicator is used to palpate the septum around the perforation to see if any cartilage remains, which is not likely if the patient has had a previous septoplasty. (©Russell W.H. Kridel, MD. Used with permission.)

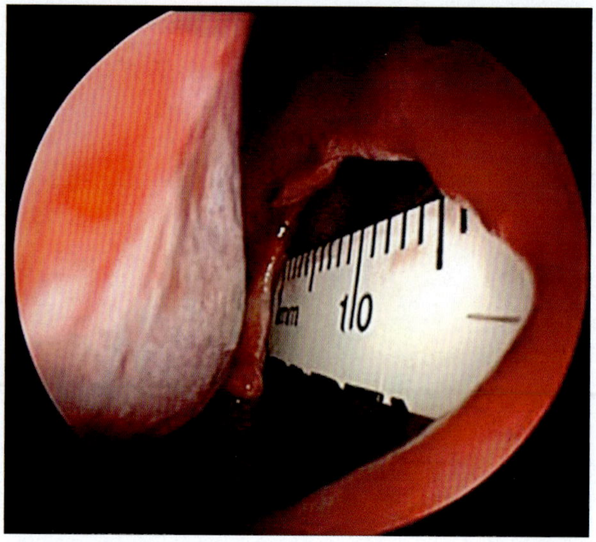

FIGURE 24.3
Endoscopic view of a septal perforation taken from the right nasal vestibule with a ruler inserted on the opposite left side to measure the size of the perforation. (©Russell W.H. Kridel, MD. Used with permission.)

noxious industrial environment, or subclinical soft tissue infection/irritation. Marked inflammation and crusting should be treated with cultures, antibiotics, and local emollients prior to any surgical intervention.

When evaluating a septal perforation (Fig. 24.3), the dimension of the perforation is a helpful determinant for the success of repair. However, it is not the absolute size of the perforation that is as important as the proportion of septal membrane remaining, especially in the vertical dimension. For example, a 1-cm perforation in a young child could be much more difficult to repair than a 2-cm perforation in an adult.

The external nose is evaluated for any evidence of a saddle deformity secondary to loss of dorsal support with a large anterior septal perforation or an active disease process. In such cases, surgical plans can be made for dorsal augmentation simultaneous with repair of the septal perforation. Evaluation and documentation of the configuration of the bony nasal pyramid is of importance in both traumatic and nontraumatic cases and may be adjusted at the time of surgery as well.

INDICATIONS

Bleeding, crusting, whistling, and nasal obstruction are indications for surgery as long as the perforation is not too large to repair. Asymptomatic septal perforations do not require surgery. The more posterior the perforation, the fewer the symptoms.

CONTRAINDICATIONS

Patients who are still using cocaine, unrelenting nose pickers, and those with underlying disease etiologies are not surgical candidates. Perforations that extend all the way to the nasal dorsum are almost impossible to repair, unless there is some small cuff of membrane to which the inferior advancement flap can be sewn. Similarly, perforations that extend all the way down onto the floor of the nose are technically difficult.

Silicone nasal buttons may be helpful in patients with a large perforation that cannot be closed surgically. Large defects usually require custom designing of a larger internal button. Although septal buttons are helpful in patients who cannot undergo surgical interventions, they can cause the perforation to enlarge, must be periodically removed for cleaning, and often worsen the patient's feeling of obstruction due to the bulk they add to the nasal airway.

PREOPERATIVE PLANNING

The major goals of surgery are to close the perforation and restore normal function and physiology to the nose. Many different techniques have been described for closure, but only those that use intranasal advancement flaps are able to achieve normal nasal physiology. However, if extensive scarring or metaplasia of the existing septal flaps is present, it may be impossible to totally restore physiologic function. Other methods that use skin grafts or buccal mucosal grafts may be effective in closing the perforation but unfortunately leave the patient with a dry nose that continues to crust because the respiratory epithelium is not restored.

SURGICAL TECHNIQUE

Surgical Approach Considerations

Although treatment of nasal septal perforations can be performed endonasally, an open approach has multiple advantages that make this the technique of choice. The open approach affords superior access to all dimensions of the perforation and provides a field without the distortion that normal intranasal retraction causes. This technique also preserves the anterior septal blood and lymphatic supply and may even improve the viability of the nasal advancement flaps. Better stated, the small transverse columellar incision is a small price to pay for the improved access to the perforation with improved outcome from the surgery.

One of the minor disadvantages of the open approach is that the medial crura are totally dissected away from each other and from the septum. The fibrous connections between the medial crura and the septum and the overlying skin are supporting attachments that normally help to preserve tip projection. It is incumbent upon the surgeon to reconstitute this support structure after the perforation is repaired; otherwise, tip-drop will almost invariably develop and create a cosmetic deformity that was not present prior to the surgical procedure. The medial crura can be sewn back together with interrupted sutures, and sometimes, a columellar strut must be placed between the medial crura to further support the nasal tip.

Bilateral bipedicled floor and dorsal (from under the upper lateral cartilages) mucosal advancement flaps require mobilization and borrowing of septal mucosa in the vertical dimensions. The upper lateral cartilages are separated from the septum, and as the membrane that is still attached to the upper lateral cartilages is pulled down for attempted closure, the upper lateral cartilages themselves will also have a tendency to be pulled inferiorly. To avoid the tendency to develop a pinched appearance of the middle one-third of the nose, spreader grafts and onlay grafting materials may be placed so as to maintain the contour of the nasal dorsum. Likewise, as the mucosal defect is closed and the bipedicled flaps are pulled into position, a certain amount of tension is placed on the mucosa of the caudal septum and the medial crura, sometimes producing a cephalad rotation of the nasal tip. If the patient has a ptotic tip, these maneuvers will actually help to improve the esthetic result. However, if the patient's nose is already overrotated or foreshortened, the problem may be worsened by the repair, and corrective methods will have to be added to the procedure to counteract these effects.

Interposition Grafts

The use of an interposition graft is necessary for successful repair. Traditionally, temporalis fascia has been used as a template for overlying mucosal tissue migration and vascularization due to its extremely thin nature and very low metabolic requirements. Additionally, the graft maintains a barrier between the corresponding repaired flaps during the healing process and decreases any risk of the incision breaking down with subsequent reperforation. If temporalis fascia is used for reconstruction, a horizontal scalp incision is made with care to bevel the incision so as to remain parallel to the hair follicles. The scalp is retracted, and the dissection is carried down to the deep temporalis fascia with wide undermining. The dimensions of the harvested graft must be significantly larger than the perforation so that its edges go far beyond the perimeter of the original perforation. The surgeon should take into account the possibility of enlargement of the perforation due to manipulation and dissection of the flaps. A large piece of temporalis fascia (5 cm) is harvested. A mastoid type pressure dressing is applied after complete hemostasis is achieved.

Because there is some donor site morbidity when temporalis fascia is used, and because these grafts are exceedingly thin and difficult to manage when they are wet, acellular dermal grafts (AlloDerm, Life-Cell Corporation, Branchburg, NJ) can be employed with success rates similar to that of temporalis fascia. Acellular dermal grafts are thicker, easier to place and suture, and may give more substance to the repaired septum.

Closure

Surgical success depends upon a tension-free closure that will prevent tissue breakdown due to postoperative scar contraction. Because there is no elastic tissue in septal mucosa, adequate mobilization of septal flaps must be performed. The open, external rhinoplasty approach affords the necessary exposure for the development of these mucosal flaps. By using sliding bipedicled flaps taken from under the inferior turbinate and advanced off the floor of the nose, and from under the upper lateral cartilages in larger perforations, the mucosal portion of the perforation can be closed with normal nasal mucosa. It is absolutely crucial that a connective tissue interposition graft be placed between the corresponding perforation repairs to act as a barrier to prevent perforation. Many authors have described this method with over 90% success rates in perforations up to 2 cm. As the size of the perforation increases, the chances of success decrease proportionately. The inferior to superior length of the perforation is the critical dimension in closure as the lines of tension from the floor of the nose to the dorsum, which is perpendicular to this axis, are the most critical in closure. As noted previously, it is also not the absolute size of the perforation that is important, but the proportion of septal membrane remaining in relation to the defect. Each of these factors must be weighed in preoperative analysis to ensure the highest likelihood of operative success.

If multiple adhesions between the remaining septal membranes and turbinates or lateral nasal wall are present, the surgeon may wish to lyse these adhesions in a separate first procedure and place Silastic sheeting along the septum for several weeks. After appropriate healing, the surgeon may return to the nasal septum for a more definitive repair. Another challenge is the limited amount of septal cartilage remaining between the residual tissue flaps. When a fairly aggressive septoplasty has been performed previously, the dissection of the adherent flaps is extremely difficult and can lead to worsening of the perforation even if a meticulous approach is applied.

Nasal Splints

Typically, thin, soft, pliable Silastic sheets are used. These are fashioned to mirror the septum and are then placed intranasally on both sides of the septum to protect the flap, keep the edges of the perforation moist, prevent injury to the mucosa during postoperative suctioning, and allow the surgeon to visually inspect the closure site in the postoperative phase. If a perforation still exists after 3 weeks, the Silastic sheets can remain in place longer to help facilitate closure. The use of hard thick nasal splints such as Doyle splints (Xomed, Jacksonville, FL) is not advocated as they are too firm, not easy to see through, and cause pain during removal.

Operative Technique

Intravenous antibiotics are administered prior to the surgical incision. General oral endotracheal anesthesia is preferred as the operation is lengthy and requires meticulous and tedious dissection and may require two different operative sites, the nose and the temporal scalp. An oropharyngeal pack is inserted to prevent any blood from entering into the esophagus and stomach, thereby helping to prevent any postoperative nausea. Infiltrative anesthesia with 1% lidocaine (Xylocaine) with 1:100,000 epinephrine is used to promote vasoconstriction. Endoscopic photographic documentation of the perforation is carried out, and diagnostic endoscopy is performed to fully examine the nasal cavity.

For those cases in which no clear etiology is documented, a biopsy, if not already performed, should be undertaken at the posterior edge of the perforation. This prevents an increase in the vertical dimension of the perforation, and if a perforation remains at the end of closure, patients better tolerate a posterior perforation than an anterior one.

A low transcolumellar incision with an inverted V configuration is outlined on the columella. The nose is opened, however, not at the columella first, but laterally inside the nostrils at the caudal marginal edge of the lower lateral cartilages. The incision is then brought medially and down the lateral sides of the columella to connect to a low inverted V transcolumellar incision. The nasal envelope is then sharply elevated off of the lower and upper lateral cartilages and nasal dorsum.

Once hemostasis is achieved, the domes and medial crura are gently retracted laterally. The fibrous attachments of the medial crura are sharply dissected to gain access to the caudal septum. Bilateral mucoperichondrial flaps are then elevated (as one would for a septoplasty staying directly on the cartilage and carrying out the elevation posteriorly toward the perforation) with a Cottle elevator (Fig. 24.4A–D). Superior mucoperichondrial pockets are developed along with the flap elevation just inferior to the junction of the upper lateral cartilages and the septum. The upper lateral cartilages then are incised sharply away from the septum leaving the mucoperichondrial flap still attached to the now laterally retracted upper lateral cartilage. As a superior pocket is made, the junction of the upper lateral cartilage to the septum can be sharply transected without compromising the pedicle of the superior flap, which remains attached to the undersurface of the lower lateral cartilages. With the superior pocket created and the nasal skin elevated superiorly, the dissection proceeds posteriorly around the perforation. Next, the inferior mucoperichondrial flap is elevated, followed by elevation of the nasal floor mucosa. Once floor pockets are made bilaterally, they are connected to the septal mucoperichondrial flaps bilaterally.

The perforation is now entered anteriorly, between the two flaps, using a broad exposure technique and careful dissection. Exceptional care is taken to avoid enlargement of the perforation at this juncture. Dissection must proceed for at least a centimeter posterior to the perforation. The two or three layers of the septum must be distinctly separated from the edges of the perforation (Fig. 24.5). If circumferential granulation tissue is present at the edges of the perforation, the edges are delicately debrided. Posterior septal deviations, if present, are corrected at this time. Care must be taken to resect only the portions of cartilage and bone necessary to correct the deviation.

Most perforations will require bipedicled advancement flaps. In order to mobilize the mucosal flap that has been elevated, freeing incisions must be made laterally from posterior to anterior along the lateral nasal wall which is the medial wall of the maxillary sinus, just inferior to the inferior turbinate (Fig. 24.6A and B). Care must be taken not to use too much force for this mucosal incision since the maxillary sinus can be entered accidentally. This incision should not be advanced the entire length of the nasal cavity to the nasal sill. Instead, an anterior and posterior attachment of mucosa must remain in order to preserve the blood supply to this flap. Lateral to medial back-cut incisions should be made at the anterior and posterior borders of the flap to allow advancement of the flap while still leaving anterior and posterior attachments which provide blood supply to the bipedicled flaps. The flap mobility is then assessed for advancement (Fig. 24.7).

If the perforation cannot be closed with bilateral nasal floor advancement flaps, bilateral superior flaps are then created. A superior flap is developed by teasing the mucoperichondrium from the undersurface of the

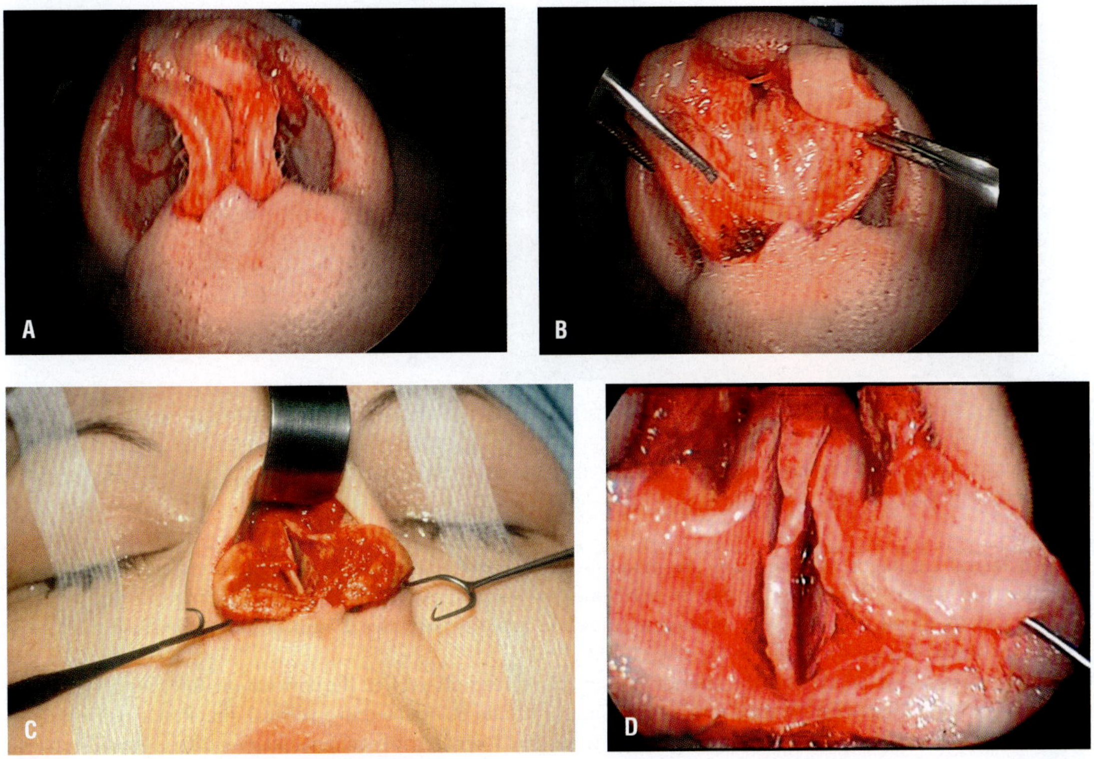

FIGURE 24.4 **A:** The open approach is used to gain access. **B:** The medial crura are separated and the caudal end of the septum is exposed. (A and B: ©Russell W.H. Kridel MD. Used with permission.) **C and D:** Dissection of mucoperichondrial flaps is carried out on both sides of the septum with care to leave the flap attached under the upper lateral cartilages which are the divided from the septum. (C: Reprinted with permission from Kridel RWH. Combined septal perforation repair with revision rhinoplasty. In: Kridel RWH, ed. Facial plastic surgery Clinics of North America. Philadelphia, PA: W.B. Saunders, 1995:462. D: Reprinted with permission from Kridel RWH, Foda H. Septal perforations. In: Papel I, ed. Facial plastic and reconstructive surgery, 4th ed. Baltimore, MA: Thieme Medical Publishers, 2016:574.)

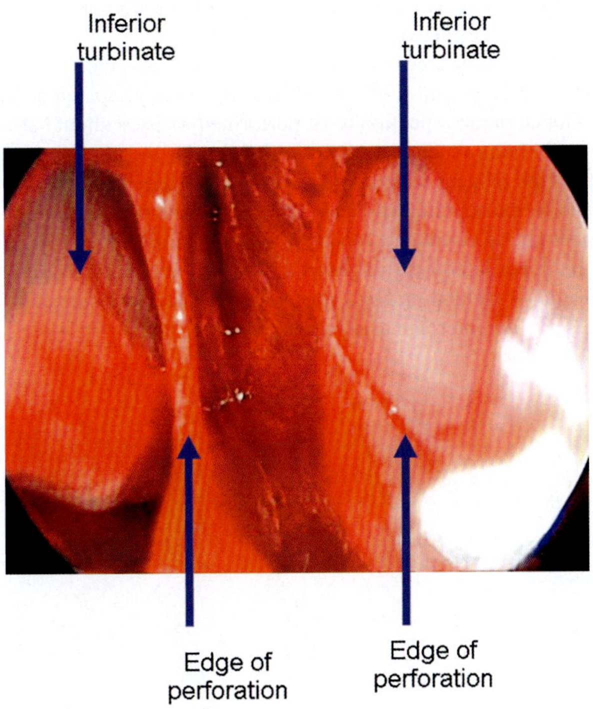

FIGURE 24.5 The septal perforation has been separated and one clearly sees the two distinct flaps, each with its own perforation (*lower arrows*). Note the absent septal cartilage. The turbinates are visible through the flap perforations (*upper arrows*). (©Russell W.H. Kridel, MD. Used with permission.)

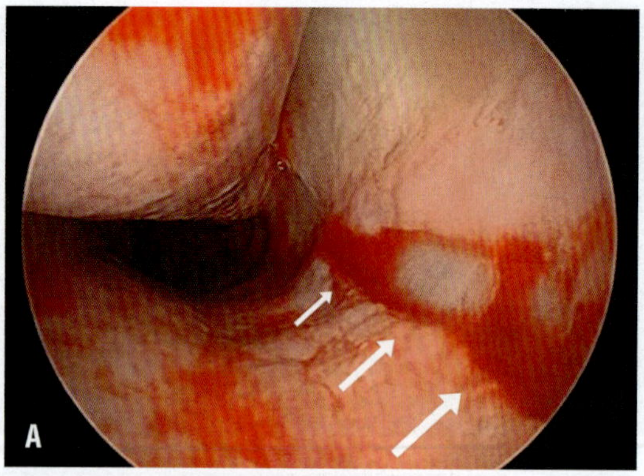

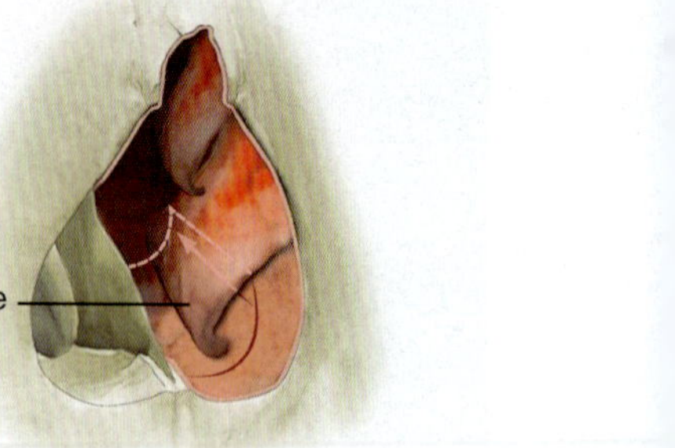

FIGURE 24.6 **A:** Endoscopic view and schematic of posterior-to-anterior incision made near the root of the inferior turbinate (*arrows*). (©Russell W.H. Kridel, MD. Used with permission.) **B:** Limited back cuts may be performed anteriorly or posteriorly to facilitate advancement of the flap. The mucosal flap from the floor of the nose can then be advanced toward the septum to close the perforation (*arrows*).

upper lateral cartilages. No incisions are made in the superior flap, since this would compromise the blood supply (Fig. 24.8). This technique can be performed on both sides without fear of stripping the cartilaginous septum of its blood supply. Every millimeter elevated actually provides 2 mm in length because the flap is dropped down. The perforation can then be closed.

The flaps are advanced from the inferior and superior directions to close the perforation. Interrupted 4-0 or 5-0 chromic or plain sutures can be used for closure. Sutures should be oriented in a vertical direction and should proceed from posterior to anterior (Fig. 24.9A and B). A piece of foil cut from suture packaging can be placed between the mucosal flaps in order to prevent catching of the contralateral flap as each individual side is sutured closed.

In some instances, the perforation cannot be closed, despite developing inferior and superior advancement flaps. In such cases, the interposition connective tissue graft prevents communication between both sides of the perforation and acts as a template for mucosal migration which may lead to closure with time. As the graft itself vascularizes, it increases the likelihood of successful closure. Anterior- or posterior-based unipedicle flaps can also be developed to aid in closure. However, this often results in further compromise in the blood supply of the mucosal flaps, which can lead to failure of the closure.

With both mucoperichondrial flaps reapproximated, the graft is now placed between the flaps. No matter the type of connective tissue barrier, the graft must be larger than the perforation, such that it overlaps the perforation peripherally. The graft is then fashioned to extend beyond the dimensions of the closed perforation and secured into place (Fig. 24.10). Because of the additional donor site morbidity associated with the harvest of the various grafts and the reduced operating room time associated with the use of acellular dermis, I often use it instead of other grafts, as it is patient friendly and cost effective.

If any cosmetic work is required, it is completed at this time. Osteotomies may be performed, dorsal humps can be reduced, or dorsal augmentation grafts can be placed (Fig. 25.12). Having already separated the upper lateral cartilages from the septum allows for dorsal hump reduction to be performed easily without harm to the continuity of the upper lateral cartilages or underlying mucosa. It also then allows for the upper lateral cartilage to be reapproximated at their new height, which reduces tension on the flap at the same time.

The upper lateral cartilages are then reattached to the septum. Spreader grafts are often used and interposed. There can be a downward traction to the upper lateral cartilages, especially if the perforation was large. To decrease tension on the flap closure, reattach the upper lateral cartilages in the normal anatomic position. Dorsal onlay and spreader grafts can help to combat any resultant pinched appearance or saddling that occurs as a consequence of the closure and can help to preserve the internal nasal valve.

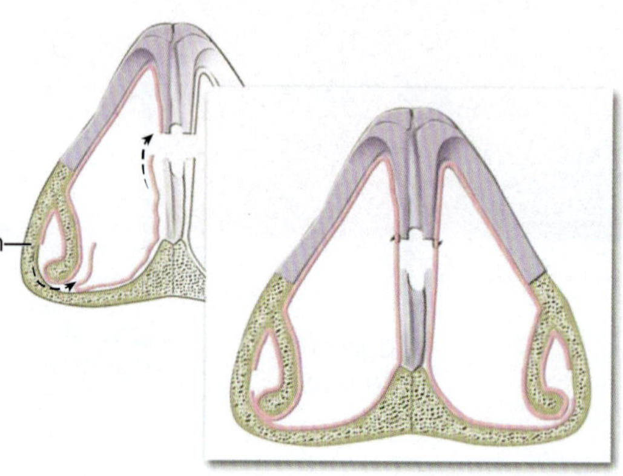

FIGURE 24.7
The inferior flap is advanced along the floor and toward the septal perforation to allow closure.

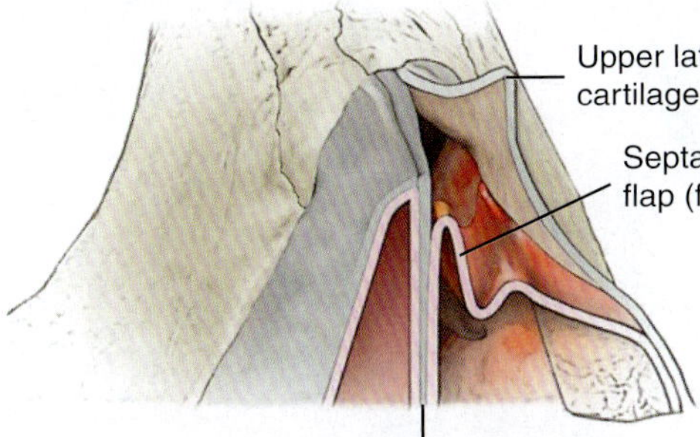

FIGURE 24.8
A superior bipedicle flap may be developed to provide more mucosal flap for closure. The mucosa is teased off the undersurface of the upper lateral cartilage.

Next, using a curved cutting needle, a 4-0 or 5-0 plain or chromic suture is used to suture the septal flaps to the interposition graft and to each other in a mattress configuration (Fig. 24.11). This helps to prevent migration of the graft and hematoma/fluid accumulation and facilitates vascularization of the graft and overall strengthening of the perforation repair.

Unwanted rotation of the nasal tip can occur as a result of closure of the perforation. Derotation of the tip can be achieved by a medial crural overlay technique or by retraction of the lower lateral cartilages to the desired point during closure of the septal perforation. Further rotation or derotation can be achieved with a columellar strut, depending on how it is fashioned and positioned. Because the medial crura have been separated completely from each other, it is important to create a pocket with sutures placed through and through the septal membranes just anterior to the caudal cartilaginous septum for a columellar strut graft to prevent posterior migration. If there is not enough remaining cartilage within the septum, cartilage from the ear or rib cartilage (autologous or irradiated) can be used for this and other grafts.

Esthetic modifications of the nasal tip may now be addressed. To prevent bossae, the domes are reapproximated with 6-0 Prolene sutures in addition to other work. The medial crura are sewn together with or without a strut with 6-0 Prolene or PDS to preserve tip projection. The nasal skin is then redraped, and meticulous closure of the columellar incision as well as marginal incisions is completed. Three individual nonabsorbable sutures anteriorly placed are used to gently approximate both Silastic sheets to the septum.

Additional light packing is placed in the nose to keep the areas of exposed bone along the nasal floor and under the inferior turbinates moist and aseptic. Absorbable gelatin (Gelfoam®Pfizer Inc., New York, NY) coated with an antibiotic cream or ointment is placed underneath the inferior turbinates, covering the sites of mucosal advancement. A light pack of nonstick dressing (Telfa™, Covidien, Dublin, Ireland) is placed to prevent collection of any clots. The nose is then taped and splinted as in a standard rhinoplasty. A drip pad is applied, as nasal discharge will continue for 24 to 72 hours. The oropharyngeal throat pack placed is removed, and the pharynx is suctioned dry, and the patient is allowed to recover from anesthesia.

POSTOPERATIVE CARE

On the first postoperative day, the nonstick dressing is removed. Gentle suctioning of some but not all of the absorbable gelatin can give some relief to the obstructed nasal cavity. Patients are instructed to use antibiotic ointment and nasal saline at least three to four times per day to keep the nasal mucosa moist and to loosen the

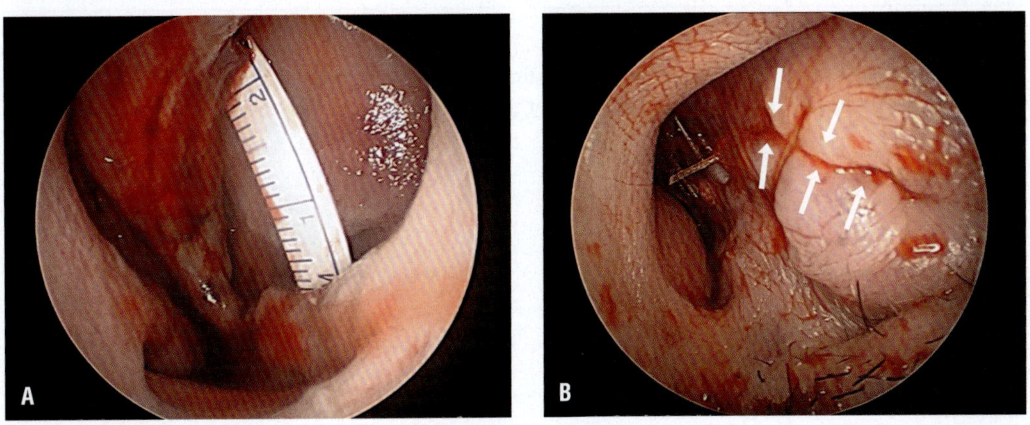

FIGURE 24.9 **A:** A large perforation prior to closure. **B:** The same perforation closed with vertical sutures from back to front. Note a small piece of acellular dermis visible through a millimeter opening in the closure line posteriorly (*arrow*). (©Russell W.H. Kridel, MD. Used with permission.)

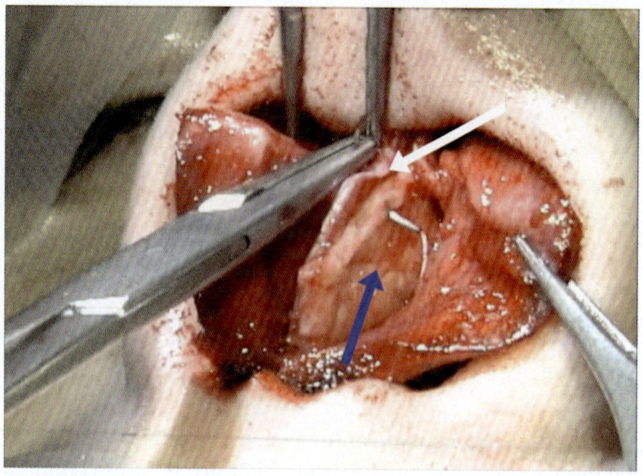

FIGURE 24.10
The connective tissue interposition graft (*blue arrow*) is secured with sutures to the remaining septal cartilage (*white arrow*). In this case, acellular dermis is used as that graft. (©Russell W.H. Kridel, MD. Used with permission.)

remaining absorbable gelatin. If the patient had a temporalis fascia graft harvested for the interposition graft, the drain is removed on the first postop day, the pressure dressing maintained for 2 or 3 more days, and the sutures are removed in 7 to 10 days.

Patients are seen frequently over the next 10 days to inspect the surgical site and gently remove the absorbable gelatin with a suction. Columellar sutures are removed on postoperative day 5. The external splint is removed on postoperative day 7, and the nose is retaped for an additional 3 to 7 days. Careful examination of the site of the perforation closure is carried out through the clear Silastic sheeting at each visit. In most cases, the Silastic sheeting may be removed after 14 days, but that time may be extended if the perforation does not appear to be fully healed. If after removing the sheeting there is still a region that is not healed, the patient is instructed to keep the area moist using antibacterial or petrolatum ointment three to four times a day along with saline drops. Crusts or scabs over the perforation closure should not be removed as they may disrupt or open the closure. It is also important to avoid aggressive suctioning of the region as well as blowing of the nose for the first month postoperatively. Patients should avoid vasoconstrictive sprays, noxious fumes, tobacco smoke, cocaine, or excessive dust. Perioperative antibiotics should be ongoing for 1 week postoperatively to prevent sinusitis secondary to inherent swelling.

COMPLICATIONS

When attempting to repair very large perforations, even with both bilateral superior and inferior flaps, total closure may not be possible. However, as long as there is an interposition graft and the perforation edges have been brought to a within a few millimeters of total closure, closure can occur over time as the mucosal edges migrate over the vascularized connective tissue graft. Moisture is very helpful in the healing process, and this can be achieved with Silastic sheeting or with topically applied petrolatum or antibiotic ointment. In the event that complete closure is not obtainable on the operative table, the perforation should be closed from anterior to posterior in order to decrease the patient's symptoms. If the perforation does not heal completely, it is often made smaller with this surgery. If necessary, a revision of this operative procedure can be undertaken 6 to 12 months later.

RESULTS

In most adult patients with an average size nose, a 1-cm perforation should be able to be closed without tension in greater than 90% of cases. Functional and esthetic appearances are interrelated when compromise of the cartilaginous framework contributes to collapse of the internal nasal airway. Some patients may only have

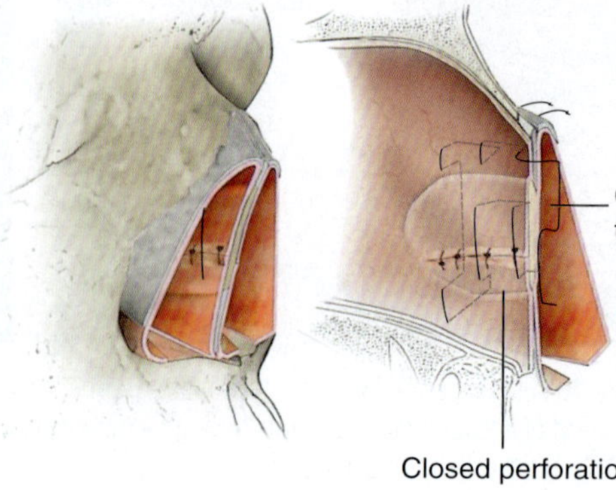

FIGURE 24.11
Once the flaps are repaired and the interposition connective tissue is placed, the septal flaps are approximated using a mattress suture.

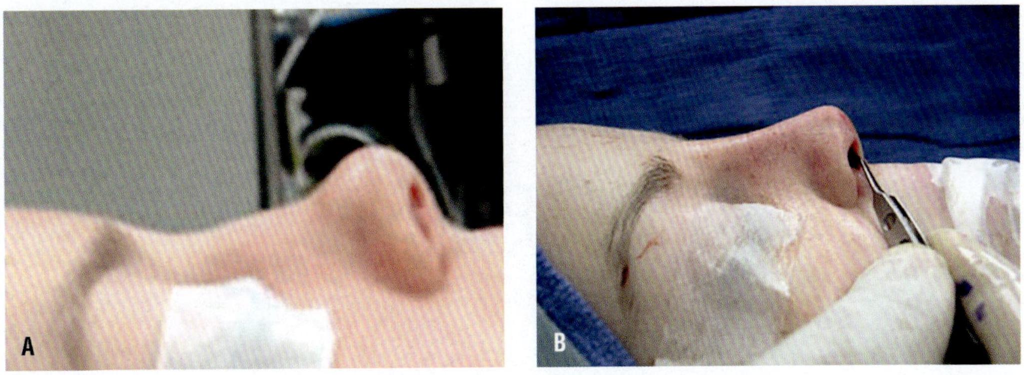

FIGURE 24.12 After closure of the perforation, rhinoplasty maneuvers may be carried out. In this instance a dorsal saddle deformity **(A)** is reconstructed with a rib cartilage dorsal sugmentation graft **(B)**. (©Russell W.H. Kridel, MD. Used with permission.)

a small perforation, while others may present with a saddle deformity (Fig. 24.12). Regardless, the essential keys in septal perforation repair are directly related to the dedicated analysis of the defect, appropriate surgical planning, and meticulous operative technique.

PEARLS

- Additional mucosa can be obtained for closure by dissecting the mucoperichondrium from the undersurface of the upper lateral cartilages and advancing the septal flaps inferiorly.
- A connective tissue interposition graft must be placed between the sewn septal flaps to enhance healing and closure as well as preventing reperforation.
- The length (from anterior to posterior) of the perforation has little bearing on the ability to obtain closure. The most important factor in perforation closure is the height of the perforation.
- Covering the perforation closure on both sides of the septum with thin Silastic sheeting maintains moisture during healing and allows the surgeon to monitor the healing process due to the transparency of the Silastic sheeting.

PITFALLS

- Failed repairs can occur when the operation is hurried or patience is lost.
- Slow, meticulous suturing is essential.
- Curved, tapered suture needles cause less damage to the tissues.
- Closing perforations in patients who continue to use cocaine is doomed to failure.
- Iatrogenic perforations are often more difficult to repair since a great deal of intervening cartilage has been removed during the previous septoplasty.
- During closure, spreader grafts may need to be considered to avoid a narrowed middle third of the nose and preserve the internal nasal valves.

INSTRUMENTS TO HAVE AVAILABLE

- Standard septorhinoplasty set
- Micro Adson tissue forceps 4¾″, 1 × 2 teeth
- Kridel delicate needle holder 6⅞″, serrated tungsten-carbide jaws (VanSickle Instruments)
- Bayonet needle holder 6½″, serrated, 14 mm fine jaws
- Castroviejo needle holder 5¾″ curved, 11 mm smooth jaws, with lock
- Castroviejo needle holder 5½″ straight, 10 mm smooth jaws, with lock

SUGGESTED READING

Kridel RK. Septal perforation presentation and reconstruction. In: Thomas JR, ed. *Advanced therapy in facial plastic and reconstructive surgery*. Shelton, CT: People's Medical Publishing House-USA, 2010:307–318, Chapter 28.

Kridel RWH. Septal perforation repair. *Otolaryngol Clin North Am* 1999;32:695–724.

Kridel RWH, Appling D, Wright W. Septal perforation closure utilizing the external septorhinoplasty approach. *Arch Otolaryngol Head Neck Surg* 1986;112:168–172.

Kridel RWH, Ashoori F, Liu ES, et al. Long-term use and follow-up of irradiated homologous costal cartilage grafts in the nose. *Arch Facial Plast Surg* 2009;11(6):378–394.

25 ASIAN RHINOPLASTY

Yong Ju Jang

INTRODUCTION

Augmentation rhinoplasty is the most commonly performed rhinoplasty in Asian countries. In addition to augmentation rhinoplasty, corrective rhinoplasty for nasal deviation and saddle, hump, and short nose deformities are also frequently conducted. In the field of Asian rhinoplasty, the main esthetic goal is to increase the size and definition of the nose. However, the unique anatomical features of the Asian nose should be seriously considered in the context of Asian rhinoplasty. Compared to a typical Caucasian nose, the typical East Asian nose tends to have thicker skin and more abundant subcutaneous soft tissue. The tip of the Asian nose is usually lower, and the lower lateral cartilages are small and weak. The nasal bones are poorly developed and thick and manifest as a low dorsum and radix. The septal cartilage is also thin and small. Therefore, the size and quantity of harvestable septal cartilage may not be adequate for complete rhinoplasty, increasing the need for harvesting grafts from other sites. The shape of the nasal tip is usually altered by tip grafting using autologous cartilage. Augmentation or camouflage of the nasal dorsum is performed using various alloplastic or biologic implant materials. Reinforcement of the septal cartilage framework is another important concept in Asian rhinoplasty used to achieve good long-term surgical outcomes.

HISTORY

When evaluating nasal obstruction, diagnostic methods such as a thorough medical history in terms of nose-related illnesses, endoscopic examination of the nasal cavity, objective airway testing, and radiologic imaging are indispensable tools for making comprehensive judgments about the cause of the ailment. For successful rhinoplasty, in addition to the above, it is critically important to also thoroughly examine the patient's personality traits. It is also extremely important to recognize in advance those patients who are more likely to experience postoperative dissatisfaction. During the preoperative consultation, the surgeon must determine whether the patient has a rational and acceptable motivation to undergo the surgery. In addition, by paying attention to minute details, the surgeon must determine whether the patient is overly anxious. It is also important to obtain information about the preexisting medical illness and history of smoking, drug abuse, or whether they are taking anticoagulants or herbal products.

PHYSICAL EXAMINATION

During the initial consultation, the shape and function of the patient's nose should be carefully examined. The overall shape of the nose, height of the nasal tip and dorsum, and thickness of the skin–soft tissue envelope should be carefully examined. Both inspection and palpation play important roles in assessing the anatomical characteristics of the nose. The nasal function and shape are closely related; therefore, a proper evaluation of nasal breathing is also important.

INDICATIONS

There are no absolute indications for cosmetic rhinoplasty. Any patient with a desire to change the shape of his/her nose can undergo rhinoplasty. However, individuals with an underprojected nasal bridge are more prone to seek rhinoplasty compared to those with a well-developed nose. A patient with a poorly defined and projected nasal tip, a consequence of underdeveloped alar cartilage combined with thick skin, is also more likely to seek rhinoplasty. Individuals with conditions such as a convex nasal dorsum, a deviated nose, a traumatic deformity, and saddle and short noses are also good candidates for rhinoplasty. However, one prerequisite for surgery is that the patient's cosmetic problem should be recognizable to others and surgically correctable.

The following are also important factors when considering rhinoplasty:

- The patient's cosmetic issue must be within the scope of the surgeon's technical skill set.
- Consensus regarding the anticipated results must be reached between the patient and the surgeon.
- The patient must be physically and psychologically fit to undergo the surgery.
- The accompanying risks of surgery must be acceptable to both the patient and the surgeon.

CONTRAINDICATIONS

Patients who are suffering from serious medical illnesses should not undergo rhinoplasty surgery. The patient's psychological fitness is a very important factor in the decision against rhinoplasty. Individuals with the following characteristics are not satisfactory candidates to undergo rhinoplasty:

- Unrealistic expectations of the surgery
- Lack of a clear understanding of the cosmetic problem
- A vague motivation for undergoing the surgery
- Displays of unreliable and exaggerated attitudes
- Communication difficulties
- Body dysmorphic disorder
- Major psychosis, such as manic-depressive illness or schizophrenia
- Excessive dissatisfaction with a prior rhinoplasty result

PREOPERATIVE PLANNING

Photo documentation of the patient's face is a critical and necessary process. During preoperative planning, the surgeon and patient should discuss the desired shape of the nose and the preferred implant or graft material. Through computer simulations, the preferred shape of the patient's external nose can be accurately determined prior to rhinoplasty; notably, this type of patient participation during the planning stage of rhinoplasty may enhance communication between the patient and the surgeon. Computer simulations also help patients who are considering rhinoplasty to gain a more realistic expectation of the surgery and to relieve anxiety. Regarding dorsal augmentation, it is important to know what type of implant or material the patient prefers. The surgeon should explain the merits and demerits of all available dorsal implantation materials and allow the patient to express his/her preference. When the surgeon anticipates the need for ear or rib cartilage harvesting, the additional morbidity and complications associated with cartilage harvesting should be explained to the patient.

SURGICAL TECHNIQUE

Nasal Tip Surgery

In my experience, the tip suture technique is not particularly useful in Asian patients, particularly those with thick nasal skin and weak alar cartilages. Instead, the tip grafting technique results in better refinement and projection in Asian patients. Septal cartilage is the preferred graft material; however, if this is insufficient, conchal or costal cartilage may also be used. In patients with extremely thick skin, costal cartilage is a useful tip grafting material.

Shield Graft

The shield graft is one of the most commonly used maneuvers for enhancing tip projection and definition in Asian patients. While carving the graft, beveling of the periphery of the graft should be performed using a knife, or the cartilage should be crushed so that the graft margin does not become visible through the skin. This procedure is particularly necessary among those with thin skin. The graft must be shaped like a shield or a ginkgo leaf, and the top part must be broad so that both ends of the top side can indicate tip-defining points. However, performing this technique may make the columellar–lobular angle blunt and infratip lobule unnaturally long, and increase the risk of excessive rotation of the tip. The leading edge of this shield graft must be slightly higher than the height of the existing dome of the tip. Usually, this technique effectively lengthens the infratip lobular segment and thereby enhances tip projection. Sometimes, the shield graft can be easily bent cephalically after skin closure, resulting in an undesired esthetic effect. To solve this problem and maintain an appropriate projection, a buttress graft should be placed immediately behind the shield graft.

Multilayer Cartilaginous Tip Grafting

Because of the diverse anatomical features of alar cartilage contours, the placement of a single shield graft is often insufficient and does not result in the desired projection and definition. To overcome the limitations of conventional tip grafting, I use multilayer tip grafting in patients with thick skin, a bulbous tip, and an underprojected shape of the tip (Fig. 25.1). Septal, conchal, tragal, and/or costal cartilage is harvested

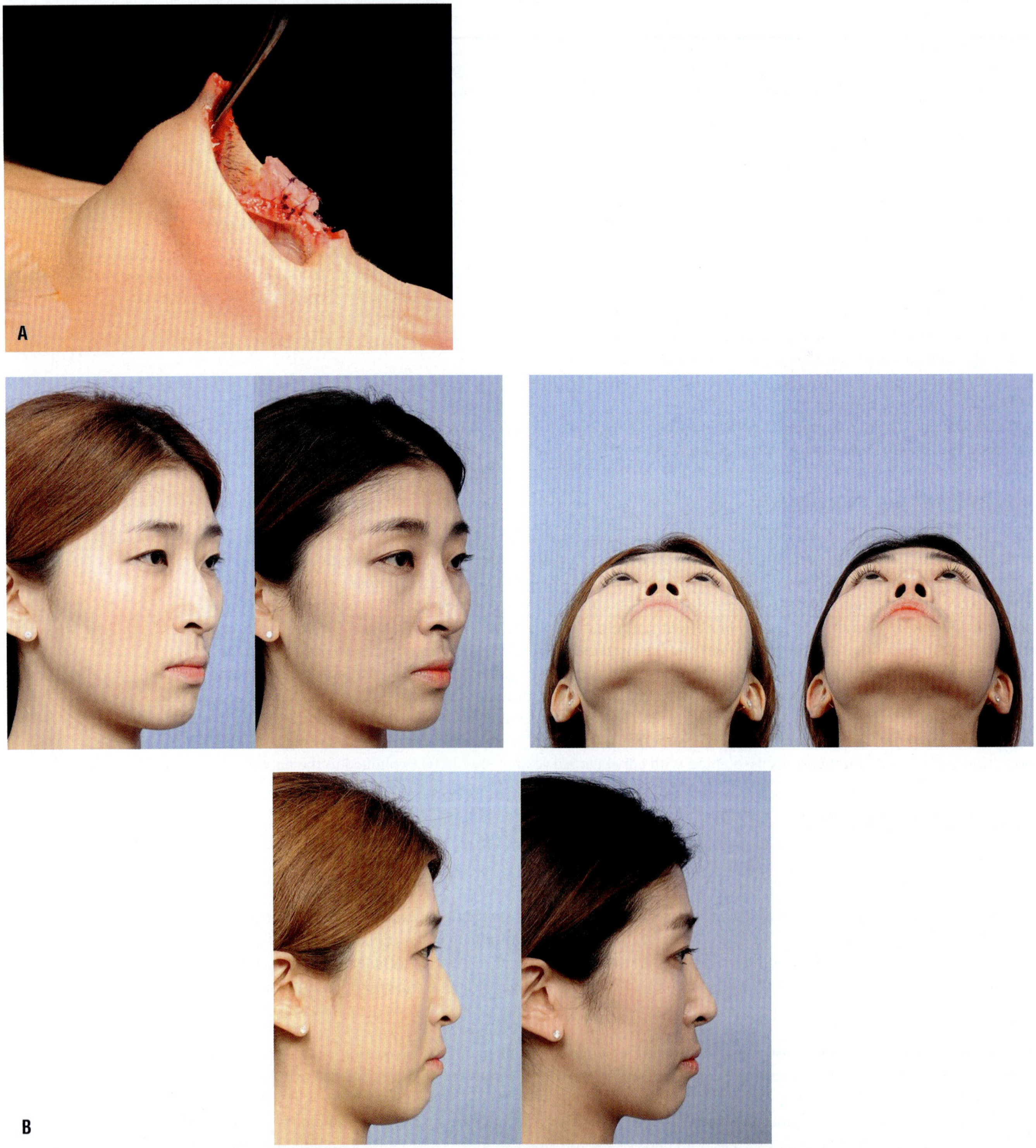

FIGURE 25.1 **A:** Intraoperative photo of multilayer tip grafting using septal cartilage. **B:** Pre- and postoperative photos of a representative case involving multilayer tip grafting.

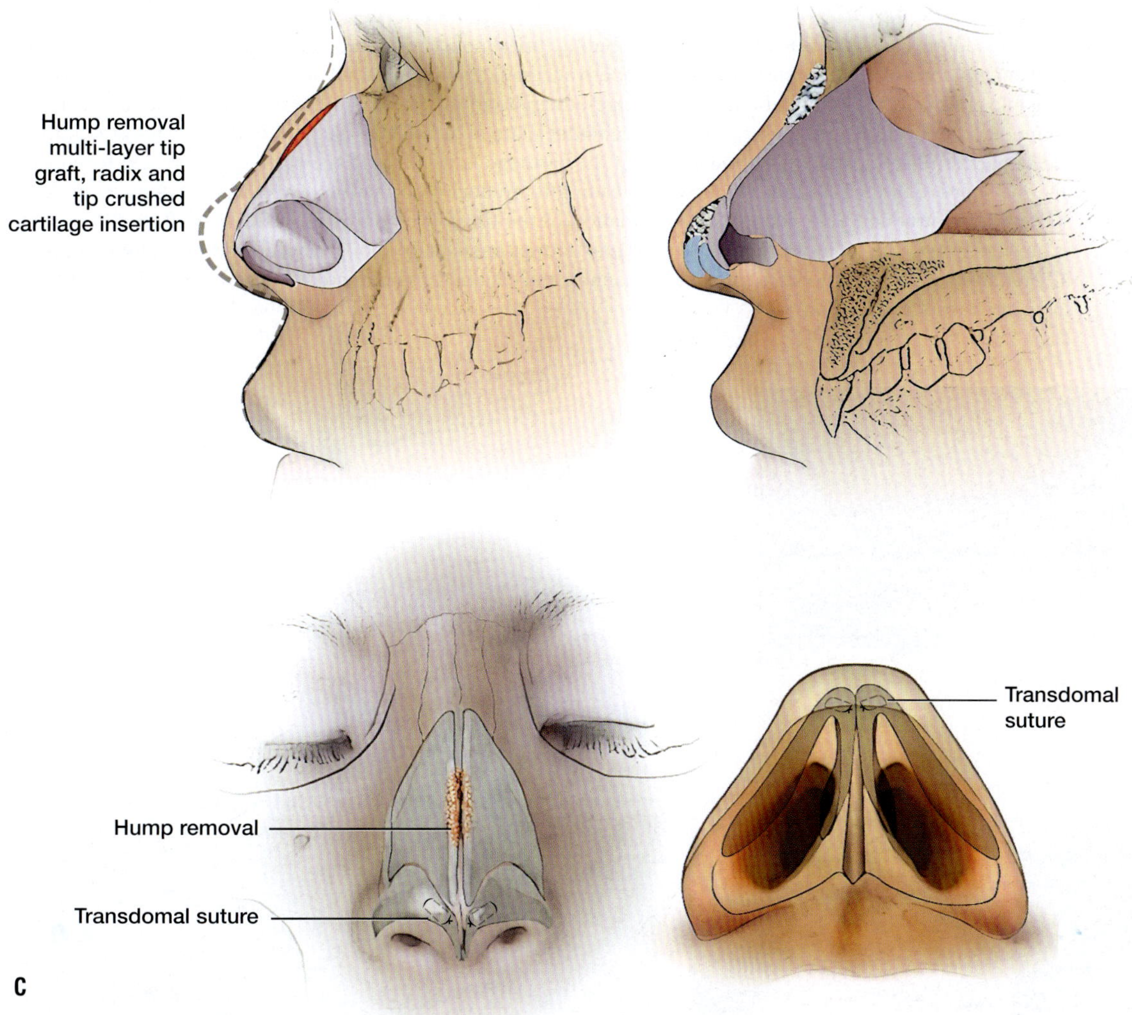

FIGURE 25.1 (*Continued*) **C:** Illustration of surgical procedures.

depending on the amount of cartilage required and the quality and amount of nasal septal cartilage available in the patient. Where necessary, caudal extension of the septum, columellar strut placement, dome suturing, and/or trimming of skin–soft tissue envelope is performed prior to the multilayer tip grafting. Following these procedures, the first cartilaginous shield graft layer is placed on the dome and secured with 5-0 PDS suture. Additional shield graft layers are then placed on top of the first layer. The more caudal layer is placed so that its leading (superior) edge is always higher than the height of the existing dome and the layer(s) beneath it. The numbers of graft layers applied depends on how much projection is required and is determined intraoperatively. The horizontal width of the shield graft is adjusted according to the thickness of the tip. For thin skin, the horizontal width should be wider to provide better tip definition. For thick skin, a narrower width provided better results. Meticulous smoothing of graft margins with gentle carving is important to provide a smooth tip. Similar to shield grafts, a buttress graft is required in many cases. This technique is fairly versatile and can easily adjust the tip projection vector, which is particularly useful for nasal lengthening. Complications associated with this technique include transient tip erythema, infection, visible graft contours with delayed-onset skin erythema, nostril deformity, and overprojection.

Onlay Tip Grafting

Onlay tip grafting is a procedure during which one or several graft layers are horizontally placed on the dome of the tip (Fig. 25.2). When performing rhinoplasty on Asian patients, stacked onlay graft placement on the domal portion of the tip is frequently combined with dorsal augmentation using an alloplastic implant material. Graft visibility is a common complication. To prevent graft visibility, the width of the graft should be almost equal to that of the domal portion of the tip and the graft margin should be properly smoothed.

Septal Extension Graft

This procedure can have various effects, including tip support reinforcement, tip projection and rotation adjustment, dorsal length extension, columellar advancement, and nasolabial angle improvement. Because this invisible graft is located within both alar cartilages, the risks of tip graft visibility or dermal thinning, which are common complications of other tip grafting techniques, are avoided. For successful septal extension grafting, the septal cartilage must be thick and strong; if the cartilage is weak, both the cartilage harvested for grafting and the supporting L-strut will also be weak, leading to gradual deformation of the septal extension graft and supporting L-strut and deprojection or deformation of the tip. 5-0 nylon or 5-0 PDS is used to fix the septal extension graft to the septal cartilage. Three to four sutures are usually enough, but a locking suture is occasionally required at the transitional area of dorsal septum and caudal septum in order to prevent rotation of the graft in an anterocaudal direction.

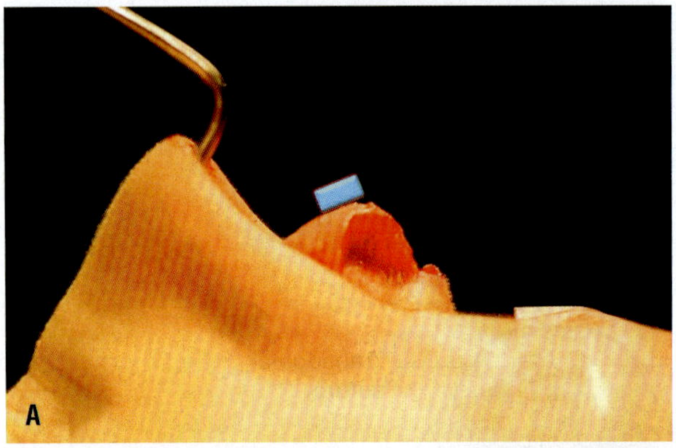

A

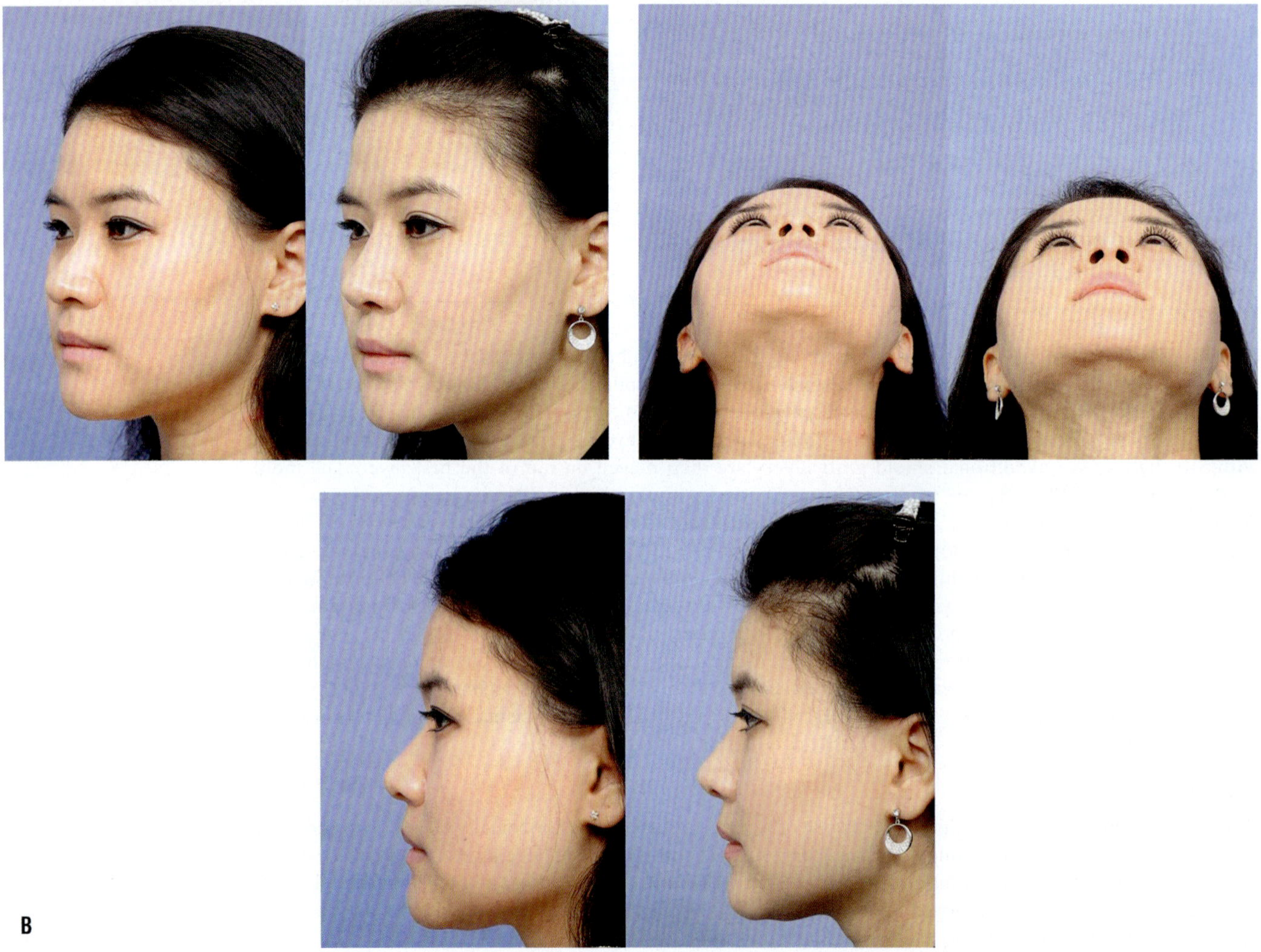

B

FIGURE 25.2 **A:** Tip onlay tip grafting. **B:** Pre- and postoperative photos of a representative case of multilayer tip grafting.

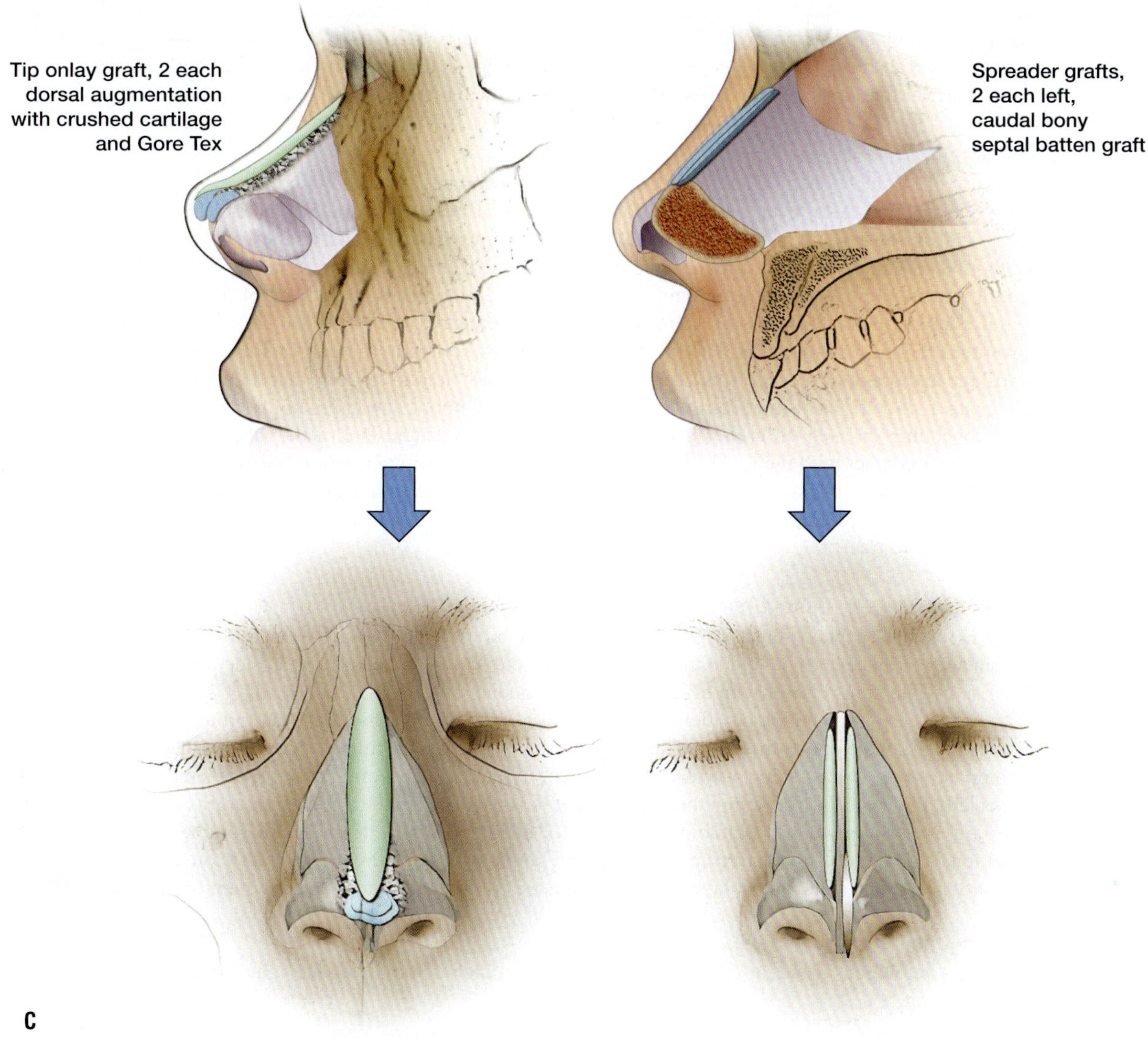

FIGURE 25.2 (*Continued*) **C:** Illustration of surgical procedures.

After suturing, the surgeon must gently press the graft with a finger to test the strength of the fixation. It is better to trim or remove parts of the graft that are not useful for fixation and may cause nasal obstruction. The caudal end of the septal extension graft is usually connected to the caudal border on both sides of the alar cartilages, but it can also be connected to the cephalic border or the middle part of the alar cartilages if needed. One or two buried sutures using nonabsorbable suture material such as 5-0 nylon are usually enough for proper fixation. Using absorbable suture such as 4-0 Vicryl at the membranous septum to further fix the graft will result in stronger fixation and can remove dead space. While the septal extension graft has many advantages, it also has many limitations. For example, this type of graft frequently creates supratip deformities. Other complications associated with the septal extension graft include nasal tip stiffness, secondary nasal obstruction, deformed nostril due to septal buckling, and tip deprojection and rotation.

Dorsal Augmentation

Dorsal augmentation is the most commonly addressed issue in Asian rhinoplasty. In all types of rhinoplasty, including simple cosmetic rhinoplasty, this maneuver is critically important for the achievement of esthetic perfection, which is determined by the height and shape of the nasal dorsum as seen from the side and front as well as harmonious alignment with the nasal tip. During dorsal augmentation, it is important to set an ideal nasal starting point that corresponds to the cephalic end of the implant. The cephalic end of the implant is ideally located near (or immediately above) the horizontal midpupillary line for women and between the upper eyelashes and eyelid crease for men. If the dorsal implant is too wide, the risk of displacement or implant visibility is relatively lower, but the dorsal line will appear masculine and esthetically less pleasing. If the dorsal implant is too narrow in the radix area, the risk of implant visibility or deviation will increase. Unlike rhinoplasty in

Caucasian patients, where the use of alloplastic implants (particularly silicone) on the nasal dorsum is avoided, alloplastic implants play an important role in Asian rhinoplasty because of differences in anatomical characteristics such as thick skin and a poorly developed cartilaginous framework. There is no single ideal implant or graft material for dorsal augmentation. However, the following materials are commonly used.

Silicone

Because of its stable chemical structure, silicone has several advantages, including easy handling and a lack of tissue reaction. Moreover, its application is convenient because of the availability of ready-made products, and its relative hardness makes it suitable for forming desired nasal shapes for application in Asians with moderate to thick skin. Silicone should preferably be trimmed to approximately 3.5 to 4.0 cm in length and 8 mm in width, with edges as thin as possible. When modifying the shape of the implant, most cases require the implant's thickness to decrease and become concave around the rhinion, because the nasal bone protrudes the most in that area. The lower part of the nasal dorsum, the part that carries through to the alar cartilage and dome of the tip, from the anterior septal angle area, is an area that requires great care in order to create a smooth, ideal line from the dorsum to the tip without any gaps. Implant design of this area differs depending on each different tip surgery technique. The caudal end of the silicone implant should not be in direct contact with the tip skin. Complications following silicone implantation include implant deviation, floating, displacement, extrusion, impending extrusion, infection, and skin contraction. Among delayed complications, contraction of the skin–soft tissue envelope, resulting in a short nose, is relatively common and difficult to treat.

Expanded Polytetrafluoroethylene (ePTFE, Gore-Tex)

ePTFE implants contain micropores that induce surrounding tissue to grow inward through the pores; the advantages of this material include increased stability and a lower incidence of capsule formation. In addition, the risk of extrusion is lower with ePTFE than with silicone

When designing a thick augmentation material of over 4 to 6 mm height, design the bottom sheet wide enough to make the entire cross-section a trapezoid shape. After stacking to the appropriate height, the sheets should be suture-fixated using 4-0 PDS, 5-0 PDS, or nylon. Good beveling of the sheet's margins is essential, especially for sheets of over 2 mm thickness. If not beveled enough, the implant's margins can be felt through the skin after surgery. One notable disadvantage of ePTFE is that it decreases in volume after insertion. In addition, it is more difficult to remove an ePTFE implant than a silicone implant from the nasal dorsum. Deviation, displacement, and delayed inflammation are complications associated with the use of this material.

Autologous Cartilage

Common autologous tissues used in dorsal augmentation include septal, conchal, and costal cartilages, fascia, and dermofat.

Septal cartilage. Because it is difficult to obtain a sufficiently long piece of cartilage (3 to 4 cm) for dorsal augmentation, it is uncommon to use a single piece of septal cartilage as the dorsal augmentation material. Usually, the remaining piece of cartilage after structural or tip grafting is crushed and used to fill regional depressions or uneven areas in the nasal dorsum or tip.

Conchal cartilage. Unlike septal cartilage, conchal cartilage has an intrinsic curvature that hinders its routine use in dorsal augmentation. In addition, conchal cartilage is usually too small to yield a single piece suitable for dorsal augmentation. Therefore, ear cartilage is frequently used in the form of diced cartilage wrapped with fascia and has thus achieved wide acceptance as the ideal dorsal augmentation technique. Another option is the use of diced conchal cartilage with perichondrial attachment (DCCP). In cases involving partial concavity or saddle in the nasal dorsum, partial dorsal augmentation can be properly achieved by dicing the cartilage to which the perichondrium of the harvested conchal cartilage remains attached, thereby ensuring attachment of the diced pieces to the intact perichondrium (Fig. 25.3). Attachment of the perichondrium

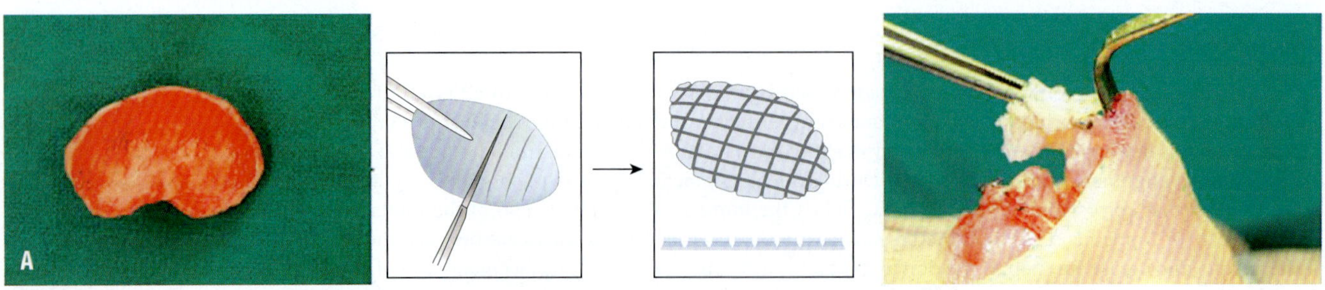

FIGURE 25.3 A: Diced conchal cartilage with perichondrial attachment.

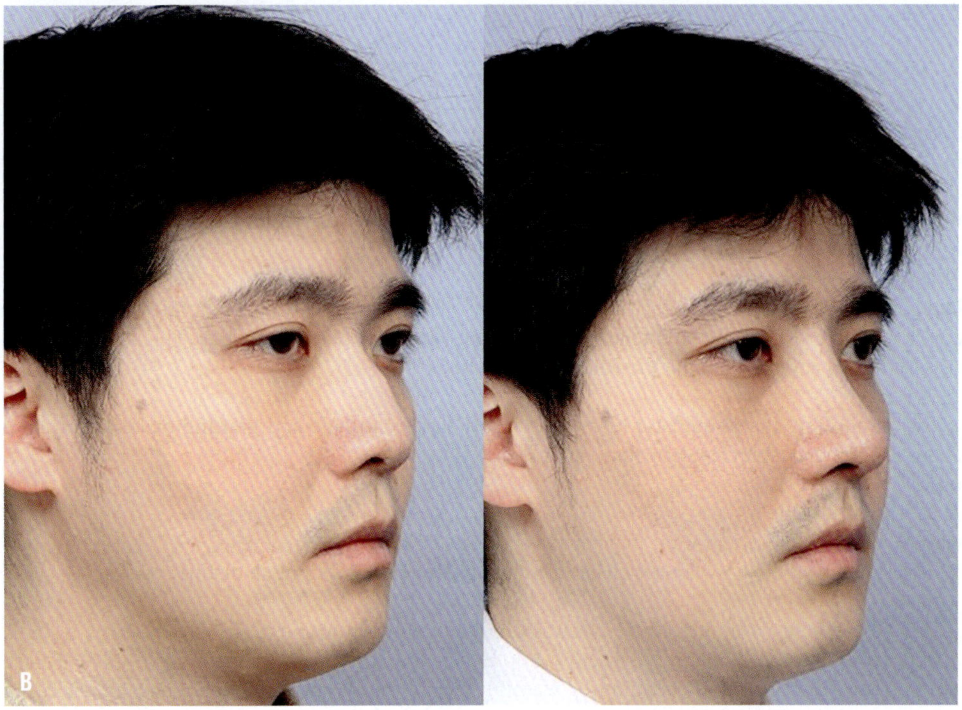

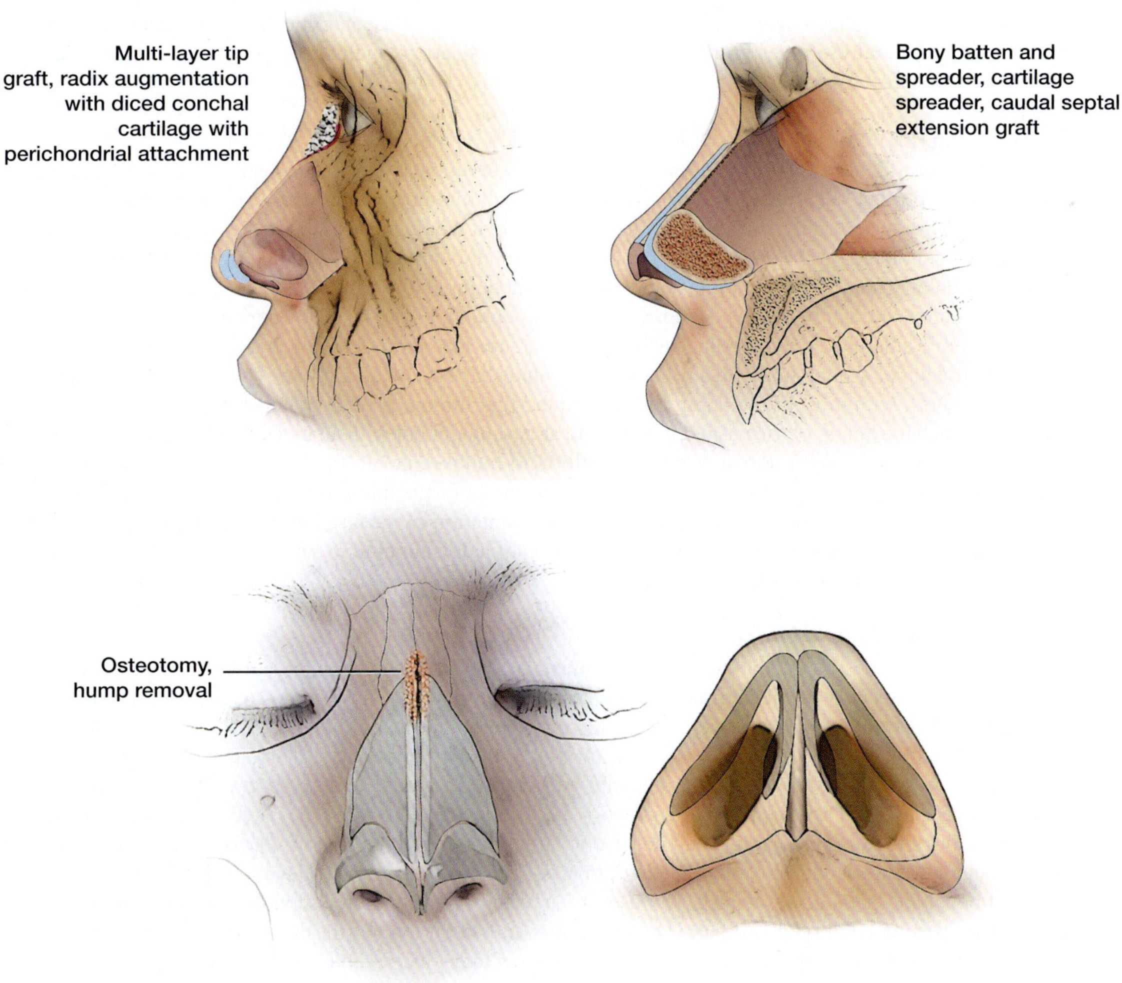

C

FIGURE 25.3 (*Continued*) **B:** Pre- and postoperative photos of a representative case involving radix augmentation using diced conchal cartilage with perichondrial attachment. **C:** Illustration of surgical procedures.

during conchal cartilage harvesting can result in an adequate graft shape and a migration-free tendency, which can be fixed and fitted without sutures onto the nasal dorsum and radix by manual molding and placement over the skin. The major limitation of DCCP is the insufficiency of material for substantial dorsal augmentation. Nevertheless, DCCP is useful and features several advantages with respect to augmenting the nasal dorsum, radix, and/or tip via rhinoplasty, including (1) autologous tissue composition, (2) soft texture, (3) easy manipulation, (4) lack of requirement for suture fixation, (5) lower risk of resorption, and (6) high resistance to infection.

Costal cartilage. Costal cartilage is one of the most useful types of autologous cartilage for patients who require substantial augmentation or who have experienced complications with alloplastic implants. This material is the primary choice for dorsal augmentation in the following situations:

- Reconstructive rhinoplasty that requires a large amount of sturdy cartilage and grafting material for nasal septum reconstruction due to severe deformation
- Saddle nose
- Short nose
- Patients who have a small nose and want major changes (Fig. 25.4)
- Patients with very thick skin who want a well-defined and projected nasal tip with distinct contours

Costal cartilage can be used in three different ways in the nasal dorsum. First, it can be used as a single piece with a well-carved form. Although this seems simple, it is not particularly easy to carve this cartilage well, and there is a possibility of graft bending or warping during the postoperative period. Second, costal cartilage can be used as a multilayered laminated form. This graft is thought to have a lower risk of warping or bending than the above-described costal cartilage dorsal graft monounit. Third, costal cartilage can be crushed to a thin, soft texture and can then be placed on the dorsum with or without fibrin sealant or fascia. In my experience, the overall complication and revision rates of rhinoplasties that use autologous costal cartilage are much higher than those that use other graft materials. These complications include warping, contour irregularities, resorption, and infection.

Dorsal Hump Reduction in Asian Patients

Although the prevalence of a dorsal hump is relatively lower among Asians than Caucasians, a fair number of Asian patients present with this unwanted feature. When examining a patient's nose, a typical dorsal hump, as well as a hump-like deformity, may be identified. Therefore, it would be desirable to define such a deformity as a convex nasal dorsum. In the Asian nose, the convex nasal dorsum can be classified into three types: generalized dorsal hump, isolated dorsal hump, and relative dorsal hump with a low tip. A generalized hump represents the typical hump commonly observed among Caucasian populations, in which the curvature of the hump begins from the bony vault and extends to the cartilaginous dorsum in a gentle curve. An isolated hump indicates an abrupt protrusion of a small hump in a triangular or round shape at the dorsal line. The total length of this type of hump is short, with most of the hump located around the rhinion. A relative hump with a low tip describes humps in which the height of the nasal dorsum is not so prominent but with an underdeveloped nasal tip, giving a false impression of a nasal dorsal hump. In addition to hump removal, tip surgery and radix augmentation are very important procedures for the successful management of the hump nose in Asian patients (Fig. 25.5). In most cases of a convex nasal dorsum, substantial augmentation of the nasal tip is a prerequisite to ensure an esthetically successful surgery. Therefore, the correction of a dorsal hump in Asian patients requires a redistribution surgery rather than simple reduction.

Correction of the Deviated Nose

The surgical principles applicable to the management of the bony and middle vaults and lower third of the Caucasian nose are also applicable to the correction of the deviated nose in Asian patients. However, one challenge associated with the management of this problem is that many patients lack a sufficient amount of septal cartilage for simultaneous use in septal framework reconstruction, tip surgery, and dorsal augmentation. In addition, the septal cartilage is generally thin and weak. Therefore, the surgeon must frequently harvest additional cartilage to ensure complete correction and reinforcement of the deviated nose. Septal bone is a particularly useful graft material that can be used to strengthen the septal L-strut. Performing a septoplasty for the deviated nose involves harvesting the central part of the quadrangular cartilage, perpendicular plate of the ethmoid bone, and parts of the vomer. The use of harvested septal bone for septal correction will reduce the need for harvesting additional cartilage. Using scissors and an otologic drill, the harvested bone is made into an appropriate size and shape. Next, a number of holes (as many as possible) are drilled using a small burr to facilitate suturing (Fig. 25.6). Prior to surgical treatment, the surgeon must carefully evaluate the presence of facial asymmetry, which could considerably limit the ability to achieve a successful surgical result. In addition, many patients undergoing correction of a deviated nose also request dorsal augmentation to enhance the cosmetic result. Accordingly, dorsal augmentation may be considered an important step in the correction of the deviated Asian nose.

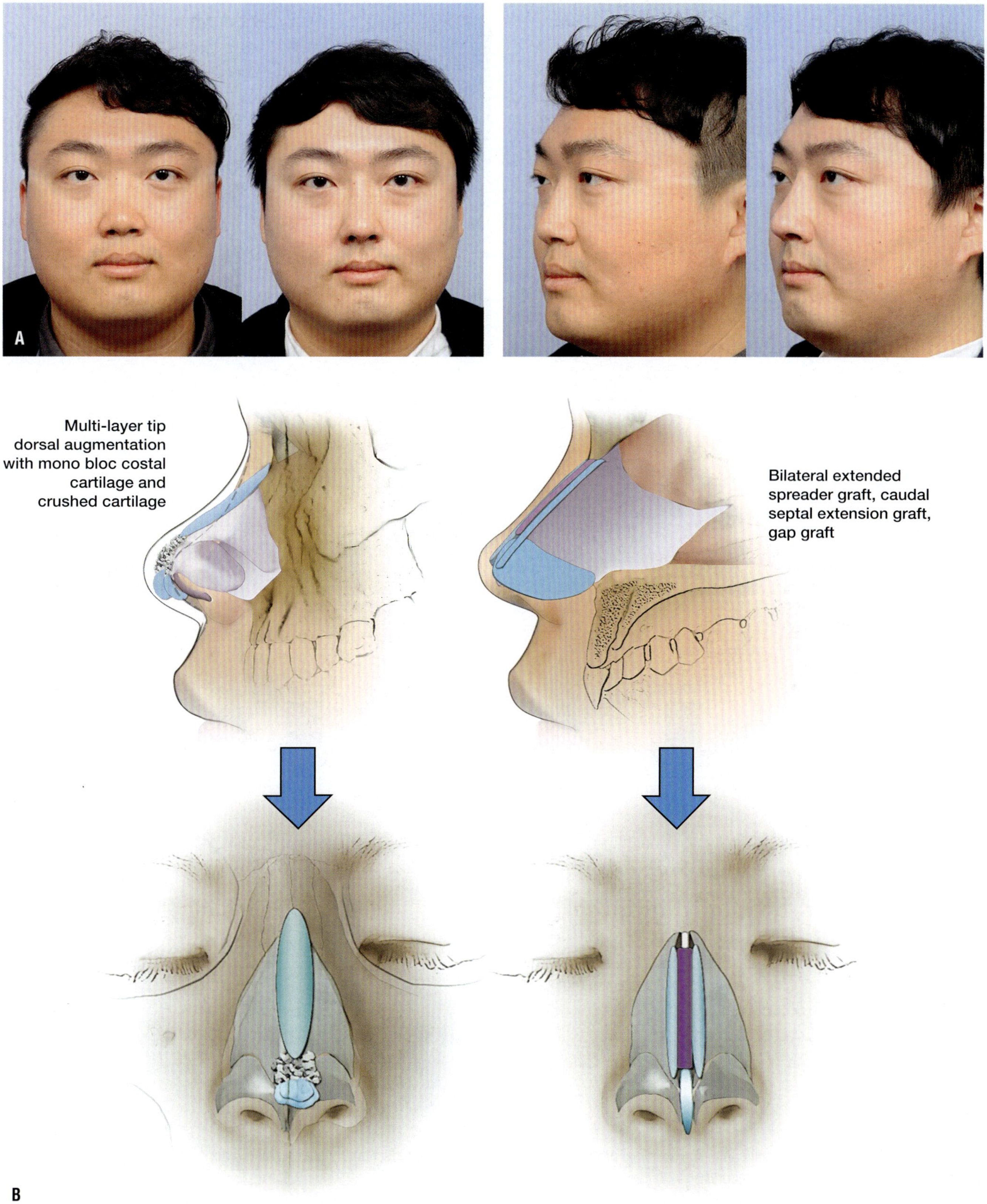

FIGURE 25.4 **A:** A patient with small nose who underwent augmentation rhinoplasty using costal cartilage. **B:** Illustration of surgical procedures.

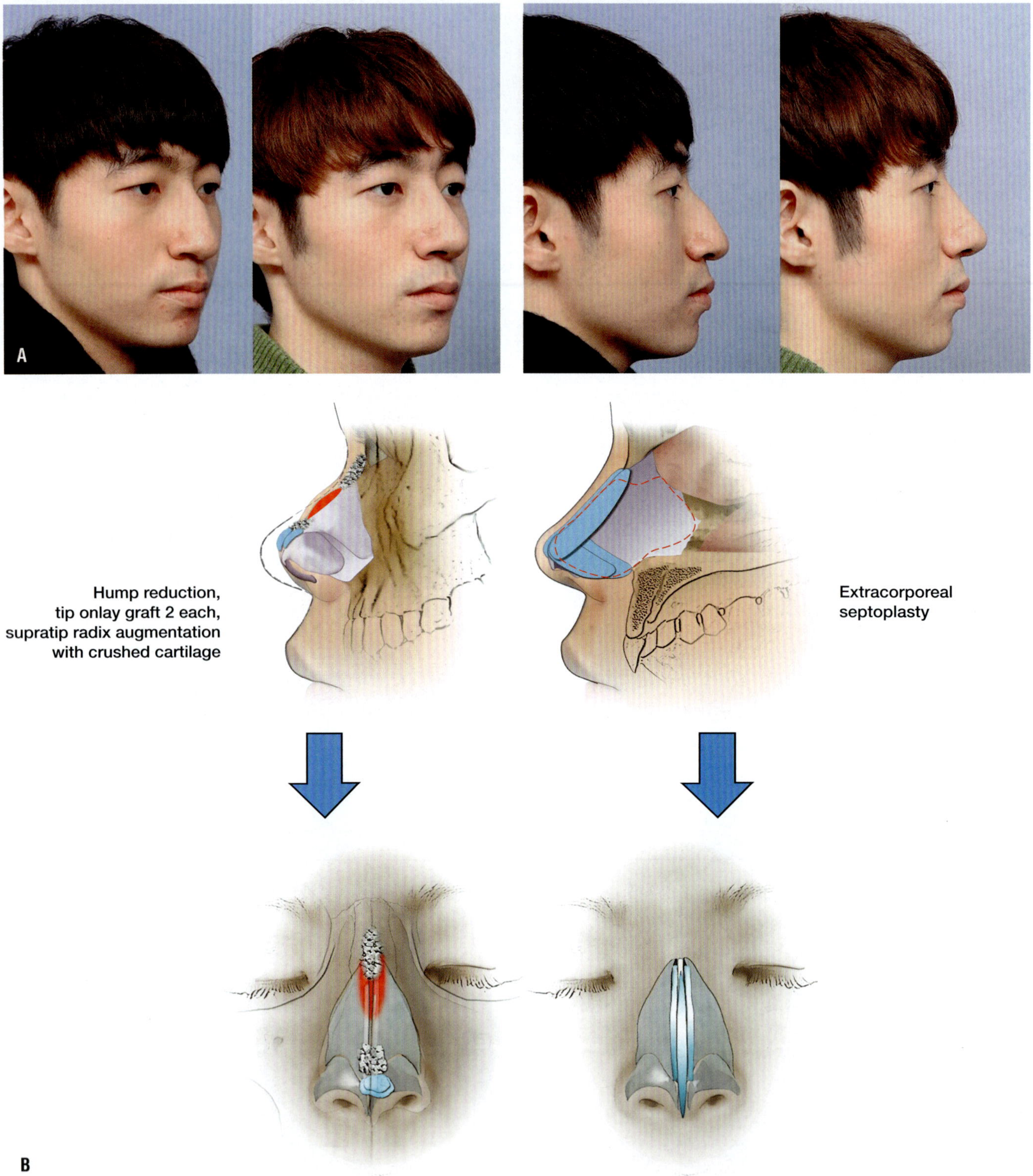

FIGURE 25.5 A patient with a dorsal hump. **A:** His dorsal profile was improved after hump reduction, tip grafting, and radix grafting. **B:** Illustration of surgical procedures.

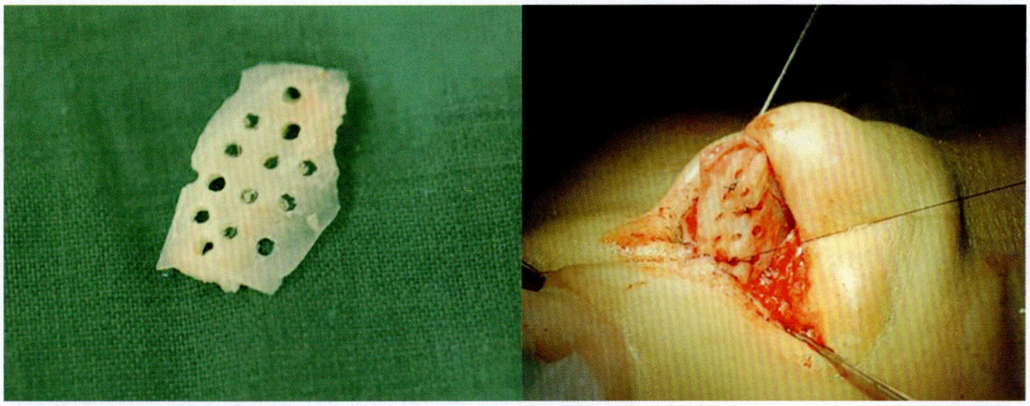

FIGURE 25.6 Intraoperative photo of a bony batten graft placed at the caudal septum.

Correction of a Short Nose

A short nose commonly occurs as a long-term complication of rhinoplasty with silicone implants or fascia grafts or the collapse of nasal supporting structures due to overaggressive removal of septal cartilage during primary rhinoplasty. Successful correction of a short nose can be achieved by extending the internal framework (internal lining) of the nasal cavity and the external soft tissue envelope. In my experience, nasal septal reconstruction using autologous or homologous costal cartilage has superior results. Among the various septal reconstruction techniques, the placement of extended spreader grafts on both sides of the dorsal strut and a caudal extension graft between the extended spreader grafts is most useful and reliable (Fig. 25.7). The nose appears to be shorter when the dorsum has a concave appearance. Therefore, dorsal augmentation is a crucial surgical procedure as the nose will appear longer after the correction of the dorsal concavity. Because many patients have a short nose resulting from silicone-related complications, the removal of the silicone implant and replacement with a different material is necessary. Nasal tip surgery also plays an important role in the final lengthening process. During correction of the short nose, if the overlying skin has become severely thickened and lost its normal elasticity because of repeated inflammation and contraction, the lengthened nasal skeleton cannot be adequately redraped with skin. In that case, secondary tip grafting or dorsal augmentation can be performed later once the incision has healed completely.

POSTOPERATIVE MANAGEMENT

At the conclusion of surgery, it is of utmost importance to verify that hemostasis is properly performed. If bleeding persists at the osteotomy site, hemostasis should be performed by applying pressure using a finger to the affected area for a few minutes. The use of an absorbable packing material can reduce the patient's discomfort and issues related to excessive packing. If a septoplasty is performed as a part of the rhinoplasty, the placement of a silastic septal splint is recommended. When skin closure and nasal packing have been completed, the exterior of the nose must be stabilized using an external splint such as plaster of Paris, Denver splint, or Aquasplint. Most patients display the maximum degree of edema and ecchymosis on the first postoperative day. To prevent severe edema, I prescribe 5 mg of intravenous dexamethasone on the day of surgery or the first day after surgery. If the edema is severe, an ice pack can be used for massage. Antibiotics are administered intravenously a few hours prior to and after surgery. Sutures of the transcolumellar incision, septal splint, and external splints are removed 5 to 6 days after surgery. If localized edema or a protruding area is discovered after the external splint is removed, the surgeon can correct the shape using gentle massage and re-taping or placing a new external splint for approximately 1 week. Despite the absence of published evidence, in cases with excessive tension on the transcolumellar suture and the use of costal cartilage grafts under a tight skin–soft tissue envelope, hyperbaric oxygen can be a helpful option for preventing postoperative wound complications and infection. Outpatient follow-up should also be performed frequently. Finally, patients should be educated to recognize the various signs and symptoms that accompany infection and should be instructed to visit the hospital at the first suspicion of infection.

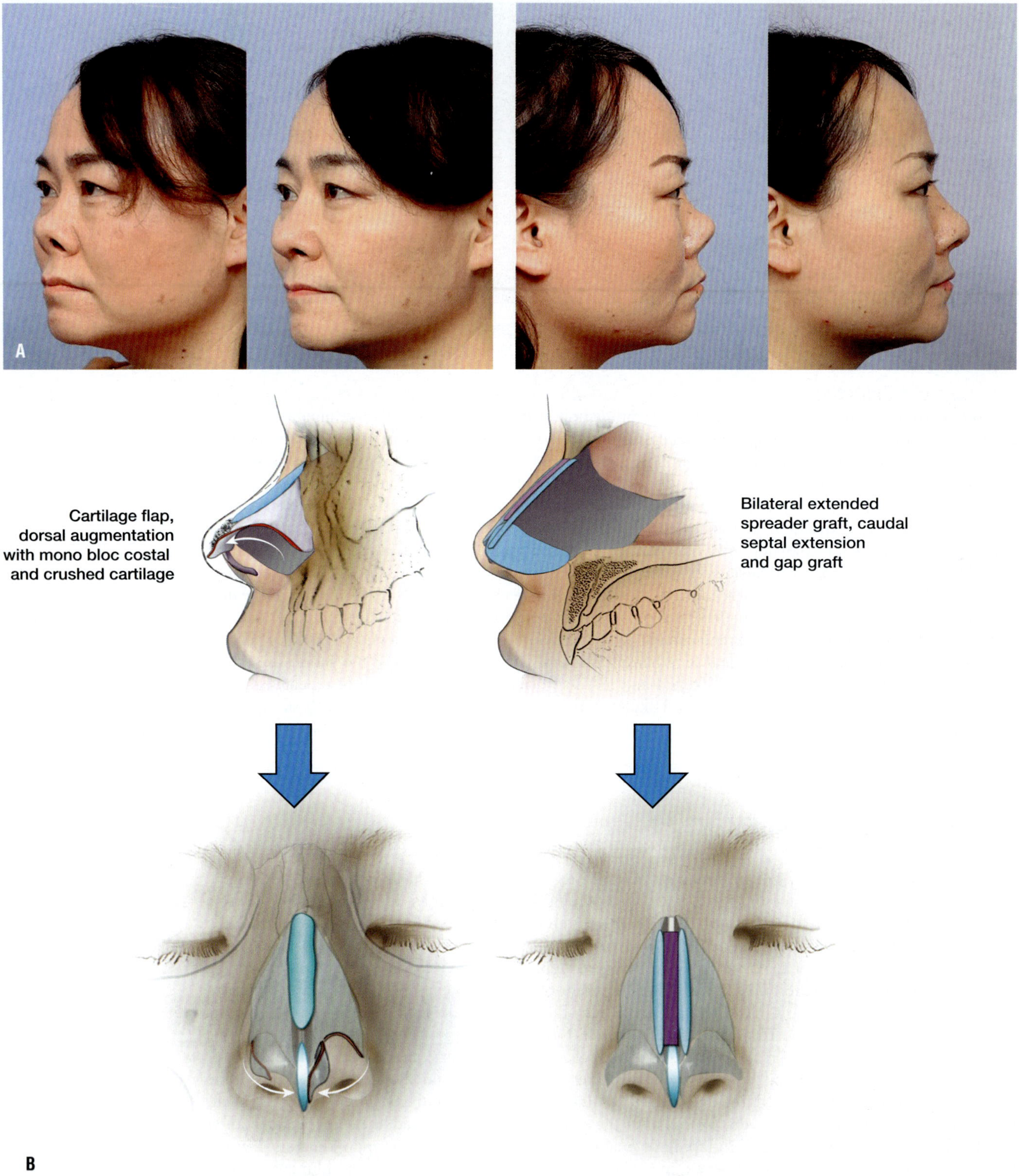

FIGURE 25.7 **A:** A typical patient with short nose caused by silicone insertion during primary surgery; this deformity was corrected by septum elongation, dorsal augmentation, and tip grafting. **B:** Illustration of surgical procedures.

COMPLICATIONS

I have experienced the following complications:

- Suboptimal cosmetic outcome
- Displacement, malposition, infection, and extrusion of the dorsal implant
- Short nose
- Warping and visible contour of the costal cartilage on the nasal dorsum
- Contour irregularity due to resorption of the fascia or cartilage on the dorsum
- Residual and recurrent deviation following correction of the deviated nose
- Minor dorsal saddle deformity
- Undercorrection of the convex nasal dorsum
- Visible tip graft contour, overprojected tip
- Tip graft infection
- Persistent or newly developed nasal obstruction

RESULTS

I recently analyzed the revision rate for my patients undergoing rhinoplasty. The determined revision rate of 8.9% includes major revisions and minor procedures for scar issues.

PEARLS

- Computer simulation for rhinoplasty is an invaluable tool that can help patients undergoing rhinoplasty gain a more realistic expectation of the surgery and can facilitate better communication with the surgeon.
- Tip grafting techniques are the mainstay of better refinement and projection of the tip in Asian patients.
- Multilayer tip grafting is fairly versatile and can easily adjust the tip projection vector, which is particularly useful for lengthening the nose.
- Alloplastic implants play an important role in Asian rhinoplasty and are widely accepted by a majority of surgeons as the first-choice implant for simple cosmetic rhinoplasty.
- Diced cartilage with perichondrial attachment is a useful dorsal implant material.
- Costal cartilage can be used at the dorsum in the following forms: well-carved monoblock, laminated multilayer, and crushed.
- The convex nasal dorsum in Asian noses can be classified into three types: generalized hump, isolated hump, and relative hump with a low tip.
- In the cartilage-deficient Asian nose, the septal bone is useful as a septal batten grafting material for the correction of a deviated septum.
- Among the various septal reconstruction techniques for correction of the short nose, the placement of extended spreader grafts on both sides of the dorsal strut and of a caudal extension graft between the extended spreader grafts is most useful and reliable.

PITFALLS

- While the septal extension graft has many advantages, it is also associated with complications such as supratip deformity, nasal tip stiffness, secondary nasal obstruction, deformed nostril due to septal buckling, and tip deprojection and rotation.
- One of the most serious complications observed in the field of Asian rhinoplasty is a short nose following capsular contracture around a dorsal silicone implant.
- The surgeon should be aware that the overall complication and revision rates are higher after rhinoplasties that use autologous costal cartilage than those that use other graft materials.
- Substantial nasal tip augmentation is a prerequisite to achieve an esthetically successful surgery in most cases of a convex dorsum.
- Before proceeding with the correction of the deviated nose, the surgeon should carefully evaluate the presence of facial asymmetry, which would considerably limit the ability to achieve a successful surgical outcome.
- During correction of a short nose, if the damaged skin–soft tissue envelope does not allow tension-free closure of the transcolumellar incision, the elongated central segment should be reshortened and a second-stage surgery should be planned.

INSTRUMENTS TO HAVE AVAILABLE

- Aufricht nasal retractor
- Converse scissors
- Joseph periosteal elevator
- Adson forceps
- Cottle cartilage crusher morselizer
- Sheen cartilage grid
- Osteotomes (curved, straight 2, 3 mm)
- Fomon rasp
- Cottle nasal speculum
- Iris scissors (curved, straight)
- Mallet
- Killian nasal gouge
- Freer elevator
- Gorney septum suction elevator
- Scalpel blades (no. 10, 11, 15) and handle
- Skin hook (single and double)
- Bayonet forceps
- Frazier suction tube (12Fr)
- Baron suction tube (5Fr)
- Nasal septum bone cutting forceps

ACKNOWLEDGMENT

The author would like to acknowledge Yeon Hee Joo, MD, for her contributions in writing this chapter.

SUGGESTED READING

Cho GS, Jang YJ. Deviated nose correction: different outcomes according to the deviation type. *Laryngoscope* 2013;123(5):1136–1142.

Jang YJ, Alfanta EM. Rhinoplasty in the Asian nose. *Facial Plast Surg Clin North Am* 2014;22(3):357–377.

Jang YJ, Kim JH. Classification of convex nasal dorsum deformities in Asian patients and treatment outcomes. *J Plast Reconstr Aesthet Surg* 2011;64(3):301–306.

Jang YJ, Moon BJ. State of the art in augmentation rhinoplasty: implant or graft? *Curr Opin Otolaryngol Head Neck Surg* 2012;20(4):280–286.

Lan MY, Jang YJ. Revision rhinoplasty for short noses in the Asian population. *JAMA Facial Plast Surg* 2015;17(5):325–332.

26 RIB GRAFTING

Christian P. Conderman

INTRODUCTION

Cartilage grafts are often required in head and neck surgery for nasal and auricular reconstruction, upper airway surgery, and primary and secondary rhinoplasty. For nasal reconstruction and rhinoplasty, septal cartilage is considered the ideal tissue for use in restoring or enhancing the structural framework of the nose. Auricular cartilage can serve as a secondary cartilage-grafting source that is readily accessed with modest donor site morbidity. Situations may arise, however, when these cartilage reservoirs do not provide a viable option, such as when larger cartilage grafts are required to provide adequate material for changes in the shape of the nose or for additional structural support. Similarly, prior surgery may have depleted an individual's septal and auricular cartilages. In these cases, alternatives must be considered, and, historically, a number of different graft materials have been used, including alloplasts, homografts, and autologous bone and costal cartilage. Nonetheless, as more experience has been gained with the use of these grafting materials, autologous costal cartilage has shown itself to be a viable and long-lasting option for functional and structural grafting in nasal surgery. Osseous grafts, such as split calvarial and iliac crest bone, have certain limitations and should not be considered as first-line alternatives. These bone grafts are prone to fracture, may lead to excessive nasal stiffness, and may resorb to a variable degree. Allografts, such as silicone and polytetrafluoroethylene (PTFE) (Gore-Tex, WL Gore & Associates, Flagstaff, AZ), may be easier to use without the attendant morbidity of a donor site, yet are associated with extrusion, infection, and foreign body reactions. As a result of the aforementioned factors, autologous costal cartilage may be viewed as the preferred grafting material when the above demands must be met.

In the early 20th century, the initial enthusiasm that accompanied the implantation of costal cartilage in nasal reconstruction and rhinoplasty waned due to the tendency of these costal grafts to warp in unanticipated ways. The problems and complications associated with warping, however, have largely been overcome as the use of cartilage has become more widespread, and approaches for harvest, sectioning, and carving have become standardized. Gibson, in 1958, described the principle of balanced cross-sections to minimize distortion of the graft and warping, and this time-honored approach relies upon harvesting cartilage grafts from the central cross-section of a rib. Similarly, Gunter has shown that a K-wire placed within the graft can be an effective means of overcoming warping, although this approach has not been widely adopted.

A variety of techniques exist for costal cartilage harvest and most have shown a long record of safe use. Moreover, the ribs provide an ample reservoir of cartilage for harvest. While the complications of this technique are well known, if performed properly, procurement of costal cartilage is a safe procedure and provides adequate graft materials for aesthetic, functional, and reconstructive operations.

HISTORY

A thorough clinical history must be obtained including a complete review of medical illnesses, previous operations, tobacco and alcohol use, current and previous medications, drug allergies, and family history. Comorbidities

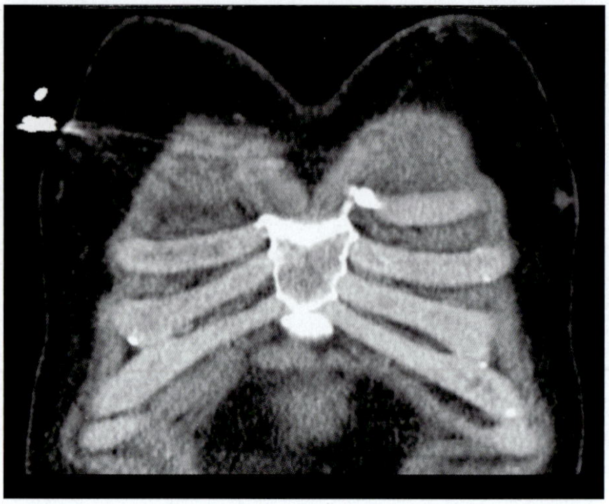

FIGURE 26.1
Normal chest CT of a 48-year-old male with minimal calcification of costal cartilage.

should also be identified at the time of the initial evaluation. During the consultation, an in-depth inquiry of any previous cardiopulmonary problems and surgery must be obtained. Patients should be queried regarding prescription and over-the-counter medications. Specifically, this should include not only prescribed anticoagulants but also herbals and over-the-counter products known to interfere with hemostatic pathways. This may include garlic, ginseng, ginkgo biloba, vitamin E, fish oil, and NSAIDs. Patients should be asked about participation in contact sports such as boxing, football, and the martial arts as thoracoabdominal trauma may lead to premature ossification of costal cartilages and may warrant a preoperative chest CT scan (Figs. 26.1 and 26.2). The operative reports of the patient's prior nasal and auricular operations should be reviewed if available. Finally, the consultation should clearly define the patient's functional (airway) and cosmetic concerns and desires.

PHYSICAL EXAMINATION

A dedicated head and neck and full physical examination should be performed prior to harvesting rib grafts. Additionally, a detailed nasal examination must be performed and particular attention should be paid to the nasal septum. This is done to evaluate the amount and quality of septal cartilage that is present. A moistened cotton-tipped applicator may be used to gently palpate the nasal septum under direct visualization with a nasal speculum to aid in the evaluation of the amount of existing septal cartilage. The posterior nasal vault may also be further examined with an endoscope, which may reveal perforations, septal spurs, and deviations that may be encountered intraoperatively and may not be evident solely on anterior rhinoscopy alone. The pinnae and periauricular area should also be examined, and the surgeon should ascertain the relative amount of auricular cartilage that may be available. While auricular cartilage is more pliable than costal and septal cartilage, it

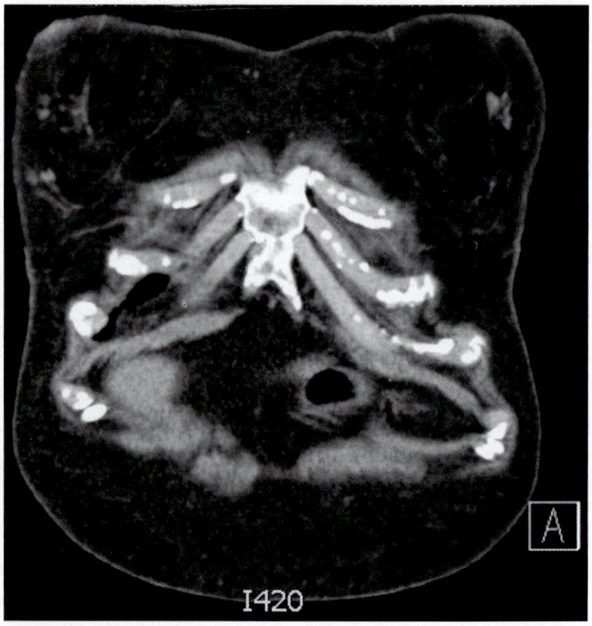

FIGURE 26.2
Chest CT showing calcification of costal cartilage seen on coronal view of a 67-year-old female.

can serve as a useful adjunctive grafting material in a variety of situations. Auricular cartilage can serve as a replacement graft for the lower lateral cartilages, especially in cases of prior overresection, overaggressive cephalic trim, and retraction of the alar margin. A thorough examination of the chest wall should also be performed. In addition to pulmonary auscultation, chest wall abnormalities should be documented at the time of the preoperative examination. Prior breast augmentation and the type of implant used should also be clarified as this may require modification of the operative plan. Obese patients may be at an increased risk for the development of a postoperative seroma and hematoma, and this should be discussed with the patient preoperatively. Lastly, patients should be made aware of the position and length of any potential incisions used for rib harvest. Generally, however, inframammary incisions on females, incisions designed to lie directly over the 6th and 7th rib in males, and incisions placed more inferolaterally on the torso/flank when composite grafts are necessary will usually heal without significant residual deformity or morbidity.

INDICATIONS

Costal cartilage is a versatile graft material and may also be used for auricular reconstruction, for pediatric laryngotracheal reconstruction, and in reconstruction of the temporomandibular joint (TMJ). I will focus mostly on its use in nasal reconstruction and septorhinoplasty. Details regarding its other uses are well described elsewhere. The indications and contraindications for its use in these procedures are as follows:

- Septorhinoplasty (SRP)
  - Cases requiring a significant increase in projection, reinforcement of tip support, or augmentation of the nasal dorsum
  - Ethnic rhinoplasty—correction of poor tip support and/or underprojection, dorsal augmentation, and premaxillary augmentation
  - Primary SRP with a need for extensive structural support with poor or limited native septal cartilage (e.g., caudal septal extension grafts, extended spreader grafts)
  - Secondary SRP
    - Cartilage-depleted individuals lacking adequate septal or conchal cartilage
    - Need for extensive structural grafting
    - Need for extensive dorsal augmentation
- Nasal reconstruction
  - Posttraumatic nasal defects
  - Nasal defects associated with cocaine abuse
  - Saddle nose deformity due to trauma, infection, or systemic disease (e.g., Wegener's granulomatosis)
  - Poor septal support and/or loss of cartilaginous L-strut
  - Rhinectomy defects requiring structural grafting
  - Septal perforation and septectomy defects
  - Total/subtotal nasal reconstruction
- Congenital nasal deformities, for example, Binder syndrome (nasomaxillary dysplasia)
- Laryngotracheal reconstruction
- Auricular reconstruction
- Temporomandibular joint reconstruction

CONTRAINDICATIONS

- Older age group
- Significant medical comorbidities
- Extensive or diffuse cartilaginous ossification as evidenced on preoperative CT scan
- History of restrictive lung disease or recent pulmonary infection

PREOPERATIVE PLANNING

The procedure should be thoroughly explained to the patient, and his/her expectations and desires should be understood prior to surgery. Complications, outcomes, risks, benefits, alternatives, and indications of the procedure should be discussed in detail with the patient. A formal surgical plan should be in place prior to proceeding to the operating room, including an estimation of the type of necessary grafts and their respective source, size, and shape. This will dictate the selection of septal, auricular, and/or costal cartilage harvest. Oftentimes, septal and auricular cartilage may adequately serve the patient's needs for grafting material and may obviate the need for costal cartilage. Furthermore, a PDS plate (Ethicon, Somerville, NJ) can be used as an adjunct during surgery to expand and supplement the use of these local reservoirs.

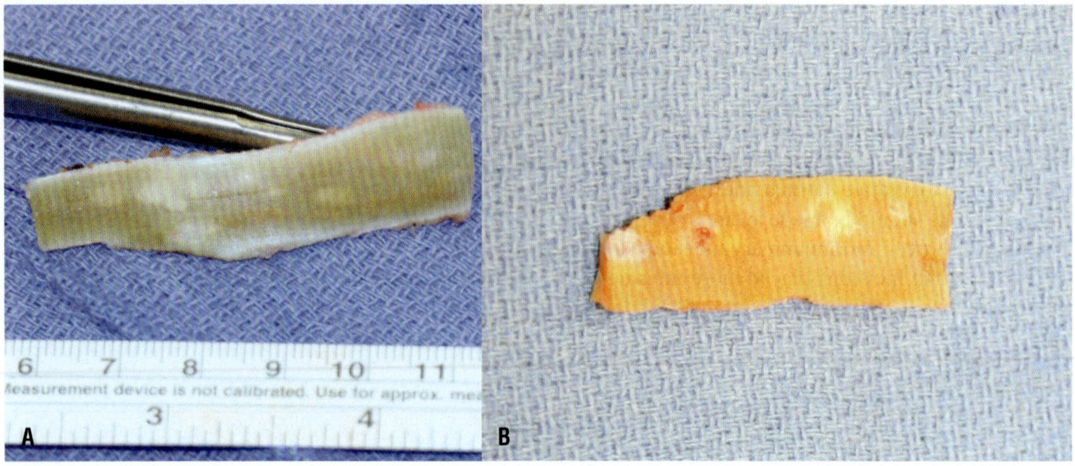

FIGURE 26.3 **A:** Calcifications seen within the central segment of harvested costal cartilage after preparation with a precision cartilage cutter. **B:** Another example of calcification seen after harvest of costal cartilage from a 67-year-old female.

A preoperative chest CT may be considered for some patients and provides information about the degree of costal cartilage calcification, and in fact, some authors advocate the routine use of preoperative CT scanning prior to costal cartilage harvest. CT imaging is of greater value in older patients or those with a history of thoracoabdominal trauma. Calcifications or mineralized costal cartilage may be more difficult to section and carve for use in structural grafting and may have a higher tendency to resorb (Fig. 26.3).

SURGICAL TECHNIQUE

Several techniques have been described to obtain costal cartilage grafts, and a number of factors must be considered prior to graft harvest. The surgeon must estimate the amount of cartilage that is required to serve a patient's functional and cosmetic needs. Additionally, the surgeon must also consider whether a cartilage-only or osseocartilaginous composite graft is desired. These decisions can dictate which rib or ribs will be selected and may dictate the use of an inframammary approach to the 5th, 6th, and 7th rib, or a subcostal/lateral approach to the 8th, 9th, and 10th ribs.

A number of factors regarding costal anatomy should be considered prior to harvesting the graft. The abdomen and thorax contain an array of muscles and fascia that are encountered during the dissection in the approach to the ribs for cartilage and/or bone harvesting. Figure 26.4 is a schematic representation of the muscular and fascial anatomy of the trunk as it pertains to this dissection. Once the soft tissue dissection has taken place and the ribs are exposed, it must be kept in mind that ribs 6 and 7 have a natural synchondrosis (Fig. 26.5) as they approach the sternum and rib. This may limit the amount of cartilage that is available for grafting purposes from these ribs. In addition, the 8th rib may become part of the synchondrosis as its cartilage approaches the costosternal junction. The 9th rib is the first floating rib and can be useful when a combined bone–cartilage graft is desired for use as a cantilevered graft for dorsal reconstruction or augmentation.

As noted above, grafting requirements will dictate which rib and approach is used for harvest. An inframammary approach to the 6th rib is oftentimes preferable as this provides a direct route to the cartilage and in most cases provides an adequate piece of straight cartilage that can then be tailored to the clinical requirements. Moreover, if additional grafting material is necessary, the rib above or below the harvested rib can be readily accessed via the existing incision. Laterality is another important consideration when performing costal graft harvesting. If a two-team approach is used, an approach to the left rib(s) may be preferable as this allows concomitant harvest of the graft while the surgeon is performing nasal surgery. Nonetheless, the differences in right and left-sided anatomy must be recognized as the pericardium lies in close proximity to the overlying synchondrosis and inadvertent entry into the pericardial space is a possible complication of left-sided harvest. Additionally, postoperative pain may mimic cardiac pain and needs to be evaluated thoroughly, especially in patients with a history of or predisposition to cardiac disease.

A number of other techniques have been described to approach rib harvest including the transumbilical approach and endoscopic harvest of the rib via a smaller incision. While these approaches may yield smaller incisions, they may add to the duration and technical difficulty of the operation and will not be elaborated upon in this text. Furthermore, microtia repair may require harvesting of a larger piece of cartilage from the synchondrosis to allow recreation of the natural shape of the pinna. This is described extensively by Brent and other authors and will not be covered in this chapter.

In females, an incision placed 1 to 2 mm above the inframammary crease is generally well concealed. In the presence of prior breast augmentation, the dissection and approach to the underlying rib must be performed in a meticulous fashion to avoid violation of the capsule surrounding the implant. While rare, rupture

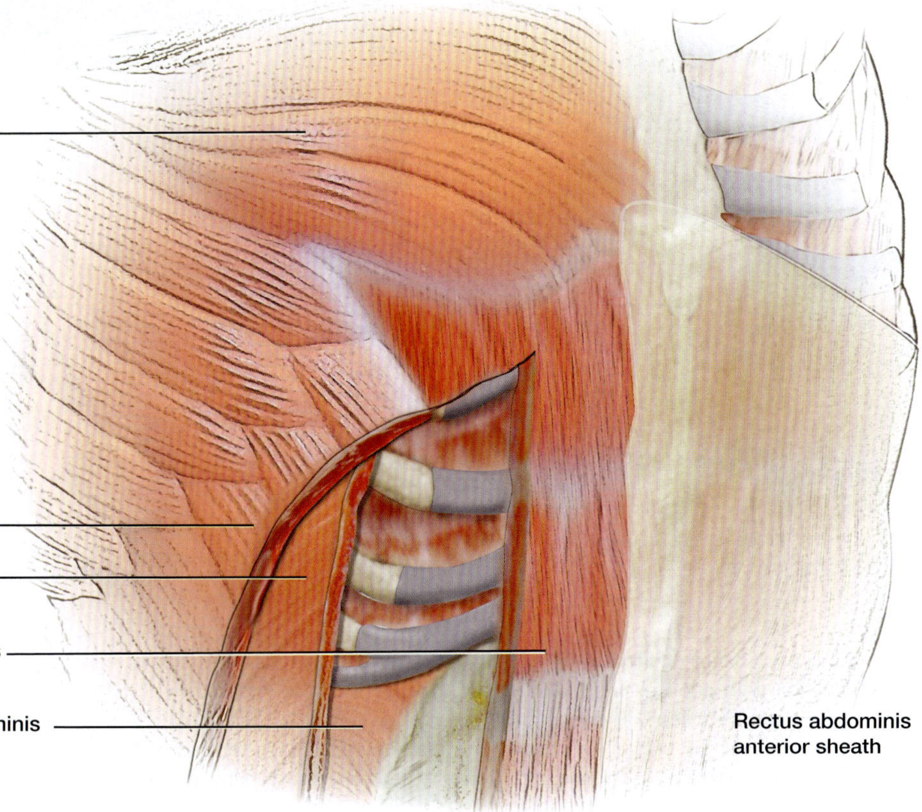

FIGURE 26.4 Schematic of the trunk musculature and muscular fascia in relation to the underlying costal anatomy.

of the implant can occur, and in cases of prior breast augmentation, patients should be advised of this possible complication during the preoperative informed consent process. In males, the incision is generally planned to lie either directly above the rib to be harvested or above an intercostal space if more than one rib harvest is anticipated.

In addition to the above anatomical considerations, certain intrinsic limitations of cartilage must also be considered. It has long been known that cartilage has an inherent propensity to warp. A variety of techniques have been described to overcome cartilage warping to obtain a straight graft for clinical use. Gibson described

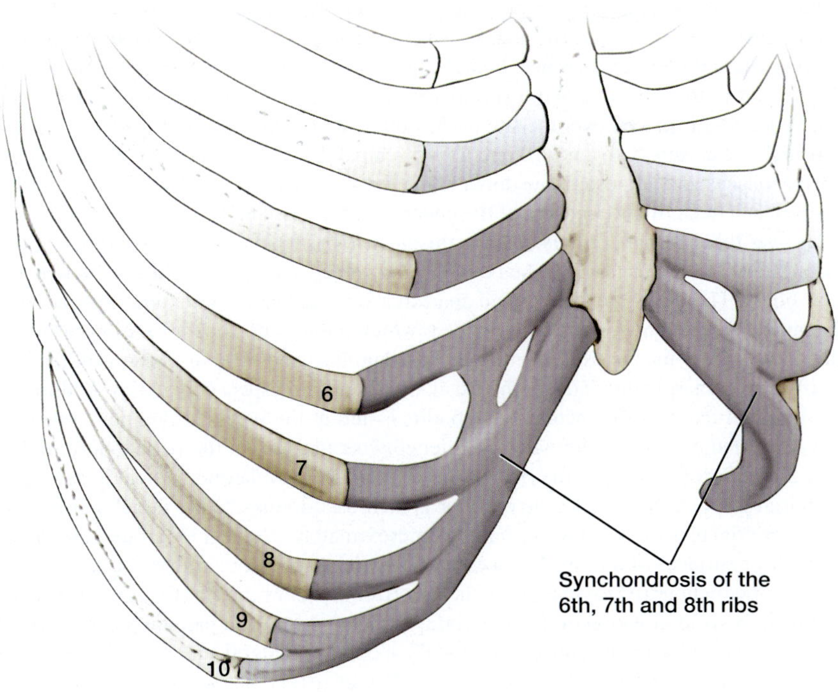

FIGURE 26.5 Schematic depicting costal cartilaginous synchondrosis of the 6th, 7th, and 8th ribs.

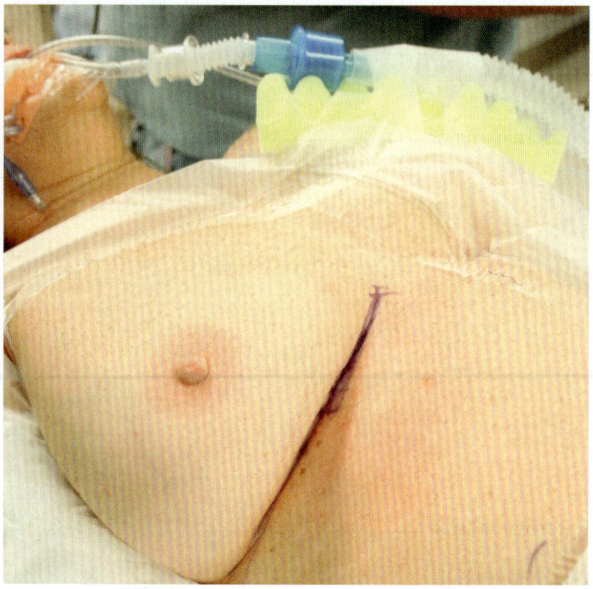

FIGURE 26.6
Patient preparation and inframammary incision design in a female. The incision lies 1 to 2 mm above the inframammary crease.

the concept of balanced cross-sections. Gunter described the use of Kirschner wires placed into the graft for stabilization with good results. Additionally, treatment of the cartilage with an infrared laser and a precise cartilage cutter have been described by Wong et al. as further means to overcome this propensity for warping. Currently, I favor the use of the precise cartilage-cutting device to readily and reproducibly obtain straight grafts of uniform thickness for use in rhinoplasty and procedures requiring costal cartilage.

Operative Technique

After induction of general anesthesia and endotracheal intubation, attention is turned to appropriate positioning of the patient. The airway circuit is then secured along the anterior chest wall, usually on the side opposite the anticipated costal cartilage harvest site, and brought down along the side of the patient to slope underneath the table. The costosternal junction is then palpated at the manubrium and the 2nd rib is identified. The intercostal spaces are then gently palpated, and the ribs are counted and marked on the skin with a pen. Specifically, the borders of the 5th, 6th, 7th, 8th, and 9th are marked on the skin. An incision is then designed to lie over the anticipated site of rib harvest. In females, this is designed 1 to 2 mm above the inframammary crease (Fig. 26.6). In males, the incision is generally designed to lie directly over the 6th rib. Once the incision has been marked, 1% lidocaine with 1:100,000 epinephrine is infiltrated into the subcutaneous tissues for anesthesia and vasoconstriction.

The patient is then draped to allow for two operative fields separated by sterile towels. A standard head drape is applied and a second sterile area is prepared around the site of cartilage harvest. The endotracheal tube will lie under the sterile towels separating the two surgical fields. In general, the preferred approach is to harvest the rib from the patient's left side as this allows a two-team approach. Additionally, an antibacterial adhesive drape (Ioban, 3M corp, St. Paul, MN) is placed over the site of the anticipated cartilage harvest.

The skin is incised through the dermis with a no. 10 or a no. 15 scalpel. Electrocautery is then used to dissect through the subcutaneous tissues and adipose tissue down to the level of the muscular fascia (Fig. 26.7A). A Weitlaner retractor is then placed to facilitate exposure of the underlying tissues. The 5th, 6th, and 7th ribs are then palpated, and the fascia over the rectus abdominis muscle (this muscle has its insertion into portions of the 5th, 6th, and 7th ribs) is identified. The rectus fascia is then divided and spread vertically to allow visualization of the underlying muscular fibers. The fibers are then spread apart in a vertical fashion to expose the underlying ribs (Fig. 26.7B). The muscular fibers are not usually divided, which reduces postoperative discomfort. A 22-gauge needle or needle tip cautery is then used to identify the cartilaginous and osseous portions of the rib. The perichondrium of the rib is then sharply divided lengthwise along its anterior aspect (Fig. 26.8). Additional vertical perichondrial incisions are made at the medial synchondrosis and at the osseocartilaginous junction to maximize the length of harvested cartilage. Alternatively, a lengthwise incision in the perichondrium can be made along the superior and inferior aspects of the rib, followed by medial and lateral vertical incisions to allow harvest of a perichondrial graft. A Freer or Cottle elevator is then used to elevate the perichondrium of the rib (Fig. 26.8). The perichondrial elevation is done initially to approximately 270 degrees around the rib on the anterior, superior, and inferior surfaces of the rib. A Doyen elevator, rib stripper, or similar instrument may then be used to complete this subperichondrial dissection on the posterior aspect of the rib (Fig. 26.9A and B). Meticulous dissection is critical to avoid violation of the underlying perichondrium and parietal pleura. A malleable retractor is then placed to protect the underlying tissues and the medial and lateral cuts through the rib are made using a scalpel or sharpened freer elevator. The harvested rib (Fig. 26.10) is then placed in an antibiotic

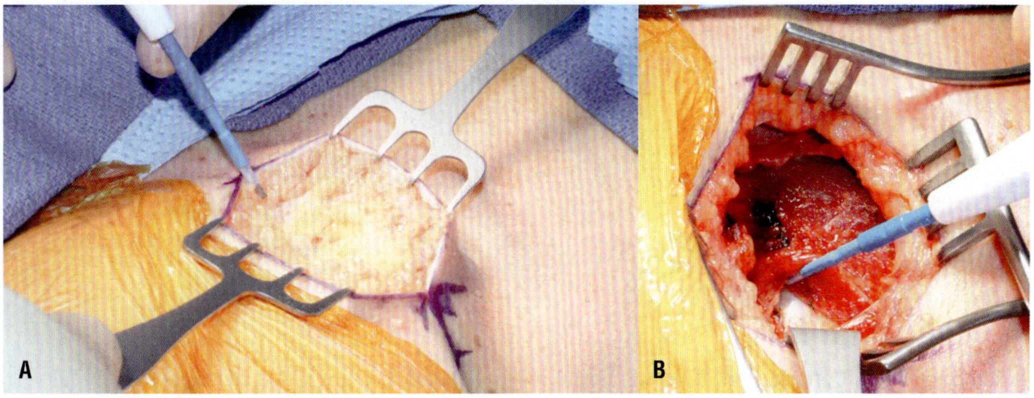

FIGURE 26.7 **A:** After the skin incision has been made, electrocautery is used to divide the subcutaneous adipose tissue and expose the underlying muscular fascia. **B:** The rectus fascia is divided vertically to expose the underlying rib. Division of the fascia in this manner minimizes postoperative pain.

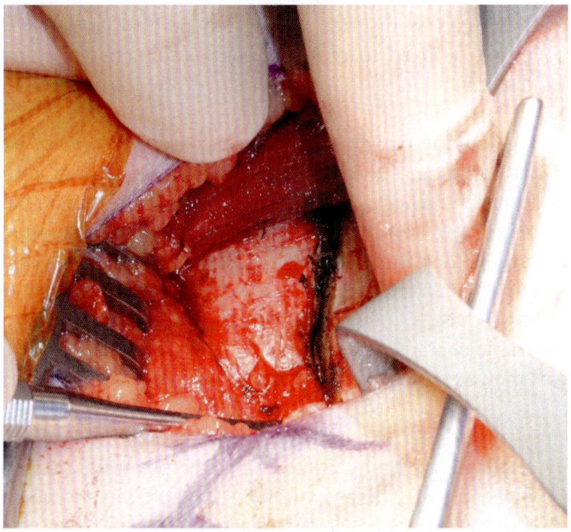

FIGURE 26.8
A lengthwise incision is made along the anterior aspect of the costal perichondrium, and dissection is performed with a Freer elevator to expose the underlying cartilage.

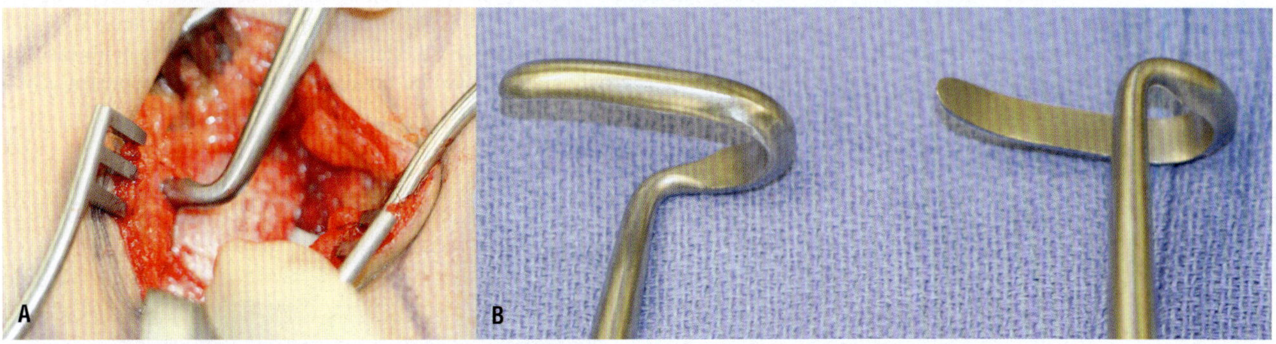

FIGURE 26.9 **A:** Intraoperative image depicting the Doyen rib elevator around the posterior aspect of the rib in a subperichondrial plane. **B:** Close-up of Doyen rib elevator.

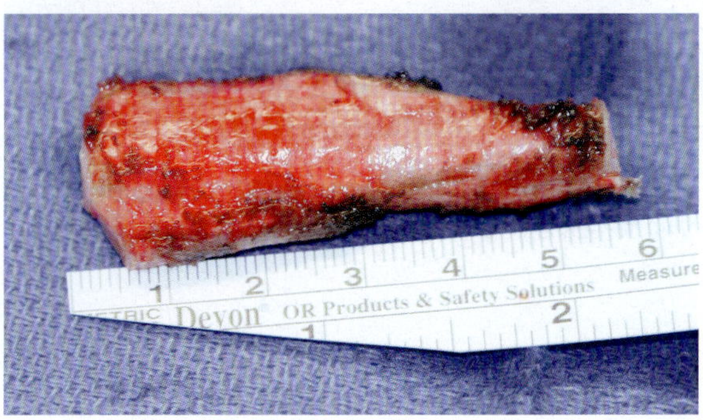

FIGURE 26.10
Rib cartilage after harvest is completed.

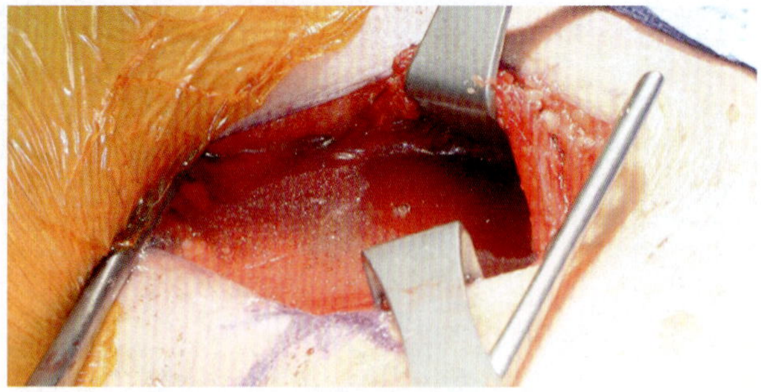

FIGURE 26.11
The operative field is irrigated with saline and a Valsalva maneuver is performed. This is done to evaluate the integrity of the pleura after rib harvest.

solution prior to graft preparation. If perichondrium is to be taken as a graft, this can be done after harvest of the cartilage has been completed.

Following harvest of the graft, hemostasis is achieved and the wound is copiously irrigated with sterile saline solution (Fig. 26.11). A Valsalva maneuver is then requested to maximally expand the lungs. The wound is then observed for air bubbles, which may indicate violation of the parietal pleura. If an air leak is not evident, the operative site is closed in layers. If an air leak exists, however, it usually involves violation of the parietal pleura only. A small Robinson catheter can be inserted through the pleural tear, and a purse-string suture of 2-0 Vicryl (Ethicon, Somerville, NJ) is used to close the surrounding muscle and tissue around the drain. A second Valsalva is then requested, and as the tube is removed, the knot is tied to repair the pleura.

After harvest of the cartilage graft, a precise cartilage-cutting device that has been described for use by Wong et al. is used to facilitate sectioning and subsequent sculpting of the harvested material for grafting purposes. The device is set to cut a piece of cartilage to a desired thickness, usually 1 to 2 mm, depending on the anticipated use of the graft. Any residual perichondrium is gently removed with a scalpel, and the harvested cartilage is placed vertically in the cutting device. A clamp is then tightened to secure the graft in place, and the cutting portion of the device is gently pushed down to obtain a graft from the straight, central segment of cartilage (Fig. 26.12A). The outer portion of the cartilage will have a larger propensity to warp, yet can be used in areas of nasal reconstruction where this may be a desirable characteristic of a graft, such as in alar cartilage reconstruction (Fig. 26.12C). The central segment can then be cut to an appropriate size depending on the patient's grafting requirements.

The perichondrium is closed with 2-0 or 3-0 Vicryl in an interrupted fashion. The rectus muscle fibers are reapproximated using 3-0 Vicryl (Fig. 26.13). Any cartilage remaining at the end of the operation may be banked by placing it into a subcutaneous pocket at the incision site. This is extremely valuable in subsequent reconstructive procedures that may require additional grafting material. The subcutaneous tissue is then also closed using 3-0 Vicryl in a buried, interrupted suture fashion. The deep dermal layer is then closed using 4-0 Vicryl, and finally, a 5-0 Monocryl suture (Ethicon, Somerville, NJ) is used to close the superficial layer in a running subcuticular fashion. Steri-Strips are then applied along the length of the incision. As in all cases of costal cartilage harvest, a postoperative chest radiograph should be obtained to assess for the presence of a pneumothorax.

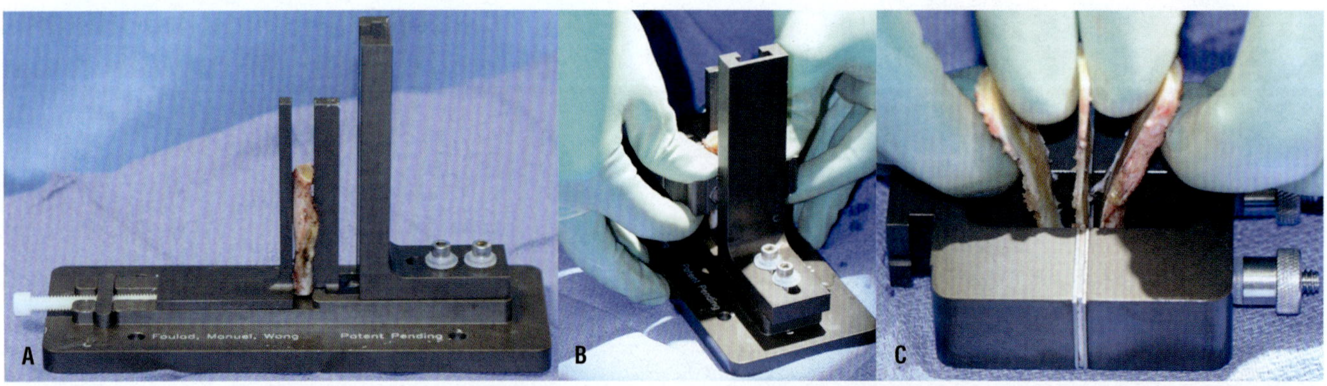

FIGURE 26.12 **A:** The piece of harvested costal cartilage is clamped into position in the cartilage-cutting device. **B:** The cutting apparatus is gently depressed to make precise cuts within the cartilage. **C:** The central and two lateral segments after the rib cartilage have been cut.

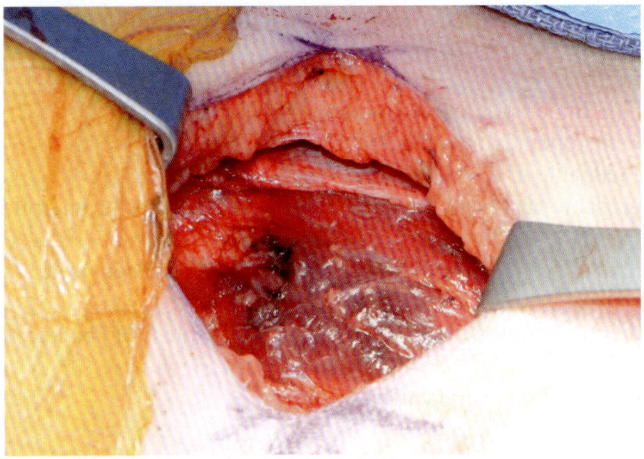

FIGURE 26.13
The rectus fascia is reapproximated prior to superficial closure.

POSTOPERATIVE MANAGEMENT

In my experience, it is prudent to obtain a routine postoperative chest radiograph in all cases following costal cartilage harvest. However, if a pleural tear is suspected or confirmed intraoperatively, a chest radiograph is mandatory. Additionally, an overnight admission to a monitored nursing unit with pulse oximetry and telemetry may be necessary. As described above, if a pleural tear is found at the time of surgery, a purse-string suture is tied over a red rubber catheter while the chest is maximally expanded. If a pleural tear occurs in this setting, it is an injury that is generally confined to the parietal pleura only and does not involve the deeper visceral pleura. A general surgery consult is obtained; however, a thoracostomy tube is not generally necessary with a tear of the parietal pleura only. The tear will usually resolve with the addition of supplemental oxygen administered via nasal cannula and should be followed with serial chest radiographs.

If the above circumstances are not encountered, and if the postoperative chest radiograph is negative, the patient can usually be discharged on the day of surgery. Admission for observation should be considered on a case-to-case basis depending on patient factors. Postoperative pain control is imperative and is usually adequately controlled using narcotic pain medications. Bupivacaine administered to the operative site after cartilage harvest via injection at the time of surgery or through a subcutaneous catheter has also been described and has been associated with less pain and a reduction in the amount of narcotic pain medication necessary to achieve adequate postoperative analgesia.

COMPLICATIONS

- Bleeding
  - Can be minimized with appropriate patient selection and discontinuation of anticoagulant medications prior to surgery and meticulous intraoperative hemostasis
- Seroma/hematoma
  - May be more prevalent with the use of the subcostal approach to rib. This complication may also be more likely in obese patients as there is more dead space that is created during rib harvest. This may contribute to seroma formation, and a closed suction drain should be considered in these patients.
- Infection
  - Uncommon given the use of peri- and postoperative intravenous antibiotics and immersion of harvested graft material in antibiotic solution prior to implantation.
  - Risk of infection may be increased with trauma to the internal nasal lining and exposure of underlying structural grafts.
  - Severe scarring of the nasal skin and soft tissue envelope may also increase the risk of infection.
- Postoperative pain
  - Bupivacaine administered after graft harvest can reduce postoperative pain.
  - Generally, pain is well tolerated and managed with narcotic pain medications (hydrocodone/acetaminophen, oxycodone/acetaminophen).
  - The perichondrium should be reapproximated with sutures to splint the wound in the postoperative period.
- Atelectasis
  - The postoperative use of incentive spirometry is encouraged in all cases.
- Scarring and adverse cosmetic outcome at the site of harvest
  - Reduced with the use of appropriate soft tissue handling and wound closure techniques. Postoperative laser resurfacing or pulsed-dye laser therapy may be considered.

  - Any history of keloid and hypertrophic scarring should be elicited from the patient prior to surgery.
  - Postoperative Kenalog injections may help to reduce scar formation.
- Pleural tear/pneumothorax
  - Meticulous surgical technique can reduce the likelihood of pleural violation.
  - See description above for management (under postoperative management).
- Chest wall abnormalities including clicking and palpable or visual defects
  - More prominent in cases where the synchondrosis is harvested for large defects and in cases of microtia reconstruction.
  - The perichondrium must be reapproximated if a subperichondrial dissection technique has been used.
- Intra- and postoperative cartilage warping
  - Proper cartilage shaping techniques should be employed following the principles of balanced cross-sectioning.
  - Graft preparation can be facilitated with the use of the precision cartilage cutter.
- Graft fracture
  - Can be reduced with appropriate fixation if a composite cantilever graft is used to reconstruct or augment the nasal dorsum

RESULTS

In my experience using autologous costal cartilage grafts in nasal surgery, I have found it to be a versatile graft material that can be used safely and effectively with a low risk of complications when appropriate surgical technique is used as outlined above. This is consistent with previously published reports that show a relatively low complication rate with good outcomes and high rates of patient satisfaction. I have found autologous costal cartilage to be especially useful in cartilage-depleted individuals and those in whom extensive structural nasal reconstruction is required. Moreover, I have found it to be an appropriate source of grafting material for a variety of structural and functional rhinoplasty grafts including the caudal septal extension graft, traditional and extended spreader grafts, lateral crural strut grafts, dorsal onlay grafts, and alar rim grafts. The accompanying figures are representative examples in which the use of costal cartilage was used to meet the patient's functional and cosmetic needs. These examples include the use of costal cartilage for cases of prior overresection in a nose devastated by multiple prior rhinoplasties (Fig. 26.14), a case of an Asian rhinoplasty requiring grafting material for enhancement of tip definition (Fig. 26.15), and a case of its use in cleft lip rhinoplasty (Fig. 26.16).

PEARLS

- Preoperative planning is essential. Prior to harvesting a rib graft, a specific and detailed plan must be in place regarding the anticipated graft (size, shape) as well as to the quantity and type (composite, cartilage only) of such a graft.
- The availability of septal and conchal cartilage must be evaluated prior to harvesting rib cartilage. This may obviate the need for costal cartilage and its attendant morbidities especially if the previously outlined indications are not met. A PDS (polydioxanone) plate may expand the reservoirs of septal and conchal cartilage.
- Consideration must be given to the anticipated location of costal cartilage harvest, that is, which rib should be harvested for a particular indication. A comprehensive understanding and knowledge of native rib anatomy is of critical importance.
- An inframammary incision is usually well concealed in a female patient and ribs 6 and 7 usually yield an adequate volume of cartilage. Furthermore, if additional cartilage is necessary, additional grafting material harvest can be taken from the adjacent rib, either above or below.
- If an osseocartilaginous graft is necessary, one may need to obtain a graft from the 9th or 10th rib via a lateral approach.
- When possible, subperichondrial dissection should be performed, especially when harvesting ribs 5 to 8 as this has been shown to have a lower risk of pleural tear and pneumothorax.

PITFALLS

- Cartilage warping must be expected and accounted for when using costal cartilage for grafting purposes in the nose. This can be minimized with appropriate graft preparation and using the central segment of the costal graft when possible. Additionally, warping may become evident if the graft is carved and sculpted 15 to 30 minutes prior to implantation.

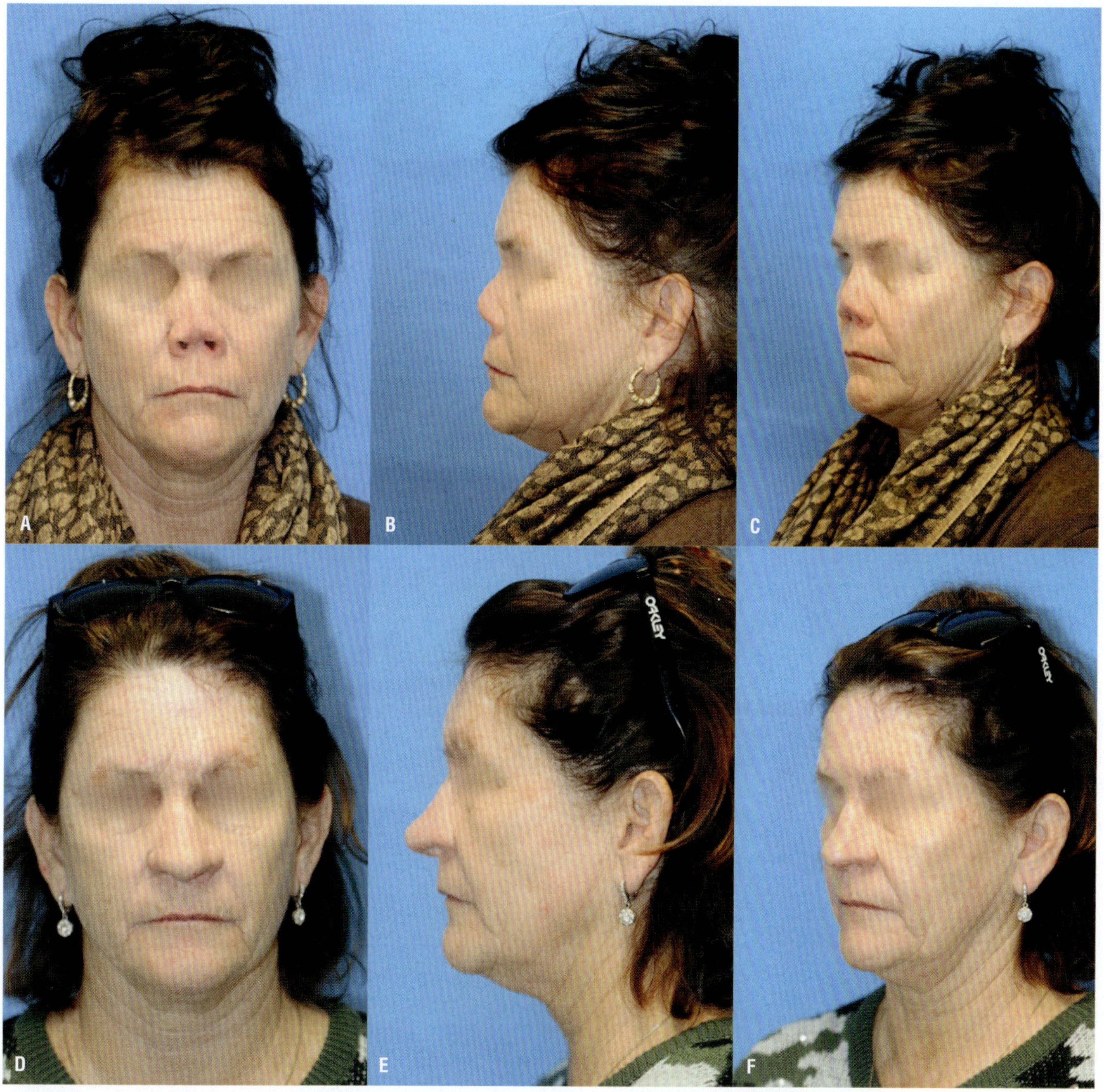

FIGURE 26.14 **A:** Preoperative frontal view of a woman with a severely contracted skin and soft tissue envelope after multiple prior rhinoplasties. **B:** Preoperative profile view. **C:** Preoperative oblique view. **D:** Postoperative frontal view after three-stage reconstruction using a paramedian forehead flap and costal cartilage grafting to reconstruct the L-strut and nasal framework. **E:** Postoperative profile view. **F:** Postoperative oblique view.

- A Valsalva maneuver should be carried out after every rib harvest, and when suspected, a pleural tear should be repaired immediately. If a pleural tear and/or pneumothorax go unrecognized, significant morbidity may result.
- The surgeon must consider circumstances (trauma, advanced age) in which a preoperative CT scan may be warranted as this may affect the choice of rib used for grafting.

INSTRUMENTS TO HAVE AVAILABLE

Medications

1. 1% lidocaine with 1:100,000 epinephrine solution
2. Betadine prep solution
3. Bacitracin ointment 30 g tube

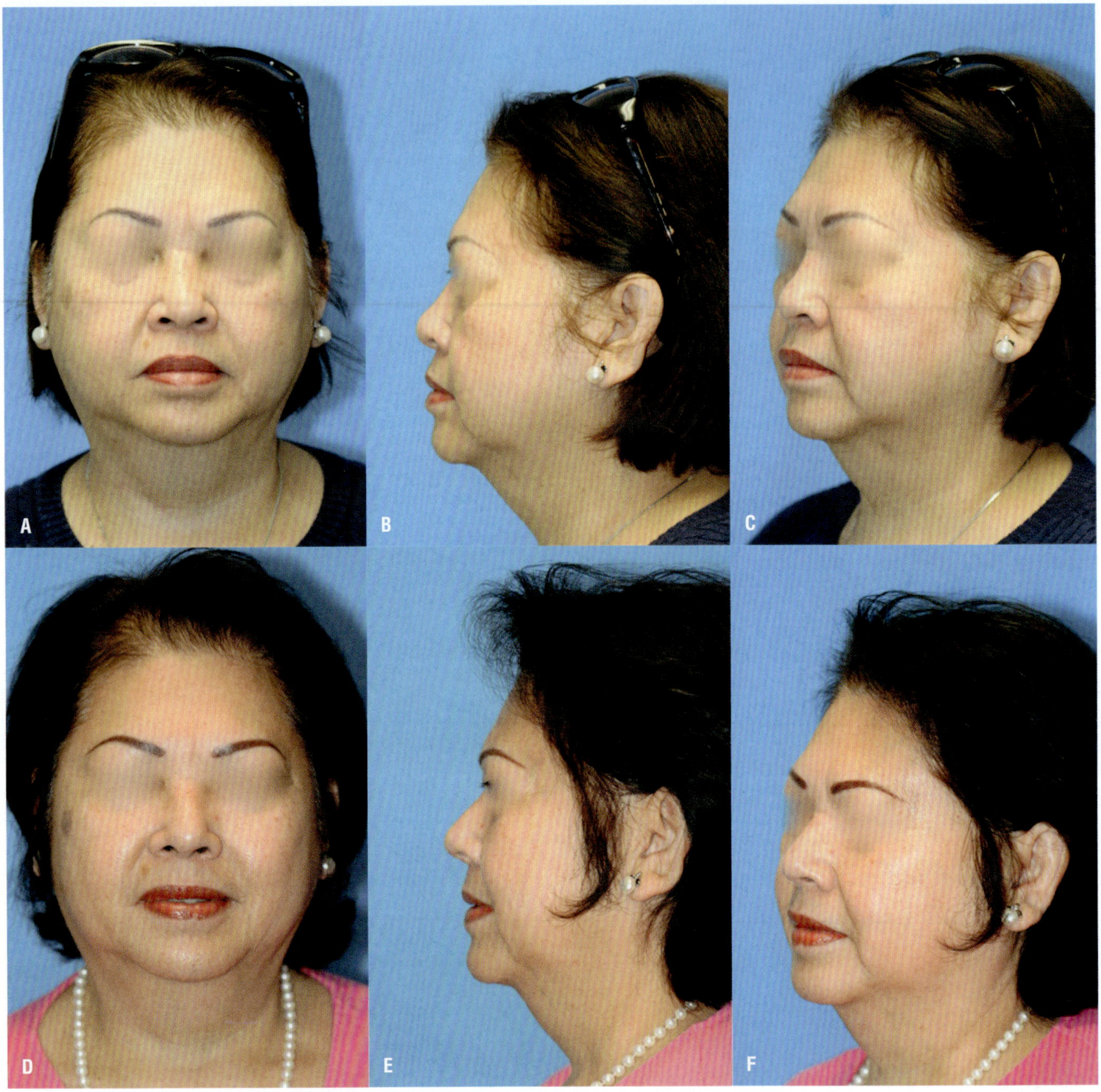

FIGURE 26.15 **A:** Preoperative frontal view of an Asian female with poor tip support and prior removal of an infected dorsal alloplast implant. **B:** Preoperative profile view. **C:** Preoperative oblique view. **D:** Postoperative view after reconstruction with costal cartilage using an open rhinoplasty approach with increased tip projection and support. **E:** Postoperative profile view. **F:** Postoperative oblique view.

Sutures

1. 3-0 Vicryl PS-2 needle
2. 4-0 Vicryl PS-2 needle
3. 5-0 Monocryl P-3 needle

Dressings

1. ¼″ × 4″ Steri-Strips
2. 5″ × 9″ Xeroform
3. 4″ × 6″ Covaderm

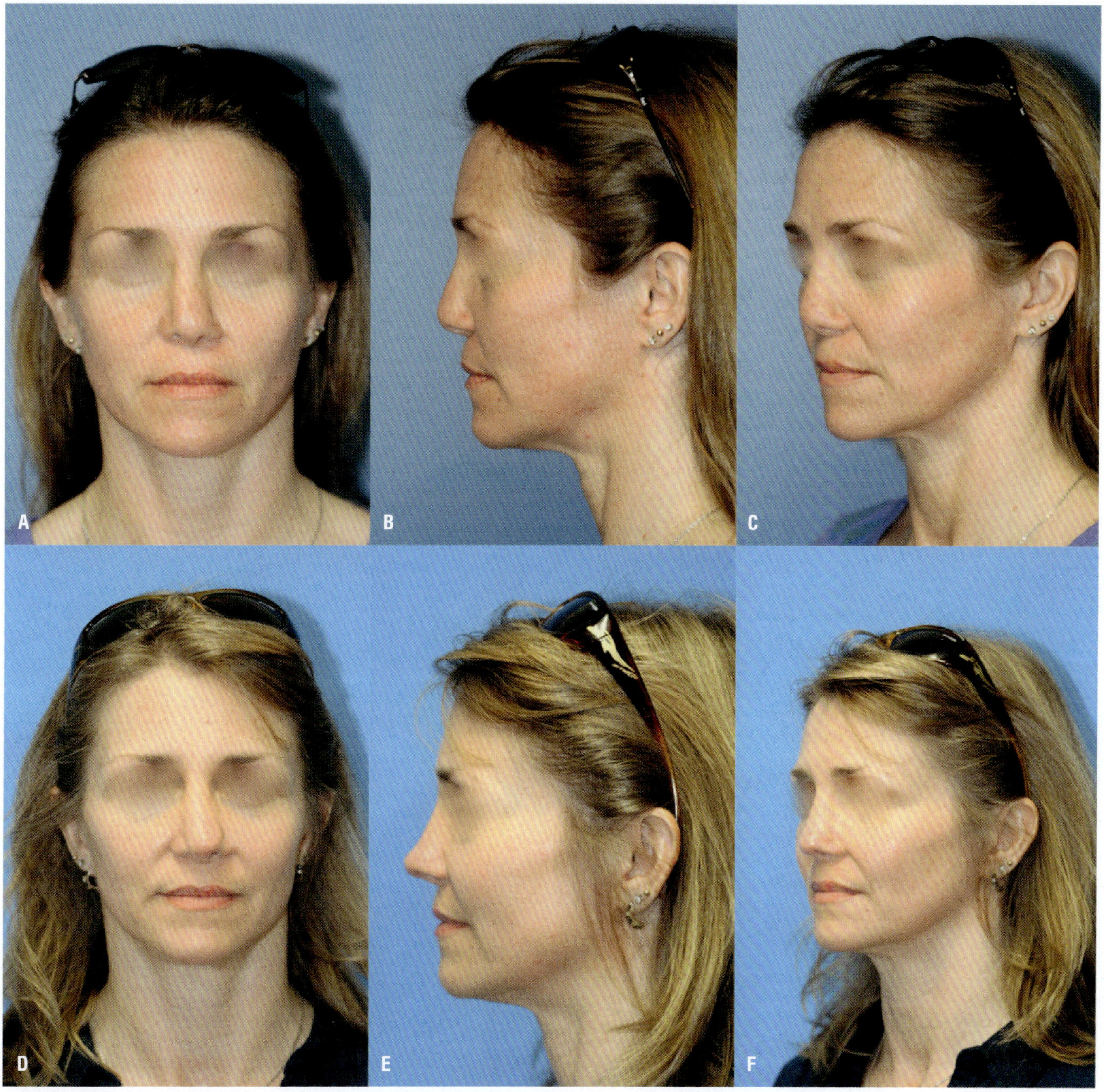

FIGURE 26.16 **A:** Preoperative frontal view of a patient following repair of cleft lip and cleft lip rhinoplasty with poor tip support and projection. **B:** Preoperative profile view. **C:** Preoperative oblique view. **D:** Postoperative frontal view after increasing tip projection and rotation using an open rhinoplasty approach. **E:** Postoperative profile view. **F:** Postoperative oblique view.

Miscellaneous

1. 27-gauge needle
2. Peanut dissector
3. Ioban drape
4. Colorado bovie needle tip
5. No. 10 and no. 15 scalpel
6. 6″ spatulated, insulated bovie tip
7. ¼″ penrose drain
8. Normal saline irrigation

Instrument tray:

1. Knife handle, no. 3 × 2
2. Adson forceps with teeth × 2
3. Brown-Adson forceps × 2
4. Heavy tissue forceps × 1
5. DeBakey medium forceps × 2
6. Cushing forceps, fine tip with Gutsch handle × 1
7. Converse single skin hook, small × 2
8. Molt no. 9 periosteal elevator × 1
9. Key ¼″ elevator × 1
10. Key ½″ elevator × 1
11. Adson periosteal elevator ¼″ (no. 2) × 1
12. Love Adson periosteal elevator 3/16″
13. Rongeur × 1
14. Leksell Rongeur × 1
15. Curved 7″ Metzenbaum scissors × 1
16. Straight Mayo scissors × 1
17. 5″ curved mosquito clamps × 5
18. Rochester-Ochsner straight hemostatic clamp × 2
19. Crile-Wood needle driver 6″ × 2
20. Doyen rib stripper, right × 1
21. Doyen rib stripper, left × 1
22. Rib cutter, adult × 1
23. Rib cutter, child × 1
24. Stille-Gertz rib shears × 1
25. Cone laminectomy sharp prong retractor × 1
26. Beckman sharp retractor
27. ½″ malleable retractors × 2
28. Malleable ribbon retractor 5/8″ × 8″ × 2
29. Malleable ribbon retractor ¾″ × 8″ × 2
30. Army/navy retractor × 2
31. Lahey thyroid retractor × 2
32. Rake brass retractor × 2
33. 4 prong sharp rake retractor × 2
34. Vascular (Andrews) suction tip × 1
35. 12 French suction tip × 1
36. Yankauer suction, large
37. Beaver knife handle
38. Weitlaner retractor, dull medium
39. Weitlaner retractor, sharp medium

ACKNOWLEDGMENT

I would like to extend my deepest appreciation and gratitude to Dr. Brian J.F. Wong for his assistance in the preparation of this manuscript and for his continued mentorship and support. He provided the intraoperative photographs for inclusion in this chapter. Additionally, he was the primary surgeon in the cases depicted in Figures 26.14 to 26.16 and provided the pre- and postoperative photographs accompanying these cases.

SUGGESTED READING

Daniel RK. Rhinoplasty and rib grafts: evolving a flexible operative technique. *Plast Reconstr Surg* 1994;94(5):597–609; discussion 610–611.

Foulad A, Hamamoto A, Manuel C, et al. Precise and rapid costal cartilage graft sectioning using a novel device: clinical application. *JAMA Facial Plast Surg* 2014;16(2):107–112.

Kim DW, Shah AR, Toriumi DM. Concentric and eccentric carved costal cartilage: a comparison of warping. *Arch Facial Plast Surg* 2006;8(1):42–46.

Marin VP, Landecker A, Gunter JP. Harvesting rib cartilage grafts for secondary rhinoplasty. *Plast Reconstr Surg* 2008;121(4):1442–1448.

Wee JH, Park MH, Oh S, et al. Complications associated with autologous rib cartilage use in rhinoplasty: a meta-analysis. *JAMA Facial Plast Surg* 2015;17(1):49–55.

27 BOTOX (FOREHEAD AND PERIORBITAL RHYTIDS AND CHEMICAL BROW LIFT)

Corey S. Maas

INTRODUCTION

Botulinum toxin is a natural polypeptide neurotoxin first described for use in glabellar lines by Carruthers and Carruthers in 1992. There are seven distinct serotypes of the toxin (botulinum toxin A, B, C, D, E, F, and G), each with unique antigenicity, binding sites, and enzymatic activity. Of the subtypes, type A has proven to be most efficacious in clinical practice. The mechanism of action of the toxin takes place at the presynaptic terminal where it effectively prevents release of acetylcholine into the neuromuscular junction thereby inhibiting muscle contraction. Although it binds irreversibly, new axonal growth allows for return of muscle function within 3 to 4 months after injection.

Since approval by the Food and Drug Administration (FDA) for cosmetic use, Botox/Botox Cosmetic (onabotulinumtoxinA; Allergan Inc., Irvine, CA), in 2002, and more recently Dysport (abobotulinumtoxinA; also known as Azzalure: Ipsen, Paris, London; distributed in the United States by Medicis Corp., Scottsdale, AZ), in 2009, neurotoxins have been a mainstay in the treatment of hyperdynamic rhytids of the upper face. Xeomin (incobotulinumtoxinA; Merz Pharmaceuticals, Germany), the most recent preparation available for cosmetic use, was approved in July 2011.

All three products contain the botulinum neurotoxin type A (BoNT-A), protein which, in its simplest form, has a molecular weight of 150 kD. The protein is made up of both a heavy chain (100 kD) and a light chain (50 kD), each with its own role in the mechanism of action of the neurotoxin. Botox and Dysport contain the active 150-kD protein along with a complex of proteins that play no role in the neurotoxin's mechanism of action. As a whole, the Botox protein complex weighs 900 kD with one active 150-kD protein per complex, while the Dysport complex, of which the biochemical composition is unknown, weighs approximately 900 kD. Xeomin contains the "naked" 150-kD protein only. Through the years, research and the widespread use of BoNT-A has shown that it has a wide margin of safety, is generally well tolerated, and has a high rate of satisfaction. Various methods of reconstitution, optimal dosage, and placement of the injections have also been described but above all a thorough understanding of the anatomy and function of the musculature of the upper face is the most important element in achieving optimal aesthetic outcomes.

RELEVANT ANATOMY

A thorough understanding of the anatomy of the upper face and muscular interactions is of utmost importance for successful treatment of hyperdynamic rhytids. For simplicity, the muscles of the upper face that are effectively treated with neuromodulators can be divided into depressors and elevators of the brow. The frontalis muscle is the sole elevator of the brow and in the classic anatomical description consists of two bellies, one on either side of the midline of the forehead. The lateral extent of the frontalis coincides with the peak of the brow, and the medial aspect of each belly lies at the medial border of the brow leaving a space devoid of muscle in the midline. More commonly, however, the muscle is found as one broad muscular band without a medial division.

Inferiorly, the frontalis interdigitates with the brow depressors and is contiguous with the galea aponeurotica superiorly. The brow depressors consist of the procerus, paired corrugators and depressor supercilii, and the medial and lateral orbicularis oculi. Medially, the procerus overlies the glabella and is flanked by the depressor supercilii, while the corrugators extend superiorly and laterally at the level of the brow. The procerus and corrugators are responsible for horizontal and vertical lines over the bridge of the nose, respectively. Although the paired nasalis muscles, which overly the upper lateral cartilages, do not contribute to brow depression, they produce horizontal lines over the lateral nasal dorsum commonly referred to when hyperactive as "bunny lines." Overall, the lateral orbicularis oculi acts as the strongest depressor of the brow and is responsible for periorbital rhytids also known as "crow's feet." Knowledge of this anatomy is important in that overzealous treatment of the frontalis with the intention of correcting all visible forehead lines could lead to significant brow ptosis.

HISTORY

A thorough history should include allergies and current medications with an emphasis on the use of anticoagulants as the procedure may need to be postponed if the patient desires minimal bruising. It is important to note previous surgical treatment of surrounding tissues as well as any past treatments with BoNT-A. Asking the patient what they liked or disliked about previous experiences with neuromodulators can be very helpful. The importance of facial expression in the patient's occupation and daily lifestyle should also be discussed. Finally, extreme caution should be taken in treatment of patients who have known peripheral neuropathies or disorders of the neuromuscular junction since they may be at increased risk of severe systemic effects such as dysphagia and respiratory compromise.

PHYSICAL EXAMINATION

During evaluation, it is important to assess the patient's goals of treatment. Evaluation of the face for any preexisting asymmetries should be performed and documented, and a thorough discussion of irregularities should take place with the patient. The patient should be asked to actively contract the glabellar, frontalis, and orbicularis oculi muscles in order to discern the amount of improvement that can be reasonably expected to guide your discussion and treatment plan.

INDICATIONS

Botulinum toxin is generally indicated for the treatment of hyperdynamic lines or furrows of the upper face that are of concern to the patient including glabellar frown lines, horizontal forehead creases, periorbital "crow's feet," and lateral nasal "bunny lines." Also, if necessary, treatment can be extended to include infraorbital lines. Though most patients present with lines or wrinkles that they wish to have treated, neuromodulators can also be used as a preventive measure prior to formation of lines in younger patients who tend to overuse their upper facial musculature. Some patients may request elevation of the lateral brow, and BoNT-A can be placed with good results into the lateral orbicularis oculi to produce what has been described as a chemical brow lift. In addition, BoNT-A can be used prior to procedures such as lower eyelid reconstruction, brow lift, scar revision, and repair of lacerations to help promote favorable wound healing. Patients may also present to the office having had a recent injection using an improper technique causing asymmetries. With a thorough understanding of the upper facial musculature, these unfortunate irregularities can be treated with small amounts of neuromodulator injected at the proper anatomical location.

CONTRAINDICATIONS

BoNT-A treatment is contraindicated in patients with active infection at planned injection sites as well as in those with known allergy or hypersensitivity to any of the formulation ingredients (botulinum toxin type A, sodium chloride, human albumin). The neurotoxin is listed as a category C drug in pregnancy meaning no adequate well-controlled studies of use in pregnant women exist, and it is unknown whether the toxin is excreted during lactation. Therefore, any patient who is pregnant or breast-feeding should not undergo treatment. It should be noted, however, that the literature contains a small number of reports of patients who underwent treatment with BoNT-A while unknowingly pregnant. Of these, one study surveyed 396 physicians of which 12 reported having injected women who were not aware they were pregnant. In this study, one miscarriage was reported in a woman with a history of previous miscarriages, but no fetal abnormalities or other adverse events have been linked to the neurotoxin.

Patients should be made aware, if present, of preexisting lid or brow ptosis and educated on the risk of exacerbation. Although careful injection technique should minimize the risk, if the possibility of worsening ptosis is unacceptable to the patient, they should not be injected. Occasionally, a patient may present with the request for further treatment although on examination they clearly have appropriate lack of muscular activity due to a recent injection. In this case, a detailed discussion with the patient should take place focusing on minimization of hyperdynamic lines as the goal of treatment rather than complete absence of muscle activity. These patients should be made aware that further injection will only place them at risk for complications and likely provide no incremental improvement.

SURGICAL TECHNIQUE

Reconstitution of Product

Reconstitution is the correct term to use when describing the method of converting dried product into solution. Using words like "dilution" or "diluted" is not accurate and can lead to a false belief by the patient that they are receiving a less-than-quality product. The "unit" (U) of measurement for Botox Cosmetic, Dysport, and Xeomin, each measured on the LD_{50} mouse test, is a proprietary measurement of the individual manufacturer. In the literature, 1 U of Botox has been shown to be closely equivalent to 2.5 to 3 U of Dysport and 1 U of Xeomin. The product is packaged in vials either vacuum dried (Botox, 50 or 100 U) or lyophilized (Dysport, 300 U, and Xeomin, 100 U) and must be kept refrigerated at 0 to 8°C (except Xeomin, which can be stored up to 25°C) until just prior to use to avoid denaturization of the protein. Since the product is packaged in powder form, it must be hydrated to make it suitable for injection, and the manufacturers package insert recommends use of preservative-free saline. In my practice, a 100-U vial of Botox or Xeomin is reconstituted with 2.0 mL of preservative-free saline to produce 5 U/0.1 mL. Similarly, 300 U of Dysport is reconstituted with 1.5 mL of preservative-free saline to give 20 U/0.1 mL. Other methods of reconstitution have been described and can be found in Table 27.1. Due to the fragile nature of BoNT-A, care is taken, in the case of Botox, to allow the vacuum property of the vial to draw in the saline rather than forcefully injecting into the container. For Dysport and Xeomin vials, which have a partial vacuum seal, the amount of saline drawn in will vary, and therefore, slow injection of the remaining saline will ensure sustained quality of the product. A gentle swirl of the vial is then performed to mix the contents. Insulin syringes with a permanently attached needle, manufactured in 50 and 30 insulin-unit capacities, are then used to carefully draw up the product. With these syringes, 10 insulin-units are equivalent to 0.1 mL allowing for ease of measurement. For Botox and Xeomin, a 50 insulin-unit syringe is utilized to draw up increments of both 0.2 and 0.4 mL, which equals 10 and 20 U, respectively. Dysport is drawn up in 30 insulin-unit syringes at increments of both 0.15 and 0.3 mL to give 30 and 60 U, respectively. When drawing up the reconstituted product, it is important to ensure that the needle does not touch the floor of the glass container as this will dull the tip and make for a more painful injection.

The following is a description of my technique for injection and dosing of both Botox and Dysport. Consensus statements on median dose ranges can be found in the literature, and Table 27.2 is provided as a guideline for treatment. The experience of the practitioner and an individualized treatment plan will

TABLE 27.1 Methods of Neuromodulator Reconstitution

Diluent Volume	Concentration in U/mL
Dysport 300-U Vial	
1.0 mL	15/0.05
1.5 mL	10/0.05
2.5 mL	10/0.08
3.0 mL	10/0.1
Xeomin, Botox Cosmetic 100-U Vial	
2.0 mL	5.0/0.1
2.5 mL	4.0/0.1
4.0 mL	2.5/0.1
Xeomin, Botox Cosmetic 50-U Vial	
1.0 mL	5.0/0.1
2.0 mL	2.5/0.1

TABLE 27.2 Median Dose Ranges

Upper Face Area	Botox Cosmetic	Dysport
Glabella	20–30 BUs	50–80 DUs
Forehead	10–20 BUs	25–60 DUs
Crow's feet	8–20 BUs/side	16–60 DUs/side
Bunay lines	5–10 BUs	10–30 DUs

The above median dose ranges are provided as a guideline for treatment. The experience of the practitioner and an individualized treatment plan will determine the appropriate dose.

determine the appropriate dose. Of note, at the time of production of this chapter, consensus dose ranges for Xeomin were not available. In my practice, patients receive the same number of units injected at examination-determined target sites during their first experience of treatment with BoNT-A. In this way, a standard of consistency can be maintained and then individualized at the patient's next treatment depending on their initial response.

- *Treatment of glabellar lines*

  The glabellar frown lines are treated by injection of the paired corrugators and procerus muscles with either 20 U of Botox or 60 U of Dysport. The patient is asked to frown and relax several times to help with identification of precise muscle location. To inject the corrugator supercilii, the substance of the muscle is pinched between the index finger and thumb at the level of the brow, first medially near its origin 0.5 to 1 cm above the orbital rim. The needle is then directed parallel to the muscle and inserted into the substance of the muscle at a slight angle. Thereupon, approximately 6 to 7.5 U of Botox or 18 to 22.5 U of Dysport is infiltrated. The muscle is then grasped more laterally 1 cm above the orbital rim at the level of the peak of the brow where the same injection technique is utilized to deposit approximately either 2 to 2.5 U of Botox or 6 to 7.5 U of Dysport. This is repeated on the opposite side. Grasping the muscle between the fingers ensures proper placement of the neuromodulator and avoids the inadvertent injection of the more superior medial frontalis muscle fibers. The remainder of product is injected into the procerus muscle at one injection point in the midline over the glabella (Fig. 27.1).

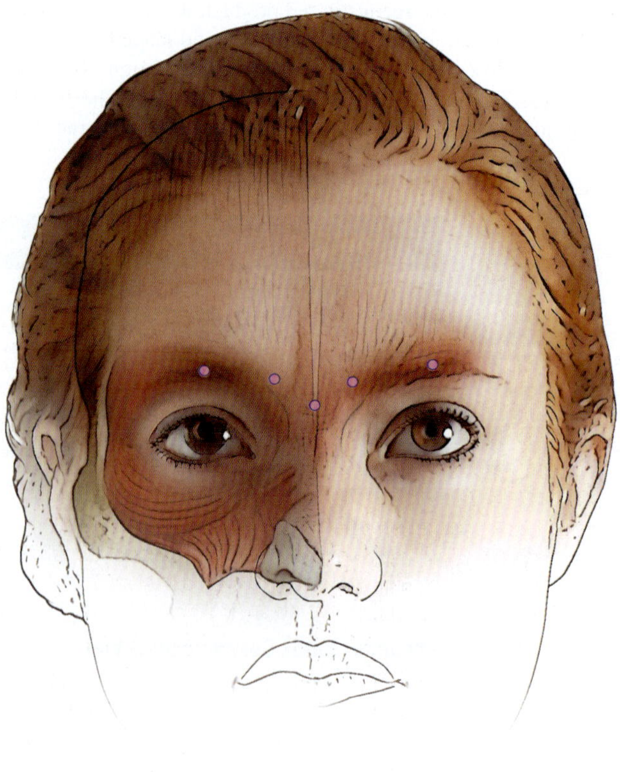

FIGURE 27.1
Magenta dots represent ideal injection sites for treatment.

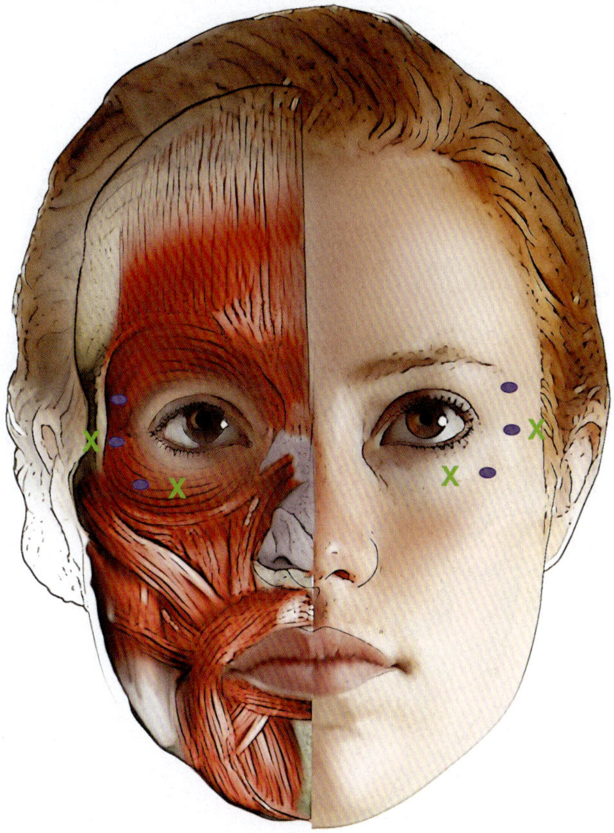

FIGURE 27.2
Blue dots represent ideal injection sites for treatment, while "X"s represent optional injection sites.

- *Treatment of periorbital rhytids ("crow's feet")*
  Periorbital rhytids are the result of contraction mainly of the lateral orbicularis oculi and sometimes to a smaller extent by the zygomatic muscles. These can be reproduced by having the patient squint or smile repeatedly. Each side is treated with either a total of 10 U of Botox or 30 U of Dysport injected perpendicular to the skin approximately 1 cm lateral to the orbital rim. Three to four injection sites are chosen to disperse 2 to 3 U of Botox or 7 to 10 U of Dysport at each site. In a recent study, conducted at my institution, treatment of the crow's feet area with abobotulinumtoxinA showed a statistically significant advantage over onabotulinumtoxinA and was also favored by the patient 67% of the time. If need be, 1 to 2 U of Botox or 3 to 6 U of Dysport can be injected slightly more inferiorly and medially below the orbital rim within the orbicularis to treat lines in this region. This should be done with extreme caution as injection too low at this site can cause asymmetries of the mouth. The lateral orbicularis oculi area has a greater amount of superficial vasculature, and therefore, care should be taken to avoid any visible vessels during injection in order to minimize bruising (Fig. 27.2).
- *Treatment of the forehead*
  The frontalis muscle is responsible for the production of horizontal lines over the forehead. To the inexperienced injector, it may seem appropriate to treat multiple sites in an attempt to eradicate all visible furrows; however, overinjection of the frontalis muscle can result in severe brow ptosis and should be avoided. With appropriate injection placement and dosage of product, a smooth appearance to the skin without brow ptosis can be achieved over time. Though it may take multiple consecutive treatments, the skin over the forehead has the ability to remodel itself once prolonged inactivity of the frontalis muscle has been achieved. Treatment across the middle of the forehead in the horizontal direction at four to five evenly spaced injection sites is ideal. A total of 10 U of Botox or 30 U of Dysport is evenly dispersed at each site (2 to 2.5 U of Botox or 6 to 7.5 U of Dysport). Injections can be extended superiorly at a level just below the hairline to treat lines in this area by infiltrating either 2 to 2.5 U of Botox or 6 to 7.5 U of Dysport at two to three evenly dispersed sites (Fig. 27.3).
- *Treatment of "bunny lines"*
  During injection of the medial brow depressors, "bunny lines," if present over the nasal dorsum, can be effectively treated with either a total of 2 to 3 U of Botox or 7 to 8 U of Dysport dispersed evenly over both nasalis muscles. Care should be taken as to not infiltrate more lateral surrounding musculature as this can cause asymmetries at the upper lip (Fig. 27.4).
- *Treatment for elevation of the brow*
  Elevation of the brow with the use of neuromodulators, also known as a chemical brow lift, as I described in 2003, requires a thorough understanding of the opposing musculature of the upper face. Careful injection

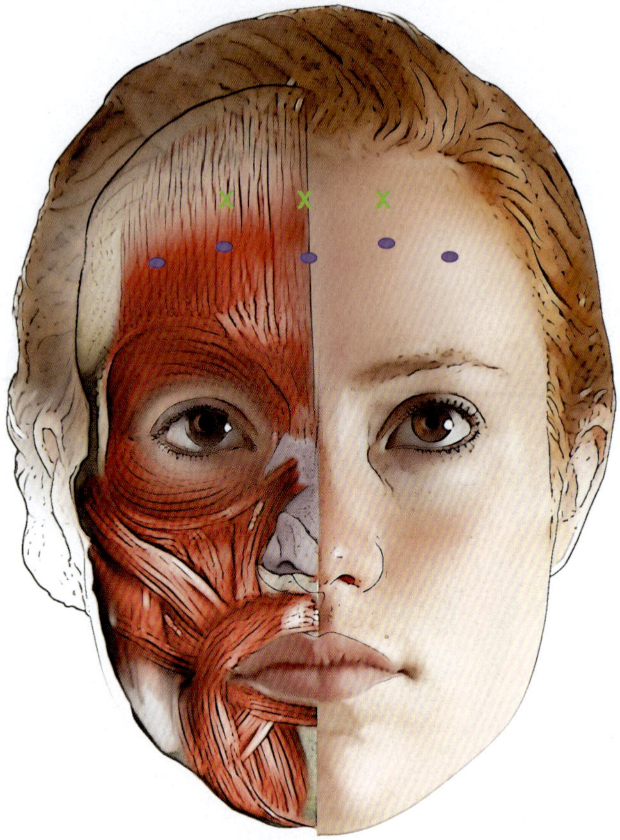

FIGURE 27.3
Blue dots represent ideal injection sites for treatment, while "X"s represent optional injection sites.

at the lateral and medial brow will allow for manipulation of brow position in a predictable and reproducible manner. To elevate the lateral brow, it is important to inject only the lateral orbicularis oculi and avoid injection of the lateral frontalis muscle fibers. The best way to identify the proper injection site is to look for thickening of the lateral orbicularis at the lateral aspect of the brow while having the patient squint. Care should be taken to ensure that this region is injected lateral to the orbital rim with the needle perpendicular to the skin and in the subdermal plane. The area is then injected with approximately 5 to 7 U of Botox or 15 to 21 U of Dysport along with injection of the crow's feet to achieve unopposed lifting of the brow by the

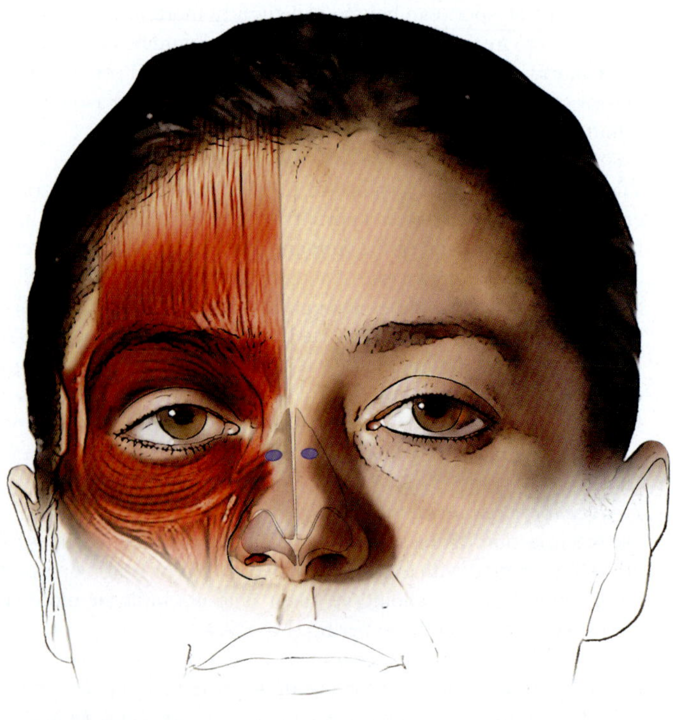

FIGURE 27.4
Blue dots represent ideal injection sites for treatment.

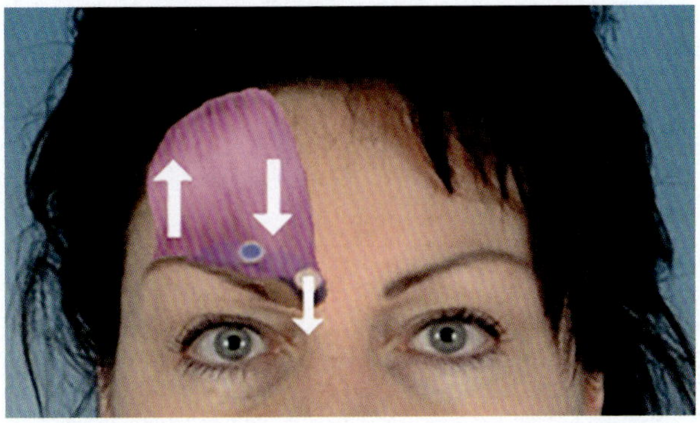

FIGURE 27.5
Arrows depict the effect of incorrect injection placement above the medial aspect of the corrugator into the lower portion of the medial frontalis muscle.

frontalis. Combining this technique with that previously described for treatment of glabellar frown lines can produce aesthetically pleasing elevation of the brow. When injecting the corrugators, especially during this procedure, it is important to inject at the level of the brow and not more superiorly into the medial frontalis muscle. In this case, the outcome will be unopposed medial brow depression and lateral frontalis elevation leading to an unnatural "surprised" look (Fig. 27.5).

POSTOPERATIVE MANAGEMENT

Minimal postinjection management is required. To help minimize bruising, ice packs can be placed over the injection sites instantly. Patients should be made aware that onset of muscle weakness is typically seen at 3 to 4 days and peaks at 3 to 4 weeks with repeat injections necessary at approximately 3 to 4 months.

COMPLICATIONS

The most common adverse events seen with the use of BoNT-A are brow ptosis and headache. Others include eyelid ptosis (Fig. 27.6), xerostomia, flu-like syndrome, ectropion, and strabismus. Proper injection technique and understanding of the anatomy of the upper face should help to prevent most adverse events. Since the effects of BoNT-A typically last 3 to 4 months, any complication should be managed appropriately during that time, for example, with α-adrenergic agonist ophthalmic drops for eyelid ptosis, while stressing to the patient that their symptoms will be short-lived.

RESULTS

Any patient who has or is predisposed to hyperdynamic rhytids and does not have a contraindication to injection with BoNT-A can expect to benefit from treatment. Proper injection technique allows for a wide margin of safety and is generally well tolerated with a high rate of satisfaction.

PEARLS

- A thorough history and physical examination allows for appropriate selection of patients who will benefit from injection while avoiding those who will likely not respond well to treatment or be placed at risk.
- A comprehensive understanding of the relevant anatomy of the upper face and muscular interactions is imperative for proper injection technique and optimal outcomes.

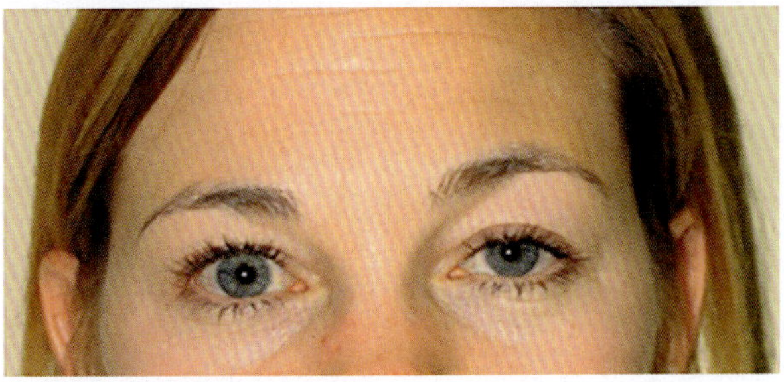

FIGURE 27.6
Ptosis of the left eyelid following BoNT-A injection.

- Injection over the glabella and at the level of the brow, while avoiding injection 1 to 2 cm above the brow, will provide optimal results and prevent medial brow ptosis, a common adverse effect.
- Small amounts of neuromodulator can be injected into the frontalis muscle to help smooth the forehead without risk of significant depression of the brow.

PITFALLS

- Eyelid ptosis is observed when treating the glabellar musculature. It is my belief that deep injection along with hydrostatic pressure near the fissures of the neurovascular bundles at the superior orbital rim allows for tracking of neurotoxin molecules toward the superior orbital fissure where the levator innervation can be affected.
- Overinjection of the medial frontalis muscle in conjunction with treatment of the lateral brow depressors will produce an unnatural surprised appearance.
- It is important to avoid overinjection of the frontalis muscle as this will lead to significant brow ptosis.

ACKNOWLEDGMENT

I would like to acknowledge my fellow, Jason P. Champagne, MD, for his assistance in the editing and final drafting of this chapter.

SUGGESTED READING

Kane M, Donofrio L, Ascher B, et al. Expanding the use of neurotoxins in facial aesthetics: a consensus panel's assessment and recommendations. *J Drugs Dermatol* 2010;9(1 Suppl):s7–s22.

Maas CS, Kim EJ. Temporal brow lift using botulinum toxin A: an update. *Plast Reconstr Surg* 2003;112(5 Suppl):109S–112S; discussion 113S–114S.

Morgan JC, Iyer SS, Moser ET, et al. Botulinum toxin A during pregnancy: a survey of treating physicians. *J Neurol Neurosurg Psychiatry* 2006;77:117–119.

Nettar KD, Yu KC, Bapna S, et al. An internally controlled, double-blind comparison of the efficacy of onabotulinumtoxinA and abobotulinumtoxinA. *Arch Facial Plast Surg* 2011;13(6):380–386.

Raspaldo H, Baspeyras M, Bellity P, et al.; Consensus Group. Upper- and mid-face anti-aging treatment and prevention using onabotulinumtoxin A: the 2010 multidisciplinary French consensus—part 1. *J Cosmet Dermatol* 2011;10(1):36–50.

28 INJECTABLE FILLERS AND FACIAL RESTORATION

Mary Lynn Moran

INTRODUCTION

Injectable treatments have been used in the face since the late 1800s following the invention of the syringe. Among the first attempts was an injection of liquid paraffin into the lips, which was disastrous. In the 1950s, liquid silicone became a popular filler for the breasts and was subsequently used in the face. A combination of complications and legal concerns ultimately forced this practice underground. Modern use of injectables in the realm of facial restoration and rejuvenation dates back to the 1980s with the FDA approval of collagen fillers. Injectables have become an important and ever-growing segment of the facial rejuvenation industry over the last two decades.

The overall growth in minimally invasive procedures between 2000 and 2016 was 180% according to the National Clearinghouse of Plastic Surgery. Cosmetic injectable neurotoxin procedures experienced a 797% growth during that period. Seven million injectable procedures were performed in 2016. This is a result of many factors. Patients hope that new less invasive technologies will eventually replace traditional surgical treatments thereby obviating the need for longer recovery and greater expense, downtime, and discomfort. New technologies have to some degree fulfilled these desires. Another element adding to the enthusiasm of physicians for injectables is our deepening understanding of the dynamic volumetric nature of the aging face. As we gain more experience with fillers, we understand more fully how they can address many of the changes that contribute to a less than desirable facial balance. The safety and straightforward nature of fillers make them an ideal choice for many indications in the face.

HISTORY

Due to the variety of applications, and the relatively low-risk nature of the filler procedure, many individuals are good candidates for filler placement. The most important element of the history is to ascertain the patient's goals. A thorough understanding of what the patient hopes to achieve should be established followed by an honest assessment by the physician of what he or she can realistically accomplish. Computer imaging is a very beneficial way of illustrating what can and cannot be achieved given the patient's desired procedure, the patient's budget, and the physician's capabilities. Once mutual goals and understanding are reached, certain elements in the patient's health history should be obtained. The patient's history with previous filler injections can be very enlightening in terms of both alerting the surgeon to any undesirable reactions and the patient's history of dealing with past disappointments. Preventative management is the best way to avoid risks. Risks for bleeding and bruising should be elicited such as a history of using anticoagulants or taking aspirin or NSAIDS. The patient with a history of perioral herpes simplex should be identified so that preventative measures can be initiated.

General health issues such as diabetes mellitus, collagen vascular diseases, or use of steroids or Accutane should also be noted. Any history of allergic reactions should be documented. If products with animal origins (such as the bovine collagen used with PMMA) are being used, any history of allergies to animal products should be established. Skin tests should be done when appropriate. Cigarette smoking and active sun exposure should be noted. It is also important to establish the patient's tolerance for bruising during the time that the patient plans to undergo treatment. If sensitive work or social events are imminent, it would be best to postpone the injections to a time when some bruising or swelling is more tolerable. Any recent facial procedures such as peels or other aesthetic treatments should be documented. Patients who are on antiretroviral therapy suffering from facial lipoatrophy will benefit from restorative fillers and were in fact the first FDA indication for fillers such as Sculptra. Patients who have congenital or acquired facial lipoatrophy also benefit greatly from fillers.

PHYSICAL EXAMINATION

Examining the patient begins when the physician first meets the patient. The seasoned facial rejuvenation surgeon is always scanning facial features and assessing which ideal modifications may best serve the patient. Before the patient has expressed his or her goals, many facial surgeons have already established their own priorities. However, during the consultation, the patients should be allowed to expresses their concerns first. After carefully listening and obtaining all of the important information, the physician should then examine the patient. This is where the computer imager can be a vital tool to objectify the physicians' observations and reflect back to the patient what he/she has just described. The physician has probably identified several other areas that could be addressed, but that the patient has not mentioned. If the physician senses that the patient is open to other suggestions, then this is an appropriate time for this discussion.

Physical findings to note are any scars from surgery, trauma, or acne. Evidence of active bacterial or viral infection, sunburn, or windburn should be discussed. Previous filler treatments, if visible, should be documented including visible Tyndall effects. Facial asymmetry needs to be documented photographically and discussed in detail with the patient. Assessment of skin type is important as different types react differently to trauma. In particular, patients with darker skin tend to have residual pigmentation after bruising that can be slow to resolve (e.g., periocular complex).

INDICATIONS

Fillers address facial changes due to a variety of causes. They can be used at nearly any depth and are being used more and more to replace lost underlying structural support. Aging causes loss of skin elasticity, weakening of ligamentous support, descent of adipose tissue, atrophy of adipose tissue, and loss of bone. These forces lead to sagging tissues and deepening creases. Essentially, the aging face is a series of shifting and shrinking vectors with a resultant cascading of soft tissue. Furthermore, repeated movement causes wrinkles, which can become quite deep. Understanding and identifying these changes is paramount in making effective improvements in the aging face. Fillers are very versatile tools to address many of these changes. They can support sagging or thinning skin, fill creases and folds, correct depressions, replace or enhance bone loss and deficiency, and replace loss of adipose tissue. The goal in treating the aging face is to restore youthful contours and facial balance.

Other conditions also respond well to treatment with filler. Atrophic or depressed scars from trauma and acne can be improved depending on the amount of tethering. Fillers can treat volume loss due to weight loss, excessive exercise, antiretroviral therapy, hemifacial atrophy, surgical removal of masses, or bony trauma.

Common treatment sites include

- Fine and deep facial lines
- Nasolabial folds
- Lip lines
- Lips (for enhancement and restoration)

Newer indications have come about as a result of greater understanding of the volumetric changes in the aging face. These include:

- Ear lobe atrophy
- Labiomental crease
- Lateral brow (orbital rim and above)
- Malar
- Malar cheek groove
- Mandibular angle/body
- Mental sulcus
- Preauricular sulcus
- Prejowl sulcus

- Submalar
- Tear trough
- Temporal hollowing

CONTRAINDICATIONS

Fillers should not be used in patients who have unrealistic expectations of what can be achieved with them. Specifically, they should be made aware of the fact that some indications require larger volumes of filler to achieve the desired result. Patients with significant lipoatrophy must be completely informed of the limitations in a chosen filler and the volume restoration that can be achieved. Elderly patients may not achieve the results hoped for by both physician and patient. It is wise with mature patients to focus on a specific limited treatment area that is most troublesome rather than attempt to achieve a great global rejuvenation.

If a patient treated elsewhere comes in already overfilled, it would be wise to discuss your observations with the patient in a tactful manner and suggest that he or she hold off on any further filler at this time. Computer imaging can also assist with this discussion. The physician can even offer reduction of the overcorrection with hyaluronidase if the filler is hyaluronic acid based. The possibility of body dysmorphic disorder should be considered, but many emotionally sound patients have fallen into the trap of not realizing the relative disproportion created by their filler treatment.

Patients who are intolerant of any bruising are not good candidates for injectable filler treatments. The likelihood of some amount of bruising during any given treatment session is high enough even in the most skilled hands that it should be considered an expected outcome.

General health concerns that would preclude using injectable fillers would apply to patients who are taking anticoagulants. In cases where anticoagulants can be discontinued prior to treatment, patients are likely to have less bruising. Patients who have active skin conditions such as rash, infection, sunburn, or herpetic outbreaks should not have this area treated until after the condition resolves. Patients who are diabetic or immunocompromised should only be treated if the physician treating their disorder clears them for the procedure. They should receive extra care during the preparation of the skin and counseled about postoperative treatment of the injection site. Patients with collagen vascular diseases should not receive collagen-based products such as polymethyl methacrylate (PMMA). Skin testing is required for most autologous collagen products, especially those of bovine origin. Clearly, any patient with a history of allergic reaction to collagen or a collagen skin test should not be considered a candidate for treatment with collagen-based products even if the reaction was in the past.

PREOPERATIVE PLANNING

Preprocedural planning begins during the consultation. Once treatment areas are identified and goals and outcomes are mutually understood, the physician should explain all of the risks to the patient and obtain a signed consent. If the patients have taken any common agents that contribute to bruising, they should be counseled that they may bruise more than average or perhaps be rescheduled. Photos should be taken of the entire face from five views as well as appropriate close-ups. Fees are thoroughly discussed in advance as are "touch-up" policies.

Filler Selection

The origins of our modern experience with fillers began with collagen. Zyplast and Zyderm were central elements in most facial rejuvenation practices. With the advent of hyaluronic acid fillers, market demand for collagen fillers diminished, and eventually production was terminated. Hyaluronic acid is a naturally occurring polysaccharide, and today's most popular product is non–animal-derived stabilized hyaluronic acid (NASHA). Other popular injectable fillers include synthetic fillers made of calcium hydroxylapatite (CaHA) and poly-L-lactic acid (PLLA). Both are biostimulatory and therefore create new collagen. CaHA also has volume replacement action. Both are temporary (see Table 28.1 for a comparison of properties). A permanent synthetic filler is PMMA. Adipose tissue and medical-grade silicone are other injectables used in facial restoration but remain outside the scope of this chapter. Another very important category of facial injectables for facial rejuvenation includes the neurotoxin family. This chapter will focus only on injectable fillers.

The choice of injectable filler is based upon operator experience and preference, location and indication, safety concerns, reversibility, patient preference, and general health factors.

The general classification of fillers is divided into the following:

- Volume replacement fillers versus biostimulatory fillers
- Short versus long versus permanent duration
- Naturally derived versus synthetic fillers

TABLE 28.1 Comparison of Properties

Hyaluronic acid	Volume replacement	Natural	6–18 mo
PLLA	Biostimulatory	Synthetic	12–24 mo
CaHA	VR and BS	Synthetic	12 mo
PMMA	VR and BS	Synthetic and natural	Permanent
Silicone	VR	Synthetic	Permanent
Adipose tissue	VR	Natural	Variable

Hyaluronic acid fillers dominate the marketplace due to the relative ease of use and low complication rate. They are also unique in that they are reversible with hyaluronidase. Hyaluronic acid is a highly hydrophilic molecule, which holds up to 2,000 times its own weight in water acting as a humectant. It is a natural, linear polysaccharide glycosaminoglycan with alternating residues of D-glucuronic acid and *N*-acetyl-D-glucosamine. It is a component of connective tissue in all mammals and so is not tissue or species specific, making it nonimmunogenic. It is found in skin extracellular matrix, synovial fluid, vitreous humor, and vocal cords, among many other locations in the human body. It exhibits isovolumetric degradation in which molecules of hyaluronic acid degrade, allowing those remaining to absorb more water. This allows the total volume of gel to remain stable over time. Currently available commercially derived hyaluronic acid is derived from strep bacterium and therefore is referred to as non–animal-derived stabilized hyaluronic acid (NASHA).

The importance of hyaluronic acid in the skin cannot be understated. Its ability to bind with water gives skin its volume and structural integrity. It interacts with intercellular lipids and regulates the mechanical properties of the stratum corneum. It maintains the viscoelasticity of the skin and its concentration diminishes with age.

Fillers are distinguished by particle size, concentration, viscosity (thickness), stiffness, rheology (flow), cross-linking, and hydration (Table 28.2).

Nonhyaluronic acid fillers are each unique in their characteristics, advantages, and disadvantages.

- *Poly-L-lactic acid (PLLA)* (Sculptra™) was approved by the FDA in 2004 for the treatment of HIV lipoatrophy. It was subsequently approved in 2009 for cosmetic use. It is different than the other fillers in that it is not a volume replacement product but rather a collagen stimulator. Volumization ensues after up to four treatments spaced at least 3 weeks apart. The results last up to 24 months. A cross-hatching layering method is used to create diffuse collagenesis as the immune response to the product takes place gradually over time. Careful technique must be used to minimize the chance of lumping or granulomas. Allergic or hypersensitivity reactions can occur. Due to its stimulatory nature and potential for lumping, it is not recommended for use under the eyes or around the mouth.
- *Calcium hydroxylapatite* (Radiesse™) was approved for cosmetic use in 2006. Upon initial injection, calcium hydroxylapatite (CaHA) acts as a volume replacer. Over time, the CaHA microspheres are slowly degraded stimulating collagen in the process. It is heralded for its ability to create significant volumization as a result of a very high G′ (which is a measure of elasticity or "push"). It is not to be used around the mouth or under the eyes for similar reasons to PLLA.
- *Artefill™* was approved in 2006 as the first nonresorbable filler for cosmetic facial use in the United States. It is comprised of 20% synthetic microspheres made of PMMA and 80% bovine collagen. A skin test is required 1 month prior to treatment. The injected collagen corrects the defect initially and is subsequently resorbed. During resorption of the injected collagen, neocollagenesis forms around the microspheres and

TABLE 28.2 Hyaluronic Acid Filler Products

Product	Particle Size	Conc./mL	Viscosity	Flow	Depth of Injection
Restylane	100k particles/mL–250 µm	20 mg/mL	High	Low	Superficial to deep
Perlane	10k particles/ml	20 mg/mL	Higher	Lower	Deep
Juvederm Ultra	N/A 9% cross-linked	24 mg/mL	High	Easiest	Superficial to medium
Juvederm Ultra Plus	N/A 11% cross-linked	24 mg/mL	Higher	Easy	Medium to deep

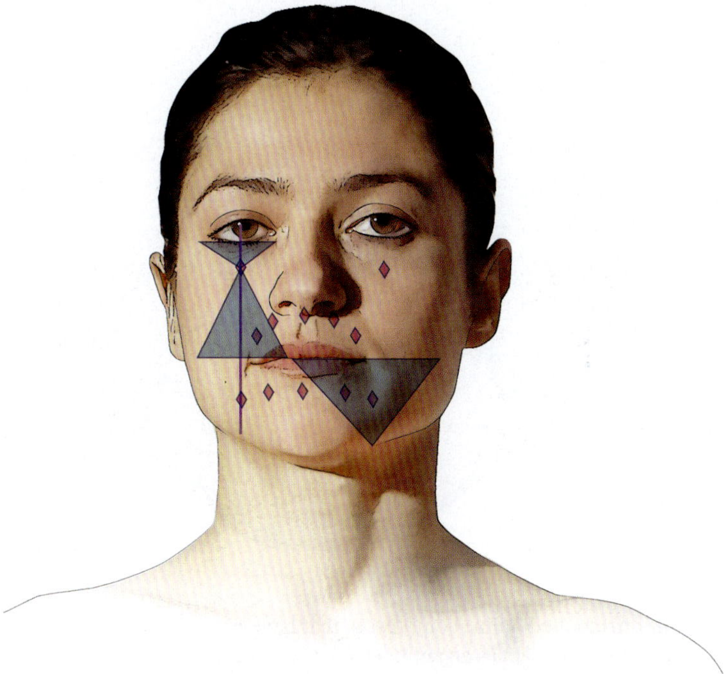

FIGURE 28.1
Infraorbital, mental, and infralabial nerve blocks.

corrects for injected collagen loss. This product is contraindicated in patients with collagen vascular diseases or a history of positive collagen skin testing. It is best used in deeper areas of the face with thicker skin. It is not appropriate for use around the eyes or lips.

For patients who are especially sensitive, nerve blocks can be employed. These are particularly helpful when the perioral area is being treated. The infraorbital and mandibular nerve blocks are helpful in addition to an infralabial block if the lips are to be injected (Fig. 28.1).

You will find that your patients are more relaxed if they are comfortable and you will be more focused as a result. Prior to beginning injections, have the patients prioritize which areas they would like you to treat. Explain which areas you believe will be successfully treated with the amount and type of filler they have chosen.

Depending on the area being treated, patient preference, and physician preference, topical anesthetic is then applied to the area to be treated. Ask if the patient has any known sensitivities to the ingredients in the chosen agent. There are many available topical anesthetic products. The most effective anesthetics are specially formulated and available through a distributor or compounding pharmacy. Care should be taken not to get any anesthetic in the eyes as it can cause corneal de-epithelialization. Also try to avoid getting any in the mouth as such products are quite bitter and numbing of the throat can make the patient feels as though he or she is having trouble breathing. Patients should be instructed not to eat or drink anything while numbing, and they should take care not to lick their lips or rub their face. After approximately 30 minutes, the physician carefully removes the topical agent. Limited surface area and nonocclusive techniques should be used to avoid absorption doses that can be toxic. Toxicity can cause seizures and death. Hypersensitivity reactions to topical anesthetics are not uncommon. Allergic reactions can also occur.

SURGICAL TECHNIQUE

Make the patient comfortable and adjust the chair to a height that is ergonomically correct for you. Cleanse the skin well with alcohol. Begin your injections using whatever methods you have become comfortable with to get the best results. There are a variety of techniques including serial puncture, linear threading, depot, fanning, cross-hatching, pinch eversion, subcision, and threading. Various techniques work best for different indications (Figs. 28.2 to 28.4).

In general, "lighter" fillers are used superficially and "heavier" fillers are used in deeper areas. Biostimulatory and permanent fillers should not be used around the eyes and mouth. Use caution near large facial vessels as occlusion can occur, especially the angular artery near the alar facial groove and the supratrochlear artery when treating the glabella.

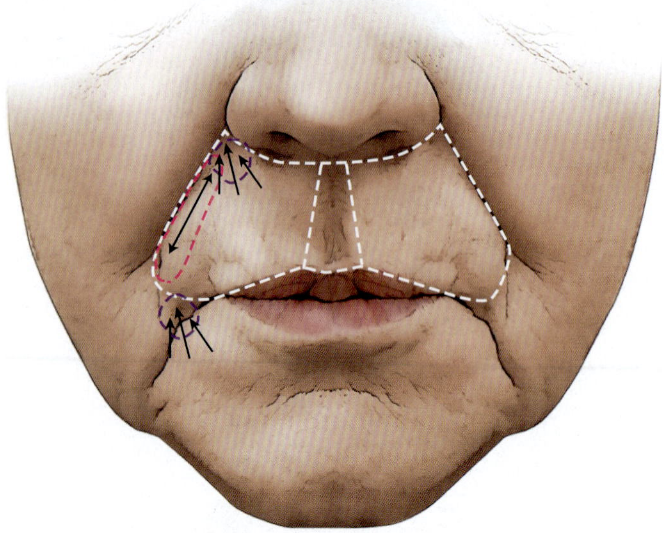

FIGURE 28.2
Techniques for treatment of the nasolabial and marionette lines.

During treatment, apply pressure with refrigerated gauze compresses that have been soaked in hydrogen peroxide and sterile saline. This will remove any blood, act as an antimicrobial, and assist in pain reduction due to the cold. Massaging the area after treatment can help smooth out any irregularities. I prefer to do this with the contents of a fresh packet of bacitracin ointment so as to temporarily coat the injection sites with antimicrobial as well as to lubricate the process.

Tear Troughs

Treatment of the tear trough should be done with great care and only after much experience with injectable fillers. The patient should be informed that this is an off-label use of the product. Also educate patients as to the multifactorial nature of their "dark circles," which may require a multimodal approach to achieve satisfactory results. Due to the proximity of the globe, and the thin nature of the skin, this procedure is fraught with challenges. There have been reports of retinal arterial occlusion and blindness as a result of retrograde embolization from periocular injections. No reported cases have occurred to this date from hyaluronic acid. When done properly, filler placement can be a very effective way to minimize the depression of the tear trough deformity, minimize pseudoherniation of the periorbital adipose tissue, and decrease the apparent darkness underneath the eye. My preferred filler is Restylane™ as it has more ideal properties in terms of viscosity, flow, and particle size compared to the other hyaluronic acid products. Other hyaluronic acid products are more likely to create excessive fullness or irregularities or cause a Tyndall effect. Nonhyaluronic acid products under the eyes carry the risk of lumping and granulomas. Unlike hyaluronic acids, they are also irreversible. A serial microdepot injection into the subperiosteal or epiperiosteal space gives the best chance of a smooth result in my hands. Others prefer a threading or more superficial technique. Nothing larger than a 30-gauge needle should be used in order to control the aliquots of material deposited as well as to

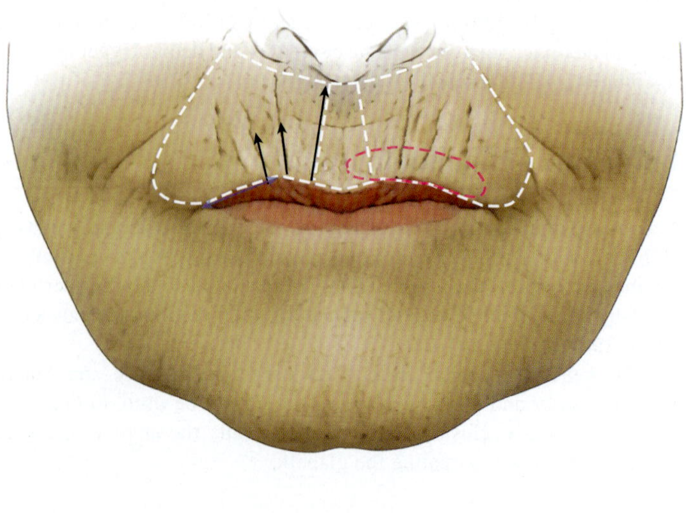

FIGURE 28.3
Techniques for perioral rejuvenation with injectable fillers.

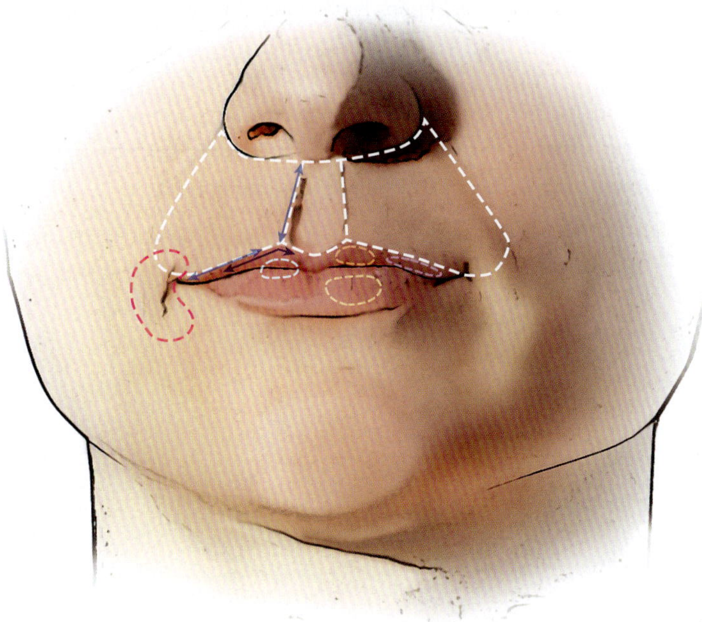

FIGURE 28.4
Lip enhancement techniques with injectable fillers.

minimize discomfort and bruising. If anything smaller than a 30 gauge (e.g., 31 gauge or 32 gauge) is used, be careful to inject with very slow and steady pressure as the high viscosity of the filler can cause the needle to dislodge and potentially cause injury to the eye. Petechiae, purpura, and ecchymosis are to be expected from this procedure due to the thin skin and location of the infraorbital vascular bundle. Massaging the area is crucial to achieve a smooth result, especially if lumps become visible during injection. Bruising in this area can be prolonged and darker than in other locations, so patients should have some "social downtime" before scheduling this procedure.

Temples

The temporal region is another indication for fillers. Treatment can create a significant difference in the aging or volume-deficient face. This therapy, like many, is also off-label. Hyaluronic acid fillers should be placed either the subcutaneous plane or in the plane between the superficial and deep fascia. PLLA is usually placed deeper under the temporalis fascia. The thin nature of the skin, lack of soft tissue in the volume depleted temple, and "minefield" of superficial blood vessels make the area prone to bruising and lumping, so careful technique should be used with rigorous posttreatment massage.

POSTOPERATIVE MANAGEMENT

Postoperative management consists of careful counseling about preventing infection, additional bruising, and when to call the office. Clean handling of the treatment areas (or ideally no handling) is strongly enforced. Patients should not put cosmetics over treated areas for 24 hours. I do not advise our patients to massage the treated areas as I would have done in the office any necessary massage to achieve an ideal result. Cool compresses are recommended for several hours after treatment to help minimize swelling and bruising. Patients are advised not to place ice or frozen products directly on the skin so as to avoid cold injury. They are counseled to avoid anticoagulants for the 2 days including NSAIDS, alcohol, vitamin E, fish oil, and flax seed oil. Hot tubs should also be avoided for 2 days as the vasodilation may exacerbate any bruising. I distribute arnica montana to patients who seem to be very likely to bruise. The less patients bruise and swell, the better their overall experience. Happy patients often become repeat patients. If the patient is highly sensitive to the possibility of swelling, then elevation of the treated area and avoidance of high-sodium foods may assist with this goal in the short term. Any patient who is prone to herpes simplex outbreaks should be given antiviral medication as well as a topical antiviral product if filler was placed in the area known to break out.

I counsel my patients to call my office if any unusual changes occur in the skin over the treatment area (darkening, blistering, weeping, redness, tenderness, discomfort). Patients who have been injected near the eye region are counseled to call immediately for any visual changes. Patients are also counseled to schedule a follow-up if they are concerned about their results, have any questions, or see any lumps or contour irregularities after 2 weeks. I inform them that they should expect to feel lumps but as long as they are not visible after 2 weeks, there is no cause for concern.

COMPLICATIONS

Complications from fillers are rarely serious and in most cases treatable or even reversible.

Minor complications include

- Bruising
- Irregularity
- Overcorrection
- Tyndall effect
- Undercorrection

Moderate and severe complications:

- Allergic reaction
- Biofilms
- Epidermolysis
- Granulomas
- HSV eruption
- Hypersensitivity reaction
- Infection
- Nodules
- Soft tissue necrosis
- Vascular embolism
- Blindness

Prevention of Complications

Careful technique, experience, and a thorough understanding of the underlying anatomy is the key to excellent results with injectable fillers. Being aware of potential pitfalls is essential to avoiding problems. Patient satisfaction starts with thoughtful communication between patient and physician. When expectations are clear, the physician is better able to deliver the desired outcome. As previously mentioned, avoidance of anticoagulants can help to minimize bruising. Proper clean handling during and after treatment will usually avoid infection. Pretreatment or immediate posttreatment can avert HSV outbreaks in those with a history. Adequate anesthesia enhances the experience and the outcome. Cool compresses during and after treatment minimize discomfort and sometimes bruising. Arnica montana orally can also mitigate bruising and swelling. Proper size needles and correct formulation for the indication lead to better outcomes with fewer complications. Conservative treatment is the best way to avoid problems including distorted facial proportions. In general, less is more to avoid "cat lip," "duck lip," "monkey lip," "trout pout," "chipmunk cheeks," or the overstuffed face.

Treatment of Complications

Overcorrection, undercorrection, and superficial placement of fillers are the leading causes of patient dissatisfaction. Fortunately, serious complications are uncommon. Since hyaluronic acid fillers make up the bulk of treatment and they are reversible with hyaluronidase, the overall risk of long-term or severely poor outcomes is quite rare.

- Overcorrection or irregularity: Sometimes, more filler is indicated to balance out or camouflage the offending area. If this is not possible or appropriate, partial or complete removal with hyaluronidase can correct the problem if a hyaluronic acid product is used.
- Tyndall effect: The phenomenon is caused by the scattering of light by particles in a colloid with resultant reflection of only blue light. Superficial placement of hyaluronic acid resulting in a bluish discoloration can be reversed with hyaluronidase.
- Hyaluronidase: This is an enzyme that is used to increase tissue permeability and therefore speed the dispersion and delivery of drugs in the tissues. It accomplishes this by degrading hyaluronan. Typical dosing to treat imperfections with hyaluronic acid is in the range of 5 to 20 U. This can be diluted with a small amount of saline and injected using a fine-gauge needle on a tuberculin syringe directly into the desired area. Undercorrection is advised since the product seems to continue to have some subtle activity for a few days.

More correction can always be achieved after the results of the first treatment are assessed at a follow-up appointment.

- Camouflage makeup: These products can go a long way to cover up bruising. My staff is trained to apply "stage makeup" for patients who request help with more significant bruising.
- "Nick and squeeze": Like its namesake, use of a needle or scalpel may be useful to extract the offending product.
- For nodules and granulomas caused by non–hyaluronic acid fillers, cautious use of injectable or sometimes oral corticosteroids, 5-FU injections, or surgical excision may be necessary. These have been reported to occur in roughly 0.1% of the patient population, mostly after the injection of permanent or semipermanent fillers. They usually occur within the first 6 months after injection, but can also occur years after. Some have reported resolution of calcium hydroxlapatite nodules by simply injecting saline into the site.

Infection

Soft tissue infections are surprisingly rare with injectables. Clean technique during treatment and clean handling of the area after treatment are very important. Single use of product on a single patient in one treatment session is imperative. Syringes are not to be shared among friends or family members. Storing partially used product for use at a later time for the same patient may introduce bacteria into the syringe as the sterile seal is now broken. Smaller dosed syringes are available in most product lines to avoid this temptation.

Infections may present as erythema, tenderness, swelling, oozing, vesicles, pustules, epidermolysis, or even a frank abscess (Fig. 28.5). Fever is not common but should be taken very seriously. These signs may present as soon as a few days or as delayed as a few weeks after treatment. Late presenting or refractory infection should raise the suspicion of atypical infections such as mycobacterium or biofilms. Empirical treatment can be initiated for normal skin pathogens if material cannot be obtained for culture. This should include an oral and a topical antibiotic with coverage for *Staphylococcus aureus* and streptococcus. Treatment with topical antibiotic ointment such as mupirocin twice/day for 7 days is very effective especially in combination with an oral antibiotic and lends coverage for some MRSA. Prompt and effective treatment of infections in the region of the face where fillers are commonly used is crucial given the possible risk of retrograde spread. Frequent follow-up is very important in patients with infection even if they seem minor. Failure of the infection to respond within a reasonable period of time should prompt further evaluation with consideration for atypical organisms. Switching to a broader spectrum antibiotic or intravenous therapy may be indicated. Never hesitate to obtain an Infectious Disease consultation. Consulting with colleagues is another valuable tool when faced with challenging complications. Inadequately treated infection can result in necrosis and sepsis.

Treatment of Vascular Occlusion

Vascular occlusion is another rare but potentially serious complication of fillers. It occurs as a result of disruption of one of the facial vessels either by obstruction of the vessel with filler, compression of the vessel, or injury (transection) of the vessel. The most commonly affected vessels include the facial or

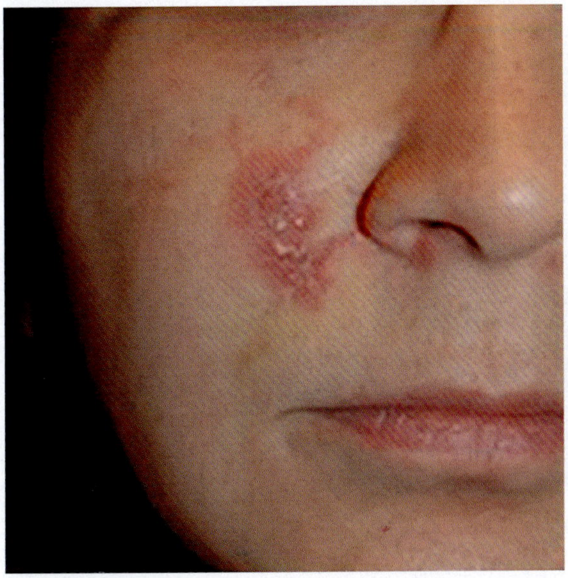

FIGURE 28.5
Infection presenting 2 days after injection of the nasolabial fold with hyaluronic acid. The patient used cosmetics the same day of treatment over the area. Topical and oral antibiotics led to resolution within 1 week.

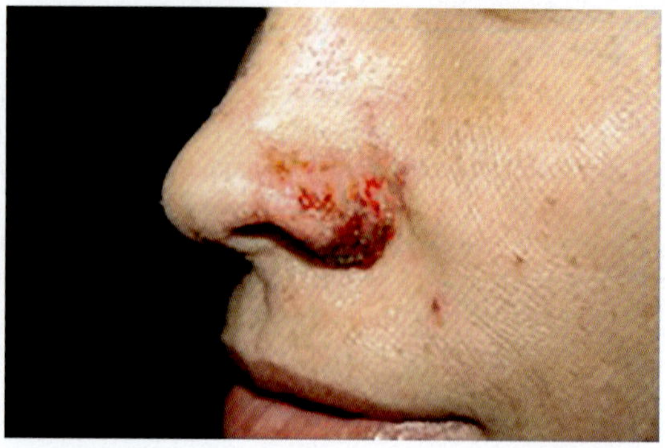

FIGURE 28.6
Alar necrosis (courtesy of Steve Dayan).

angular artery, supratrochlear artery, and labial arteries resulting from treatments in the alar–facial region, glabella, and lips, respectively (Fig. 28.6). Awareness and caution must be employed when treating these areas. If blanching or duskiness is seen during the course of treatment or reported by the patient after treatment, immediate treatment with hyaluronidase should be given if hyaluronic acid was used. Other treatments, regardless of filler, include massage, nitropaste, warm compresses, and oral antibiotics. The patient needs to be followed closely, and topical wound care should be initiated. If necrosis ensues, then steroids, hyperbaric oxygen, and lasers may be needed to assist in the healing process. Surgical reconstruction may be required in extreme cases.

RESULTS

Filler treatments are among the most rewarding treatments we offer our patients (Figs. 28.7 to 28.10). They deliver instant results and high satisfaction when done properly. Given the relative affordability and lack of downtime, they are in increasingly higher demand. While complication rates are relatively low, this should still be viewed as an invasive medical treatment.

The tendency in recent years is to commoditize filler injections, which is alarming. Practitioners need to be well trained, and if the procedure is delegated to physician extenders, both the supervising physician and supervisee need to be thoroughly experienced. The supervising physician needs to perform the appropriate prior medical examination and obtain consent before the prescription for the filler can be administered.

PEARLS

- Hyaluronic acid fillers have the greatest ease of use and are reversible.
- CaHA, PLLA, and Artefill are not recommended for use around the eyes or mouth.
- Injection is to be performed only after the needle has been advanced or while it is withdrawn.

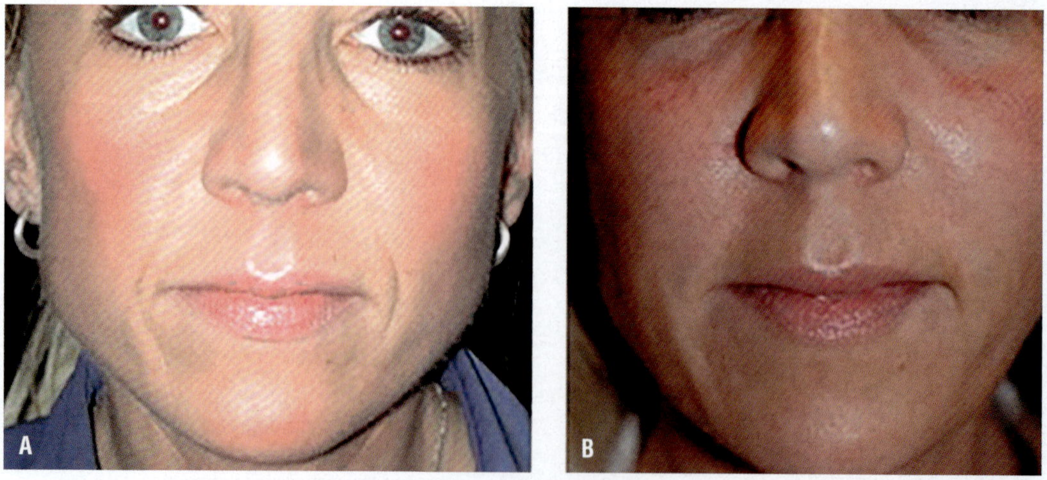

FIGURE 28.7 Before **(A)** and after **(B)** treatment of nasolabial folds tear trough with hyaluronic acid.

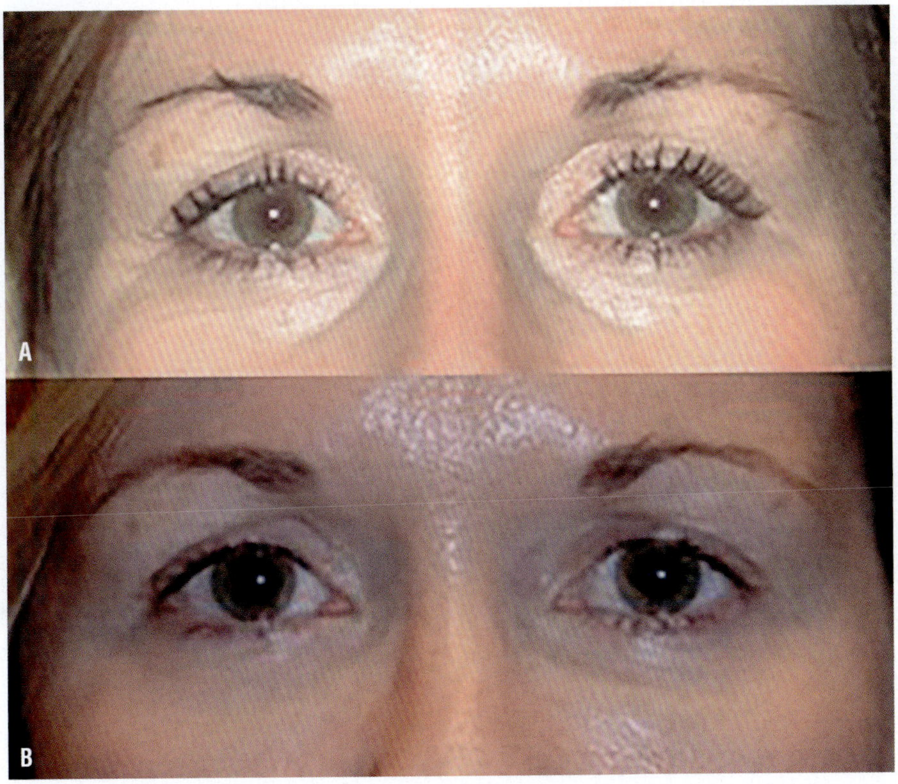

FIGURE 28.8 Treatment of tear troughs before **(A)** and after **(B)** with hyaluronic acid.

- Review of pricing prior to treatment is imperative in preventing "sticker shock."
- Any filler from the non-US distributor is not FDA approved in the United States.

PITFALLS

- Blanching or duskiness seen during the course of treatment or afterward is to be treated as a vascular insult.
- Resistance and patient discomfort while advancing a needle for deep injections commonly represent a vessel or nerve. Repositioning is recommended.
- Undercorrection is easier to treat than is overcorrection.

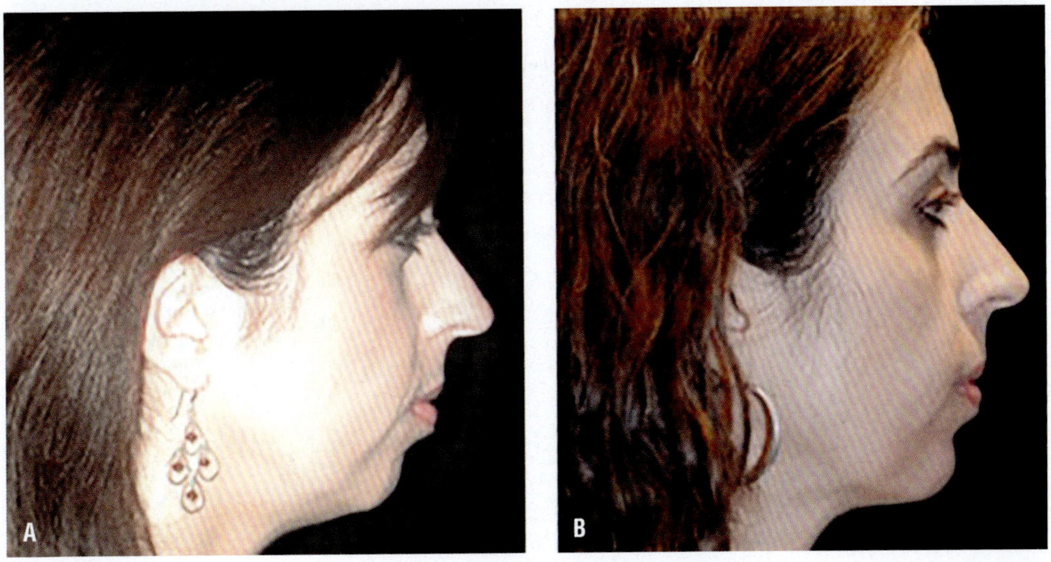

FIGURE 28.9 Chin augmentation before **(A)** and after **(B)** with hyaluronic acid.

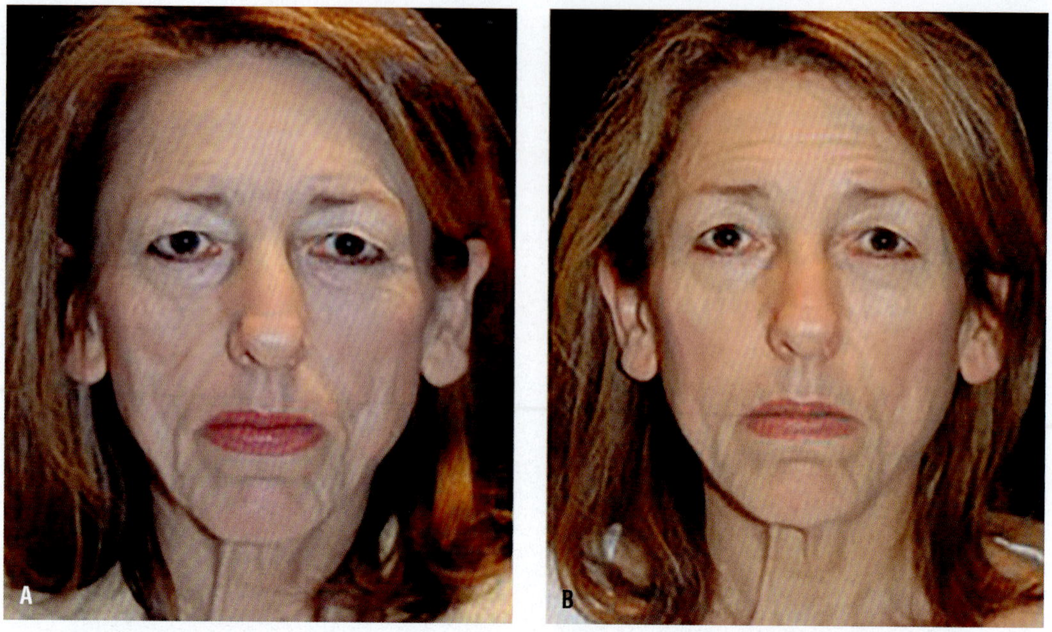

FIGURE 28.10 Treatment of facial volume loss after significant weight loss with hyaluronic acid to the malar and submalar regions before **(A)** and after **(B)**.

INSTRUMENTS TO HAVE AVAILABLE

- Antimicrobial cleanser
- Isopropyl alcohol swabs
- Hand mirror for patient
- Gauze soaked in refrigerated sterile saline and hydrogen peroxide
- Injectable filler of choice
- Needle or cannula of choice
- Hyaluronidase if using hyaluronic acid filler

SUGGESTED READING

Fitzgerald R, Graivier MH, Kane M, et al. Discuss injectable shaping agents within the context of the established and emerging concepts of facial aging. *Aesthet Surg J* 2010;30(Suppl):36S–45S.

Lambros V. Observations on periorbital and midface aging. *Plast Reconstr Surg* 2007;120:1367–1376.

Rohrich RJ, Pessa JE. The fat compartments of the face: anatomy and clinical implications for cosmetic surgery. *Plast Reconstr Surg* 2007;119:2219–2227.

Shaw RB Jr, Kahn DM, Koltz PF, et al. Aging of the facial skeleton: aesthetic implications and rejuvenation strategies. *Plast Reconstr Surg* 2011;127:374–383.

29 AUTOLOGOUS ADIPOSE TISSUE GRAFTING

Richard A. Gangnes

INTRODUCTION

The ability to enhance facial contour and structure using autogenous adipose tissue has been one of the most important adjuncts in the facial plastic surgeon's armamentarium to have been popularized in the last 20 years. I now use adipose tissue to provide volume and shape to the aging face during facial surgery and as a stand-alone procedure. It is used to restore traumatic or iatrogenic soft tissue defects; it is used for acquired or congenital facial contour abnormalities or asymmetries; to improve the quality and texture of severely actinically damaged skin; and to help restore facial shape, symmetry, and eyelid closure after facial nerve dysfunction secondary to eighth cranial nerve tumor surgery. The ability to graft adipose tissue to the face precisely, easily, and effectively should be in every facial plastic surgeon's skill set, along with the knowledge of its benefits, limitations, and risks.

Aesthetic surgery of the aging face has traditionally focused on excisional techniques. Surgery was aimed at counteracting the natural descent of facial structures and removing redundant soft tissue. In recent years, however, the concept of volume restoration has increasingly become recognized to be of vital importance in treatment of the aging face. A look back into history reveals that plastic surgeons of the previous century understood the need of volume restoration. Reports from the literature of the early 20th-century describes efforts to augment tissues with a wide array of injectable substances, such as paraffin, petroleum jelly, latex, gold, silver, ivory and cow horn.

Different types of face-lifts were popularized and promulgated as ways to lift and elevate with the consequence of thinning and flattening the face. As we have learned more about the aging face, we know that the changes involve more volume changes than a falling or laxity, particularly after the recognition that part of the aging process involves a shrinking of the underlying bony skeletal framework. What appears as facial laxity is not just intrinsic laxity of the soft tissue and the skin envelope but it is having the envelope reside over a shrinking skeletal support. With the realization that volume restoration alone, as Dr. Coleman demonstrated in the early nineties with structural adipose tissue grafting, achieved in many cases a remarkable youthful enhancement without the tightening, elevation, or tissue removal, we began to see the value of volume restoration as an important adjunct to surgery of the aging face. What began as an either–or proposition evolved into a simultaneous operation with ever-improving results and with greater patient and surgeon satisfaction. Now, volume restoration is an important part of the surgical and nonsurgical treatment of both the aging face and other facial abnormalities. In fact, with the increasing numbers of injectable fillers with varying characteristics that have been brought to the cosmetic market in the last 10 years, both surgeons and nonsurgeons have seen the volumizing of the face as an increasingly important part of their practice. With that, however, we are seeing an increasing number of patients "overvolumized" as patients, surgeons, and nonsurgeons choose to use volume enhancers instead of surgery for a variety of reasons, when the best outcomes are more often achieved with a blend of both volumizing and surgery. It is clear that the medical profession has recognized the importance of volume restoration in the treatment of the aging face, and now the dilemma is to choose the most appropriate way to achieve those soft, round, energetic, and beautiful contours of the youthful face. After using nearly all of the facial fillers including injectable collagen introduced over 20 years ago, adipose tissue remains one of the most valuable volume- and contour-enhancing materials that we use both as an adjunct to surgery and as a procedure by itself.

A review of the past efforts to rejuvenate the aging face reveals that excisional-based surgery has not provided sufficiently good results for facial rejuvenation. These traditional excision-only approaches do little to improve cheek or temporal hollowing. Indeed, the tightening and lifting procedures may accentuate volume loss by flattening facial contours. Adipose tissue and skin removal during a blepharoplasty may even worsen the hollowed-out, aged appearance of the eyes. Many contemporary aesthetic surgeons now routinely employ adipose tissue transfer or injectable fillers to enhance their outcomes. Several types of commercial fillers have been used with varying degrees of success and longevity. On the other hand, adipose tissue grafting has demonstrated excellent availability and biocompatibility as well as improved overall skin quality in treated areas for reasons that are unknown. Early criticisms of adipose tissue grafting were the variable and seemingly high degrees of adipose tissue graft loss. However, today, with more experience and improved understanding of atraumatic tissue handling and refined harvest and injection techniques, graft retention has improved significantly. Autologous adipose tissue transfer is now well regarded as an invaluable tool in the plastic surgeon's armamentarium that can be used either alone or in combination with traditional excisional techniques in facial rejuvenation.

Volume loss has been studied by many and is understood to be a fundamental component of the aging process. Coleman, one of the most influential pioneers of adipose tissue grafting, regarded atrophy of adipose tissue as the primary factor in aging. He also proposed that a significant amount of volume loss was due to colloidal fluid loss with aging. Gonzalez-Ulloa described facial aging as volume loss involving all the structures of the face, including the muscles, bone, skin, and adipose tissue. Lambros singled out specific areas (the brows, the tear trough, the cheeks), and demonstrated how the addition of volume may give results better than traditional methods. A radiologic study by Pessa demonstrated the effect of bony changes on volume loss in the aging process. More recently, the anatomic cadaver work by Rohrich and Pessa illustrated the loss of adipose tissue in specific compartments of the face. While the mechanism for age-related volume loss continues to be investigated, the role of volume restoration in facial rejuvenation is well accepted.

As more research and study has been conducted into the basic science, biology, and technique of grafting over the last 20 years, autologous adipose tissue grafting has assumed an important role in nearly every facial plastic surgeon's practice. Just as the explosion in popularity of liposuction of the body and the face in the early eighties resulted in many patients having contour irregularities that subsequently required correction with adipose tissue and other techniques, we will be seeing problems related to autologous adipose tissue grafting because of the marked increase in the number of procedures performed in the last few years. Just as we saw in the eighties the increasing numbers of complications that tempered our enthusiasm for liposuction and forced a critical look at the science and technique behind this new procedure, we are beginning to see similar problems with adipose tissue grafting as the techniques have become more commonly used by plastic surgeons. It is now more important than ever to adopt a judicious approach to structural adipose tissue grafting; learn what has worked, what problems we have seen, and where this valuable procedure benefits our patients; and learn about ideal facial shape and contour in both the youthful face and the aging face so that we can bring both science and art to the benefit of those entrusted to our hands.

HISTORY

As with any surgical procedure, a history of previous surgery, medical problems, medications, previous fillers, cosmetic surgery, and allergies, must be obtained. It is also important to ask questions about expectations, goals, and, if previous surgery was performed, whether the patient was satisfied with the results. Expectations and psychological suitability are important parts of the assessment based on history and are explained additionally later. The patient's age and body habitus as well as the degree of regular physical activity has a direct impact on the long-term results of adipose tissue grafting, the degree of overcorrection that one should consider, how to counsel the patient with regard to expectation, and the location and amount of donor adipose tissue. The patient's menstrual history in the case of female patients and whether they are pre-, post-, or perimenopausal will impact one's decisions as to patient suitability and the volume of adipose tissue to be used at any one time.

PHYSICAL EXAMINATION

Initial Consultation and Evaluation

For any consultation regarding evaluation of the aging face, we ask that the patients bring in photos of themselves smiling and not smiling from 10 to 15 years ago including their twenties and thirties. This is particularly important and pertinent in the evaluation of patients for adipose tissue grafting for several reasons. It allows an illustrative discussion on the aging process in general and the volume loss that occurs over time to specific areas of the face. It is educational for the patient to see the changes that have occurred over time and relate that to what we are seeing now and can form a basis of discussion regarding the utility of fat to restore these softer, rounder, more energetic contours of their more youthful face. We find that in the discussion of adipose tissue grafting with patients, it is just as much a matter of educating the patient about this procedure as it is evaluating the patient for technique, amount, and location of the area to be grafted. The two common misperceptions among patients with regard to adipose tissue grafting in that "it doesn't last" or "all goes away" or that their face will look puffy and overdone as they see now more increasingly with the widespread injudicious use of fillers by so many specialties.

Part of the educational process is aided by the use of photographs during these times of one's life. We now consider much of facial aging resulting from changes in the soft tissue envelope of the face, which include the progressive changes involved in connective tissue support and bony support and skin changes. Part of the change we experience in the volume loss is depletion and change of the adipose tissue, but also a considerable portion of the deflation is a decrease in the extracellular fluid space consisting mostly of glycosaminoglycans. It is also well established that bony changes occur that accentuate these soft tissue changes including a loss in vertical dimension of the midface accompanied by an increase in size and volume of the orbit along with a shrinkage in the height and projection of the both midface and mandible. Photos at several ages help us illustrate these changes as part of the educational process of the patient.

As we evaluate facial volume and shape through the decades of life with photos and assess these changes in the context of the patient's ideal proportions, most patients would say, and we would generally agree, that the refinement of more juvenile adipose tissue contours and bony maturation of our 30's represent the optimal appearance with regard to facial volume. By bringing in photos during these decades of life, it gives us an idea of contours that patients generally like and would be worthwhile pursuing. It is also important to bring in photos both smiling and in repose as the facial musculature during animation lifts and alters adipose tissue contours that hide areas of hollowing that can be seen in repose. They may also disclose areas where one may need to be more cautious such as the crowding of the eye that can occur in some patient's with smiling. Photographs remain very helpful for both planning and education.

The face is typically assessed in terms of volume as consisting of two major components. Because the eyes are truly the focus of conversation and the most beautifying segment of the face, it is evaluated as a complex involving the periorbital area and adjacent contours of the temple and forehead. The second major component for preoperative assessment is the lower face, which includes the neck. Both of these components are assessed preoperatively for volume, contour, and profile considerations to determine the location, amount, and insertion site of the grafted adipose tissue.

The periorbital area includes the lateral and inferior orbital rims, medial orbital rim, part of which is described as the tear trough, and also an area that is termed the anterior triangle, which will be discussed further. Preoperative evaluation of the inferior orbital rim segments involves the assessment of the degree of depression along the rim or degree of hollowing and the amount of adipose tissue that may be required to soften these areas of volume depletion. The aesthetic unit of the brow and upper eyelid is assessed together as the insertion site for adipose tissue grafting for both areas is within the brow just lateral to the notch or foramen of the supraorbital nerve. The amount of adipose tissue grafted here is dependent on the degree of hollowing and deflation of the upper lid infrabrow and supratarsal fold area medially, in addition to the shape, height, and convexity of the brow laterally. The degree of temple fullness or hollowing, shape of the forehead, and the degree and depth of horizontal frontalis and vertical glabellar lines completes the preoperative evaluation of the upper face and eye aesthetic unit. The preoperative evaluation of this complex involves not only the degree of deflation and hollowing that exists but also whether there is a negative, neutral, or positive vector of the globe as adipose tissue grafting is able to change the relative vector by changing the soft tissue volumes that contribute to this characteristic. The areas of adipose tissue grafting for the eye complex that require preoperative evaluation are

- Tear trough or medial orbital rim
- Inferior orbital rim
- Anterior triangle
- Lateral orbital rim
- Medial infrabrow
- Lateral infrabrow
- Temple subcutaneous
- Temple subfascial
- Suprabrow laterally
- Suprabrow medially
- Forehead

The lower face is likewise treated as a unit and further divided into the component regions to determine whether grafting is necessary and in what volumes. This is particularly done in the context of both the patient and the surgeon's sense of aesthetics in conjunction with previous photos in an effort to maintain the essence of the face to which we have been entrusted. Photographs of patients in their 20s and 30s are very helpful in the decision-making process when adipose tissue-sculpting the aging face. It helps the patients understand the aging process and allows them a better understanding of the value of volume augmentation. It also helps the surgeon in the preoperative analysis of where and how much adipose tissue is grafted particularly in the lower face. The lower facial segments that require evaluation for adipose tissue graft consideration are

- Medial cheek below the anterior triangle
- Upper nasolabial fold to the deep nasal fat pad
- Malar eminence
- Medial zygomatic arch or lateral cheek
- Lateral zygomatic arch at light reflex point
- Nasolabial fold
- Subcutaneous cheek
- Prejowl sulcus
- Lateral mandible, angle of mandible
- Later subcutaneous cheek
- Chin
- Oral commissure
- Lips
- Premaxilla

INDICATIONS

The Periorbital Complex

Adipose tissue used as an augmentation material to the inferior orbital rim area is used primarily to decrease orbital hollowing in those patients without significant orbital adipose tissue pseudoherniation. It can camouflage prominent orbital adipose tissue while filling the orbital rim and thereby shortening the effective vertical height of the lower eyelid and can be used as an adjunct to either adipose tissue removal or adipose tissue repositioning blepharoplasty to accomplish those same goals. We have also used adipose tissue successfully to improve lower lid malposition and dystopia from previous blepharoplasty and have used it to improve dry eye syndrome in patients with facial nerve injury from tumor removal and Bell's palsy.

The orbital rim area consists of the evaluation of four primary areas for grafting:

- The tear trough
- Inferior orbital rim
- Lateral orbital rim
- Anterior triangle

The *tear trough or nasojugal* groove is one of the most widely talked about area of periorbital rejuvenation with a number of different surgical techniques, implants, and fillers used to soften the appearance of this area. Most of the widely used injectable fillers have been tried in this area with differing degrees of success and with some complications. It is generally agreed that the lower molecular weight and less hydrophilic hyaluronic gel fillers are safe in this area, while the more highly cross-linked fillers are fraught with problems although experienced injectors have used the more viscous and highly cross-linked hyaluronic acids in this area with local anesthesia or saline dilution with good success. One needs to be careful with any injectable filler here, including adipose tissue as vascular complications have occurred with retrograde embolic phenomenon causing both vascular compromise to the retina vessels with subsequent visual disturbance and necrosis of the periorbital skin. The anatomy of the orbicularis muscle medial to the infraorbital nerve needs particular attention when injecting adipose tissue. Contour irregularities are more likely to occur here than other areas of the orbital rim. The orbicularis is firmly attached to the periosteum in this location with no subcutaneous adipose tissue or areolar tissue, and the orbicularis tends to be thinnest in this area, corresponding to the tear trough.

Upper Eyelid, Brow, and Temple

Adipose tissue grafting to the area below the brow, the *medial infrabrow and lateral infrabrow*, has been one of the most important adjuncts to blepharoplasty and forehead surgery to beautify the eye. An evaluation of female eyes that are considered beautiful in Western culture reveal infrabrow fullness with a convexity that causes light to be reflected particularly beneath the lateral half of the brow. It is this light reflex that highlights the eye and makes it look more energetic and youthful and which makeup artists try to simulate with white highlights. As orbital hollowing occurs with aging along with some descent of the brow, the lateral brow becomes shadowed and deflated, and the light reflex can be lost. In addition to loss of infrabrow fullness laterally, we frequently see medial infrabrow hollowing, also termed deepening of the "A" frame, that becomes more pronounced as the orbit enlarges with age and relative volume loss occurs. I now perform adipose tissue grafting as a simultaneous procedure in the majority of both upper lid blepharoplasty and endoscopic forehead lifts. Adipose tissue as part of upper lid blepharoplasty allows us to resect less tissue, create a subtler supratarsal fold that is more beautiful, and produce a smooth convex contour from the brow to the supratarsal fold. This is what patients are really asking for when they complain of "too much skin on the upper eyelid." We also find that infrabrow adipose tissue grafting can create a lateral brow lift without surgery as the increased volume below the brow pushes the tail of the brow up. Adipose tissue grafting to this area can be performed either simultaneously with lid or forehead surgery or as an independent procedure depending on the patients' needs.

The *temple injection* is designed to soften the temporal concavity if hollowing is present and to smooth a skeletonized lateral orbital rim. This is accomplished using both a *subcutaneous* plane and a *subfascial* plane depending on the degree of temporal hollowing. Deflation in the temple both produces a skeletonized look and tends to cause some descent of the tail of the brow.

Adipose tissue placed in the *forehead* over the frontalis is done less often than to other areas but can be done as an isolated procedure or simultaneously with a forehead lift. Its primary benefit is to soften horizontal lines of the forehead caused by an active frontalis muscle usually the result of frontalis compensation for a low brow configuration and can be of benefit for very deep horizontal furrowing in patients with weathered skin with active frontalis function.

The Lower Face and Neck

The preoperative evaluation of the lower face and neck area begins as a continuation of the *periorbital complex*. I generally perform my adipose tissue grafting starting with the periorbital complex and upper face and then continue inferiorly similar to how our preoperative evaluation is done. As part of that progression and as a continuation of the periorbital complex, the area of the anterior cheek above the nasolabial fold, the malar eminence, and the anterior segment of the zygomatic arch are then evaluated as well as the interzygoma distance and ideal point of lateral cheek light reflex.

The *anterior cheek* tends to flatten and lose volume with age as the orbicularis and cheek pads descend so that on the profile view, there is a more vertical orientation of the anterior cheek below the orbital rim. Anterior projection of the cheek can be accomplished with adipose tissue grafting below the *anterior triangle*. Adipose tissue grafted here helps to augment the anterior triangle and improve profile balance in those patients and can also assist in changing a prominent globe, negative vector patient to a neutral or even slightly positive vector depending on volumes used. Too much adipose tissue to this area however can be problematic as it produces an operated look. One must be careful then to assess the anterior cheek just above the superior aspect of the nasolabial fold, and it is particularly useful to look at the profile view to assess this area.

Volume augmentation to the *deep nasal adipose tissue pad* just lateral to the nasal ala can accomplish softening of the *nasolabial fold* when adipose tissue is placed in the supraperiosteal plane. I have been using adipose tissue in this area for the last decade with good success in achieving reflation and softening of the nasolabial fold. The *malar prominence*, *submalar* area, and *anterior zygomatic* arch can be one of the most beautifying contours of the female face with nearly 60% of adipose tissue grafted patients receiving adipose tissue in this area. The artistic approach required here is dependent on one's sense of aesthetics in addition to the patient's sense of aesthetics, as one can achieve an increase in the intermalar distance and elevate the prominence of the lateral cheek that many patients desire. One, then, must assess the intermalar distance, overall shape of the face, and one's artistic assessment of the patient, helped in part by previous photographs of the patient to determine whether the lateral malar area should be augmented.

Softening and rounding of the *malar eminence* and anterior *zygomatic arch* and cheek pad are achieved through two approaches. The first approach is accomplished through the lateral nasal alar insertion site. Sculpturing of the cheek, including intermalar distance and lateral cheek, is accomplished using the 7-cm × 1.2-mm curved cannula to course over the curvature of the zygoma. The adipose tissue may also be placed in a *submalar* location for those patients with submalar hollowing in much the same plane that submalar implants have been used for the last 20 years. In adipose tissue grafting, one must take into consideration both to the orbital rim and into the malar cheek area, the patient's preexisting dynamics during smiling. Some patients appear to be hollow in repose, but upon smiling have a mild degree of eye and eyelid encroachment as the zygomaticus muscles and orbicularis muscle elevate the cheek adipose tissue pads crowding the eye. One must always assess this dynamic preoperatively and be careful to avoid putting too much volume both in the orbital rim and over the zygoma as it may cause crowding of the eye during smiling or facial animation. When this occurs, the patient will complain of eyes that have been made smaller by the procedure. Adipose tissue grafting to the malar area requires experience and a conservative approach until experience has been gained, but the results can be very rewarding to the surgeon and the patient.

The second insertion approach to the zygoma and lateral cheek area is through a stab incision with an 18-gauge needle that is lateral and below the body of the zygoma inferior to the zygomatic arch. This allows for access with the long curved cannula to the inferior malar area, malar area, lateral orbital rim, and lateral zygoma. Generally, the amount of adipose tissue that is placed through this approach is less than that placed through the lateral nasal alar approach, but can achieve additional volume and with the crossing of tunnels that occurs with these two approaches and together can aid in softer contours with a smaller chance of contour irregularities.

Patients who have hollowing in the submalar area as described above may achieve softening with injections below the zygoma on the anterior face of the maxilla in the supraperiosteal plane in addition to adipose tissue placed in the subcutaneous plane from above through that lateral nasal alar approach. The long 7-cm × 1.2-mm cannula is employed for this injection while being able to achieve softening down to the mandible. By fanning this injection out from the malar eminence down to the mandible, several things can be accomplished. The submalar hollowing that is seen in some patients can be reduced, but also patients who have deep rhytids in the anterior cheek with degradation of the dermal support of the skin from actinic damage can be improved. Patients who have hollowing in the *submalar* area as described above may achieve softening with adipose tissue with a subcutaneous injection using the long cannula. Normally, this is an injection using the lateral nasal alar approach in a fanning pattern using the longer cannula. In fact, we find that patients who have significant deep rhytids achieve their best results when a combination limited dissection face-lift along with adipose grafting in the subcutaneous plane and fractional CO_2 laser is employed in a simultaneous procedure. Therefore, the subcutaneous injection of adipose tissue in the cheek is a valuable tool to achieve several goals.

As we evaluate the patient from superior to inferior, the *prejowl sulcus and mandibular* contour require assessment. As mandibular bony changes occur with loss of height and volume in the anterior mandible, accentuation of the jowl and jowl adipose tissue occurs. I have used adipose tissue over the last decade to augment the prejowl sulcus and anterior mandible producing softening and reduced prominence of jowl fat. Adipose tissue grafted to this area includes the triangle limited by the oral commissure, the prejowl sulcus, and the chin pad with the mandible. Adipose tissue grafted to this area can accomplish not only reduction in the prominence of the jowl but also reduction of the prominence of the labiomandibular or marionette line and some elevation of the oral commissure.

Likewise, *the lateral mandible* can be augmented with grafted adipose tissue as one loses prominence of the angle of the mandible sees flattening in this area. The choice and decision for adding volume to the posterior mandible and *angle of mandible* is most frequently dependent upon whether or not a limited dissection face-lift or an extended face-lift is performed simultaneously. Generally, if one is contemplating simultaneous surgery with adipose tissue grafting with a limited dissection or extended face-lift dissection, prominence and definition of the angle can be created with the surgical rotation and folding of the platysma at the angle, but increasing definition of the angle can also be achieved by placing adipose tissue under the platysma along the mandible if the subplatysma dissection is limited in this area. Most of the adipose tissue grafts that I perform in this area are done as an independent procedure in an effort to improve contour along the jaw in that area. I have seen a number of patients, including a few of my own, who appear to have had SMAS face-lifts who have lost volume in the posterior mandible and cheek corresponding to thinning and volume loss of the SMAS from wide SMAS undermining and tension placed on its closure. This may be a less recognized problem of SMAS face-lifts, but I think it is not uncommon if one specifically looks for volume loss over the posterior jaw and parotid area that would correspond to a SMAS dissection. Adipose tissue grafted into this area can provide an improved mandibular contour when volume loss has occurred from previous surgery. The insertion sites for the cannula can be both posterior and anterior with the posterior being toward the base of the ear lobule and the anterior closer to the jowl area, the same location of the prejowl sulcus insertion site. I generally use the 7-cm × 1.2-mm cannula for this purpose, and with its curved configuration, it allows me to nicely follow the contour of the mandible from both anterior and posterior approaches.

Likewise, when volume loss is seen in the *lateral cheek* from causes that include aging and previous surgery, this approach using the insertion site from the area below the lobule can be utilized to graft the preauricular cheek in a subcutaneous plane to add volume. Again, the 7-cm × 1.2-mm cannula is employed. The preoperative evaluation relies on the need for volume in these areas and whether or not simultaneous surgery with fat grafting is contemplated.

As much of adipose tissue grafting is aesthetic, artistic, and individual, the profile view is useful in assessing anterior projection of the different facial segments. One can achieve anterior projection of the *chin* with adipose tissue grafting without the use of chin implants although the amount of anterior projection achieved with adipose tissue is limited to about 3 to 4 mm. This can be achieved through an insertion site created with the 18-gauge needle on the anterior aspect of the prejowl triangle using the 1.2-mm or 0.9-mm cannula, and one can sculpture the projection of the chin in the subcutaneous plane. The adipose tissue can also be placed deeper into the mentalis muscle and even in the supraperiosteal plane. This is generally done through a bilateral approach using each side working toward the midline. Also, through this approach, one can augment the sub labial sulcus.

As the assessment continues from the upper part of the face to the lower face, I then evaluate the *neck*. As Coleman has shown, volume augmentation with adipose tissue to the neck can soften prominent platysma bands, can soften and decrease submandibular hollowing between the platysma bands in the midline, can support thin inelastic skin, can soften deep horizontal neck creases, can decrease the noticeability of submaxillary glands, and can have an overall softening effect of the neck skin. With the introduction of facial liposuction in the 1980s, I began to see patients with a very skeletonized platysma as surgeons became increasingly more aggressive with liposuction in an effort to produce a more contoured neck. Adipose tissue in the neck, however, produces soft contours, supports the skin, and allows for the gliding of the platysma under the skin without depressions or irregularities. I have used adipose tissue grafting to the neck for patients who have had previous aggressive submental liposuction producing contour irregularities along the jaw, skeletonization of the platysma producing noticeable striations of the muscle below the skin, or contour irregularities in the lower neck from previous thyroidectomy scars. It can soften submental hollowing during face-lifting when an anterior approach to the platysma is not contemplated. It can also soften the noticeability of the platysma in thin patients with little to no subcutaneous adipose tissue during a face-lift when minimal undermining of the skin from a posterior approach is considered best because of the lack of subcutaneous adipose tissue.

Generally, the last area to be grafted in the face is the *lips* because of the need to reduce oral cavity contamination. I like to graft clean areas first followed by a manipulation of the lip. We find that the persistence rate of grafted adipose tissue in the lips is lower than any other place in the face. It is estimated that we achieve only a 20% to 25% take rate of the grafted adipose tissue in the lip. Patients are given the option of having a conservative or moderate approach with regard to the amount of adipose tissue that is grafted, with a conservative approach limiting the amount of adipose tissue to about seven-tenths of a cc to each quadrant of the lip. The patient is informed that adipose tissue grafted in this amount will achieve a nice short-term result, but the amount of adipose tissue that persists long term will provide very little improvement in volume over the preoperative appearance. This still may be useful, however, for those patients who are unsure, unclear, or anxious about the possibility of grafted adipose tissue producing an unnatural or overdone look. This is probably the most common source of anxiety when talking about lip augmentation. Patients overwhelmingly do not want an overdone look or look that draws attention to a lip that may look surgical. The moderate approach requires nearly twice as much adipose tissue in each quadrant of the lip, injected through this lateral upper lip insertion site using a 0.9-mm cannula. The lips will look overdone for at least 2 weeks with a moderate approach, but we find that the long-term result produces a noticeable but not substantial increase in lip volume. Most patients would prefer this approach rather than a more aggressive approach, which may produce an abnormal or overdone look for 3 to 4 weeks after surgery, but have a long-term greater volume enhancement. These are issues and questions that are explored at the time of the consultation or preoperative evaluation and documented so that the intraoperative decision has already been made based on the patient's desire and requirements regarding healing and downtime.

CONTRAINDICATIONS

Relative contraindications include the following:

- Pain syndrome or autoimmune connective tissue disease
  One must be careful about patient selection and counsel patients appropriately. Some have experienced increased postoperative inflammation in both the donor and recipient sites in patients with active Raynaud's syndrome (Coleman, 2001). Patients with chronic fatigue or pain syndromes may have more difficulty with postoperative pain and swelling at both the donor and recipient sites.
- Preoperative facial asymmetry
  One must counsel appropriately if a patient has a facial asymmetry as this may become enhanced with the addition of adipose tissue grafting. For instance, a minor asymmetry of the lip may turn into a sneer after upper lip augmentation. Efforts should be put forth to create a symmetric and favorable result in these cases.
- Weight instability
  The surgeon should also inquire about any expected weight gain. It may be in the patient's best interest to wait until his or her weight is stable. In our experience, grafted adipose tissue can hypertrophy or contract with weight gain or loss, respectively. Grafted adipose tissue in a patient with significant weight gain can sometimes become visible and lead to contour irregularities or disproportions.
- Premenopausal women
  Particular caution is needed while adopting a more conservative approach in premenopausal women because of the hormonal changes that will occur with age affecting weight changes and changes in lean body mass that will sometimes have an adverse impact on facial volumes that may look overdone with age and weight gain.

PREOPERATIVE PLANNING

The preoperative assessment of both the periorbital complex and the lower facial segments is marked and documented on a facial diagram sheet, and it is discussed with the patient extensively at the preoperative visit, with the help of both photos taken at the preoperative visit and photos that the patient brings in taken a number of years prior. Along with the preoperative assessment and surgical plan, a discussion regarding the benefits of adipose tissue grafting is undertaken along with potential risks and complications, adipose tissue take rates, what the patients can expect in the days and few weeks following adipose tissue grafting, and what one can expect as a long-term result.

Adipose tissue transfer can be performed with any level of anesthesia, from only local infiltration to general anesthesia. Sterile techniques are employed. There are several possible sites for adipose tissue harvesting: lateral thigh, inner thigh, abdomen, flank, knees, buttock, lower lateral back, and triceps. The harvest site depends on ease of access in the supine position, availability of adipose tissue stores, ability to enhance body contour, and surgeon preference. As a facial plastic surgeon interested more in the ease, availability, and quantity of adipose tissue from various donor sites than the body contouring that can be achieved from the harvest site, the lateral thigh began as an early favorite for donor adipose tissue. I initially harvested from the upper lateral greater trochanteric area of the thigh but found that this area was more likely to produce contour irregularities that patients did not like given the amount of adipose tissue needed for most cases. Although I have used adipose tissue from all areas of the trunk and legs, the posterior lateral thigh adipose tissue is currently my preferred site of harvest. This adipose tissue seems to be superior for viability, longevity, and take rate, but has the added advantage of harvest with the least amount of connective tissue that may result in small cannula blockage during injection. It is easily accessible and is usually abundant in most women, with evidence to suggest that it is different adipose tissue from other donor sites possibly explaining and supporting my clinical observation. In order of preference for the donor site, posterior lateral thigh is first followed by medial thigh, flank, and abdomen, with other areas used when body contouring is needed or if the preferred sites have little adipose tissue.

Regarding viability of adipose tissue, a study by Rohrich demonstrated no differences in adipocyte viability among abdominal adipose tissue, thigh adipose tissue, flank adipose tissue, or knee adipose tissue donor sites (Rohrich, Sorokin et al. 2004) although other authors have disputed this assertion, and my clinical observation supports the use of lateral thigh adipose tissue. Regarding the quality of the adipose tissue, our experience reveals better and less fibrous adipose tissue quality in the lateral thigh donor site. Other authors have had similar experience (Tzikas 2004). Given the favorable accessibility, adipose tissue stores, and adipose tissue quality, the lateral thigh constitutes my favorite donor site.

SURGICAL TECHNIQUE

Donor Site Anesthesia

Depending on surgeon's preference, anesthetic administration can be performed in several ways with differing rationale for each method:

- High-volume tumescent technique: This is my preferred method. 25 mL of 1% lidocaine with 1:100,000 epinephrine is mixed with 500 mL of lactated Ringer's in a commercially prepared I.V. bag. Using extension tubing attached to a one-way valve and 10-mL syringe, the solution is injected with a 22-G needle or multiport injection cannula. The multiport cannula is preferred and used with an infiltration pump because of ease of use and its greater comfort in the awake patient. Approximately 250 mL is injected into each posterior lateral thigh or other harvest site as needed (Fig. 29.1).
- Medium-volume, blunt infiltration tumescent technique: This is the method described by Coleman and others. A stab incision is made at a previously anesthetized site. A 12-French liposuction cannula with a tapered tip and two side ports is attached to a 20-mL Luer-Lok syringe and is used to infiltrate tumescent solution (1 mL 1% lidocaine with 1:100,000 epinephrine, 4 mL 1% plain lidocaine, and 15 mL saline). The solution is injected in a fanning fashion into both the central and deep planes of the adipose tissue pad. Typically, 40 mL of solution is injected into each lateral thigh. The same cannula is then used later for the harvest.
- Low-volume, nontumescent technique: A 20-mL syringe with a mixture of 15 mL of normal saline and 5 mL of 1% lidocaine with 1:100,000 epinephrine is infiltrated into the donor site using a 7" spinal needle in a fanning fashion. Half the volume is distributed in the deep aspect of the fat pad, and half is distributed superficially in the subcutaneous plane. If the patient is under local anesthesia only, one can use 10 mL NS and 4 mL 1% lidocaine with 1:100,000 epinephrine.

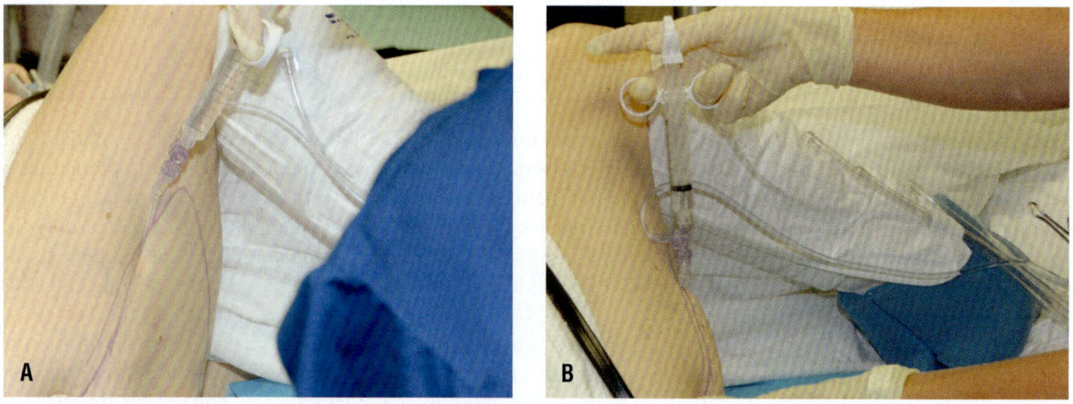

FIGURE 29.1 **A:** Fluid is injected into the posterolateral thigh. **B:** Tubing system for fluid injection is visualized.

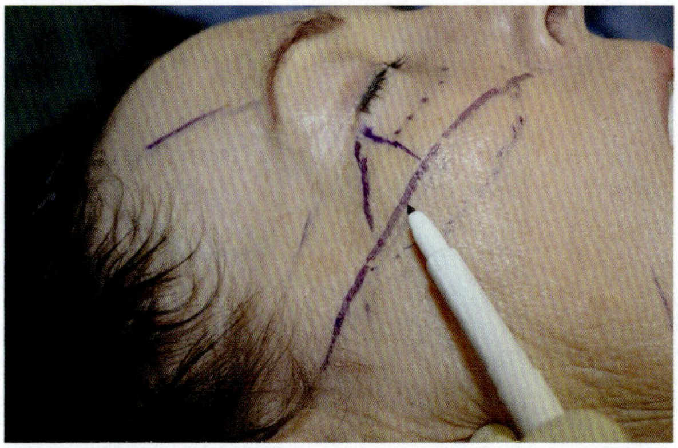

FIGURE 29.2
Face is marked out to identify areas that are volume depleted.

Recipient Site Anesthesia

After marking the anatomic areas that will be grafted (Fig. 29.2), the insertion sites are then determined and infiltrated with lidocaine with 1:100,000 adrenaline. Usually, only the insertion sites are injected if the patient is under general anesthesia, but if local or local with sedation is employed, additional anesthesia nerve blocks need to be considered. An attempt is made to minimize the amount of local anesthetic used to the recipient bed to decrease the distortion produced by larger amounts of local anesthetics.

Harvesting Technique

After infiltration of local anesthesia to the donor site, a 2- to 3-mm stab incision is made in the lower lateral posterior thigh and dilated with a hemostat. A two-holed 3-mm Coleman harvesting cannula is attached to a 10-mL Luer-Lok syringe. The donor adipose tissue pad and overlying skin are grasped firmly with the nondominant hand and the cannula introduced into the deep aspect of the donor adipose tissue pad (Fig. 29.3). The syringe plunger is gently retracted to create a minimally traumatic negative pressure. The plunger needs only to provide 1 to 2 cc of negative pressure space in the barrel of the syringe. I do not recommend machine or wall suction that may have a greater tendency to disrupt adipocytes. Depending on the amount of adipose tissue needed and the degree of adipose tissue stores present, either one or both lateral thighs are used. If more adipose tissue is needed, an easily accessible adjacent area is the medical thigh adipose tissue above the knee, although there is usually more fibrous connective tissue from fat harvested here.

Preparation of Adipose Tissue: Strain and Wash Technique

After harvest, the syringes full of adipose tissue are emptied into a strainer. Most of the infiltrative solution, blood, and free lipid and liquid portion of the harvested material are allowed to drain into a recipient cup under the strainer, and only minimal actual washing of the adipose tissue is accomplished using lactated Ringer's. Gauze sponges placed in contact with the undersurface of the strainer remove both residual liquid adipose tissue and aqueous fluid by capillary action. I remove prominent pieces of fibrous tissue or fascia that may cause plugging of the cannula during the adipose tissue injection into the recipient sites. The resultant processed adipose tissue appears smooth and homogeneous, ready for application. This refined adipose tissue may be used with good results without centrifugation. Because centrifugation for 2 minutes at 3000 rpm results in both a supernatant of a small amount liquid adipose tissue from lysed cells and a small amount on infranatant representing lactated Ringer's and some red cells, I routinely centrifuge. Adipose tissue that is destined for use in the periorbital area or temple in the subcutaneous plane will be diluted with a 5:1 dilution with lactated Ringer's to allow for injection pressures to be less and as an attempt to decrease

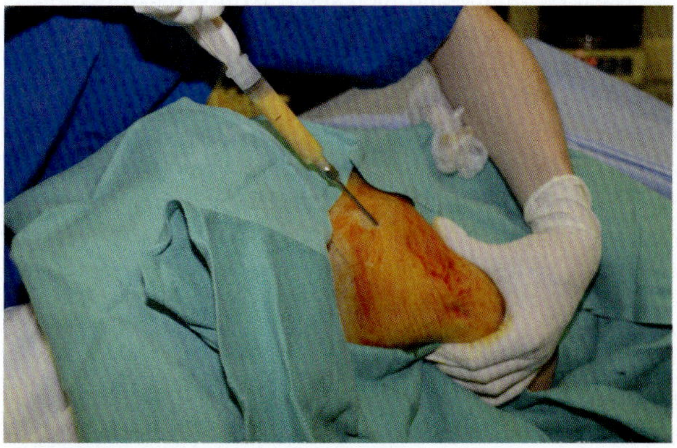

FIGURE 29.3
A cannula is introduced into the thigh using nondominant hand to grasp skin.

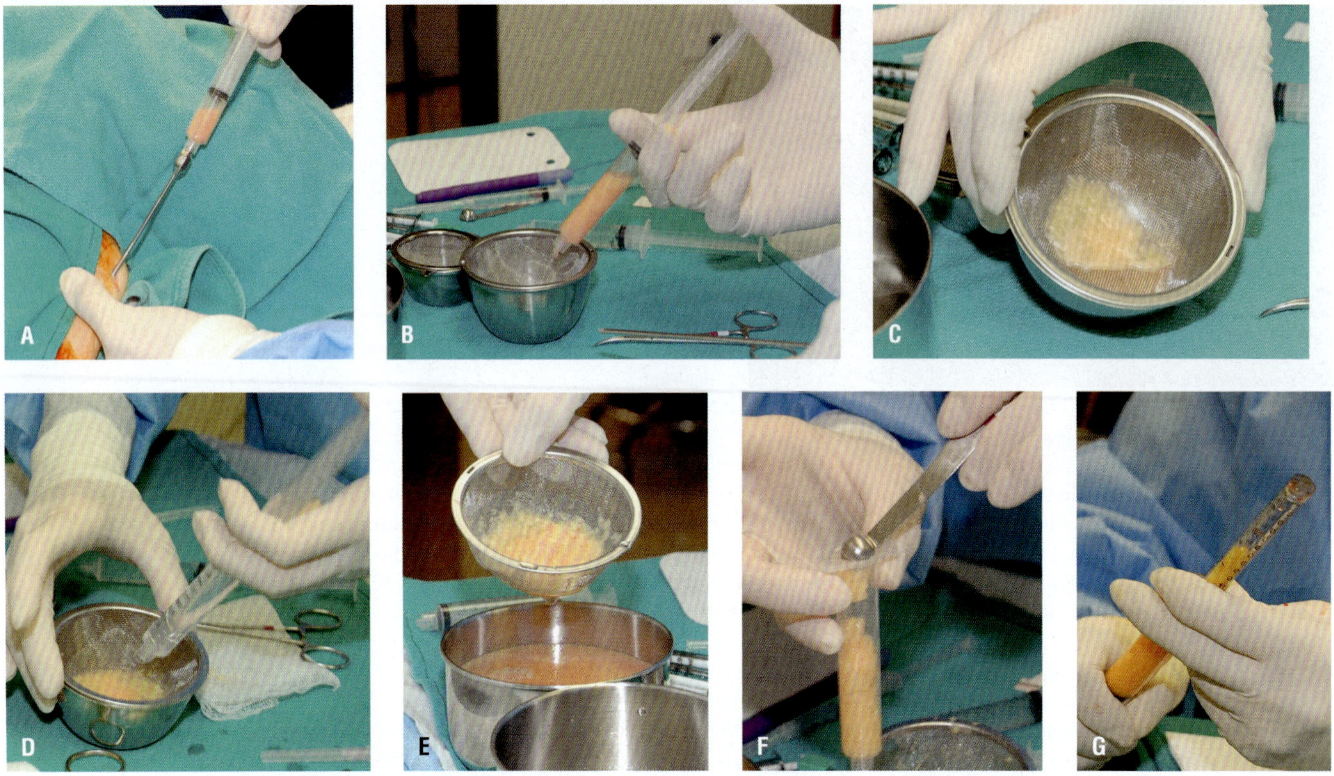

FIGURE 29.4 **A:** Harvesting of adipose tissue. **B:** Adipose tissue that is harvested is then strained. **C:** Strained adipose tissue. **D:** Addition of lactated Ringer's helps to create less lumpiness. **E:** Visualization of lactated Ringer's and adipose tissue combination. **F:** Combination is then scooped into the syringe for injection. **G:** Adipose tissue is transferred from a 10-cc syringe into one that is suitable for injection.

the risk of contour irregularities in this thin tissue area. The adipose tissue is loaded into 1-mL syringes attached to 0.9-mm and 1.2-mm cannulas of various lengths depending on the injection site. Of note, I find that it is easier to first load the adipose tissue into 10-mL syringes with subsequent transfer into the 1-mL syringes. I fill each syringe with only 0.7 mL of adipose tissue as this allows for ergonomic and controlled injection. See Figure 29.4 for stepwise approach on adipose tissue preparation.

It should be noted that a wide range of opinions exists on how to prepare adipose tissue, including, but not limited to, strain only, strain and wash, gravity separation, wicking, or centrifuge only. Other surgeons support keeping the adipose tissue in a closed system to avoid contact with air. Centrifugation techniques typically use a speed of 3000 rpm for 3 minutes. This separates the contents into three layers: bottom, blood/water/lidocaine; middle, viable parcels of adipose tissue; and top, oil from ruptured adipose tissue cells (Coleman 2004). The infranatant bottom layer is pushed out of the syringe, and supernatant top layer is decanted and wicked away.

I began using the strainer and wash technique of adipose tissue preparation in an effort to simplify the process and after transitioning from the syringe and ratchet device of the early 90's to the small cannula injection technique described by Coleman, I continued with straining and washing as it precluded the need for additional equipment, was simple, and I had good experience with its use. I now avoid washing or flooding the adipose tissue to minimize potential loss of colloidal proteins that may have an effect on changing oncotic pressures of the graft. To assess the degree of refinement from only a strain and wash technique, adipose tissue was treated with the usual strain and wash technique and then subjected to centrifugation at 3000 rpm for 3, 5, and 10 minutes and found that in a 10-mL syringe of adipose tissue, there was .2 to .3 mL of aqueous solution in an infranatant and very little free lipid, blood, or connective tissue was found (Figs. 29.5 and 29.6). Although controversy exists as to which is the best technique for adipose tissue preparation, I know of no convincing study to suggest which technique produces the greatest longevity or persistence. I have seen continued, good, long-term results both with this simple approach and with the combined approach straining and centrifugation approach so that either can be easily adapted to any practice, easily, inexpensively, and with good outcomes. My preferred technique, however, continues to be the combination technique as it allows us to dilute the adipose tissue as necessary and remove most remaining red cells.

Injection

If the patient is not under general anesthesia or deep sedation, a local nerve block is beneficial as it reduces excess contour changes from the local infiltration itself. Infraorbital and supraorbital regional nerve blocks are

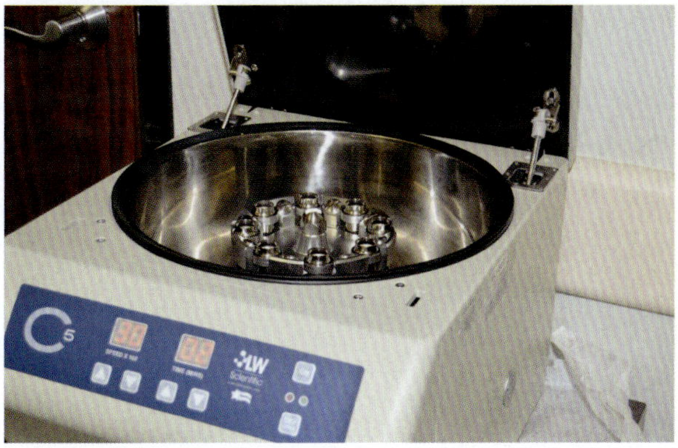

FIGURE 29.5
Machine that is used for centrifuge.

often used. Additional local anesthetic infiltration may be added as needed. For full face injection, the following port locations are typically created using an 18-gauge needle: superior brow, temporal hairline, medial cheek, zygoma, lateral upper lip near the commissure, prejowl sulcus, chin, ear lobule, submental sulcus, and neck (Fig. 29.7). All parts of the face are accessible through a combination of these ports (Fig. 29.8). The skin and soft tissue are stabilized with the nondominant hand, and the cannula is inserted and advanced through the tissues to the appropriate plane. Adipose tissue can be injected with an anterograde movement of the cannula toward the recipient area and on the withdrawal motion of the cannula depending on location. Thinner tissue or subcutaneous injections are usually best injected as the cannula is withdrawn, but operator experience and preference are the determining factors. Once the cannula has reached the desired location, the plunger of the 1-mL syringe is gently pushed while the cannula is withdrawn depositing between .01 and .05 mL per pass in most cases. This retrograde injection of adipose tissue allows for a more controlled and safer application of adipose tissue and reduces the risk for contour irregularities. One should be very judicious in applying pressure on the plunger, and if the adipose tissue does not exit the syringe with minimal pressure, it should be withdrawn and checked for obstruction. This smooth, incremental placement allows for optimal surface area contact with

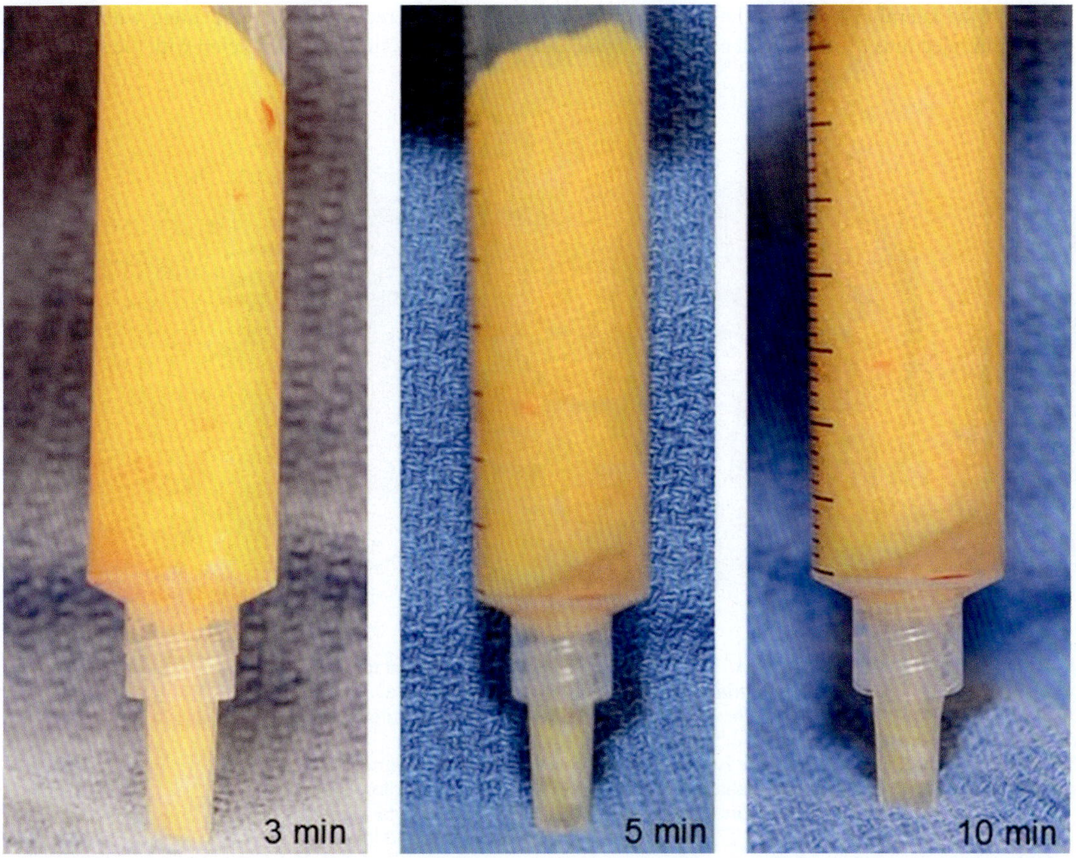

FIGURE 29.6 Adipose tissue is centrifuged at 3, 5, and 10 minutes to see how much infranatant is present. There is concern that centrifuge greater than 3 minutes may be linked with less viability of adipose tissue.

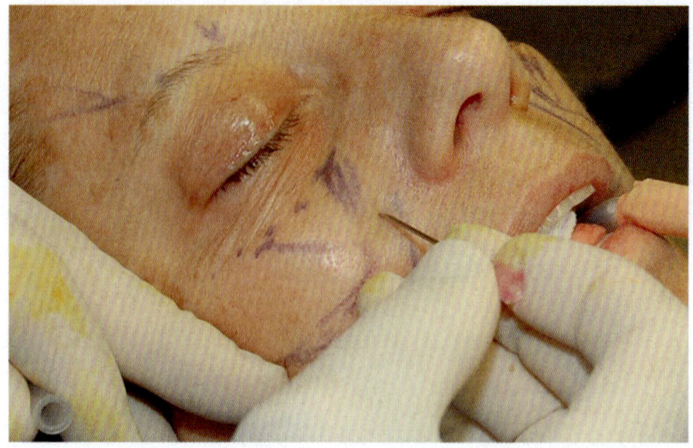

FIGURE 29.7
An 18-G needle is inserted to allow for injection of adipose tissue into the anterior triangle. Through this, one can also access the entire cheek area.

native tissues and increased nutrition and neovascularization. It also reduces the risk of large lumps or other surface contour irregularities. I typically dilute the adipose tissue by 20% by adding 2 mL of lactated Ringer's to 8 mL of adipose tissue to be used in the periorbital region and temple of other areas of thin tissue in a subcutaneous plane.

A major goal of the technique is to achieve the distribution of adipose tissue parcels into multiple tissue planes, moving from deep to superficial, using a fanning technique when appropriate:

- Deep: above the periosteum
- Middle: within the muscle and deep subcutaneous plane
- Superficial: within the subcutaneous plane

During the injection, the surgeon must be committed to rigorous assessment and reassessment in order to achieve augmentation to the desired effect. The tear trough injection is usually performed first through the lateral nasal ala insertion site followed by the central lower orbital and lateral orbital rim through the same insertion site (Fig. 29.9). I use adipose tissue thoroughly free of connective tissue and diluted for these and the infrabrow injection because of the need for precise placement with no force and smooth application (Fig. 29.10). If the lateral approach to the orbital rim and cheek is considered, it is also done along with the other orbital rim injections using fat with no fibrous tissue. The periorbital complex is completed with the suprabrow

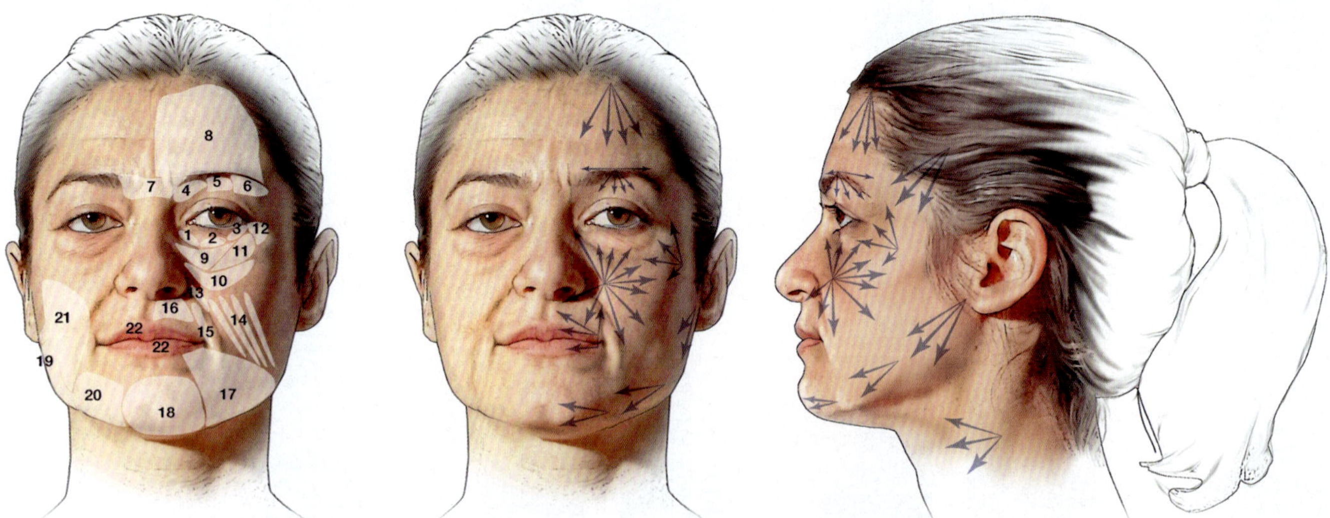

1. Tear trough
2. Mid inferior orbital rim
3. Lateral orbital rim
4. Medial infrabrow
5. Central infrabrow
6. Lateral infrabrow
7. Glabella
8. Forehead
9. Anterior triangle
10. Submalar
11. Malar
12. Anterior zygomatic arch
13. Deep nasal fat pad
14. Subcutaneous cheek
15. Nasolabial fold
16. Premaxilla
17. Prejowl sulcus
18. Chin
19. Lateral mandible
20. Mid mandible
21. Preauricular cheek
22. Upper and lower lip

FIGURE 29.8 Various insertion sites and areas that can be augmented.

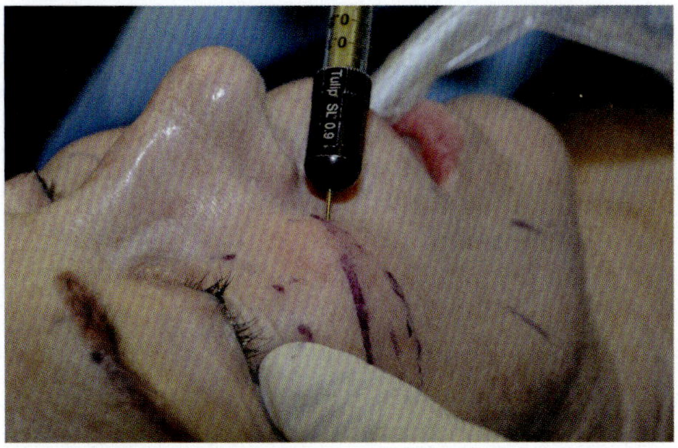

FIGURE 29.9
Tear trough injection is usually performed first through the lateral nasal ala insertion site.

subcutaneous injection to sculpture the brow followed by the temple using both planes, if desired (Fig. 29.11). The medial forehead subcutaneous injection is performed through the brow insertion site from each brow with the last area of the periorbital complex being the subcutaneous forehead injection from the hairline insertion site if it is being done.

The adipose tissue grafting sequence continues inferiorly with the lower face beginning with the anterior triangle then medial and lateral cheek, through the same lateral ala insertion site. The cheek contour deep to superficial is sculptured and any submalar adipose tissue added also through this site. The deep nasal adipose tissue pad, subcutaneous cheek, nasolabial fold and premaxilla if, needed, then complete the grafting from the lateral nasal insertion site (Figs. 29.12 and 29.13).

Attention is directed to the jowl and prejowl sulcus and labiomandibular crease for grafting. The insertion site is posterior to the marionette line and anterior to the jowl for lateral chin, prejowl augmentation. By directing the cannula superiorly toward the oral commissure in a subcutaneous plane, one not only softens the marionette line but a slight elevation of the corner of the mouth can be achieved. An opening anterior to the marionette line will allow access to the chin and mandible, with the posterior mandible and preauricular cheek accessed through a stab incision at the base of the lobule.

The neck and anterior mandible is accessed through insertion sites at the lateral portion of the submandibular sulcus area. The longer 7-cm and 1.2-mm cannula can be used to extend down to the midneck and along the inferior border of the mandible if needed. For those patients receiving low neck adipose tissue, the long cannula is used through an insertion site in the midneck along the anterior border of the sternocleidomastoid muscle.

The lip is the last area of grafting and both upper lip and lower lip may be augmented through an insertion site on the lateral upper lip (Fig. 29.14). I generally put more adipose tissue in the lower lip than upper lip, but lip balance, structure, and shape are very individualized decisions by both the surgeon and patient. An overdone lower lip rarely looks operated, but an overdone upper lip almost certainly does. I like to maintain normal lip architecture by recognizing the three masses of the upper lip and two masses of the lower lip with relatively little to no adipose tissue injected into the upper lip central mass. All of my adipose tissue grafting is done as the initial phase of surgery if surgery is being done simultaneously. This precludes surgical interruption of tissue planes so that the more precise grafting can be achieved in undisturbed, native tissue. Some patients benefit from volume enhancement of the angle and body of the mandible. This may be achieved through a subcutaneous plane or during a face-lift may be placed under the platysma and SMAS

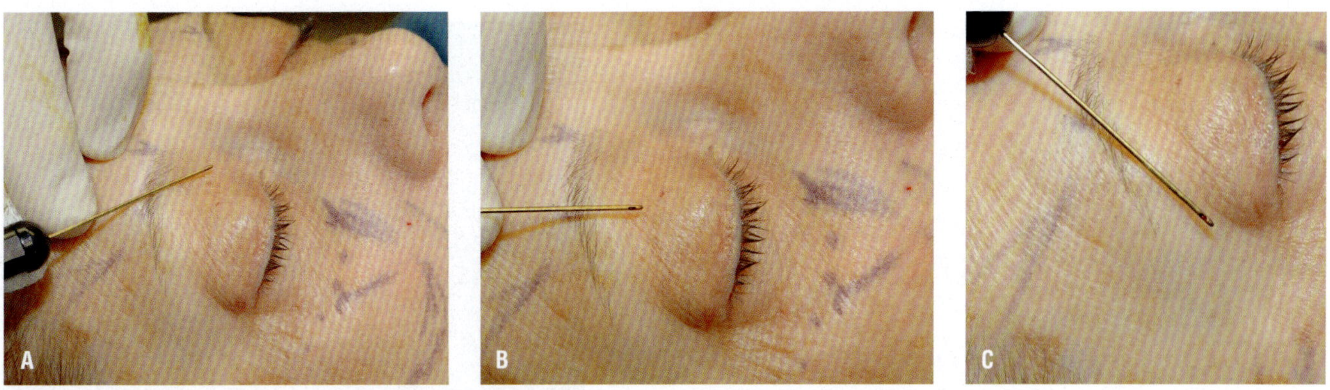

FIGURE 29.10 Infrabrow injection has three potential vectors (**A, B, and C**).

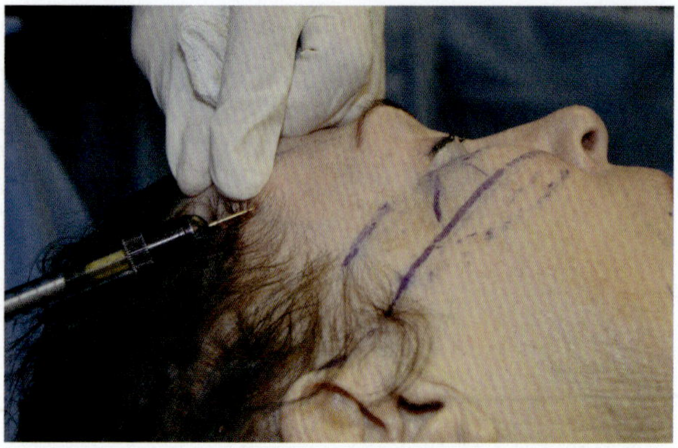

FIGURE 29.11
Temple injection is used for the lateral periorbital complex.

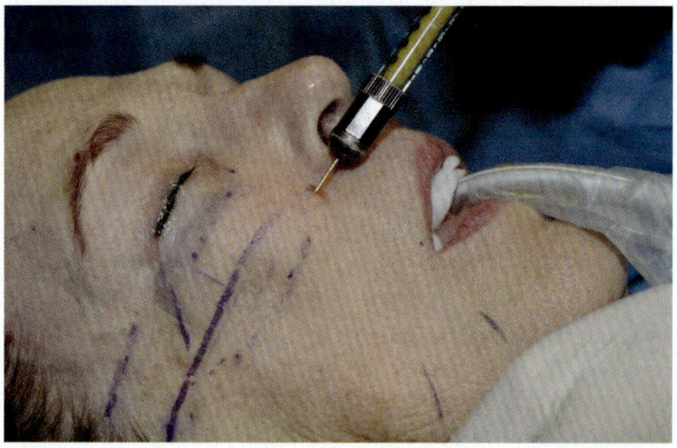

FIGURE 29.12
One can inject along the malar eminence with a 7-cm × 1.2-mm cannula, all the way to the zygoma.

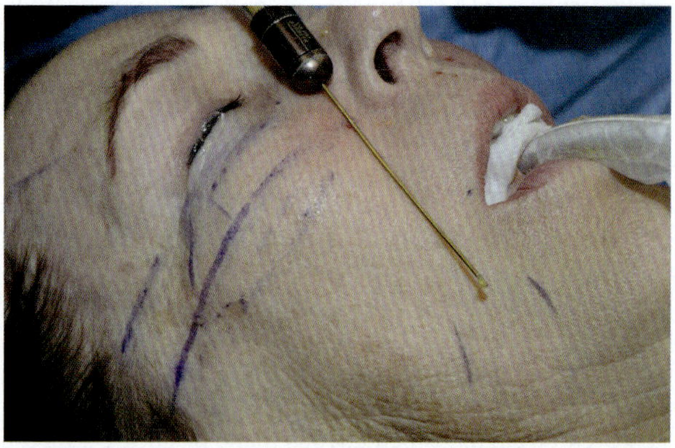

FIGURE 29.13
Injection along nasolabial fold.

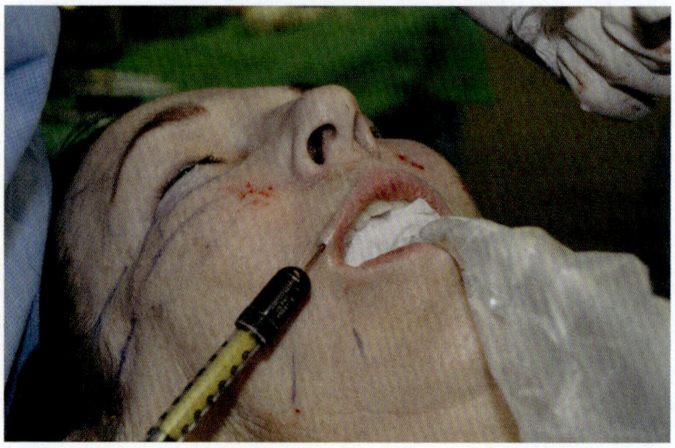

FIGURE 29.14
Lateral access for injection into the upper lip.

TABLE 29.1 Amount and Cannula Gauges for Various Sites of Autologous Adipose Tissue Transfer

Adipose Tissue Transfer Facial Area	Cannula Gauge and Length (Tulip)	Injection Site Access/Aliquot Amount (mL) per Side
a. Orbital rim:	0.9 mm	
Tear trough		Medial cheek port: 0.1–0.2 cc (limit 0.5)
Inferior orbital rim		Medial cheek port: 2.5; zygoma: 1.5 cc
Lateral orbital rim		Zygoma port: 0.7–1.5 cc
Anterior triangle		Medial cheek port: 1–2 cc
b. Brow:	0.9 mm	Superior brow port: 0.5–2 cc total
Medial infrabrow		
Lateral infrabrow		
Suprabrow lateral		
Suprabrow medial		
c. Temple:		
Subcutaneous plane	7 cm × 0.9 or 1.2 mm	Temporal hairline port: 3–3.5 cc
Subfascial plane	7 cm × 1.2 mm	Temporal hairline port: 3–4 cc
d. Forehead	Curved 7 cm × 1.2 mm	Superior brow port: 3–3.5 cc
e. Nasolabial fold	7 cm × 1.2 mm	Medial cheek port:
Subfascial plane		0.7–2 cc
Subcutaneous plane		0.7–1.5 cc
f. Deep nasal fat pad	7 cm × 1.2 mm	Medial cheek port:
Subfascial plane		0.7–2 cc
g. Premaxilla	7 cm × 1.2 mm	0.7–1.5 cc
h. Cheek or Periorbital complex:		Medial cheek port:
Malar prominence	Curved 7 cm × 1.2 mm	3–10 cc total
Subfascial	Curved 7 cm × 1.2 mm	3–10 cc
Subcutaneous and fibromuscular	Curved 7 cm × 1.2 mm 7 cm × 1.2 mm	2.5–4 cc
Submalar area	Curved 7 cm × 1.2 mm	2–3.5 cc
Anterior zygomatic arch	7 cm × 1.2 mm	1.5–3 cc
Lateral mandible	Curved 7 cm × 1.2 mm	2–5 cc
Anterior or medial cheek	7 cm × 1.2 mm	2–5 cc
Lateral cheek	7 cm × 1.2 mm	1.5–3 cc
i. Prejowl sulcus	7 cm × 0.9 or 1.2 mm	Upper lip port: 1.5–2 cc Prejowl sulcus port: 1.5–2 cc
j. Chin	7 cm × 0.9 or 1.2 mm	Prejowl sulcus port:
Subcutaneous plane		1.5–2 cc
Subfascial plane		1.5–2 cc
k. Neck	Curved 7 cm × 1.2 mm	Prejowl sulcus port: 1.5–2 cc Submandibular sulcus port: 3–6 cc
l. Lips	7 cm × 0.9 mm	Upper lip port:
Submucosal		0.7–1 cc to each quadrant

when a sub-SMAS plane is developed. (See Table 29.1 for detail regarding amount and cannula gauges for various sites of autologous fat transfer.)

POSTOPERATIVE MANAGEMENT

- Antibiotics are generally given for 3 days.
- Ice compresses are not used.
- Steroids are usually used for 4 days if adipose tissue is combined with lasers or surgical procedures.
- The patient must be told not to manipulate the facial tissues for 7 to 10 days.
- Head elevation and avoid side sleeping.
- Follow-up in the office in 24 hours.

COMPLICATIONS

- Inaccurate volume

  Careful preoperative discussion is imperative for understanding the amount of facial fullness the patient wishes to achieve along with comparison of photos taken at a younger age. Once the desired goal is established, there are still many factors that can affect the outcome of the grafting. Although often difficult to achieve, one of the key goals of adipose tissue transfer is to have predictable adipose tissue graft survival. Some of the factors that may affect volumes that can be achieved are as follows:

  A. Excess volume of local anesthetic

  First, excess infiltration of local anesthetic to the recipient site should be avoided, as this can produce transient volume excess that makes intraoperative assessment of facial contours difficult. Peripheral nerve blocks are beneficial in reducing the volume requirement of local anesthetic and should be used whenever possible.

  B. Intraoperative edema

  The surgeon should be aware of the presence of acute soft tissue edema when assessing facial contours during fat injection, as this produces transient bulk that can mislead the surgeon into grafting insufficient volume. Alternatively, one should also resist the urge to overcompensate. It is common for patients to complain about too much or too little fullness after resolution of swelling.

  C. Low viability of injected adipose tissue

  Whichever refinement technique is used (gentle wash, no wash, centrifuge, no centrifuge, closed system with no exposure to air), the goal is to minimize trauma to the fat in order to increase survival of adipose tissue cells. Too much negative pressure during harvest may theoretically rupture the cells. Too much positive pressure and forcing the adipocytes through cannulas that are too small may also cause mechanical trauma. There has been discussion of the importance of maintaining interstitial components and colloid for maximizing the viability of fat cells. Some advocate the addition of human serum albumin to the harvested adipose tissue to improve the colloid component. Again, a wide range of opinions exists on how to prepare adipose tissue for grafting. I have found good take rates and long-term volume enhancement even with just a simple harvest and strain technique.

  D. Low purity of injected adipose tissue

  Local anesthetic from the tumescence at harvest and blood and oil are all present to some degree even after the adipose tissue is processed and refined. Excesses of local anesthetic and blood can be avoided with good peripheral nerve blocks and good harvest technique, respectively. Blood remnants within the adipose tissue stimulate macrophage activity to eliminate adipose tissue cells. Proponents of adipose tissue washing aim to remove excess blood and reduce macrophage activity.

  E. Necrosis

  If grafted adipose tissue does not have access to adequate nutrition, some degree of necrosis may occur. Theoretically, this can happen if fat is injected too thickly in a single tissue plane or if adipose tissue is injected adjacent to a synthetic implant. This can lead to calcification and subsequent contour irregularities or nodules.

- Persistent malar edema

  This is described as a persistent boggy, edematous appearance of the malar mound that may fluctuate in severity after grafting. It is thought to be exacerbated by smoking, alcohol consumption, and increased salt intake. Resolution of mild malar edema requires time and reassurance. For cases that do not spontaneously resolve, Lam et al. advocates steroid injection between 2 and 4 months postoperatively. In extreme cases, staged excision may be required.

- Overcorrection

  This situation is highly unusual and occurs when too much adipose tissue was grafted to a given area. Postoperative edema usually resolves, and many surgeons recommend waiting a duration of at least 6 months before proceeding with any intervention. Correction would be performed by targeted liposuction to the area. I have used monopolar RF devices with some degree of improvement in patients referred to me who have had overzealous grafting.

- Undercorrection

  After resolution of the expected postoperative edema, the patient or surgeon may find that the desired degree of facial "fullness" was not fully achieved. This situation is easily approached with additional adipose tissue grafting or injectable fillers, which can be performed at anytime; however, I recommend waiting until at least 6 months if the under correction is mild.

- Contour irregularities of the recipient site

  Lumps may result from injection of too much volume of adipose tissue or injection of adipose tissue too superficially in the skin. Even at the subdermal level, excess volume can sometimes manifest as a contour irregularity. If the injection cannula has a side port, it is a good technique to have the port face deep so that infiltration of the adipose tissue is delivered deep to the cannula and not superficially. If a nodule persists, unchanged in size after 2 to 3 months, a steroid injection may be of benefit and occasionally may need to be removed with direct excision or liposuction.

- Contour irregularities of the harvest site
  Placement of the cannula too superficially during the harvest may cause contour deformities. This is difficult to correct and should be avoided. Adipose tissue transfer back to the harvest site from a new donor site may be required. Scar band formation of the skin to the deeper tissues may result in a dimple at either the harvest site or the recipient site. These can be softened with a dry cannula dissection technique using a 3-mm spatula cannula.
- Adipose tissue migration
  Subtle migration of adipocytes may occur with muscle contraction and movement particularly superficial muscles such as the orbicularis oculi and orbicularis oris. For instance, adipose tissue injected into the orbicularis oris demonstrates poor longevity and suboptimal effect since the adipose tissue is then subject to the constant movement of the lips. Also, when adipose tissue is injected into muscle, the subsequently displaced adipose tissue can sometimes create unintended contour irregularities at locations adjacent to the injected sites. I and others have noted this phenomenon when augmenting the glabella. Immediately after adipose tissue infiltration into the glabella, the skin contours appear favorably smooth. However, when the patient begins moving his or her face, the robust movement of the corrugators recreates the unwanted native depression or furrow and enhances the adjacent tissues with the displaced adipose tissue. One way of subverting this issue is by using neurotoxin to the procerus and corrugator muscles 2 weeks prior to the adipose tissue transfer procedure. Facial manipulation theoretically may also displace adipose tissue so we encourage patients to avoid applying digital pressure to the face for at least a week.
  Injection of adipose tissue into areas of thick or dense scar has a similar issue. Like anything else, grafted adipose tissue will take the path of least resistance, and if it encounters significant pressure from an area of scar, the adipose tissue will tend to displace to adjacent areas.
- Nerve injury
  Although possible, this is rare with the use of blunt cannulas. While others have reported anecdotal incidents of sensory or facial weakness, the issues are transient and mild. I use blunt cannulas, and I have never encountered nerve injury in my experience.
- Vascular injury
  Ecchymosis or hematomas may occur from venous injury. These complications are mild and without major sequelae. If, however, a hematoma is large, it may impede the surgeon's ability to make an accurate intraoperative assessment of facial volume. Blood in the soft tissue may decrease adipose tissue survival so that gentle pressure applied to an area for several minutes if one sees any significant blood from the insertion sites might help to mitigate the formation of a hematoma.
  Anecdotal reports of patients with arterial occlusion due to injection with sharp cannulas or needles or using frozen adipose tissue have been discussed and are extremely rare. Arterial occlusion can cause skin necrosis and usually presents with significant pain on injection. Blindness from central artery occlusion involving the ophthalmic artery while possible is also extremely rare. It too is avoided by the use of blunt cannulas.
  Using blunt cannulas instead of sharp needles helps reduce the risk of any vascular injury.

RESULTS

Autologous adipose tissue grafting should be an integral part of the facial plastic surgeons practice. With experience, one can achieve facial contour improvement unavailable with other techniques. My goal in the next few years is to improve predictability of grafted adipose tissue volumes over time. A number of adjunctive procedures have been advocated to achieve this end that are under current investigation.

I generally see very little bruising with adipose tissue grafting, but with the trauma and swelling combined with some overcorrection attendant with adipose tissue grafting, and the effect of local anesthesia, the patient will look a degree overcorrected for 1 to 4 weeks depending on the area grafted and the amount of volume the surgeon decides to use in each area. After the first 8 weeks after adipose tissue grafting the volume appears to diminish with a trough in volume occurring between 10 and 16 weeks. I find that volume in many cases begins to recover and increase over the next 6 to 9 months, so that many patients have better contours and volumes at 1 year than at 3 to 4 months (Figs. 29.15 and 29.16). The reason for this is conjectural at this point but is worth noting so that a discussion with the patient about the dynamics of this process is undertaken to avoid having an unhappy patient. The need for a second adipose tissue session may also tempered by the notion of gradual, subtle volume increase over time in many cases but not all.

PEARLS

- Educate the patient about the benefits and more importantly limitations of adipose tissue grafting.
- Use previous photos as part of this educational process and to help determine where to put adipose tissue and how much.
- Document amounts and in what location for your critical review.
- Use minimally traumatic technique for harvest and preparation.
- Remove blood from prepared adipose tissue.

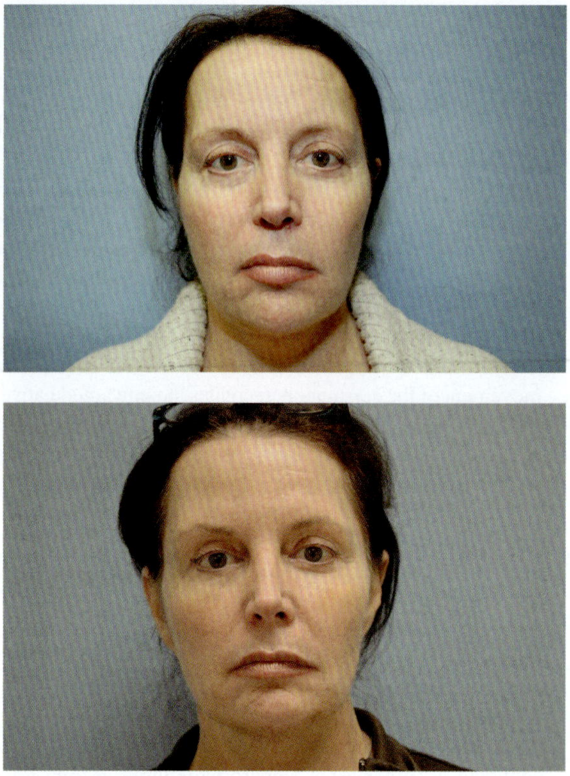

FIGURE 29.15
This patient underwent autologous adipose tissue grafting to tear trough, infrabrow, temples, cheeks, prejowl sulcus, mentoplasty, and liposuction of jowl and neck. Top photo is preoperative, while bottom is 1-year postoperative results.

- Develop an efficient process to minimize time from harvest to injection.
- Inject using small cannula techniques with small volumes with each pass.
- Treat adipose tissue grafting as a surgical, sterile technique.

PITFALLS

- Don't allow adipose tissue to dry or desiccate.
- Minimize local anesthesia at recipient site.
- Avoid being aggressive in thin tissue.
- Avoid iced compresses post-operative.
- Overdoing is worse than having to redo.

INSTRUMENTS TO HAVE AVAILABLE

- Several 10-mL syringes
- 250-mL or 500-mL bag of lactated Ringer's for tumescent infiltration
- One-way valve with extension tubing
- 22-G spinal needle
- 3-mm Coleman basket harvesting cannula
- Tea strainers of various sizes to fit over stainless steel cups
- Lactated Ringer's as a washing agent
- Small spatula
- Small mosquito clamp
- Scalpel with a no. 11 blade
- Multiple 1-mL Luer-Lok syringes
- Injection cannula, coated Tulip 0.9 mm × 1.2 mm of various lengths including curved 7 cm
- Gauze sponges
- Suture for harvest site closure
- Variable speed centrifuge with horizontally opposed baskets
- Sterilized syringe holders

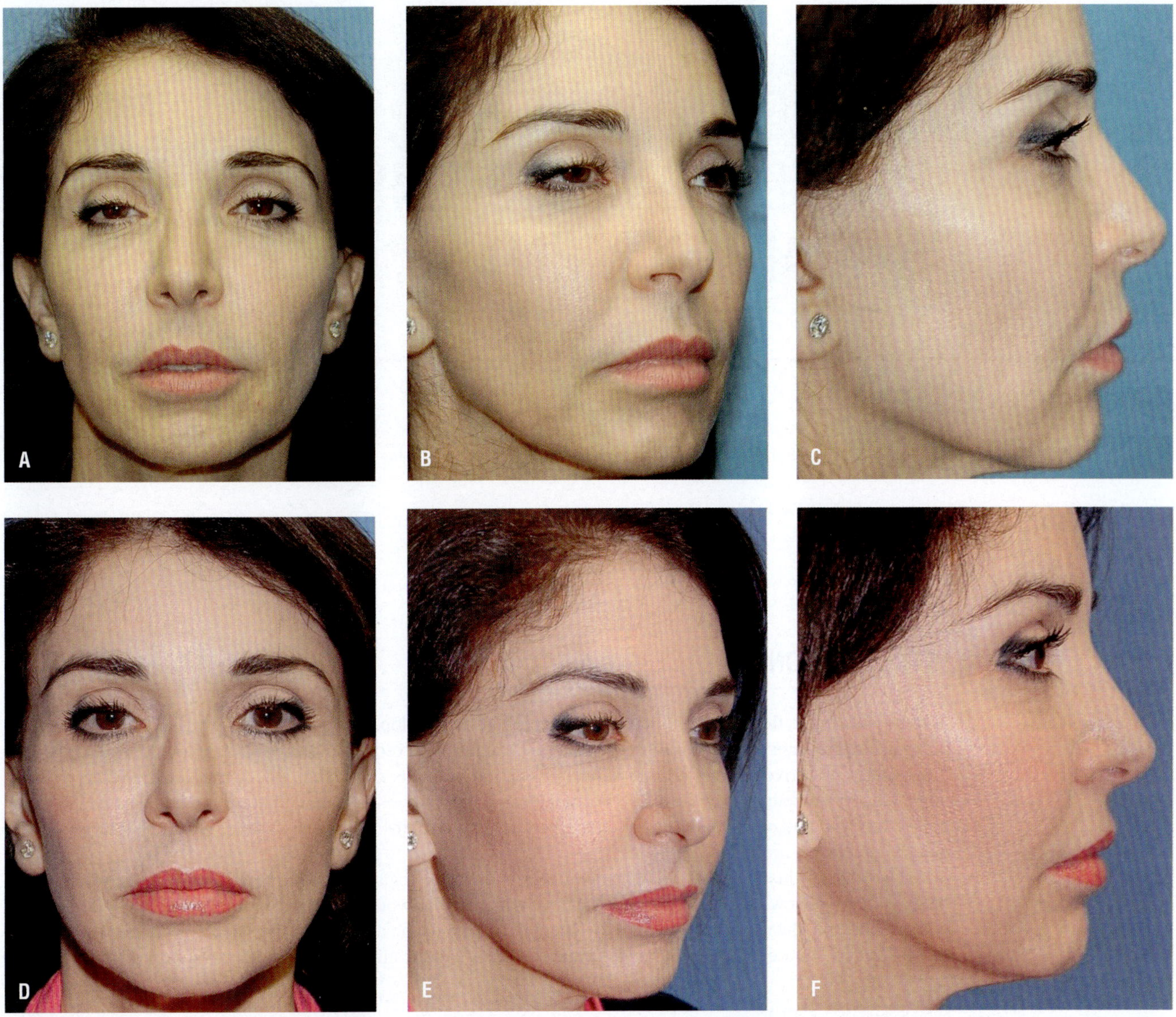

FIGURE 29.16 This patient underwent adipose tissue grafting alone; comparison of preoperative photos **A, B,** and **C** with postoperative photos **D, E,** and **F** shows improvement in supraorbital sulcus hollowing, softer cheeks, and better brow configuration.

ACKNOWLEDGMENT

Lynn Chiu-Collins, M.D., for assistance in manuscript preparation.

SUGGESTED READING

Coleman S. *Structural fat grafting*. St. Louis, MO: Quality Medical Pub., 2004.

Lam SM, Glasgold MJ, et al. *Complementary fat grafting*. Philadelphia, PA: Wolters Kluwer Health/Lippincott Williams & Wilkins, 2007.

Lambros V. Models of facial aging and implications for treatment. *Clin Plast Surg* 2008;35(3):319–327; discussion 317.

Minton TJ, Williams EF. Lipotransfer in the upper third of the face. *Facial Plast Surg* 2010;26(5):362–368.

Shiffman MA. *Autologous fat transfer: art, science, and clinical practice*. Berlin, Germany: Springer, 2010.

30 CHEMICAL PEELS: EVALUATION AND COMPREHENSIVE MANAGEMENT

Devinder S. Mangat

INTRODUCTION

As advances in the field of aesthetic medicine continue to develop, so does the desire of the general public to postpone and reverse the undesirable, age-related changes observed in our outward appearance. Unfortunately, this impetus has driven a multitude of skin rejuvenation products and techniques to market that often promise unrealistic or unattainable end results. Fortunately, chemical peeling has withstood the harshest of critics in both safety and outcome standards for over a century and remains as the standard by which new technologies and advancements are judged.

The goal of this chapter is to enhance one's knowledge regarding both the art and science of chemical peeling and to review the overall management for patients who would benefit from this procedure. After proper patient selection, the necessary depth of the chemical peel must be determined. The depth is defined by the level of penetration, nature of epidermal and dermal treatment, and resultant inflammatory response.

Superficial Peels

Alpha hydroxy acids (AHAs) are natural fruit, carboxylic acids that are nontoxic. Due to their relatively high safety profile, they have become the most popular technique, not only of plastic surgeons and dermatologists but also of the cosmetic therapists and aestheticians. Glycolic acid or 2-hydroxyethanoic acid is the most commonly used AHA. Glycolic acid is derived from sugar cane and is typically used in concentrations of 20% to 70%. Other commonly used AHAs are lactic acid (2-hydroxypropanoic acid), found in sour milk and tomato juice, and citric acid (2-hydroxy-1,2,3-propanetricarboxylic acid), found in citrus fruit. Salicylic acid, in concentrations of 20% to 30%, are also used for superficial chemoexfoliation. AHAs affect both the epidermis and most superficial layer of the dermis by creating a loss of cohesion of keratinocytes of the stratum granulosum. This allows sloughing of the abnormal cells and affords thinning of a thickened stratum corneum. These benefits can last for 2 to 3 weeks.

The Jessner's solution, composed of 14 grams (g) of salicylic acid, 14 g of lactic acid, and 14 g of resorcinol in 100 mL of ethanol, can be used safely as a superficial peeling agent. Its depth is coat dependent and applying one to three coats, exfoliation, or removal of the stratum corneum, can be achieved. However, by applying 5 to 10 coats, the depth of penetration extends to the basal cell layer. Similarly, a simple 50% resorcinol solution, applied for up to an hour, can result in a superficial peel.

A false sense of safety should be avoided with AHAs. For example, without neutralization, glycolic acid can penetrate deeply. Its time-dependent action should be neutralized with water. By leaving glycolic acid unneutralized, dermal penetration will ensue and healing problems, crusting, and scarring can result. The desired endpoint of an AHA peel should be erythema and light peeling of the epidermis.

Medium-Depth Peels

Medium-depth peeling agents are those that create injury through the depth of papillary dermis and create some inflammation in the upper reticular dermis. The recent gold standard of the medium-depth peel has been trichloroacetic acid (TCA). This agent has no systemic toxicities, and in its crystalline form, it lacks light sensitivity and does not require refrigeration for stabilization. However, it has a narrow margin of error, and the risk of scarring is much higher than with phenol-based solutions. TCA concentration is based upon a strict weight by volume standard (g/100 mL distilled water). There have been anecdotal accounts of miscommunication between the physician and the pharmacist in which the pharmacist instead used a weight-to-weight concentration. The results ended with patients being exposed to concentrations greater than 50% TCA with resultant scarring. For clarification, scarring has also been reported when using TCA concentrations of 50%. No emulsifiers, additives, or surfactants have been found to lessen this risk.

Combining TCA 35% solution with another less potent agent allows practitioners to achieve the same effects of a 50% TCA without the aforementioned risks. The additional agent is applied first as an epidermolytic to allow the TCA solution to penetrate more deeply into the dermis.

Monheit has written extensively regarding the combination of the Jessner's peel solution and 35% TCA. The Jessner's peel destroys the epidermis and is followed by an immediate application of a 35% TCA solution. This allows for even application of the TCA solution and affords a deeper penetration. In contrast to the phenol peels, the frost does not form immediately and an adequate time of 3 to 4 minutes must be allowed for the full frost to appear. Additional applications can be made to the desired depth. This combination has shown to produce an increase in type I collagen deposition, increased fibroblast activation, and decreased elastic fibers relative to 35% TCA alone. Application of multiple layers of the 35% TCA solution has an additive effect, which can cause a deeper peel leading to hypopigmentation and scarring.

Similarly, the combination of glycolic acid with 35% TCA increases the depth of the peel. Histologic biopsies have proven that this is a slightly deeper level peel than Monheit's Jessner/35% TCA combination peel and was found to cause more neoelastogenesis, neovascularization, and papillary dermal fibrosis. The mentioned combination peels have a risk of scarring of less than 1%, which is similar to that of CO_2 laser resurfacing and phenol–croton oil–based peels.

Deep Peels

When medium-depth peels do not afford enough penetration to treat the deepest of rhytids, specifically the "crow's feet" and perioral region, a deeper treatment is considered. The deep peel relies on injury to the reticular dermis to affect change to these areas. The Baker-Gordon peel (Table 30.1) provides considerable improvement of deeper rhytids; however, the irreversible hypopigmentation risk and widely discussed phenol cardiac and renal toxicity shifted resurfacing practices away from this once popular formulation. While the papillary dermis heals through reorganization, the reticular dermis is thought to heal through the process of scarring. Further, with additional healing time due to the depth of treatment, additional risks and complications rise. Despite these well-known risks, in selected patients and situations, the Baker-Gordon formulation provides an effective treatment option for those patients with Fitzpatrick type I and II skin who present with deepened rhytids in discrete anatomic subunits. It is then combined with medium-strength peel solutions throughout the rest of the face. Conservative and even application with awareness of frost development will further help to avoid potential complications.

Modified Phenol–Croton Oil Peels

Croton oil is pressed from the seeds of *Croton tiglium*, a small shrub found in India and Ceylon. The oil consists mainly of oleic, linoleic, myristic, and arachadonic acids. Less than 5% of the oil is made up of a resin, which has been known since 1895 in scientific literature to possess irritant and toxic properties. When applied to the skin, this toxic resin creates severe vesiculations of the skin and a resultant wound taking almost 3 weeks to

TABLE 30.1 The "Classic" Baker or Baker-Gordon Formulation Published in 1962 Following His Original Initial Formulation from November, 1961

Ingredients	Baker-Gordon Solution	Original Baker Formulation
Phenol USP 88%	3 cc	5 cc
Distilled water	2 cc	4 cc
Croton oil (27 guttas = 1 cc)	3 guttas	3 guttas
Septisol	8 guttas	8 guttas

heal. In order to better understand the role of croton oil, Hetter performed multiple chemical peels of different concentrations of phenol and croton oil. He found that phenol penetrated more deeply with increased concentrations, that higher concentrations of phenol (88%) without Septisol penetrated more deeply than lower concentrations (50% and 35%), and that increasing the concentration of croton oil added to peel formula resulted in a more profound dermal effect and deeper peel. It should be noted that multiple coats will increase the depth of injury. Finally, 1% croton oil solutions were noted as the upper threshold for safe use to avoid serious risk of hypopigmentation.

Today, it is optimal to have a more standardized means of measuring the croton oil concentrations, instead of relying on droppers, which are inherently inconsistent. Drops are now converted to cubic centimeters by having 25 drops equal one cubic centimeter. Using this conversion, a stock solution of 0.04 mL of croton oil per 1 mL of phenol, from which one can make varying croton oil concentrations of 0.4%, 0.8%, 1.2%, and 1.6% in a constant phenol concentration, needing only Septisol, phenol, and water. Using these formulations, the practitioner can decide between a phenol concentration of 35% or 48.5%.

Due to the differences in skin throughout the face, it is common practice to apply different depths of peeling for individual subunits of the face. This can also be translated into the use of varying concentrations of croton oil in different regions of the face. While the lower nose can tolerate croton oil concentrations up to 1.2%, the cheeks and forehead only tolerate concentrations up to 0.8%, and the upper nose, temple, and lateral brow can only withstand concentrations up to 0.4% before the risk of complications arise.

While the depth of penetration is dictated not only by the components of the peeling solution but also by the concentrations of these components, the application of these varying concentrations must be controlled to create desired results. For example, Stone's work revealed that varying the concentration of phenol and croton oil produced equivalent levels of fibrosis when applied with 50 rubs. However, when fewer strokes were used, thus increasing the concentration of phenol, a greater depth of peel was observed. This was again confirmed with the use of a lower phenol concentration and found that increasing concentrations of croton oil lowers the threshold number of applications needed to achieve the same depth of peel. This work emphasizes that the technique and application of the peel formula to the skin is as important as the formula used. This is where we feel the experience of the peeler and the "art" of peeling become critical to achieving a successful outcome.

HISTORY

Excellent results in skin resurfacing begin with proper patient selection. A history and physical examination is required for each patient undergoing chemical peeling. More advanced investigations are standard for deep peels, which would include cardiac, pulmonary, hepatic, and renal profiles. The medical history should include the completion of a Fitzpatrick scale, while the subsequent clinical examination affords the opportunity to complete Glogau classification (Tables 30.2 and 30.3). Attention is dedicated to the review of any personal and/or familial history of abnormal wound healing (delayed, keloid, or hypertrophic), dermatologic conditions (allergy, autoimmune, chronic inflammatory, infectious, collagen), herpes simplex, melasma, surgical and non-surgical interventions, sun exposure, hyperpigmentation, hypopigmentation, and photosensitivity.

PHYSICAL EXAMINATION

Knowing who would benefit from more invasive resurfacing procedures directly relates to the interpretation of clinical findings. The clinical examination should include a complete examination of the head and neck as well as a comprehensive dermatologic examination. Skin quality, color, type, thickness, complexion, rhytids, photodamage, dyschromias, telangiectasias, keratosis, lesions, and scars should be noted and documented accordingly. Rhytids and photodamage must be distinguished from age-related gravitational changes, jowling, and

TABLE 30.2 Fitzpatrick Classification Scale

Skin Type	Skin Color	Characteristics
I	White; very fair; red or blond hair; blue eyes; freckles	Always burns, never tans
II	White; fair; red or blond hair; blue, hazel or green eyes	Usually burns, tans with difficulty
III	Cream white; fair with any eye or hair color; very common	Sometimes mild burn, gradually tans
IV	Brown; typical Mediterranean Caucasian skin	Rarely burns, tans with ease
V	Dark brown; mid-eastern skin types	Very rarely burns, tans very easily
VI	Black	Never burns, tans very easily

TABLE 30.3 Glogau Classification Scale

Skin Class	Description

I	"Early Wrinkles"
	• Patient age: 20s–30s
	• Early photoaging
	  • Mild pigment changes
	  • Minimal wrinkles
	  • No "age spots"

II	"Wrinkles in Motion"
	• Patient age: 30s–40s
	• Early to moderate photoaging
	  • Appearance of smile lines
	  • Early brown "age spots"
	  • Skin pores more prominent
	  • Early changes in skin texture

III	"Wrinkles at Rest"
	• Patient age: 50s and older
	• Advanced photoaging
	  • Prominent brown pigmentation
	  • Visible brown "age spots"
	  • Prominent, small blood vessels
	  • Wrinkles, even at rest

IV	"Only Wrinkles"
	• Patient age: 60s or 70s
	• Severe photoaging
	  • Yellow-gray skin color
	  • Prior skin cancers
	  • Precancerous skin changes (actinic keratosis)

loss of the volume of facial adipose tissue. The findings should also be reviewed with the patient in order to establish their expectations for proposed treatments. The use of standardized, high-resolution photo documentation should be employed prior to any treatment.

INDICATIONS

Defining the patient's suitability for a chemical peel is of paramount importance. It is necessary to determine that each patient is both physically and mentally fit for his or her desired peel. In general, facial resurfacing, and the degree thereof, is determined by the presence and severity of facial rhytids, keratosis, scarring, atrophic changes, hyperpigmentation, melasma, and dysplastic lesions. The ideal candidate for a chemical peel is one with fair skin, fair eyes, and mild, shallow rhytids. However, this only represents a minority of the patients who will seek treatment for rhytids and photodamage.

CONTRAINDICATIONS

Relative contraindications for any resurfacing procedure include history of cutaneous radiation, smokers, active or frequent herpes simplex virus (HSV) infections, diabetes, hypertrophic scar, or history of keloids. Birth control pills, exogenous estrogens (including soaps and cosmetics containing lavender oil), or photosensitizing drugs are to be avoided due to risks of hyperpigmentation. Due to elevated estrogen levels of pregnancy, the patient should not have plans to become pregnant within the first 6 months after the chemical peel for the same reason.

It is important to address lifestyle and habitual activities of all patients being considered for a chemical peel. Smoking causes significant microvascular damage that could hinder tissue healing and lead to a poor cosmetic outcome. Practitioners should be honest and frank regarding the risks, and a cessation program should be recommended. Smokers should stop smoking 1 month prior to and should avoid smoking for at least 6 months after the peel. A patient's habitual sun exposure should be assessed prior to proceeding with the peel. Ultraviolet (UV) light exposure can be equally problematic in the postoperative period. The patient should be advised that chronic or frequent sun exposure should be avoided after the chemical peel. The practitioner should consider other options and not perform a peel if these lifestyle changes are unacceptable to the patient.

Isotretinoin (Accutane) use is an absolute contraindication to chemical peeling or any other resurfacing procedure. Postpeel reepithelialization relies upon the epidermis within hair follicles and sebaceous glands. Isotretinoin prevents reepithelialization from these locations. Most recommendations include a cessation period of 12 months prior to the peel. Also, patients with unrealistic expectations place the practioner in an unreasonable professional and personal circumstance. These patients are appropriately counseled and even referred for psychiatric evaluation when reasonable.

PREOPERATIVE PLANNING

Once the patient has been defined as a suitable patient, proper skin preparation must begin. This skin preparation helps to prevent complications and allow the best outcomes. Sunscreens, including both UVA and UVB block, should be started to prevent prepeel burns or tanning. This helps to decrease melanocyte activity prior to the peel. Ideally, sun protection should begin 3 months prior to the peel in combination with minimizing sun exposure.

Topical tretinoin (Retin-A) is recommended for 6 to 12 weeks prior to the peel. Synergistic qualities of pretreatment tretinoin and TCA peels have been shown to sustain the effects of the chemical peel. Tretinoin aids in reepithelialization and leads to increased melanin distribution. Tretinoin treatment results in a thickened epidermis that displays decreased corneocyte adhesion, decreased stratum corneum thickness, and neocollagen production, all of which are beneficial to the postoperative outcome. The thickened and uniform epidermis also aids in the uniform application of the peeling agent.

Tretinoin should be applied at nighttime 6 weeks prior to the peel and should be continued after the postpeel reepithelialization is completed. The dose range recommended is between 0.025% and 0.1%. However, there is no literature describing an improved benefit with the higher dosing, indicating that the lower concentrations may be just as effective. Some patients may be sensitive to tretinoin use, and a lower dose may be better tolerated. Potential side effects that each patient should be warned about include irritation, erythema, and flaking of the skin. If this occurs, the dose should be decreased or the tretinoin should be discontinued altogether.

Hydroquinone is also beneficial in the pretreatment of all peel patients, especially those with lentigos, dyschromias, and Fitzpatrick skin types III to VI, due to the higher risk of postinflammatory hyperpigmentation (PIH). Hydroquinone blocks the conversion of tyrosine to l-Dopa by tyrosinase, thus decreasing melanin production. Hydroquinone, in a concentration of 4% to 8%, should be started 4 to 6 weeks prior to resurfacing. Like tretinoin, hydroquinone should be started after the peel as soon as the patient's skin can tolerate its application.

All patients should be warned of the possibility of a HSV outbreak in response to the peel, even if they have no recollection of prior herpetic vesicle occurrence. Patients can have a latent infection even in the setting of a negative history. A common and advisable practice is to start any patient with a negative history on a prophylactic dose of antivirals, acyclovir 400 mg three times a day, 3 days prior to and continued for at least 7 days after the peel. For those patients with a positive history of active HSV infections, a therapeutic dose of antivirals should be used, such as valacyclovir 1 g three times a day for the aforementioned time period. Postpeel herpetic infections can be unnerving for the practitioner, but devastating for the patient; hence, all precautions should be taken to avoid them.

The skin, especially the relatively resistant epidermis, is the main infectious barrier for the human body. Resurfacing procedures reduce this barrier and can lead to infections by cutaneous bacterial flora, especially staphylococcal and streptococcal species. Appropriate antibacterial coverage should be initiated prior to the peel as prophylaxis. I prescribe cephalexin, 250 mg four times a day, 1 day prior to the peel and continue it for 7 days in the postoperative period, and feel that this is sufficient for prophylaxis. For those patients who are beta-lactam sensitive, a macrolide (i.e., erythromycin 250 mg q.i.d.) with similar coverage can be used.

There is limited evidence that supports the clinical safety of combining resurfacing procedures with rhytidectomy. The compromised blood supply and healing from these procedures creates too great a risk to advocate stacking these procedures in a single therapeutic window. Some authors combine resurfacing procedures with the deep-plane rhytidectomy, due to preservation of the cutaneous perforating blood supply. However, there is a great degree of variation in the surgical techniques of a "deep-plane" face-lift and for this reason we do not recommend a combined protocol. Additionally, in order to maintain appropriate and uniform depth of penetration of the peeling agent, I recommend the avoidance of waxing, dermabrasion, and electrolysis for 3 to 4 weeks prior to peeling.

SURGICAL TECHNIQUE

The peeling solution should always be applied on sufficiently prepared skin. This preparation begins with a pretreatment regimen and ends with a vigorous cleaning, with Septisol or an acne wash, the evening before and the morning of the procedure. Upon arrival to the office, and after completion of procedural consents, preoperative oral sedation (10 to 15 mg of diazepam and 100 mg of Dramamine) is administered to relieve the patient's anxiety regarding the intravenous (IV) catheter placement and the upcoming procedure. Further, the antihistamine reduces oral secretions and helps to protect the patient's airway during periods of deeper sedation.

It is important that the patients are adequately hydrated prior to beginning the chemical peel. Intravenous fluids should be initiated prior to bringing the patient to the operating room in order to replenish overnight loss of intravascular volume. Additional IV benzodiazepine can be administered at this point if the patient continues to be anxious.

After being placed in a seated position, the patient's submandibular shadow is marked. This step is important to avoid obvious postoperative delineation between peeled and nonpeeled areas at the jawline. The patient is then placed in the supine position. After administering a sedating dose of propofol, the nerve blocks (supraorbital, infraorbital, mental) and field blocks are performed with an equal mixture of 2% lidocaine and 0.5% bupivacaine. Avoid the use of epinephrine, even in the nerve blocks, to allow maximal clearance of phenol, if being used. While waiting for maximal anesthesia to occur, the face is thoroughly degreased with an acetone-soaked gauze. Any residual oil on the skin will cause an uneven peel. Repeat the acetone cleaning throughout the procedure if necessary.

I support the standard use of 2- × 2-inch cotton gauze that is adequately wrung out to remove excess solution when applying the peeling agent; however, I feel that wide cotton-tipped applicators offer superior control of the peel application. As discussed above, the depth of the peel is dependent upon the uniform application of the solution, the amount of solution utilized on the cotton tip, and the number of strokes applied. The immediate frost that occurs with phenol-based peels represents precipitation of the keratin by the phenol. This indicates a completed reaction, and there is no need for neutralization of solution. The immediate frost is one of the benefits of using a phenol-based solution is compared to TCA peels. With a TCA peels, practitioners need to wait three to four minutes before assessing a peeled area for needed repeat applications. With the phenol–croton oil peel, the quality of the depth is quickly and readily apparent, and areas in need of reapplication can be immediately treated. Medium-depth peels should give you a level II to level III frosting, described in Table 30.4.

The subunits of the face should be divided by degree of rhytids, lentigos, and photodamage as well as inherent thickness. My experience has been to use 0.8% croton oil Hetter solution in areas of deeper rhytids (Glogau III and IV) and thicker skin, such as the perioral, glabellar, and lateral periorbital areas. The intermediate areas (Glogau II and III) are treated with 0.4% croton oil Hetter solution. In order to even the appearance of the face, a simple 88% USP phenol solution is used for all other areas. In the case of severe Glogau IV rhytids in the upper lip, in patients who are Fitzpatrick I or II, a classic Baker formula can be used.

To avoid cardiac toxicity, approximately 10 to 15 minutes must be allowed between each subunit peeled to allow for proper clearance of the phenol. The entire face should be peeled over 90 to 120 minutes. In the event that a minor supraventricular arrhythmia occurs, the peel should be stopped and the practitioner should wait for a return to normal sinus rhythm. The peel should be carried into the hairline, as phenol and croton oil will not affect pigment of the hair follicles. The edge of each peeled area will have a line of reactive hyperemia. This does not represent peeled skin, but rather it represents an unpeeled skin reaction.

When treating adjacent areas, this line of hyperemia (Fig. 30.1) should be included and adequately peeled so as to not create obvious lines of demarcation. Similarly, the peel should be carried over the vermillion border. The practitioner can stretch wrinkled skin to allow an even peel over these areas. For deep perioral rhytids, the cotton tip applicator can be broken and the wood edge used to apply the peeling agent in the rhytid. Great care must be taken around the lower eyelid margin. The peel should be performed to within 3 mm of the ciliary line and stopped. There should be no excess solution on the lower lid. The patient may develop tearing during the procedure. Any tearing should be dried to avoid the tears pulling the peeling solution into the eye.

If not adequately anesthetized, the patient will experience an immediate burning sensation for 15 to 20 seconds. However, this sensation will return in 20 minutes and can last 4 to 8 hours later. The longer-lasting effect of the bupivacaine will greatly aid in minimizing this burning sensation in the postoperative period. Therefore, it is essential to perform adequate nerve and field blocks.

Even with all precautions in place, accidents may happen. In the case of excess phenol exposure to the patient or the staff, propylene glycol, glycerol, olive oil, castor oil, or cottonseed oil should be poured onto the site to solubilize the phenol. If exposure to the eyes occurs, mineral oil should be immediately applied to the eyes using a dropper.

TABLE 30.4 Reaction to the Peel
Level I: erythema with stringy or blotchy frosting
Level II: white coat with erythema showing through (should be used for eyelids, and areas of bony prominences, i.e., zygomatic arch, malar, chin, higher rate of scarring)
Level III: solid white frost with little or no background erythema

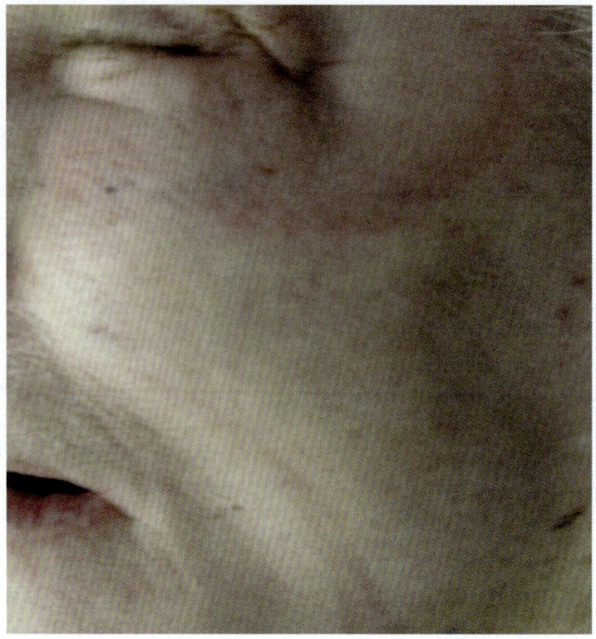

FIGURE 30.1
This demonstrates the clear line of hyperemia that occurs at the periphery of a peeled area. This hyperemic skin has not been peeled. Care must be taken to peel this area so as to not leave a discrete line of unpeeled skin.

POSTOPERATIVE CARE

Postoperative care begins immediately after the last subunit is treated. The patient is once again reminded of the burning sensation that may last up to 8 hours after the procedure as well as the expectation of facial edema, erythema, and eventual desquamation. When the frost subsides and only erythema persists, a thick layer of bland emollient should be applied to all treated areas, leaving no peeled skin exposed. I prefer Eucerin cream, but Elta or bacitracin ointment may be used. None of these act as an occlusive dressing, and they will not increase the depth of penetration. Starting with postoperative day one, the patient will then apply the cream to those areas that are exposed three to four times a day. By using the emollient, the peeled skin can be monitored with greater ease on a day-to-day basis.

There are four stages to the healing process. First, inflammation occurs and increases during the first 12 hours. Next, the epidermis will begin to change in appearance, becoming leathery, and will separate from the dermis. The underlying dermal injury will become necrotic and slough. The emollient will aid in clearing this necrotic tissue from the underlying dermis, which is then covered with the emollient. Desquamation will occur over 4 to 7 days, exposing the underlying erythematous dermis. Depending on the depth of the peel, the reepithelialization process usually begins 48 to 72 hours after the peel and is completed by 7 to 10 days (Fig. 30.2). This reepithelialization will be represented by a conversion of bright red erythema to a lighter shade of pink. The benefit of the peel is born out of the fourth and final stage. This stage involves fibroplasia, which begins during the first week and continues for 12 to 16 weeks after the peel. This period is marked by neoangiogenesis, neocollagenesis, and collagen reorganization.

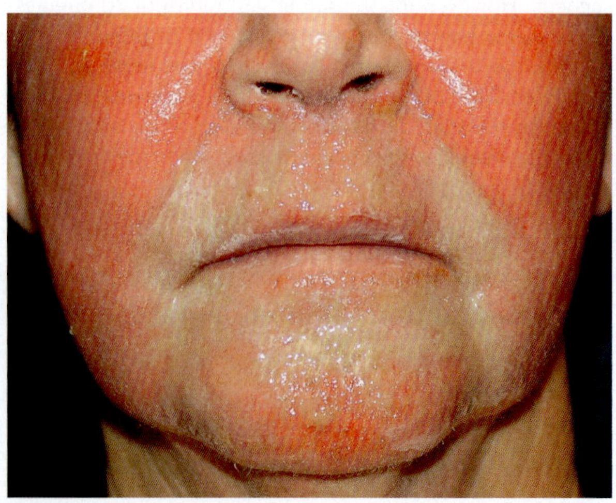

FIGURE 30.2
This photo demonstrates the erythematous neoepithelialization that has replaced the sloughed chemoexfoliated skin, postoperative day 6.

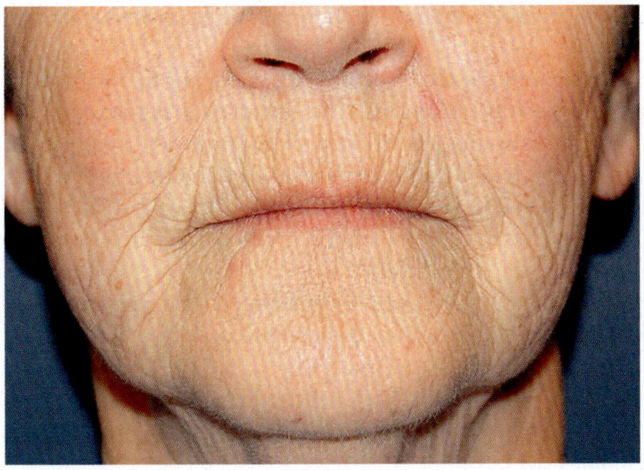

FIGURE 30.3
This patient underwent chemoexfoliation with Hetter formulas for significant wrinkles and dyschromias from photodamage.

The preoperative and postoperative photographs demonstrate the marked improvement that can be seen at 6 months following the peel (Figs. 30.3 and 30.4).

During the first 12 weeks after the peel, the patient is susceptible to UV light exposure and a resultant hyperpigmentation. Strict avoidance of direct, prolonged sun exposure should be encouraged for that 12-week period. It has been my experience that sunscreens should also be avoided for the first 6 weeks. Paraaminobenzoic acid, found in many sunscreen preparations, can cause an undesirable reaction, including irritation, increased erythema, and induration. Women of childbearing age should avoid birth control pills or pregnancy. Increased circulating estrogens can result in hyperpigmentation following chemoexfoliation.

COMPLICATIONS

Despite taking all necessary preoperative precautions and measures, the busy practitioner can encounter a number of postoperative complications. Early identification and management of these adverse events, both minor and major, will make the difference between undesirable and optimal results.

- *Cardiac arrhythmia*: Probably the most feared complication of phenol peels is cardiac arrhythmias. Though no death due to phenol peeling has been described in the literature, an appropriate caution regarding the use of phenol is advised. Even in well-hydrated and appropriately screened patients, a reversible arrhythmia can occur, especially in those with undiagnosed myocardial sensitivity. These patients will develop a supraventricular tachycardia within 30 minutes of the onset of the peel, which, if exacerbated, can progress into paroxysmal ventricular contractions, paroxysmal atrial tachycardia, ventricular tachycardia, and, possibly, ventricular fibrillations. The key is to not allow this progression to take place. Once an irregular rhythm is noted, the peeling should be halted, adequate hydration continued, and the patient's rhythm will return to baseline as the phenol is cleared. At this point, the chemical peeling can proceed, but with vigilant observation of the cardiac rhythm. In the extremely rare case that a heart rate does not return to normal, proper measures should be employed for the aberrant rhythm.
- *Delayed healing*: Prolonged healing times are a nuisance for both the patient and the practitioner. Prolonged healing is defined by any area that does not reepithelialize by day 10. This is more common with medium-depth TCA and deeper phenol peels. These wounds should be checked daily. The practitioner must rule out the presence of infection, contact irritants, patient noncompliance, and

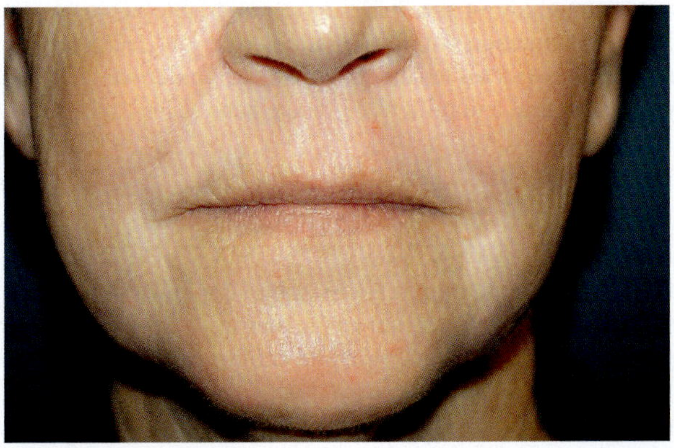

FIGURE 30.4
This photo demonstrates the results 6 months following the peel.

nighttime scratching. These areas should be treated promptly with protective measures, or they can possibly result in scarring.

The most common site for scarring to occur is the perioral area, specifically the upper lip. Scarring is most often the result of too deep a peel or from poor postoperative care. The risk of scarring is increased in isotretinoin users. Again, after discontinuing isotretinoin, the practitioner should wait until the patient is clearly developing skin oil. These scars can be treated with Silastic (cross-linked polydimethylsiloxane polymer) sheeting and intralesional steroid injections (Kenalog 20 mg/mL) every 2 to 3 weeks. Overuse of steroids can result in dermal atrophy; therefore, judicious use is recommended. If these scars are erythematous, multiple treatments with a flashlamp-pumped dye laser are helpful.

- *Infection*: A bacterial pyoderma can aggravate wound healing and lead to scarring. In the rare case of a bacterial or fungal infection, appropriate antimicrobials should be initiated and continued for a 7- to 10-day course.
- *HSV activation*: A herpetic infection can be devastatingly uncomfortable for the patient. If this infection occurs, despite adequate pretreatment prophylaxis, a maximal antiviral course should be used. Valacyclovir 1 g three times a day for 10 days is a typical regimen.
- *Prolonged erythema*: The postoperative erythema that is typical in all peeled patients may last longer than expected. This is more prevalent with patients with sensitive skin or in cases of contact dermatitis. Topical hydrocortisone (2.5%) lotions are helpful for accelerating the resolution of this erythema.
- *Hyperpigmentation*: As the erythema is subsiding, some patients, as result of inadvertent sun exposure or from darker skin type, will develop PIH. This usually occurs weeks after the peel. This is more common in the Fitzpatrick III to VI skin types and is most commonly seen in the skin overlying bony prominences, such as the lateral malar regions. A combination of 0.05% retinoic acid, 8% hydroquinone, and hydrocortisone cream is affective at reducing or eliminating this pigmentation. Glycolic acid lotion has been noted to be effective as well.
- *Hypopigmentation*: Classically, this is a more common and irreversible complication related to phenol-based peels, but many facets of skin resurfacing can cause this unwanted event. Phenol is thought to eliminate the melanocytes ability to produce melanin. Peeling single facial subunits makes this complication much more noticeable. The concentration of the phenol and croton oil, the skin type and taping are all factors contributing to the risk of hypopigmentation. Patients should be counseled regarding the possible need for makeup use as there is no treatment to reverse this complication.

RESULTS

In general, patients with a fair complexion, thin skin, and fine wrinkles represent the ideal candidate for resurfacing in relation to procedure outcomes and potential adverse events. Further, patients with realistic expectations, as well as a firm understanding of the recovery timeline and postprocedural discomfort, also benefit exceptionally well. For those patients with mild actinic damage, superficial lentigos, and fine, mild rhytids, a superficial peel may be safely used with few complications. The superficial peel extends through the depth of the epidermis and results in epidermal sloughing. The superficial peel will also create an inflammatory response in the uppermost portion of the papillary dermis.

For those patients included in the Glogau III and IV classification and who are Fitzpatrick type I or II, typically in the perioral areas, a deep peel can be carried out, such as the classic Baker formulation. The deep peel creates sloughing of the epidermis and the papillary dermis and creates an inflammatory response in the reticular dermis. Although effective in minimizing deep rhytids, the deep peel solutions result in a much higher risk of complications, such as scarring and hypopigmentation. With the superficial and deep peels being the two extremes of peeling, in terms of effectiveness and risk, the medium-strength peel balances great results with decreased risk.

The medium-strength peel is where application technique becomes tantamount and also the "art" of peeling becomes a factor. The medium-depth peel creates sloughing of the epidermis and variable necrosis and inflammation of the papillary dermis. Minimizing the inflammation within the reticular dermis decreases the common risks of the deeper peels. The medium-depth peel provides a reliable treatment for epidermal growths, moderate photoaging skin (Glogau II), pigmentary dyschromias, and mild to moderate acne scars.

PEARLS

- Careful patient selection and preoperative evaluation is critical to minimize the risk of complications.
- Pretreatment regimen is essential in the reduction of adverse events and optimization of outcomes. This includes use of UVA/UVB sunscreens, tretinoin, hydroquinone, and antiviral and antibiotic prophylaxis.
- Use different depths of peels for the individual subunits of the face.
- The technique and application of the peel formula to the skin is just as important as the formula used.

- To avoid cardiac toxicity, approximately 10 to 15 minutes must be allowed between each subunit peeled to allow for proper clearance of the phenol.
- Close postoperative care is critical to minimizing complications through early identification.

PITFALLS

- Avoid the use of epinephrine, even in the nerve blocks, to allow phenol and croton oil to clear.
- To avoid obvious lines of demarcation, be sure to include the line of reactive hyperemia when peeling the adjacent subunits.

INSTRUMENTS TO HAVE AVAILABLE

No unique instrumentation required

ACKNOWLEDGMENT

My sincere gratitude is extended to Jessica L. Kulak, MD, for her contributions to the writing of this chapter. Her work in the writing, editing, and figure creation for this chapter is greatly appreciated.

SUGGESTED READING

Brody HJ. Complications of chemical resurfacing. *Dermatol Clin* 2001;19(3):427–438.

Glogau R. Aesthetic and anatomic analysis of the aging skin. *Semin Cutan Med Surg* 1996;15(3):134–138.

Hetter GP. An examination of the phenol-croton oil peel: part IV. Face peel results with different concentrations of the phenol and croton oil. *Plast Reconstr Surg* 2000;105(3):1061–1083.

Monheit GD. Medium-depth chemical peels. *Dermatol Clin* 2001;19(3):413–425.

Stone PA, Lefer LG. Modified phenol chemical face peels: recognizing the role of application technique. *Facial Plast Surg Clin North Am* 2001;9(3):351–376.

31 VASCULAR LESIONS TREATED WITH LASER THERAPY

Jonathan W. Boyd

INTRODUCTION

Laser treatment of vascular lesions requires a complete understanding of the various cutaneous vascular diseases as well as the means by which they can be treated using laser technology. Once previously considered untreatable, cutaneous vascular lesions of the head and neck can cause significant morbidity and facial deformity. The use of lasers in the treatment of these lesions has become a historic step in the fields of both facial plastic surgery and applied laser technology.

The word LASER is an acronym for "light amplification by the stimulated emission of radiation," as proposed in Albert Einstein's landmark 1917 article, "Quantum Theory of Radiation." In 1963, Solomon et al. introduced the use of lasers for the medical management of cutaneous vascular lesions, such as port-wine stains (PWS) and cavernous hemangiomas. By the early 1980s, laser therapy became the first effective treatment for PWS based upon the work of Anderson and Parrish and their theory of selective photothermolysis. This theory describes how light energy is used to target a specific light-absorbing chromophore residing at a particular depth within tissue while not injuring normal adjacent structures. Target selectivity is based upon each chromophore's preferential absorption of a light at a specific wavelength(s). The overall parameters of laser therapy depend upon light wavelength, pulse duration, and energy density used. This is of critical importance as the precise control of thermal energy/injury is just as important as optical and tissue factors. One measure to maximize the spatial confinement of heat is to use a laser with pulse duration on the order of the thermal relaxation time (T_r) of the target chromophore. T_r is defined as the time required for the heat generated by the absorption of energy within the target chromophore to cool to 50% of the original value immediately after the laser pulse. During longer laser exposures, a more generalized heating, and less spatial selectivity, are produced and result in nonspecific thermal damage to adjacent structures. However, if the laser pulse is suitably brief, the energy is invested in the target chromophore before thermal diffusion extends out of the exposure field. Simply stated, shorter laser pulse durations confine the energy to smaller target regions with more spatial selectivity and less collateral damage.

The final consideration in selective photothermolysis is energy density, defined as transmitted light energy per unit area. The absorption of light in a specific region is attenuated by competing chromophores as well as the normal scattering of the optical beam. These factors must be considered in order to achieve an energy density adequate to induce selective destruction of the targeted chromophore/region. Additionally, the effect of spot size on energy density is an inverse and squared relationship. If the spot size is decreased by a factor of two, energy density increases by a factor of four. In similar fashion, doubling of the laser spot size results in a fourfold reduction in energy density.

With these central concepts in mind, there are a variety of lasers approved by the Food and Drug Administration (FDA) for the treatment of cutaneous vascular lesions. Recognition and understanding of the most common devices provides a necessary foundation for appropriate clinical therapy.

- **Flashlamp-Pumped Pulsed Dye (PDL) Laser:** The common chromophore of cutaneous vascular lesions is hemoglobin (i.e., oxyhemoglobin). For these reasons, the pulsed dye laser (577 to 595 nm) has been the mainstay of treatment in children and adults for multiple cutaneous vascular lesions as there is adequate tissue penetration, less injury and heating to surrounding tissues, and directed therapy to the blood vessels of interest. Wavelengths and pulse durations are fixed with several manufacturers producing devices with wavelength emissions ranging from 585 to 595 nm with pulse durations of 450 μs to 40 ms.
- **Neodymium: Yttrium-Aluminum-Garnet (Nd:YAG) laser:** Light penetration into skin is very deep (4 to 6 mm) resulting in a large volume of coagulated tissue (substantially larger than that created by the PDL). Photons are emitted at a wavelength of 1,064 nm and are poorly absorbed by hemoglobin, melanin, water, and other skin chromophores. Deeper light penetration with increased risk for scar formation.
- **Potassium Titanyl Phosphate (KTP) Laser:** The green light (532 nm) produced by the frequency-doubled Nd:YAG laser (KTP laser) is preferentially absorbed by hemoglobin. The KTP laser has been approved by the FDA for many of the same procedures as the PDL. Melanin absorption is higher and light penetration into human skin is less at this shorter wavelength. This laser can create an average power up to 160 W per pulse and can be adjusted to pulse durations of 1 to 100 ms at repetition rates of 1 to 10 per second.
- **Alexandrite Laser:** Produces red light at a wavelength of 755 nm that targets deoxyhemoglobin, which absorbs light at 760 nm. Deeper penetration into tissue is achieved and useful for the treatment of thicker, hypertrophic vascular lesions.
- **Intense Pulsed Light (IPL):** Unlike the single wavelength method of previously described systems, this technology allows for the use of a broad spectrum of visible light ranging between 515 and 1,000 nm at 1 to 3 pulses per utilization. Filters limit the spectrum of light to the desired wavelengths, while a larger spot size apparatus delivers treatment to a broader area.

HISTORY

A complete general history is a requisite for each patient undergoing laser therapy. The history should include the location, dimensions, and duration of each lesion, as well as the growth rate and previous interventions undertaken. It is also important to identify any symptoms attributable to the lesions including mass effect, bleeding, sensation change, and pruritus. Specific attention must be paid to any direct or family history of similar lesions as well as aberrant scarring (i.e., hypertrophic scar or keloid formation), dermatologic diseases (e.g., allergic, immunologic, inflammatory), allergies, past complications in wound healing, degree of sun exposure, bleeding disorders, and prior skin procedures or surgery over the area to be treated. Complicating factors for wound healing, such as smoking, diabetes, and use of the isotretinoin should also be identified.

PHYSICAL EXAMINATION

The physical evaluation should consist of a comprehensive examination of the head and neck as well as a dermatologic examination. The thickness, quality, and tone of the skin should be assessed in addition to a complete/standard examination of the cranial nerves. The proximity of each lesion to adjacent and sensitive structures must be thoroughly evaluated. The size and location of the lesion are directly correlated to the success of the treatment. For example, PWS lesions involving cranial nerve V_2 distribution are generally more difficult to achieve lightening or clearance despite multiple comparable treatments. The depth of each lesion should be assessed, since deeper lesions may require alternative treatments including intralesional injections, cryotherapy, sclerosing therapy, or surgical excision and debulking. All pertinent abnormalities found on examination should be clearly explained to the patient and representative family members in order to establish rapport and determine expectations. Patients need to understand that laser treatment does not always entail complete resolution of the lesions or a lack of potential risks, as may be insinuated from patient research or advertisement. Such therapy may also involve serial treatments and follow-up visits with incremental benefit. Photography must be used to record the findings of the initial physical examination and throughout treatment. Standard facial views should be employed as well as specific images focusing on the target lesion. The visualization and documentation of normal adjacent tissue are also of clinical and therapeutic importance.

INDICATIONS

Cutaneous vascular lesions of the head and neck are easily recognized and difficult to conceal. These lesions may compromise the function of vital structures or remain purely cosmetic in their impact. Commonly a negative psychological impact develops, including a perceived cosmetic deformity, decreased in self-esteem, and significant emotional stress, resulting in a compromised quality of living. When laser therapy is effective, it can lessen the patient's physical and emotional burden. These findings coincide with the benefits of early therapy (fewer treatments to achieve an improved response with fewer complications) when compared with treatment initiated at a later age.

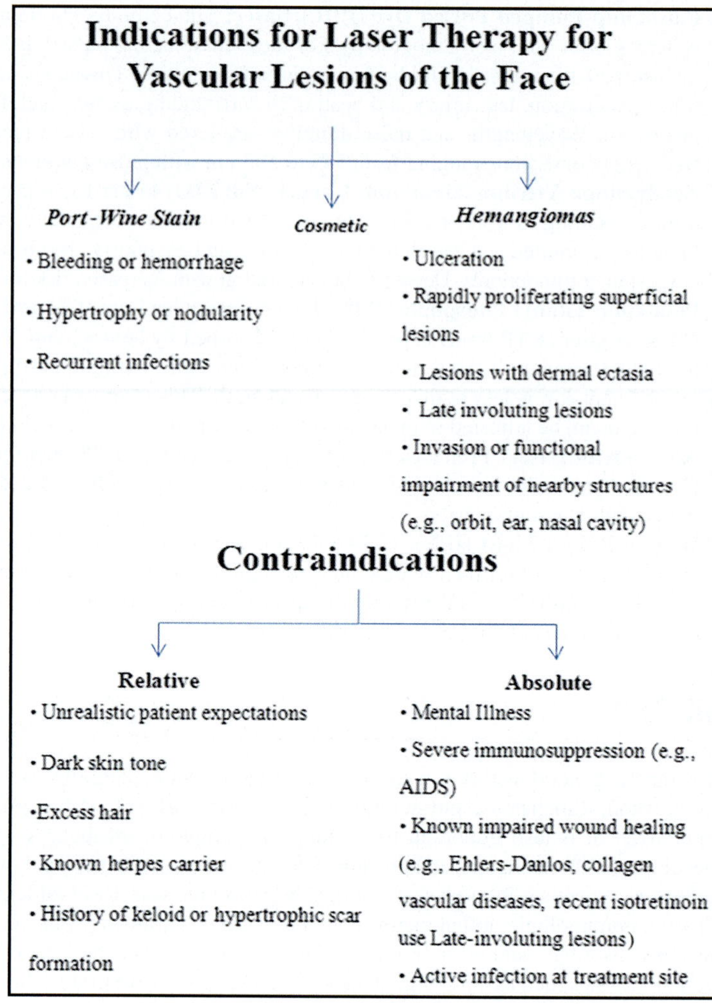

FIGURE 31.1
Most common vascular lesions and the indications and contraindications for laser therapy.

While clinical observation may be appropriate for lesions of the extremities and trunk, facial hemangiomas should be treated early and aggressively. Periorbital hemangiomas may impair vision due to obstruction of the visual axis and potentially cause permanent vision loss due to impaired development of the visual cortex (amblyopia). Perioral hemangiomas can lead to recurrent hemorrhage and ulceration with the possibility of infection. High-output cardiac failure can develop due to the circulatory demands of an enlarging vascular tumor. Nasal obstruction as well as conductive hearing loss may develop when vascular lesions are located along these sensitive facial structures. Alterations of the nasal and auricular cartilage may occur from the weight and growth of such lesions, as well as abnormal development of the bony facial skeleton. A review of indications may be found in Figure 31.1 along with contraindications, as noted below.

CONTRAINDICATIONS

While there are a wide variety of indications in the treatment of cutaneous vascular lesions, there are equally important reasons to withhold or delay therapy. The following represent relative and absolute contraindications:

- **Skin tone and hair:** Patients with a darker skin tone (higher epidermal melanin content) should be counseled carefully on the increased risks of burn injury and pigmentary changes following laser therapy. The Fitzpatrick scale may serve as a guideline, with increasing risk of pigmentary changes noted at levels III and greater. Hydroxyquinone, alpha hydroxy acids, and azelaic acid may be used to reduce epidermal melanin concentration. Hair should be removed from any treatment site, as direct radiation of hair may interfere with the delivery of laser energy or surface coolant. For some patients, covering the lesion with hair is more aesthetically satisfying compared to being shaved and having a visible lesion that treatment may not fully resolve. Patients with an excess amount of vellus hair in the treatment region also have an increased risk of laser-related burns and should be counseled of this risk prior to laser therapy.
- **Infection:** Similar to standard surgery, any infected facial vascular lesion should not be treated using laser therapy until the infection is resolved as the infection may interfere with proper healing and produce undesired scarring. Of note, herpes simplex virus (HSV) has a known propensity for reactivation following laser

therapy, particularly around the eye and mouth. All patients are questioned about previous HSV infection. Active HSV infection in close proximity to the site of the lesion is a cause for treatment delay. Valacyclovir and famciclovir prophylaxis against herpes reactivation is well described. Immunosuppressed patients with skin infections should be treated with appropriate antibiotics, and the treatment site should be kept clean and protected. Therapy is absolutely contraindicated in severely immunosuppressed patients (e.g., AIDS) due to an unacceptably high rate of infection.

- **History of scar formation:** Patients with a history of keloid or hypertrophic scar formation may not be suited for laser therapy, as healing may be erratic and lead to undesirable and/or unpredictable outcomes. Despite a variety of preventive measures available for abnormal scars, efficacy remains controversial and reported results are often conflicting.
- **Dermatologic conditions:** Patients with abnormalities in wound healing or skin integrity, such as Ehlers-Danlos, Marfan, scleroderma, collagen vascular diseases, and previous radiation therapy, should not undergo laser therapy. Patients who have taken isotretinoin within the last 6 to 12 months should avoid laser therapy, as adverse wound healing and keloid formation have been reported. Patients should adequately protect their skin from the sun following laser therapy, as even short exposures may cause dyspigmentation or skin irritation and impact the effectiveness of future treatments. A patient who anticipates significant sun exposure after laser therapy should delay treatment. If photoprotection cannot be achieved, then patients should be counseled on applying sunscreen with a sun protection factor (SPF) of at least 30 that contains a physical barrier component (zinc oxide, titanium oxide) and a sweat proof formula.
- **Psychological condition:** In evaluating candidates for laser therapy, the clinician must be prudent in patient selection as patients with psychological issues and/or unrealistic expectations may require extensive counseling and education. Careful screening in order to acquire an adequate understanding of each patient's psychological and emotional status is highly recommended. For those individuals with more complex issues, referral for psychiatric evaluation is appropriate.

PREOPERATIVE PLANNING

Approximately 60% of all vascular tumors and malformations involve the region of the head and neck. Vascular tumors, such as hemangiomas, are benign proliferations of endothelial cells found within the skin or mucosa with a spontaneous regression rate of 40% over a 12-year period. Vascular malformations, by comparison, originate from congenitally dysmorphic vessels that hypertrophy and never involute. Based on the vasculature involved, malformations are anatomically classified based on the prevailing vessel—capillary, lymphatic, venous, or arterial. These may be further divided into high- or low-flow lesions. Since these malformations occur during embryogenesis, vascular malformations may include combined channels (e.g., arteriovenous malformations). For clinical and therapeutic reasons, it is important to determine the classification of the vascular lesions being evaluated (Fig. 31.2).

- **Hemangioma:** These tumors are the most common vascular tumors, presenting as early as the first week of life. These tumors are well circumscribed and may be isolated or in a constellation. There is a predilection for hemangiomas to occur in premature infants and those with first-degree relatives who have vascular

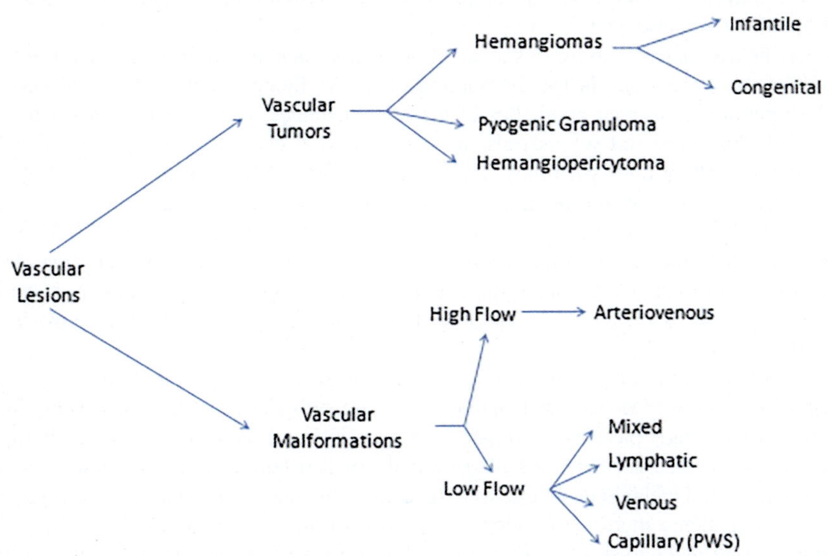

FIGURE 31.2 Vascular lesions. (Adapted from Mulliken JB, Glowacki J. Hemangiomas and vascular malformations in infants and children: a classification based on endothelial characteristics. *Plast Reconstr Surg* 1982;69:412–422.)

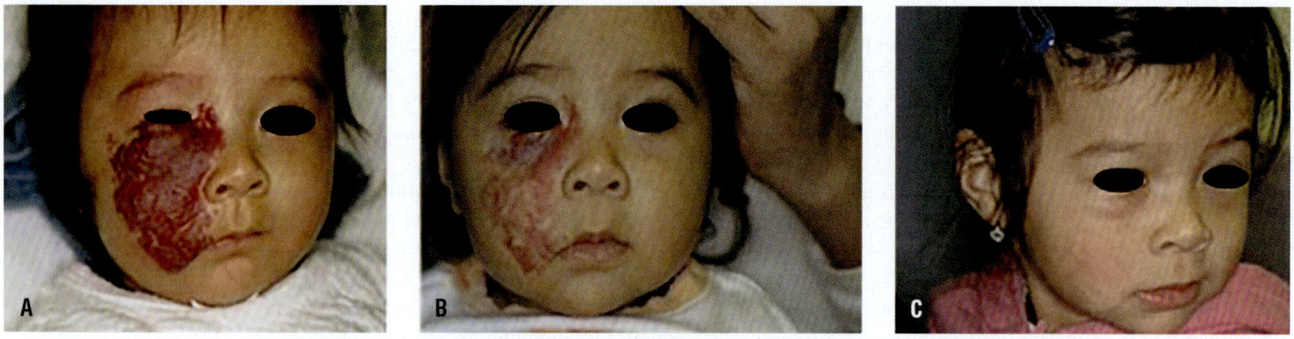

FIGURE 31.3 Serial treatment pulsed dye laser therapy of a large facial hemangioma. Photodocumentation occurred pretreatment **(A)**, after the fourth treatment **(B)**, and after the eighth treatment **(C)**.

lesions. While spontaneous involution commonly occurs in childhood, involution is not always synonymous with resolution. Atrophic scarring, fibrofatty degeneration, and telangiectatic vessels commonly remain in the superficial and deep dermis after involution, creating residual aesthetic concerns for affected individuals.

The initial medical treatment for hemangiomas threatening vital structures is pharmacologic. Propranolol (2 mg/kg/day) offers tremendous resolution in severe lesions. Despite such dramatic clinical results, side effects such as transient bradycardia, hypotension, bronchospasm, hypothermia, and hypoglycemia have been reported, particularly in those infants less than 3 months of age. Patients should have pretreatment electro- and echocardiograms and screening for asthma. All patients should be admitted for observation when propranolol therapy is started in order to identify and limit side effects.

Another therapeutic option is intralesional steroid injection. Such treatment has been found to arrest proliferation but carries the risk of local thrombus formation as well as the concern for blindness when treating periocular lesions. Systemic prednisone is the preferred route of administration when steroid treatment is contemplated. Adherence to treatment schedules and appropriate dose tapering are necessary to ensure risk reduction with adequate therapy. Laser treatment has an important role in the very early treatment of flat, superficial hemangiomas when the lesions are less than 1 to 2 mm thick. Figure 31.3 portrays a large hemangioma treated by serial pulsed dye laser. Based on a treatment algorithm developed by Williams et al., laser treatment is specifically indicated for ulcerative lesions, rapidly proliferating superficial lesions, and lesions with dermal ectasia. Deeper subcutaneous lesions do not respond as well to laser therapy as do superficial lesions.

- **Port-wine stains:** PWS, also referred to as nevus flammeus, are cutaneous vascular malformations involving the postcapillary venules. PWS appear as pink to violaceous patches on the skin and can have potentially devastating physical and psychological ramifications. They occur in 0.3% of newborns but may be acquired secondary to trauma in rare cases. While PWS may be localized anywhere on the body, most involve the head and neck region and classically follow a trigeminal nerve distribution. The exact mechanism of PWS development is unknown. It has been hypothesized that there is a deficiency of regulatory neurons controlling blood flow through the ectatic postcapillary venules resulting in permanent dilation of the blood vessels.

PWS may be associated with serious medical problems, such as Sturge-Weber syndrome, which consists of capillary malformations in the distribution of the V_1 branch of the trigeminal nerve, glaucoma, choroidal hemangiomas, vascular anomalies of the leptomeninges with potential for seizure activity, and potential cognitive impairment. PWS may also be an indicator of other associated problems such as Klippel-Trenaunay-Weber (PWS, limb hypertrophy, venous and lymphatic malformations) and Cobb (PWS, spinal angiomas) syndromes. Spontaneous hemorrhage and infection often cause additional complications.

Growth of PWS is commensurate with the growth of the child and do not have a tendency to involute. If left untreated, PWS progress from flat macules to thick papules or nodules by adulthood leading to disfigurement from hypertrophy of the underlying soft tissue and complications such as spontaneous bleeding. Treatment of PWS is recommended at an early age to prevent the development of hypertrophic change and complications.

Aggressive treatment of infants and young children is well tolerated and improves clearance. The most successful outcomes are seen in patients less than 1 year old with PWS smaller than 20 cm^2. Since PWS are generally smaller in younger patients, clearance is more easily achieved at an earlier age. Furthermore, with the variations in blood vessel diameter (30 to 300 μm), depth distribution (100 to 1,000 μm), epidermal thickness (50 to 150 μm), and melanin concentration, there are many optical advantages to treating patients early as well. In younger patients, there is less epidermal melanin to compete for laser light absorption; less dermal collagen, which contributes to light backscatter; and a thinner dermis and lower fractional blood volume that allows for more light to penetrate the skin. Finally, beyond optical advantages, it is easier to immobilize infants rather than more resistant toddlers during uncomfortable procedures (Fig. 31.4).

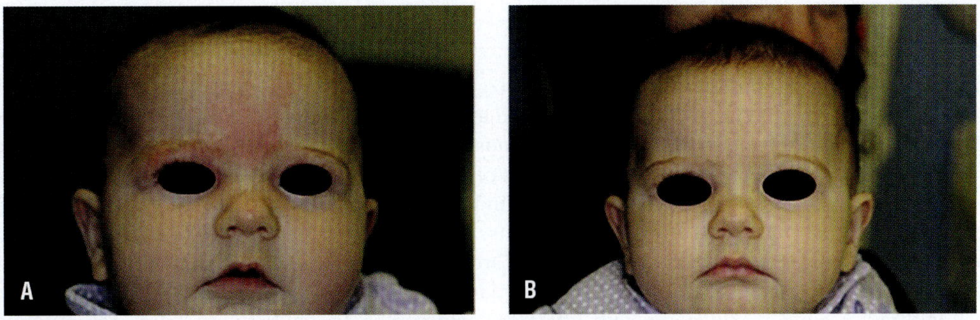

FIGURE 31.4 Port-wine stain before **(A)** and after **(B)** treatment with pulsed dye laser.

- **Telangiectasia:** Representing a dilated venule, capillary, or arteriole, these superficial cutaneous vessels are classified based on their clinical appearance—simple or linear, arborizing, spider, and popular. Telangiectasias of the face are usually linear and often seen in patients with lighter skin types. Occurrence is commonly on the nasal alae, nasal body, and midface. They are usually arteriolar and exhibit vasodilation due to vessel wall weakness, becoming more noticeable with sun exposure, trauma, and hormonal changes. Additionally, telangiectasias are associated with collagen vascular disease and a variety of genetic conditions, such as hereditary hemorrhagic telangiectasia (aka. Osler-Weber-Rendu), Bloom syndrome, and ataxia-telangiectasia.
- **Rosacea:** Rosacea is a complex cutaneous vascular disorder related to *Demodex folliculorum* and brevis mite infestations within the facial hair follicles. These mites contribute to the inflammatory processes that produce the characteristic nontransient erythematous feature of rosacea and the constellation of telangiectasias, papules, pustules, and rhinophyma. Additional manifestations include facial flushing, temperature changes, and sebaceous gland hypertrophy. Patients are often distressed both by the physical findings of the condition as well as the social stigma that results from rosacea's association with alcohol consumption.

  Treatment of rosacea is generally pharmacologic with topical agents (e.g., metronidazole, benzoyl peroxide, sulfacetamide) plus oral antibiotics (e.g., tetracycline, doxycycline, erythromycin). Therapy is targeted toward colonized *Staphylococcus* species, which are purported to be related to the altered skin temperatures of rosacea patients. Along with mites, bacteria are thought to compound the pervasive facial inflammation indicative of this condition. As a result, topical acaricides (pesticides to eliminate mites) have shown some benefit.

A variety of additional vascular lesions are well described and Figure 31.5 offers an extended list of such conditions.

Vascular Malformation	Vascular Tumor
	Hemangioma
Single-Vessel Type	Hemangioma of infancy
Capillary	Congenital hemangioma
Venous	Rapidly involuting congenital hemangioma (RICH)
Lymphatic	Noninvoluting congenital hemangioma (NICH)
Combined/Complex Malformations	Lobular hemangioma (pyogenic granuloma)
Arteriovenous	Vascular Neoplasm
Lymphaticovenous	Kaposiform hemangioendothelioma
Capillary-venous	Angiosarcoma
Capillary-lymphaticovenous	Hemangiopericytoma
Capillary-arteriovenous	Miscellaneous
	Tufted angioma

FIGURE 31.5 Binary classification of vascular lesions based upon the workshop of the International Society for the Study of Vascular Anomalies (ISSVA) in 1996. (Adapted from Enjoiras O, Wassef M, Chapot R. *A color atlas of vascular tumors and vascular malformation.*)

SURGICAL TECHNIQUE

Safety is of paramount importance and a standardized protocol for the benefit of all patients and health care providers is necessary. A stepwise table is provided to maintain attention to detail and a consistent work flow (Table 31.1). With each procedure, the surgeon must confirm the availability of the laser and its function, access to protective devices, and the chosen means of tissue cooling. The patient is then greeted and a review of the operative consent along with the physical findings is performed. The patient is then brought into the operating room and positioned appropriately. Conscious sedation may be required and is based upon individual patient needs. Tetracaine ophthalmic drops are instilled bilaterally and metal eye shields are inserted. The treatment area is sterilely prepped and allowed to completely dry. Anesthesia is provided, generally via local infiltration using 1% lidocaine with 1:100,000 epinephrine diluted 9:1 with 8.4% sodium bicarbonate. Confirmation of appropriate and sufficient local anesthesia is performed. The patient is then draped appropriately, and moist towels are used to cover exposed nontreatment sites.

With the patient positioned and adequately anesthetized, the operating laser is brought into position. Power settings are done at this time, the spot size is determined (generally 7 to 12 mm), and intraoperative alterations are performed as needed. Before laser application, safety procedures are once again reviewed and implemented. Protective eyewear is worn by all team members, appropriate signs are posted, and a procedural "time out" is performed. A dedicated assistant is in charge of controlling the laser settings and laser operation throughout the procedure.

Cryogen spray is used to cool the epidermis prior to laser use. The target area is then lased, followed by treatment of the adjacent regions. Multiple passes may be necessary. Preservation of facial subunit boundaries is achieved with the use of a smaller laser spot size. Uniformity in energy delivery is essential. Meticulous application of energy with the fiber tip, in close proximity to the skin, is essential in preventing checker and skips regions. If encountered, skip regions are also treated with a smaller spot size. The laser wavelength, spot size, pulse duration, energy density, and total number of pulses delivered are recorded. The laser is then turned off. The wound is dressed with a thin layer of antibiotic ointment and the operative drapes are cleared. Protective eye shields are removed, counts are verified, and the patient is transferred to the postoperative care area. Vision and pain are assessed. Photography is used with permission, and the patient is discharged after meeting the required postoperative protocol.

Specific operative considerations are as follows:

- Port-wine stains: PWS in infants and young children can be treated effectively by PDL using energy densities of 5 to 10 J/cm^2 with a larger spot size at 595 nm. Adults may be treated with a similar approach although higher energy densities and longer pulse durations may be helpful (Fig. 31.6). More mature and hypertrophic malformations require a greater depth of penetration and higher energy, such as with the alexandrite laser at 755 nm and 40 to 60 J/cm^2. Several treatment sessions spaced at 4 to 8 week intervals may be required for maximum efficacy. However, the number of treatments required for maximum PWS fading can be variable and unpredictable. Changing the wavelength or pulse duration of the laser can result in substantial PWS fading not previously observed with single device therapy.

TABLE 31.1 Technical Work Flow

Preoperative	Operative	Postoperative
1. Laser selected	1. Position patient	1. Postoperative care
2. Power established	2. Prep surgical site	2. Assess pain and vision
3. Cooling selected	3. Demarcate lesion	3. Provide antibiotic ointment
4. Examination reviewed	4. Anesthesia	4. Establish follow up
5. Consent reviewed	5. Patient eye protection	5. Contact patient postoperatively to reassess
6. Discuss flow with patient	6. Drape patient	6. Follow up visit in 2 weeks
7. Photograph lesion	7. Confirm staff eye protection	7. Photograph wound healing
	8. Cool surgical site	8. Establish distal follow up in 4–6 weeks
	9. Treat lesion to demarcations	9. Determine need for retreatment
	10. After laser settings as needed	
	11. Withdraw laser and confirm off	
	12. Dress wound	
	13. Clear drapes	
	14. Assess pain and vision	
	15. Verify counts	
	16. Photograph wound	

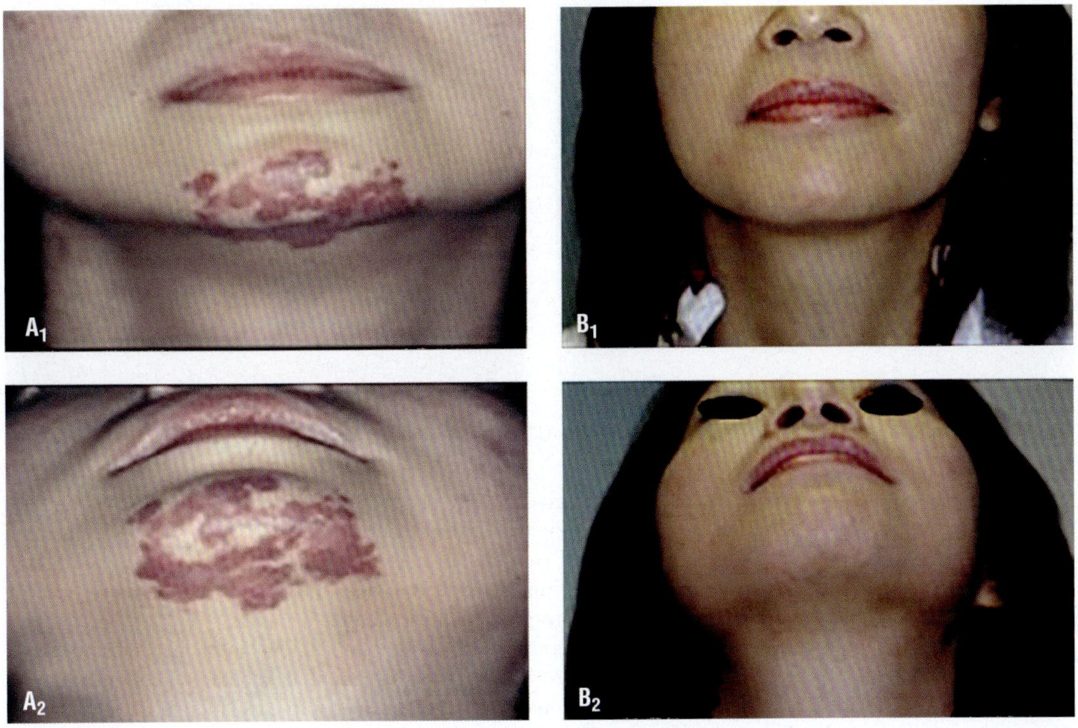

FIGURE 31.6 Port-wine stain before ($\mathbf{A_1}$ and $\mathbf{A_2}$) and after ($\mathbf{B_1}$ and $\mathbf{B_2}$) treatment with pulsed dye laser.

- Telangiectasia: The standard treatment of telangiectasia is PDL with low energy densities of 7 to 12 J/cm^2, pulse durations of 6 to 40 ms, and spot sizes ranging from 7 to 10 mm (Fig. 31.7). Vessel tracing using lasers is a common surgical technique unique to telangiectasia due to its linear, easy-to-follow presentation. In spider angiomas, the central vessel is targeted with settings mentioned above for linear telangiectasias (Fig. 31.8). The branching peripheral capillaries may be treated in a subsequent visit if they persist.
- Rosacea: Over the last 25 years, rosacea laser therapy has been primarily performed with PDL, KTP, and IPL. Their efficacy relates to vessel destruction, which lowers skin temperature and alters the environment of *Staphylococcus* and mite colonization. For PDL, energy densities of 6 to 10 J/cm^2, pulse durations of 3 to 20 ms with 10 to 12 mm spot sizes provide effective treatment. Retreatment may be necessary both in the postoperative period and at yearly intervals.

POSTOPERATIVE MANAGEMENT

The "success" of laser therapy as in any aesthetic procedure is contingent upon the patient's appearance after healing. This healing period constitutes a significant portion of the surgeon–patient relationship. The effect of laser therapy often takes weeks to months to evolve. This is an important point that will need to be mentioned to patients prior to initiating any treatment.

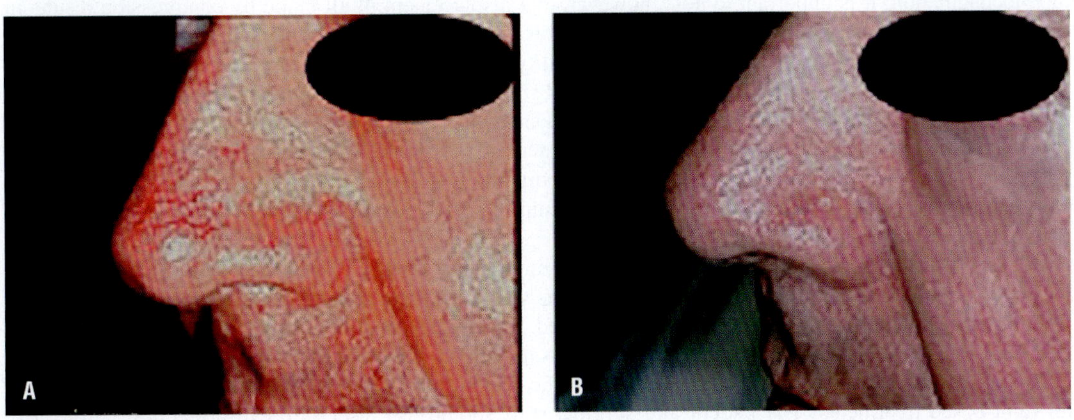

FIGURE 31.7 Single treatment pulsed dye laser therapy of nasal telangiectasia with before **(A)** and after **(B)** photodocumentation.

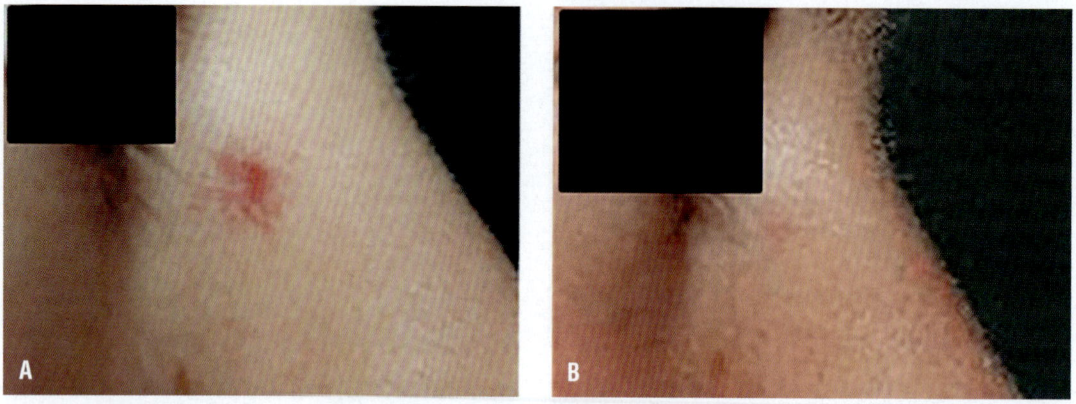

FIGURE 31.8 Single treatment pulsed dye laser therapy of nasal angioma. Before **(A)** and after **(B)** are marked.

In general, pain is limited during recovery, but given the potential need for serial treatment, the patient's degree of discomfort should be addressed. Pharmacologic treatment for pain should rarely result in the need for narcotics. Pain of this caliber should be evaluated for significant infection or thermal injury. Cold compresses are beneficial in the immediate postoperative period for the reduction discomfort and swelling. Evidence of blistering or crusting is indicative of injury, and antibiotic ointment should be provided.

Reassessment determines the need for further therapy and allows for adjustments in fluence, duration, spot size, and other parameters. Follow-up also allows for the evaluation of patient satisfaction. There is a known risk of recurrence, making remote follow-up a reasonable component in complete patient care. Immediate postoperative follow-up should be within 1 to 2 weeks with another at 4 to 6 weeks to determine the need for additional treatments.

COMPLICATIONS

The use of laser devices in the treatment of vascular skin lesions carries the potential for complications. This may involve the lesion of interest or the adjacent tissues. As previously discussed, understanding the Anderson and Parrish theory of selective photothermolysis is paramount in the reduction of collateral injury. Once an appropriate device is selected, complication containment is well underway.

The most common complications include purpura and pigmentary changes. Purpura may be noted in the immediate postoperative period and is a result of intravascular coagulum and limited ecchymosis. These purple lesions remain for 1 to 2 weeks and were traditionally regarded as evidence of effective treatment. However, current practice has determined that is not the case, especially for patients seeking primarily cosmetic treatment, for telangiectasia or rosacea. Short pulse durations should be avoided in such patients as this tends to increase the incidence of purpura.

A persistent challenge in the treatment of vascular lesions is minimizing injury to surrounding nontarget tissues. Epidermal injury/burns are prevented by active cooling of the skin surface prior to irradiation. The extent of cooling is controlled by varying the cooling time, termed "dynamic cooling." Cooling may be administered via convection system, cryogen spray, or contact materials such as gels, compressive hand pieces, or ice. Contact cooling adds a compressive effect, which can be used to manipulate the amount of blood available for thermocoagulation. It is important to note, however, that displacement of all blood by compression results in the loss of the target chromophore, oxyhemoglobin. This is of particular importance with fine vessel treatment, where slight compression induces inaccuracy as visibility of the target vessel is lost.

Cryogen spray cooling (CSC) offers a well-established barrier to thermal injury, while being tailored easily to individual patient needs. CSC uses tetrafluoroethane, which has a low boiling temperature (−26.2°C) and relatively high latent heat of vaporization to extract latent heat from the skin surface by its rapid evaporation confining the cooling to the epidermis. A further important advantage in CSC use is the ability to electronically control the timing of the cryogen spray. This feature offers a predictable cooling effect and reliable safety margin when preventing thermal injury.

Careful planning can reduce thermal injury by limiting the energy density and clearly delineating the lesion by surgical marking. This creates visible borders so that erythema due to the laser treatment is not mistaken for the vascular lesion and inappropriately treated. Infection is an additional concern, but local treatment with antibiotic ointment is generally sufficient. Serious infections are rare events.

Complications are not necessarily a threat to the patient alone. Ocular injury is a significant risk in all light-based treatments. The patient and surgical staff should use laser safe eye protection before use, even when the device is not currently in use. Multiple reports of patient and practitioner ocular injury have been cited in the literature from laser and intense pulse light therapy, despite the relative safety of such devices. The iris and retina contain a high density of melanin, making these structures susceptible to laser injury. Closed eyelids are insufficient protection, as high wavelength lasers such as Nd:YAG (1,064 nm) and Alexandrite (755 nm) may easily pass through the thin skin and conjunctiva to affect the globe. Bell's phenomenon, which is generally considered a protective reflex of the globe, may bring the iris closer in line with laser therapy, placing it at significant risk. Any concern for ocular injury after photodynamic therapy, including vision changes, new onset floaters, photophobia, pupil irregularity, or ocular pain should prompt urgent ophthalmology consultation.

RESULTS

Vascular lesions may be treated through a variety of methods, with laser therapy offering both an effective and efficient means of treatment. Several lasers are available with individual utility based on the characteristics of the target lesion. Laser selection additionally depends on the surgeons skill, available technology, patient skin coloring and thickness, comorbidities, risk of infection, and scar formation. With this in mind, the results of laser surgery for cutaneous vascular lesions can be significant and commonly afford full lesion resolution. The therapeutic examples shared in this chapter reveal the transformative effects of laser therapy. Many lesions may be treated in a single setting, such as flat superficial hemangiomas and telangiectasias, providing excellent outcomes to patients with either cosmetic or functional concerns. While many lasers have been discussed, the utility of the PDL should been stressed as it remains the treatment of choice for many vascular lesions. The PDL is well studied, has an excellent safety margin, and should be the laser with which initial expertise is developed and further employed.

The treatment of cutaneous vascular lesions requires the surgeon to master a broad array of therapeutic options. The outcomes of laser therapy depend upon attention to detail, with fine adjustments and judicious treatment yielding the best results. Comprehensive preoperative planning, close follow-up, and a thorough understanding of laser technology and its medical applications are necessary for successful treatment. Once achieved, laser therapy offers a powerful and effective tool in the management of vascular lesions, a group of conditions known for their tenacity and resistance to therapy.

PEARLS

- Always use a standard system for photo documentation.
- Establish expectations of the patient and/or family at the time of initial consultation.
- Although several vascular lesions can be treated with a single visit, be prepared for the possibility of repeat therapy.
- Use lasers familiar in your practice.
- Most lesions can be treated by PDL.
- PDL has an important role in the treatment of early, flat and superficial hemangiomas.
- PWS require the most auxiliary care and can significantly impact a patient's development.
- Cryogen cooling provides unparalleled protection from undesired epidermal injury.
- Laser safety is a necessity and should never be compromised.

PITFALLS

- Lasers are tools, not cures.
- Larger lesions need to be staged by facial subunits.
- Though limited, significant hemorrhage can result from laser treatment.
- Inadequate preoperative discussion can significantly damage the physician–patient relationship.
- Purpura is unacceptable in the laser treatment of cosmetic vascular lesions.
- While effective, propranolol has the potential for serious side effects. A complete evaluation of the patient prior to treatment is necessary, and preparation for hospital admission should be expected.

INSTRUMENTS TO HAVE AVAILABLE

- Laser eye shields
- Protective eyewear
- Laser signs
- 4 surgical towels, moist
- Two 100-mL syringes
- Two 27-gauge needles
- Cryogen spray

ACKNOWLEDGMENTS

The author would like to thank J. Stuart Nelson, MD, PhD, and Edward Kuan, MD, MBA, for their contributions to the writing of this chapter.

SUGGESTED READING

Anderson RR, Parrish JA. Selective photothermolysis: precise microsurgery by selective absorption of pulsed radiation. *Science* 1983;220:524–527.

Mulliken JB, Glowacki J. Hemangiomas and vascular malformations in infants and children: a classification based on endothelial characteristics. *Plast Reconstr Surg* 1982;69:412–422.

Tanzi EL, Lupton JR, Alster TS. Lasers in dermatology: four decades of progress. *J Am Acad Dermatol* 2003;49:1–31; quiz 31–34.

Williams EF III, Stanislaw P, Dupree M, et al. Hemangiomas in infants and children. An algorithm for intervention. *Arch Facial Plast Surg* 2000;2:103–111. (official publication for the American Academy of Facial Plastic and Reconstructive Surgery, Inc and the International Federation of Facial Plastic Surgery Societies).

Zide BM, Levine SM. Hemangioma update: pearls from 30 years of treatment. *Ann Plast Surg* 2012;69(1):99–103.

32

SURGICAL HAIR RESTORATION: THE TREATMENT OF HAIR LOSS

Jeffrey S. Epstein

INTRODUCTION

Over the past 22 years, the time I have been fortunate to practice in the field, few plastic surgery procedures have evolved as extensively in terms of overall success and aesthetic outcomes as surgical hair restoration. Driven by the collective, usually collaborative and at times competitive, efforts of the leaders in the field, in spite of (or perhaps as a result of) their various backgrounds ranging from dermatology, emergency medicine, cardiology, urology, family practice, and, of course, plastic and facial plastic surgery, surgical hair restoration has earned its position as a true plastic surgical procedure.

Prior to the relatively rapid evolution of aesthetic hair transplant techniques starting in the early 1990s, there was an almost 30-year period in which hair transplantation was essentially limited to the simple production of cornrows or doll's hair configurations. This started with Norman Orentreich's 1959 explanation of donor dominance and posited how transplanted hairs maintain their genetic basis to continue growing, no matter where transplanted, whether on the bald scalp, face, chest, or anywhere on the body. Unfortunately, these plug grafts were 3 and 4 mm in diameter, contained 15 to 20 hairs, and produced rather unnatural results. Appearances could be somewhat improved when the hair was held together with gel or creatively styled. Using Donald Trump–like hairstyles, these 4-mm plugs could, to the benefit of some patients of more creative surgeons, create a more natural appearance when they were divided in half or even quarters before transplanting.

Because of the relative shortcomings of plug grafting, even after the development of subdividing these larger grafts, alternative hair restoration techniques were developed. Scalp flaps and bald scalp reductions became viable and reasonable alternatives in comparison to plug grafting. The temporoparietooccipital scalp flap, also called the Juri or Fleming-Mayer flap, involved the rotation of a 3- to 4-cm wide by 25- to 30-cm long flap of scalp from the side and back of the head into the hairline. These flaps created an unsurpassed density of hair along the anterior hairline. However, a constellation of new aesthetic problems was created, not only due to the usual posterior direction of hair growth, and that occurred where there was further progression of hair loss. Bald scalp reductions were enthusiastically embraced for their ability to reduce the size of the bald scalp, especially along the crown, but at the price of frequent scar widening, stretch-back, thinning along the sides of the scalp, and misdirection of hair growth. Perhaps the most important downside of this technique is its namesake: bald scalp reduction. In the end the bald scalp is not eliminated, and with progressive hair loss, the bald area eventually returns and possibly to even greater dimension. The only surgical procedure that has retained its usefulness is the surgical hairline advancement, or forehead reduction surgery. In the appropriate patient with a stable hairline and very good scalp laxity, the entire hairline can be brought forward by 3 to as much as 5 cm, permitting the shortening of the height of the forehead. As shown in Figure 32.1, female patients tend to be the most appropriate, as they are much less likely to lose hair in the future, something that makes the procedure contraindicated in most men.

In the early 1990s, with the advent of micro- and minigrafting, hair transplantation became the preferred technique of surgical hair restoration. Through a combined placement of minigrafts (3 to 6 hairs) and micrografts (1 or 2 hairs) along the anterior hairline, a reasonable cosmetic result could be achieved. Procedures of

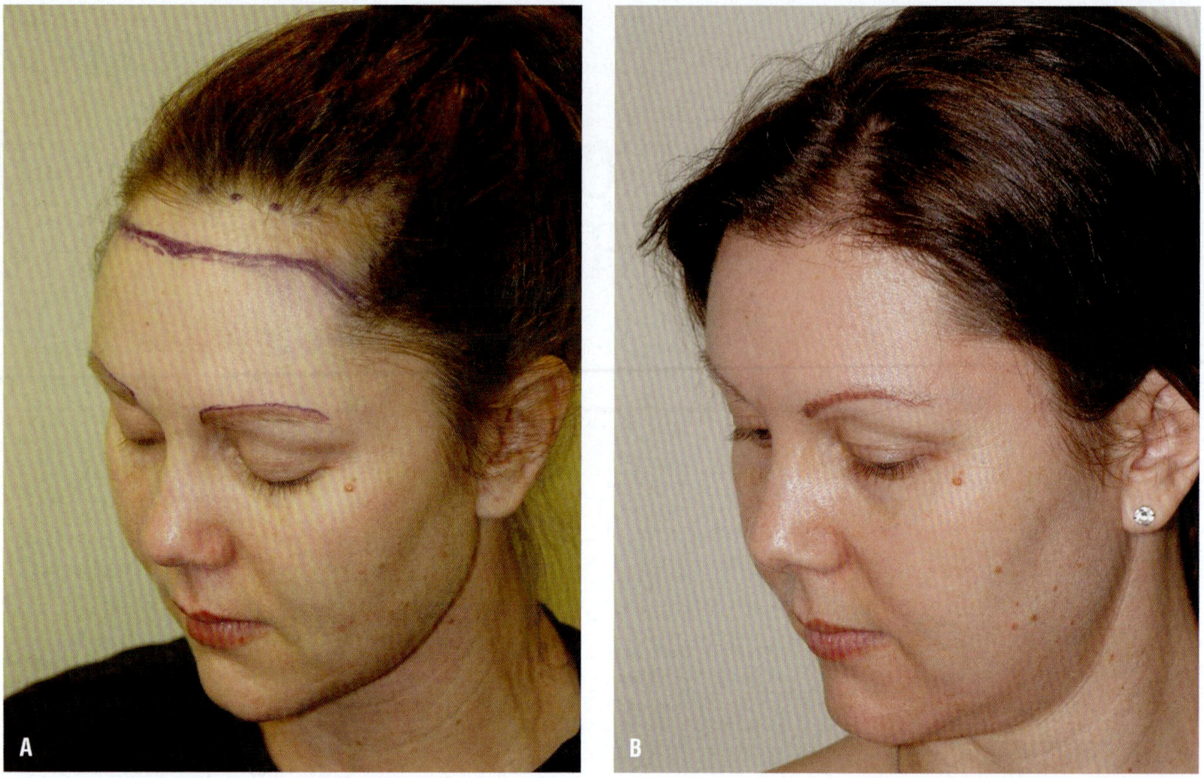

FIGURE 32.1 A and B: Before and after the surgical hairline advancement/forehead reduction surgery in a female, which allows the hairline to be brought forward as much as 5 cm in a single procedure.

500 to 1,200 grafts were the standard of care for nearly the next 10 years. Heavy marketing by several corporate chains further defined the understanding of hair transplantation and hair transplantation evolved into one of the most commonly performed plastic surgical procedures.

Follicular unit grafting (FUG) was developed in the late 1990s and transformed hair restoration into a true aesthetic procedure capable of consistently creating natural-appearing results. FUG involves the transplanting of as many as 2,000 to 3,000 or more grafts in a single procedure. Each graft contains a single follicular unit, which is the natural grouping of hairs in the scalp, and is composed of one to four hairs. As described below, the grafts are dissected out under microscopic visualization from a single donor strip obtained from the back and sometimes sides of the head. The grafts are then placed one at a time into recipient sites made in areas where hair is desired. The other technique outlined in this chapter is follicular unit extraction (FUE). This is a more recently introduced procedure in which the hair grafts containing a single follicular unit are obtained not from a donor strip but rather by their individual extraction using 0.9- to 1-mm punches. The FUE approach is a more labor-intensive technique but confers the advantage over FUG with the absence of a linear donor site scar. As a result, this technique allows patients to cut their hair as short as they wish since camouflage is unnecessary.

Both FUG and FUE are based on the original principle of donor dominance in hair growth. Each approach uses hair from more permanent/stable regions of hair growth for the treatment of the balding scalp and other areas devoid of hair.

HISTORY

Appropriate expectations must be established, and this is the most important in determining patient candidacy for a procedure. Additionally, it is important to anticipate for the progression of hair loss. This first means taking a family history and learning of the patient's hair loss progression up to that point and then explaining the progressive nature of hair loss. Younger men, particularly those under the age of 30, must realize that lowering of the hairline and/or filling in of the frontotemporal recessions, as well as filling in of any crown loss, may not make sense as the donor supply could eventually be depleted, making it not possible to further fill in areas of loss in the future. For most young men, filling in of the frontal forelock may be the best and most appropriate procedure. Also, particularly in the younger male patient, for a number of reasons (the greater risk of widened donor site scars, the potential for the desire to shave his head in the future), but ultimately in any man who does not have to ever worry about cutting his hair short, FUE is the preferable technique to FUG.

In women, in addition to taking a thorough family and personal history, inclusion of questions about hormonal and nutritional health is essential. Blood testing should include thyroid function tests, total iron, ferritin, total and free testosterone, and DHEA-sulfate if there is a history of abnormal menses. Trichotillomania should be considered when the pattern of hair loss is atypical. A biopsy of the scalp may be necessary in the differentiation of androgenic alopecia (female pattern hair loss) from alopecia areata, telogen effluvium, and a variety of scarring alopecias including lichen planopilaris. The density of hairs in the donor area and the caliber of these hairs, as well as the color contrast between the scalp and hairs, are of particular importance in determining candidacy for a transplant procedure in women. For most women, it is not possible to completely fill in all areas of thinning; therefore, it must be explained that only those areas of greatest cosmetic importance can be restored and that the degree of improvement is better in cases of thick donor hairs and lower color contrast between the scalp and these hairs. Also, in women, there is a greater risk than in men of shock hair loss right after a transplant, particularly in cases of hair loss characterized by diffuse thinning and miniaturization versus when the hair loss is more patchy, the latter a situation more appropriate for hair grafting.

Usually, the FUE procedure is not indicated in women because of the need for shaving a large area of scalp for the procedure, except in the case of a woman who wants to avoid altogether any linear donor site scar. As it is, one of the key challenges in women is obtaining a sufficient amount of donor hairs, a challenge made greater by the use of the FUE technique. Other indications for hair procedures in women in particular include eyebrow restoration (a procedure also done in men), filling in of lost sideburns or of scarring from prior plastic surgery, and advancement of the overly high hairline. There are two techniques for advancing the hairline, the more common of which is hair grafting, the other the surgical hairline advancement procedure, a single-stage technique where the entire frontal hairline is advanced and the forehead shortened through a hairline incision, as discussed in the prior section. In the highly motivated patient with an immobile scalp, tissue expanders can be used to advance the hairline as desired.

Generally, while a medical evaluation is not indicated, options in medical therapy should be presented. Finasteride, a 5-alpha reductase blocker that prevents the conversion of testosterone into dihydrotestosterone, the hormone that causes miniaturization and eventual loss of the hair, is only to be used in men. Other therapies include minoxidil 5% and laser light therapy, the latter which can be particularly effective in slowing down or stopping altogether shedding and in some cases cause partial reversal of the miniaturization that can be seen in male and female pattern hair loss.

PHYSICAL EXAMINATION

The physical examination complements the detailed patient history with emphasis upon the scalp and any associated hair abnormalities. This relates to the pattern of hair loss as well as the potential mechanism (hormonal, traumatic, burn, iatrogenic). A small test spot of hair pulling is also performed to evaluate hair breakage versus removal of hair from the follicle. Evaluation for traction alopecia, which is more common in African American women, and in relation to hair weaving and treatments, is also necessary. Assessment for the presence of patchy hair loss and/or changes to the skin, best seen by dermoscopy, is suggestive of one of several types of cicatricial alopecias and can be confirmed on biopsy.

The hairline is perhaps the most important element to an aesthetic restoration and must be defined during evaluation. Elements of the hairline that must be incorporated into the physical examination and surgical planning include the overall position and shape, as well as the specific pattern and angulation of the hairs. Adding a degree of challenge is the need to plan for future hair loss and the recognition that once restored, a hairline is permanent, and needs to be age appropriate especially as the patient gets older. This must be explained and accepted by the male patient, something which can be particularly difficult for younger patient who will likely want a lower and/or less receded hairline to match those of his peers.

INDICATIONS

The majority of patients, who have reasonable expectations and no medical contraindications, are appropriate candidates for a hair restoration procedure. This is particularly true in males, nearly all of whom present with male pattern hair loss (MPB). It is essential to evaluate all prospective patients with regard to the hair loss at presentation as well as their future hair loss. Continued progression of hair loss occurs in most cases of MPB and is critical in long-term outcomes.

CONTRAINDICATIONS

Medical contraindications include soft tissue infection, skin cancer (untreated), active autoimmune disease, alopecia areata/totalis, scarring alopecias, and a general health status that is inadequate to undergo an elective procedure. Unrealistic expectations of surgical results or the social rewards of undergoing a hair restoration procedure are definite contraindications of any elective procedure.

PREOPERATIVE PLANNING

Hair Design

The position of the male hairline is typically placed so that the central-most area is approximately 8.5 to 10 cm above the glabella, usually at the junction of the vertical forehead with the horizontal scalp. Extended laterally, there is some degree of frontotemporal recession, best observed on the Frankfurt horizontal plane as the hairline appears to get higher as it proceeds posteriorly. A widow's peak can be aesthetically desirable in some patients, particularly those with a more oval-shaped face.

Perhaps no single factor is more important for making a difference between a good and a truly natural-appearing hair restoration than the forward angulation of hair growth throughout the frontal half to three quarters of the scalp. In no area is this angulation more important to achieve than along the anterior hairline. More advanced hairline designs recognize that there is a varied direction of hair growth. For example, along the widow's peak, the hairs do not grow directly forward but actually toward one side with the change in angulation more dramatic and varied. Along the temporal sides of the head, the angulation of hair growth is usually downward and slightly posterior.

A natural-appearing distribution of hair growth is achieved with the exclusive use of single hair grafts along the front two to three rows of the hairline. The hairs are arranged in an irregularly, irregular pattern of thicker and thinner small triangle-like extensions and recessions. Two to three rows back from the single hair grafts, along the base of each triangular-like extension, is the desired placement of two-hair grafts that further accentuate variation in follicular density. This is best demonstrated in Figure 32.2 and in several close-up hairline photos. While some authors describe these alternating extensions/recessions like a "snail's trail," I prefer to create a more angular insetting that results in a more natural appearance.

Nearly all the elements described above apply to both male and female hairline designs, with a few exceptions. In women, the hairline is usually placed in a more anterior location, as low as 6.5 to 8 cm above the glabella, to uphold the aesthetic ideal of the facial thirds. Extending from the central-most point, the female hairline does not typically recede but "rounds out" into the temporal side hairline. In cases of sideburn restoration, gender differences also exist. Whether indicated due to a previous facelift surgery or genetic determination (more common in men), women's hairs usually grow posterior toward the ears, while the male hairs usually grow downward to blend naturally with the facial beard.

Along the crown, hair growth direction is typically in a swirl pattern with the vortex of the swirl typically off to one side, most commonly the right. The hairs then radiate out from this point, with the posteriormost hairs actually growing toward the back of the head, while those on the side grow laterally. It must be explained to the patient that crown restoration is more challenging for a variety of reasons. First, the appearance of hair density achieved in the crown is typically less than that which can be achieved in other areas of the scalp. This is due to the radial direction of hair growth, the convex shape of the scalp, and what typically turns out to be a lower percentage of hair regrowth likely due to a more tenuous blood supply. Second, patients should be advised that with age, the crown area will likely increase in size, thus potentially requiring additional grafting procedures in the future. For these reasons, in younger patients, conservative filling or withholding of crown transplantation may be advisable.

SURGICAL TECHNIQUES

Sedation and Anesthesia

Most procedures are performed under oral sedation, such as 10 mg of diazepam and Ambien®, adjusted as necessary. Local anesthesia is first infiltrated very slowly along the back of the scalp, with one or two assistants comforting the patient with hand-holding. To allow the procedure to proceed smoothly, an iPad® is given provided to each patient, offering a large choice of downloadable movies that can be viewed during the procedure that can last from three to as long as 8 hours.

Anesthetic infiltration along the hairline is performed once the donor hair has been removed. On the rare occasion, a supraorbital and supratrochlear nerve block is performed, but usually, local infiltration just below the planned hairline is adequate. The initial injection is with 2% lidocaine with 1:100,000 epinephrine. Subsequent injections are performed with bupivacaine 0.25% with 1:200,000 epinephrine so as to maintain a longer period of anesthesia.

Follicular Unit Grafting

The first step is the removal of the donor strip with the patient sitting up in the OR chair. This strip, depending on the anticipated number of grafts and the flexibility of the scalp, has a width ranging from 8 to 15 mm and a length best limited to no longer than 12 to 14 cm, so that it is limited to within the occipital protuberances to assure the best healing. In the average patient, 60 to 70 grafts (each containing a follicular unit) can be

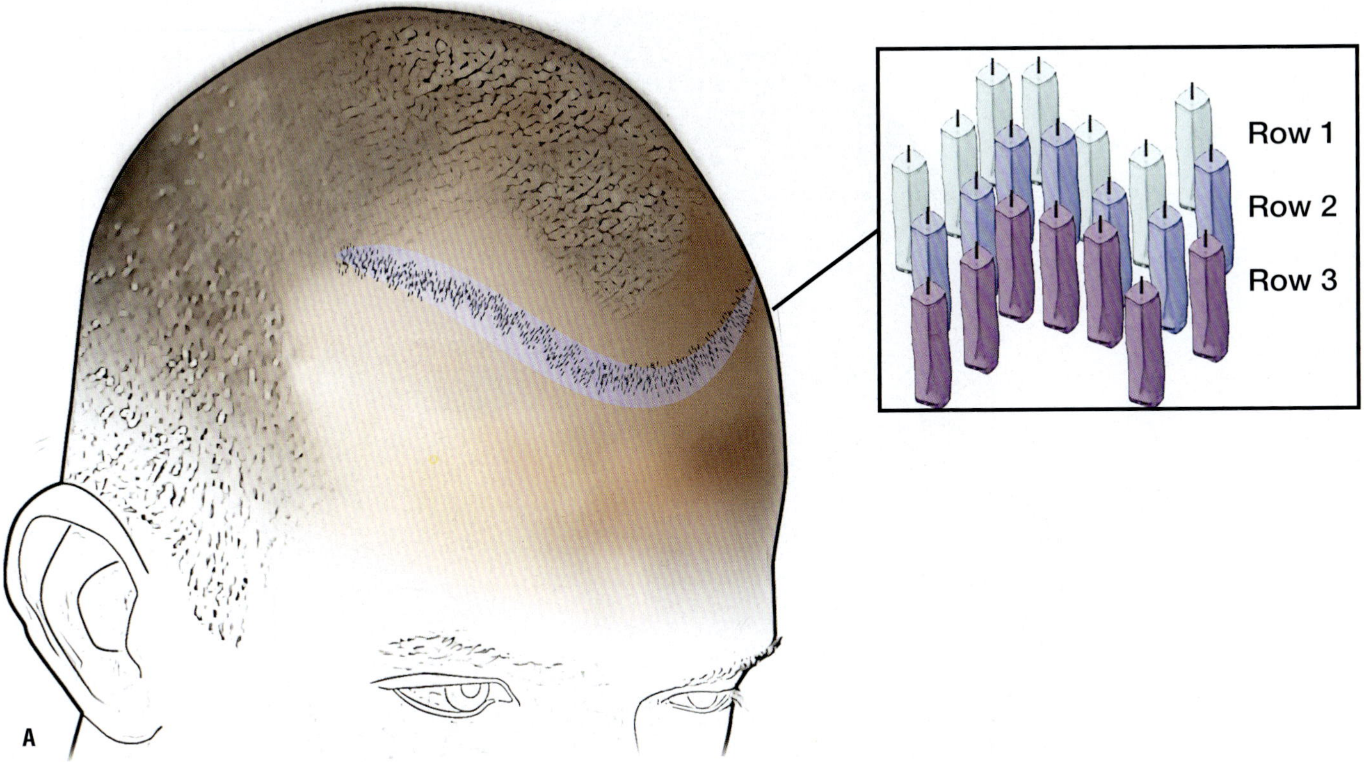

A

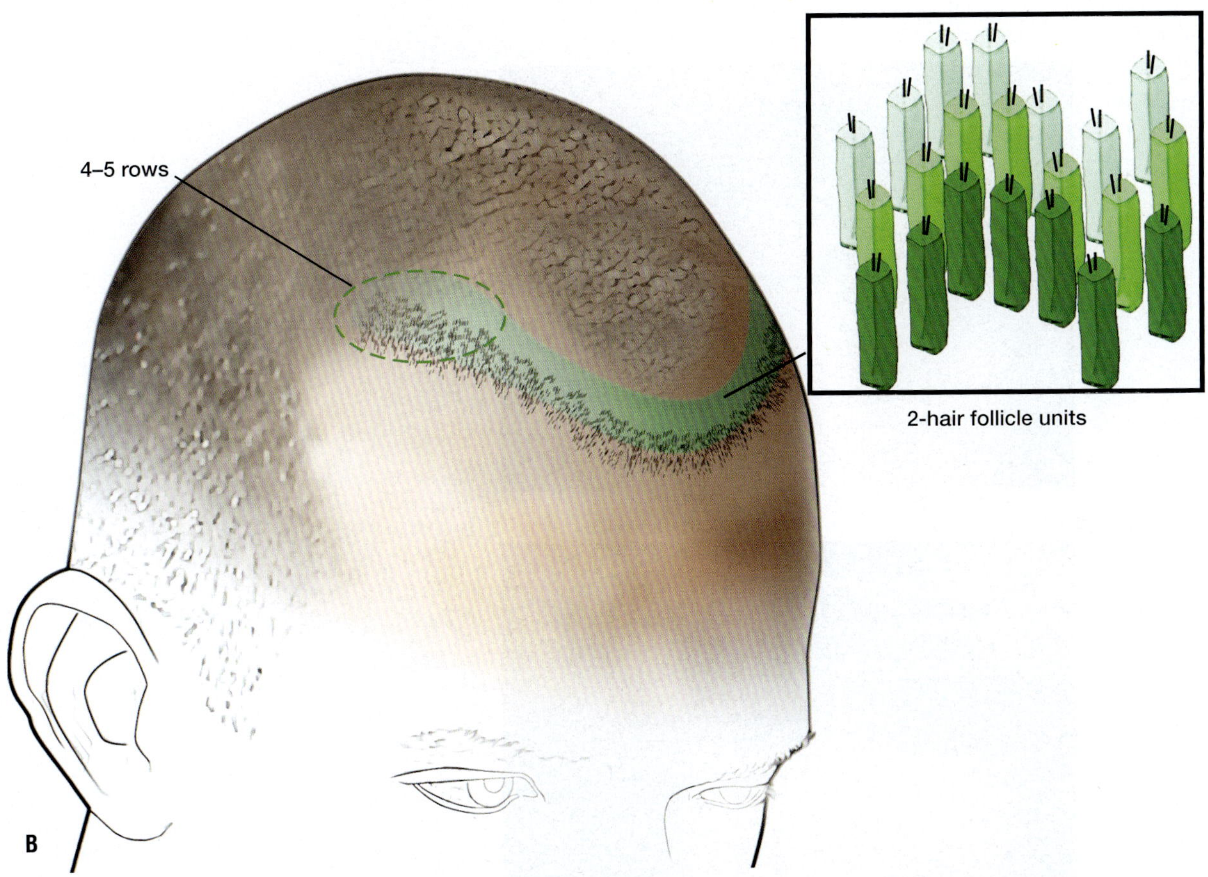

B

FIGURE 32.2 **A–C:** The frontal restoration is created by **(A)** the frontal two to three rows of irregularly distributed "triangles" consisting of single-hair grafts followed by **(B)** two to four rows of two-hair grafts that reinforce these "triangles" as well as go along the posterior border of the restoration, with lastly **(C)** the central core of the restoration achieving maximal density through the use of three- and four-hair grafts. **D and E:** Before and 1 year after 1,300 grafts to restore a female hairline.

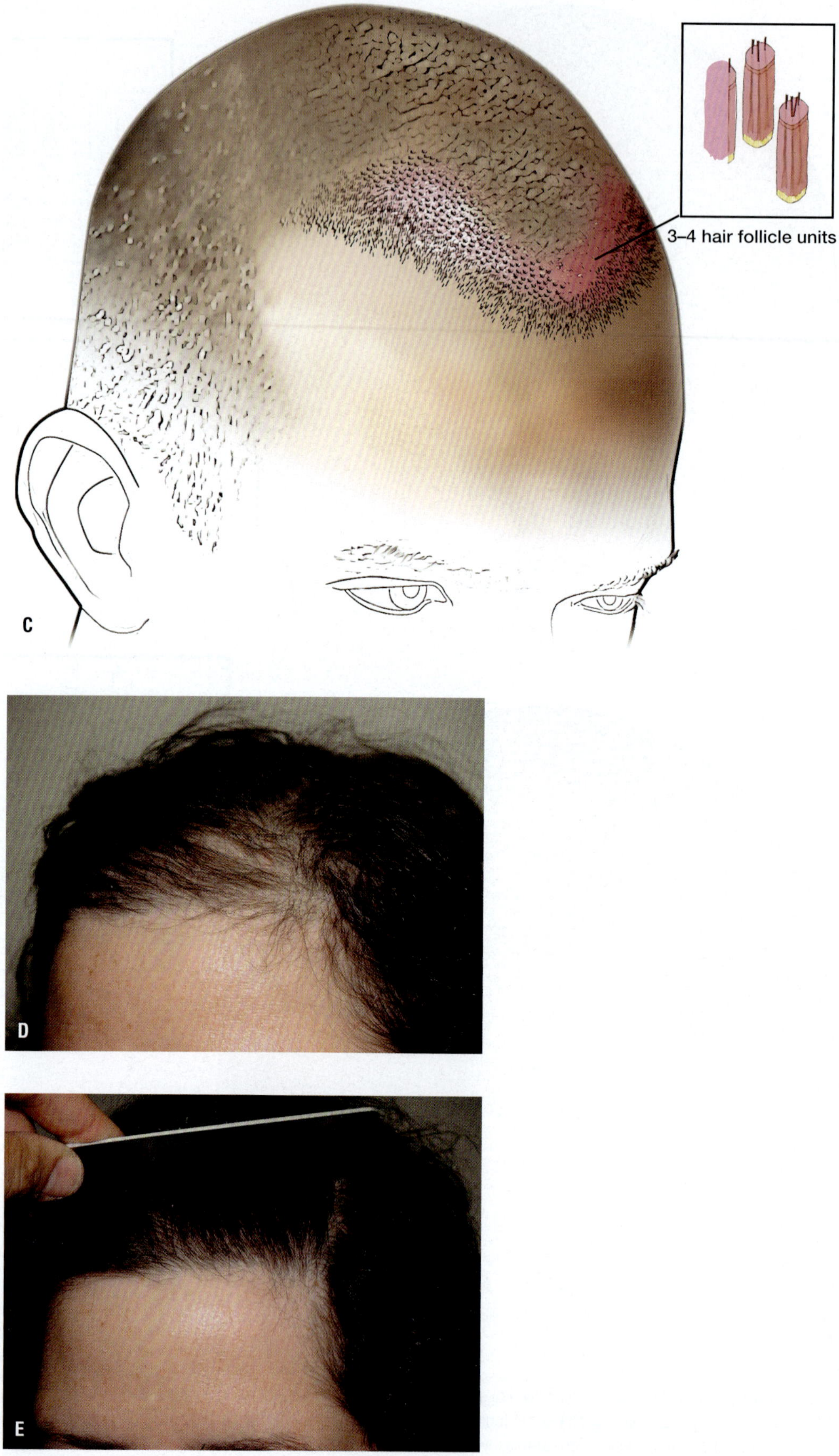

FIGURE 32.2 *(Continued)*

obtained per 1 cm^2 of donor strip. However, it is important to note the variability that exists in hair density among individuals. It is critical for the surgeon to determine hair density to correctly match the size donor strip necessary to the number of follicular units required for restoration. With larger procedures, grafts removed by the FUE technique from the lower back of the head and/or the sides of the head can complement the grafts that can be obtained from the strip, in what is called the "hybrid" approach. A single blade is used to incise the donor strip parallel to the hair follicles to minimize accidental trauma. The strip is then extracted by gently cutting through the adipose tissue just deep to the follicles. Closure of the donor incision is usually done with a simple running suture, taking small bites to stay superficial to the follicles. This closure seems to work as well as any more complex closure technique. This is usually sutured with a 3-0 Prolene® suture, but for patients from out of town, Caprosyn® 3-0 is a very good choice. Once removed, the donor strip is handed off to the technicians for dissection and the patient is placed in a recumbent position for the remainder of the procedure.

Graft dissection is performed under microscopic visualization, which is best done with the binocular Mantis® scope. A team of as many as four to six technicians dissect out each graft containing a single follicular unit, free of the non–hair-bearing tissue, and with a small cuff of adipose tissue around the follicles. The graft material must be kept moist and stored in chilled saline or PlasmaLyte® or Hypothermosol® transplant solution. Desiccation of the grafts is the number one reason for decreased hair regrowth. Careful handling of the grafts to avoid physical damage is also of critical importance. Better stated, the technical role of graft dissection and planting is paramount to having a successful result.

Graft dissection and recipient site creation are conducted at the same time. The grafts are test planted to determine the ideal recipient site size. Appropriate sizing affords a snug, but atraumatic placement. These recipient sites are usually 0.5, 0.6, and 0.7 mm in size for one-, two-, and three-hair grafts, respectively. When indicated, slightly larger recipient sites can be used to prevent any damage to the grafts during placement. Generally, the smaller the blades, the quicker the healing, the less risk of damage to existing hairs, and the closer the grafts can be packed.

To expedite the process, graft planting begins as soon as several hundred recipient sites are made on one side of the scalp, while recipient sites continue to be made on other areas of the scalp. These grafts are carefully placed into the recipient sites using jewelers' forceps, leaving a small cuff of skin of the graft just above the surrounding scalp to prevent pitting. Each graft is inserted according to an individualized pattern made for each patient, which is explained to the planting assistants. The process of planting and recipient site formation continues throughout the procedure.

Follicular Unit Extraction

Using this approach, the anticipated donor area is shaved, with the size of the area dependent upon the number of grafts to be harvested. The back of the scalp, with the patient lying face down, is the first area harvested, where 1,000 to 1,400 grafts can be obtained in the first 2 hours or less. Later on in the procedure, 300 to 500 grafts can be extracted from each side of the head if indicated.

There are a variety of graft extraction techniques. We prefer the use of a 0.9-mm sharp punch on a hand-held drill. It is a two-person approach, with the surgeon or primary assistant doing the drilling with a second assistant gently pulling out the grafts that have been freed up from the surrounding skin attachments. Several other devices are available for graft extraction, including one that is more automatic, with its computer determining which follicular units are to be extracted.

To minimize the time the grafts spend ex vivo, the patient is usually placed supine within 2 hours to allow the making of recipient sites and then the placement of the grafts. With FUE, because the grafts can have a bit less surrounding fat, slightly larger recipient sites are used, typically 0.6 to 0.9 mm, to assure the least traumatic insertion of the grafts.

POSTOPERATIVE MANAGEMENT

Postoperative care is the same for both FUG and FUE. No dressings are used, other than antibiotic ointment placed on the FUE donor areas, and a saline spray is applied to the transplanted grafts hourly for the first 3 days to accelerate healing (Fig. 32.3). Most patients return to the office on the first postoperative day for a hair wash. On the 3rd postoperative day, the patient performs gentle hair washing if permitted, with normal hair washing at 5 days. Analgesics and 3 days of antibiotics are provided.

Sutures of the FUG donor area are removed on the 8th to 10th day, unless dissolvable sutures were utilized. Normal exercise and activity, with the exception of swimming, are permitted after 6 days. For most patients, the tiny crusts start to fall off by 5 to 6 days and should all be gone by 10 days. Hair growth will begin around 4 months after the procedure with the transition from fine to more course hair during this process. Ultimately, the quality of each hair transplanted matches the site from which it was obtained.

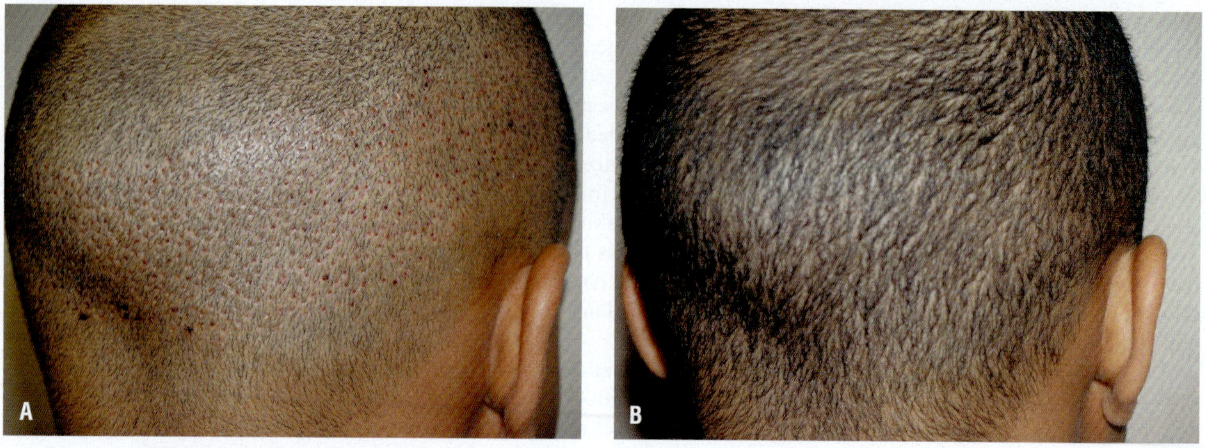

FIGURE 32.3 A and B: FUE donor area 3 days and 4 months after 1,400 grafts.

COMPLICATIONS

Considerable efforts are undertaken to prevent the most common complications in hair transplantation: graft failure, scar formation, recipient site irregularity, and inadequate density. The greatest enemy of graft failure is desiccation. It is critical to place the grafts in chilled saline, or another preferred suspension medium, from the moment they are harvested to the moment of implantation. Chilled saline is also the preferred liquid for cleaning of the scalp during the procedure.

Scar formation is minimized at both donor and recipient sites using several measures. The closure of all donor site wounds is performed in a tension-free manner. Sutures are placed superficial to the follicles. The width of the donor site FUG strip is minimized (10 to 12 mm) to prevent tension and confined to the central back of the head. If the donor site is above the horizontal plane along the top of the ears, the risk of scar widening is reduced due to the diminished influence of the occipitalis muscle during postoperative healing. Recipient site scarring and hypopigmentation are avoided by minimizing the amount of grafted skin but maintaining a cuff of protective adipose tissue. Recipient site irregularity (dimpling) is prevented by not inserting the graft tissue below, or to the level of, the recipient site skin. The skin of each graft should sit just above the surrounding tissues. In the event of grafting into scarred tissues, I recommend using larger, three- to five-hair grafts since smaller grafts do not reliably grow in fibrotic tissues. Lastly, realistic expectations can help make sure that patients are satisfied with the density achieved.

RESULTS

The tiny transplanted hairs fall out by week three, at which point the scalp essentially looks just like it did preoperatively, with the possible exception of some minimal thinning of the original hairs. The incidence of clinically detectable "shock" loss or the falling out of original hairs within the first 6 weeks due to the trauma (physical, vascular, anesthetic agent) of the procedure is quite low, less than 1% in men and 2% to 5% in women. To help accelerate the regrowth, not only of hairs lost to shock loss but also to the transplanted hairs, patients are instructed to apply minoxidil 5% (in women 2%) several times weekly starting 3 weeks postoperatively. This seems to lead to hair regrowth in as soon as 4 months or less.

Regrowth of the donor hairs is the single most important factor in determining patient satisfaction. Fortunately, in most cases, there is a +90% regrowth with both FUE and FUG transplanted hairs. Regardless of whether the procedure is done by FUE or FUG, the goal is the achievement of the ideal combination of density, naturalness and irregularity, and can lead to superior results and satisfied patients (Figs. 32.1, 32.3 to 32.7).

PEARLS

- Hair loss is progressive; therefore, all patients should be treated accordingly, anticipating for future hair loss.
- Medical therapies like finasteride and minoxidil, as well as laser light therapy, have varying degrees of efficacy and are particularly valuable in younger men.
- Forward angulation of grafts and irregularly irregular distribution of these grafts are valuable aesthetic steps when transplanting a hairline.
- FUE is far and away the more popular procedure, particularly in men.

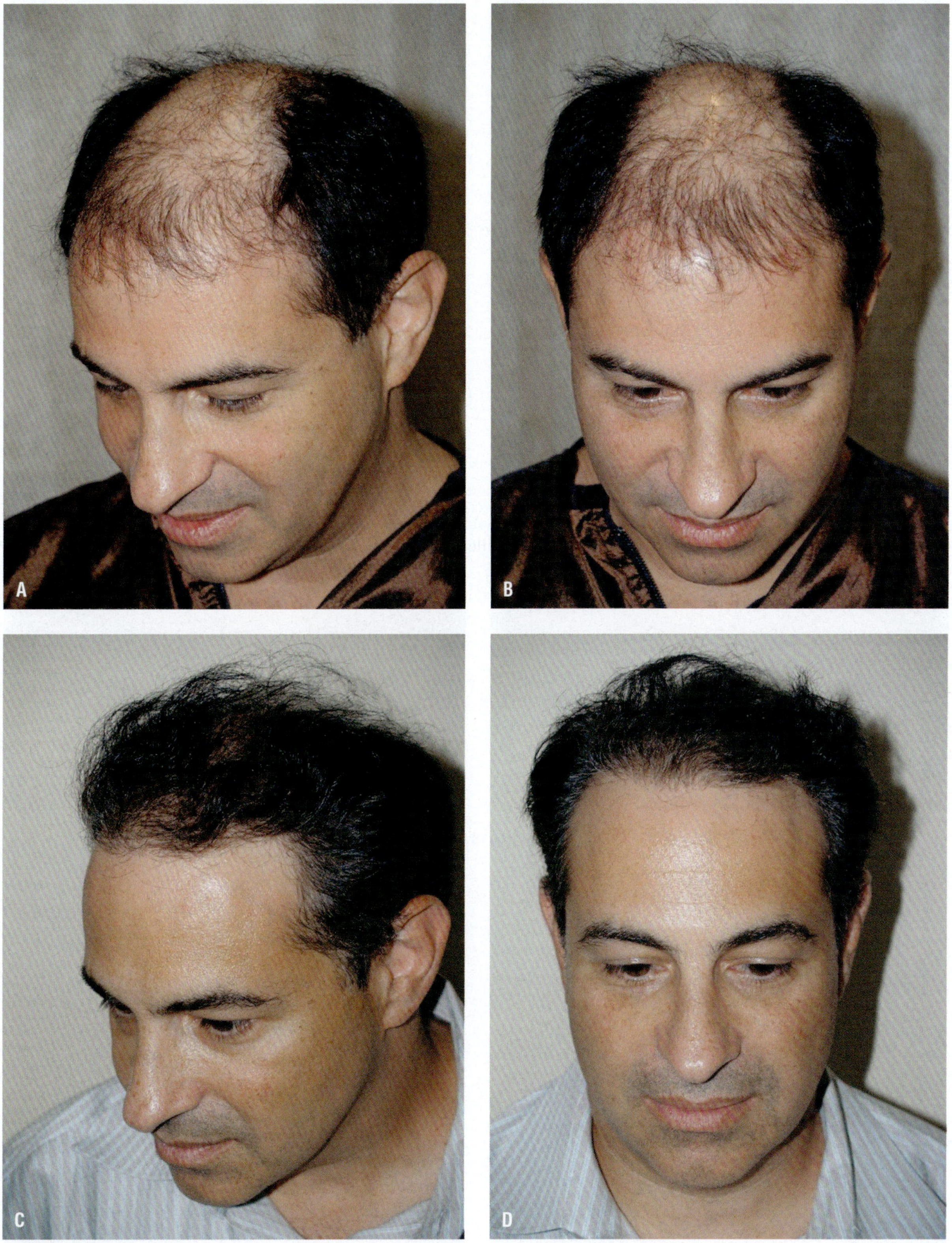

FIGURE 32.4 **A–D:** Before and after 2,500 grafts.

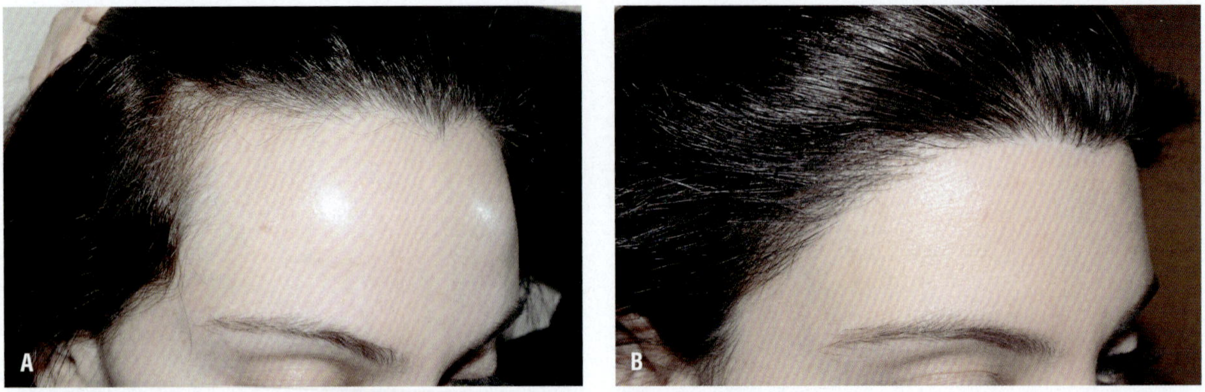

FIGURE 32.5 A and B: Before and after 1,600 FUE graft procedure.

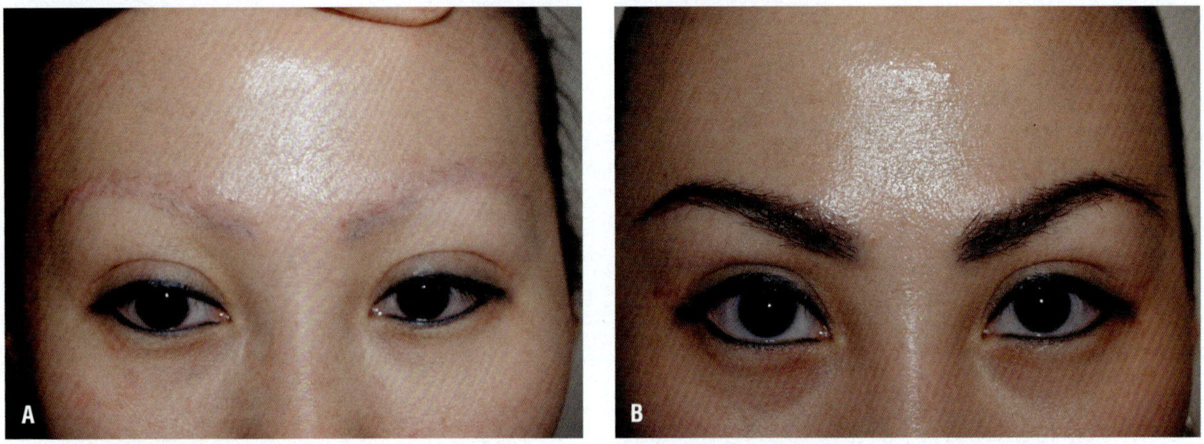

FIGURE 32.6 A and B: Before and 1 year after eyebrow transplant.

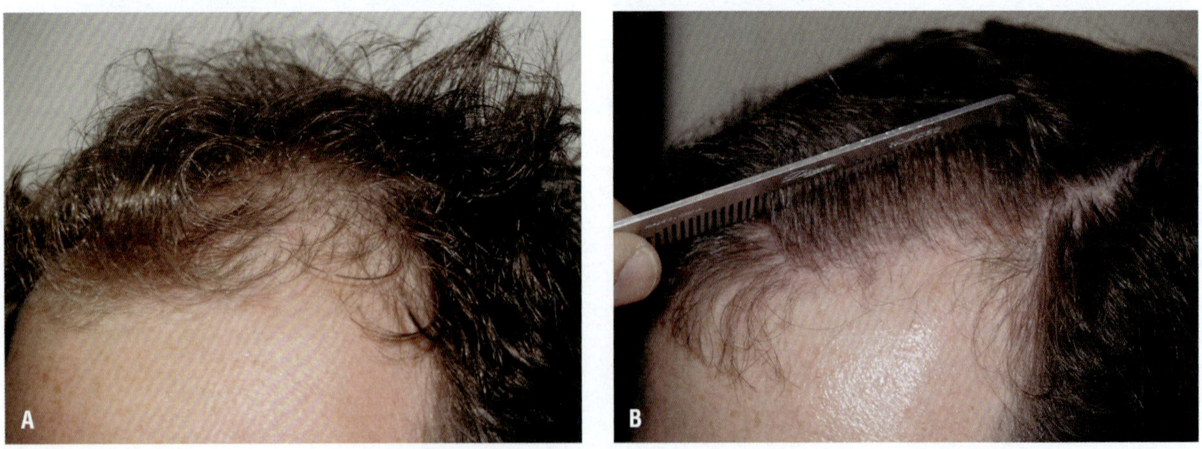

FIGURE 32.7 A and B: Before and after 2,400 grafts to lower a genetically high female hairline.

PITFALLS

- Underestimation of time, team, and practice commitment. The development of a hair practice complements a facial plastic surgery practice but requires a substantial paradigm shift in treatment in comparison to other common procedures.
- Oversimplification or "cookie-cutter" approach to hair design. The lack of an individualized approach and disregard for angulation are the most common "tell" of a hair transplant procedure.
- Grafts desiccation will compromise operative result of any procedure.
- Rough and crush treatment of human tissue produces scarring and graft failure.

INSTRUMENTS TO HAVE AVAILABLE

- Standard plastic surgery set
- Jewelers' forceps, curved and straight, depending on each planter's preference
- Binocular microscope
- Micro Beaver-type blades, cut 0.5 to 0.9 mm, with blade handle
- FUE drill system

SUGGESTED READING

Epstein JS. Follicular-unit hair grafting: state-of-the-art surgical technique. *Arch Facial Plast Surg* 2003;5(5):439–444.

Epstein JS. The treatment of female pattern hair loss and other applications of surgical hair restoration in women. *Facial Plast Surg Clin North Am* 2004;12(2):241–247.

Epstein JS. Evolution of techniques in hair transplantation: a 12-year perspective. *Facial Plast Surg* 2007;23(1):51–59.

Gandelman M, Epstein JS. Hair transplantation to the eyebrow, eyelashes, and other parts of the body. *Facial Plast Surg Clin North Am* 2004;12(2):253–261.

Swerdloff J, Kabaker S. The state of the art: donor site harvest, graft yield estimation, and recipient site preparation for follicular-unit hair transplantation. *Arch Facial Plast Surg* 1999;1:49–52.

PART V: IMPLANTS AND AUGMENTATION

33 THREE-DIMENSIONAL ALLOPLASTIC MIDFACE VOLUMIZATION

Edward O. Terino

INTRODUCTION

Public demand and expectations for aesthetic facial surgery, in both males and females, have increased dramatically over the last two decades. This has challenged surgeons and scientists to develop more natural and longer-lasting enhancements that are safe, ethical, and scientifically validated. Today's augmentation technology far exceeds earlier fads such as the well-publicized 1970s silicone injections to accentuate "cheekbones" and facial contours. Such interventions resulted in horrific complications and ultimately led to the necessary medical advances seen today.

At the turn of century, the search for safer and more durable alloplastic materials continued to develop out of necessity in the treatment of contour defects secondary to congenital (e.g., cleft deformities) or traumatically acquired (e.g., modern warfare, automobile accidents) facial skeletal deformities. Among the first materials used successfully were nonreactive metals such as stainless steel and Vitallium. The past four decades of scientific research in solid-state synthesis, material sciences, and facial contour aesthetic theory have yielded a new applied clinical science with an armament of tools that are reliable, reproducible, and minimally invasive. These surgical techniques can be permanent, but are easily reversible, if required.

Effect of Altering the Facial Skeleton

When we look at a person, our attention inevitably focuses on the eyes, lips, eyebrows, and hair. Yet, these are merely the adornments of the underlying facial framework. What determines the full extent of a person's facial physical appearance is the unique volumetric contour created by their underlying skeletal architecture. The skin is the canvas of the face. When distributed over the facial framework, in a smooth and attractively contoured manner, it presents a youthful and aesthetically pleasing appearance. As years go by, this canvas becomes coarse and wrinkled, while the underlying soft tissues and bone atrophy in accordance to the genetically programmed process of aging. Every face takes on the stigmata of advancing age.

When a surgeon strategically augments the underlying bony architecture of the aging face, a new and dramatic visage can be achieved. Although people are clearly identifiable by their individual facial features, a more general and youthful appearance can be achieved with the purposeful augmentation of their underlying bony architecture. Stated differently, balance in facial volume is what gives the face its maximum harmony, which is perceived as beauty.

Interrelationships of the Facial Promontories

There are three major facial promontories of volume and mass. In order of importance, they are the nose, the two zygomatic–malar eminences, and the chin–jawline (Fig. 33.1). The supraorbital ridges constitute a fourth promontory, which is of lesser significance and will not be discussed in this chapter. By altering the

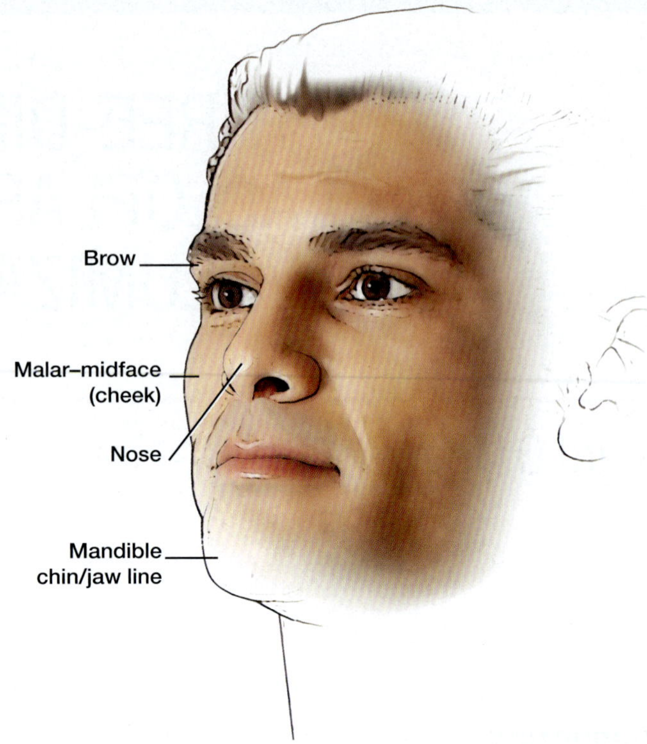

FIGURE 33.1
Artist's rendering of facial architecture illustrating major promontories of mass and volume: the nose, malar–midface, and mandible jawline.

interrelationships of these three major promontories, a surgeon can uniquely create or restore facial harmony, balance, and beauty. By mathematical law, the diminution or enhancement of any one of the three promontories directly and inversely affects the aesthetic importance of the others (Fig. 33.2). Over the decades, facial surgery has evolved dramatically. Surgical procedures that were once simple skin-tightening techniques now entail the complementary restoration of anatomic suspension and facial volumization.

The restructuring of the various facial layers still has limitations. Patients who display round, full, fleshy facial contours with an abundance of subcutaneous adipose tissue rarely typify the aesthetic ideal placed forward by contemporary standards. This is also observed among exceptionally lean individuals who display a longer facial contour with inadequate skeletal promontories in the malar and/or mandibular regions. It is within these extremes of facial types, as well as innumerable patients who have combinations of volume deficiencies in varying anatomic locations, that significant improvements in facial harmony can be achieved with targeted alloplastic augmentation techniques. Furthermore, contour surgery of the facial skeleton should also be complemented by a wide variety of other sound coordinated facial procedures (Fig. 33.3).

Zonal Anatomy of the Malar–Midface Region

The region of the facial skeleton that, when appropriately augmented, produces an aesthetic change in the midfacial contour can be called the "malar–midface space." To determine the most aesthetic augmentation of this region, it is useful to partition the midface into five distinct anatomic zones (Fig. 33.4). By understanding these five zones, and their interrelationships, the surgeon can vary cheek and midface shapes to accommodate each unique patient.

Zone 1, the largest area, includes the major portion of the malar bone and the first third of the zygomatic arch. Augmentation of this entire zone produces the greatest volumetric filling of the cheek and also maximizes the projection of the maxillary eminence (Fig. 33.5).

Zone 2, the second most important site, overlies the middle third of the zygomatic arch. Enhancement of this zone along with zone 1 increases accentuation of the cheekbone laterally, giving a broader dimension to the upper third of the face and creating a high-arched appearance. This change in contour is particularly useful for individuals with a narrow upper face or a long-face syndrome. When, however, zones 1 and 2 are augmented in excess, an abnormal and unattractive protuberance may result (Fig. 33.6).

Zone 3 is the paranasal area, which lies medial to the infraorbital foramen. A line drawn vertically down from the infraorbital foramen marks the medial extent of the usual dissection for malar augmentation. This line also represents the lateral border of zone 3. When paranasal augmentation in zone 3 occurs, medial fullness of the face is created, often in the upper nasolabial area, which can be highly unattractive. The skin and

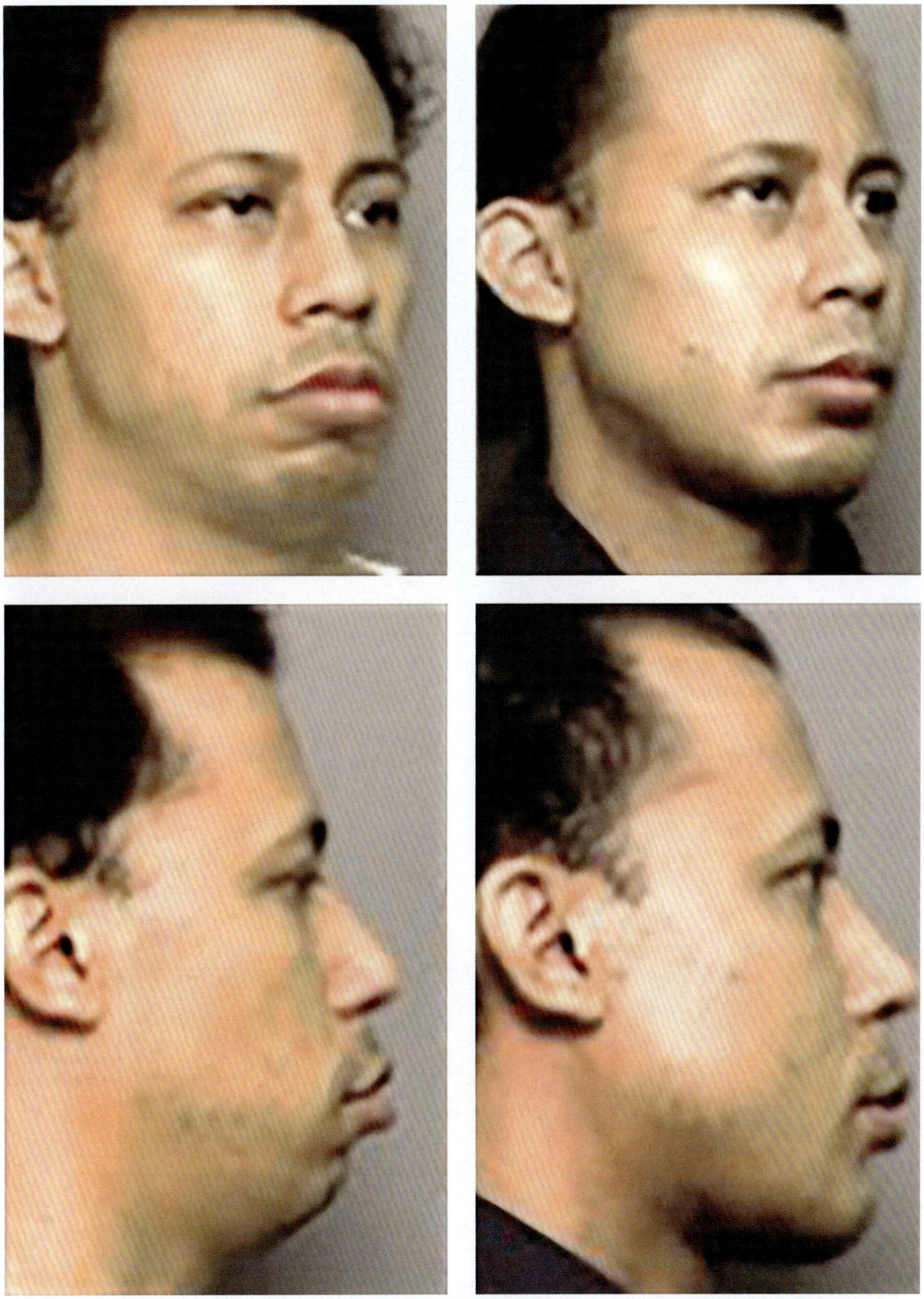

FIGURE 33.2 Example of a 36-year-old male with disproportion and imbalance of malar midface to the mandibular chin–jawline aesthetic segment. A dramatic improvement in facial harmony was created by augmenting the central mentum, mandibular angles, and malar region.

subcutaneous tissues are notably thin, and any implant placed there must be carefully sculptured and tapered. Augmentation of zone 3 is indicated for certain reconstructive purposes, following trauma or other heredity deficiencies (Fig. 33.7). Often this deficiency is accompanied with adjacent zone 1 and 2 deficiencies, which commonly need volume correction.

Zone 4 overlies the posterior third of the zygomatic arch. Augmentation in this area is never needed, as it would produce an unnatural appearance. Moreover, dissection here may be dangerous, since it is very possible

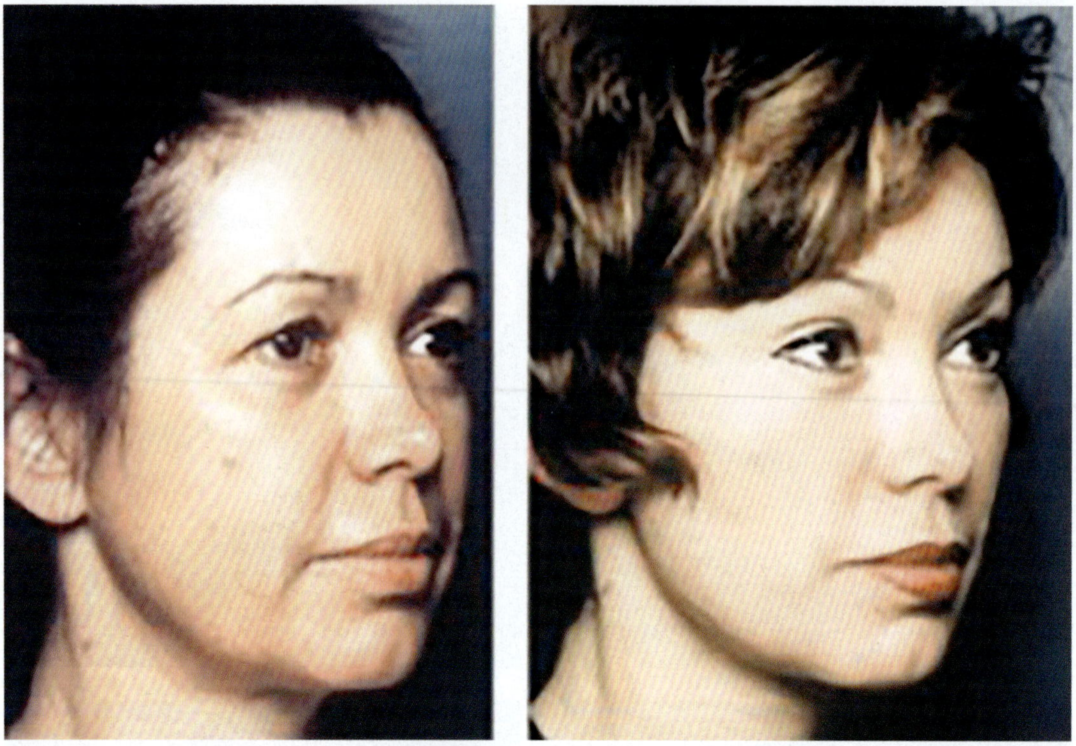

FIGURE 33.3 A 56-year-old female who demonstrates the significant benefits from upper midface suspension, malar–submalar augmentation, and rhytidectomy techniques.

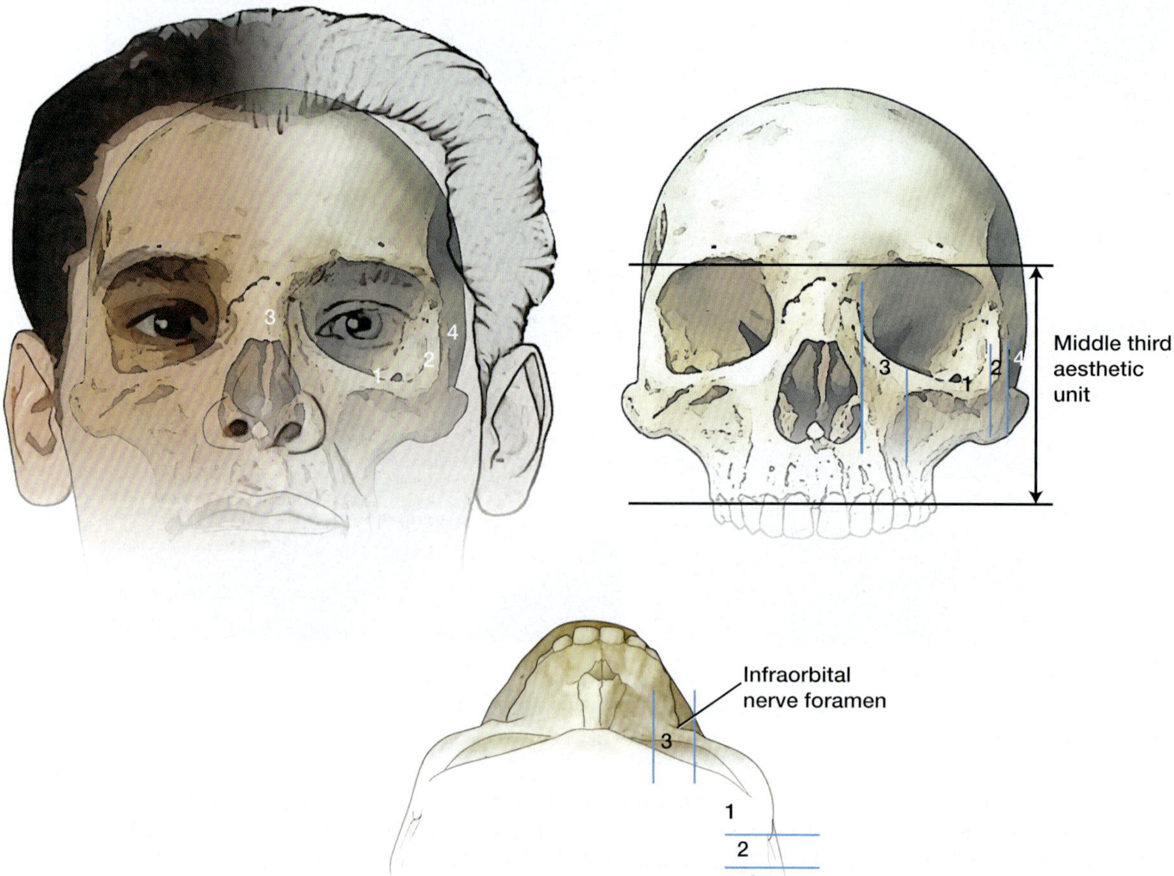

FIGURE 33.4 Anatomic facial contour zones of the midface. These are critically important in understanding the aesthetics of the face when choosing the proper location to place an implant to achieve a desired appearance.

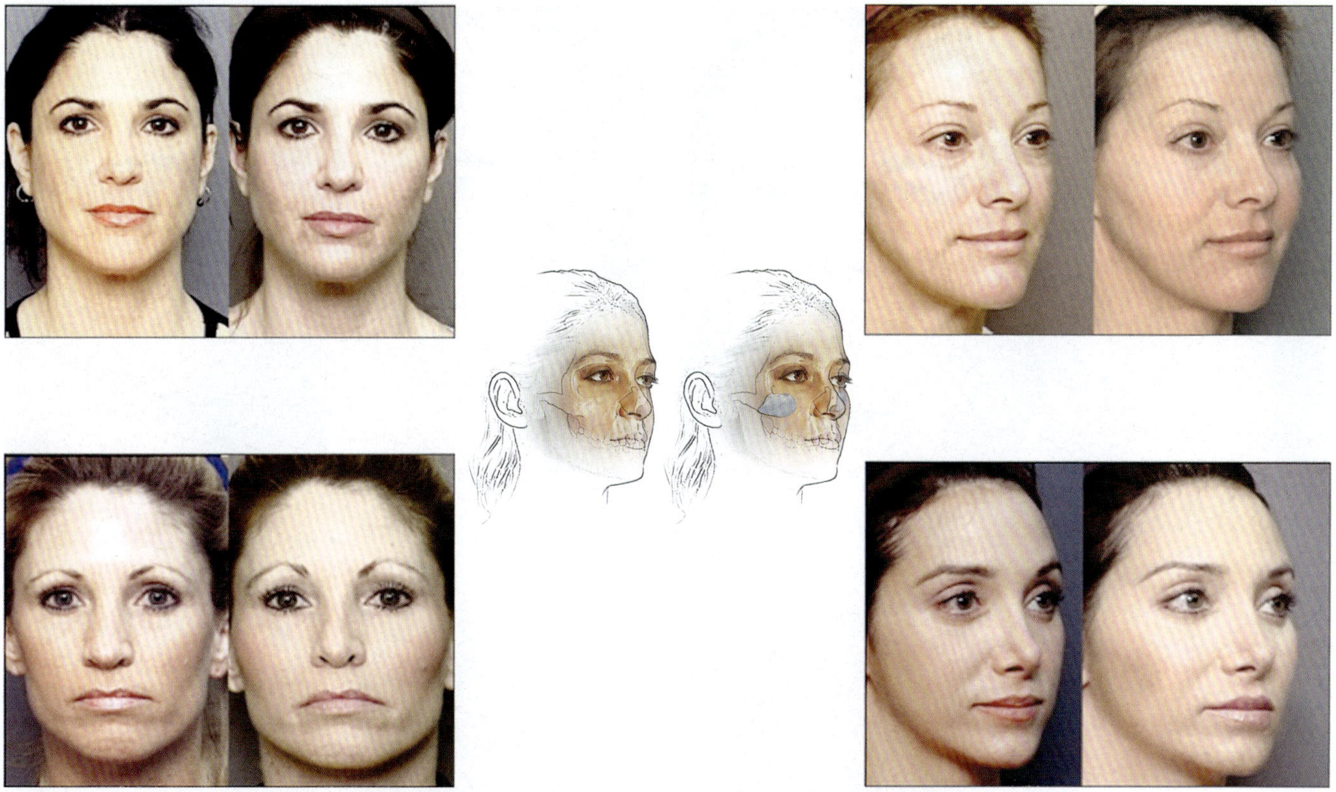

FIGURE 33.5 Three examples of type 1 face with relative or absolute malar–zygomatic deficiency. Postoperative views show attractive malar–midface contour from zone 1, 2 malar volume enhancements.

to injure the zygomaticotemporal or orbicularis oculi branches of the facial nerve. Infrequently, deformities have been observed that resulted from operations in this area.

Zone 5, the submalar zone or "submalar triangle," is bounded posteriorly by the tendinous surface of the masseter muscle and anteriorly by the canine fossa region of the maxilla. The superior boundary of zone 5 is the inferior margin of the malar bone, which constitutes the first two-thirds of the zygomatic arch. The medial

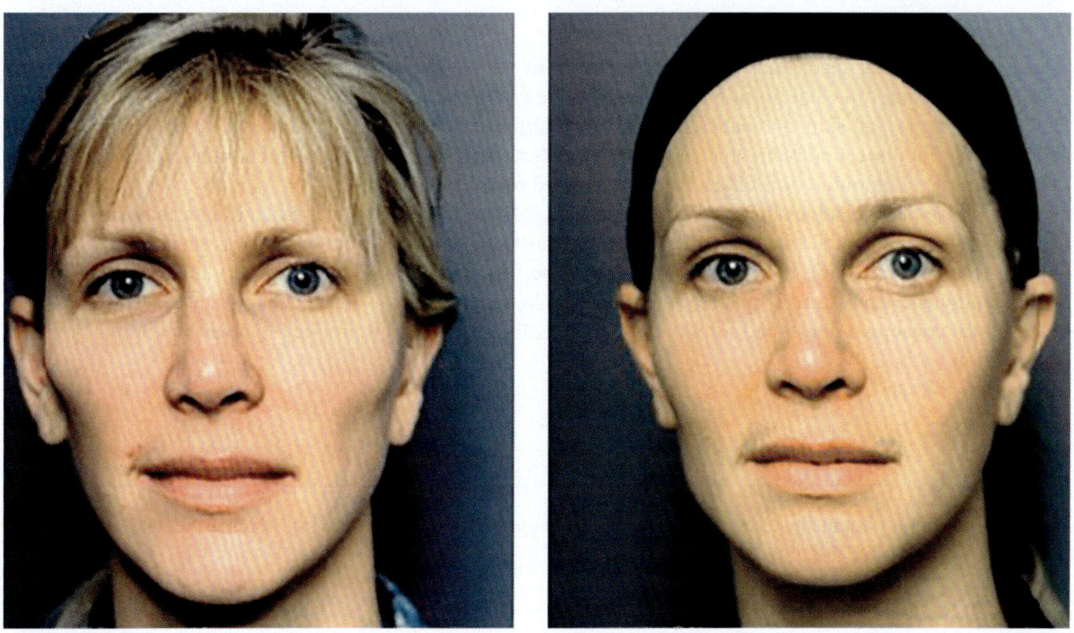

FIGURE 33.6 A 35 year-old model whose postmalar–zygomatic implant appearance that is too strong and skeletal looking due to the wrong implant size, shape, and position. Postoperative view shows significant improvement by using a generous malar shell in zone 1 and SM5.

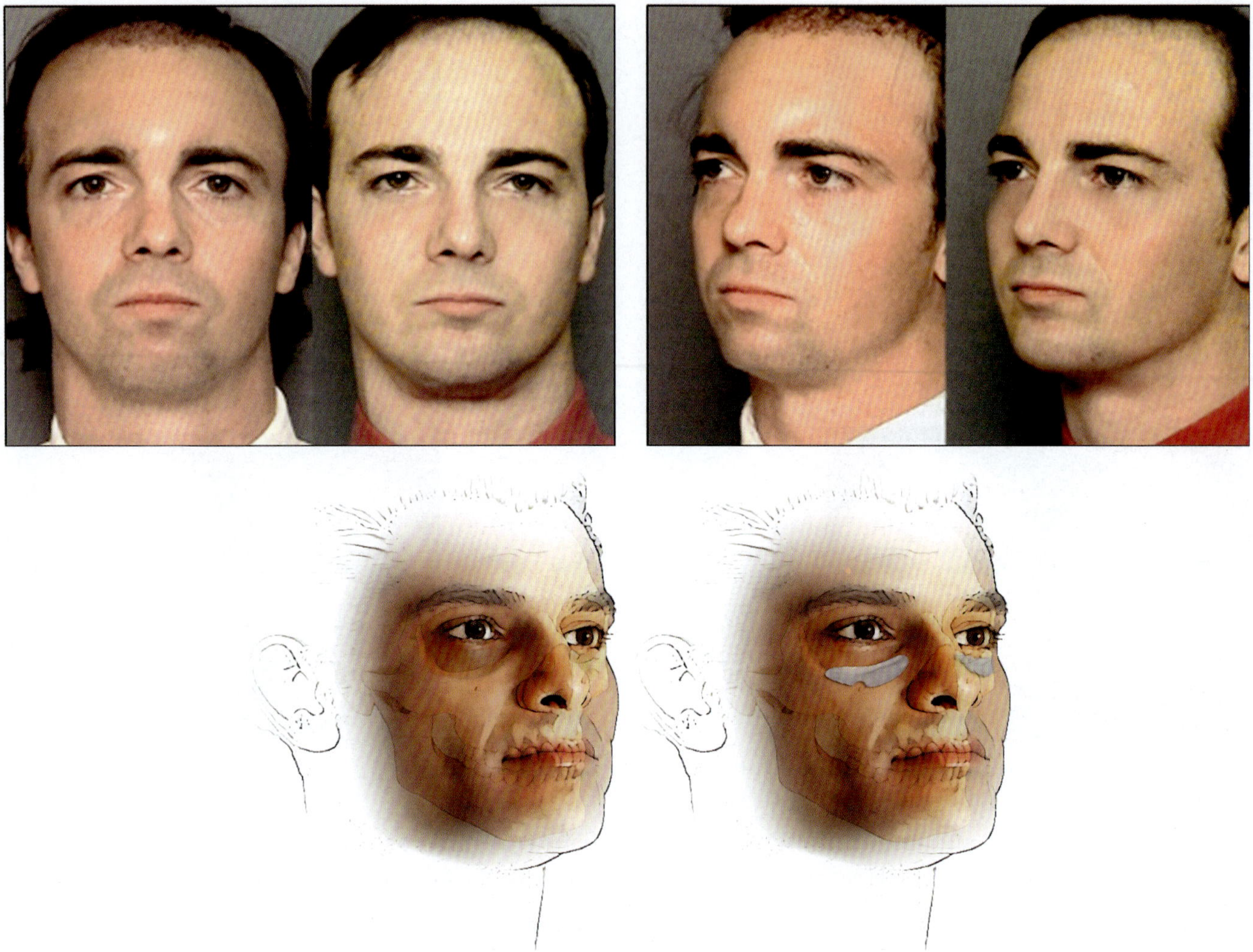

FIGURE 33.7 A 41-year-old male, with extreme suborbital volume deficiency. Postoperative view taken 1 year following correction with a combined tear trough–malar implant (large size with 5-mm tear trough thickness and a malar thickness of 4 mm projection (placed through a transconjunctival approach).

extent of the submalar space ends at the lateral border of the nasolabial mound and sulcus. Its anterior limit is bounded by the inferomedial portion of the roof of the entire malar–midface space. It contains the overlying facial musculature, fat, skin, and subcutaneous of the midface region. The inferior limit is selected by the surgeon, the natural dissection plane that separates the masseter from the overlying facial musculature according to the desired configuration of midface fullness selected by the patient.

Today, we find ourselves in a new era of facial augmentation with an ever-expanding armatorium including classical tissue transfer, injectable fillers, and alloplastic implants. Recent history has seen the introduction of silicone rubber (Silastic), Proplast I and II, Mersilene, Teflon, Dacron, Gore-Tex, acrylic, methyl methacrylate, polyethylene, and hydroxyapatite, among others. We will endeavor in this chapter to describe the facial architectural concepts I developed for a more anatomically precise and reproducible result in alloplastic facial rejuvenation.

HISTORY

When evaluating a patient for total alloplastic facial augmentation, the following items are used in the history of the patient as part of the global assessment:

- What problem does the patient want you to solve?
- Get the patient's verbal description of his/her "*ideal scene*" appearance of facial change.
- Patient "homework assignment": Bring magazine photos of specific "**do's and don'ts**" on desired anatomic part changes.

- Have older patients bring a variety of earlier personal photos
- Use computer face photos (5 views) and imaging technology to do the consultations.
- Use an anatomic facial zone model and facial type analysis as an integral part of the physical exam.

Additionally, for each patient, a comprehensive past medical and surgical history is obtained. By nature, surgical facial augmentation is an elective procedure, and each patient is to be assessed with regard to suitability to undergo a general anesthesia. Conditions including diabetes, coagulopathy, autoimmune, congenital, and syndrome are evaluated on a case-by-case basis. Questions regarding previous surgical interventions and radiation treatments are of importance and can have considerable surgical repercussions.

PHYSICAL EXAMINATION

Understanding of the facial contour according to one of the following facial types can facilitate the process of physical examination:

Type 1 facial aesthetic consists of a deficiency in the upper malar bone segment of the malar–midface. This specific contour weakness encompasses zones 1 and 2. Augmentation of zone 1 creates upper cheek fullness that pleasingly simulates bony contour. When a large implant is used to augment zone 2, as well as zone 1, widening of the upper midface occurs, which shortens the appearance of a long and narrow face.

The transverse dimensions of the malar bone in the upper malar–midface measure from 4.5 to 6.5 cm from the infraorbital foramen to the posterior third of the zygomatic arch. Vertically, there is, on average, 3.0 to 4.0 cm in distance from the lateral canthus to the inferior margin of the malar bone. Overaccentuation of zone 1 in females may result in a masculine, sharp, angular, harsh, or skeletal appearance.

Type 2 facial aesthetic deficiencies consists of a soft tissue contour depression specifically in the lower aspect of the midfacial aesthetic unit called the submalar zone 5 (SM5) or submalar "triangle." This deficiency resides over the masseter tendon and the canine fossa lying under the inferior border of the malar bone and zygomatic arch. A large malar shell implanted over the inferior aspect of the malar bone in zone 1 and extending into the submalar space below the border of the malar bone creates the illusion of a round, full "apple cheek" in females.

The soft tissues overlying the skeleton of the midface, malar, and submalar areas undergo environmentally influenced predetermined genetic-based atrophy. A modest 3- or 4-mm implant thickness can augment and rejuvenate an aging face.

Augmenting the submalar region creates the youthful appearance of soft tissue fullness in the midface as well as the illusion of a larger malar bone. This is especially useful in the aging face where atrophy and the midface soft tissue descent create a more pronounced nasolabial fold. The inferior limit of the submalar zone space is variably created by dissecting the soft tissue roof (buccinator, zygomaticus muscles, and superficial musculoaponeurotic system [SMAS]) from the masseter tendon. As the SM5 space is dissected and augmented in a more inferior direction, a larger, rounder cheek contour is produced, which simulates both bony and soft tissue fullness. This type of midface contour is exemplified in the images of actresses Bo Derek and Linda Evans or today's Angelina Jolie.

By definition, a comprehensive augmentation of the entire malar–midface unit may require an implant shell with maximal transverse dimensions of 5.5 cm across and 4.5 cm vertically. A type 2 face has adequate malar bone prominence but is deficient in similar soft tissue volume. This creates a flat, older, midface contour. This frequently occurs in the aging face of both males and females. In a young individual with strongly defined cheekbones and yet deficiencies in the midface soft tissues, a similar augmentation produces aesthetic softness and adds youthful fullness to the face. Some people feel strongly that a similar implant can lift the nasolabial sulcus and give the illusion of facial tightening that will postpone the perceived need for rhytidectomy. The authors have not observed this occurrence and favor volume filling of the midface just posterior to the nasolabial mound in order to de-emphasize the appearance of fullness and simultaneously correct the soft tissue volume deficiency in the midface.

Type 3 facial aesthetic deficiencies consist of a very strong malar–zygomatic superstructure and a very sunken submalar infrastructure. Such faces often have thin skin and subcutaneous support requiring a generous submalar augmentation with a projecting implant thickness (5 to 8 mm). This facial type occurs with aging as well as from ancestry (Fig. 33.8). The appearance is that of an emaciated, drawn, haggard, and even sick countenance. This can result from soft tissue disease states such as Romberg's hemifacial atrophy and HIV lipodystrophy. The remedy, for any etiology, is the same: a generous volume filling of the SM5 (Fig. 33.9).

Type 4 facial type consists of extreme volume deficiency in both malar zones 1 and 2 and the SM5 regions and may also include the suborbital and paranasal zone 3 areas. It is more common in men than in women. It is identified by a "flat face" appearance. It also has been described as the "polar bear" syndrome because of a suborbital skeletal deficiency, which contributes to a proptotic, bulging appearance of the globe

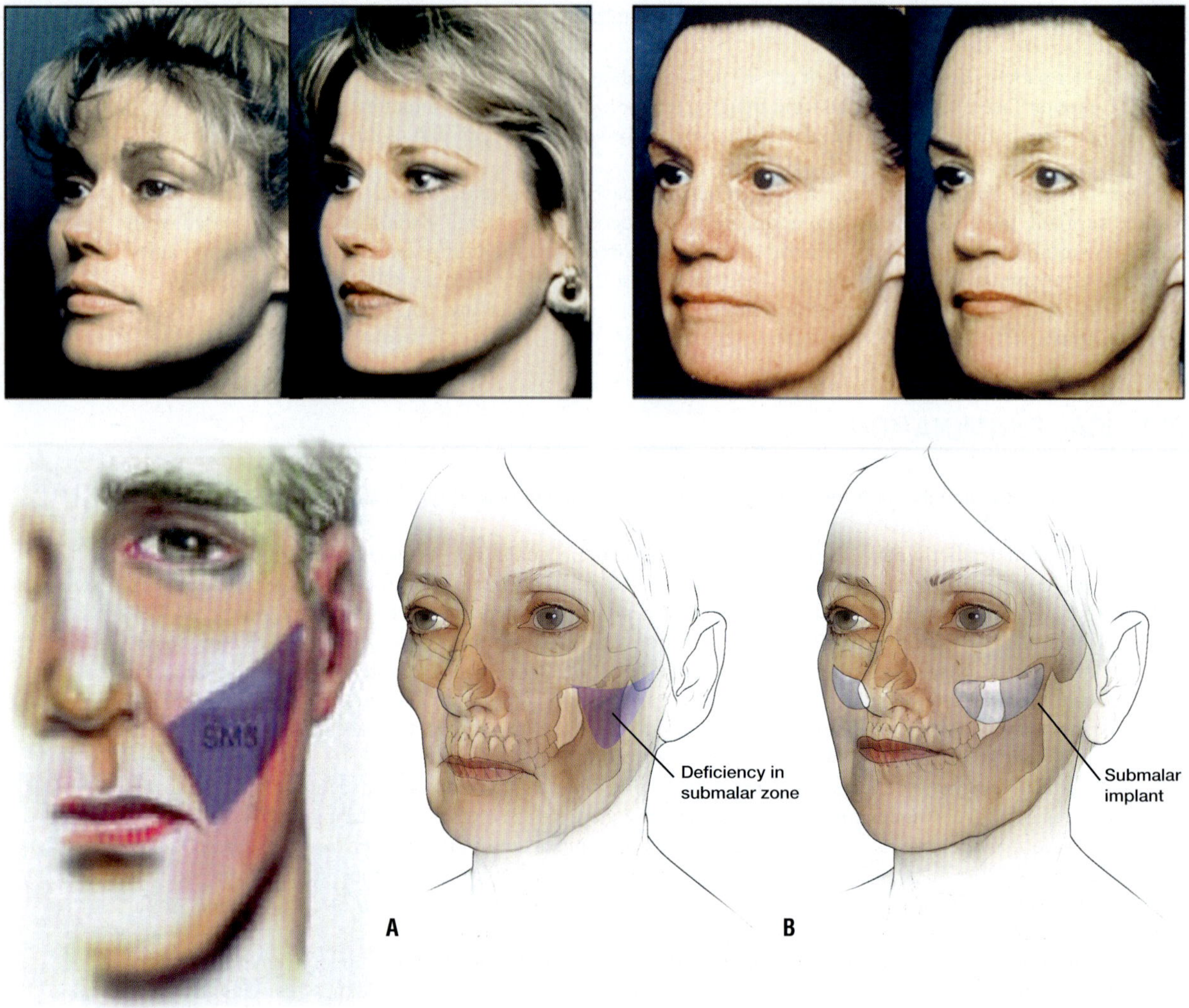

FIGURE 33.8 Upper left photo **(A)** shows a 28-year-old female who disliked her inherited submalar soft tissue recession, while **(B)** demonstrates a 47-year-old female with aging midfacial atrophy resulting in a tired haggard emaciated look. Submalar zone 5 is anatomically below the lower border of the malar bone. It may be volume deficient either by heredity **(A)** or from aging atrophy **(B)**. An appropriate submalar implant placement provides excellent aesthetic improvement.

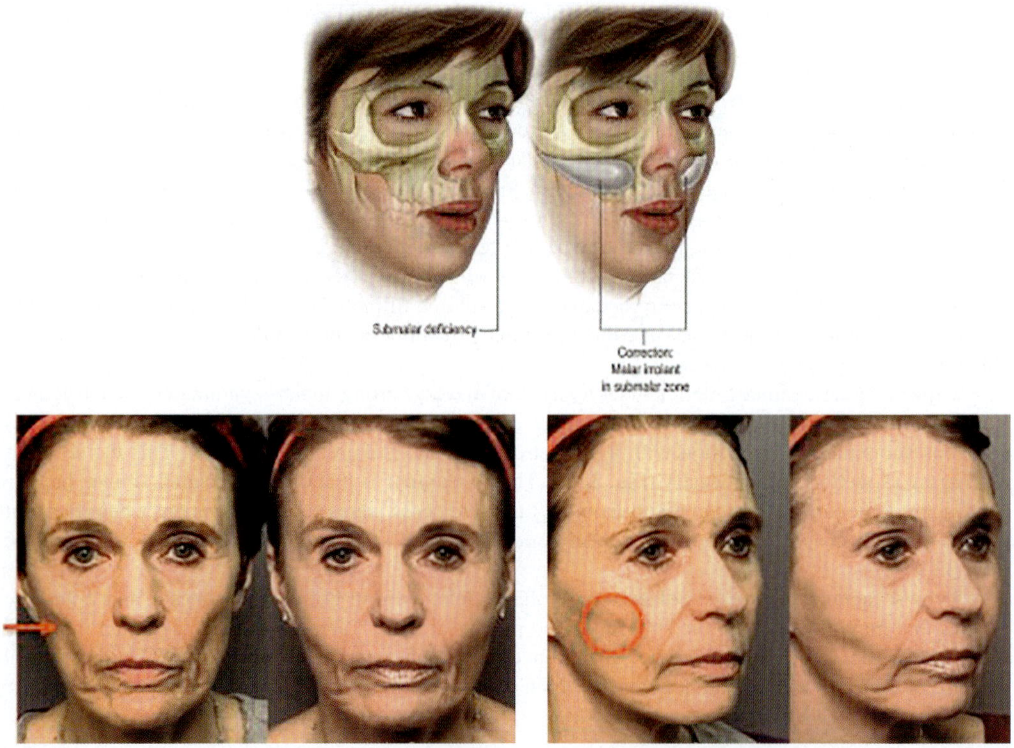

FIGURE 33.9 Tissue atrophy occurs universally with the aging face. When there is adequate malar bone prominence in a type 2 or type 3 face, a large malar shell placed in the submalar region (SM5) restores a youthful fullness to the face.

of the eye. Due to bony deficiency of the infraorbital region, a downward or vertical descent of the lower eyelid may result in scleral show.

A comprehensive shell implant that fills the medial tear trough, the suborbital rim, and the upper malar zones improves this aesthetic imbalance significantly. For some patients, a large shell implant to fill malar zones 1 and 2 as well as SM5 is all that is necessary. Theoretically, the shell implant may also add support and elevate the eyelid into a more attractive horizontal position. However, lateral canthopexy techniques may be necessary to benefit patients with this facial type.

Type 5 aesthetic facial deficiency exists as a weakness of facial structure in the suborbital "tear trough" region. This creates a tired and "hollow" appearance around the eyes, especially in the lower orbital region. There may also be a tendency for the eyeball itself to look proptotic due to the "negative vector" orbit (Fig. 33.10).

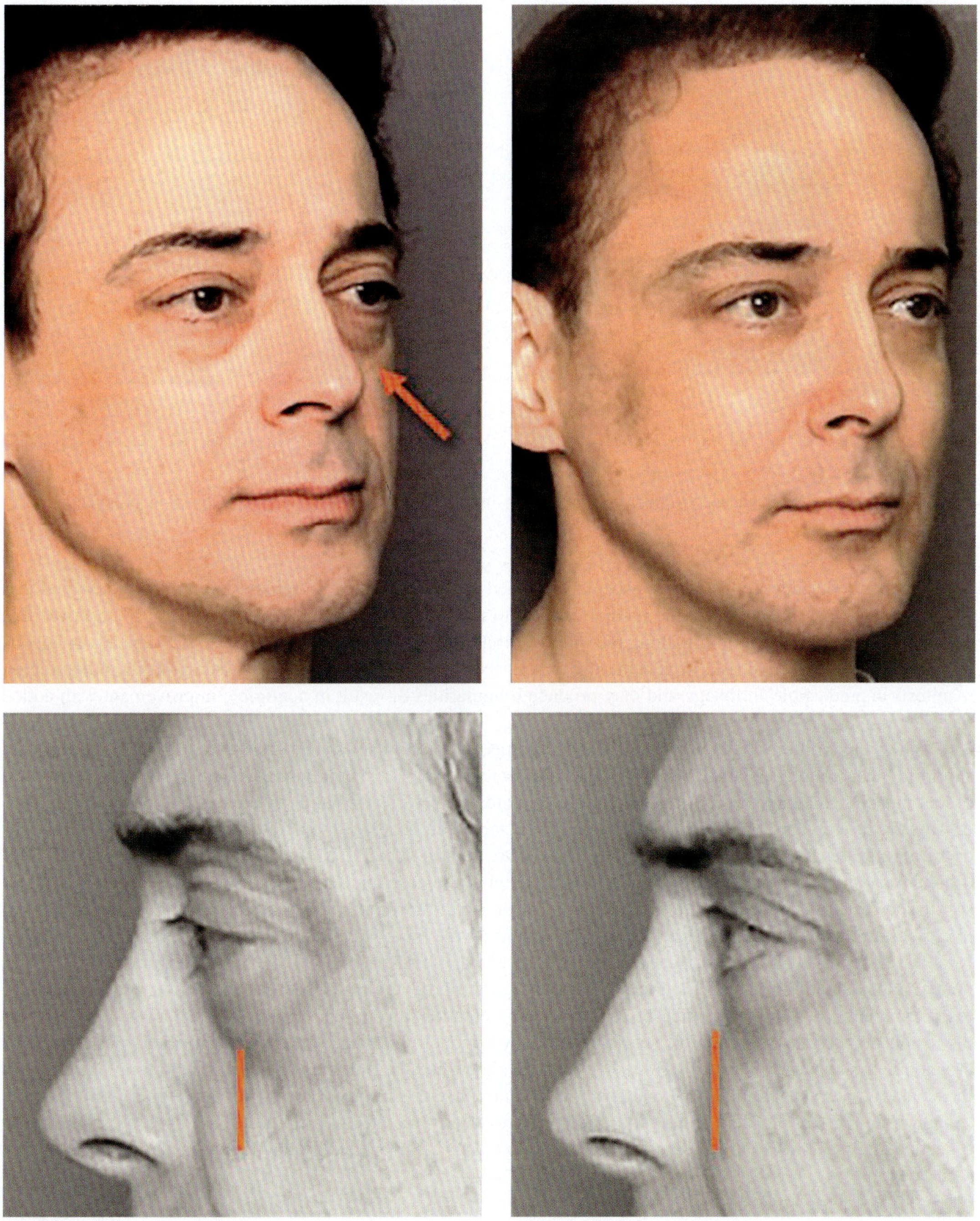

FIGURE 33.10 Before and after pictures of a patient with a type 4 face demonstrating the improvement of an extreme volume deficiency of the entire maxilla and a "negative" vector suborbital bony rim using a comprehensive extended tear trough–malar shell. This helps to correct a flat or dish-face appearance.

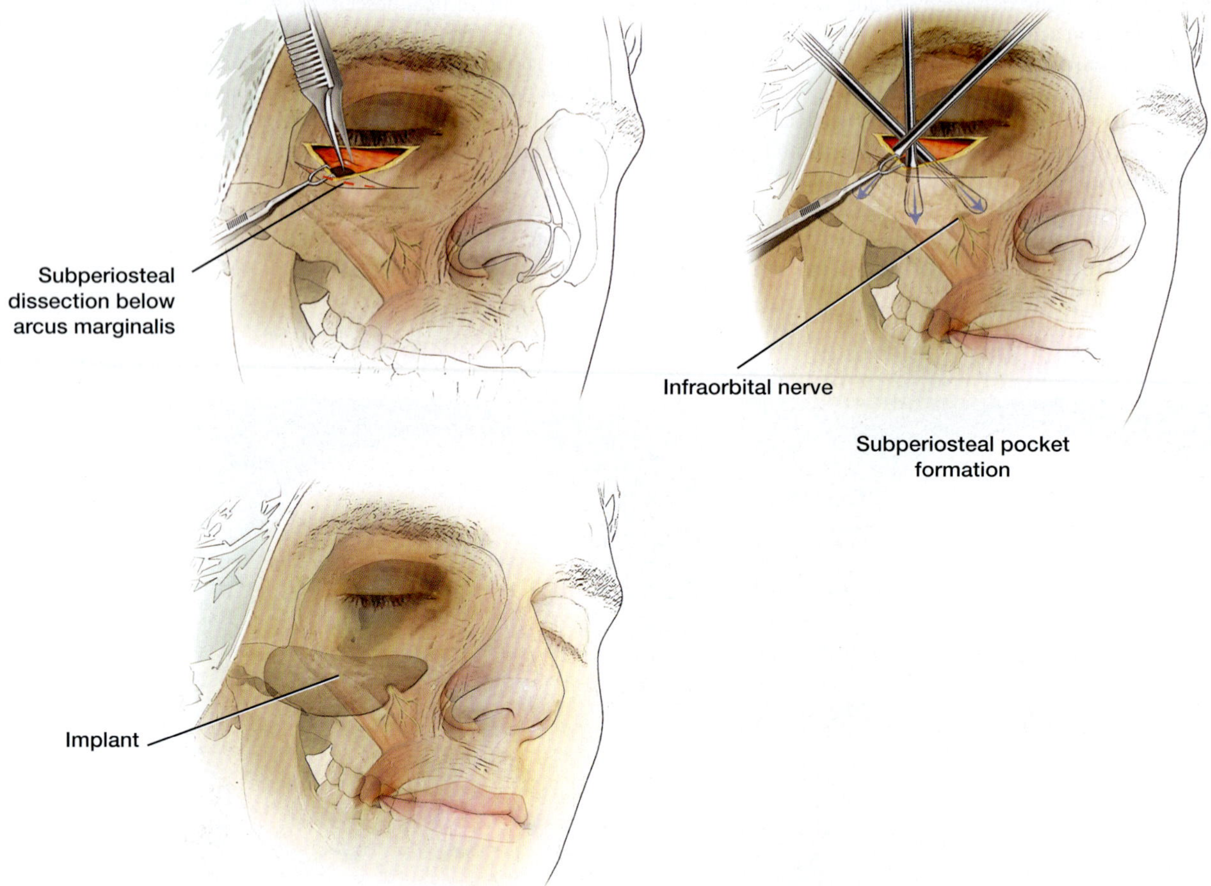

FIGURE 33.11 Illustration showing a suborbital tear trough–malar implant and the technique for insertion around the infraorbital nerve.

Volume deficiency in this area is especially viewed to be unattractive in females. A uniquely designed tear trough implant that extends from the medial canthus to the lateral orbital malar rim considerably improves this deficiency. Adipose tissue grafting along the inferior orbital rim has been considered by some to be advantageous but by others to be of high risk. In general, my experience is that all autologous soft tissue grafting in this region manifests unpredictable shrinkage and may produce irregularities or result in negligible improvement with added risks.

When this volume deficiency is also accompanied by significant malar–zygomatic hypoplasia, the new suborbital tear trough–malar shell (SOTTM) is indicated (Fig. 33.11). Autogenous tissue transplants of adipose tissue, muscle, galea and temporalis fascia into this area by a variety of authors have been only partially successful because all autologous grafts, due to unpredictable cell death, demonstrate variable shrinkage and contour irregularities. Their success and complication rate are still debated. More recent techniques for suborbital orbicularis oculi fat (SOOF) infraorbital dissections which release and elevate the suborbital cheek and malar soft tissue structures beneath the orbital rim and transpose intraorbital adipose tissue exist are more successful in correcting this deficiency but still remain dependent on the locally available tissue mass.

Tissue repositioning techniques whether "Deep Plane," "FAME," "SOMME," or "Subperiosteal" are still undergoing evaluation for their long-term persistence and reproducibility. Used in conjunction with the guaranteed permanence of alloplastic malar or suborbital augmentation, this tissue repositioning achieves optimum aesthetic appearances and reproducible surgical results. A silicone rubber implant has been specially designed to fit around the lower pyriform aperture. It is easily placed either directly onto the bone through intraoral or intranasal incisions. Its natural anatomic shape and posterior contour provide stability when positioned properly (Fig. 33.12).

In my practice, physical examination is conducted with the aid of computer imaging to provide a more objective analysis of the patient's anatomic contours. Using a mirror held by the patient is also necessary.

Facial Asymmetries

One of the most important points in the physical examination is to identify precisely the various asymmetries, which the patient's face has both bone and soft tissues. It is imperative to get the patient to understand the severe limitations in correcting them. Natural facial asymmetry is universal. A form of hemifacial microsomia occurs

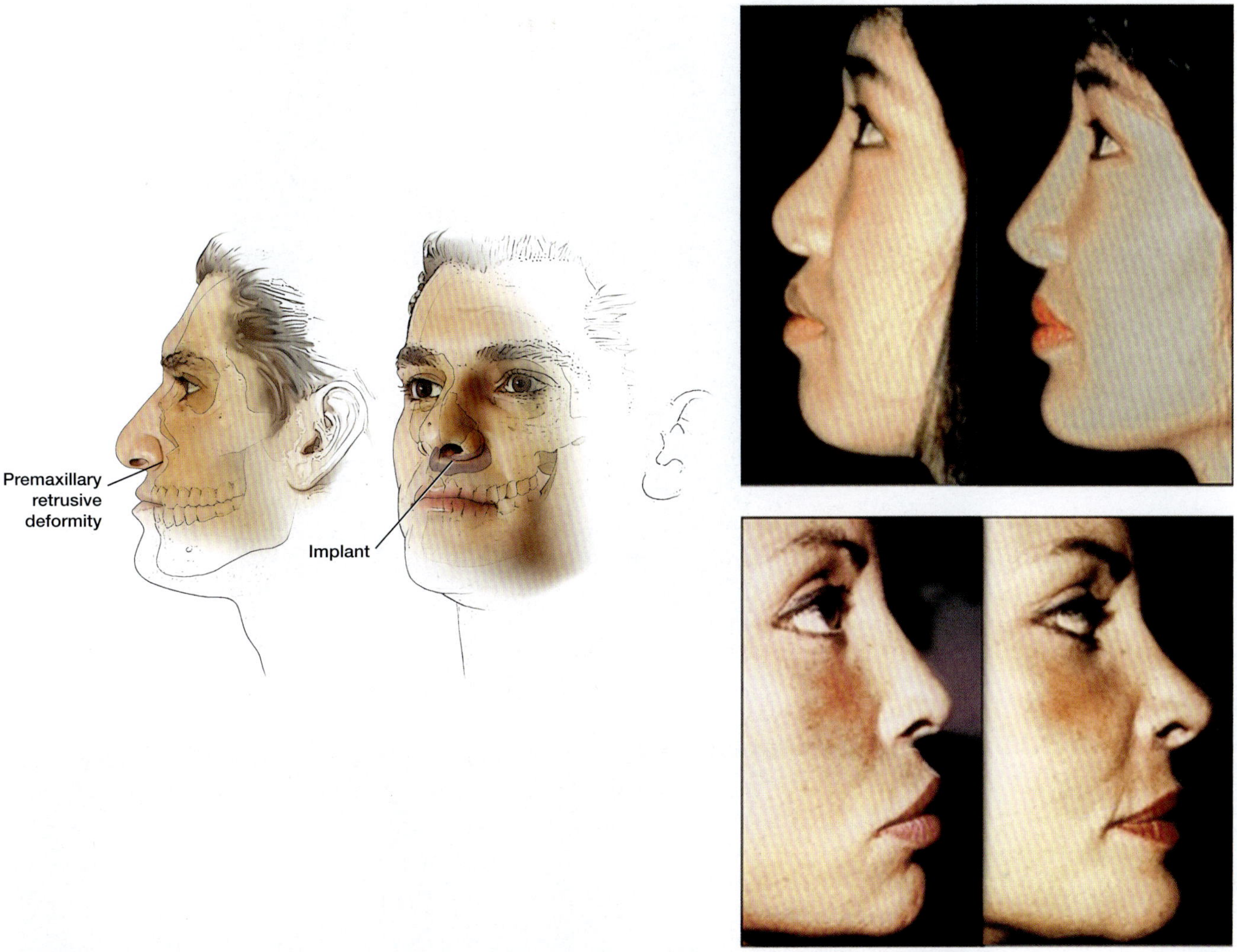

FIGURE 33.12 Example of two patients in whom premaxillary retrusive contour deformities were corrected using a peripyriform premaxillary contemporary design implant. Preoperative photos are on the left.

in more than 90% of patients. On careful examination, the left and right side of the face are usual quite different in size, shape, or volume. One side is wider and has a greater volume of bone and soft tissue. Also, one orbit, eyebrow, and eye complex is usually lower than the other (Fig. 33.13).

Patients can be very particular and obsessed with asymmetries. Such asymmetries frequently go unnoticed before facial implant contouring. It is imperative, therefore, to evaluate facial asymmetries meticulously, note them in the medical records, and explain them in detail to the patients. It is also necessary to warn patients that asymmetries will always still be present to some degree following surgery, even when implants of different sizes are chosen and positioned to compensate for the variations in volume and shape that already exist (Fig. 33.14). In my practice, asymmetries are documented in the patient's chart by computer imaging or photographic modalities. Documentation helps to prevent criticism postoperatively if the asymmetry is still apparent to the patient, even in the slightest degree.

INDICATIONS

Alloplastic facial implants are fundamental in all aspects of facial surgery. Implants are able to restore, augment, and rejuvenate facial contours by building a better three-dimensional foundation on the underlying skeletal framework of the face. Since most facial implant procedures are performed by an intraoral or transconjunctival approach, there is almost no need for external incisions except perhaps for the chin region.

In the realm of reconstructive surgery, implants can improve facial asymmetries after fundamental craniomaxillofacial treatments. Implants are also used for restoration of facial balance in adult patients with hereditary regional deficiencies and congenital anomalies or for establishing more attractive facial harmony in conjunction with orthognathic surgery.

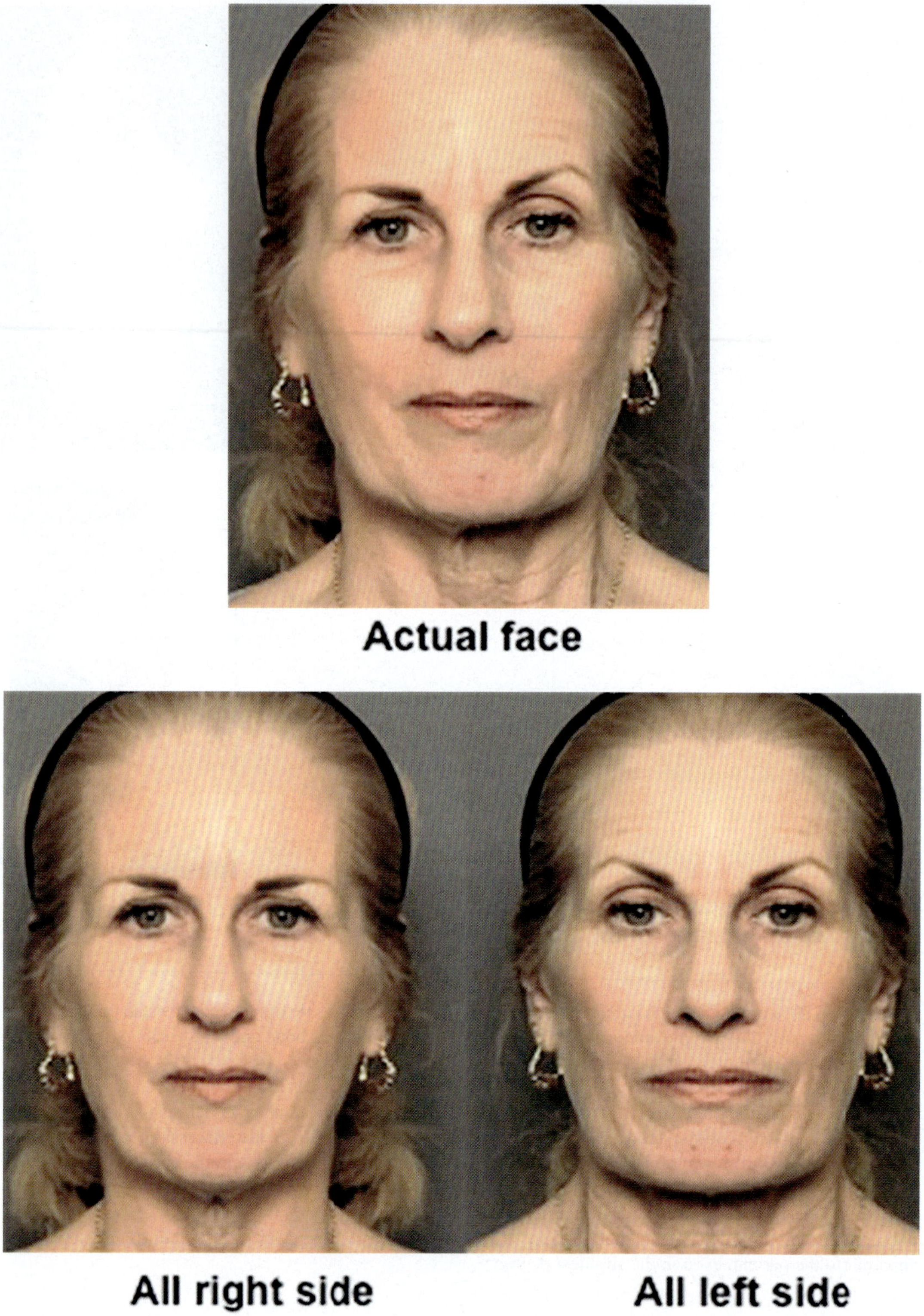

FIGURE 33.13 A 61-year-old female whose natural inherited facial asymmetries are easily revealed with a computer imaging tool.

Facial rejuvenation with implants is an essential component for achieving optimum surgical improvements of facial aging. Recent studies have demonstrated dynamic skeletal changes that occur with aging and the applicability of implants in such circumstances.

As the face ages, the orbital aperture area and width increase. The soft tissue envelope atrophies and is subsequently affected in multiple planes so that facial features are repositioned accordingly. The orbit appears more hollowed and enophthalmic, while the lateral palpebral fissure loses its youthful upward slant and the lower lid vertical distance increases. These changes result in a more noticeable and unattractive lid cheek junction.

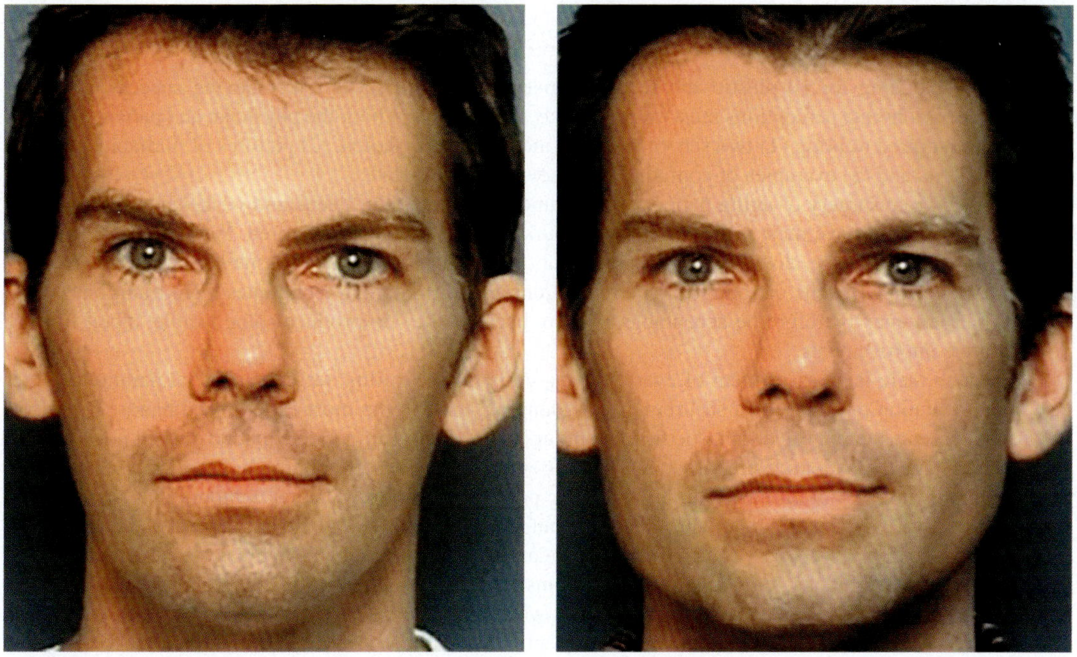

FIGURE 33.14 A 38-year-old male, with posterior lateral zone (PL) deficiency of the premandible region, desiring mandible augmentation. Postoperative view taken 1 year following mandibular angle augmentation using 12-mm implant size on the smaller right side and a 10-mm implant on the larger left to improve preoperative facial asymmetry.

Significant changes are also seen in the malar–midface region with an increase in midface concavity and malar flattening. The mandible undergoes atrophic changes: shrinking and thinning of the mandibular body, shortening of the rami vertical height, and an increase in the mandibular angle, causing it to be more obtuse. This measurable loss of volume affects the development of jowling, marionette lines, and facial rhytids.

Facial implants are the most powerful tool in restoring the volume of more youthful facial contours to an aging face. During a rhytidectomy procedure, infraorbital, malar, paranasal, and mandibular implants can be placed in the affected sites to dramatically improve the appearance of the face. Implants also serve as the underlying foundation or scaffold for the resuspension and repositioning of the laxed soft tissues.

The last category of patients who present for facial augmentation are young adults with no significant signs of aging, previous trauma, or severe disfiguring hereditary deformities. Some patients are displeased with a specific facial feature such as a certain bony or soft tissue deficiency, while others may desire a change in their overall facial skeletal disharmony.

CONTRAINDICATIONS

There are almost no absolute contraindications to the use of facial alloplastic implants. Some of the more common concerns preoperatively are as follows:

1. The possibility of infection. This is similar to any other plastic surgery procedure, which introduces a foreign material into the body. Therefore, placement of facial implants in the presence of facial infection or an unknown inflammatory process is not recommended. If an infectious process has affected the implant and the production of a biofilm around the implant has taken place, removal of the implant is likely to be necessary. Porous implants become infiltrated with fibrous tissue ingrowth, which prevents easy removal.
2. Unreasonable patient expectations. Preexisting natural inherited asymmetries are universal and frequently persist postoperatively even after attempts are made to correct them with differential implant choice and/or placement. This is the cause of over 90% of patient dissatisfactions with their implant surgery. Therefore, the surgeon must point out these asymmetries and explain to the patient the shortcomings of any procedure that aims to correct them. Patients should have some form of basic psychological assessment by the surgeon in order to rule out individuals with body dysmorphic disorder. Those patients are unlikely to be happy with the outcome and should be discouraged from having the procedure done.
3. Previous radiation exposure. Often patients who have undergone external beam radiation treatments have undergone surgical treatment as well. The dimensions of the remaining defect, integrity and redundancy of the overlying skin, and location to be corrected all play into the associated risks. Although there are notable benefits in the treatment of such patients, there are also considerable complications that can unfold with wound breakdown and soft tissue erosion.

PREOPERATIVE PLANNING

Preoperative planning for all plastic and reconstructive surgery is critical for achieving successful results. Patient expectations and perceptions must be completely understood by both the physician and patient alike. All patients are required to bring (1) two sets of standard medical facial photos, (2) pictures of midfacial contours they do not like, and (3) examples of contour ideals they want to emulate.

For traditional surgery of aging patients, communication about their needs and wishes may be relatively simple. They wish to have their prior youthful contours and facial features restored. With the passing years, individuals acclimate to the slow, gradual changes that take place along the soft tissue contours of their faces. The limited technical results of routine tissue repositioning and tightening techniques from traditional facial aesthetic surgery may therefore be acceptable to them, because they do produce some visible, albeit limited, postoperative improvements.

Although there is an assortment of ever evolving tools for measuring aesthetic skeletal parameters, precise implementation of facial form still remains challenging, even in the most experienced hands. Therefore, before the surgeon attempts an alloplastic facial contour alteration, it is imperative that he or she knows exactly what facial image the patient desires. I request my patients to either modify photographs of themselves, bring in photos of themselves at an earlier time period, or provide examples of facial contours that they admire, namely, faces that they feel look similar to their own but are more attractive in the pertinent skeletal areas (Fig. 33.15). Although this process may run contrary to standard teaching in residency, it creates an understanding of patients' expectations by providing invaluable visual insights and imagery to discuss. Most patients have very precise ideas about the images of facial contours they wish to emulate. Therefore, when they do not, it is easy to discover that their expectations cannot be met. In elective operations, surgeons must not undertake what they are not sure they can accomplish, especially when the patient's own visually described goals are poorly defined. Overall, I find computer-imaging technology to be indispensable in this process.

Patient Education and Patient Consent

In my practice, patient education begins with the requirement that patients who desire facial contour alterations must describe, not only verbally but also in writing, the specific details of their desired contour changes. This must include their perception of the contour deficiencies that they feel they possess. This written statement must be accompanied by standard professional photographs of the patient in 5 views: frontal, 2 profile and 2 oblique views. These facilitate analyzing their perceived contour deficiencies and are used along with photographs they choose from magazines and other sources to demonstrate the "ideal scene" they would like surgery to create. Photos of the patient at earlier times of life are also requested to use as the "model image" to strive to recreate in the operating room (Fig. 33.16)

I use several excellent instructional tools to explain concepts of facial balance as they relate to the basic interrelationship of the three major promontories: the malar–midface, the nose, and the chin–jawline (Fig. 33.17). I also use videos and photos that demonstrate the zones as well as computer imaging of the

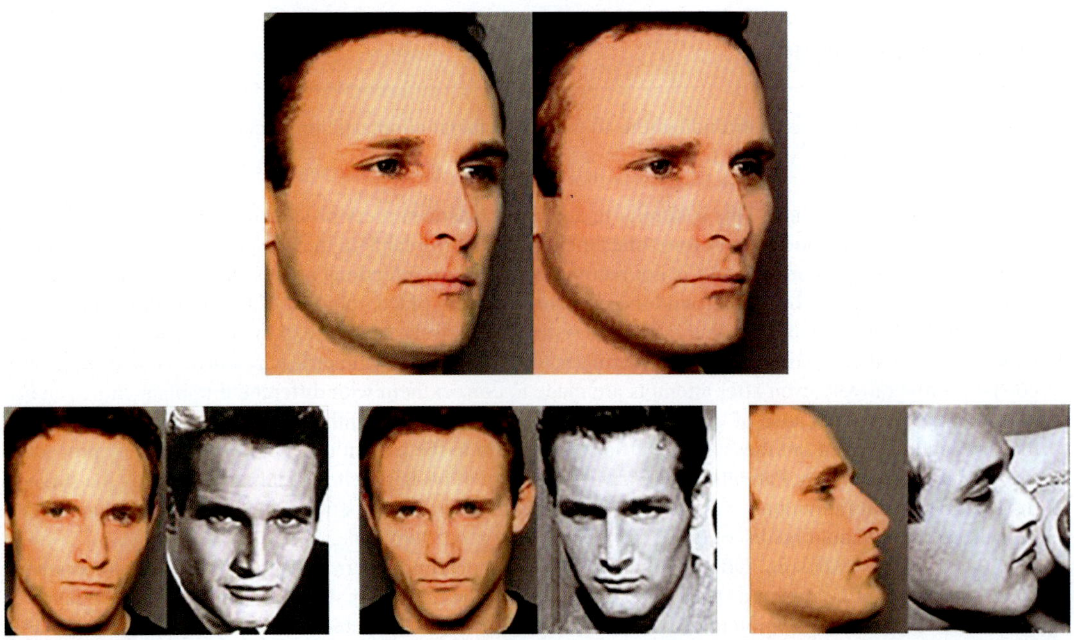

FIGURE 33.15 A 32-year-old aspiring actor who desired to improve his resemblance to Paul Newman by acquiring malar and chin implants.

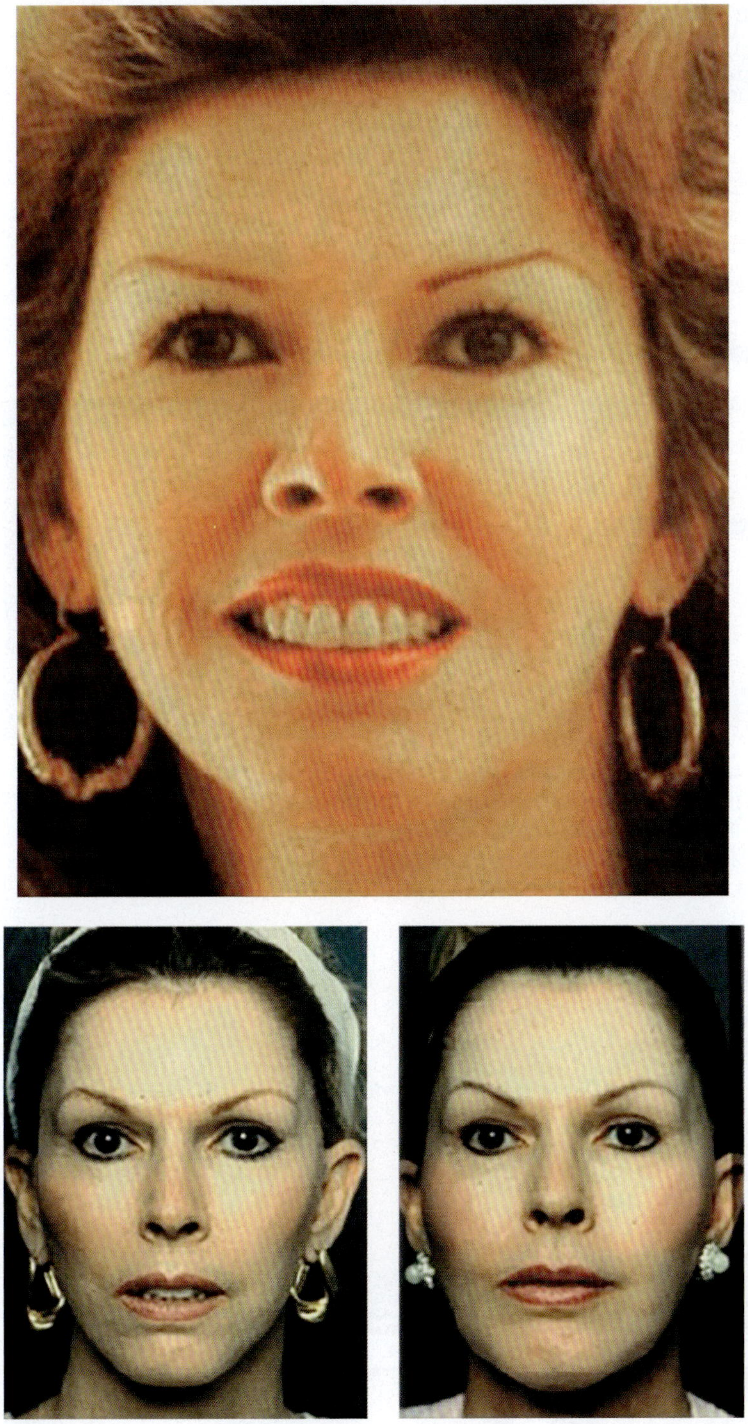

FIGURE 33.16
All patients wish to have youthful fullness return to their faces. This can be accomplished by alloplastic augmentation. Patients are asked to bring photographs of themselves in a more youthful time of life in order to try to recover their earlier "ideal scene."

malar–zygomatic zonal contours of the facial skeleton on the patient's face. This illustrates how specific positioning of various size and shape implants alters the three-dimensional balance of the midface in different ways (Fig. 33.18).

Computer imaging is an invaluable tool to assist the surgeon. Not only can changes be made that simulate desired volume and shape alterations, but these can be compared using a side-by-side pre- and postimage of the patient's presurgical image. When used cautiously and conservatively, the final result of surgery 1 year postoperatively is photographically superior to the image alterations made in the examining room during the consultation (Fig. 33.19).

Final planning is done on the morning of surgery before the patient is taken to the operating room or given any form of preoperative medication. The surgeon sits with the patient before the image computer and with the selected magazine photographs brought by the patient and reviews his imaging agreements with the patient. Markings are made on the patient's face to outline the borders of the bony architecture and designate the facial zones of the midface (Fig. 33.20). Similar markings can be made on the magazine photographs. An interactive process then occurs whereby the patient is asked to identify which specific zones he or she wants altered by

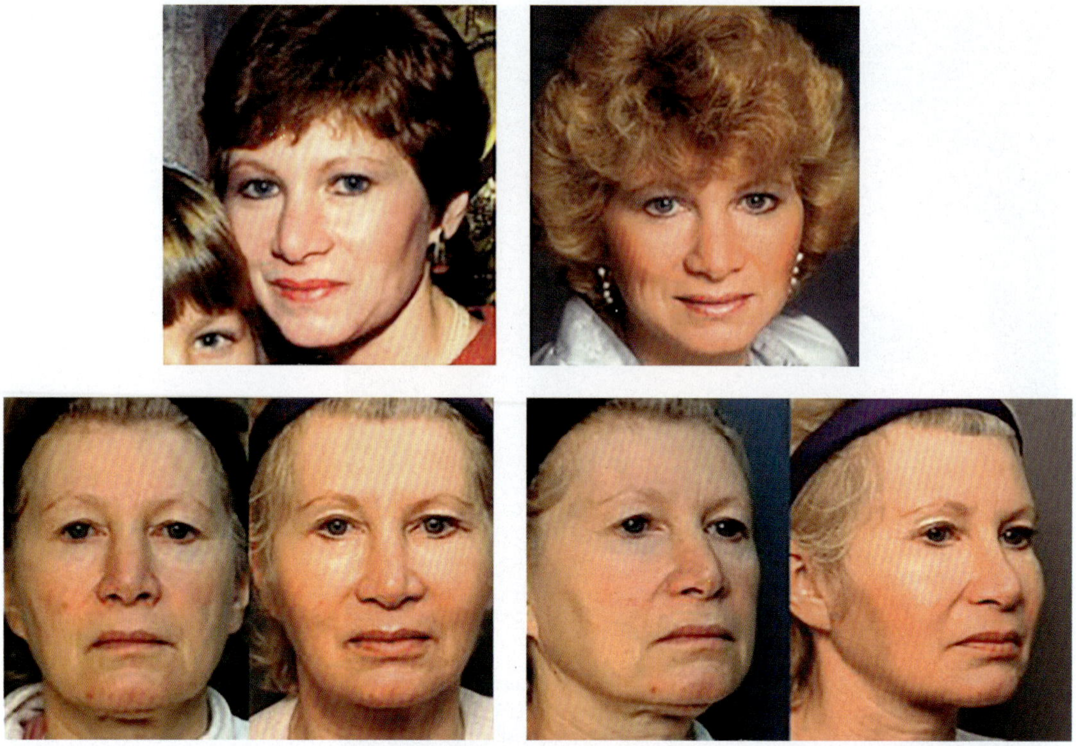

FIGURE 33.17 A 59-year-old female, with relative midfacial atrophy from aging, who desired a return of youthful fullness as well as contouring of the lower face, neck, and jowls. *Top left* view shows the patient at age 41, with right view at age 50. *Bottom* views, preoperative view on left and postoperative view on right 1 year following upper midface suspension, with lateral temple brow contouring. Submalar midface augmentation, lower zone 1 and submalar zone (SM5), using large Terino malar shell of 4 mm, and lower face and neck rhytidectomy with SMAS and platysma plication.

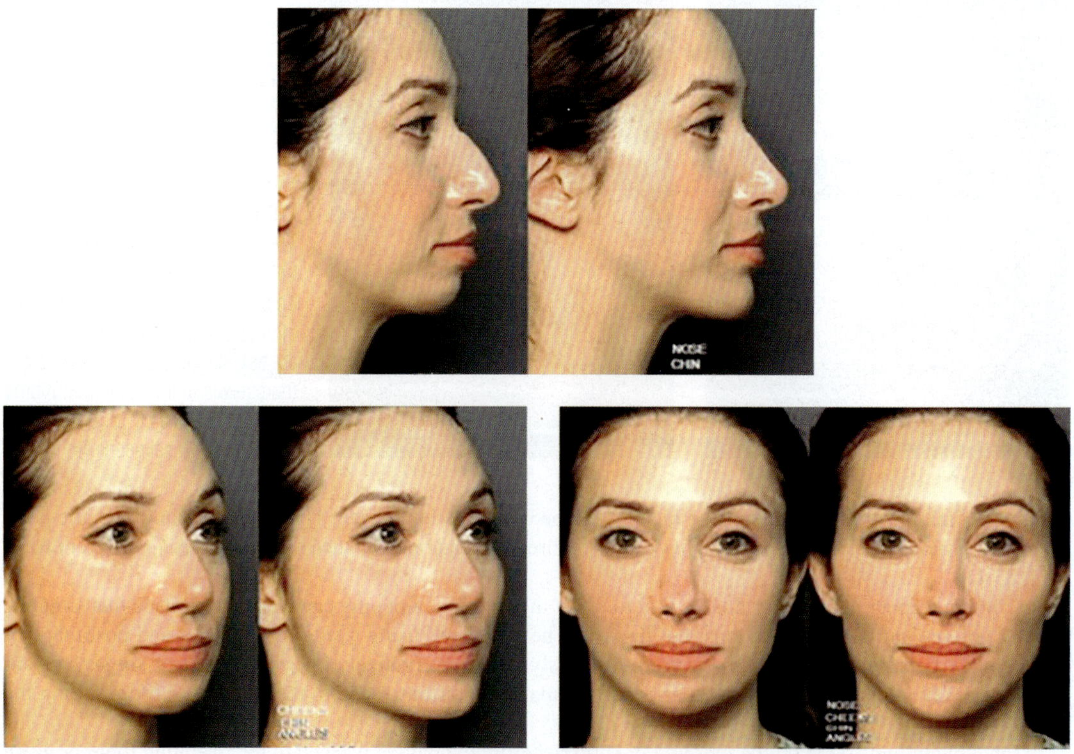

FIGURE 33.18 Computer images demonstrating facial balance and the interrelationship of different regional facial volume augmentations. *Top* images reveal volume augmentation of the chin producing a diminishing effect on the volume of the nose. *Bottom left* demonstrates the effect of augmentation of the cheeks, chin, and angle of the mandible without rhinoplasty. *Right bottom* left shows the effect of using rhinoplasty in addition to malar, chin, and angle of mandible augmentation.

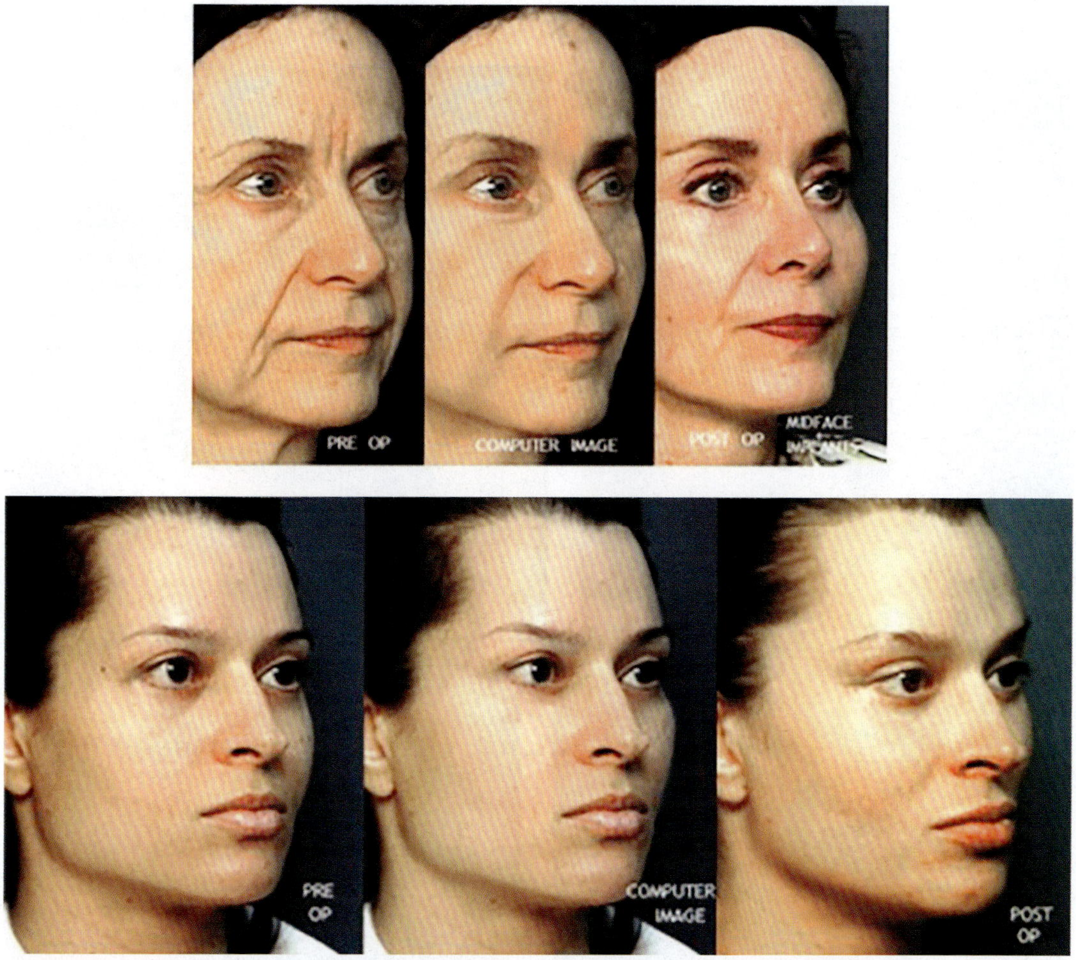

FIGURE 33.19 These patients demonstrate the final effects of facial surgery 1 year postoperatively (*right view*) versus the best computer imaging at the time of original consultation (*middle view*). The 1-year postoperative results nearly always prove better than the consultation image modifications.

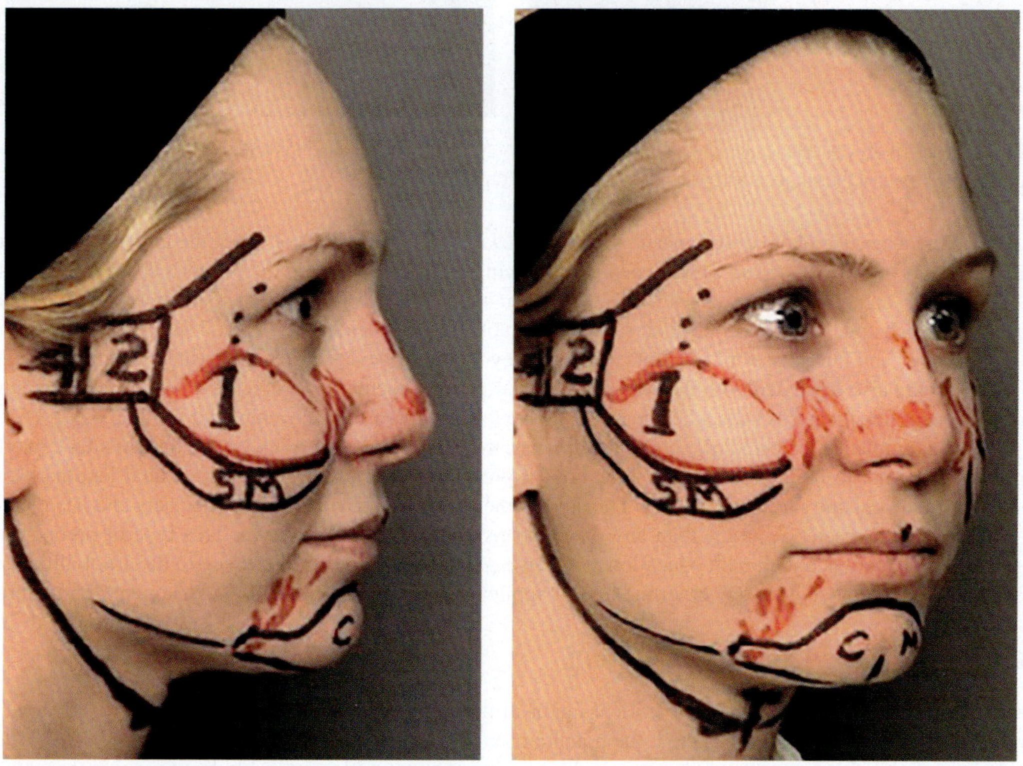

FIGURE 33.20 Preoperative markings are made on all patients' faces the morning of surgery to outline their zonal anatomy and bone structure.

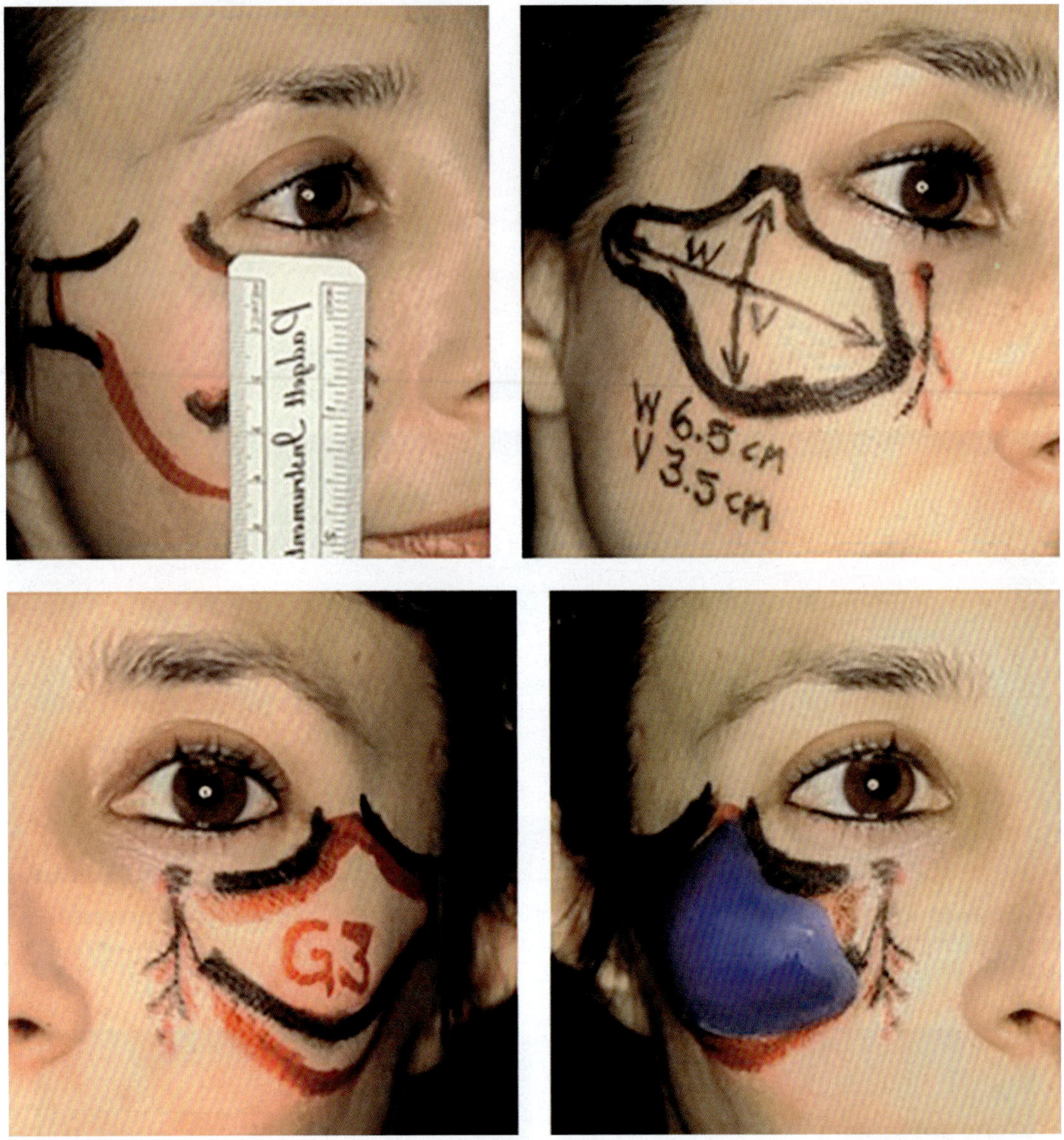

FIGURE 33.21 A 28-year-old female preoperatively with malar–zygomatic facial markings and different "sizer" implants being applied to assist the surgeon and patient make final decisions.

looking at the magazine photo drawings and their own facial markings in a mirror. Then the implant size, surface area, and projection are discussed with the patient by placing implant "sizers" on the patient's cheek over the skin markings of the anatomic zone or zones which the patient has selected. In this way the patient assists in the decision about which zone area and implant size is most suitable for his "ideal scene" (Fig. 33.21). The implications of various sizes and thicknesses of implants and how they would achieve subtle, conservative or more dramatic appearances are also discussed with the patient. A similar patient–doctor communication session with the computer and magazine images is used when augmenting the lower third of the face, chin, and jawline.

Once an implant is selected, the outline of its margins is drawn with red ink on the patient's face overlying the facial zone to be altered. During the surgical procedure, the inside anatomic skeletal landmarks are compared to the outside surface markings. This allows the surgeon to place implants precisely and is a method of ensuring much greater accuracy than any other means that the author has used. This type of preoperative assessment, evaluation, and patient education provides a greater precision and accuracy to the art of alloplastic facial augmentation than does any other method. It applies equally in either primary or secondary procedures.

Selection of the Ideal Facial Implant

The anatomic shape of implants is the critical factor in imitating aesthetic facial contours. In practice, when appropriate implants have been selected, the potential for mobility and malposition is almost negligible. Ideal implants should be easily implantable, nonpalpable, readily exchangeable, malleable, conformable, acceptable to the body, resistant to infection, and easily modifiable by the surgeon (Table 33.1).

TABLE 33.1 Optimum Qualities for Facial Implants

Ideal Qualities	Silicone Rubber	Gore-Tax® Soft Form	Porex Medpor®	Hydroxyapatite
Biocompatible	4	3	4	4
Modifiable	4	2	3	3
Exchangeable	4	2	1	1
Resistant to infection	3	1	3	2
Anatomic contours	4	1	2	2
Visible, palpable	3.5	1	2	2

Note: 4, most optimum; 1, least optimum.

When placed directly on bone, smooth silicone implants become rapidly fixed and securely surrounded by capsular fibrosis because this creates a space well demarcated, they can be removed readily and exchanged when necessary or desirable. On the other hand, porous implants that permit tissue ingrowth such as high-density polyethylene (e.g., Medpor), fenestrated implants, and implants with Dacron backing have a low but consistent, predictable, and clinically significant incidence of infection. They are also significantly more difficult to exchange or modify due to bone sequestration and other locally induced tissue interactions. Perhaps the most pertinent finding is the recognition that Medpor is also more likely to extrude when placed under thinner tissue coverage. By contradistinction, silastic implants can survive the onset of inflammation and even gross purulence, whereas infected porous implants may require removal.

The success of recent anatomic facial implants is also, in large part, due to their conformability to the facial skeleton. Implants are being produced whose posterior aspects are accurately molded to the shape and form of the facial skeleton (Fig. 33.22). The evolution of implants volumetrically to fit the dimensions of the face effectively minimizes implant mobility and malposition. A second achievement has been the increased malleability and compressibility of facial implants, which enable the insertion through smaller apertures. With the currently expanding use of larger implants, these two qualities have become even more critical. Often implants of 10 to 20 square cm need to be placed onto the malar bone of the facial skeleton. Silicone rubber implants, fabricated into a suitable medium-grade consistency, make it possible to perform this procedure with ease. Finally, the ready modifiability of silicone implants works in the surgeon's favor when a formidable

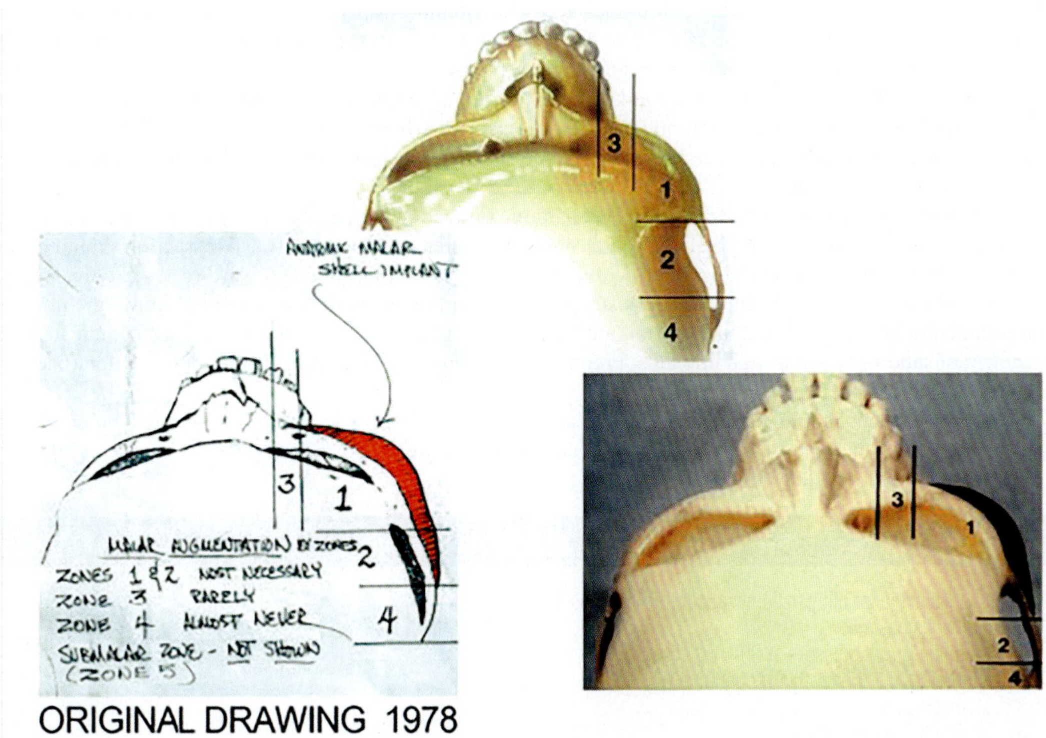

FIGURE 33.22 Anatomic design implants are contoured posteriorly to securely fit the bony surface of the facial skeleton like a glove.

barrier is encountered during the operation. Instead of enforcing a traumatic dissection upon an area of anatomy where nerve damage may be imminent, the surgeon can easily diminish the implants or alter their configuration with a scalpel without affecting the resulting contour.

SURGICAL TECHNIQUE

General Considerations

Patient Positioning

In all facial contouring surgery the patient is supine on the operating table.

Anesthesia Strategies

General anesthesia is indicated in order to control the blood pressure adequately. Clondine (0.2 mg) is given preoperatively for vasosympathetic stabilization. The systolic blood pressure is maintained by the anesthesiologist at a level of 90 to 100 mm of mercury. Local anesthesia is also generously infiltrated into the tissues. A volume of 20 mL is injected into each malar region and each premandible region. This lidocaine solution contains 0.2% concentration with an epinephrine concentration of 1/800,000. An attempt is made to place the anesthesia solution beneath the periosteum. The above actions enable the surgeon to execute facial implant surgery in a nearly bloodless field (Table 33.2).

Operation

Incision Placement

The various routes for entering the malar space, including the submalar region, are as follows: (1) intraoral, (2) lower blepharoplasty (subciliary), (3) rhytidectomy, (4) zygomaticotemporal, (5) transcoronal, and (6) transconjunctival.

Intraoral Route

The intraoral route has been the traditional and most frequent approach to maxillary malar and midface augmentation. I use an incision that is L shaped with 1 cm limbs, made through the mucosa only and in a vertically oblique direction. It is located over the anterior buttress of the maxilla, just above the canine tooth and approximately 2.5 cm medial to the orifice of Stensen's duct.

A spatula-shaped elevator with a 1-cm-wide blade is thrust directly under the periosteum and under the orbicularis oris muscle in a vertical orientation at the inferior base of the maxillary buttress, in the apex of the gingival–buccal sulcus. The overlying soft tissues are swept obliquely upward over the maxillary eminence by maintaining the elevator directly on bone. The elevator should always remain on the bony margin along the inferior border of the malar eminence and zygomatic arch (Figs. 33.23 and 33.24).

Manual palpation of the previously marked zonal design of the malar space anatomy on the skin is performed, while the underlying elevator mobilizes the tissues directly from the bone. This maneuver includes palpating the orbital rim and the upper and lower borders of the zygoma as the elevator dissects the subperiosteal space within these areas (Fig. 33.25).

A fiberoptic Aufricht retractor confirms the anatomic dissection. Once bony margins are reached, further space expansion is performed only by means of a rounded, blunter spatula elevator. No dissection should occur into the soft tissues with a penetrating and forceful motion. No dissection should occur directly into the area of the infraorbital nerve. When desired, the periosteum may be mobilized, both lateral and inferior to the infraorbital foramen, with a careful scraping motion until the nerve and foramen are visualized. This is indicated for placement of suborbital tear trough implants. Frequent irrigation is performed with antibiotic solution (bacitracin, 50,000 U/L or Ancef 1 g/L of normal saline).

Once the space is mobilized, the chosen implant is introduced with a long, curved, serrated clamp placed transversely across the upper end of the implant and inserted into the posterior zygomatic tunnel while two

TABLE 33.2 Anesthesia Strategies

The ideal anesthesia for alloplastic facial contouring is as follows:

1. General anesthesia
   A. Maintain blood pressure at 90–100 systolic
   B. Clonidine, 0.2 mg orally preoperatively
2. Local anesthesia
   A. Lidocaine solution 0.2%
   B. Adrenalin 1:800,000
   C. Generous tissue infiltration into malar or premandible space (20–30 mL each area)

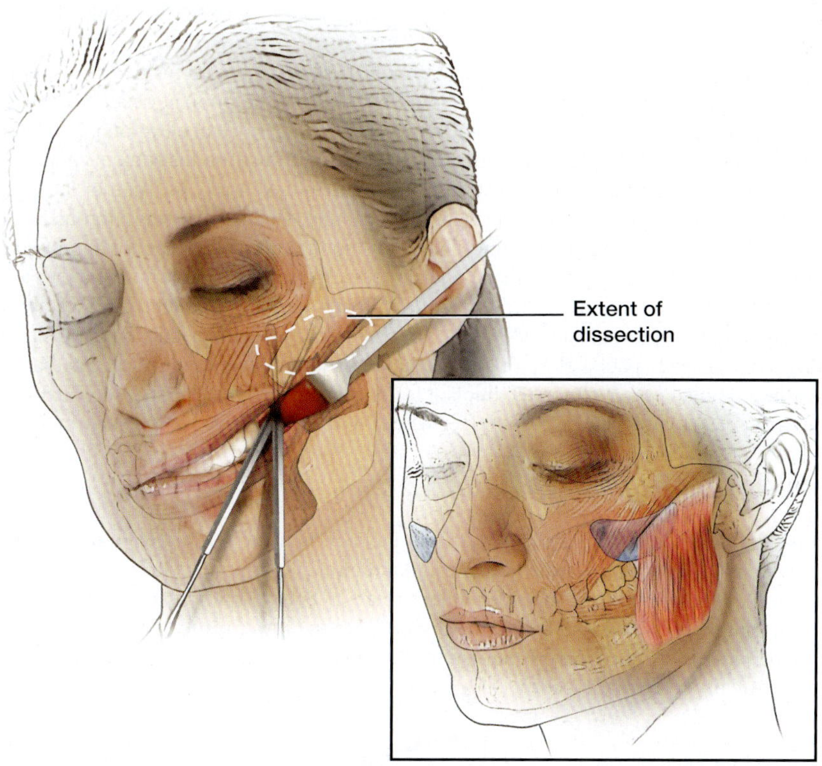

FIGURE 33.23 Artist's rendering of the actual surgical dissection for intraoral introduction of malar–submalar implants. The dissection is subperiosteal, through the lower border of the incision beneath the muscles, and always remains on bone.

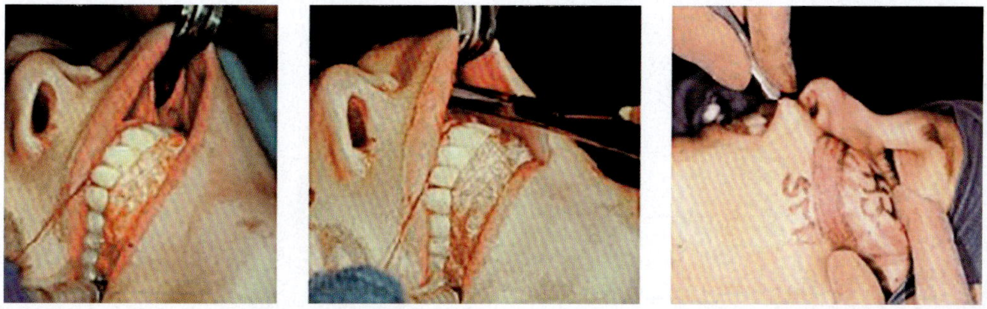

FIGURE 33.24 Intraoperative photos of intraoral approach with manual guidance to placing malar zone 1 and 2 implants.

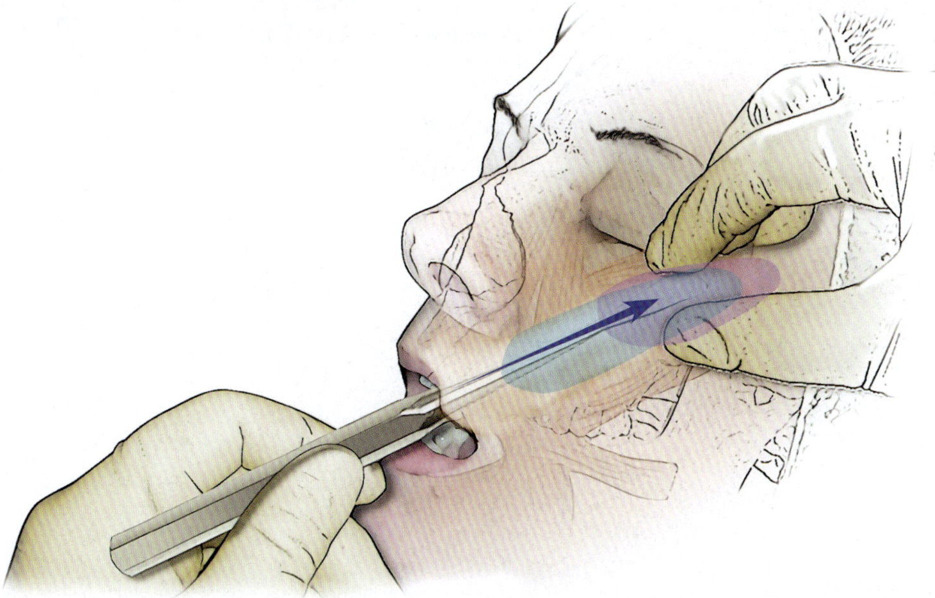

FIGURE 33.25 Illustration and actual photo showing manual guidance of an elevator beneath the previously marked malar anatomy while creating an accurate subperiosteal space for malar shell placement.

10-inch needles swedged on a 2-0 Prolene suture (Ethibond) are placed from inside to outside in the temporal region and then tied over a large bolster sponge. Should buckling of the implant occur, correct positioning can be ensured by using Russian forceps, in combination with a spatula periosteal elevator, passed both anterior and posterior to the implant. Fiberoptic Aufricht retractors or other illuminating instruments are used to illuminate the interior of the space, reveal the internal anatomy, and confirm the correct position of the implant.

In the submalar zone, the soft tissues are swept off the shiny, white, glistening, fibrous tendon of the masseter muscle in an inferior and outward direction. This opens up the submalar space for approximately 1 to 2 cm, depending on the desired choice of cheek shape and the corresponding implant necessary to achieve it. When adequate anesthesia techniques are used, the intraoral approach permits excellent visualization of the skeletal anatomy and musculature. This exposure allows accurate implant placement into zones 1, 2, and 5 (SM5). It permits the surgeon to place a spatula elevator above and below the implant to make certain that its edges are not buckled or that the zygomatic extension of the implant is not curled. It is not necessary to visualize the infraorbital nerve, but it is rather easy to do so when required, or when an implant is used for the suborbital region.

Subciliary and Transconjunctival Approaches

In the standard subciliary blepharoplasty approach, an incision is made 3 mm below the lash line and limited in its lateral extension to avoid scars in the lateral canthal region. This approach may be used either in conjunction with routine blepharoplasty or as an independent route of entry for a malar implant. A skin–muscle flap or a transconjunctival incision can also be used to dissect onto the lower orbital bony margin and penetrate the SOOF layer in the lateral aspect of the orbit down to the bone. In this manner, the midface zone 1 area can be dissected subperiosteally from that location (Fig. 33.26).

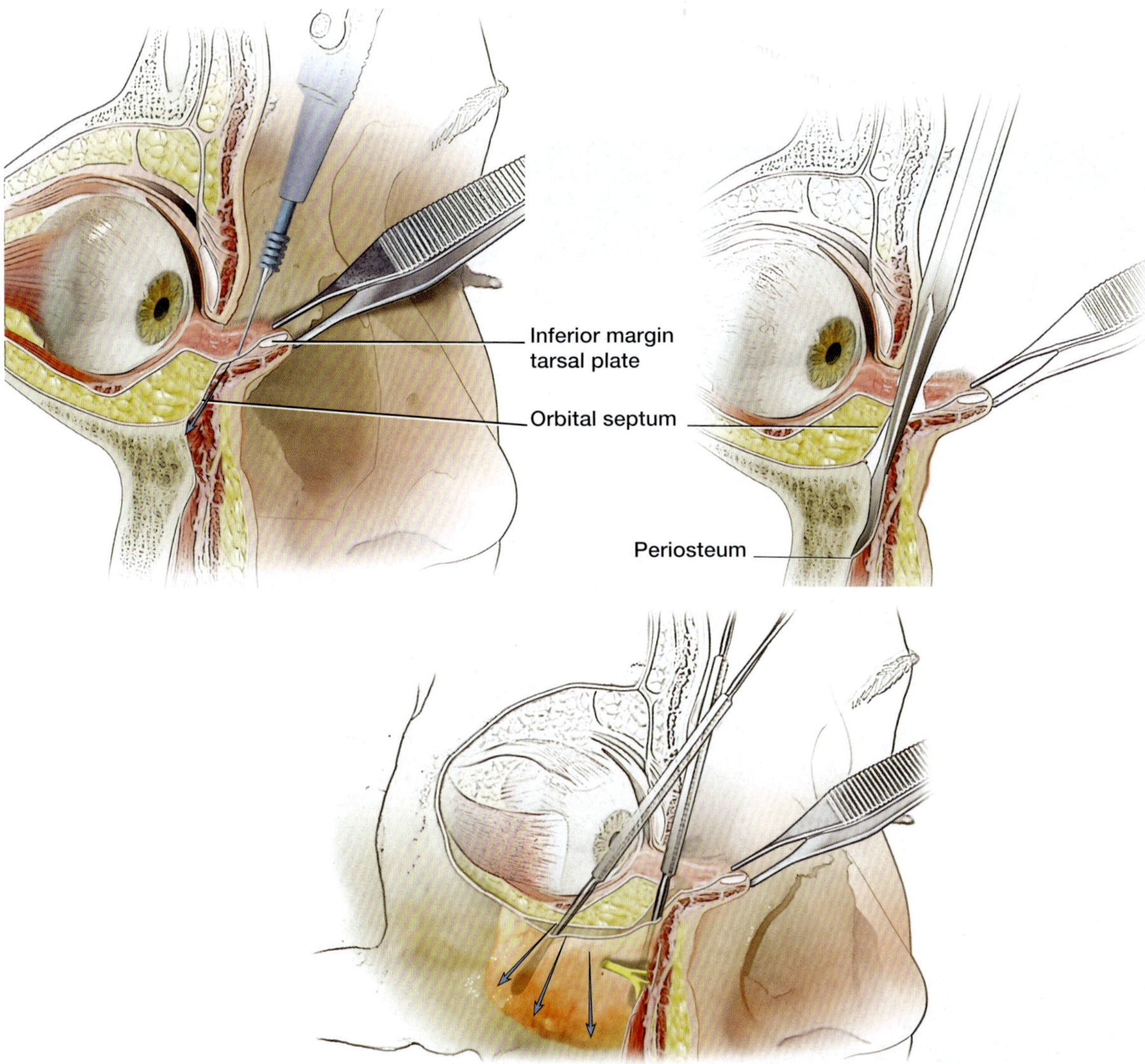

FIGURE 33.26 Shows a transconjunctival approach to dissect down to the inferior orbital bony margin and penetrate the periosteum and SOOF layer 4 mm below the orbital rim in order to elevate all midfacial soft tissue layers and facilitate placement of any type of midface implant.

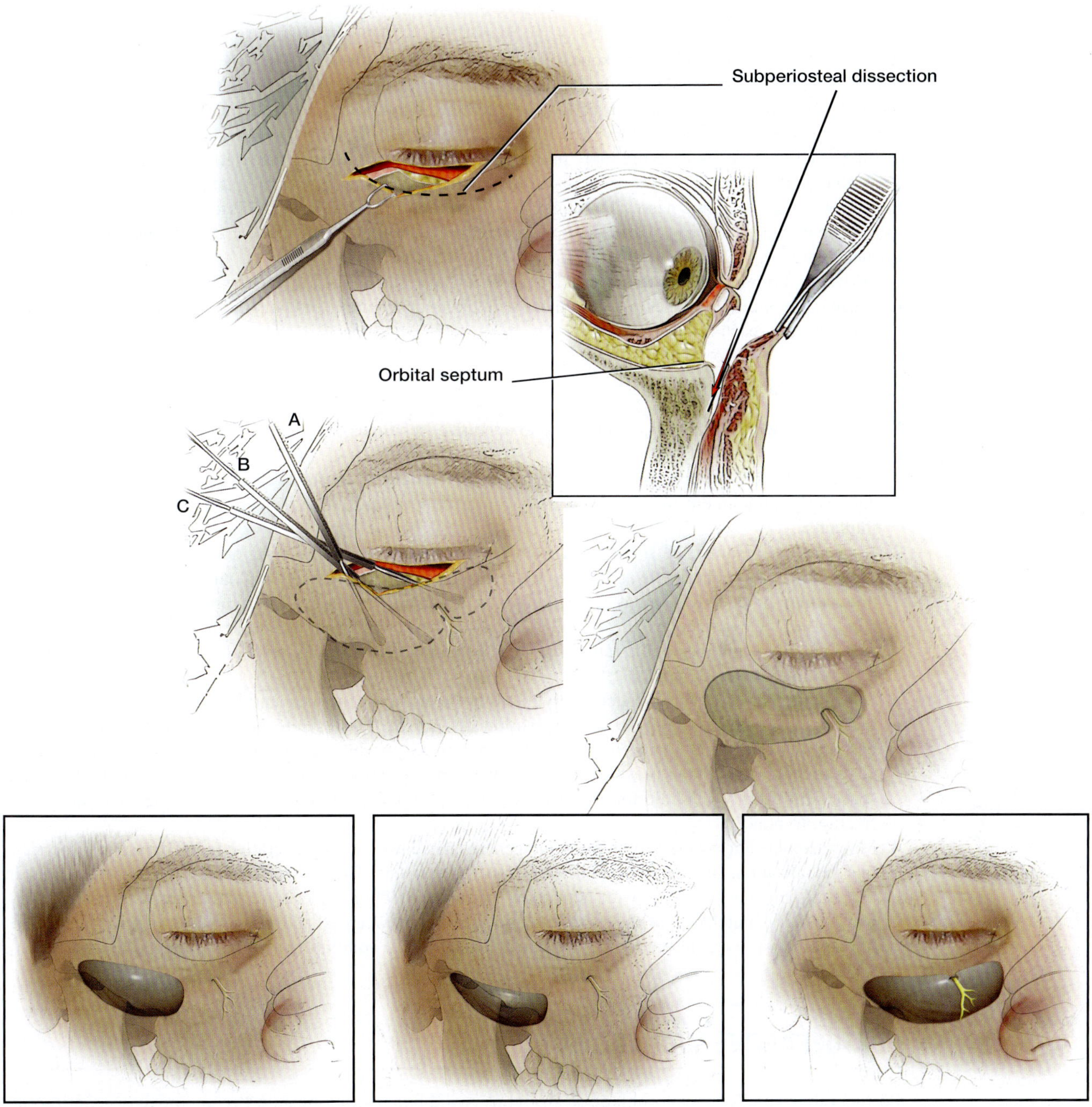

FIGURE 33.27 Shows the external limited lateral lower eyelid skin–muscle flap approach to exposing zones 1 and 2 and submalar 5 for placing any style midfacial implant.

When used for implant placement alone, the incision is limited to a length of 10 to 15 mm. It is designed only in the middle to lateral third of the lower eyelid, in the subcilial region. Moreover, the dissection inferiorly provides a sturdy shelf upon which the implant rests. A midfacial implant for any purpose can be inserted using a subcilial or a transconjunctival approach (Fig. 33.27).

If a rhytidectomy insertion is intended, a small penetration is made through the soft tissues over the lateral aspect of the malar bone at the junction with the zygomatic arch. This provides entrance into the subperiosteal malar space easily and in an area where no major facial nerve branches are endangered.

Tear trough implants can be placed through an external subciliary blepharoplasty incision, a transconjunctival incision, or an intraoral route. The tear trough implant is placed after cutting out a segment, which allows it to surround the main trunk of the infraorbital nerve. If desired, it can be secured by one or two sutures to the medial orbicularis muscles or to the inferior orbital rim.

The greatest advantage of the subcilial blepharoplasty approach is the opportunity for correct positioning because the surgeon is able to directly observe the relationship of the implant to the inferior orbital arcus marginalis.

Rhytidectomy Approach

Zone 1 of the malar region is a safe zone for penetration through the SMAS into the malar space. There are no named branches of the facial nerve in that region. Once the rhytidectomy flap is elevated over zones 1 and 2, the roof of the malar space can be directly penetrated through the SMAS with a small, sharp elevator onto the malar bone. This may be done either medial or lateral to the zygomaticus origins. The seventh nerve branches leading to the frontalis muscle run more proximal over the middle third of the zygomatic arch, and the motor nerve to the orbicularis oculi is more superior. By creating a transverse aperture that parallels the fibers of the facial nerve, the risk to the nerve is minimal. It is important to remember that dissection backward along the zygomatic arch is necessary to position a malar shell implant comfortably and correctly without a buckling of the lateral tail.

Rhytidectomy insertion offers two advantages: (1) a sterile and readily accessible entry wound and (2) a reasonable opportunity for accurate placement with direct observation and palpation. This being stated, I have not used this approach frequently.

Points of Emphasis

I offer the following suggestions with regard to operative technique:

1. Stay directly on the bone and the periosteum. Placement of implants directly on bone creates a firm and secure attachment to the skeleton. Capsular contracture has not been seen with facial anatomic implants.
2. Be gentle in elevating the soft tissues from the malar and premandible regions. When there is adequate infiltration of local anesthetic agents, the tissue planes separate easily and without need for force. Excessive trauma may produce trigeminal nerve symptoms, transient or prolonged, but rarely permanent. Paresis or paralysis of the zygomaticus, the orbicularis oculi, and even the frontalis muscle may also occur. Such damage is usually temporary, but in rare cases it can be permanent. This has never occurred in my series of over 3,500 chin implants.
3. Expand the dissection space adequately in either the malar or the premandible regions to accommodate the chosen prostheses comfortably. Elevation of the soft tissues into areas adjacent to bone should be done with a blunt-edged elevator and as gently as possible. Anatomically contoured implants of adequate size and shape present very few problems in malposition or mobility because they fill the space comfortably and hold their position by virtue of their contoured posterior surface and their rapid fixation to bone.
4. Minimize bleeding by using both local and general anesthesia. A "dry operative field" is essential for accurate visualization, precise dissection, and proper placement. These three critical factors are essential in avoiding potential problems with hematoma, seroma, infection, inaccurate placement, and nerve injury. Once again, maintenance of the systolic blood pressure between 90 and 110 provides optimal hemostasis in combination with infiltration of a dilute lidocaine 0.2% solution containing epinephrine (Adrenalin), 1:800,000.

POSTOPERATIVE MANAGEMENT

Postoperative care for facial implants is straightforward and uncomplicated. Perioperative oral antibiotics are used. At the present time, cephalosporins are favored. Prior to the start of surgery, the anesthesiologist gives 1 to 2 g of Ancef intravenously. 10 mg of Decadron are also given intravenously during the surgery to control postoperative edema. During the postoperative period a 5-day diminishing course of steroid in the form of a Medrol dose pack is taken orally. For the first 12 hours, cold compresses are applied intermittently to the operative site. No bandages are used. Removal of intraoral mucosal and external subcuticular sutures is unnecessary. A soft diet is maintained for 10 days. It is highly recommended that the patient recline at a 45-degree angle and in the supine position for at least 1 week. *Vigorous physical activity is not permitted for 4 weeks.* After this time period patients may engage in any and all types of exercise activities.

COMPLICATIONS

There are several major disadvantages when using alloplastic materials:

1. Possibilities of severe infection, especially with porous materials that become infiltrated with fibrotic ingrowths or bone sequestrum that complicates easy removal.

2. Contour abnormalities of an unattractive or even disfiguring nature when implants do not have the proper shape, size and positioning.
3. Possibilities for damage to the facial nerve and musculature due to excessive and inappropriate trauma during dissection to introduce or to remove the implant materials.
4. Complications from the intraoral approach include dysesthesias from damage to the infraorbital nerve or motor dysfunction of the orbicularis oris musculature. Nerve symptoms may be attributed to transection of small branches in the lip during the incision or direct damage to the major nerve bundle during dissection or pressure impingement on the nerve from an implant. These complications, however, are rare and almost nonexistent when the previously stated guidelines to dissection are applied.
5. Use of traditional transverse incisions through the muscle pillars of the zygomaticus produce traumatic transection, resulting in transient and perhaps even permanent damage to muscle function. This can inhibit normal lip elevation.
6. During the subciliary dissection, the infraorbital nerve is also intentionally avoided. An incision is made in the periosteum 3 to 4 mm anterior to the orbital rim along its lateral aspect, to obviate potential adhesions that may result in ectropion and lower lid contracture. A skin flap should *never* be used, because it always shrinks and predisposes to eyelid retraction and ectropion. By using a skin–muscle flap approach, however, there should be no trauma to the orbicularis muscle.
7. Excessive muscle damage, with bleeding into lid tissues, stimulates fibrosis and contracture within the middle lamella of the lower eyelid, producing ectropion. Standard lateral canthopexy techniques are used to minimize this possibility. Resection of skin and muscle flap should be conservative (i.e., minimal to no excision) because of additional traction exerted on the lower eyelid from the volume expansion caused by the implant under the malar tissues.

RESULTS

Alloplastic facial implantation is reliable, safe, and easily reversible. The improvement of facial contours by augmentation of the appropriate facial zones yields consistent results in facial rejuvenation and restoring a youthful appearance. The determination of the proper augmentation, implant selection, active involvement of and open dialogue with the patient including clarification of patient goals results in a successful surgery and a highly satisfied cosmetic patient (Table 33.3).

PEARLS

- Infection and cellulitis around facial implants made of silicone rubber (Silastic) can almost always be resolved by antibiotics and/or drainage procedures when necessary.
- Smooth-surfaced silicone rubber (Silastic) implants have a thin overlying capsule immobilizing them. They are easy to insert and easy to remove or replace.
- Implants placed in a subperiosteal location directly on bone or a stable base such as the masseter muscle will be fixed and nonmobile. Nonsubperiosteal placement will result in mobility.
- Bone remodeling or erosion occurs to a degree with all implant materials. With my more than 50 years of experience, no significant number of malar–zygomatic–suborbital bone erosion problems.
- Except for complete transactions or major damage, nearly all nerve injuries completely recover with time.

TABLE 33.3 Surgical Treatment Plan Malar—Midface Augmentation Regional Volume-MASS Deficiencies Anatomic Zone Augmentation Size

Facial Type	Anatomic Augmentation Zone	Size (Depends on Skull Size)
1	1 and 2	3 or 4 mm (occasionally 5 or 6 mm)
2	SM5	4 or 5 mm (possibly a combined shell)
3	SM5	5 or 6 mm (large or extra large)
4	1, 2, SM5	5 or 6 mm malar shell (large or extra large)
5	3	Tear trough implant (small, medium or large)
6	Premaxilla	Various premaxilla Implants Brink implant[a]

[a]IMPLANTECH Corp., Ventura, California.

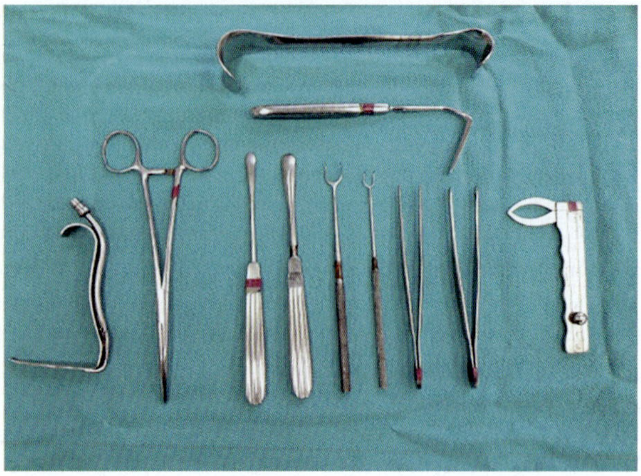

FIGURE 33.28 Surgery instruments used in performing facial implant insertions.

PITFALLS

- Not analyzing and discussing with patients their preexisting asymmetries and the impossibility of predicting total correction thereof.
- Attempting reoperations, improvements, or corrections during the interval of 17 days to 1 year following initial procedures when reactivation of scar contracture is restimulated and/or density of scar adherences can predispose to nerve damage.
- Letting a patient convince the surgeon that the implants are too big or out of a desired position before 6 months to 1 year when nearly all swelling has subsided.
- Making a subperiosteal implant space too big or too small.
- "Forcing" a dissection in areas around the infraorbital nerves. This is of particular concern in the midface–submalar and malar–zygomatic areas when trying to expand the space more posterolaterally, where the main trunks and branches of the facial nerve reside.

INSTRUMENTATION

Using alloplastic techniques and facial surgery requires very few special instruments (Fig. 33.28):

- Goulet mouth retractor to expose incision sites
- Two Aufricht retractors with 2-cm-wide blades and blunt teeth (5- and 7-inch-long blades)
- Two Obwegeser periosteal elevators (8- and 12-mm-wide blades)
- A long curved clamp to insert implants
- Two 2-cm-wide sharp double hooks
- Cushing retractor
- Russian forceps, medium length
- One pair of dressing forceps, medium length

With these few instruments, any implant insertion in the face may be performed with relative ease.

ACKNOWLEDGMENTS

The author would like to thank Ron Hazani, MD, and Alicia Sanderson, MD, for their contributions in the writing of this chapter. Their work in the writing, editing, and figure creation for this chapter is greatly appreciated.

SUGGESTED READING

Binder WJ, Shire JR, eds. Custom designed facial implants. *Facial Plast Clin North Am* 2008;16(1):133–146.

Carboni A, Gasparini G, Perugini M, et al. Evaluation of homologous bone graft versus biomaterials in the aesthetic restoration of the middle third of the face. *Minerva Chir* 2002;57(3):283–287.

Rubin LR, Walden RH. A seven year evaluation of polyethylene in facial reconstructive surgery. *Plast Reconstr Surg* 1955;16(5):392–407.

Sevin K, Askar I, Saray A, et al. Exposure of high-density porous polyethylene (Medpor) used for contour restoration and treatment. *Br J Oral Maxillofac Surg* 2000;38(1):44–49.

Terino EO. Alloplastic facial contouring: surgery of the fourth plane. *Aesthetic Plast Surg* 1992;16(3):195–212.

34 MENTOPLASTY

Harry Mittelman

INTRODUCTION

While facial aesthetics has evolved over time, the balance of facial proportions is a common and universal aesthetic ideal. A straight and central mentum with smooth transitions to the lateral mandible defines an aesthetically pleasing and youthful chin. Augmentation and contouring of the chin and mandible are essential procedures in addressing age or congenitally related conditions. These procedures have become increasingly popular due to the improved understanding of changes in the mandible over time as well as the continued evolution of alloplastic implants. Many materials are used for augmentation including Gore-Tex, Medpor, Acrylico, Mersilene mesh, and solid flexible silicone. In my opinion, the silicone implants are by far the implants that are easiest to work with and least reactive. These implants are anatomically and artistically designed to deliver a significant improvement in what is commonly a relatively straightforward procedure. Alloplastic implantation is also completely reversible—a feature that may help broaden its appeal to prospective, but anxious patients. The size of the implant can also be adjusted to specific patient and surgeon desires.

The variety of materials that are available for augmentation of the mandible may, at first, be overwhelming. This perception is further heightened with the diversity of injectable fillers used to augment the facial soft tissues. It has become possible to achieve "surgical results" with the materials available, but such changes commonly require additional interventions and maintenance. With an erudite understanding of the morphologic differences between individual mandibles, and the aging process as it applies to them, permanent implant selection becomes much more clear-cut. More simply stated, a small number of alloplastic extended mandibular implants can fulfill the vast majority of the facial plastic surgeon's clinical challenges. Few other procedures in the surgeon's repertoire yield as much benefit for as little time and effort expended as augmentation of the mandible with a properly chosen alloplastic implant.

HISTORY

As with all patients pursuing cosmetic surgery, the history should begin by evaluating each patient's motivation and emotional state to ensure that these are appropriate. Pertinent points in a patient's history should include previous surgeries, facial trauma, dental/orthognathic procedures, bleeding problems, and anesthetic risk factors. Medical issues such as osteoporosis, previous cancer of the oral cavity, history of intravenous (IV) bisphosphonates, or radiation treatment should be evaluated and the results documented. Once a detailed medical history is completed, the surgeon should focus on the patient's prior history of cosmetic procedures, including injectable fillers, as these are often directly or mistakenly omitted by the patient when completing standard preoperative questionnaires. It is critically important to identify any signs of functional mandibular problems, dysplasia, malocclusion, or temporomandibular joint dysfunction. These conditions are not directly addressed by chin augmentation and should prompt a referral to the appropriate specialist for further evaluation.

PHYSICAL EXAMINATION

Relevant Anatomy

While the basic anatomy of the mandible is familiar to the facial cosmetic surgeon, some points about the mental nerve are worth emphasizing. The mental foramen transmits the mental nerve, which exits in a superior direction and supplies sensation to the lower lip and chin. The expected location of the mental nerve is inferior to the second mandibular premolar on either side, although significant variability can exist in up to 50% of patients, with slight displacement of the mental foramen either anterior or posterior to this. In the typical young adult mandible, the mental foramen is located approximately halfway between the alveolar ridge and the inferior border of the mandible, and approximately 25 mm lateral to the midline, within a range of 20 to 30 mm. In children, the mental foramen lies closer to the inferior border of the mandible and slightly more anterior. During the aging process, atrophy of the alveolar ridge causes the foramen to lie in a relatively more superior position, since the distance to the inferior border of the mandible remains fairly constant. Even in the aging mandible, there is generally a distance of more than 8 mm between the mental foramen and the inferior border of the mandible at the site of the muscular attachments.

The surgeon must dissect carefully when creating a pocket for the implant that is below the mental foramen yet immediately above the muscular attachments at the inferior border of the mandible. Generally, one has approximately 10 mm of space in this area. Properly designed implants should have a vertical height of 6 to 8 mm when placed into this area. The facial nerve is unlikely to be damaged with the use of extended Silastic mandibular augmentation.

Care should be taken to avoid injury to the mentalis muscle. The mentalis muscle is a fan-shaped muscle separated in the midline by a firm septum. From an intraoral approach, one should take care not to strip the mentalis muscle from its origin.

Aesthetic Analysis

The basic tenets of facial aesthetic proportions have been summarized by Powell and Humphreys and include both a frontal and a lateral assessment. The frontal view of the face may be divided into thirds, with the lower third extending from the subnasale to the menton. This lower third can be subdivided so that the upper third is occurring from the subnasale to the stomion superius and the lower two thirds occurring from the stomion inferius to the menton. There is loss of the vertical height and anterior projection of the mandible with advancing age, resulting in a loss of the ideal proportions. Simultaneously, during this aging process, the soft tissues covering the mandible often display some atrophy as well as laxity. On lateral view, the method of Gonzalez-Ulloa may be applied to define a hypoplastic mentum. In this technique, a line is dropped from the nasion perpendicular to the Frankfort horizontal plane. The ideal chin projection should be at this line. However, when the chin is posterior to this line and the patient has a Class I occlusion, then a hypoplastic mentum is present. Another frequently used method is to simply drop a line from vermilion of the lower lip perpendicular to the Frankfort horizontal plane. Once again, the ideal chin projection should be at this line and a chin posterior to this line with Class I occlusion is considered hypoplastic. While a man's ideal pogonion position is tangential to this line, a woman's ideal position may lie 1 to 2 mm posterior to it.

Physical Examination

While assessing a patient for chin augmentation, the surgeon should be attentive to both the patient's individual anatomy and his/her appearance in relation to that patient's aesthetic ideal. More importantly, the surgeon should evaluate for any functional disturbance of the mandible (malocclusion, temporomandibular joint dysfunction). One must evaluate both the underlying skeletal structure as well as the overlying soft tissue envelope, as these elements contribute to the aesthetic lines of the jaw and cervicomental angle. The mentalis muscle and overlying soft tissue pad should be evaluated and palpated, and any pathology should be noted. Patients with a severely hypoplastic mentum and strong mentalis strain leading to lip incompetence should be considered for osseous advancement.

Although the development of a hypoplastic mentum is largely determined by genetic factors, the development of a prejowl sulcus is primarily the result of aging. However, the prejowl sulcus, or antigonion notch, may also be congenital and be present from childhood. A combination of progressive soft tissue atrophy and gradual bony resorption of the inferior mandibular edge between the chin and the remainder of the body of the mandible results in the development of the anterior mandibular groove, as named by the author in 1981. This area is known as the prejowl sulcus (Fig. 34.1). With continued aging, the prejowl sulcus may merge with the commissure–mandibular groove, or "Marionette line," further accentuating the aging jawline.

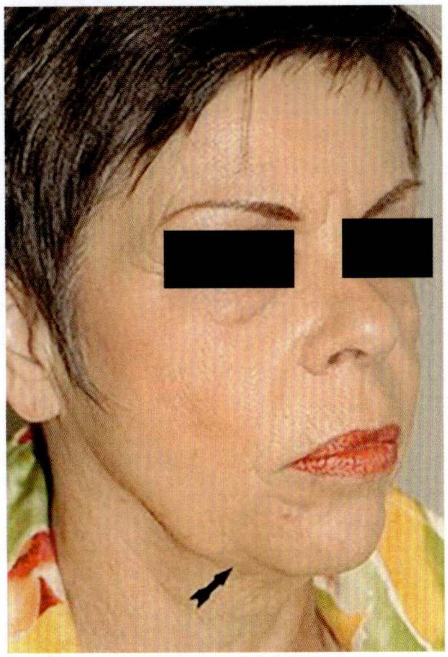

FIGURE 34.1
Patient with a hypoplastic mentum and prejowl sulcus (*black arrow*) secondary to aging.

INDICATIONS

The main indication for chin augmentation is mild microgenia. As described above, there are a number of different methods to describe the appropriate relationship of chin position to the rest of the face. I prefer to use a straight line perpendicular to the Frankfort horizontal dropped from the vermillion to estimate appropriate anterior projection.

The presence of a prejowl sulcus is an indication for prejowl augmentation. While deficiency of volume in the prejowl area may be related to bony deficiency or to soft tissue deficiency alone, it is often multifactorial. Mild soft tissue deficiency in the prejowl area may suggest that the patient may benefit from injection of soft tissue filler injection only.

CONTRAINDICATIONS

Severe microgenia is a contraindication to augmentation mentoplasty as is a patient with unrealistic expectations. Other relative contraindications include labial incompetence, lip protrusion, shortened mandibular height, severe malocclusion, and periodontal disease.

PREOPERATIVE PLANNING

Chin augmentation is frequently done in conjunction with other procedures, such as rhinoplasty or rhytidoplasty. Since chin projection is best viewed in profile, many patients are unaware of deficiencies when seeking consultation to improve their submental or nasal appearance. It behooves the astute facial plastic surgeon to always consider the importance of chin projection or irregular mandibular contour and explain the importance to the patient in order to obtain an optimal, balanced result (Fig. 34.2).

Preoperative photography with a minimum of frontal, lateral, and oblique views, ensuring that the patient is placed in the Frankfort plane, is essential for photodocumentation of the preoperative appearance and for implant sizing. Computer simulation is a useful tool to demonstrate the benefit of chin augmentation, especially for those patients who do not seek improvement in this area during their initial consultation (Fig. 34.3). Preoperatively, it is critical that the surgeon identify, document, and discuss with the patient any existing asymmetry, which otherwise may be noticed by the patient only after surgery. Also mandatory are preoperative assessment and discussion of occlusion with the patient, since alloplastic implants will not affect the patient's occlusal status. Any desire by the patients to functionally improve their occlusion would be more appropriately addressed in orthognathic surgery.

It is most important to fully discuss the risks of surgery, especially paresthesia of the chin and lower lip. These are frequently resolved within 6 weeks of surgery but can persist for months. Rarely, some numbness of a portion of the chin and/or lip may be permanent.

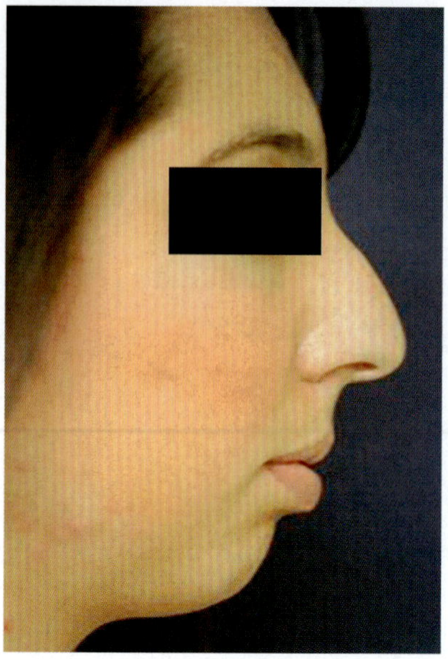

FIGURE 34.2
Preoperative view of a patient presenting for cosmetic rhinoplasty, with a severely hypoplastic mentum in addition to a dorsal hump nasal deformity. She would likely be an excellent candidate for augmentation mentoplasty at the time of rhinoplasty.

Implant Selection

An ideal approach to chin augmentation requires an understanding of alloplastic implants, autologous augmentation materials (adipose tissue, fascia), and injectable fillers. Often, the use of a single modality can produce an acceptable outcome. However, taking advantage of the synergy between multiple modalities of chin augmentation can produce the most natural and long-lasting results. While a thorough discussion of adipose tissue grafts and their applications are beyond the scope of this chapter, adipose tissue grafts can be placed in such a way that they are long lasting, integrated, and natural in appearance. However, variable resorption, growth, and migration of injected adipose tissue grafts can lead to unpredictable clinical results with undesirable contours and bulges that are difficult to correct.

Hyaluronic acid (HA) fillers can be used alone to augment the mentum or to fill the soft tissue deficits of a prejowl sulcus, thus returning the contour of the jawline to a more youthful, straight, configuration (Fig. 34.4). The added safety profile of these fillers provided by the potential use of hyaluronidase to reverse, alter, or refine the HA injection provides a degree of safety not previously possible. Other injectable alloplastic materials, including poly-L-lactic acid (Sculptra, Dermik-Bridgewater, NJ) can be used to serially augment the soft tissues of the mentum and prejowl area to soften contour irregularity and increase projection.

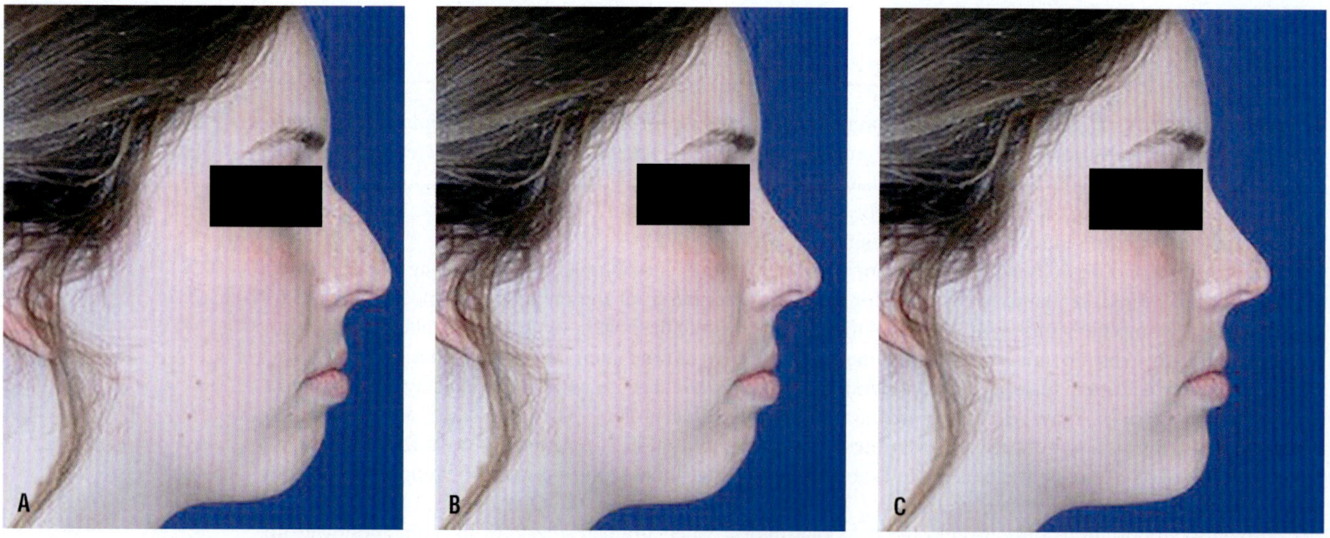

FIGURE 34.3 **(A)** Preoperative photograph and computer-imaging photographs showing the potential changes to facial balance with **(B)** rhinoplasty alone or **(C)** rhinoplasty with chin augmentation implant.

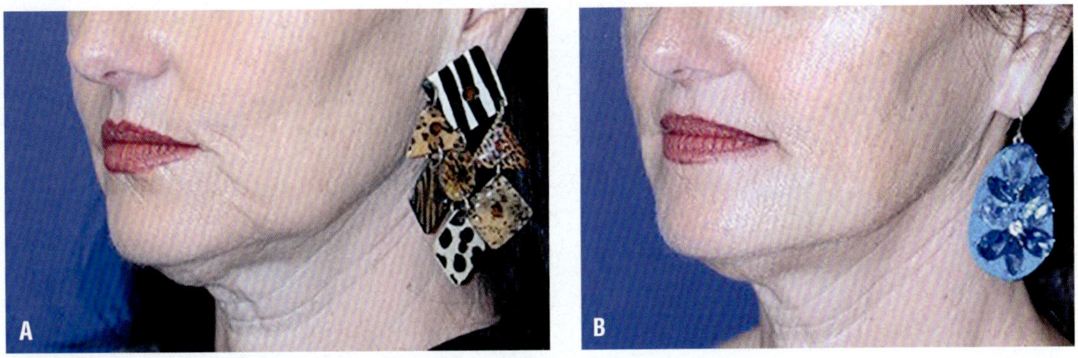

FIGURE 34.4 **A:** Pretreatment photograph illustrating development of mild jowling and prejowl sulcus. **B:** Posttreatment photograph after treatment with 1 syringe of hyaluronic acid filler, with excellent improvement in prejowl sulcus and reestablishment of a youthful jawline contour.

The ideal mandibular implant should have the proper consistency, flexibility, and firmness for facile implantation. Moreover, it should be nonreactive and resistant to infection and should maintain a stable shape and position after placement. If the need arises, it should be readily removable. The ideal implant should also be easily manufactured and reproducible so that minimal intraoperative modification is required. In my judgment, the alloplastic material that best meets these criteria is a solid, but flexible, silicone elastic polymer (Silastic).

Silastic is a polymer that can be chemically altered to modify its consistency with the goal of achieving an optimal balance of stability, natural feel, and flexibility. Within the body, Silastic is nonreactive and becomes enveloped with a nondistorting fibrous capsule. Fenestrated Silastic implants may be further stabilized by tissue ingrowth. If indicated, the surgeon may further modify Silastic implants by trimming the edges with conventional instruments.

Selection of one of the many commercially available Silastic mandibular implants can be confusing. The first decision must be the use of an extended mandibular implant rather than a central chin implant. Central chin augmentation alone can result in an unnatural, nonanatomic, pointed chin and poorly defined jawline. Central chin implants frequently migrate, creating asymmetry (Fig. 34.5). Properly designed extended mandibular implants have tapered ends that provide a smooth transition from the central mentum to the lateral mandible, preserving the natural jawline.

Some of the most commonly used implants are the extended anatomical mandibular implant, the Mittelman Pre Jowl Chin implants, the Mittelman Pre Jowl implants, the Terino Square Chin implants, and the Flowers chin implants. Each variety of implant is available in a number of sizes and configurations. While these implants provide a slightly different configuration and philosophy, all can provide excellent results. The extended anatomical mandibular implant provides uniform augmentation of the prejowl area with varying degrees of central chin augmentation. The Flowers mandibular implants provide a variation in the tilt of the implant at the central mentum with a tapered extension along the mandible beneath the mental foramen.

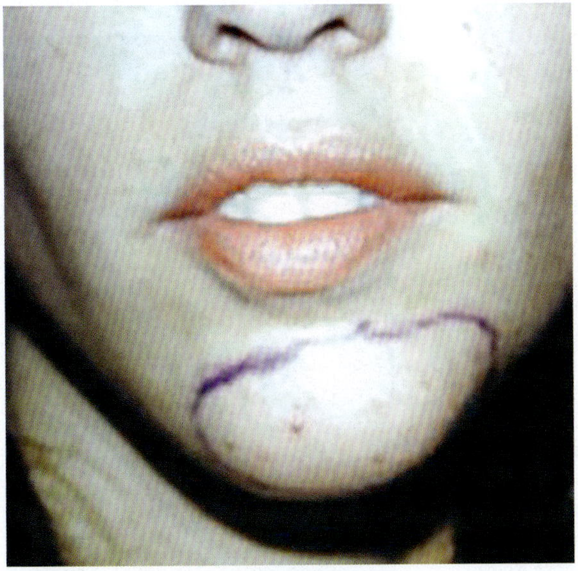

FIGURE 34.5
Patient with a central chin implant which has migrated. The position of the implant has been marked.

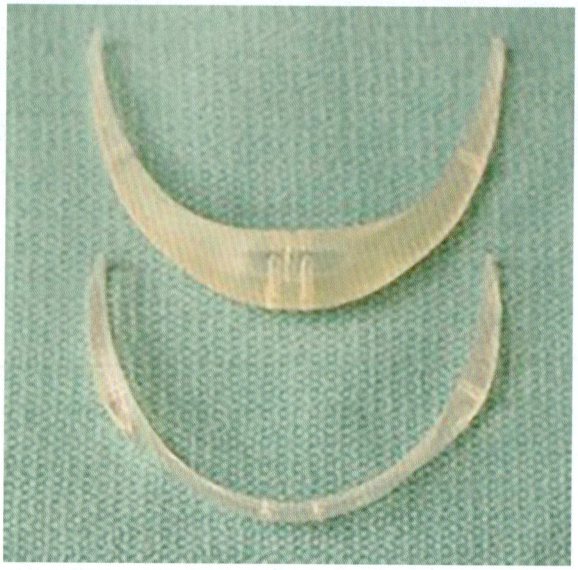

FIGURE 34.6
The Mittelman Pre Jowl Chin implant (*above*) and the Mittelman Pre Jowl implant (*below*). Note the thin profile in the central segment of the prejowl implant.

The extended prejowl–chin implant provides four progressive variations in size of central mentum augmentation with a comparable increase in thickness in its lateral extensions, which provide augmentation to the prejowl area. In addition, the extended mandibular prejowl implant (without chin/mentum augmentation) is designed to provide stable augmentation of the prejowl area, without affecting chin projection (Fig. 34.6). In my hands, this implant has proven invaluable for the facelift patient who has adequate chin projection but a significant prejowl sulcus. In another modification of the extended anatomical chin implant, Dr. Terino has a more squared anterior projection, which can be especially suitable for some male patients.

SURGICAL TECHNIQUE

This procedure can be performed either under local or general anesthesia. If the patient is placed under general anesthesia, the endotracheal tube is secured to the central incisors with either 0 silk suture or dental floss. The incision is marked with a surgical marking pen. The submental incision is generally placed immediately anterior to the submental crease, since placement of the incision within the crease may result in a more depressed scar and an accentuated submental crease. The soft tissue midline is then located and marked on the pogonion for reference (Fig. 34.7). Approximately 5 mL of local anesthetic (the author prefers a 1:1 mixture of 1% lidocaine and 0.5% bupivacaine, with 1:100,000 epinephrine) is injected into the skin and soft tissues of the submental crease. The instruments and implant are soaked in a solution of gentamicin (20 mL of 40 mg/mL IV gentamicin solution in 300 mL saline) in preparation for use.

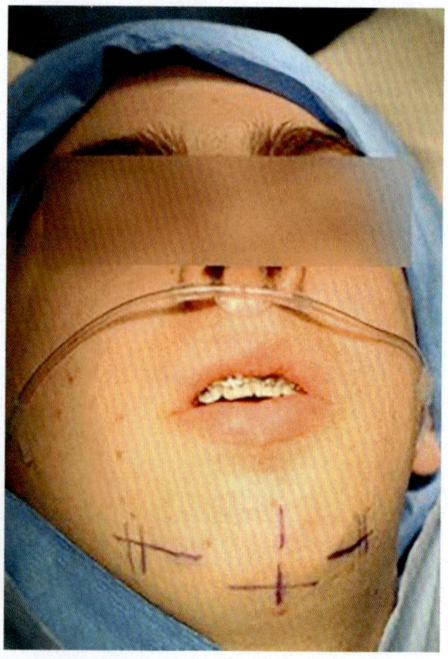

FIGURE 34.7
The surgical patient is a 16-year-old male with a severely hypoplastic mentum. His occlusion is normal (Class 1). Note that in patients who are functionally comfortable with their Class II or Class III malocclusion but want cosmetic improvement, mandibular augmentation with Silastic implants is ideal.

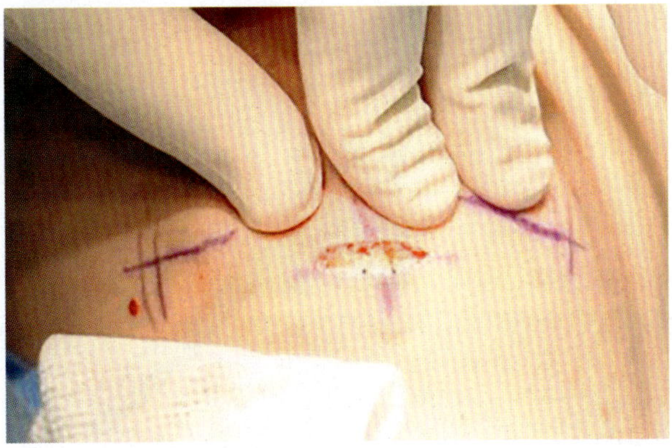

FIGURE 34.8
The submental incision is generally placed immediately anterior to the submental crease, since placement of the incision within the crease may result in a more depressed scar and an accentuated submental crease.

A 1- to 2-cm transverse incision is made with a 15-blade scalpel. The middle of the incision should line up with the soft tissue midline as well as the center of the lips, central incisors, nasal columella (Fig. 34.8). Dissection then proceeds in the same transverse plane with a monopolar cautery and cold steel through the subcutaneous tissues and mentalis, until the anterior periosteum is identified (Fig. 34.9). The periosteum is then incised with a scalpel in a transverse direction. A small periosteal elevator is used to elevate the periosteum superiorly until an appropriate periosteal flap is created that can accommodate the superior–inferior dimension of the chosen implant (Fig. 34.10). The inferior periosteal flap is also elevated, but to a lesser degree (approximately 2 to 3 mm). Some authors advocate leaving a central portion of intact periosteum on the mandible, placing the central portion of the implant supraperiosteally with the lateral thirds of the implant placed subperiosteally, in the belief that mandibular resorption in the central area of the implant may be decreased. However, I generally undermine the periosteum throughout. Resorption does occur but does not appear to be clinically significant.

Attention is turned to the creation of the right-sided subperiosteal tunnel. This is done with a small periosteal elevator in the surgeon's dominant hand while at the same time the other "smart" hand is placed with the thumb and first finger grasping the mandible at the estimated location of the mental foramen (Fig. 34.11). Care is taken to dissect along the inferior border of the mandible, raising a precise subperiosteal pocket that is just wide and long enough to accommodate the implant, avoiding the location of the mental foramen and nerve. Because the neurovascular bundle is encased in a strong, connective tissue sheath and exits the mental foramen in a superior direction, the use of an elevator in this space may touch the sheath and may stretch it to some degree. Once the right-side pocket is created, a small volume of antibiotic-containing saline is poured into the dissection pocket, and attention is turned to the left side. An identical procedure is performed, with creation of a subperiosteal pocket of appropriate dimensions to accommodate the lateral extension of the implant.

Attention then turns to placement of the implant. The surgeon and assistant bathe their hands in antibiotic-containing solution. The implant is then grasped on its right lateral end with a straight Kelly clamp and placed into the right subperiosteal pocket. It is often helpful to ask the assistant to grasp the left end of the implant and prevent its contact with skin, as this helps maintain the sterility of the implant (Fig. 34.12). The implant should slide with relative ease into the pocket. It is then grasped on the left lateral end, folded acutely on itself, and the implant is guided into the left subperiosteal pocket (Fig. 34.13). While performing these maneuvers, it is helpful to maintain the nondominant "smart" hand over the location of the mental foramen and nerve, which helps prevent dissection of a false passage by the implant itself. Proper positioning of the implant is confirmed by palpation of its lateral extensions, and midline positioning of the central portion is confirmed by lining up the blue mark on the implant with the previously marked soft tissue midline (Fig. 34.14). If difficulty is encountered during insertion of the implant after a pocket was created,

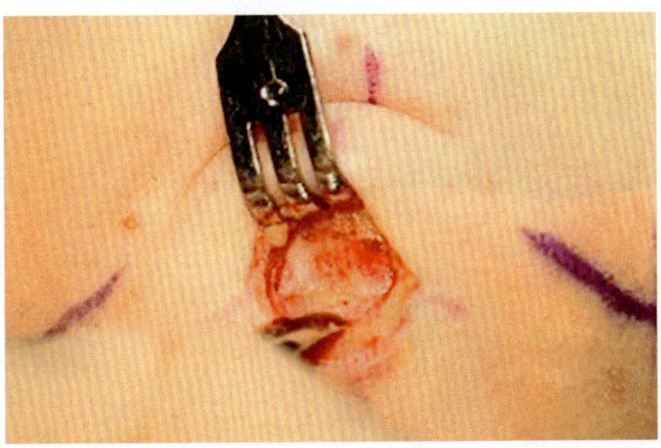

FIGURE 34.9
Dissection proceeds through the mentalis muscle to reveal the periosteum of the mandible in the central portion.

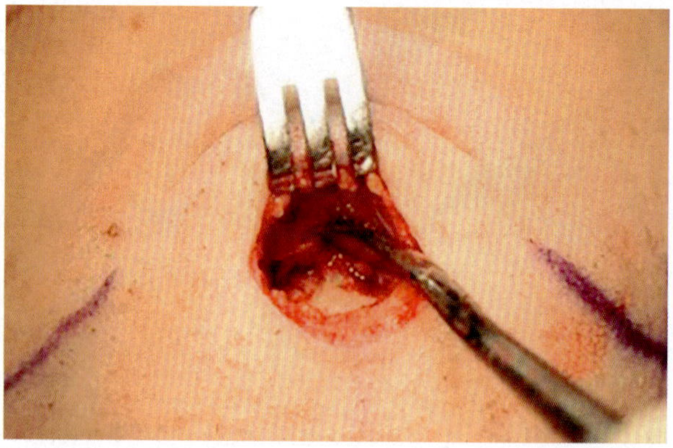

FIGURE 34.10
The periosteum is undermined for several millimeters inferiorly and approximately 2 cm superiorly to expose the central mentum.

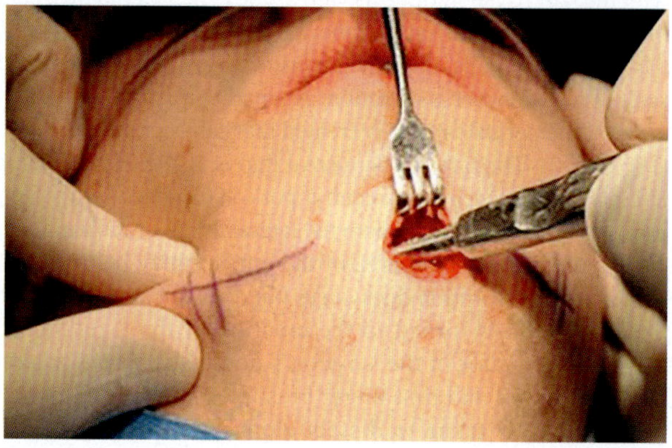

FIGURE 34.11
The dissection continues laterally in the subperiosteal plane between the muscular attachments at the inferior border of the mandible and the mental nerve superiorly. Note the surgeon's right hand holding the periosteal elevator, while the left "smart" hand protects the nerve of the mental foramen and assists in guiding the elevator along the anteroinferior border of the mandible. This helps to prevent excursions above the intended dissection pocket. Lateral dissection should extend approximately 6 to 7 cm from the midline, depending on the size of the implant.

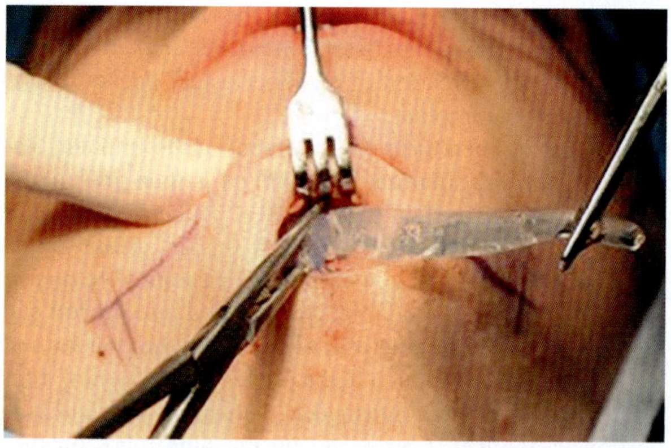

FIGURE 34.12
The implant is removed from the gentamicin solution and placed in the subperiosteal pocket. Two straight clamps are used to guide the implant into the right lateral pocket first. Note that the assistant holds the left half of the implant to help prevent contact with and potential contamination by the skin.

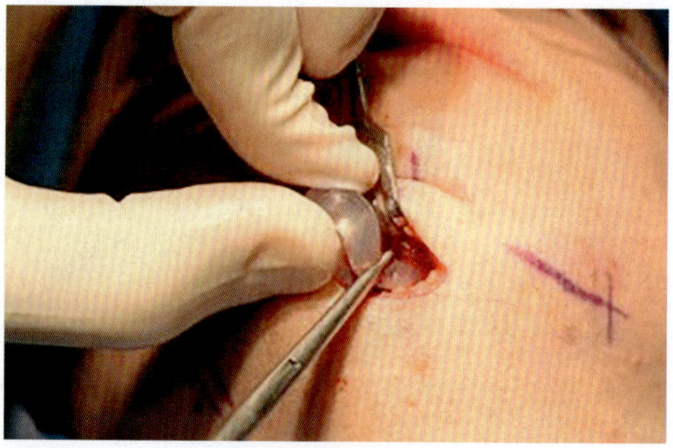

FIGURE 34.13
After the right one-half of the implant is placed in the pocket, the implant is folded acutely on itself and the left half of the implant is guided with clamps and retractors into the left pocket.

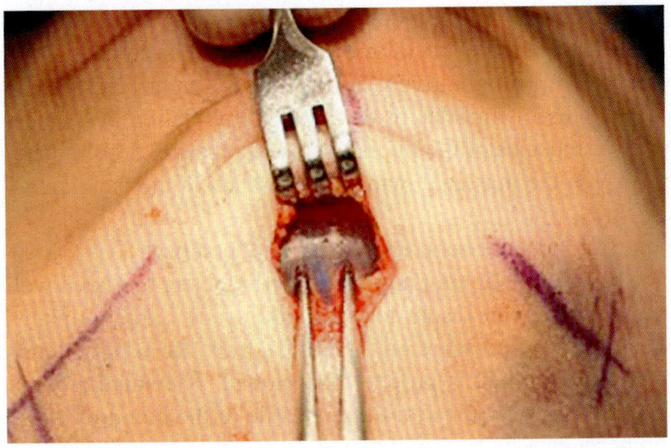

FIGURE 34.14
Midline placement of the implant is confirmed with the implant's vertical *blue line*. The *blue line* should line up with the previously marked central point of the mentum. The implant is then secured with a suture, and layered closure is then completed.

the surgeon must identify where the obstruction lies. This may be due to failure of extending the dissection far enough laterally. More commonly, the obstruction is found immediately lateral to the central dissection zone, since the implant is still prominent in its vertical height in that location as it tapers from the center to the lateral extensions. This is the location of the anterior mandibular ligament, which is somewhat resistant to elevation in most patients.

The implant is then secured to the inferior periosteum with 3-0 Prolene suture to prevent migration. The superior periosteum is then reapproximated with the inferior periosteum and sutured with interrupted 3-0 Prolene sutures. The overlying muscle and soft tissues are then closed with inverting sutures in layered fashion using 4-0 Prolene, and the skin is closed in a meticulous single layer closure with the surgeon's preferred suture.

POSTOPERATIVE MANAGEMENT

Patients receiving alloplastic implants are always placed on intraoperative and postoperative antibiotics. In those patients without allergy, IV cefazolin 1,000 mg is given 30 minutes prior to incision. The patient continues on cephalexin 500 mg twice daily for 5 days postoperatively. A light compressive dressing is used when chin augmentation is performed concurrently with rhytidectomy or submentoplasty and is removed 24 hours after surgery. This dressing is generally unnecessary when chin augmentation is performed as a stand-alone procedure. During the healing period, the patient is instructed to avoid manipulation or any trauma of the chin or prejowl area. Sutures are removed by 7 days postoperatively, and the incision is reinforced with Steri-Strips for 1 week following suture removal.

COMPLICATIONS

Fortunately, the number of complications from placement of alloplastic mandibular implants is small, and most are temporary. When complications occur, they are usually easily treatable. In the case of improper implant selection or patient preference, the implant may be exchanged for a different size or removed in a relatively simple procedure.

- **Infection:** Risks with mandibular augmentation implants is similar to many other facial plastic surgical procedures. However, this can be minimized by the use of meticulous technique and the incorporation of intraoperative gentamicin solution to bathe all instruments, the alloplastic implant, and the surgically created subperiosteal pockets prior to implantation. It is also important to place the patient on prophylactic antibiotics before and after the procedure. I have not experienced an infection since using perioperative gentamicin solution. If infection were to occur, it usually entails an aggressive regimen of oral antibiotics. This should resolve the problem, but if infection persists, then removing the implant, waiting for proper healing, and consideration of replacement of the implant at a later time would be appropriate.
- **Sensory alterations:** These are more common occurrences and are the most important negative sequelae of this procedure. Twenty to thirty percent of patients may expect some hypoesthesia of the mental nerve distribution on one or both sides. Hypoesthesia is almost always temporary and must be discussed with the patient preoperatively. A period of observation for many weeks is indicated before taking any action if the implant was placed properly. Often, a "tingle" or "pins-and-needles" sensation will herald the return of sensation. Occasionally, a longer lasting hypoesthesia may be the result of improper dissection of the lateral pocket and placement of the implant superior to the mental nerve foramen. In such a case, removal of the implant with or without replacement must take place.

- **Motor Nerve Impairment:** Very infrequently, the smile may be temporarily altered as a result of surgical trauma to mentalis muscle or stretch injury of marginal branch of facial nerve. A very small percentage of patients may exhibit very temporary speech dysfunction postoperatively, usually intermittent lisping, secondary to the effects of swelling or bruising to the depressor muscles of the lip. A combination of hypoesthesia of the lip and injury to the mentalis or depressor muscles of the lip may cause temporary drooling and difficulty with proper enunciation. Motor nerve injury to the marginal mandibular branch of the facial nerve is extremely rare and is typically temporary.
- **Hematoma:** This is a very uncommon complication and has not been observed in my practice.
- **Bone resorption** of the outer mandibular cortex associated with chin augmentation implants has been well described. The firmer Silastic implants tend to promote more bone resorption than softer ones. Larger implants may cause greater resorption due to the greater dimension of pressure on the bony cortex. Resorption tends to occur in the first 12 months but is self-limiting if the implant is properly positioned. The small amount of bone resorption that typically occurs is not expected to affect the soft tissue profile of the mentum. If the implant is removed, the area of bony resorption may regenerate to some degree.
- **Palpable Implant:** Visual or palpable projections along the lateralmost portion of the extended mandibular implants may occur due to capsular formation around the implant or possibly as a result of infolding of the edge of the implant. This is especially true of the extremely thin, pliable edges of the extended anatomical chin implants. Frequently, gentle massaging over these areas will resolve the problem. Rarely, the implant will need to be removed and repositioned.
- **Asymmetry:** This may occur due to improper identification of the patient's preoperative mandibular asymmetry or due to improper placement of the implant. The surgeon must be aware of any preoperative asymmetry and discuss this with the patient before the procedure. If asymmetry is due to improper placement, the lateral pocket can be dissected and the implant repositioned into proper position.
- **Other:** Migration or extrusion of extended mandibular implants has not been reported. Also, neither has skin necrosis from the external approach nor allergy to the Silastic component of the implants.

RESULTS

Mandibular contouring with alloplastic implants is a valuable tool that allows the facial aesthetic surgeon to improve balance and restore youth to the patient's jawline. While techniques and technologies are sure to evolve, alloplastic chin augmentation and prejowl augmentation have been readily established as safe and straightforward procedures. As illustrated in Figures 34.15 to 34.21, these procedures provide a tremendous amount of aesthetic improvement.

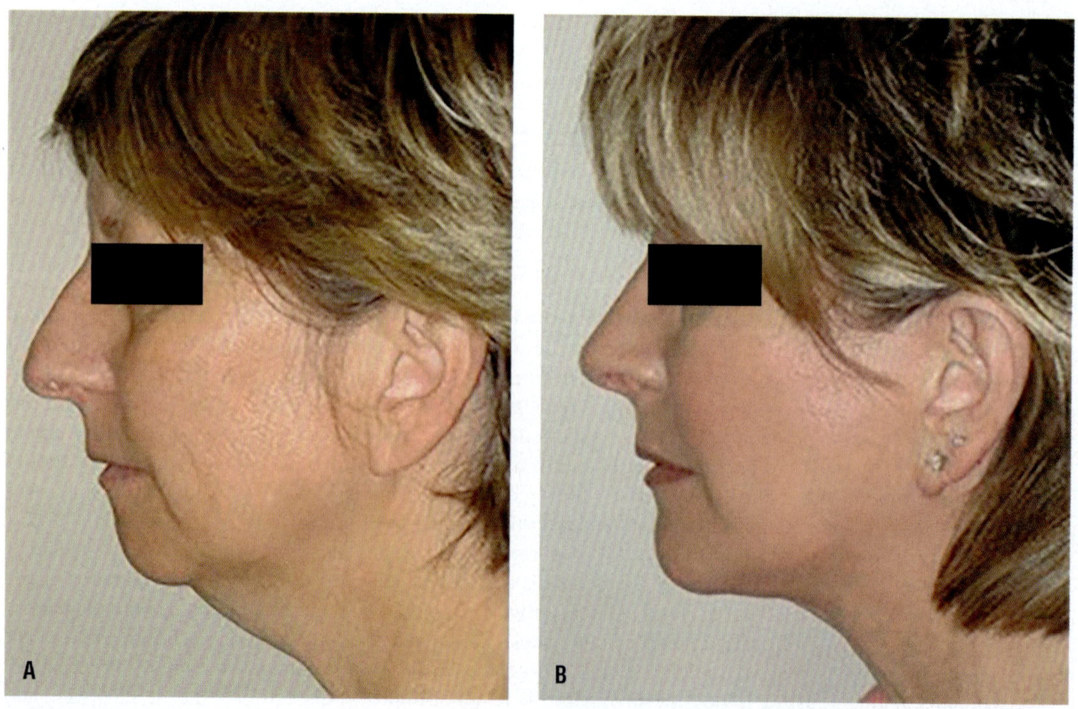

FIGURE 34.15 **(A)** Preoperative and **(B)** postoperative photographs of a patient with microgenia who underwent chin augmentation concurrent with cosmetic rhinoplasty. Note improved facial balance and aesthetics.

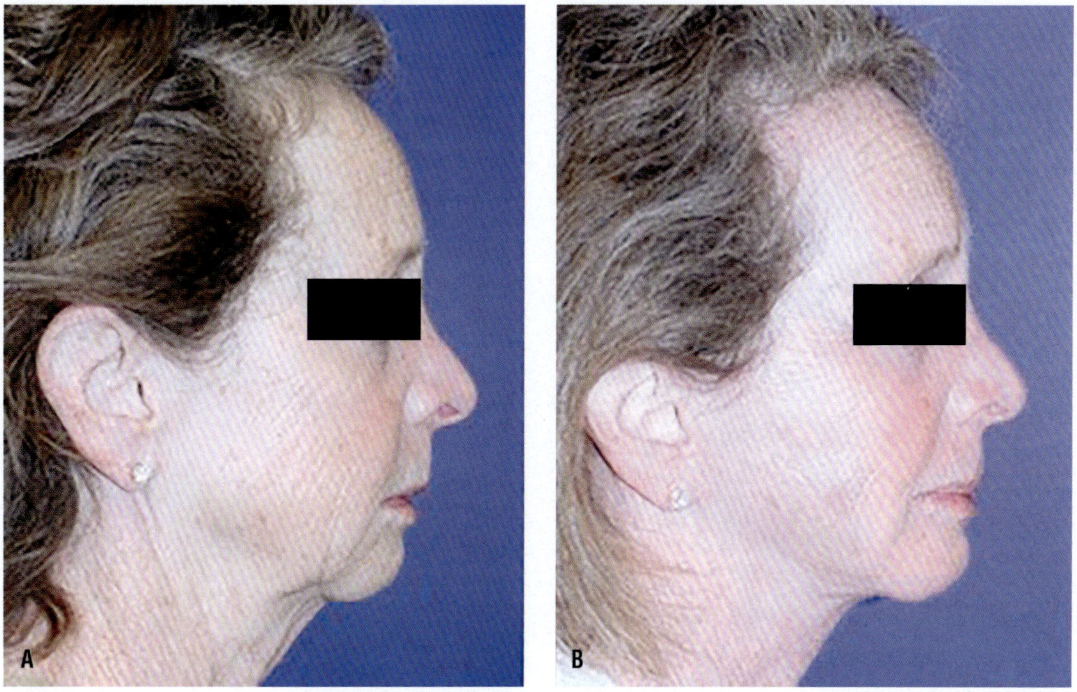

FIGURE 34.16 **(A)** Preoperative and **(B)** postoperative photographs of a patient with aging face and moderate microgenia with prejowl sulcus. Note improvement in facial proportions and balance after rhytidectomy with chin/prejowl augmentation.

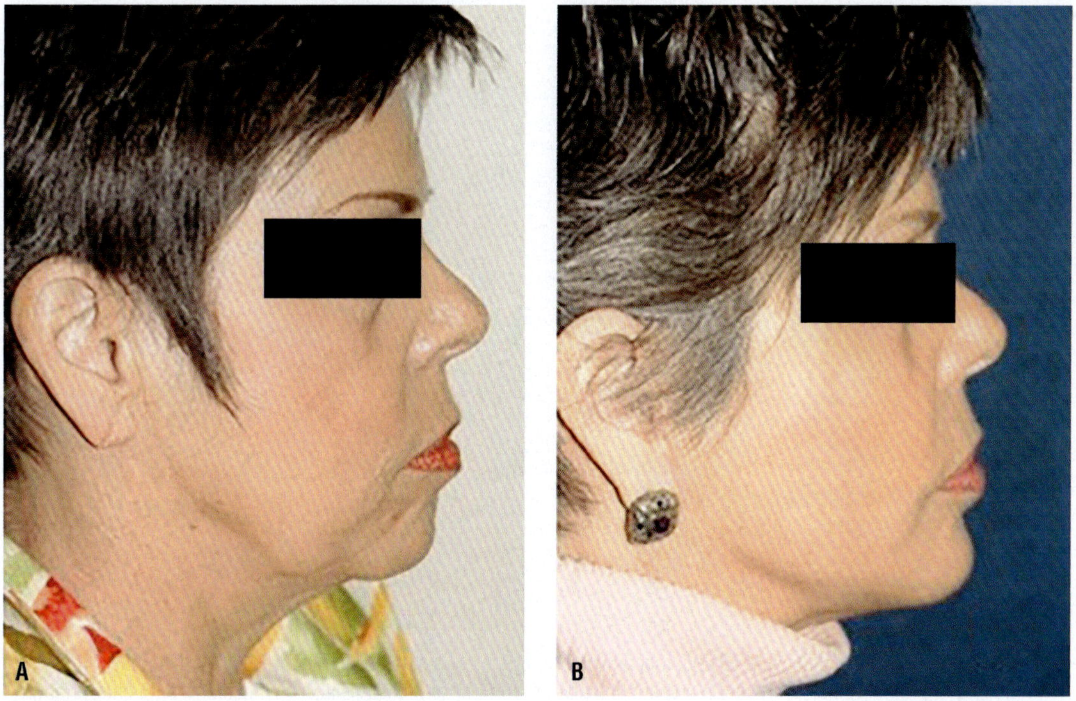

FIGURE 34.17 **(A)** Preoperative and **(B)** postoperative photographs of a patient with microgenia who underwent chin/prejowl augmentation alone.

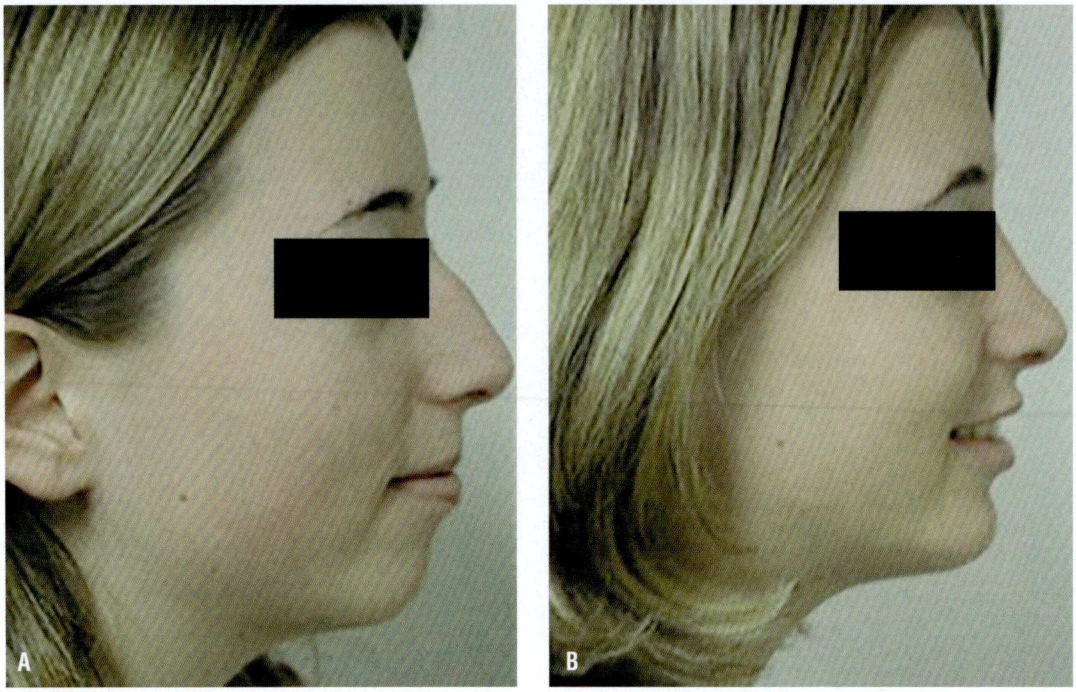

FIGURE 34.18 **(A)** Preoperative and **(B)** postoperative photographs of a patient with microgenia who underwent chin augmentation concurrent with cosmetic rhinoplasty.

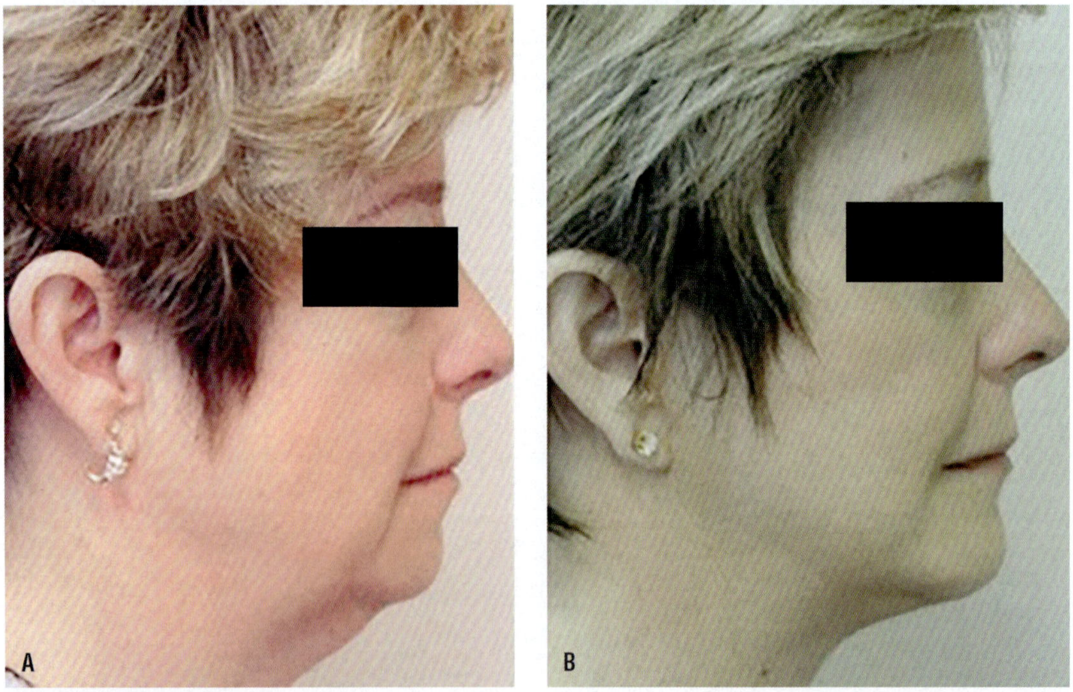

FIGURE 34.19 **(A)** Preoperative and **(B)** postoperative photographs of a patient with aging face and moderate microgenia with prejowl sulcus. Note improvement in facial proportions and balance after rhytidectomy with chin/prejowl augmentation.

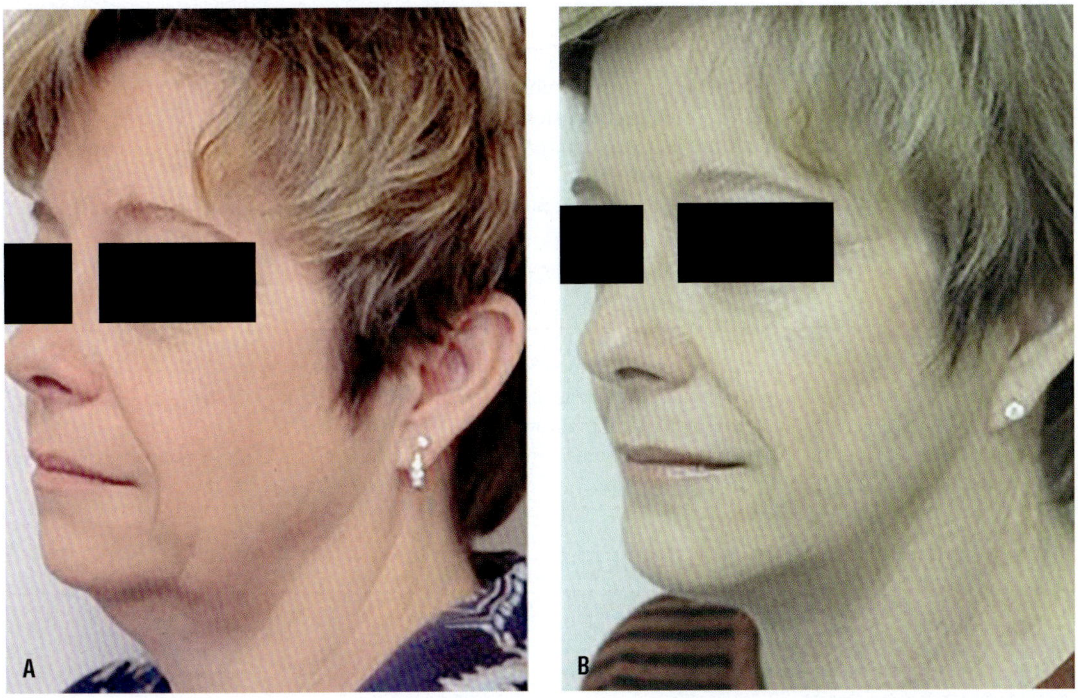

FIGURE 34.20 **(A)** Preoperative and **(B)** postoperative photographs of a patient with aging face and moderate microgenia with prejowl sulcus. Note improvement in facial proportions and balance after rhytidectomy with chin/prejowl augmentation.

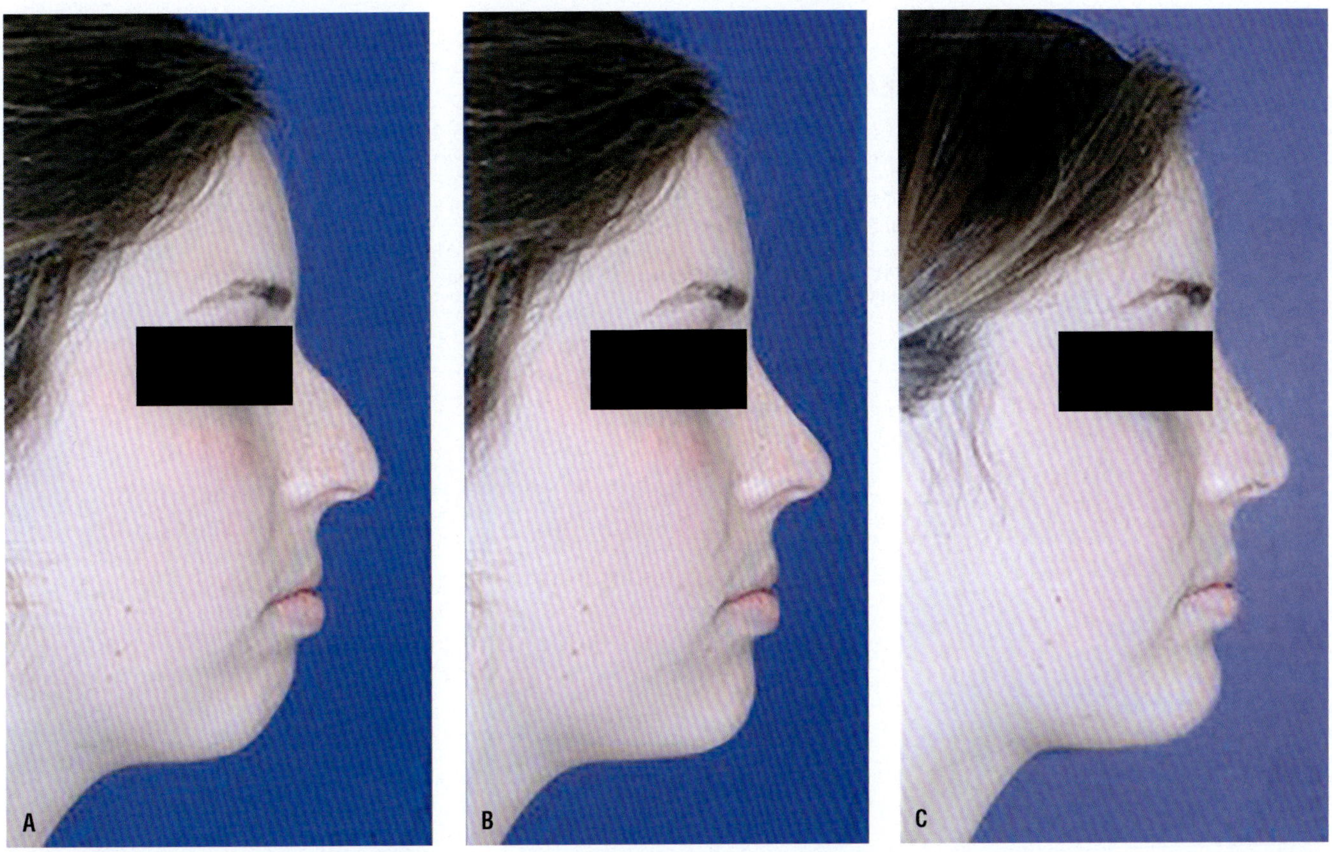

FIGURE 34.21 **(A)** Preoperative, **(B)** computer imaging, and **(C)** actual postoperative result of chin augmentation at the same time as cosmetic rhinoplasty. Computer imaging can be a valuable tool in communicating the planned surgery with the patient, and the cosmetic outcome can often closely approximate the patient's predicted final appearance.

PEARLS

- Carefully observe for contour imperfections of the chin and prejowl sulcus.
- The wider the incision over the periosteum, the easier the placement of the implant.
- Always use extended mandibular implants for chin/prejowl augmentation, never a central chin implant.
- Careful, three-layered closure is important.
- Temporary bone bleeders are commonly encountered during subperiosteal dissection.

PITFALLS

- Do not elevate the pocket above the mental foramen to help avoid paresthesias.
- Paresthesias or even total anesthesia unilaterally is a significant clinical warning. Observe the patient carefully for return of sensory function in the chin and lower lip.
- Judgment in selecting the proper size of implant is important and, if not correct, may result in exchanging one size for another in a subsequent procedure.

INSTRUMENTS TO HAVE AVAILABLE

- Standard plastic surgery set

ACKNOWLEDGMENT

The author would like to thank Dr. Maxwell Furr for his contributions to the writing of this chapter. His work in the writing, editing, and figure creation for this chapter is greatly appreciated, without which this chapter would not have been possible.

SUGGESTED READING

Choe KS, Stucki-McCormick SU. Chin augmentation. *Facial Plast Surg* 2000;16:45–54.

Mittelman H, Jen A. Aesthetic mandibular implants. In: Papel I, ed. *Facial plastic and reconstructive surgery*. New York: Thieme, 2002.

Mittelman H, Spencer JR, Chrzanowski DS. Chin region: management of grooves and mandibular hypoplasia with alloplastic implants. *Facial Plast Surg Clin North Am* 2007;15(4):445–460.

Powell N, Humphreys B. *Proportions of the Aesthetic Face*. New York: Thieme-Stratton, 1984.

Zide BM, Pfeifer TM, Longaker MT. Chin surgery: I. Augmentation—the allures and the alerts. *Plast Reconstr Surg* 1999;104(6):1843–1853.

35 SLIDING GENIOPLASTY

Edward W. Chang

INTRODUCTION

Patients seeking advice about facial cosmetic surgery often focus on structures such as the nose, the eyes, and the laxity of their skin, while the surgeon's assessment frequently identifies areas of the face that could be surgically modified to improve overall appearance and harmony. When considering facial augmentation, the lower third of the face can have a profound influence on other facial structures, such as the nose. The smaller the chin, the larger the nose appears, and augmenting the chin gives the nose a diminished appearance (Fig. 35.1). These relationships are critical to facial symmetry. The patient profile can be significantly altered with chin augmentation, which can have significant effects on the overall facial aesthetics.

Surgical goals include creating an aesthetically pleasing facial contour and establishing proportionate facial height. This may entail the reduction of a prominent chin or the augmentation of a poorly projected chin. Ideally, the augmentation procedure should be performed with minimal morbidity.

Several surgical options exist for the augmentation of the chin. Alloplastic implants and the sliding genioplasty are the most common methods of augmentation. While both modalities may be used in chin augmentation, the sliding genioplasty has the advantage of changing the vertical height of the chin, correcting asymmetry of the chin and reducing chin projection. In the sliding genioplasty, the cut segments of bone can be moved to a new position and rigidly fixated. This can be performed alone, or used along with placement of autologous bone grafts. The sliding genioplasty is technically demanding, and is time consuming, but yields excellent cosmetic results.

In the 1940s, surgeons started using various osteotomy techniques to address the retruded mentum. Currently, the sliding genioplasty is performed by several surgical specialties. Correction of poor projection of the mentum is desirable in approximately 20% of patients undergoing rhinoplasty and about 25% of patients having a rhytidectomy. However, the patient often must be educated that this deficiency exists and that, with appropriate surgery, an overall balanced cosmetic result may be achieved.

In general, alloplastic implants are not technically demanding and have a low complication rate. Furthermore, these implants may be placed easily under local anesthesia. This well-accepted technique is generally used in the correction of the chin that has only mild-to-moderate microgenia and a shallow labiomental fold.

The sliding genioplasty has been reported to have similar rates of success. Additionally, this technique can address abnormalities in three dimensions of asymmetry, including vertical microgenia with and without retrogenia as well as vertical macrogenia with retrogenia and prognathia, making it a more versatile procedure (Fig. 35.2).

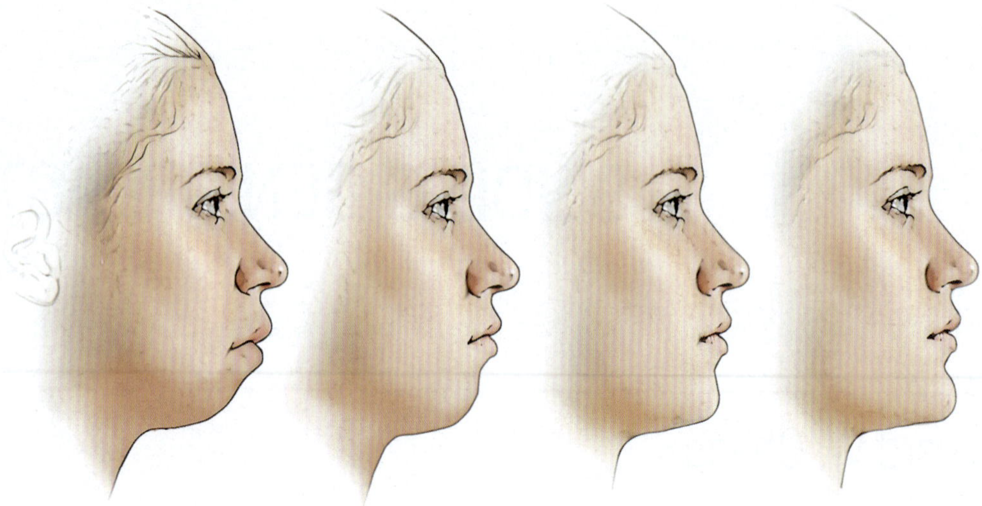

FIGURE 35.1 The position of the chin has a profound influence on the perceived projection of the nose. Only the chin position is changed. Notice the effect on nasal projection.

HISTORY

A comprehensive medical and surgical history is necessary in all patients. The use of a standardized questionnaire is helpful in documentation. Specific attention is given to congenital, developmental, and traumatic events involving the face, in particular the facial skeleton and teeth. Discussions with regard to dental alignment, corrective interventions, and temporomandibular joint disorders are reviewed as well. A listing of all medications, vitamins, and supplements is made to determine risks of bleeding. Drug and anesthetic allergies/intolerances are also noted. A social history of tobacco use, alcohol consumption, and illicit drug use is obtained.

PHYSICAL EXAMINATION

The preoperative consultation should include a complete history and physical examination, including dental evaluation, along with standard facial photographs. Assess asymmetry in the transverse dimension by using standard photographs on frontal view. Asymmetry may exist for various reasons, and it is crucial to appreciate asymmetry preoperatively. Asymmetry in the chin can be corrected easily with an offset (transverse) sliding genioplasty.

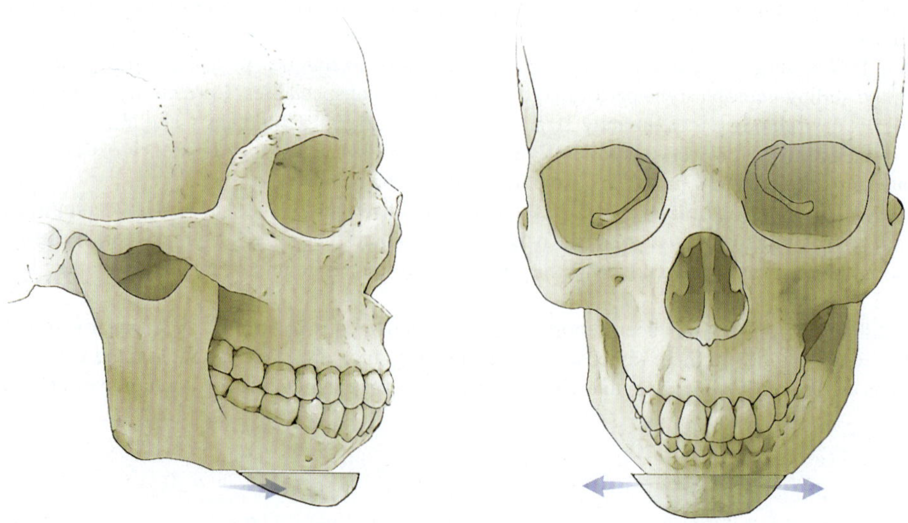

FIGURE 35.2 Versatility of the sliding genioplasty; treats abnormalities in three dimensions.

INDICATIONS

When facial analysis identifies a patient's profile with facial disharmony in the lower third of the face, one must determine whether there is an underlying dental and skeletal deformity or if the mentum (chin) is merely under- or overprojected. When the poor projection is skeletal in nature, the situation is considered an Angle's Class II skeletal deformity. Angle's skeletal classification is based on the relational position of the upper and lower first molars (Fig. 35.3).

In retrognathia, the mesiobuccal cusp of the maxillary first molar is mesial (or anterior) to the buccal groove of the mandibular first molar. If only a hypoplasia of the mandible exists, the term micrognathia is more accurate and should be used. When there is no skeletal malformation, the terms for a recessed chin include retrogenia, microgenia, retruded chin, hypoplastic mentum, and horizontal mandibular hypoplasia. In chin augmentation, genioplasty usually implies an osseous movement, whereas mentoplasty suggests the use of an alloplastic implant. However, the two terms currently are used synonymously.

CONTRAINDICATIONS

There are few situations that would preclude the use of a sliding genioplasty. Severe dentoskeletal deformities will generally require more than just advancement of the chin and will require consultation for one with expertise in this field. Additionally, the teeth and mandibular height may not be favorable for an osteotomy to be performed. When considering a mandible reduction or a sliding osteotomy, carefully evaluate the teeth and the height of the mandible prior to surgery. Having long teeth with a short mandibular height is a relative contraindication for an osseous genioplasty or aggressive bone reduction. Imaging, which may be plane films or CT, will help to define issues that would dissuade the surgeon from the use of the bony genioplasty.

PREOPERATIVE PLANNING

For a sliding genioplasty, dental occlusion and skeletal structures are evaluated with the aid of preoperative photography as well as a lateral cephalometric soft tissue study and panoramic radiographs. The cone beam CT is also useful in accessing the bony anatomy of the face. Dental models should be fabricated and are used to evaluate the patient's dental and maxillofacial situation. Functional and cosmetic goals should be discussed with the patient.

Cephalometric tracings and measurements should be done for patients undergoing a sliding genioplasty. The cephalometric evaluation includes measurements of sella–nasion–subspinale A-point of the maxilla (S-N-A) and sella–nasion–supramentale B-point of the mandible (S-N-B) angles to provide information on the sagittal relationship between the anterior skull base and the maxilla and mandible, respectively (Fig. 35.4). The soft tissue and lip profile yields a tremendous amount of information on the chin projection. As with the midface, the evaluation of the chin prominence can be accomplished many different ways. Ricketts draws a vertical line tangential to the nasal tip and pogonion. The upper

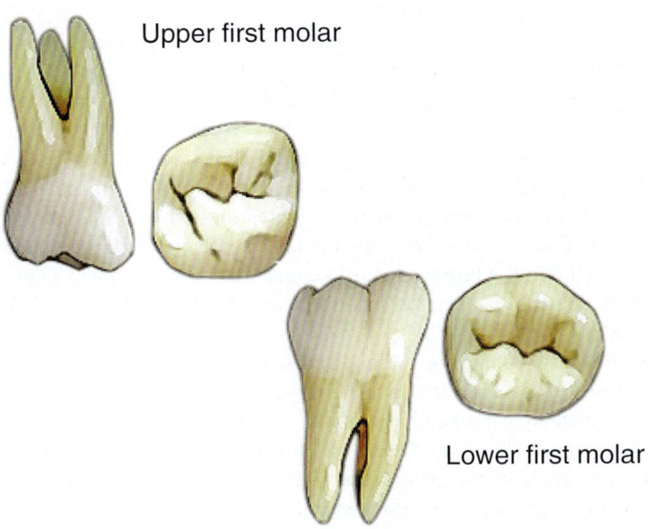

FIGURE 35.3
Upper and lower first molar teeth.

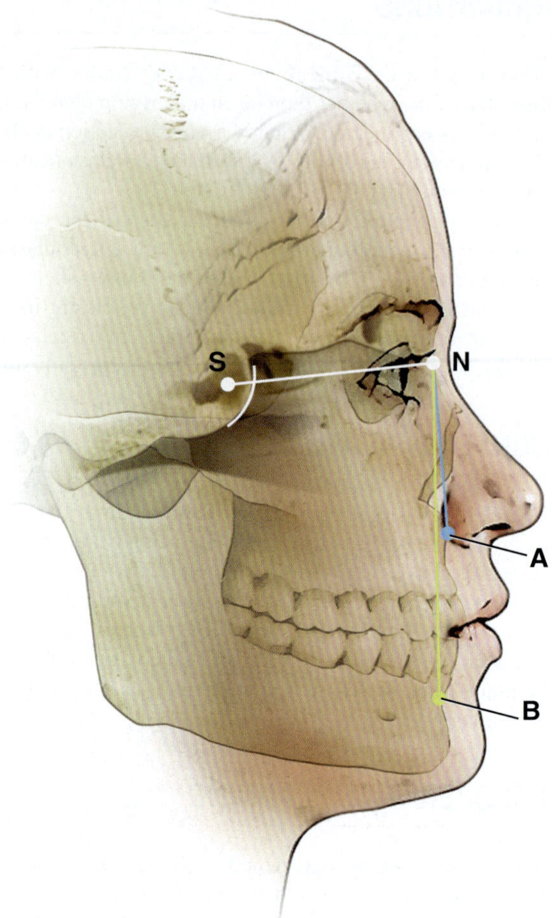

FIGURE 35.4
Sella–nasion–subspinale A-point of the maxilla (S-N-A) and sella–nasion–supramentale B-point of the mandible (S-N-B) angles.

lip should rest 4 mm behind this line, and the lower lip at 2 mm. Gonzalez-Ulloa uses the Frankfurt plane and a line designated as the zero-degree meridian. The Frankfurt plane is a horizontal line from the upper external auditory canal to the infraorbital rim. The zero-degree meridian is perpendicular to the Frankfurt plane and is started at nasion. If the chin is behind the zero-degree meridian, it is considered retruded. Another method drops a line perpendicular to the Frankfurt plane through subnasale. The upper lip should be at this vertical +/– 2 mm, the lower lip should be behind this line by 2 mm and +/– 2 mm, and the chin should be 4 mm posterior (Fig. 35.5). Once deficiencies have been measured, plan the movement. The literature shows that the ratio of correlation from bone to soft tissue movement is 1:0.6 to 1. More recent studies show the ratio to be about 1:0.9 for horizontal movements up to 8 mm. Beyond this length, muscular and soft tissue forces are thought to cause resorption. The literature suggests less predictability in vertical movements.

Determine the vertical height of the face, by employing the method described by Powell and Humphreys. The face is divided into horizontal thirds, from the hairline to the glabella, the glabella to the subnasale (where the nasal columella meets the upper lip), and subnasale to the menton. Vertically, the face is divided into fifths. The eyes and the nose are generally equal to a fifth. There are alternative ways to evaluate the face, especially if the hairline is missing. The lower two-thirds of the face are evaluated alone, the midface is 43% of this region, and the lower third is 57%. This information is used to advise the patient of the choices available for obtaining the best result. If a skeletal abnormality exists, one can suggest orthodontic realignment and orthognathic surgery as a surgical alternative. This would address function, as well as form. If the patient desires a purely cosmetic correction, options include alloplastic implant augmentation and a sliding genioplasty. Recommendations on which surgical modality to use are based on the severity of the deformity and concomitant facial procedures being considered.

Detailed preoperative counseling allows the surgeon and the patient to discuss and evaluate the desired changes. Computer imaging often provides a useful teaching tool and helps the discussion. A caveat is to emphasize to the patient that a digitally altered image may not be representative of the actual surgical changes.

For an augmentation, the depth of the labiomental fold may dictate which technique is used. Alloplastic implants tend to deepen the sulcus, which may be particularly unattractive in the female patients. With osseous genioplasty, the fold generally increases with advancements and/or vertical shortening and becomes more effaced with vertical lengthening.

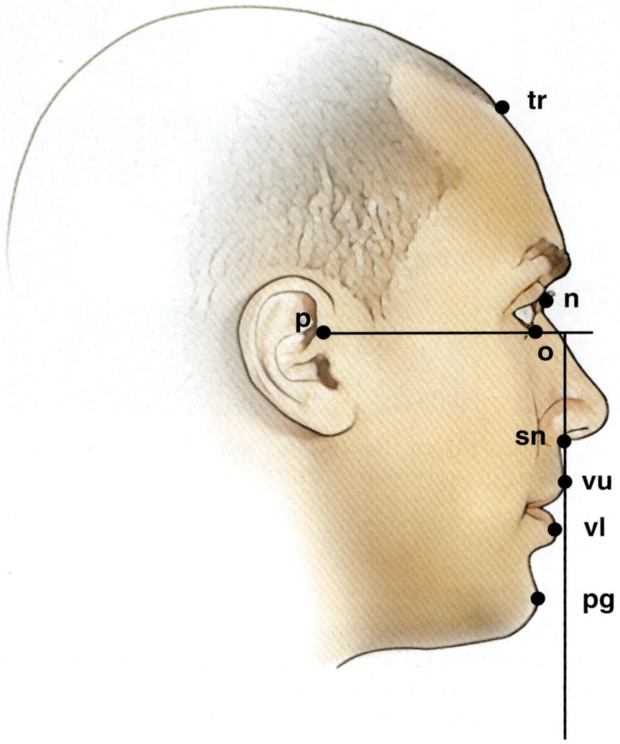

FIGURE 35.5

Profile of soft tissues in relation to cephalometric imaging. TR, trichion; N, soft tissue nasion; SN, subnasale; O, porion; P, porion; VU, vermillion of the upper lip; VL, vermillion of the lower lip; PG, soft tissue pogonion. Lateral osteotomies should be 4 to 5 mm below the foramina to compensate for the path of the inferior alveolar nerve. Bone forceps help mobilize the distal segment.

SURGICAL TECHNIQUE

The sliding genioplasty can be performed under local anesthesia in an outpatient setting with good results; however, general anesthesia is most commonly used with this procedure. Patients are more comfortable and the airway is better protected under general anesthesia. Unless a rhinoplasty is performed concurrently, nasotracheal intubation is preferred.

Injection of 0.25% bupivacaine with epinephrine (1:200,000) mixed in equal part with 1% lidocaine with epinephrine (1:100,000) locally in the mental foramen region can reduce operative bleeding and provide long-lasting anesthesia. Perioperative and postoperative antibiotics should be administered. Access is through the gingivolabial sulcus incision. An intraoral incision will transect the mentalis muscle, which elevates and protrudes the chin. It attaches the chin to an area just beneath the tooth roots. It is crucial to leave an adequate cuff of mucosa along with a good part of the mentalis muscle to allow for later resuspension; this technique leads to avoidance of lower-lip ptosis.

Subperiosteal dissection is carried out laterally to identify the mental nerve. The surgeon should always be cognizant of the location of the mental foramen. The mental foramen lies on the same vertical line defined by the pupil. The foramina of the nerve are generally found between the first and second premolar teeth at the level of the origin of the mentalis muscle or 2 to 4 mm below the level of the bicuspid teeth apices. The foramina are situated deep to the midportion of the depressor anguli oris. Dissect inferolaterally to allow for a longer osteotomy preventing unsightly mandible notching. Leave the periosteum intact at the inferior rim. Align the skeletal midline with the overlying soft tissue corollary. Use a sagittal saw with a 30-degree bend to facilitate an even osteotomy while minimizing soft tissue trauma (Fig. 35.6). A cadaver dissection shows the osteotomy going under the mental foramen and extending posterior to help avoid a step-off (Fig. 35.7). Angling of the osteotomy in a more acute manner will decrease the vertical height of the chin.

Perform double osteotomies in the same manner and plan asymmetric osteotomies well in advance. Fixation can be achieved with wires or plates. Of note, wire fixation may lead to increased resorption due to greater periosteal dissection and a possible drop of the anterior segment from muscle pull. Great success has occurred using a single, 4-hole, titanium plate with 12-mm screws for males and 10-mm screws for females (Fig. 35.8). Each plate is marked with the amount of movement obtained on the face of the plate.

Closure is accomplished in multiple layers. Resuspension of the mentalis muscle is performed with 3-0 interrupted buried Vicryl sutures and closure of the mucosa is conducted with a running 3-0 chromic suture. Redraping of the skin is done at the level of the labiomental fold with Mastisol (Ferndale Laboratories, Ferndale, MI) and paper tape. The surgical time for the osseous genioplasty procedure ranges from 15 to 105 minutes, with an average surgical time of about 45 minutes. The alloplastic implantation is roughly 25% shorter in operative time. Schedule a follow-up visit with the patient on postoperative days 7 and 14. Each of the procedures described has its own unique advantages, disadvantages, and complications.

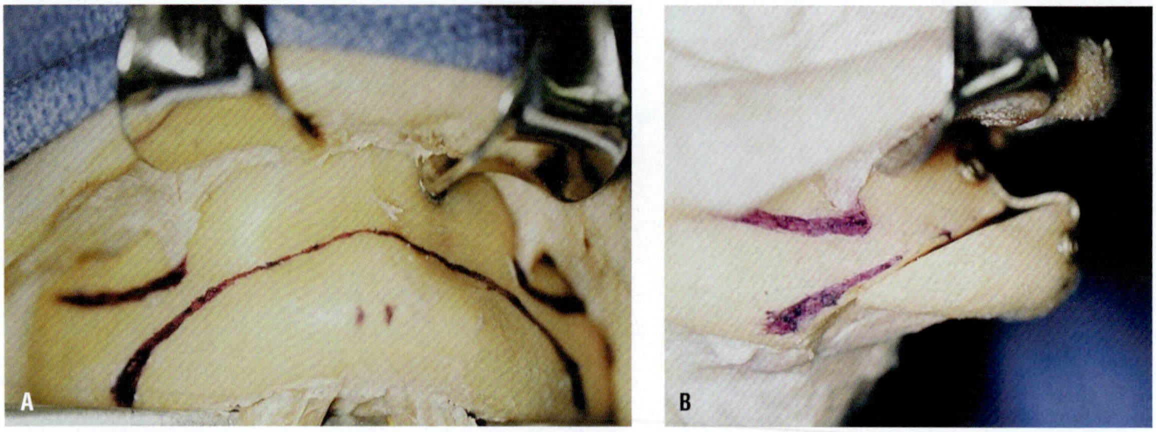

FIGURE 35.6 Cadaveric demonstration of the osteotomy in anterior **(A)** and lateral **(B)** views. Note extension 5 mm below the mental nerve foramen and posterior to prevent nerve injury and to avoid step-offs.

POSTOPERATIVE MANAGEMENT

The patient undergoing sliding genioplasty is admitted into the hospital only if orthognathic surgery is performed. Otherwise, the procedure can be performed in an outpatient setting even when concomitant procedures, such as rhinoplasty or liposuction, are performed. After the surgery, patients are advised to stay on a soft diet and to rinse their mouth frequently with saline solution until the first postoperative visit. Strenuous activity should be avoided, and physical contact to the chin should be delayed for 4 weeks.

COMPLICATIONS

There are associated complications with the sliding genioplasty procedure. Mental nerve and vascular injury, malunion, nonunion, contour irregularities, step-type deformities, lip drop, and overcorrection or undercorrection have been reported. Of note, undercorrection is better accepted than overcorrection because the chin placed forward to the lower lip can yield a disharmonious profile.

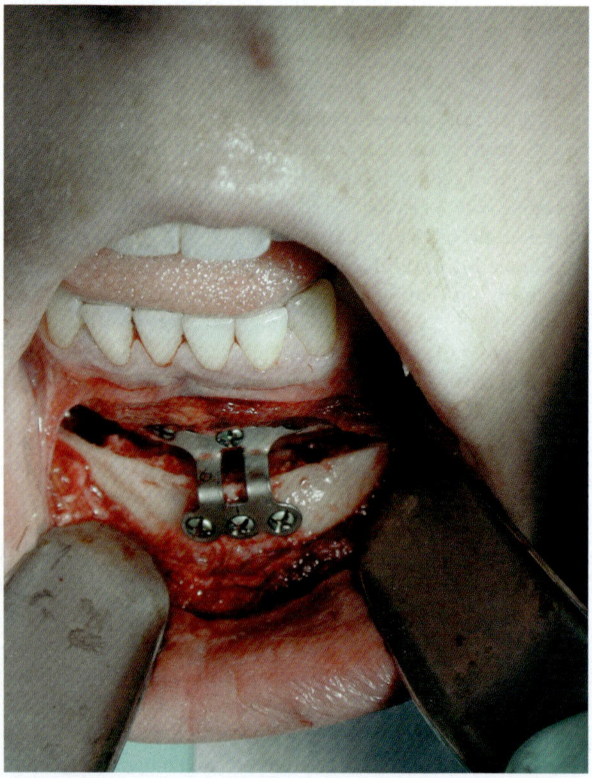

FIGURE 35.7
Fixation can be done with preformed plates or with wires.

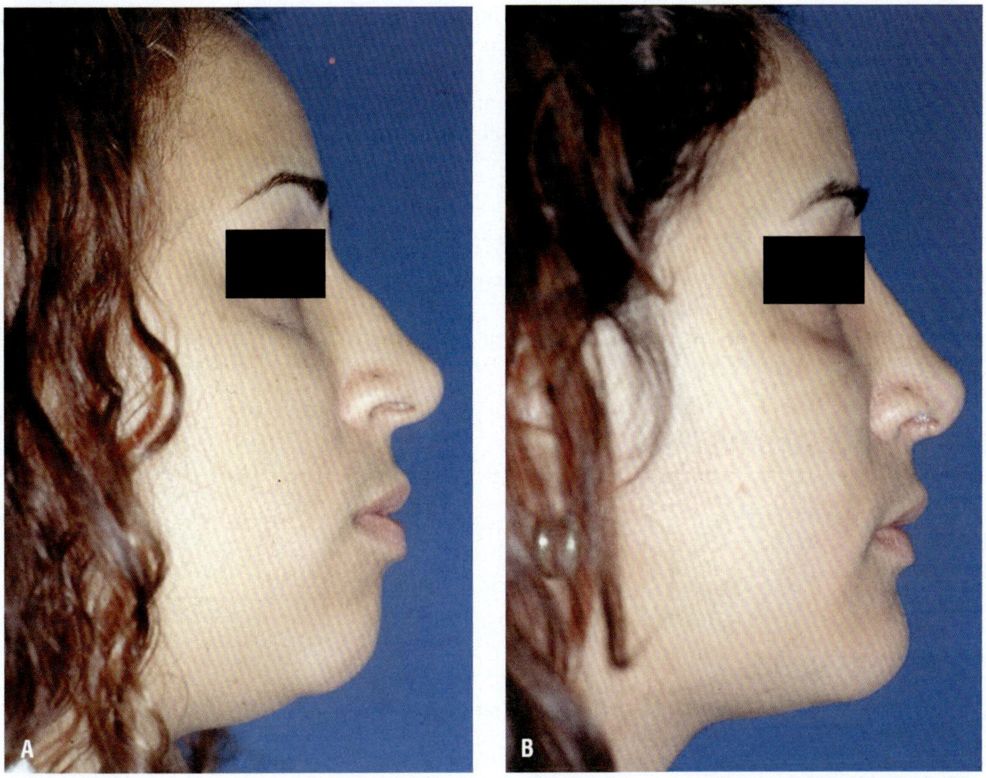

FIGURE 35.8 **A, B:** Pre- and postoperative photographs of a patient who had undergone sliding genioplasty.

Whether an alloplastic implant or an osseous implant is used, more than 90% of the patients are satisfied with their results. Complications observed with the sliding genioplasty are minimal, and benefits are readily evident to both patient and surgeon.

RESULTS

With appropriate preoperative planning, excellent results are obtainable, surgical time is acceptable, and high patient satisfaction can be achieved with the sliding genioplasty. This surgical technique has its own advantages and disadvantages, and these should be balanced with the desires of the patient, along with the experience of the surgeon to achieve harmonious and cosmetically pleasing aesthetic results (Fig. 35.9).

PEARLS

- The sliding genioplasty is a highly versatile in correcting chin abnormalities in every dimension and its relative ease of use in comparison to a standard chin implant.

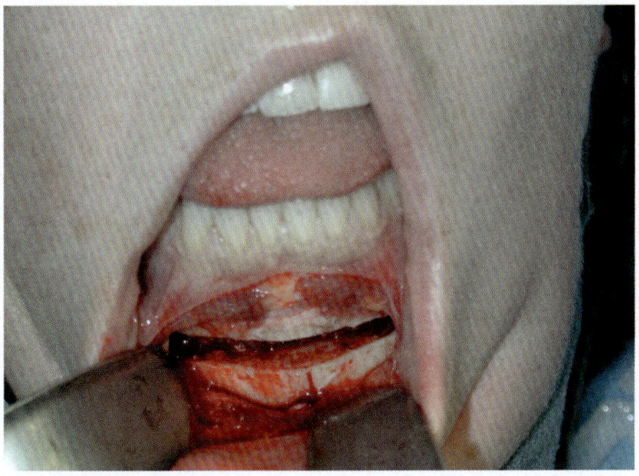

FIGURE 35.9
Augmentation and asymmetry correction were performed.

- A detailed facial analysis is critical in evaluating the proportions of facial structures with the nose, malar, and chin regions contributing the most balance to the face.
- Dental occlusion and skeletal structures need to be evaluated and documented with digital photography, lateral cephalometric soft tissue studies, and panoramic radiographs.
- Skeletal asymmetries or deficiencies may result in suboptimal aesthetic situations.

PITFALLS

- Not appreciating the skeletal path of the mental nerve and thus causing permanent paresthesia in the chin region is the most significant pitfall.
- Aesthetic pitfalls include too large of an advancement resulting in a notched appearance of the mandibular border or undercorrection.

INSTRUMENTS TO HAVE AVAILABLE

- Standard plastic surgery set
- Molt elevator
- Minnesota retractors

SUGGESTED READING

Chang EW, Lam SM, Karen M, et al. Sliding genioplasty for correction of chin abnormalities. *Arch Facial Plast Surg* 2001;3(1):8–15.

Frodel JL, Sykes JM. Chin augmentation/genioplasty: chin deformities in the aging patient. *Facial Plast Surg* 1996;12(3):279–283.

Grayson BH. Cephalometric analysis for the surgeon. *Clin Plast Surg* 1989;16(4):633–644.

Guyuron B, Kadi JS. Problems following genioplasty. Diagnosis and treatment. *Clin Plast Surg* 1997;24(3):507–514.

Rosen HM. Aesthetic guidelines in genioplasty: the role of facial disproportion. *Plast Reconstr Surg* 1995;95(3):463–469; discussion 470–472.

36 CLEFT LIP AND PALATE

Travis T. Tollefson

INTRODUCTION

Comprehensive management of the patient with a cleft lip and palate requires a collaborative multidisciplinary team of specialists, typically including facial plastic or general plastic surgeons, otologists, speech and language pathologists, nurses, geneticists, orthodontists, dentists, oral surgeons, audiologists, pediatricians, and social workers. Orofacial clefting is the most common craniofacial birth defect; surgical management of this issue requires meticulous soft tissue technique, in which mere millimeters of error in infancy may result in permanent cleft stigmata. Producing a satisfactory aesthetic result depends upon careful attention to the skin and soft tissue, nasal cartilages, teeth, and skeletal components, which must be addressed sequentially during the child's growth and development. Concomitantly, speech and swallowing function are rehabilitated through painstaking restoration of dental and palatal structures.

An orofacial cleft represents failure of fusion of the lip, nasal sill, alveolus, or palate, which may occur in a spectrum of combinations of unilateral or bilateral deformities. The etiology of orofacial clefting is not well understood, but the condition results from an interruption in the complex craniofacial developmental pathway. Clefts may develop as complete or incomplete lip defects, complete or incomplete palate defects, or a combination that may span all the way from the nasal sill to the uvula (Fig. 36.1). Lesser manifestations of orofacial clefting are termed "microform," "occult," "minor," or "forme fruste" (aborted form).

A variety of classification schemes have been suggested, the first in 1938 when Veau described his system: group A includes defects of the soft palate l only; group B includes defects of the hard and soft palate not extending anterior to the incisive foramen; group C includes defects extending through the entire palate and the alveolar ridge; and group D includes complete bilateral cleft lip. This general framework may be useful in discussion; however, further understanding of the developmental pathways that lead to orofacial clefting has simplified classification of the palatal cleft based on whether the primary palate (structures anterior to the incisive foramen, including the lip, premaxilla, and anterior septum) or the secondary palate (structures posterior to the incisive foramen, including the lateral palatine shelves, soft palate, and uvula) is involved.

A comprehensive classification scheme should identify involvement of the primary and secondary palates as well as lip and nasal deformities so that these areas may be addressed specifically during management. I prefer to determine initially whether the cleft is typical or atypical. The atypical craniofacial clefts were described in the landmark 1976 article by Tessier, who outlined a classification scheme for orofacial clefts that present with atypical orientations, such as the number 7, macrostomia due to a cleft at the commissure of the lip (Fig. 36.2). Extension of these clefts through the soft tissues may involve the maxilla, orbit, and skull base. For example, a bilateral Tessier number 4 cleft extends from the upper lip through the nasolacrimal duct and into the lower eyelid at the medial canthus (Fig. 36.3).

Typical orofacial clefts are described by laterality of the lip cleft (unilateral or bilateral) and its degree. The cleft lip may be complete (through the lip and nasal sill), incomplete (orbicularis oris and skin are intact for at least three-fourths of the length of the lip), or microform (characterized by a philtral skin

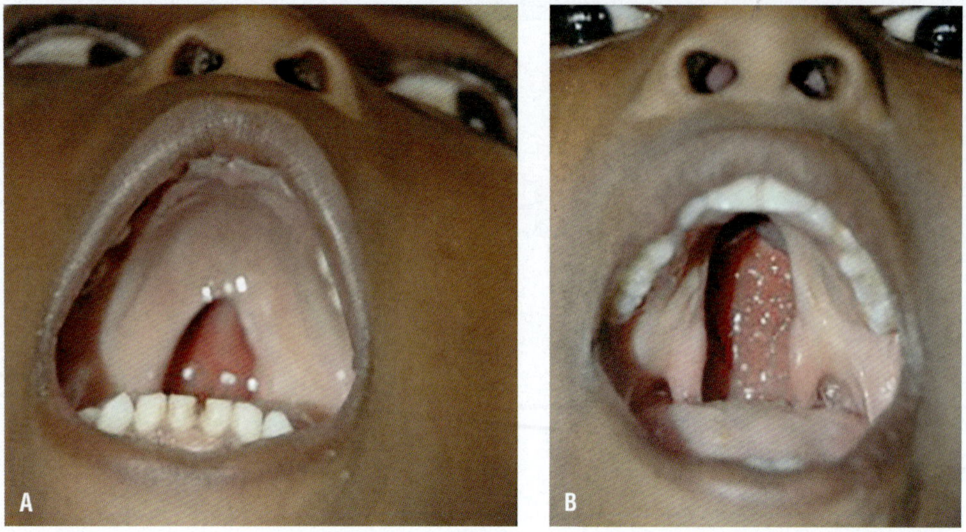

FIGURE 36.1 The spectrum of incomplete cleft palate includes defects ranging from isolated uvular bifidity to palatal clefting as anterior as the incisive foramen: **(A)** intraoral view of an incomplete soft palate cleft shows extension just to the hard palate; **(B)** another child's unrepaired cleft palate extends through the hard palate. The adenoid pad is seen between the two sides of the cleft uvula.

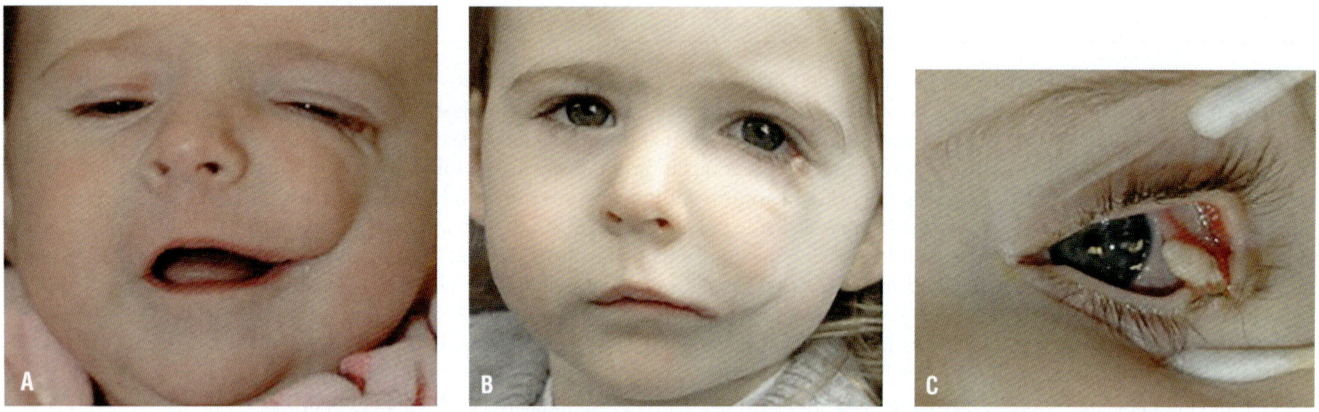

FIGURE 36.2 Atypical orofacial cleft, Tessier No. 7, demonstrating macrostomia **(A)** preoperatively, **(B)** after soft tissue repair, and **(C)** left lower eyelid coloboma and ocular dermoids prior to removal.

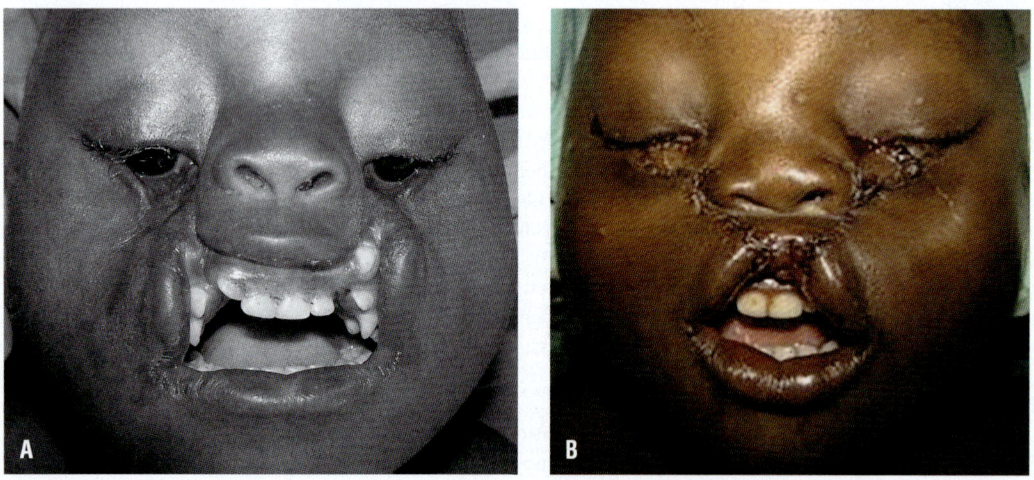

FIGURE 36.3 Photograph of a child with bilateral Tessier No. 4 orofacial clefts **(A)** preoperatively and **(B)** after subunit repair to recreate lower eyelids and continuity of the mouth; maxillary clefting will require future bone grafting.

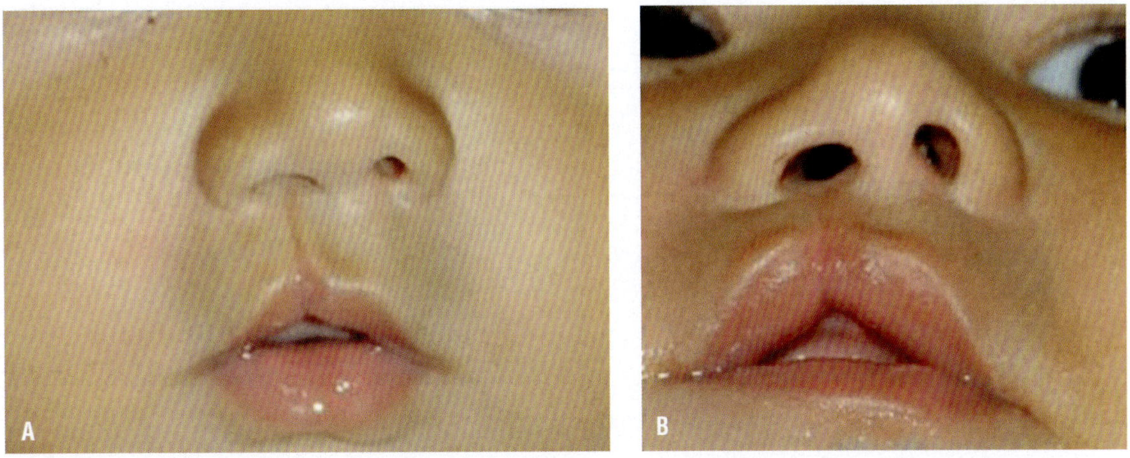

FIGURE 36.4 The features of a typical right microform unilateral cleft lip shown in **(A)** frontal view and **(B)** base view, including notched mucosa, elevated Cupid's bow peak, furrowing of the philtral column, thinning of the dry vermilion medially, widening of the nasal base, hypoplasia of the orbicularis oris muscle, and asymmetry of the nostril.

groove, minor nasal deformity, orbicularis oris discontinuity, and a notched vermilion–cutaneous junction with disruption extending to no more than one-fourth of the labial height, as measured from the normal peak of the Cupid's bow to the nasal sill) (Fig. 36.4). The cleft alveolus may be complete or notched. Independent of the cleft lip type, the cleft palate is described as unilateral (one palatal shelf is attached to the nasal septum) or bilateral.

In this chapter, I will outline the following: multidisciplinary management of cleft lip and palate, physical examination findings, and potential associated syndromic and nonsyndromic comorbidities. Preoperative planning will be reviewed, along with presurgical nasoalveolar molding (PNAM), and the indications and contraindications for repair of the surgical cleft. Preferred techniques for unilateral and bilateral cleft lip repair and palatoplasty will be described. Postoperative management will be reviewed with emphasis on prevention of complications.

HISTORY

The role of a multidisciplinary team is to address the conditions that coexist with orofacial clefts, ranging from difficulties with speech and swallowing to Eustachian tube dysfunction and audiologic issues to orthodontic, dental, and orthognathic problems. Care of the child born with a cleft lip and/or palate begins with a consultation soon after birth, during which the multidisciplinary team focuses on teaching the mothers effective feeding techniques and emphasizes the importance of appropriate weight gain. In each patient, a comprehensive history is obtained that includes familial, prenatal, and delivery events. Attention is dedicated to the presence of additional physical findings as well as the possibility of a syndromic or sequence event. Consultations with neonatal intensivists, geneticists, and additional specialists are made on a case-by-case basis. With each patient, specialized care commonly continues through the teenage years and into early adulthood, involving regular team meetings and sequential intervention, both operative and nonoperative.

PHYSICAL EXAMINATION

The presence of an orofacial cleft may be identified on routine prenatal ultrasound at 18 to 20 weeks of gestation. Three-dimensional ultrasound technology has increased the detection rate of cleft lip, but not isolated cleft palate. Because of this, expectant parents with a positive ultrasound are now presenting for prenatal facial plastic surgery consultation. Preparation for and understanding of the surgical repairs through educational consultation may help allay parental concerns. Prenatal consultation also allows the surgeon to begin assessment for preoperative therapies, such as PNAM, which requires frequent clinic visits and significant parental commitment.

The neonate is examined for cleft lip and cleft palate immediately after birth. Identification of the subtle microform cleft lip or submucous cleft palate is facilitated with training and experience in identifying muscle abnormalities that lack obvious epithelial defects. A thorough examination of the head and neck begins with assessment and palpation of the continuity of the upper lip and nares. The maxillary alveolus is palpated for a notch or cleft.

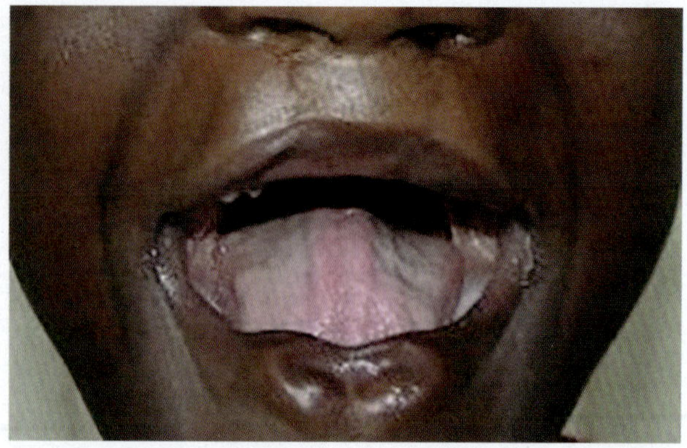

FIGURE 36.5
Lower lip pitting seen in Van der Woude's syndrome.

Improved visualization of the soft palate may be achieved by placing the child supine in the parent's lap and carefully extending the neck. The neonate often opens his or her mouth and spontaneously protrudes the tongue, giving a good view. A tongue depressor and light should also be used to assess the palate and uvula. A bifid uvula or zona pellucida in the soft palate should prompt palpation for a hard palate notch. The lower lips are inspected for nodular lip pits as seen in Van der Woude's syndrome (Fig. 36.5). The oral commissure and cheeks are evaluated for atypical clefting or auricular remnants found in oculoauriculovertebral spectrum (Fig. 36.6). The shapes and positions of the ears are inspected, looking for microtia or other features of hemifacial microsomia. The eyelids may also demonstrate colobomata or notches.

INDICATIONS

The typical indications for proceeding with repair of the cleft lip are difficulty feeding, poor weight gain, and airway obstruction. Although poor weight gain may indicate feeding difficulty, the surgeon and pediatrician must also consider cardiac or other defects leading to failure to thrive. Breastfeeding is encouraged, though formula supplementation is common. Postnatal weight loss of up to 10% of birth weight is normal, but should be regained in 2 weeks. Thereafter, at least 1 ounce of weight gain per day indicates adequate feeding. Nasogastric tube feeding is seldom required if a feeding nurse specialist can counsel the mother effectively. Neonates with cleft palate have difficulty creating suction; they should be positioned upright to limit nasal regurgitation. Specialized nipples, such as the Haberman nipple (Fig. 36.7), control the flow rate from a bottle and may limit the infant's fatigue while feeding.

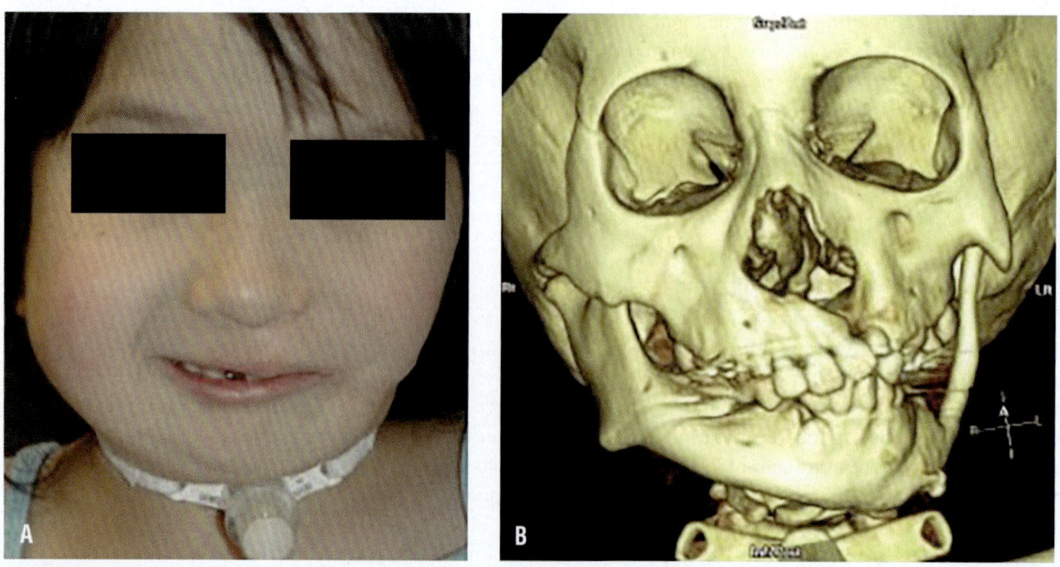

FIGURE 36.6 Oculoauriculovertebral spectrum, demonstrating hemifacial microsomia, left anotia, and **(A)** a repaired unilateral complete cleft lip and palate, **(B)** 3-D CT scan showing the left unrepaired alveolar cleft and left mandibular ramus reconstruction with rib grafting.

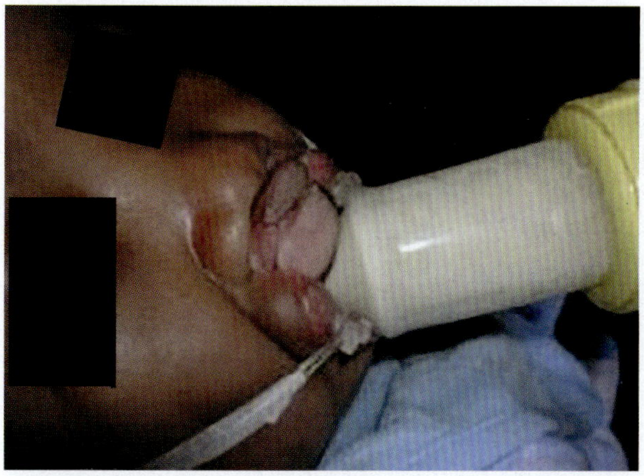

FIGURE 36.7
Infant with a bilateral cleft lip and palate feeding with a Haberman nipple, while the PNAM appliance is in place. The cylindrical nipple on the bottle may be squeezed to control flow.

CONTRAINDICATIONS

Repair of an orofacial cleft may be contraindicated until airway obstruction is addressed. Airway obstruction due to the tongue is seen in a small proportion of infants with orofacial clefts, with Pierre Robin sequence being the most common cause (Fig. 36.8). Initial treatment includes prone positioning, nasopharyngeal trumpet, nasal continuous positive airway pressure, or endotracheal intubation. Definitive surgical intervention may include tracheostomy, mandibular distraction osteogenesis, or tongue–lip adhesion.

PREOPERATIVE PLANNING

The typical timeline for each of the discrete steps of orofacial cleft management is shown in Figure 36.9. Cleft lip repair is often performed at 3 to 5 months of age. For infants with cleft palate, bilateral myringotomy and tympanostomy tube placement is followed by behavioral audiometry prior to the cleft palate repair, performed between 10 and 14 months of age. Speech and language pathology assessment and therapy are initiated after vocabulary develops (3 to 5 years old) with emphasis on identifying velopharyngeal dysfunction. A secondary speech surgery may be required to address hypernasality at this time. Superiorly based flap pharyngoplasty, sphincter pharyngoplasty, and Furlow double-opposing Z-palatoplasty are procedures frequently used to limit nasal air escape; when employing these techniques, the surgeon must be aware of the potential to produce obstructive sleep apnea from excessive nasal obstruction.

In the presence of a typical unilateral or bilateral cleft lip and palate, dental and orthodontic care should be initiated early. Prior to the eruption of the maxillary canines at around 7 to 10 years of age, an orthodontist will begin dental preparation for the alveolar bone graft. The bone graft is often harvested from the iliac crest at approximately 10 years of age. Orthognathic surgery for correction of dentofacial malocclusion is delayed

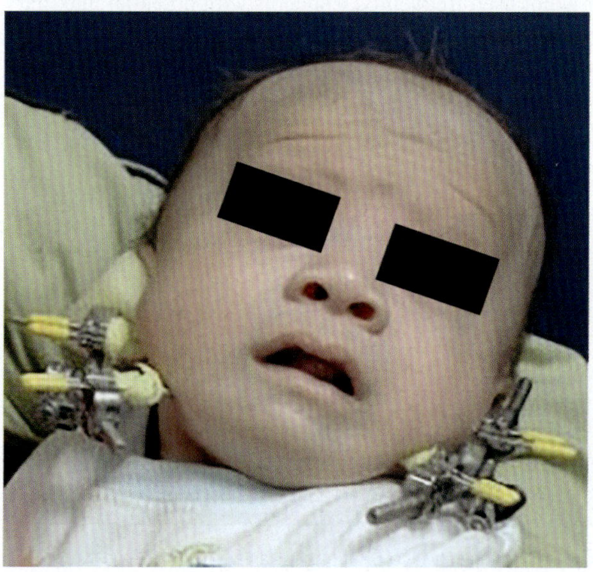

FIGURE 36.8
Infant with Pierre Robin sequence demonstrating microgenia, glossoptosis, and cleft palate with external mandibular distraction device.

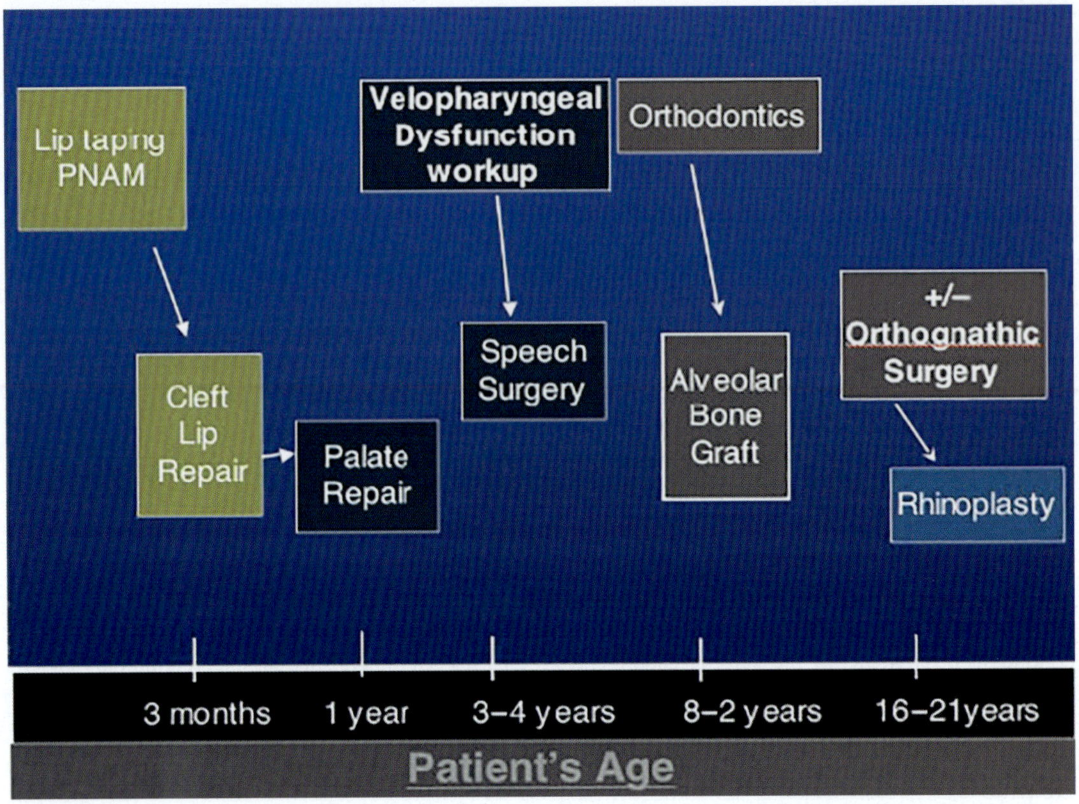

FIGURE 36.9 Timeline for comprehensive management of cleft lip and palate showing surgical procedures on the bottom and nonsurgical treatment above, from birth to adulthood.

until skeletal growth is complete, which occurs earlier in females than in males. Subsequently, definitive cleft septorhinoplasty will address the nasal deformity in the teenage years.

Cleft Lip Repair

During the initial consultation, weight gain and feeding are assessed. The upcoming surgical procedures and future multidisciplinary management are discussed. Wide cleft lips may require one of several presurgical preparations including: lip taping, oral appliance use (Latham device), PNAM, 2-staged repair with a primary lip adhesion, or delayed repair to allow tissue growth. Daily lip taping may affect soft tissue expansion. Standard protocols use an adhesive strip or tape to appose the lip edges. The cheeks are protected with a skin barrier that requires routine replacement due to lip wetting from feeding (Fig. 36.10). The Latham appliance actively repositions the premaxilla but is not used frequently. Concerns with potential maxillary growth inhibition continue to fuel the debate regarding the appropriate use of presurgical premaxillary positioning.

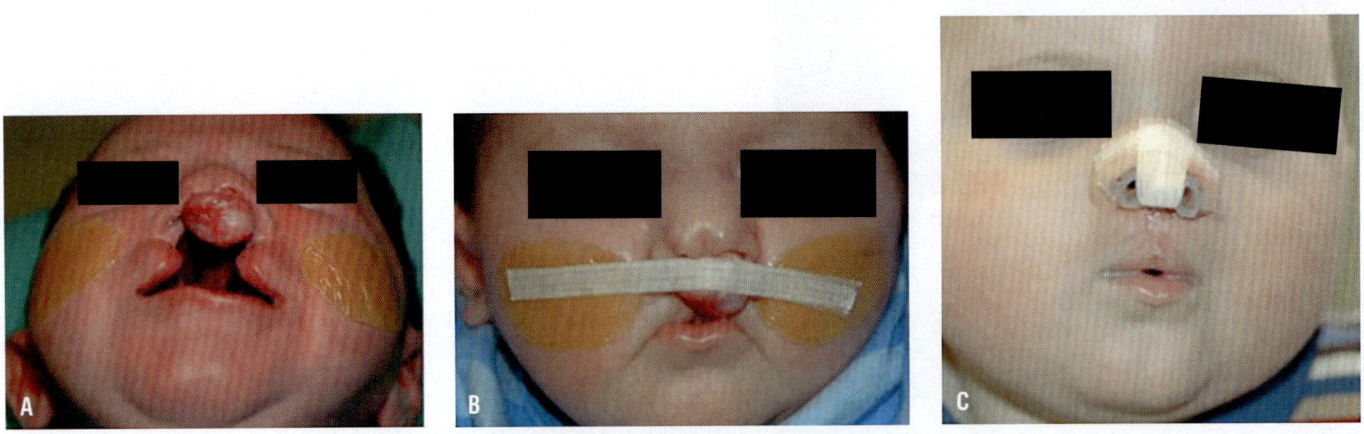

FIGURE 36.10 Infant with bilateral cleft lip and palate shown **(A)** preoperatively, **(B)** during lip taping, and **(C)** 1 week after surgical repair, with silicone nasal stents taped in place.

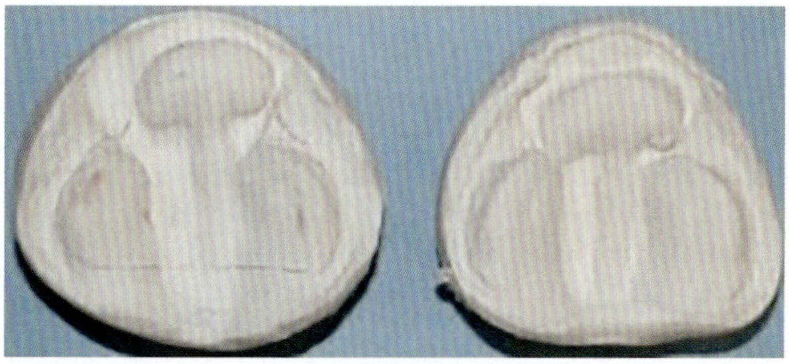

FIGURE 36.11
Intraoral impression of the maxilla of an infant with a bilateral cleft lip and palate shown before (**left**) and after (**right**) nasoalveolar molding repositioned the premaxilla posteriorly.

Presurgical Nasoalveolar Molding

Greyson and Cutting introduced and developed the principles of PNAM, including the addition of nasal prongs to the traditional intraoral alveolar molding device. Alveolar molding will bring the maxillary alveolar segment or segments into contact with the premaxilla in both unilateral and bilateral cleft lip and palate. Further objectives of the PNAM technique are to bring the cleft lip segments closer together, expand the columellar mucosa and skin, and improve symmetry of the nasal tip. Parental compliance should be assessed before initiating a PNAM treatment program, which should begin within the first several weeks after birth.

In cases of a wide unilateral or bilateral cleft lip, alveolus and palate, presurgical orthodontic treatment with PNAM is started at the second office visit (Fig. 36.11). A specialized orthodontist fabricates the PNAM appliance; a maxillary impression is taken around the third postnatal week, after which, the mold is used to create an acrylic nasoalveolar molding appliance. The orthodontist adjusts the appliance every week by removing hard acrylic and adding soft acrylic (Permasoft denture liner, Dentsply International, Chicago, IL). Nasal prongs may be added to the appliance and positioned just under the soft tissue triangle of the nostril (Fig. 36.12). The stents are adjusted by adding soft acrylic to help create a tissue-expanding effect on the columellar skin, simultaneously reorienting the nasal tip. The orthodontist adapts the appliance over the next several months to reposition the alveolar arches, delaying the definitive cleft lip repair until approximately 4 to 5 months of age. The alveolar segments may be repositioned to come in contact prior to lip closure, potentially allowing closure of the alveolar cleft with a gingivoperiosteoplasty.

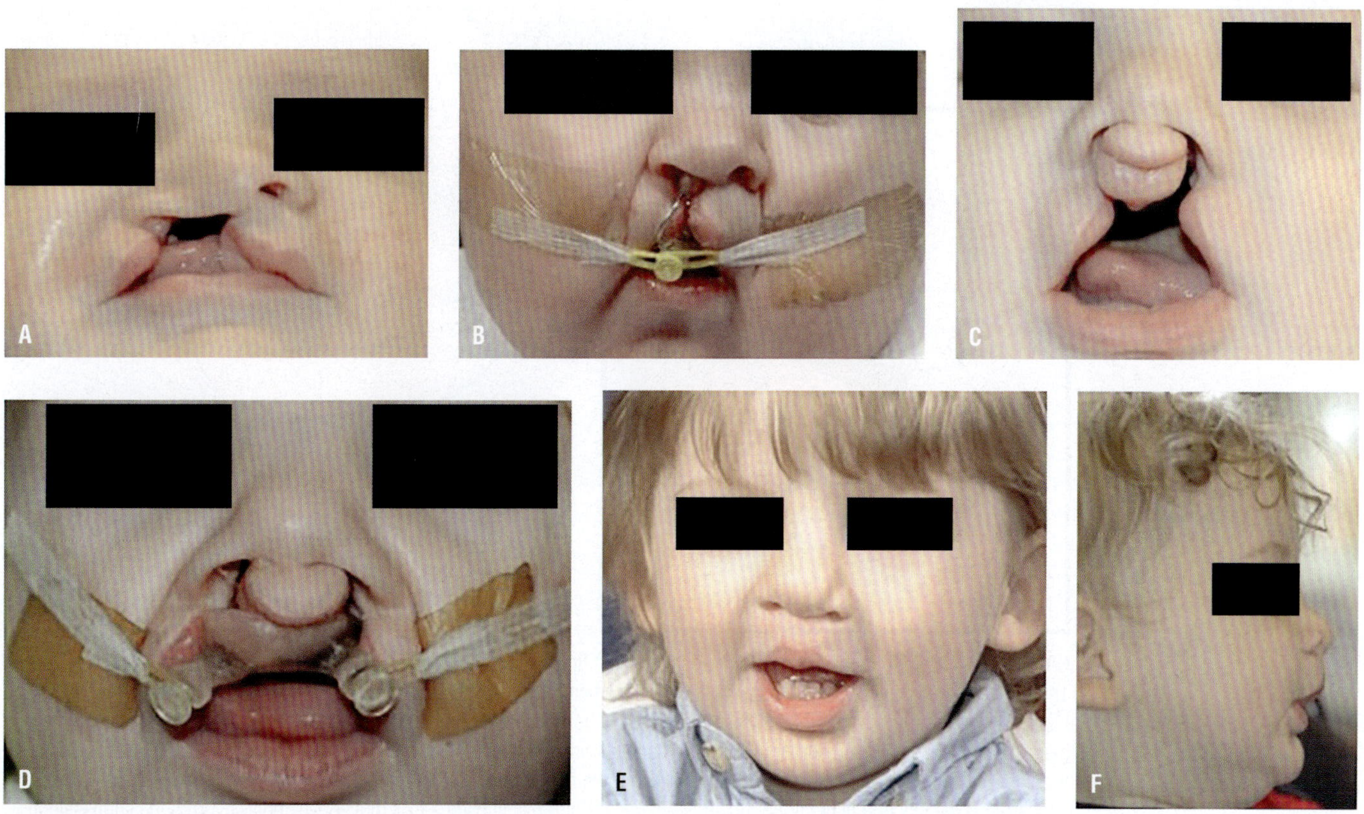

FIGURE 36.12 Infant with a right complete unilateral cleft lip and palate **(A)** preoperatively and **(B)** during PNAM with the appliance and nostril prong in place; **(C)** another infant with bilateral cleft lip and palate shown preoperatively, **(D)** with PNAM appliance, and **(E)** after repair in a frontal view showing the enhanced medial lip tubercle and **(F)** profile view showing the effect of primary rhinoplasty on the nasolabial relation.

Staged Repair

In the severely wide cleft lip, some surgeons choose to use a lip adhesion technique to bring the mucosa and lip skin together without dissection of orbicularis oris muscle. The second-stage definitive cleft lip repair is then delayed for several months until the orthopedic forces created by the lip adhesion move the lip and alveolar segment into closer proximity. Another way to stage repair of the bilateral cleft lip deformity is to address each side individually. The main drawbacks to this approach are the increased potential for asymmetry and difficulty in reconstituting an intact orbicularis oris sphincter over the premaxilla.

SURGICAL TECHNIQUE

Unilateral Complete Cleft Lip

After induction of general endotracheal anesthesia, the tube is taped to the midline of the chin to avoid distortion of the upper lip and nasal tip, and the eyes are protected with occlusive dressings. Local anesthetic (1% lidocaine with 1:100,000 epinephrine) is infiltrated under the upper lip, into the supraperiosteal planes of the maxilla, in order to block the infraorbital nerves. The oral commissures and midline buccal sulcus are injected, taking care to avoid edema at the lip edges. Low volume injection into the plane between the lower lateral cartilages and skin–soft tissue envelope (SSTE) of the nasal tip is performed through standard marginal injection sites.

Lip Markings and Flap Design

Initial markings are placed at the subnasale and lateral alar base, by tattooing with a 30-gauge needle and methylene blue (Fig. 36.13). The junction of the columella and the upper lip is marked, followed by the midline

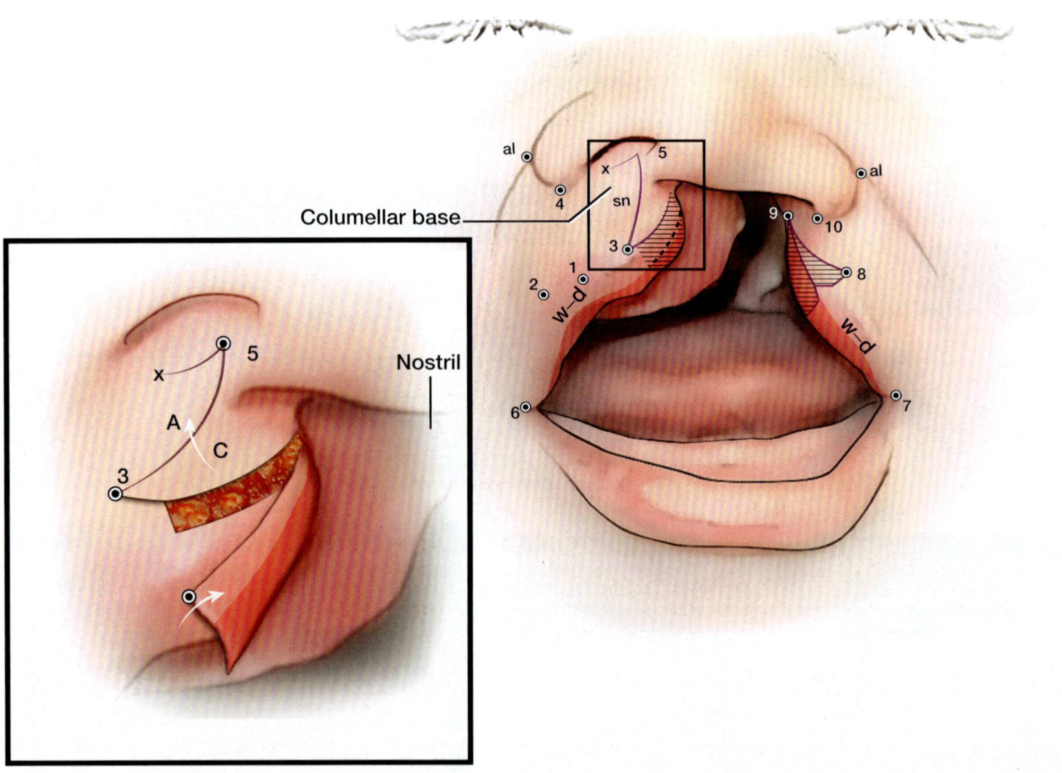

FIGURE 36.13 Cleft lip markings for the unilateral cleft lip repair using a modified Mohler rotation–advancement technique. The five flaps are visualized as the rotation, the advancement, the columellar, the medial mucosal, and the lateral mucosal flaps. The wet–dry (*w–d*) junction is where the wet vermilion and dry vermilion meet. The triangle flap of the left lateral lip is marked just below point *8* to add dry vermilion mucosa to the medial lip. The numbered points include the following: point *1* is center of Cupid bow, with point *2* the Cupid peak on the noncleft side and point *3* the Cupid peak on the cleft side. The subnasale is the junction of the upper lip and columella. Point *5* is chosen 2 to 3 mm above and away from the subnasale in the highest point of the rotation flap. Points *3* to *5* are lengthened with a back-cut made to point (see **inset**). Points *6* and *7* are the commissures of the lip. Points *4* and *9* are the junction of the ala to the columella in the nasal sill. Points *8* and *9* make up the advancement flap height, which should equal line *3-5-x*. **Inset:** The columellar flap (*C*) is elevated deep to the dermis and rotated into the donor site of the rotation flap (*A*).

philtral column at the vermilion–cutaneous (v–c) junction. Approximately 2 to 3 mm lateral to this, the Cupid's bow peaks on the cleft and noncleft sides are marked.

The modified Mohler rotation–advancement markings place the rotation flap incision up onto the columella, approximately 1 to 1.5 mm above the subnasale and toward the noncleft side, approximately two-thirds to three-fifths of the width of the columella away from the cleft side. This additional length of skin on the columella adds to the rotational component of the rotation–advancement closure, and a back-cut may be added to extend the rotational flap length. Attention is then directed to the columellar ("c" flap) markings, which follow the lateral cleft edge of the prolabium at the junction of the cutaneous component of the columella and medial oral mucosa. Great care should be taken to not include any mucosa in the "c" flap to ensure that mucosal edges are not involved in the skin closure.

The most important consideration when restoring cutaneous lip height is proper marking and adjustment of the position of the lateral advancement flap. This is necessary to create lip length symmetry between the cleft and noncleft sides. Using a caliper, the first measurement is taken from the subnasale to the Cupid's bow peak on the noncleft side. This measurement is recorded in a simple "tic-tac-toe" chart, which includes left and right on the vertical columns and lip and nose on the horizontal rows (Fig. 36.14). The distance from the subnasale to the Cupid's bow peak on the cleft side is then measured. The design of the flaps permits lengthening of the cleft side to equal the height of the noncleft side. The difference in lip height between the cleft and noncleft sides may be reduced by rotation–advancement and/or a small triangle flap from the lateral lip segment inserted into the inferior-most medial lip v–c junction.

Using the noncleft side lip height as a guideline, the lateral lip advancement flap is drawn. Starting where the triangular-shaped dry lip mucosa begins to taper, the length of the advancement flap should be designed to equal the noncleft side lip length. This flap occasionally extends too far inferior and lateral toward the commissure and may sacrifice excessive lateral lip. One key step is to look at the wet–dry lip junction on both the lateral lip segment and the noncleft side. If the dry vermilion height on the cleft side is more than 1 mm deficient compared to the noncleft side, then a triangle flap may be created on the dry vermilion from the lateral lip segment and inset into the medial lip dry vermilion.

If the cleft side rotation flap height is insufficient, the advancement flap may be modified with a triangle flap placed just above the cutaneous roll. Using this lateral lip triangle to add additional length to the advancement flap side is similar to the Fisher subunit principle for cleft lip repair. The lateral triangle will be inserted into a back-cut on the medial lip, resulting in an additional 1.5 to 3 mm of lip height. A triangle greater than 3 mm is not recommended, as abnormal scarring outside of the lip subunits may result. Examples of advancement flap markings on a very short lateral lip segment are shown in Figure 36.13.

Skin Incisions and Flap Creation

The lip segments are grasped with the thumb and index finger, and a #11 blade is used to incise the red lip's lateral mucosal "l" flap. A #15C blade is then used to incise the cutaneous aspect of the lateral lip segment with a minimal back-cut. The "l" flap mucosal edge is incised down to the buccal sulcus. This buccal sulcus incision allows for a supraperiosteal dissection over the maxilla using gentle dissection with a cotton-tipped applicator or gauze-covered fingertip. The "l" flap, which has been elevated off the edges of the orbicularis oris, is retracted inferiorly so that dissection may extend to the piriform aperture. This permits the alar base to be released sharply from the underlying, aberrant attachments. The mobilized alar base may then be repositioned superomedially.

The orbicularis oris muscle is dissected free from the overlying dermis and the underlying mucosa. Retraction using a double-prong hook and Adson-Brown forceps provides countertension during sharp undermining, but only to the extent necessary for closure. A wider cleft will require dissection for up to 5 to 7 mm, while a narrower cleft may only require 3 to 4 mm of subcutaneous dissection of the advancement flap.

The rotation flap incision is facilitated using a double-prong hook under the nostrils to pull cephalad, while downward finger tension is applied during incision from the columella down to the Cupid's bow peak on the cleft side. The perpendicular dry vermilion incision at the distal end of the "m" flap is made with a #11 blade. The "m" flap is dissected free from the underlying orbicularis oris muscle, and then the buccal sulcus and frenulum are incised and separated from the premaxilla, releasing the orbicularis oris fibers from the nasal spine region bluntly. The back-cut at the base of the columella is made with a #11 blade. The "c"

	Right	Left
Lip	14	9
Nose	16	29
	in millimeters	

FIGURE 36.14 Measurements are recorded to establish the advancement flap height using the noncleft side lip height, the distance from subnasale to the Cupid's bow peak. The nasal base width is measured from the subnasale (sn) to the alare (al) on the left and right.

flap is then incised and separated from the orbicularis oris fibers. A pair of round-tipped scissors is used to dissect between the medial crural footplates of the lower cartilages and the subcutaneous soft tissue envelope. The dissection of the SSTE off the lower lateral cartilages and nasal tip is performed just deep to the columella and extended laterally. The dissection pocket is created as atraumatically as possible, extending over the upper lateral cartilages.

To reconstruct the floor of the nose, an incision through the mucosa extends the "c" flap posteriorly along the inferior aspect of the nasal septum. The septal mucosal edge is bluntly dissected and rotated laterally to contact the lateral lip and nasal base. The nasal floor is closed with 5-0 chromic gut sutures, using the columella and nasal ala junction on the noncleft side as a guide. The alar base "cinching" suture is passed through the cleft side alar base and suspended to the level of the nasal spine and caudal septum with a 3-0 polyglactin suture. If the alar base appears inferiorly malpositioned, cephalad placement of the suture may reposition the alar base more symmetrically with respect to the contralateral side. Calipers are used to achieve symmetry in this maneuver by measuring from subnasale to the alar base tattooed marking points. Meticulous closure of the floor of the nose is essential in order to prevent nasolabial fistula formation. In a wide, unilateral cleft lip and palate, the "l" flap may be transferred to the prolabium and secured to the "m" flap in a side-to-side fashion to add additional mucosal closure or may be passed into the buccal sulcus. However, the skin edges of this flap leave epithelialized lining in the buccal sulcus, and this is rarely needed.

The inner lining of the lip mucosa is approximated between the cleft and noncleft sides using 5-0 chromic gut suture. Closure of the lateral lip mucosa to the premaxillary mucosa is performed, but undone if it distorts the cutaneous lip closure. Usually, one 5-0 chromic gut suture is used to advance the lateral lip segment to the premaxilla differentially, leaving the lateral-most aspect of the buccal sulcus incision without sutures. To create symmetric fullness in the red lip, the orbicularis oris flap from the rotation side is sutured to the advancement side in a horizontal mattress fashion using buried, 4-0 polyglactin or polydioxanone suture. The inferior-most aspect of the orbicularis oris is reconstructed using a vertical mattress suture to evert the tubercle region. Additionally, 3 to 4 sutures in the orbicularis oris are usually required.

Primary Rhinoplasty

Previously, the subcutaneous soft tissue envelope was released from the lower nasal cartilages in preparation for cartilage repositioning. The neonatal period provides a unique opportunity to reorient the lower lateral cartilages surgically. Circulating maternal hormones responsible for softening cartilage are theorized to create plasticity in the neonate's nasal cartilage, potentially permitting reshaping in the early neonatal period. Two approaches should be considered: a transcutaneous plication approach and an intercartilaginous approach. A transcutaneous suture may be used to reorient the cleft side dome of the lower lateral cartilage in a cephalic direction. While cephalically positioning the cleft side nasal dome, full-thickness triangular fixation sutures may be placed with the knot in the nose, using absorbable suture. Alternatively, through an intercartilaginous incision, a 5-0 polydioxanone suture may be used to grasp the cephalic border of the cleft side lower lateral cartilage, reorienting it more cephalically and medially to the upper lateral cartilage and dorsal septum, similar to Skoog's description.

Lip Closure

Skin closure requires attention to the key area of the v–c junction, with the white roll first being reapproximated using 5-0 polydioxanone suture on a P-2 needle, allowing precise matching of dermal height on either side of the wound. If a lateral lip triangular flap was designed, insertion is completed in a back-cut mirroring the vertical position of the inferior-most base of the triangle flap, usually just above the cutaneous roll. Subcuticular closure continues superiorly. The "c" flap is rotated into the defect of the columella rotation flap site with deep 5-0 polydioxanone and 6-0 fast-absorbing gut. The distal tip of the "c" flap may be trimmed to improve contour and symmetry. The lateral lip segments may require an additional fast-absorbing gut suture to ensure exact dermal height matching of the skin edges. Mucosal reconstruction will begin with buried 5-0 polydioxanone suture to approximate the dry vermilion triangle flap from the lateral lip segment into a back-cut on the medial lip segment, and 5-0 chromic gut is used to reapproximate the mucosal edges, with care taken to maintain the symmetry of the wet–dry junction. The skin edges are closed with surgical glue.

Once the mucosal closure is completed, and the dermal glue has been applied, a silicone elastomer nasal stent is placed into the nostrils and secured with 4-0 silk for 7 days (Fig. 36.15). When the stent is removed, it is cleaned and taped into position to maintain the nostril's shape for up to 6 weeks postoperatively.

Bilateral Cleft Lip

A modified Mulliken bilateral cleft lip and nasal deformity repair consists of concentric orbicularis oris reconstruction, midline tubercle reconstruction, alar base narrowing, and primary rhinoplasty (Fig. 36.16). Markings and presurgical planning are of the utmost importance. Precise lip markings, after local anesthetic has been infiltrated, are possible only if the injections are performed in the deep mucosal layers, under the lip and up to the infraorbital nerves, thereby avoiding distortion of the soft tissues.

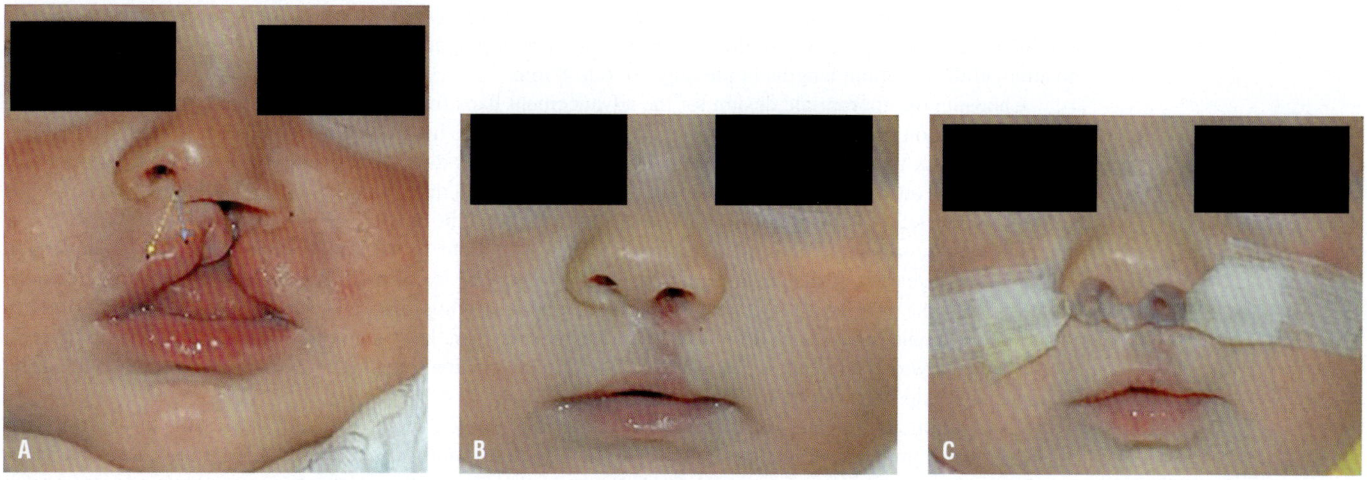

FIGURE 36.15 Infant with a left complete unilateral cleft lip and palate **(A)** preoperatively, showing the simplified markings, which demonstrate that the left *blue line* needs to be elongated to the length of the *yellow line*, **(B)** 1 week after repair; and **(C)** nasal silicone conformers are taped either to the cheeks or nasal tip for up to 6 weeks after repair.

Lip Markings and Flap Design

Landmarks are temporarily tattooed with methylene blue, using a 30-gauge needle and a cotton-tipped applicator for hemostatic compression. Initial markings include the midline of the subnasale (Sn, the junction of the lip and the columella) and the lateral-most aspects of both nasal alae (al). The alar base width (al-al) and each distance from subnasale to alar base are recorded. The v–c junction in the midline of the philtrum is also marked.

The new philtral column will take the shape of a necktie. As suggested by Mulliken, the width of this in most 3- to 5-month-old infants should be no more than 3 to 4 mm at the Cupid's bow peaks. At the base of the nose, however, the philtral flap may be as narrow as 2 mm. Creating a narrow philtrum accounts for widening

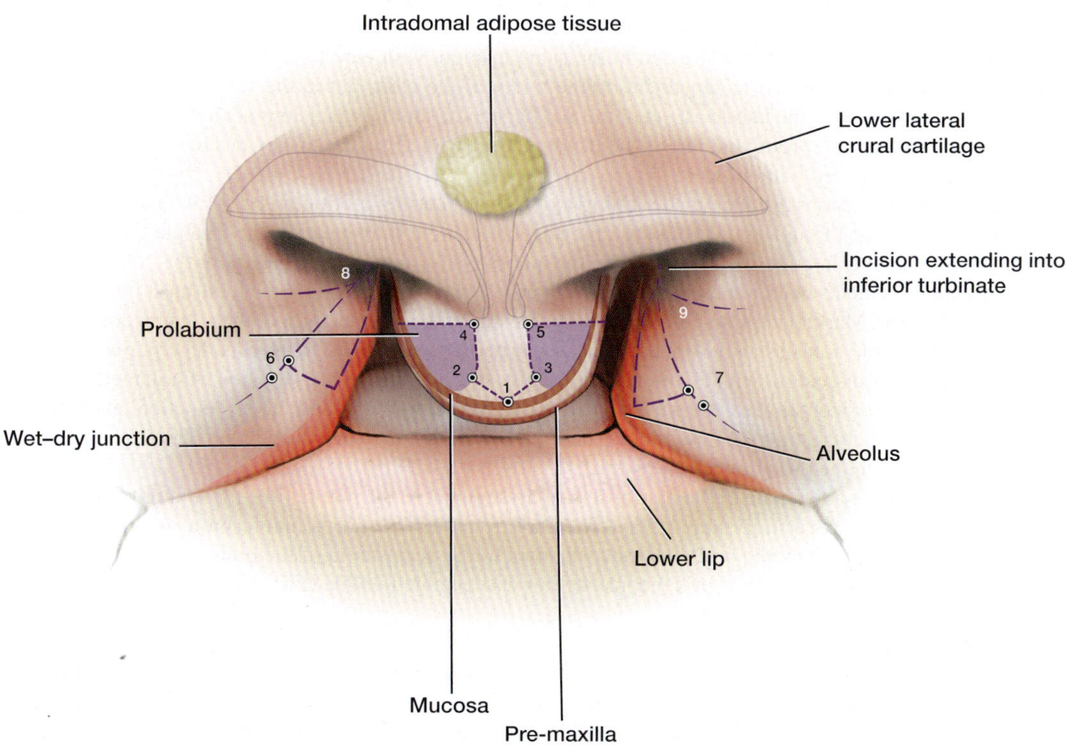

FIGURE 36.16 Illustration of a bilateral cleft lip repair using a modified Mulliken technique. Labels are the same as in Figure 36.13 except that the lowest point of the midphiltrum makes up a necktie shape to account for wound tension and growth of the philtral column. The inferior-most philtral triangle has two points (*2* and *3*), which are 2 to 3 mm lateral to the center. The lateral segments of the prolabium are de-epithelialized (*shaded purple*). The nasal marginal incisions provide access for the primary rhinoplasty.

that inevitably occurs during the healing process. Differential growth patterns of the lip and nose must also be considered during flap design in order to produce a more normal appearance. At this stage, the goal should be to attain philtral column lengths in the range of 6 to 8 mm.

Choosing the appropriate design for the advancement flaps from the lateral lip segments is the most difficult consideration in preoperative marking, as several factors are involved. First and foremost, the v–c junction separates the dry red lip and the cutaneous lip. The white roll is directly above this v–c junction. The wet–dry junction of the vermilion lip is identified and marked where the dry lip mucosa begins to narrow as it extends into the upper cleft. The height of the advancement flaps should be equal to or slightly longer than the length of the philtral column, roughly 8 mm, which has been marked on the prolabium. If necessary, a triangular portion of the superior margin of the advancement flap lip skin may be excised during the final lip closure. However, in most cases, the priority is to create enough lip length by drawing this advancement flap incision inferiorly to where the v–c junction and dry lip mucosa widths are symmetric between both sides. The midline lip tubercle will be created with the lateral lip dry mucosa. The "l" flap incisions are started 2 to 3 mm proximal to the distal advancement flap height (Fig. 36.16).

Restoration of the alar base requires anatomic reconstruction of the nasal sill through identification of the point at which the columella extends down onto the premaxilla. Making these markings symmetric preoperatively preserves the soft tissue of the nasal sill and alar base, preventing future nostril stenosis.

Lip Incisions and Flap Mobilization

The lateral lip segment incisions and release are performed first because of their dependent positions, so that any bleeding from prolabium incisions will not compromise visualization. Using a #15C blade, the advancement flaps are incised from the alar base down to the cutaneous roll. The incision across the dry mucosa is made approximately 2 to 3 mm proximal to the distal-most point of the advancement flap incision. This allows the dry vermilion mucosa to be rotated outward as it comes in contact with the prolabium, facilitating creation of a tubercle. The incision results in a classic "l" flap, or lateral mucosal-type flap, which then is extended along the buccal sulcus under the lip to allow for release of the orbicularis oris muscle attachments from the alar base. Supraperiosteal dissection extends laterally onto the maxilla, with the amount of dissection being dependent on lip width. To account for the increased wound tension in a wider cleft lip repair, more dissection along the face of the maxilla will be required. The lateral lip soft tissue is released from the piriform aperture, extending to the level of the inferior turbinate. Using cautery for this component may be helpful because of the vascularity of turbinate tissue.

The contralateral segment is addressed in the same fashion, with care to make only a minimal alotomy. The length of alotomy required is dependent on the width of the cleft, but in the vast majority of cases, the alotomy does not extend to the lateral aspect of the ala. In general, alotomy incisions are avoided because suture track marks may become prominent and difficult to conceal with growth, and the desired nasal architecture generally may be achieved without them.

The prolabial incisions are then made. Using a downward cutting motion with a #15C blade, the philtral column is incised just through the dermis in a pie-shaped fashion, thus creating the triangle tip at the distal edge of the prolabial skin but not extending onto the mucosa. This flap may be narrow at the columella as the lateral prolabial segments maintain their strong vascularity. The skin overlying the lateral-most prolabium will be de-epithelialized. Markings for de-epithelialization are made along the margin of the v–c junction. Incisions are made down to the soft tissues just superficial to the periosteum of the premaxilla. The periosteum is an easy plane for blunt dissection with a cotton-tipped applicator and allows preservation of columellar vessels. The superior-most horizontal nasal sill incisions are made lateral to the columella–lip junction, extending 90 degrees laterally to help restore the nasal floor. These incisions are made just deep to the dermis so that vascularity is maintained in the prolabium.

To prevent future adherence of the new prolabial lip segment to the premaxilla, the mucosa from the prolabium is trimmed to size; usually, approximately 50% is removed in a horizontal fashion, and then 5-0 chromic gut suture is used to tack the prolabial mucosa down to the periosteum of the premaxilla, thus creating a sulcus across which the orbicularis oris reconstruction will be able to slide (Fig. 36.17).

Primary Rhinoplasty

The primary rhinoplasty technique is modified depending on the severity of the cleft lip nasal deformity. For a severe bilateral deformity, the philtral incisions are extended into marginal incisions just anterior to the caudal-most aspect of the lower lateral cartilages. This allows dissection over the dysmorphic lower lateral cartilages in a plane just deep to the superficial musculoaponeurotic system. Circumferential incisions are contraindicated due to the potential for causing nasal stenosis. Intradomal fat may be repositioned cephalically, but removal is not recommended. The lower lateral cartilages are apposed to the upper lateral cartilages with 5-0 polydioxanone suture, using Skoog's technique. Intradomal suturing increases tip projection as the domes are created from the lateral crura. The SSTE must be manipulated atraumatically to prevent scarring or pigmentation changes. Careful marginal incision closure and excision of nasal rim soft tissue hooding is performed later in the procedure.

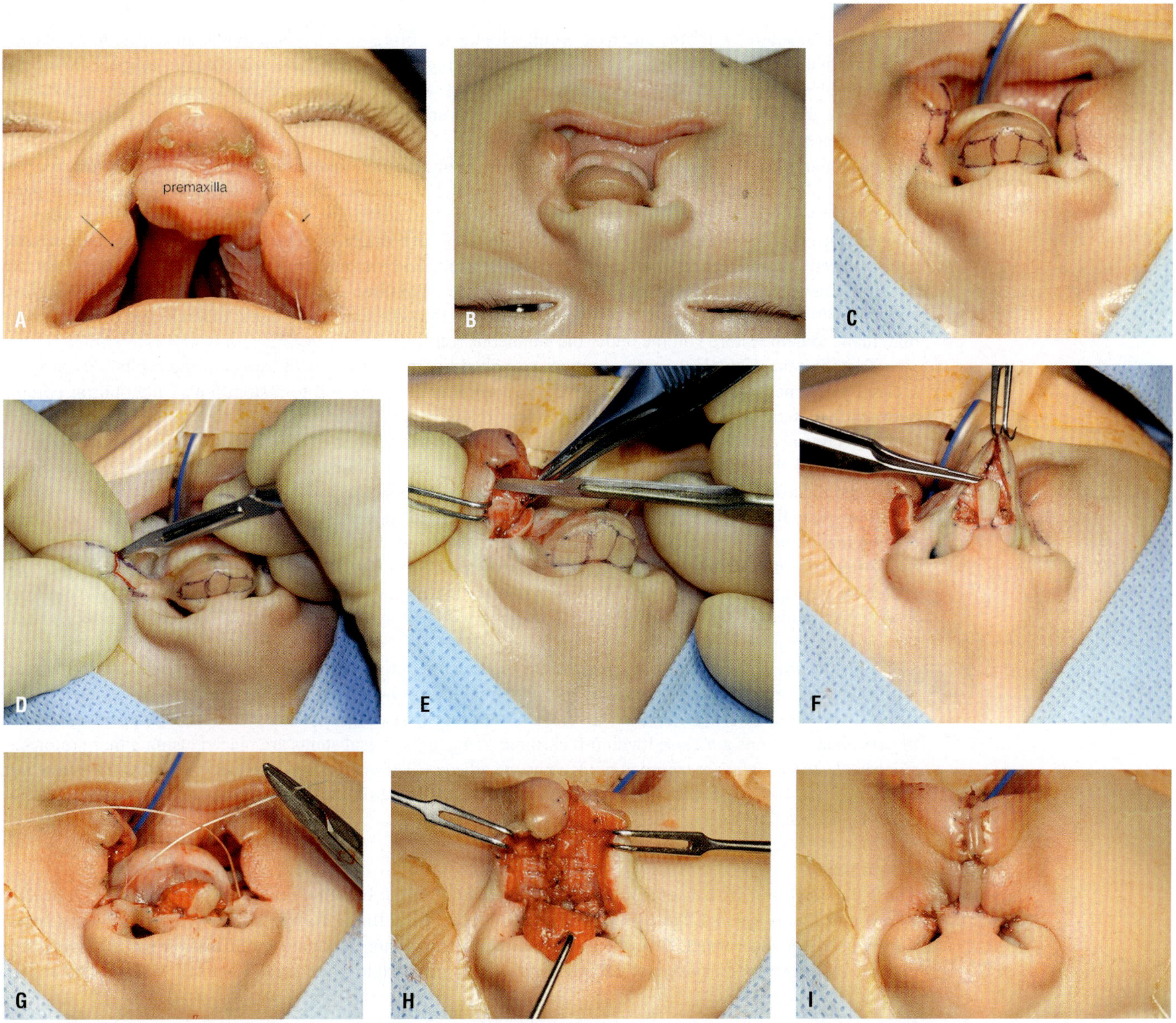

FIGURE 36.17 Sequence of steps for repair of this bilateral cleft lip and palate shown in **(A)** base view with wet–dry junction of the vermilion (*long arrow*), cutaneous roll (*short arrow*), and prolabium just superior to the premaxilla; **(B)** operative view, **(C)** lip incisions markings, **(D)** incision for the left lateral flap, and **(E)** elevation of the skin from the underlying orbicularis oris; **(F)** the prolabial incisions are made and the philtrum created by removing lateral epithelium; **(G)** the alar base suture is tightened to near 25 mm in width; **(H)** the orbicularis oris muscle edges are sutured in the midline, and **(I)** the philtrum is secured into position with the lip mucosa everted to accentuate the tubercle.

Muscle Dissection

Orbicularis oris dissection from the overlying dermis of the lateral lip segments is then performed with traction and countertraction applied to the overlying skin. Careful soft tissue handling includes avoidance of skin edge pinching. Using a small double-prong hook, the skin edge is rolled outward and the dermis is elevated with a #15 blade. Release from the orbicularis oris is performed for approximately 3 to 4 mm laterally, while the muscle is grasped with Adson-Brown forceps to provide countertraction. In the case of a wide cleft, the dissection should extend further, to a maximum of approximately 1 cm. To preserve orbicularis oris pars marginalis a 90-degree change in plane is made at the vermilion as the double-prong hook is applied to the vermilion and retracted upward. The orbicularis oris is released from the lip mucosa in the plane of the minor salivary glands. This allows a rectangular orbicularis oris flap to be dissected free from the skin and mucosal linings. The flap is then advanced over the prolabium to secure it to the contralateral side after the exact same dissection is performed on the contralateral lip segment.

Lip Closure

The key initial suture "sets" the alar base width with the use of a 3-0 or larger polyglactin suture. After placing the suture symmetrically through the alar bases and passing under the new philtral column, calipers are used to set the width at around 25 mm. Suture tension is adjusted accordingly. The previously recorded sn–al distances are used for reference. Difficulty may arise in cases with an asymmetric or very wide bilateral cleft as one may encounter preoperative alar base widths up to 45 mm.

Although a 25-mm alar base may seem narrow during closure, this intraoperative width accounts for tension on the alar base and widening during wound healing. Avoidance of an unsightly, wide alar base is paramount to preventing the stigmata of the bilateral cleft lip nasal deformity. After the alar base width has been set, a concentric orbicularis oris is reconstructed. The muscles are brought together with a 3-0 or 4-0 polydioxanone suture placed just under the v–c junction. The needle is placed orthogonal to the muscle fibers to orient the two lateral segments symmetrically. After the sutures are placed in three equally divided spaces of the lip length, a vertical mattress suture is placed to promote eversion of the orbicularis oris in the tubercle and orient the pars marginalis to help restore volume under the cutaneous roll.

To define the nasolabial angle, a suture is applied to the superior-most aspect of the orbicularis oris and secured to the periosteum of the nasal spine. Attention is then directed to restoration of the philtral column between the lateral skin segments using a 6-0 absorbable monofilament suture on a small needle. The knot is buried to prevent dermal suture granulomas. Meticulous approximation of the cutaneous aspects of the philtrum to the area just above the cutaneous roll allows the triangular inferior aspect of the philtrum to be suspended within the mucosa of the tubercle. The dry mucosa edges are sutured with vertical mattress 5-0 chromic gut suture to create the midline tubercle. Reapproximation of the superior-most lateral lip segments to the philtral column may require triangular skin excisions to form the nasal sills.

After subcuticular closure of the lip, any irregularities in epithelial heights are repaired with 6-0 fast-absorbing gut suture. Surgical glue is applied in two thin layers to the skin edges, to avoiding causing track marks. Alternatively, skin closure may be performed with 7-0 nylon sutures, but this requires a brief sedation for suture removal in 5 to 7 days.

The closure of the rhinoplasty component requires meticulous attention to reapproximation of the marginal incisions using 5-0 or 6-0 chromic gut. Potential excess hooding of the medial-most soft tissue triangle skin may be trimmed using a Tajima "inverted-U" approach. The alar rims are symmetrically positioned when the marginal incisions are closed with 6-0 chromic gut sutures. Nasal stents are placed, using either preformed silicone elastomer stents or trimmed red Robinson catheters. These are sewn into place with 4-0 silk suture and left in position for 7 days with attentive cleansing using saline droplets to maintain patency, as infant patients are obligate nasal breathers.

Palatoplasty

The 2-flap palatoplasty is useful for most cases of unilateral or bilateral complete cleft palate (Fig. 36.18). The vomer flap is opened like a book to reconstruct the nasal lining for the latter, while a unilateral septal flap is used for the former. Overall goals include establishing adequate mobilization for a tension-free closure in three layers, posterior lengthening of the soft palate with levator muscle release and repair,

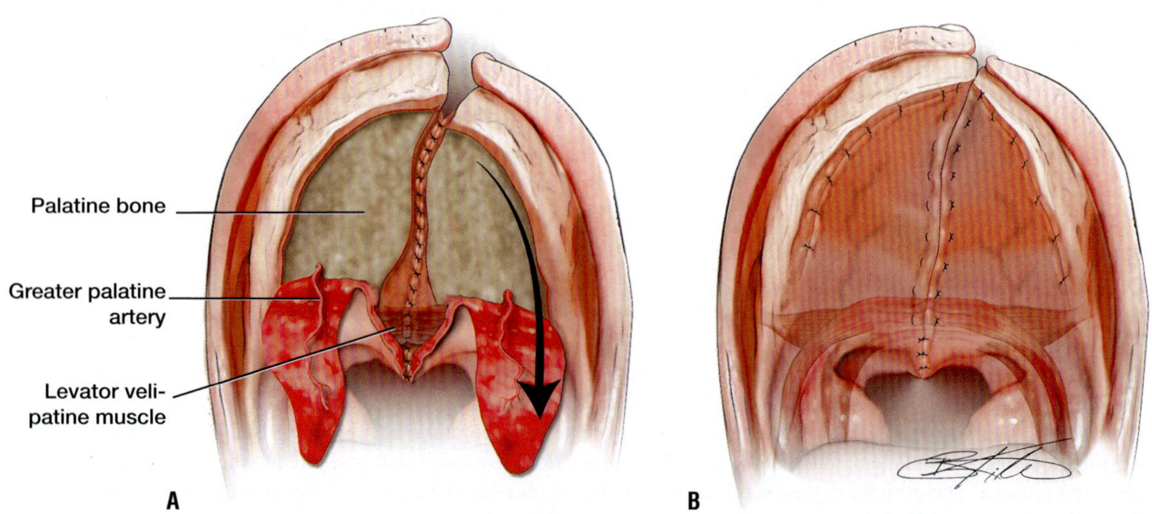

FIGURE 36.18 Two-flap palatoplasty technique. **A:** Unilateral cleft palate repair with flaps based on the greater palatine artery are used. The levator veli palatini is released from the palatal bones and from the oral and nasal flaps. If the muscle is moved posteriorly (intravelar veloplasty), the levator sling is created. **B:** After.

and closure of the anterior nasal floor, if possible. After induction of general endotracheal anesthesia, a shoulder roll is placed and the eyes are protected with occlusive dressings. Preoperative cefazolin and dexamethasone are given.

A Dingman retractor is used to expose the palate, and a repeating 20-minute timer is set to prompt regular release of the tongue, thereby decreasing postoperative edema. Using a 27-gauge needle, 1% lidocaine with 1:100,000 epinephrine is injected around the greater palatine vessels and incisive foramen. The medial uvular mucosa is excised with tenotomy scissors to address uvular bifidity. A #15 blade is used to incise the periosteum of the medial cleft margin from the uvula to the border of the posterior palatal shelf, leaving a 2-mm mucosal edge for closure. The incision extends to the posterior premaxilla and medially along the alveolar cleft. If this was not previously addressed during cleft lip repair, the incision is then extended medial to the tooth-bearing maxilla from the posterior maxillary tubercle. Scoring of the periosteum facilitates flap elevation. A Beaver blade may be used to make the anterior horizontal incision, completing the U-shaped flap.

A Hurd elevator is used to mobilize the flap posteriorly up to the greater palatine vessels, working in a subperiosteal plane. Elevation medial to the vessels reveals the posterior extent of the palatal shelf. The aberrant levator veli palatini aponeurosis is released from the posterior palatal shelf, allowing medialization for future closure. Blunt dissection with a Freer elevator is performed lateral to the greater palatine neurovascular bundle until the space of Ernst is entered behind the vessels. Gentle, controlled upward traction releases the pedicle. Occasionally, periosteal release is required for adequate mobilization. The tensor veli palatini is either released from the hamulus or gentle infracture of the bone may be performed in those cases where excess flap tension is noted. The flap edges are gently cauterized, and Surgicel (Ethicon, Somerville, NJ) is applied for hemostasis. A Woodson elevator is used to release the nasal mucosa from the undersurface of the palatal shelf along the entire extent of the bony margin.

The soft palate dissection is completed with the release of the levator veli palatini from the nasal layer, thereby eliminating traction between the oral and nasal layers. Intravelar veloplasty is performed by some authors, but I feel that it may diminish vascularity and increase scarring as a result of additional dissection. In a unilateral cleft palate, any septal mucosa on the vomer is incised where the oral mucosa and septum converge. The submucoperichondrial flap is elevated for adequate mobilization but minimized in order to respect the potential septal cartilage growth centers. The nasal layers are closed with buried 5-0 chromic gut sutures. Uvular reconstruction is completed with a traction suture placed at the apex, allowing the uvula to be pulled forward while the posterior surface is sutured. Fine 6-0 polyglactin sutures are used to reorient the uvular muscle during closure. The two sides of the levator muscle sling are approximated in the midline with 4-0 polyglactin sutures, taking care to avoid sawing of the sutures through the friable mucosal edges. The oral layer is then closed using a combination of vertical mattress and simple interrupted 4-0 polyglactin sutures. Three tacking sutures are applied between the oral and nasal layers to minimize dead space. The anterior and lateral flap margins are then apposed to the maxillary mucosa with 3-0 polyglactin sutures. Cautery and digital pressure provide hemostasis prior to the patient's emergence from anesthesia.

Other Techniques

Incomplete and submucous cleft palate may be addressed using similar approaches, but varying the incisions and flap design. The von Langenbeck palatoplasty is a variant of the 2-flap technique in which the anterior-most flap is left attached to the posterior maxillary arch. Transposing these two bipedicled flaps to the midline closes the cleft. The Furlow double-opposing Z-plasty is a useful technique for closing the incomplete cleft palate or for subsequent lengthening of the palate. The majority of the levator veli palatini muscle is included in the posteriorly based flaps. When the limbs of the Z-plasty are completed for the nasal and oral flaps, the amount of palatal lengthening is determined by the angle of the flap design (Fig. 36.19).

POSTOPERATIVE MANAGEMENT

Cleft Lip Repair

The goals of postoperative care are to provide analgesia, promote early feeding, and protect the repair from infection or trauma. The use of intermittent soft arm restraints for up to 2 weeks postoperatively should be considered when the patient is not under direct observation. Feeding with a catheter-tipped syringe for the first 3 to 7 days will minimize orbicularis oris motion and tension on the skin sutures. However, in my experience in international work where breast-feeding may be the only available option, I have found that breast-feeding does not result in a higher rate of wound complications.

A nasal Merocel (Medtronic, Mystic, CT) maybe used to maintain a dry postoperative wound and can be placed in the cleft side nostril instead of the silicone conformers. A light coating of bacitracin ointment over the mucosal closure and nostrils may also be applied. Of note, the ointment should not contact the surgical glue as it may cause premature degradation of the adhesive.

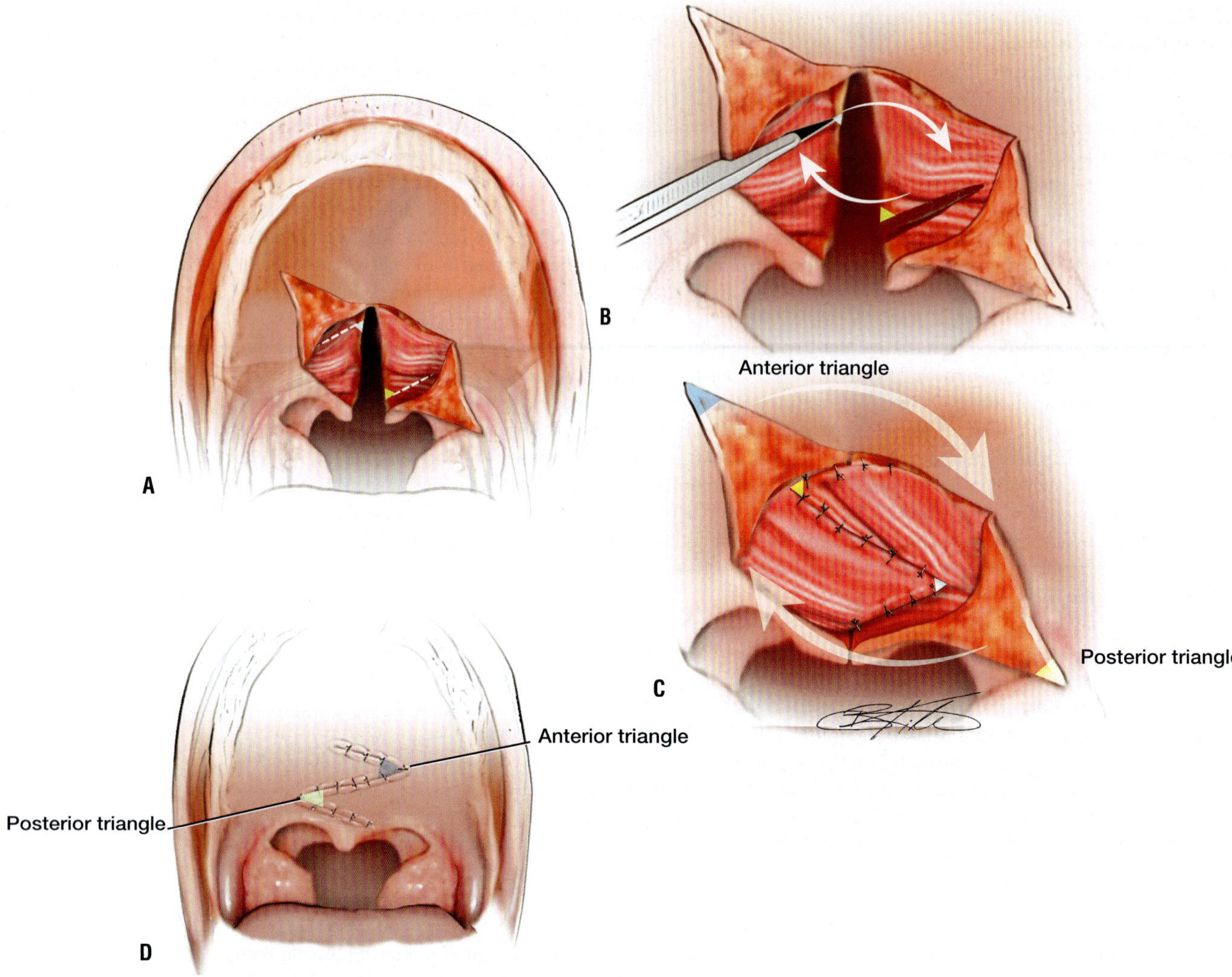

FIGURE 36.19 Furlow palatoplasty (double-opposing Z-plasty) technique. **A:** The posteriorly based oral myomucosal layer on the right is rotated posteriorly, whereas the left nasal mucosal layer is rotated anteriorly. **B:** Conversely, opposing flaps are oriented to avoid suture lines that are directly over one another. **C:** The Z-plasty increases palatal length and creates a levator sling. **D:** Nasal mucosal flaps are closed first maintaining the myomucosal flap posteriorly.

Pain management usually requires acetaminophen, with or without codeine, and may be augmented with bupivacaine nerve blocks at the conclusion of surgery. The use of intravenous antibiotics (cefazolin, 25 mg/kg) and steroids (dexamethasone 0.5 mg/kg) is limited to a single preoperative dose and then two postoperative doses.

On postoperative day 6 or 7, the silicone nostril conformers are removed and washed. The surgical glue is released with petroleum jelly and the wound cleansed with saline. The silicone nasal conformers are taped into the nostrils, and either silicone gel sheeting or paper tape covers the incision for the next 3 to 4 weeks.

Cleft Palate Repair

Although a tongue suture may assist with airway maintenance, this is rarely needed. Positioning the patient in the lateral decubitus position allows secretions to drain from the mouth and opens the airway. Perioperative antibiotics include one preoperative and two postoperative doses. Analgesia is achieved with acetaminophen and codeine, quickly transitioning to acetaminophen alone when possible. Ibuprofen is allowed 48 hours after surgery.

The initial postoperative period requires oxygen saturation monitoring and parent teaching for feeding with a catheter-tipped syringe. For 2 weeks after cleft palate repair, no bottles or nipples should be introduced into the mouth, and soft foods served with a spoon should be allowed only with proper parent counseling on preventing the child from placing fingers or foreign bodies into the mouth.

COMPLICATIONS

Cleft Lip Repair

With appropriate preoperative planning, few complications should arise after cleft lip repair. Inadequate weight gain and nutrition may lead to a prolonged hospital course, possible anesthesia difficulties, or wound healing impairment. Aesthetic outcomes after cleft lip and palate repair are difficult to measure objectively. When unsatisfactory results are seen after cleft lip repair, the deformity is categorized as the following:

- Cupid's bow peak "creeping" into the cutaneous lip height
- Vermilion deficiency or excess
- Orbicularis oris discontinuity

Subtle minor deformities may be addressed at the time of planned operations in the future, but major revisions should be performed before the child enters school.

- Decreased lip height may result when the medial cleft lip is inadequately rotated. This may be rectified using a revision rotation–advancement and/or a laterally based triangle flap. A vermilion mismatch between the two sides of the cleft lip may be addressed with a triangle flap Z-plasty and redistribution of mucosal volume. More sophisticated revision techniques are employed in areas of deficiency, such as reorientation of buried flaps or application of free dermal grafts to the lip.
- Dynamic lip examination may reveal that the orbicularis oris was inadequately released or repaired. Repairing this defect requires complete division of the lip, removal of any central scar, dissection of functional muscle, and creation of a concentric orbicularis oris sphincter. A common site for this problem is the nasal sill, which may also be the site of a fistula due to inadequate nasal floor reconstruction. Although direct access through the nostril may be effective, closure of the nasal floor and fistula is often better approached through complete division of the lip repair and thorough revision closure.
- Lip dehiscence, though rare, occurs more frequently in the setting of patient-centered problems (e.g., poor nutrition or infection) or surgeon error (e.g., excessive wound tension or a lack of layered closure). Delaying a cleft lip repair for weeks or months may allow maxillary repositioning or soft tissue taping, as well as improvement in nutritional status.
- The risk of an undiagnosed cardiac defect is also higher in patients with cleft lip and palate. Delaying surgical repair permits additional time to identify associated comorbidities that may affect the patient's recovery.

Palatoplasty

Complications following palatoplasty may present both in the immediate postoperative period and in a more delayed fashion.

Common Immediate Complications

- Hemorrhage
- Airway obstruction related to anatomic compression (e.g., Pierre Robin sequence)
- Narcosis: Oxygen saturation monitoring and careful attention to the patient's level of consciousness are imperative.

Late Complications

- Palatal dehiscence
- Palatal fistula
- Tooth bud injury
- Midface growth inhibition

Palatal fistulas may be repaired primarily, with a tongue flap or with a facial artery myomucosal flap. Even with proper palatal reconstruction, approximately 10% of patients will have velopharyngeal insufficiency despite speech therapy. These patients will require a thorough multidisciplinary speech evaluation and treatment program including consistent and carefully directed speech therapy, nasopharyngeal fiberoptic endoscopic examination, and possible nasometry or lateral fluoroscopic videography. The latter has lost favor due to the radiation exposure required for the study. Surgical correction may include double-opposing Z-plasty, sphincter pharyngoplasty, or superiorly based flap pharyngoplasty.

RESULTS

While it is nearly impossible to erase completely the stigmata of orofacial clefting, the well-executed repair should achieve middle and lower facial symmetry with a normal lip contour, adequate nasal tip projection, and

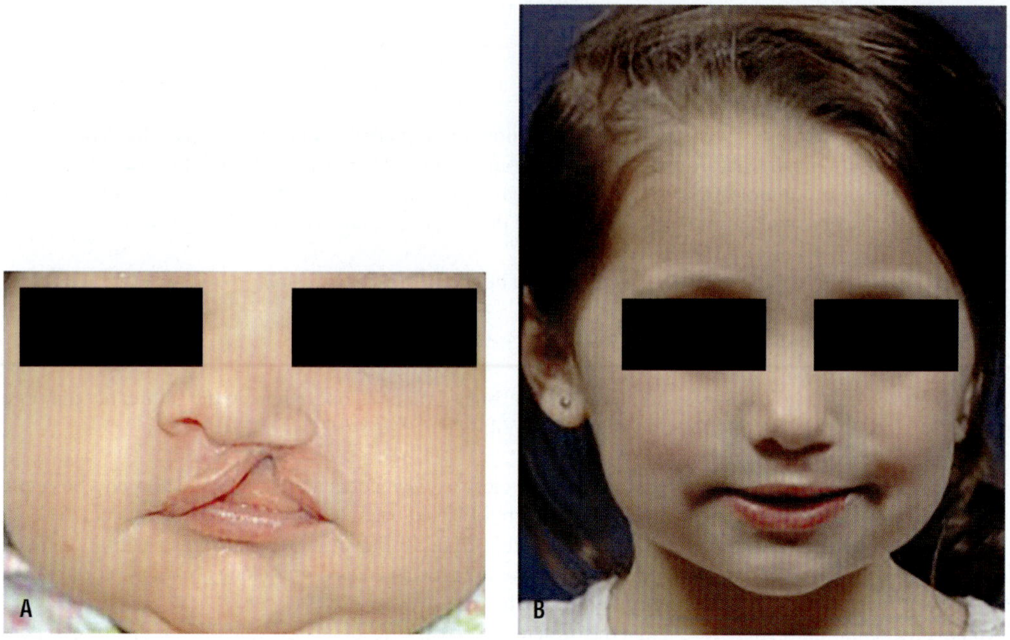

FIGURE 36.20 Patient with an incomplete unilateral cleft lip preoperatively **(A)** and 3 years after surgery **(B)**.

minimal scarring. Velopharyngeal reconstruction should permit normal phonation and minimize nasopharyngeal reflux, without causing upper airway obstruction. Examples of cleft lip and palate repairs are illustrated in Figures 36.20 to 36.23.

PEARLS

- Management of cleft lip with or without cleft palate is best accomplished by a multidisciplinary team.
- The nasal deformity seen in both unilateral and bilateral orofacial clefts should be addressed with the primary lip repair.

Unilateral Cleft Lip

- Creation of adequate medial lip height with either a rotation flap or inset of a triangle flap is imperative.
- Orbicularis oris undermining from the cutaneous lip dermis is limited on the medial side in order to produce a philtral dimple.
- The nasal floor is created from septal mucosal dissection and lateral nasal mucosa divided from the piriform aperture.

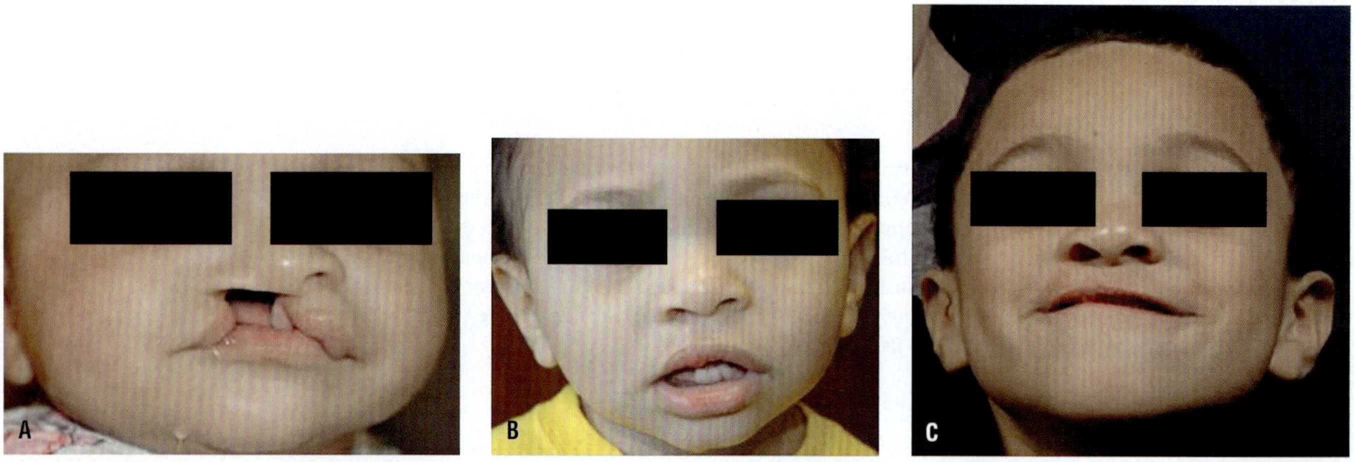

FIGURE 36.21 Patient with a complete unilateral cleft lip and palate preoperatively **(A)**, 6 months postoperatively **(B)**, and at 4 years **(C)** after surgery.

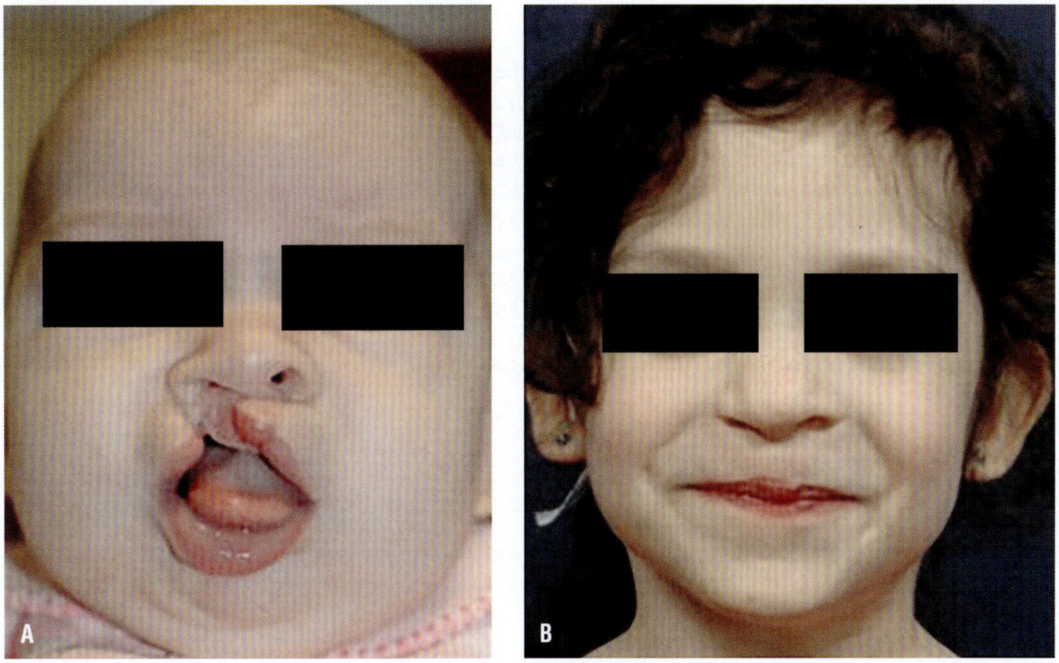

FIGURE 36.22 Patient with an asymmetric bilateral cleft lip and palate preoperatively **(A)** and 4 years postoperatively **(B)**.

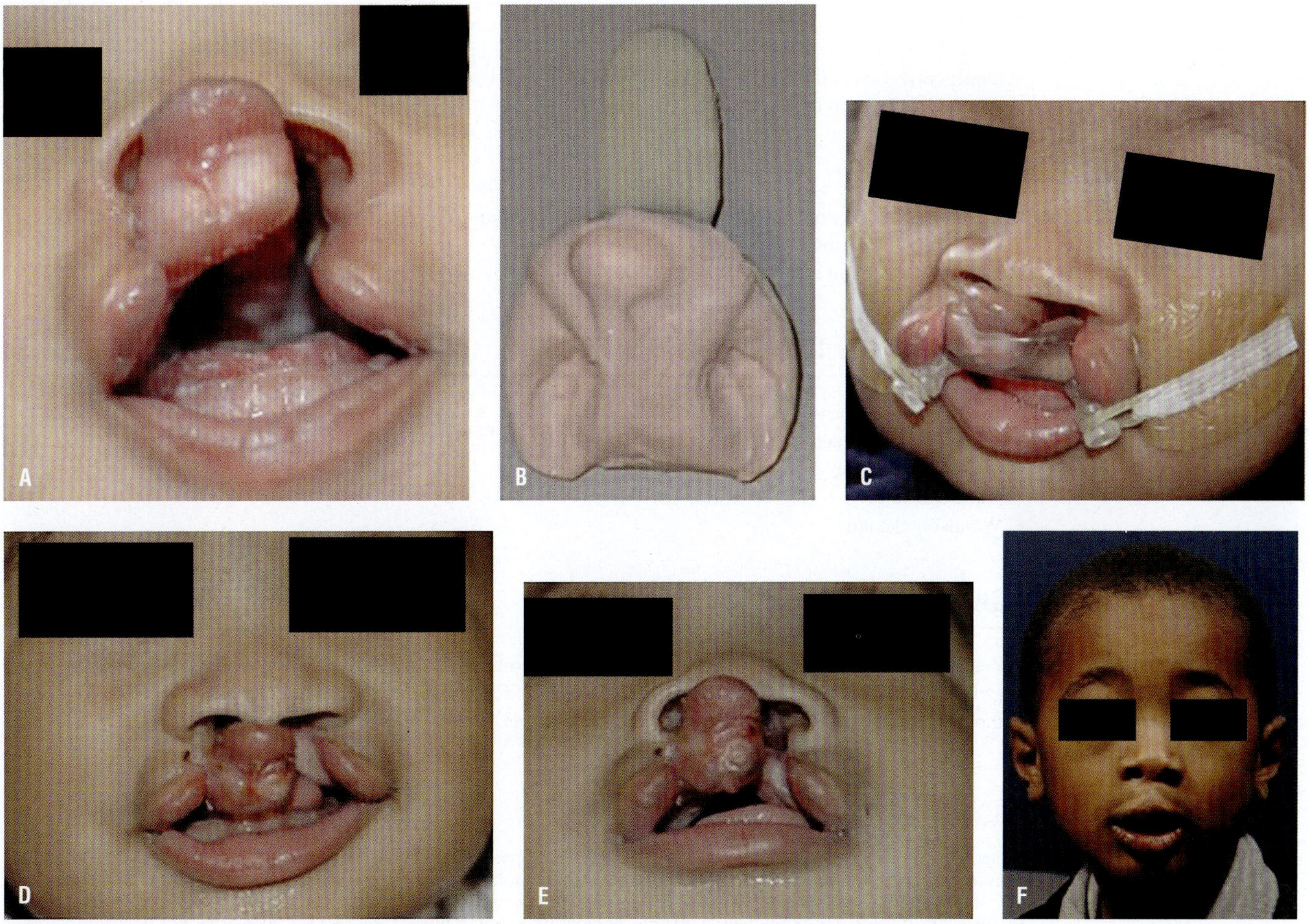

FIGURE 36.23 Patient with incomplete bilateral cleft lip and palate. Imaging during the first week of life **(A)**, of the PNAM molding **(B)**, with the application of the PNAM molding **(C)**, 7 months after PNAM molding **(D and E)**, and 3 years after surgical correction **(F)**.

Bilateral Cleft Lip

- Presurgical molding and lip taping may help prepare the lip for tension-free repair.
- The use of primary rhinoplasty and PNAM may obviate the need for secondary columellar skin lengthening.
- The philtral column should be made necktie shaped and as narrow as 4 mm at the Cupid's bow peak.
- The narrow philtrum will survive due to vascularity from the de-epithelialized prolabium.
- Suturing the superior-most orbicularis oris to the nasal spine may help emphasize the nasolabial angle.

Palatoplasty

- Complete dissection and release of the palatoplasty flaps allows tension-free apposition and three-layered closure.
- The greater palatine neurovascular bundle may be released bluntly from the periosteum to maximize mobility of the flaps.

PITFALLS

- Poor soft tissue handling techniques compromise tissue viability and lead to scarring, hyperpigmentation, tears, and compromise of the end aesthetic outcome.

Unilateral Cleft Lip

- Daily lip taping may affect soft tissue expansion.
- Nasal alotomy is not necessary with modern cheiloplasty techniques.

Bilateral Cleft Lip

- Under correction of the alar base width is common. One should set made as narrowly as possible, around 25 mm.
- Wound healing forces will widen a philtral column flap making it excessively wide.

Palatoplasty

- Incomplete dissection and release of the palatoplasty flaps leads to a greater incidence of palatal dehiscence and fistula formation.
- Failure to close the anterior-most nasal flaps can lead to a nasolabial fistula.

INSTRUMENTS TO HAVE AVAILABLE

- Cleft lip and palate set
- Standard plastics set
- Dingman retractor
- Hurd elevator
- Woodson elevator

ACKNOWLEDGMENT

The author would like to recognize Maj. Marc H. Hohman, MD, for his exceptional contributions to the writing of this chapter. His work in the writing, editing, and figure creation of this chapter is greatly appreciated, without which this chapter would not have been possible.

SUGGESTED READING

Fisher DM. Unilateral cleft lip repair: an anatomical subunit approximation technique. *Plast Reconstr Surg* 2005;116:61–71.

Grayson B, Cutting C. Presurgical nasoalveolar orthopedic molding in primary correction of the nose, lip, and alveolus of infants born with unilateral and bilateral clefts. *Cleft Palate Craniofac J* 2001;35:193–198.

Mulliken JB. Primary repair of bilateral cleft lip and nasal deformity. *Plast Reconstr Surg* 2001;108:181–194.

Skoog T. A design for the repair of unilateral cleft lips. *Am J Surg* 1958;95:223–226.

Tessier P. Anatomical classification facial, cranio-facial and latero-facial clefts. *J Maxillofac Surg* 1976;4:69–92.

37 CLEFT LIP RHINOPLASTY

Jonathan M. Sykes

INTRODUCTION

All patients with a cleft lip deformity have an associated deformity of the nose. The surgical repair of the cleft nasal defect is performed at the time of the primary cleft lip operation at approximately 10 weeks of age. The goal of the primary rhinoplasty is to lessen the secondary deformity and to allow the nose to grow in a symmetric fashion. A secondary rhinoplasty is sometimes required, and is preferably performed in late adolescence, after facial skeletal growth is complete. Successful cleft rhinoplasty requires a structural approach that rebuilds the nasal infrastructure. The deformity associated with congenital clefting of the lip and nose requires restoration and repositioning of multiple layers of tissue. The nose must be reconstructed on a stable foundation to achieve symmetry, to preserve function, and to correct facial deformity.

In order to properly treat the cleft lip nasal deformity, one must understand the characteristic defects of the nose associated with a unilateral or bilateral cleft lip. This chapter describes the nasal abnormalities associated with cleft lip and outlines the operative techniques and timing of the surgery to correct the cleft nasal deformity.

HISTORY

Ultrasound techniques and advances in perinatal medicine allow many children with a cleft lip and nasal deformity to be diagnosed in utero. Early detection of facial irregularities helps the surgeon counsel the child's parents and plan for surgical treatment. It is important for families to understand prenatal and hereditary risk factors that may have resulted in the cleft deformity. A geneticist can elicit a family history of any craniofacial abnormalities or syndromes, evaluate genetic risk factors, and provide counseling to families.

Upon learning that their child has a cleft lip and nasal deformities, many parents are anxious to expedite reconstructive surgery. Prenatal, birth, and postnatal histories are of considerable importance in the evaluation of a patient who may undergo future surgical interventions. Further, ensuring adequate growth and weight gain before surgery is paramount. The goal weight prior to surgery is 10 pounds. Cleft lip and cleft nasal deformity are often associated with a cleft palate, which may cause difficulties with nursing. Specialized feeding techniques using bottles with customized nipples, such as the McGovern nipple, facilitates nursing and subsequent improvement in nutrition and weight gain. Nurses especially trained in working with cleft lip and palate patients are a good resource for parents and the surgeon.

PHYSICAL EXAMINATION

The physical examination of a patient with a cleft lip nasal deformity should include an assessment of the severity of the cleft lip along with any other associated defects, such as the presence of an associated cleft palate or cleft alveolus. Additionally, it is important in any child with a congenital cleft malformation involving the lip,

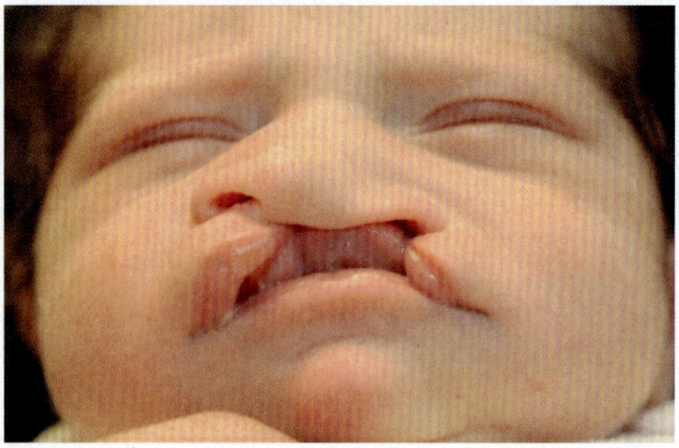

FIGURE 37.1
Unilateral cleft lip nasal deformity. An infant is shown with a complete left cleft lip, cleft palate, and cleft nasal deformity. The left nostril is displaced inferiorly, laterally, and posteriorly; the nasal tip is flattened, asymmetric, and poorly defined; the floor of the nose is absent.

nose, or palate to examine the patient for any associated syndromes, abnormalities, or deformities. Patients who have syndromic clefting should be carefully examined by a knowledgeable pediatric geneticist to identify any potential systemic anomalies.

Patients who have undergone primary surgical treatment for clefting of the lip with an associated nasal deformity may require a secondary nasal surgery, usually in late adolescence. The nature of the secondary cleft rhinoplasty operation depends on the identification of nasal deformities that have persisted following the original repair. Several nasal features must be noted in the physical exam, including alar position, columellar height, tip definition, symmetry, nasal tip projection, and the position of the nasal septum.

Unilateral Cleft Lip Nasal Deformity

A unilateral cleft lip nasal deformity results from a lack of bony support for the nasal base. Depending on the severity of the defect, a cleft nasal deformity can include a common cavity from the nasal floor into the mouth, depression and widening of the ala on the cleft side, flattening of the nasal dome, underprojection of the nasal tip on the cleft side, and deficient bone in the alveolus and maxilla (Fig. 37.1). The features of a unilateral cleft lip nasal deformity are summarized in Table 37.1.

Bilateral Cleft Lip Nasal Deformity

Patients with a bilateral cleft lip deformity have a range of severity in their oral and nasal defects. The common sequelae of a bilateral cleft lip nasal deformity are a shortening of the columella; a wide, flattened appearance of the nasal tip; and a substantial loss of nasal tip support (Fig. 37.2). Clefting and bone loss in the maxillary eminence and bilateral alveolar ridges are important to note. Dentition and alignment of the incisor and canine teeth can be significantly impacted by clefting of the alveolus. Stunted midfacial growth can occur in patients with bilateral cleft lip deformities. Nasal symmetry is often present if the severity of the bilateral cleft lip deformity is equal on both sides. The features of the bilateral cleft lip nasal deformity are summarized in Table 37.2.

Secondary Nasal Deformity

Although the original nasal deformity associated with congenital cleft lips are characteristic, secondary cleft nasal deformities exhibit more variability. Secondary cleft nasal deformities are related to three factors: (1) the original congenital malformation, (2) any repositioning and surgical scarring resulting from prior surgical intervention, and (3) alterations of the nose related to growth. At the time of evaluation for secondary rhinoplasty,

TABLE 37.1 Physical Examination Findings of the Unilateral Cleft Lip Nasal Deformity

Nasal tip	• Medial crus of lower lateral cartilage is shortened on cleft side • Lateral crus of lower lateral cartilage is lengthened on cleft side • Total length of the lower lateral cartilage on the cleft side equal to the noncleft side • The nasal tip on the cleft side has a flattened appearance and is displaced laterally
Columella	• Appears shortened on the cleft side • Columellar base is deflected to noncleft side (from orbicularis oris muscle contraction)
Nostril	• Has widened, flattened, horizontal appearance
Floor of the nose	• Occasionally absent
Nasal septum	• Deviated caudally to the noncleft side and posteriorly to the cleft side • Deviation typically does not cause nasal airway obstruction
Alar base	• Displaced laterally, inferiorly, and posteriorly

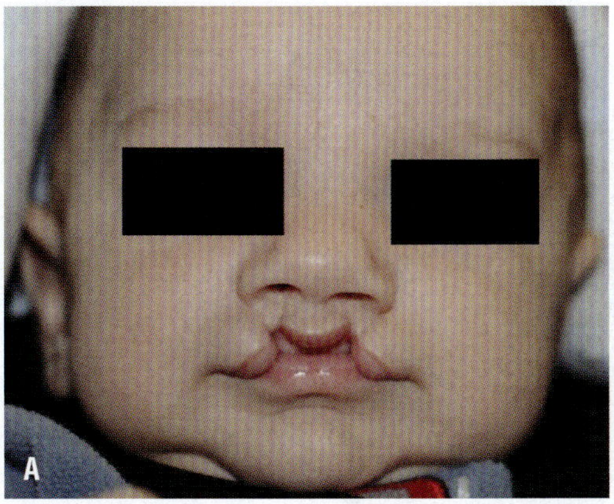

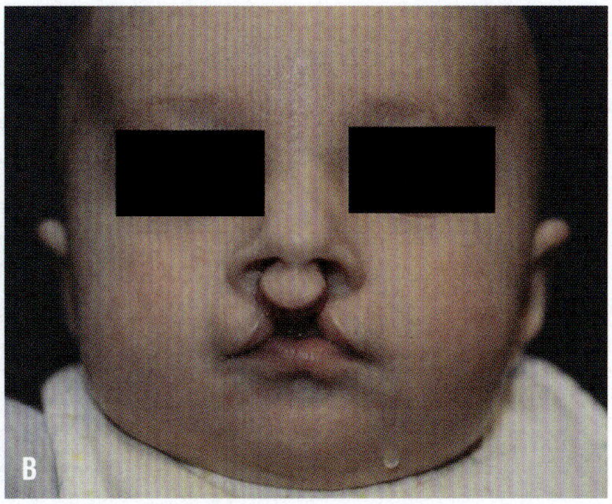

FIGURE 37.2 Bilateral cleft lip nasal deformity. **A:** A male infant is shown with a congenital bilateral symmetric cleft lip in addition to clefting of the secondary palate. He has a mild nasal deformity associated with his bilateral cleft lip deformity and a notched alveolus. **B:** A male infant with a complete bilateral cleft lip and cleft in the anterior palate is shown. The patient has a more severe nasal deformity than the patient shown in **(A)** and suffers from a shortened columella, absent nasal floor bilaterally, and an overly protruding premaxilla.

the septum has not typically been corrected with a previous procedure and has characteristics associated with either the unilateral or bilateral cleft lip deformity. In the unilateral cleft lip nasal deformities, the septum is caudally deviated to the noncleft side and posteriorly deviated to the cleft side. In symmetric bilateral cleft lip nasal deformities, the septum is often wide but is relatively in the midline.

Secondary deformities of the septum and nasal tip can be addressed during definitive septorhinoplasty. In a unilateral cleft lip patient, the nasal tip is underprojected on the cleft side. In bilateral cleft lip nasal deformities, the tip is underprojected bilaterally. The underprojection of the nasal tip is often associated with a deficiency of internal and external skin. Because the underlying deformity is deficient bony skeleton on the cleft side, there is typically inadequate support to the alar base (Fig. 37.3).

INDICATIONS

Patients with a cleft lip will often require surgery to correct associated deformities of the nose that are not addressed primarily with the initial cleft lip repair. The goal of initial repair is to create symmetry and improve nasal tip projection, in addition to closing connections between the floor of the nose and the mouth.

Secondary cleft lip rhinoplasty is performed to correct aesthetic and functional problems of the nose. Indications for revision surgery include a widened nasal base, persistent columellar shortening, poor tip definition, a flattened nasal dorsum, alar asymmetry, and the desire for scar revision. Timing for secondary rhinoplasty is preferably when a patient's facial growth is complete. Performing an intermediate rhinoplasty before the completion of facial growth may be warranted in school-age children or adolescents with severe nasal deformities that are socially hindering and a source of ridicule.

CONTRAINDICATIONS

Infants who are underweight or malnourished or who suffer from global illness or syndromic sequelae may not be good candidates for any elective primary surgery on a cleft lip nasal deformity. Secondary definitive

TABLE 37.2 Physical Examination Findings of the Bilateral Cleft Lip Nasal Deformity

Nasal tip	• The medial crura portion of the lower lateral cartilage is shortened bilaterally • The lateral crura portion of the lower lateral cartilage is shortened bilaterally • The lateral crura are caudally displaced • The domes are widened, leading to a flat tip with poor definition
Columella	• Short • Wide columellar base
Nostril	• Horizontal shape bilaterally
Floor of the nose	• Usually absent bilaterally
Nasal septum	• The septum is midline if the severity of the bilateral cleft lip is equal; if one side is more severe, the septum deviates to the less affected side
Alar base	• Widened with excess show of internal nasal lining

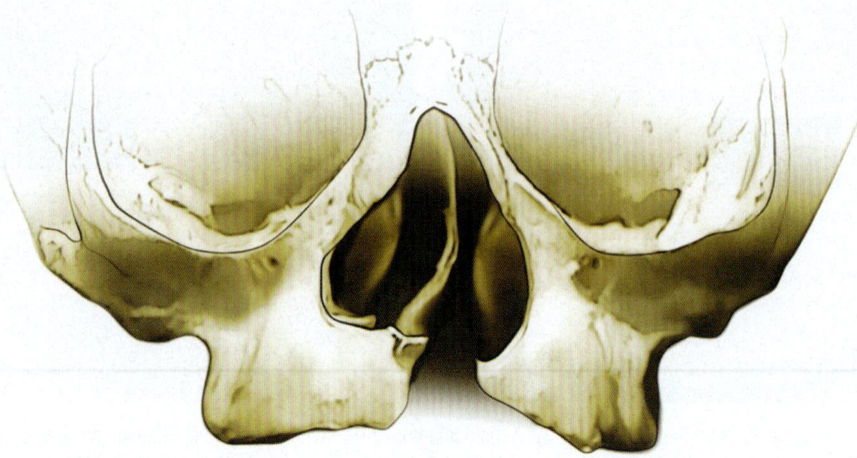

FIGURE 37.3 Skeletal changes in a unilateral cleft deformity. The septum is deviated caudally to the noncleft side and posteriorly to the cleft side. The nasal floor is absent, and there is a common cavity between the mouth and the nose.

rhinoplasty, including major revisions, should be avoided in children and young adolescents who are expected to have further facial growth. Operating on the nose too early in children and adolescents may damage growth plates and create problematic scarring, stunting midfacial growth or nasal growth. If Class III malocclusion is present in patients who have a cleft lip and nasal deformity (Fig. 37.4), orthognathic surgery for malocclusion should precede their planned definitive secondary cleft rhinoplasty.

PREOPERATIVE PLANNING

Patients with a cleft lip nasal deformity may also have a cleft palate, middle ear effusion and hearing loss, speech delay, and significant dental, orthodontic, and orthognathic issues. A team approach to patients who suffer from any craniofacial abnormality is important. Any planned procedure on a patient with multiple surgical concerns should be coordinated with all involved team members. Patients with a cleft nasal deformity in addition to a cleft lip and palate are expected to undergo a sequence of procedures at different ages (Table 37.3).

Before any surgery is performed, patients with a unilateral cleft lip and nasal deformity may benefit from the use of nasal alveolar molding (NAM). NAM is a nonsurgical technique that uses a custom-fit prosthesis to guide and reshape nasoalveolar segments of tissue (Fig. 37.5A and B). The alteration of tissue using NAM can shorten a wide cleft, improve nasal tip symmetry, and lengthen the columella in a bilateral cleft deformity.

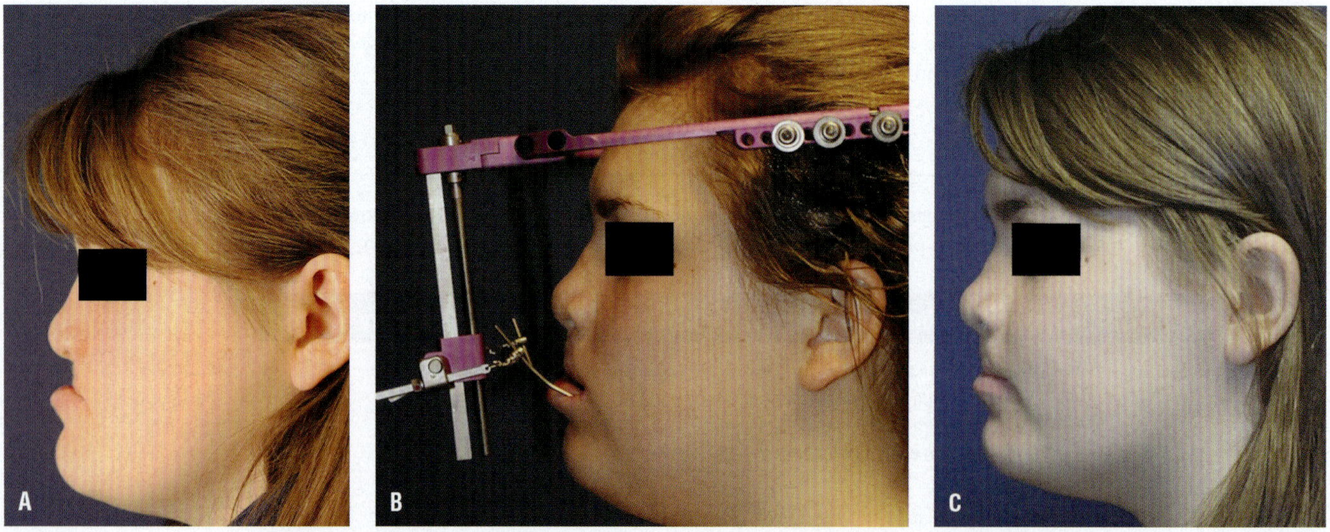

FIGURE 37.4 Class III malocclusion treated with Le Fort I osteotomy and maxillary distraction. The teenage patient shown has undergone a bilateral cleft lip repair and palate repair when she was a child. She subsequently developed maxillary hypoplasia and Class III malocclusion. A preoperative photograph is shown on the left, prior to any maxillary distraction **(A)**. The central photograph **(B)** shows the titanium halo and maxillary distraction device in place following a Le Fort I osteotomy. The postoperative result after plate fixation of the distracted maxillary segment is shown on the right **(C)**.

TABLE 37.3 Surgical Interventions for Cleft Lip, Cleft Palate, and Cleft Nasal Deformity

Primary cleft lip repair and cleft rhinoplasty, bilateral myringotomy tubes	• 10 wk of age
Palatoplasty (repair of cleft palate)	• ~1 y of age
Alveolar bone grafting	• Between ages 9 and 11 year old
Secondary cleft rhinoplasty	• Completion of facial growth; 15 year old in males and 17 year old in females

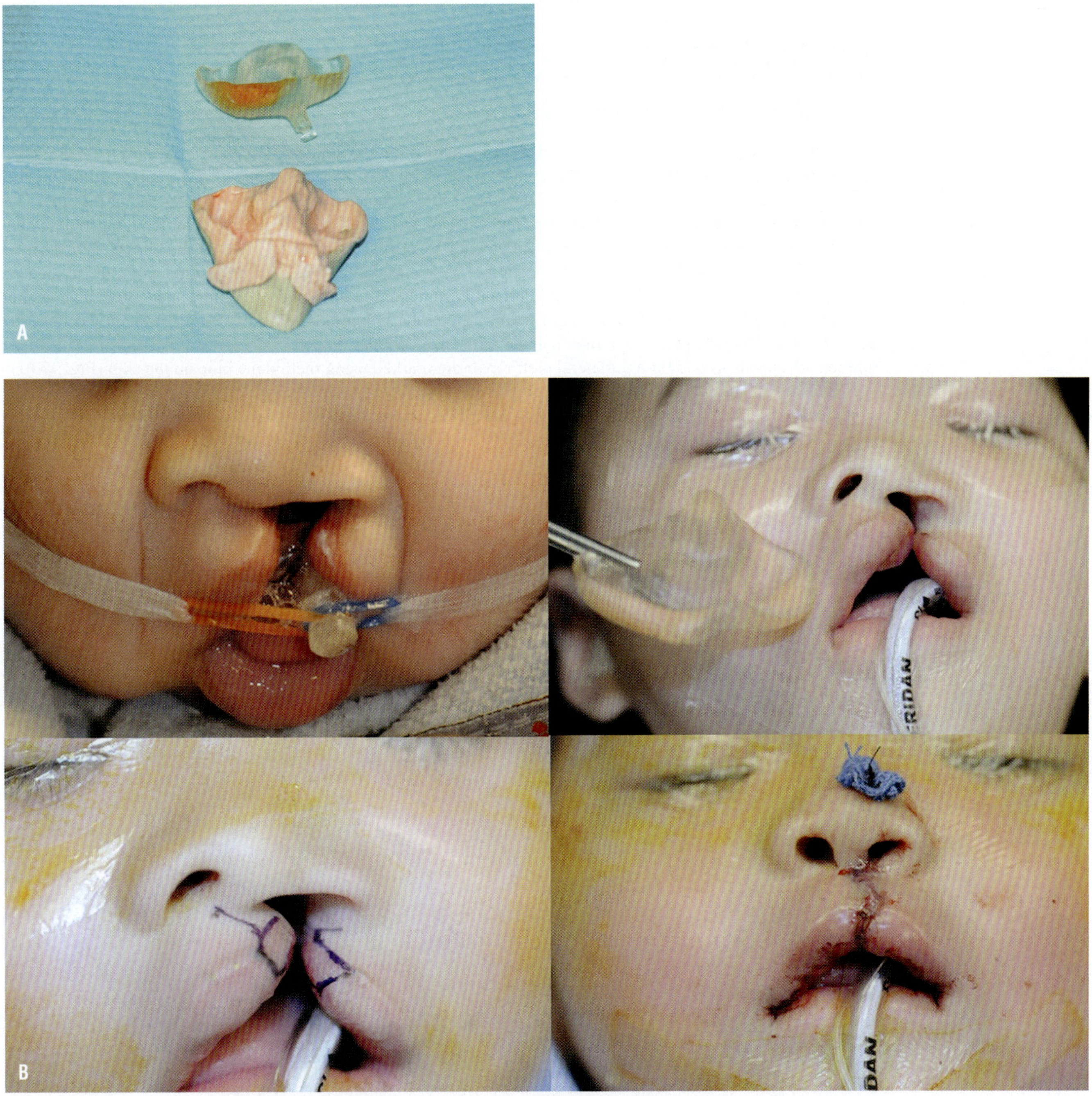

FIGURE 37.5 **A:** Nasal alveolar molding (NAM). By placing a malleable synthetic material into the unilateral cleft lip and palate defect of a patient, a custom NAM has been made. The custom mold is shown in the lower part of the image. From the custom mold, a firm prosthesis can be made for nasoalveolar molding. The final NAM device is shown in the superior aspect of the photograph. **B:** Preoperative use of NAM prior to primary unilateral cleft lip repair and cleft rhinoplasty. *Upper left*: A nasoalveolar molding device is taped in place. *Upper right*: The device has been removed after extended preoperative use, and the patient is intubated for a primary cleft lip repair and cleft rhinoplasty. *Lower left*: The skin markings for a Millard advancement rotation unilateral cleft lip repair are made. *Lower right*: The immediate postoperative result following cleft lip repair and cleft rhinoplasty is shown.

Surgical planning for primary cleft lip rhinoplasty includes performing a careful three-dimensional assessment of the cleft nasal deformity and the confluent cleft lip. Anticipated challenges, such a wide cleft, should be included in the operative plan. Proper instruments and materials must be available for the procedure, such as Silastic nasal conformers and arm restraints to prevent manipulation of the wound in the postoperative period. Consistent and thorough communication with the parents of an infant undergoing surgery helps to manage expectations in the postoperative period.

Patients undergoing secondary cleft rhinoplasty may require auricular or costal cartilage for nasal reconstruction. Contingency plans for graft material should be considered, including the possibility of cartilage and tissue harvest from multiple sites or the use of alloplastic materials. Preoperative photography helps the surgeon to analyze the nasal deformity and communicate the surgical plan with the patient.

SURGICAL TECHNIQUE

Unilateral Cleft Lip Rhinoplasty

At 10 weeks of age, infants with a unilateral cleft lip deformity may undergo a repair of the cleft lip and associated nasal deformity. A primary cleft rhinoplasty is performed at the same time as the lip repair with no extra incisions. Patients are placed under general anesthesia and incubated with an oral RAE endotracheal tube. The operating room table is turned 180 degrees. The eyes are protected with Tegaderm. The gingivolabial sulcus, periphery of the cleft lip, and nasal sill are injected with Xylocaine 1% with 1:100,000 epinephrine. Care is taken to avoid distortion of the tissues with the injection of local anesthetic. The landmarks of the cleft lip are marked for planned incisions using a 1-cc syringe filled with a small amount of methylene blue and a 30-gauge needle. The most critical marks made on the skin help to guide the reapproximation of cupid's bow on the noncleft and cleft side. The patient's face is then painted with Betadine and draped. The planned incisions for a Millard rotation advancement flap for a unilateral cleft repair are marked using methylene blue on the skin (Fig. 37.6).

Incisions made for a primary cleft lip repair provide access for primary cleft rhinoplasty. Once the incisions for a Millard rotation advancement flap have been made, the lower lateral cartilage on the cleft side is

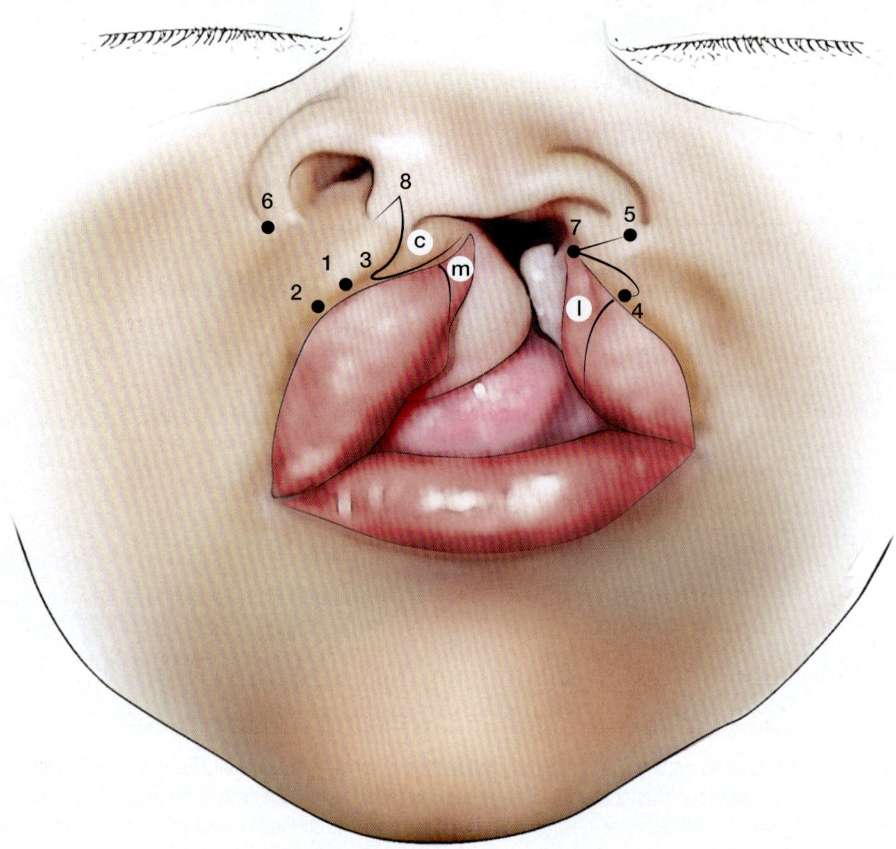

FIGURE 37.6 Skin markings and landmarks for a Millard advancement–rotation flap repair of a unilateral cleft lip. M, medial mucosal flap; L, lateral mucosal flap; C, central cutaneous flap. (From Hopper RA, Cutting C, Grayson B. Cleft lip and palate. In: Thorne C, ed. *Grabb and Smith's plastic surgery*. Philadelphia, PA: Lippincott Williams & Wilkins, 2007:201–225.)

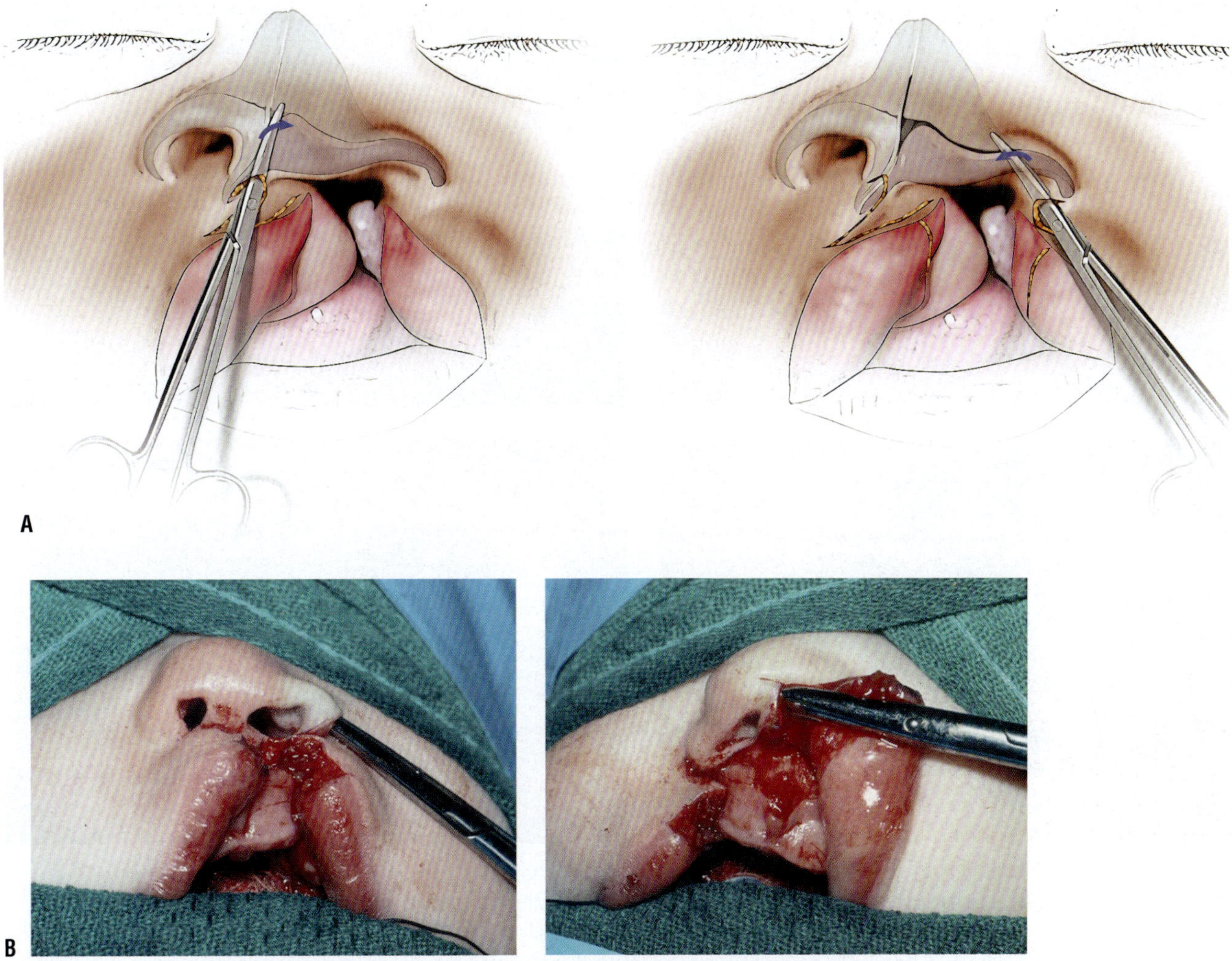

FIGURE 37.7 **A:** Approach to the lower lateral cartilage on the cleft side during primary cleft rhinoplasty. Dissection superficial to the lateral (*left*) and medial (*right*) crura is shown. Access to the lower lateral cartilage is achieved through the cleft lip incisions. Dissection takes place superficial to the cartilage and beneath the nasal skin envelope. **B:** Intraoperative dissection of the lower lateral cartilage on the cleft side. Incisions for a left-sided unilateral cleft lip repair have been made. *Left*: Scissors are inserted deep to the skin and superficial to the lateral crura. *Right*: In a similar fashion, the medial crura are dissected to enable tip refinement in this primary cleft rhinoplasty.

mobilized by performing a subcutaneous dissection of the medial and lateral crura. Scissors are introduced caudally beneath the columellar skin to access and free the medial crura and to release the dome of the cleft side of the nose (Fig. 37.7A). In a similar fashion, the lateral crura on the cleft side is accessed through an existing incision and released from the overlying skin (Fig. 37.7A). Dissection takes place superficial to the lower lateral cartilage on the cleft side and beneath the skin (Fig. 37.7B).

Following dissection of the lower lateral cartilage on the cleft side of the nose, sutures are placed full thickness through the skin and nasal lining. The nasal sutures placed during a primary cleft rhinoplasty are intended to raise the nasal tip on the cleft side, narrow the tip, and improve nasal symmetry. Nasal sutures are tied externally over a bolster made of a cut laparotomy sponge tape. Soft Silastic nasal conformers are then placed in both nostrils (Fig. 37.8). The nasal conformers are secured with a through and through 4-0 nylon suture through the nasal septum. Arm restraints ("No-Nos") are placed to prevent the patient from manipulating the surgical site.

Bilateral Cleft Lip Rhinoplasty

The bilateral cleft is usually symmetric. In isolated cases, a bilateral cleft deformity can be asymmetric (Fig. 37.9). In most instances where asymmetry is not significant, the goal of the primary rhinoplasty is to increase nasal tip projection and to improve columellar length. Improvement in tip symmetry as well as tip projection is the goal when asymmetry is severe. In cases of severe asymmetric bilateral cleft asymmetry,

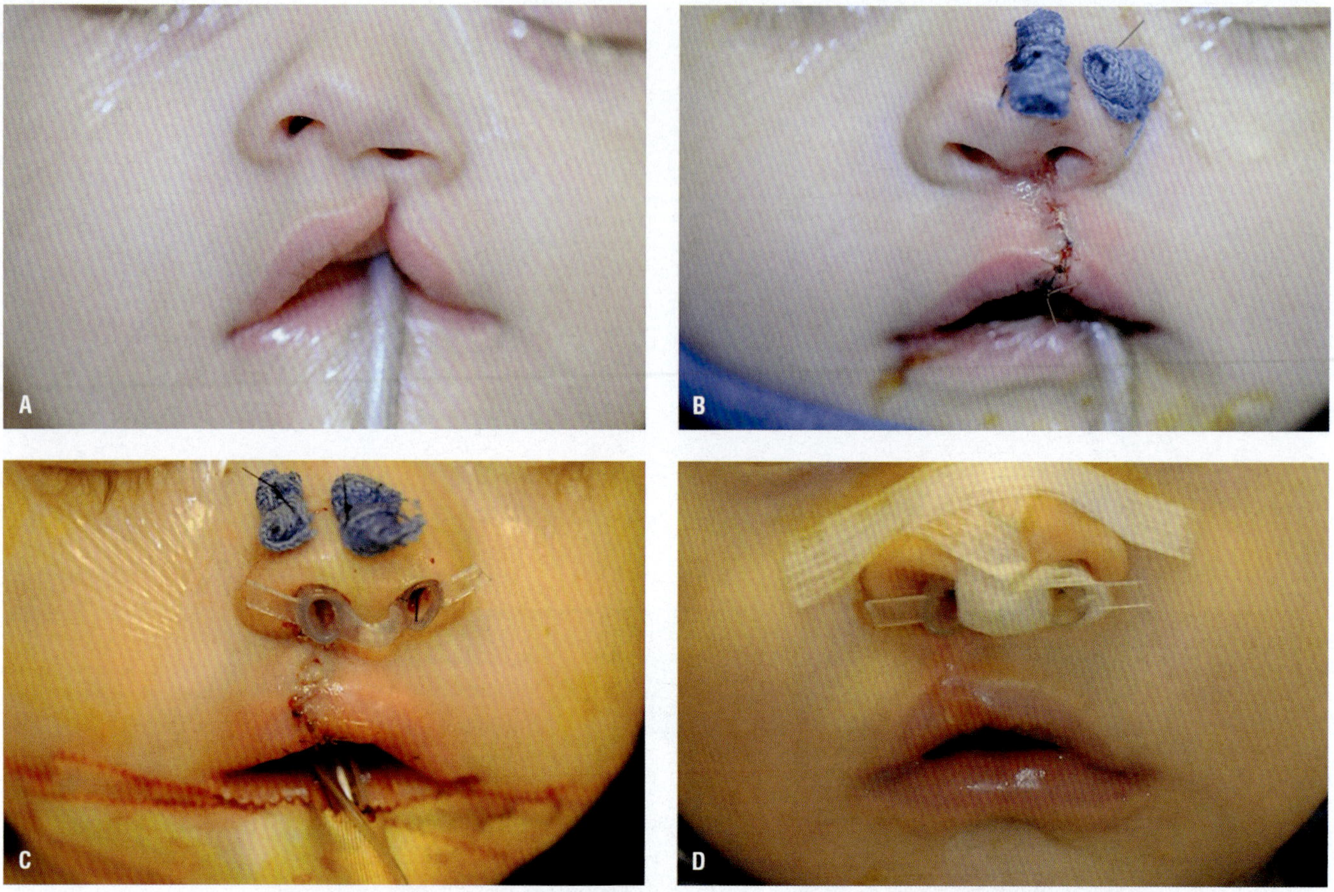

FIGURE 37.8 Nasal bolsters and Silastic nasal conformers following unilateral cleft rhinoplasty. **A:** A preoperative photograph is shown of a left unilateral incomplete cleft lip with an associated nasal deformity. **B:** The patient with the incomplete left cleft lip has undergone a primary repair, including a cleft rhinoplasty and the placement of nasal bolsters and sutures. **C:** A patient with a right complete cleft lip has undergone primary cleft lip repair and rhinoplasty, with nasal bolsters and conformers shown in place. **D:** A postoperative photograph showing nasal conformers taped in place.

patients should be treated similarly to a unilateral cleft deformity. The operative goals are then to close the nasal floor, create a normal nasal sill on each side, reposition the alar base, and increase nasal tip projection.

In the bilateral (symmetric) deformity, the operative goals are to reconstruct the nasal floor and nasal sill, to reposition the alar base into a more normal position, and to increase nasal tip symmetry bilaterally (Fig. 37.10). Repositioning the nasal base is accomplished by freeing up the alar base from its attachments to the maxilla. This is done by releasing the soft tissue fibers from the pyriform aperture that attach the alar base to the deeper soft tissue structures and bony skeleton. After these soft tissue attachments are divided with a curved tenotomy scissor, the alar base can be repositioned by recreating the muscular sling at the superior aspect of the lip. Reapproximation of the muscle is accomplished with a 4-0 clear monofilament long-acting absorbable suture.

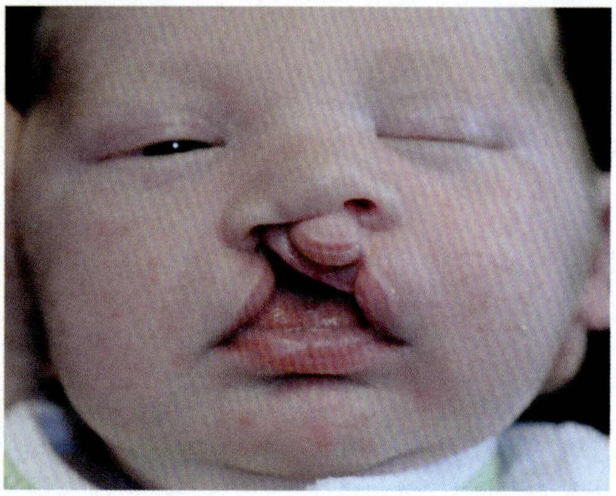

FIGURE 37.9
Asymmetric bilateral cleft lip deformity. A patient is shown with an asymmetric bilateral cleft lip in which the right side is more severely affected than the left.

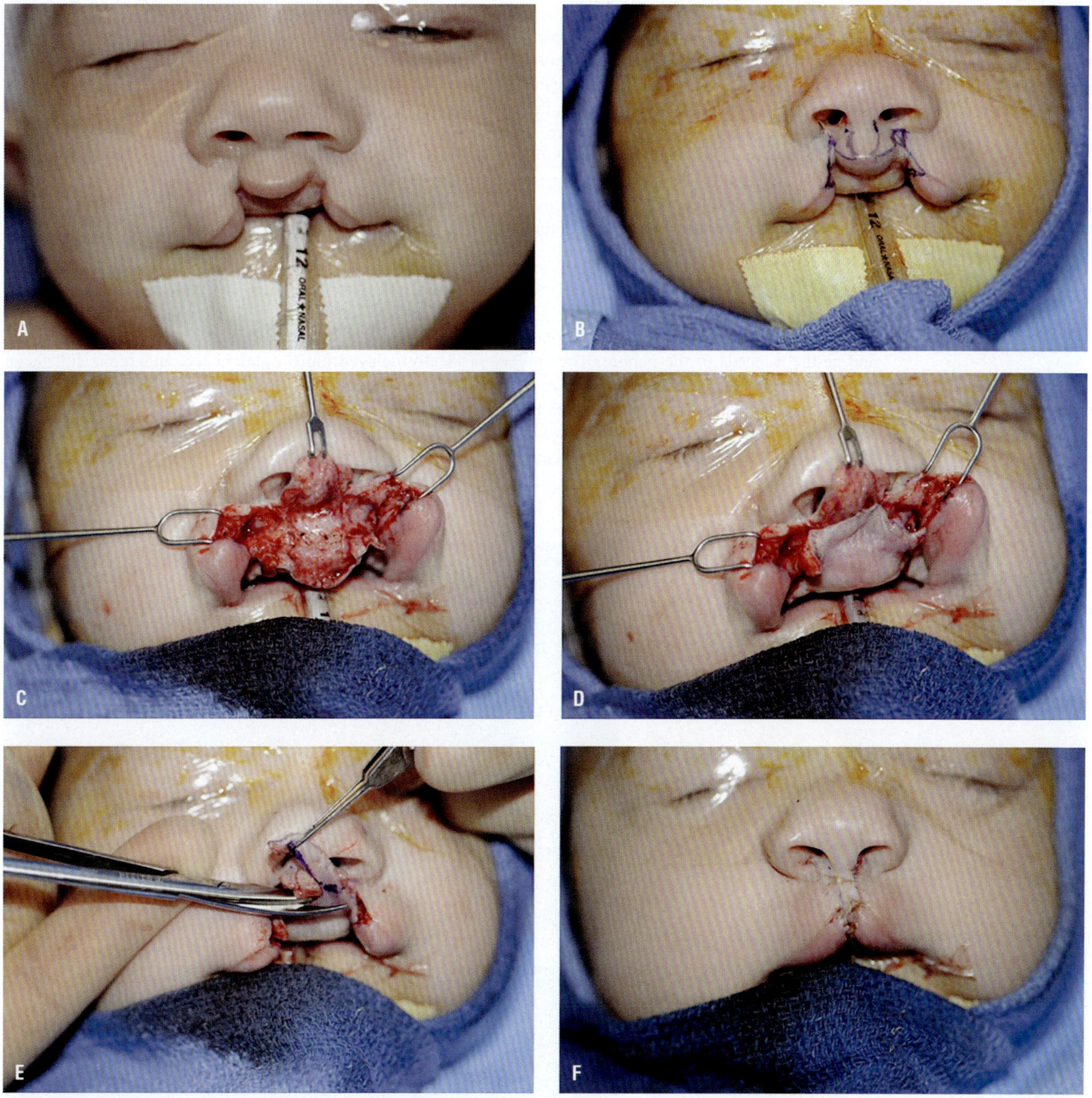

FIGURE 37.10 Primary bilateral cleft lip repair with tip rhinoplasty. **A:** A patient with an incomplete symmetric bilateral cleft lip deformity is shown. **B:** Skin markings are made in preparation for cleft lip repair and primary cleft rhinoplasty. **C and D:** Flaps are dissected, and mucosal closure is planned. **E:** Excess skin is removed. **F:** The immediate postoperative result is shown, including narrowing of the nasal base. The nasal base was narrowed by placing sutures through the deep alar tissue bilaterally during the lip repair dissection.

Reapproximation of the muscular sling at the base of the nose provides volume to the superior aspect of the lip and support to the floor of the nose and nasal sill. Reapproximation of the muscle must be performed in a symmetric fashion so that reconstruction of the nasal sill does not differ from one side to another. Because of the absence of muscle in the central prolabium in the bilateral cleft lip deformity, the muscle provided to the base of the nose must come from the lateral lip segments. Therefore, muscle dissection in the lateral lip segments is performed to advance the orbicularis oris muscle across the midline of the lip. The muscular reapproximation should be performed throughout the entire height of the lip. It is crucial to advance the upper portion of the muscular sphincter of the lip to provide sufficient volume to the central lip segment while recreating the muscular sling that supports the base of the nose.

The standard bilateral upper lip incisions are used to gain access to the nasal tip. Dissection between the lower lateral cartilages and skin of the nasal tip is performed in a blind fashion. The external skin is carefully freed from the lower lateral cartilage, centrally over the medial crus and laterally over both lateral crura. After the skin is freed from the lower lateral cartilages, the lip is closed in a standard layered fashion. This is performed by first closing the mucosal layer, then the muscular layer (as mentioned above), and finally the external skin in a bilateral fashion. After lip closure, sutures are placed within the nasal domes to achieve more definition and projection of the nasal tip. The new domes are refined with bolsters and sutures. Medial advancement of the lateral crura is used to obtain improved medial crural projection. Two to four domal bolster sutures are placed lateral to the preexisting dome. At the conclusion of this procedure, Silastic nasal conformers are sutured into position with 4-0 monofilament nylon suture.

Secondary Rhinoplasty

The operation performed during a secondary cleft rhinoplasty is completely dependent on the functional and aesthetic needs of the patient. The surgery is ideally delayed until a patient has undergone full facial growth. Goals of the operation may be to improve airway function, define the nasal tip, achieve nasal symmetry, increase nasal projection, lengthen the columella, and narrow the nasal base (Fig. 37.11). Principles of secondary rhinoplasty combine the known underlying tissue defects present in a cleft nasal deformity with the structural and grafting techniques of revision rhinoplasty (Fig. 37.12A and B).

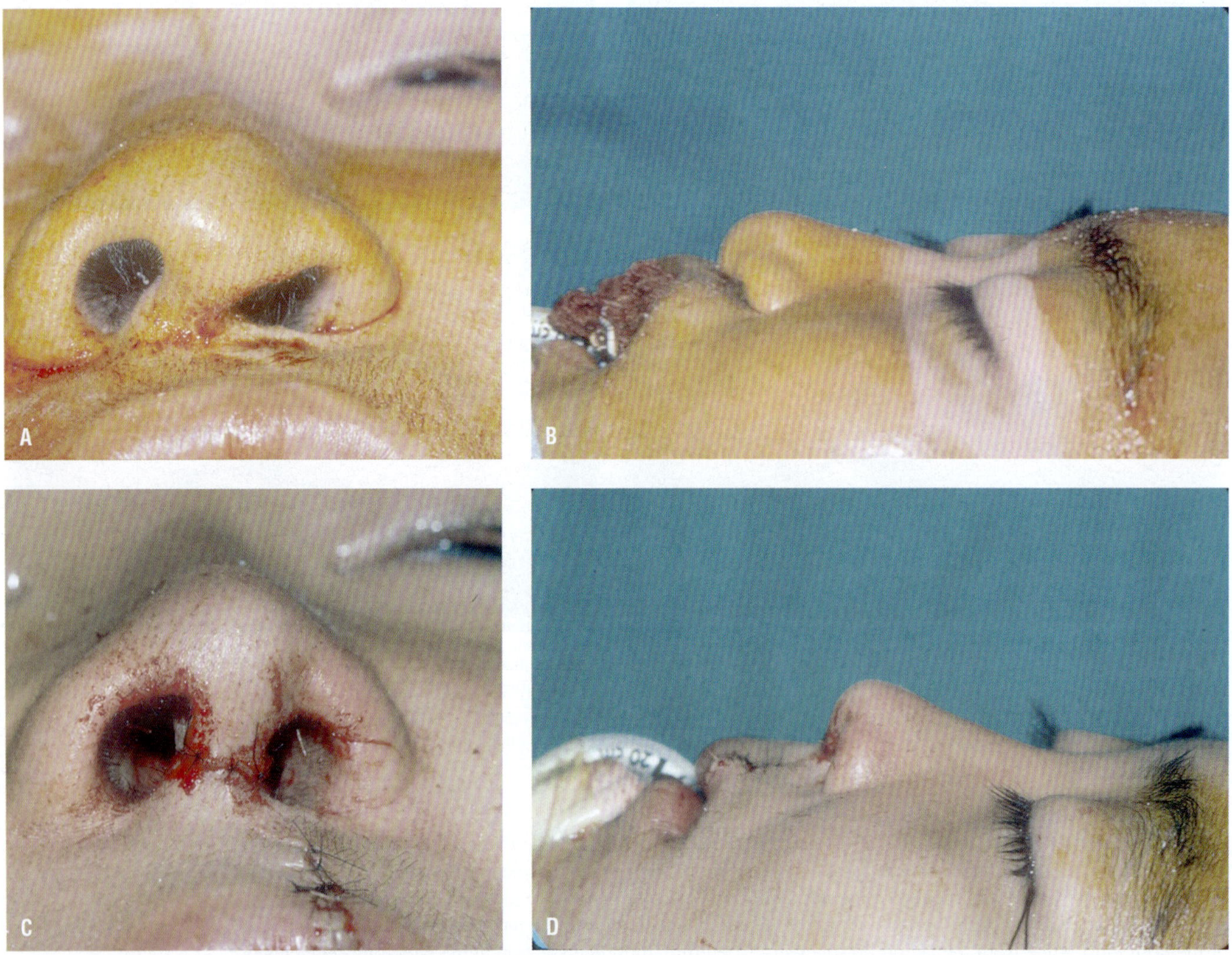

FIGURE 37.11 Secondary cleft rhinoplasty. **A:** A preoperative base view is shown of a patient with a left unilateral cleft lip and associated nasal deformity. **B:** A sagittal view of the same patient reveals a flattened and underprojected nasal tip. **C:** A postoperative base view is shown following secondary rhinoplasty and lip revision. The tip has more definition, and there is improved projection and symmetry. **D:** The immediate postoperative sagittal photograph, demonstrating improved projection, rotation, and definition of the nasal tip.

The surgery is performed with the patient under general anesthesia intubated with an endotracheal oral RAE tube secured to the midline lower lip and chin. The table is turned 90 or 180 degrees, and the nasal septum and nasal dorsum are injected with Xylocaine 1%, 1:100,000 epinephrine. It is of critical importance to perform a careful and thorough injection with local anesthetic to minimize bleeding. An open approach is frequently used when extensive tip work and grafting is expected. For an open approach, standard columellar and marginal

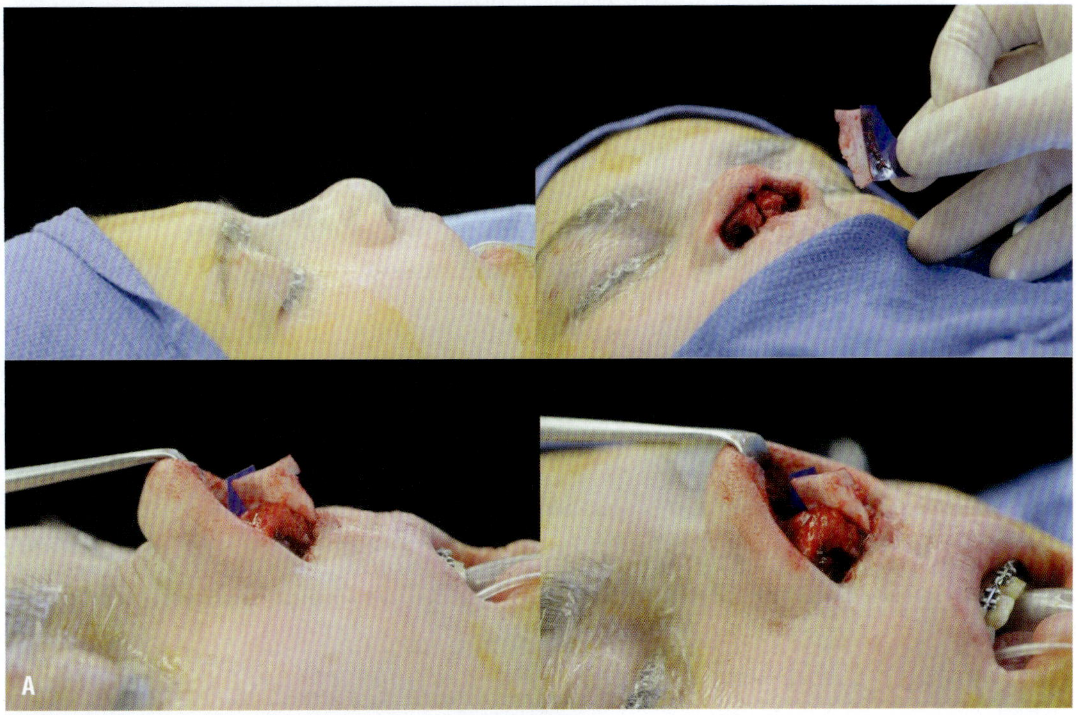

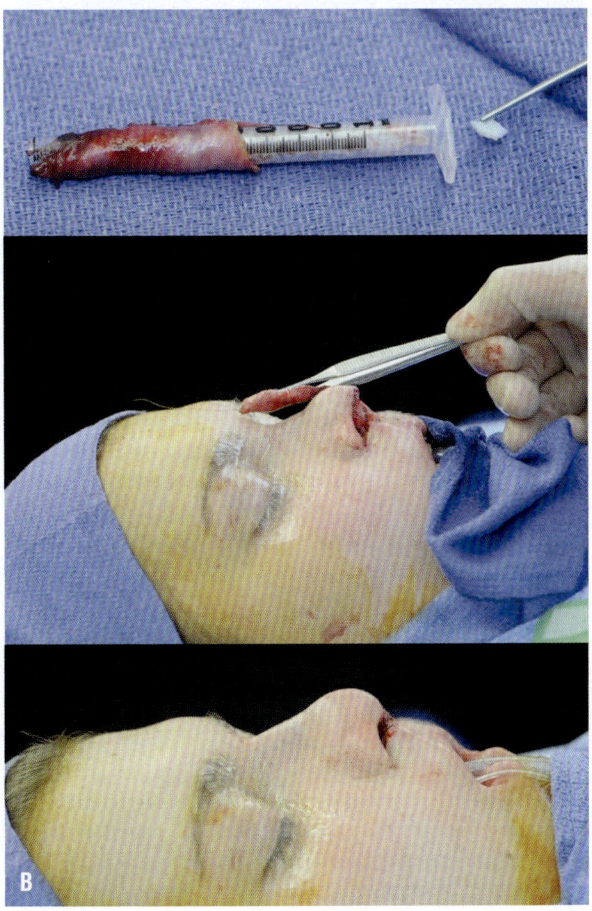

FIGURE 37.12

A: Bilateral cleft lip definitive rhinoplasty. *Upper left*: A photograph of patient with a bilateral cleft lip nasal deformity is shown. Definitive secondary rhinoplasty is planned to correct a low dorsum, to lengthen the nose, and to increase tip projection. An intraoperative lateral view of the nose is shown prior to any surgical intervention. *Upper right*: The nasal tip skin envelope has been elevated with standard marginal and columellar incisions and an open approach. To increase nasal length and projection, a caudal septal extension graft is used. The graft consists of PDS foil (*blue*) secured with 5-0 PDS suture to a thin carved rib cartilage graft. *Lower left*: A lateral view of the caudal septal extension graft is shown. *Lower right*: An oblique view of the nasal tip shows the caudal septal extension graft in place and secured to the short caudal native septum and placed between the medial crura. The graft is then trimmed, and the medial crura are secured to the caudal septal extension graft in a tongue-and-groove fashion. **B:** *Top*: Following the placement of a caudal septal extension graft **(A)**, dorsal augmentation is planned in a patient with a bilateral cleft lip nasal deformity. Temporalis fascia is secured in a tubular fashion with interrupted 5-0 chromic suture around a 1-cc syringe after the Luer-Lok tip is cut off. The syringe is then filled with diced rib cartilage. The native syringe plunger is then used to gently fill the tubed temporalis fascia with the diced cartilage while gently pulling the fascia off of the syringe. *Middle*: The temporalis fascia filled with diced cartilage is held above the nasal dorsum and will be used for dorsal augmentation. *Bottom*: Immediate postoperative photograph following the placement of diced cartilage–filled temporalis fascia for dorsal augmentation, in addition to the placement of a caudal septal extension graft.

TABLE 37.4 Problem-Based Operative Techniques in Secondary Cleft Rhinoplasty

Functional nasal obstruction	• Septoplasty • Correction of vestibular or nasal scarring/stenosis
Poorly defined nasal tip	• Columellar strut for projection and stabilization • Tip-defining suture techniques • Cartilage tip or shield graft
Middle third deficiency/collapse	• Spreader grafts to internal nasal valve • Onlay grafts • Flaring sutures
Nasal tip asymmetry	• For unilateral cleft patients: lateral crural steal on the cleft side with interdomal sutures • Possible vertical dome division
Shortened columella	• For unilateral cleft rhinoplasty patients, consider V–Y lip skin advancement • Columellar strut graft • For bilateral cleft rhinoplasty, consider central V–Y skin advancement or bilateral "forked flaps"[a]
Widened alar base	• Alar base reductions
Malpositioned ala	• Excision of concave lower lateral cartilage and replacing it in convex fashion[a]

[a]Sykes JM, Jang YJ. Cleft lip rhinoplasty. Facial Plast Surg Clin North Am 2009;17:133–144.

incisions are used. Any donor graft site is injected with local anesthetic, prepped, and draped. Grafting material used in secondary cleft rhinoplasty includes the nasal septal cartilage, auricular cartilage, costal cartilage, temporalis fascia, costal perichondrium (harvested simultaneously with cartilage), or alloplastic. A summary of operative techniques to address the cleft nasal deformity in secondary rhinoplasty is presented in Table 37.4.

POSTOPERATIVE MANAGEMENT

Following primary cleft rhinoplasty, infants and children are typically kept in the hospital for 1 or 2 days to ensure adequate oral intake and pain control. The patient's arms are restrained to avoid manipulation of the wound. Soft Silastic nasal conformers are kept in place with a nylon suture, and the suture is removed at 1 week postoperatively. The conformers are then kept in for 6 weeks postoperatively to help stent the nostrils open and support the ala and tip on the cleft side. The Silastic conformers can be secured to the nose with tape, if needed. Nasal suture bolsters are removed at 7 to 10 days postoperatively.

Secondary rhinoplasty patients often require wound care from the donor site used in cartilage grafting in addition to nasal incisions. All incisions are kept clean and antibiotic ointment is applied three times a day for the first postoperative week. The avoidance of vigorous activity for 3 weeks and contact sports for up to 6 months can help prevent trauma to the healing nose.

COMPLICATIONS

Wound dehiscence and infection are potential complications in the early postoperative period following a cleft lip repair and primary cleft rhinoplasty. Long-term and unsightly scarring may occur as a result of poor wound healing. In patients who lack a nasal floor on the cleft side, an oronasal fistula may persist after attempted surgical repair. Overaggressive narrowing of the nostril on the cleft side during primary cleft rhinoplasty can cause vestibular and nasal stenosis. Secondary rhinoplasty patients have preexisting scar that may persist or worsen after surgery.

RESULTS

All patients with a cleft nasal deformity and associated cleft lip or palate are expected to have a sequence of operations to address underlying functional and aesthetic problems. Patients with an isolated cleft lip and nasal deformity may achieve acceptable symmetry and cosmesis with a primary surgery. Patient's families are always counseled, however, that major or minor interventions may be necessary in the future, depending on the needs of the patient and the desires of the parents. It is important to temper the expectations of the patient and their families. The goal of performing major secondary interventions after full facial growth has been achieved and following any orthodontic or orthognathic interventions should be communicated.

PEARLS

- A team approach is necessary in the treatment of patients with craniofacial abnormalities.
- Parent and family compliance is critical for the success of primary cleft rhinoplasty.
- Avoid making the nostril too small during primary cleft rhinoplasty; it is easier to narrow the nose at a later stage than to correct a nasal stenosis.
- Secondary rhinoplasty should take place after orthodontic and orthognathic issues have been addressed.

PITFALLS

- A wound dehiscence or infection in the early postoperative period can lead to long-term scarring of the lip and nose.
- Aggressive intermediate rhinoplasty may impede nasal growth in children and young adolescents.

INSTRUMENTS TO HAVE AVAILABLE

- Basic rhinoplasty set
- Basic plastic soft tissue set
- Soft Silastic nasal conformers
- Nasoalveolar molding device

ACKNOWLEDGMENTS

The author would like to thank Drs. Christina K. Magill and Gregory C. Park for their contributions in the writing of this chapter. Their work in the writing, editing, and figure creation for this chapter is greatly appreciated, without which this chapter would not have been possible.

SUGGESTED READING

Grayson BH, Santiago PE, Brecht LE, et al. Presurgical nasoalveolar molding in infants with cleft lip and palate. *Cleft Palate Craniofac J* 1999;36(6):486–498.

Hopper RA, Cutting C, Grayson B. Cleft lip and palate. In: Thorne C, ed. *Grabb and Smith's plastic surgery*. Philadelphia, PA: Lippincott Williams & Wilkins, 2007:201–225.

Sykes JM, Jang YJ. Cleft lip rhinoplasty. *Facial Plast Surg Clin North Am* 2009;17:133–144.

Sykes JM, Senders CW. Surgery of the cleft lip and nasal deformity. *Oper Tech Otolaryngol Head Neck Surg* 1990;1:219–224.

38 OTOPLASTY

James D. Sidman

INTRODUCTION

Otoplasty is a surgical technique that is commonly performed for the child or young adult who has protruding ears. Although parents often seek advice early for a child with prominent ears, it is frequently the young adult who independently presents for clinical evaluation. In the case of a child who is brought in for otoplasty consultation, there are two lines of consideration regarding the timing of surgery. One school of thought suggests that the children should reach an age in which they are able to participate in the decision of whether or not they wish to have otoplasty performed. This timing further allows the parents to see whether this is a social issue for the child among the peer groups. The other school of thought feels that it is better to perform the operation correcting protruding ears before the child is aware of this as an issue and before social pressures are encountered. Unfortunately, there have been no definitive studies to current date to determine the proper timing of the otoplasty procedure.

From a purely surgical point of view, the tradition is that otoplasty should not be performed before the age of 6. This is based upon two general concepts: The first is that the auricle is 80% to 90% of the adult size by the age of 6 and anticipated future growth is of minimal concern. The second is that most 6-year-old children will cooperate with the postoperative care and will wear their dressings and headbands for weeks after the surgery without putting up too much of a fuss.

This chapter is devoted to the treatment of the protruding ear with an absence of the antihelical fold and a deep conchal bowl and does not address issues such as microtia or a constricted or lop ear, which occurs when the ear is foreshortened and the vertical dimension is folded over the helical edge. Techniques for this type of reconstruction can be found in other sections of this textbook.

HISTORY

As with all surgical patients, the usual questions about the onset of the condition, past surgical interventions, trauma, and hereditary factors are reviewed. The history of the patient's general health is obtained and includes cardiac, pulmonary, hepatic, and renal systems. Two key points of a child or young adult undergoing surgery should focus on a family history of bleeding disorders and/or connective tissue disorders. These two elements are of considerable importance with regard to the quality of healing.

The most important lines of questioning are directed toward the social aspects of the protruding ear. One must be certain that the family or the young adult patient has appropriate expectations and reasons for doing the surgery and does not consider the surgery a completely life-changing event. There is no reason to delay or avoid surgery on patients who wear eyeglasses as the eyeglasses can be worn postoperatively except for 1 or 2 days during the postoperative period. Even then, bandages can be tailor-made so that eyeglasses can be incorporated into them.

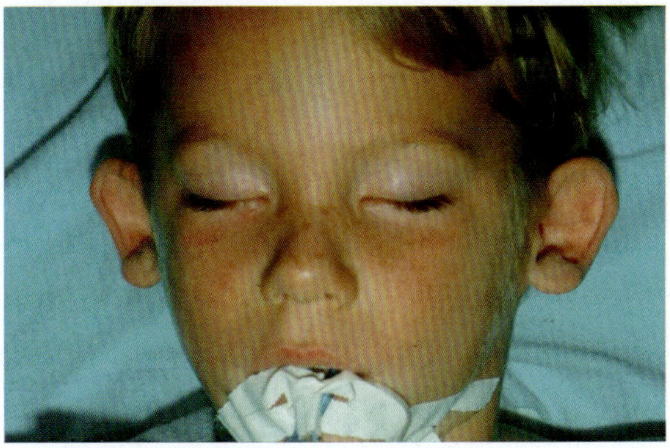

FIGURE 38.1
Prior to starting the operation, appropriate photographs should be taken. Both ears should be examined to analyze the presence and dimension of the antihelical fold, the superior and inferior crura of the antihelix, and the size, shape, and protrusive qualities of the conchal bowl (with permission by Peter Hilger, MD).

PHYSICAL EXAMINATION

The physical examination of the patient with protruding ears is not complex. The position of the ear on the head, the vertical dimension of the ear, and development of normal landmarks should be identified and documented. Frequently, measurements are made of the distance from the mastoid skin to the superior, middle, and lobule of the external ear. Although many authors discuss the angle of the ear from the head, I do not make those measurements due to relative biologic variation in the shape of the head.

Care should be taken to analyze the presence and dimension of the antihelical fold, the superior and inferior crura of the antihelix, as well as the size, shape, and protrusive qualities of the conchal bowl (Fig. 38.1). Other abnormalities such as a Darwin's tubercle or a slightly constricted superior helix should be noted. The presence of a protruding lobule should be noted and discussed as its presence can have significant implications for surgical and aesthetic outcomes if not recognized.

INDICATIONS

Patients and their families who present with the desire to correct protruding ears and who harbor realistic expectations regarding the surgical treatment are considered surgical candidates.

CONTRAINDICATIONS

Contraindications to this surgery are a bleeding disorder, inability to cooperate with postoperative care, or other external or middle ear conditions that would take higher priority (canal atresia, middle ear disease). As noted above, a patient or family with unrealistic expectations as to the outcome is a contraindication to surgery.

PREOPERATIVE PLANNING

Photographs are to be taken of all patients preoperatively. Anterior, posterior, lateral, and oblique views should be taken with the hair pinned back. A submental view can also be quite helpful. Measurements of the distance between the mastoid skin and the superior, middle, and lobular portion of the ear should be recorded preoperatively for each ear so that these measurements can be compared with postoperative and intraoperative findings. The external ear should be examined for any obstruction to the ear canal and tympanoscopy should be accomplished to rule out middle ear disease. Although an actively draining ear would be a contraindication to surgery, the presence of ventilating tubes or recurrent otitis media is not a contraindication to otoplasty.

SURGICAL TECHNIQUE

This procedure may be done under local for adults, MAC, or general; the latter is typically reserved for children. Long hair is placed into multiple small ponytails or braids without shaving the hair. The ears and face are prepped and draped in standard sterile fashion. The surgical prep is to include both ears and the face so that the head can be turned side to side during the procedure without reprepping and draping. Preoperative broad-spectrum skin antibiotic prophylaxis is given.

Measurements are made on both sides of the distance from the mastoid skin to the superior portion of the auricle, the middle portion, and the lobule. These recordings are labeled right and left side on the back table or by the circulating nurse. Using a sterile marking pen, a dumbbell-shaped incision is marked on the medial

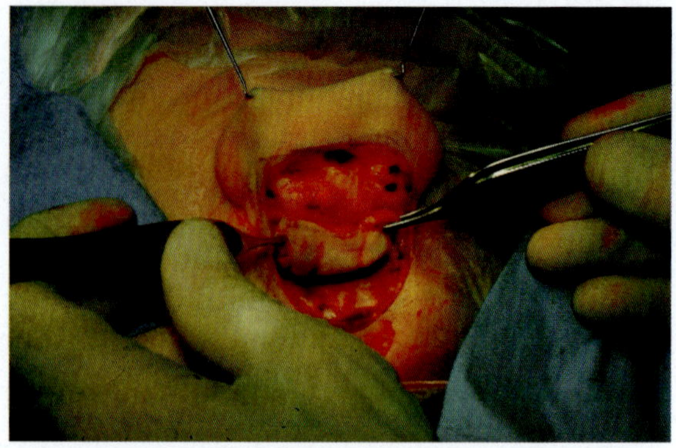

FIGURE 38.2
Illustration depicting excision of the postauricular skin onto the perichondrium.

surface of the auricle. A fusiform excision can also be performed, but this does not give as much skin resection at the superior and inferior portion of the ear as the dumbbell excision does. The skin excision is completely on the medial surface of the auricle and does not go into the postauricular crease, nor does it extend up to the helical rim. The wide portions of the dumbbell excision inferiorly and superiorly are about 1 to 1.5 cm and the narrow neck in between is about 0.5 cm. The postauricular skin is injected with 1% lidocaine with 1:100,000 epinephrine and allowed to set for 8 minutes. The skin and underlying tissues that were marked are excised down to the level of the perichondrium and the surrounding soft tissues are raised from the helical rim to the mastoid underneath the postauricular crease (Fig. 38.2). When dissecting down to the mastoid bone, one must incise the postauricular muscle and it is common to find mastoid emissary veins that must be cauterized.

Once wide exposure has been accomplished, attention is directed to marking the antihelical fold. This is done by creating an antihelical fold by folding the ear in its proper fashion and taking a 25-gauge, 1.5-inch needle and inserting it from laterally to medially through the middle of the antihelical fold so that the needle comes out into the surgical incision area (Fig. 38.3). The assistant then takes a Q-tip dipped in methylene blue and puts some methylene blue on the tip of the needle before it is withdrawn. As the needle is withdrawn, it leaves a blue mark on the medial surface of the antihelix in the surgical field. By doing this repeatedly inferiorly and superiorly, and marking out the superior and inferior crura of the antihelix, the apex of the antihelical fold can be marked carefully in the surgical field. A line including the inferior and superior crura can then connect these dots.

I do not recommend any cartilage weakening techniques to recreate the antihelical fold. No scoring in the cartilage or full or partial thickness or removal of cartilage by any method is recommended. Simple Mustarde sutures have always worked, and the key is to place at least three or possibly four sutures and not put too much tension on any single suture.

Attention is next paid to the conchal bowl. If the conchal bowl is deep and conchal setback needs to be performed, then the conchal cartilage can be weakened by taking shaved discs of partial-thickness cartilage out of the conchal bowl using a #10 blade, or simply conchal–mastoid sutures can be placed without taking the discs out. This depends on the thickness and the malleability of the conchal bowl cartilage. In my experience, it is rare to perform Mustarde sutures alone for otoplasty. Almost all patients receive a conchal setback in addition to Mustarde sutures. The conchal setback is completed prior to the creation of the antihelix with Mustarde sutures. Once the discs have been shaved off in three or four spots of the concha, 4-0 Mersilene suture is used for the conchal setback. These are simple sutures taken through the conchal cartilage, but not through the skin. This maneuver can be easily performed by the operating surgeon by putting the forefinger in the conchal bowl as the suture is driven from laterally to medially. By palpating with the finger in the skin of the conchal bowl, one can feel the needle pass through the conchal cartilage, but not through the skin. This suture is then passed down to the periosteum of the mastoid, which has been exposed by the previous dissection. Two or three sutures are placed, and then all are tied down together. One should take care not to pull the conchal bowl too

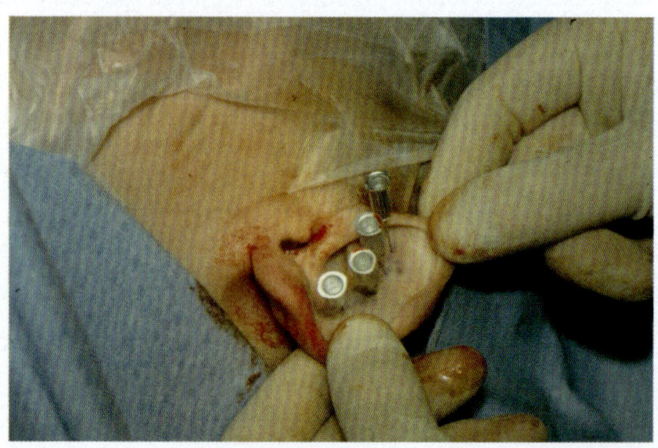

FIGURE 38.3
Illustration depicting use of 25-gauge needles inserted from lateral to medial through the middle of the proposed antihelical fold so that the needle comes out of the surgical incision area.

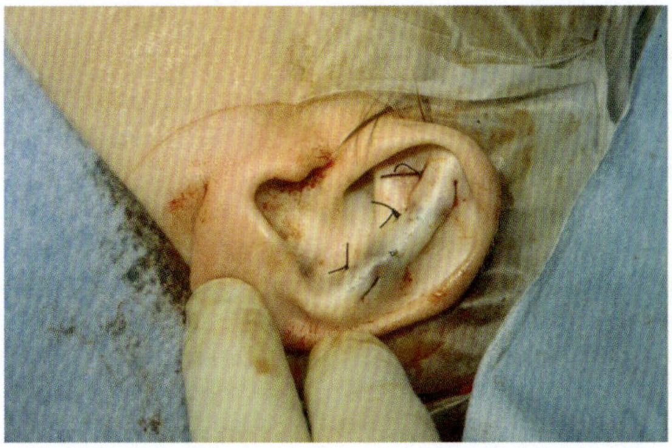

FIGURE 38.4
Evenly dispersed Mustarde sutures used to recreate the antihelical fold.

far posteriorly or too far anteriorly, as this will cause distortion and occlusion of the external ear canal. One can easily look in the ear canal as these sutures are being placed to determine if the ear canal dimension is being compromised.

Once the conchal–mastoid setback sutures have been placed and tied. I proceed to the Mustarde sutures to recreate the antihelical fold (Fig. 38.4). At least three Mustarde sutures must be placed to disperse tension and to prevent a broken or tented suture. Each suture should be placed as a mattress suture that is essentially in a "square" configuration. The limbs of the square should be about 6 to 8 mm apart, and each limb of the horizontal mattress suture should be about 3 to 4 mm from the antihelical fold line that has been previously drawn with the percutaneous tattooing. One suture should be placed at the superior crus and the other two or three sutures along the antihelical rim. Each one of these square mattress sutures is placed using the 4-0 Mersilene suture; no suture is tied until all sutures are placed, and then all sutures could be tied. By using a surgeon's knot with each mattress suture, the exact tension can be tailored so that a pleasing antihelical fold can be created. All of the sutures then are tied appropriately and cut. At this point, if the lobule is somewhat intrusive, then the cauda helicis must be cut and a Mustarde suture must be placed to pull the lobule into position. This is an uncommon step.

At this point, prior to skin closure, measurements should be taken again as this is truly the final result that the patient will live with for the rest of his or her life (Fig. 38.5). Care should be taken to take measurements now just like at the beginning of the procedure and compare the change in distance from the mastoid skin to the ear at all three positions. Closing the skin will result in even a tighter appearing ear, but this skin will relax over time, hence the relapse that many authors describe. At this point, deep 4-0 or 5-0 Vicryl sutures are placed in the skin, and the superficial skin is approximated with a running 6-0 fast-absorbing gut suture. Mineral oil–soaked cotton balls are placed in the conchal bowl and in the scapha. Then, cotton bolsters are placed behind the ear, and a nonstick dressing is placed over the postauricular skin. A formal mastoid dressing is placed with fluffs and stretch gauze wrapped around both ears.

POSTOPERATIVE MANAGEMENT

The dressing is removed on the second to fourth postoperative day and the patient is encouraged to wear a wide sports headband over both ears, all day and all night, for 2 weeks. Dressings are then continued at nighttime for another 3 weeks for a total of 5 weeks of postsurgical dressing care. Local wound care includes daily cleaning with 1:1 concentration H_2O_2 mixed with water as well as the application of an antibiotic ointment. Pain management consists of short-term oral narcotics and nonnarcotic oral analgesics. Postoperative antibiotics are not mandatory and generally not prescribed.

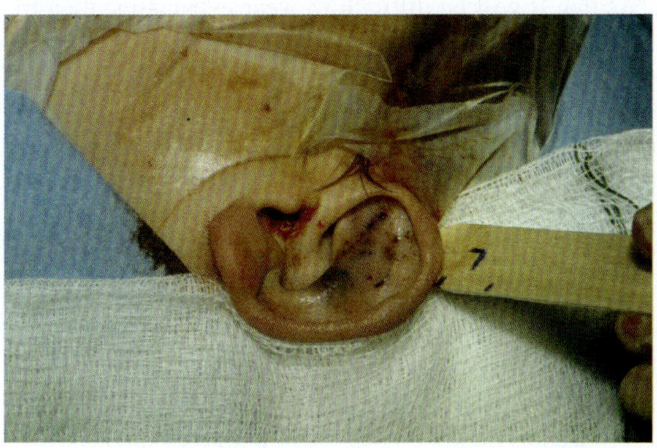

FIGURE 38.5
Final measurements to be taken after conchal–mastoid setback and Mustarde sutures have been placed, but before skin closure (with permission by Peter Hilger, MD).

COMPLICATIONS

- Bleeding/hematoma: It is very common to have some pain and swelling over the auricle postoperatively, but there should be no palpable fluid accumulation. This is rare, but if it does occur, it would require immediate drainage to eliminate a nidus for infection or unsightly scarring.
- Infection: Any developing signs of infection (redness, irritation, fluid drainage, excessive swelling) should be treated aggressively with antibiotics.
- Suture break: The breaking of a suture, which can occur through accident or error, requires replacement 4 months to 1 year postoperatively (not immediately).
- Suture placement: The placement of too much distance in the horizontal mattress Mustarde sutures, or placing them too close to the mastoid, so that there is a bridge of tissue like a bowstring between the antihelix and the root of the ear, or even the mastoid. Each of these circumstances represents a problem due to inappropriate placement of the Mustarde or conchal setback sutures and should be avoided.

RESULTS

The outcome of this operation should be a naturally curving antihelical fold and an auricle that sits closer to the calvarium. Symmetry is important both in terms of contour and the projection of the auricle from the postauricular scalp. The projection should also be consistent between the superior pole of the auricle and the ear lobule. In fact, when it is done properly, nobody should ever be able to tell that this person has had an otoplasty unless they see a scar on the medial surface of the ear (Fig. 38.6).

PEARLS

- Preoperative asymmetries: They are a normal biologic variation and are to be addressed with regard to differences in dimension, shape, rotation, protrusion, and general location (height on head). If these findings are not discussed, they are commonly attributed to the surgical procedure.
- Relapse over time: Many authors describe a 30% to 50% relapse in the distance of the auricular setback. I feel that this is due to a lack of understanding of the different elements of the operation. The measurements taken at the end of the cartilage-placed sutures should be permanent. The Mustarde and conchal setback sutures should not relapse at all. The relapse that does take place is the distance the ear is brought back due to skin closure. Skin stretches over time, and any auricular setback that is accomplished by skin closure will not last. Therefore, if the surgeon takes care to take measurements of the ear preoperatively, intraoperatively after all cartilage sutures have been placed but before skin closure, and postoperatively after the skin sutures have been placed, there will be three different sets of measurements. The middle set taken intraoperatively with only the cartilage sutures being placed is in fact the true final measurements. If the ear still looks protrusive at this point, it will look protrusive in a few months when the skin stretches. If the ear distance is pleasing at this point, and if it is symmetrical, then the final result should be excellent.
- Natural appearance (helix and antihelix relationships): Many surgeons are taught that the helical rim should always be the lateralmost landmark of the ear and not the antihelix. Some teach that the antihelix should never protrude beyond the helix. In fact, this is not true naturally. At least 20% of humans have an antihelix that protrudes further than the helix, and this is natural for them. This is true for unoperated patients, and so the same is true for many postsurgical patients. This is not a complication of the operation.

PITFALLS

- Cartilage sutures should not be able to be palpated through the skin.
- If there is a bowstring feel or appearance or it appears that it will be difficult to wear eyeglasses, then the cartilage sutures have not been placed properly.
- If the sutures are placed too close to the antihelical rim, it will result in a very tight-looking antihelix; but if they are placed too far away, then this bowstring results will become apparent.
- If the ear canal has changed in shape, review the placement of the conchal–mastoid suture and adjust accordingly.
- When placing a mattress Mustarde suture, please note that 6 mm from the antihelical rim on each side is enough. Anything more than this can be excessive and can result in "tenting" of the skin.

INSTRUMENTS TO HAVE AVAILABLE

- Soft tissue set
- Bipolar cautery
- Mastoid dressing (Kerlix fluffs and 2- to 4-inch Kling dressing) to apply pressure over the surgical site

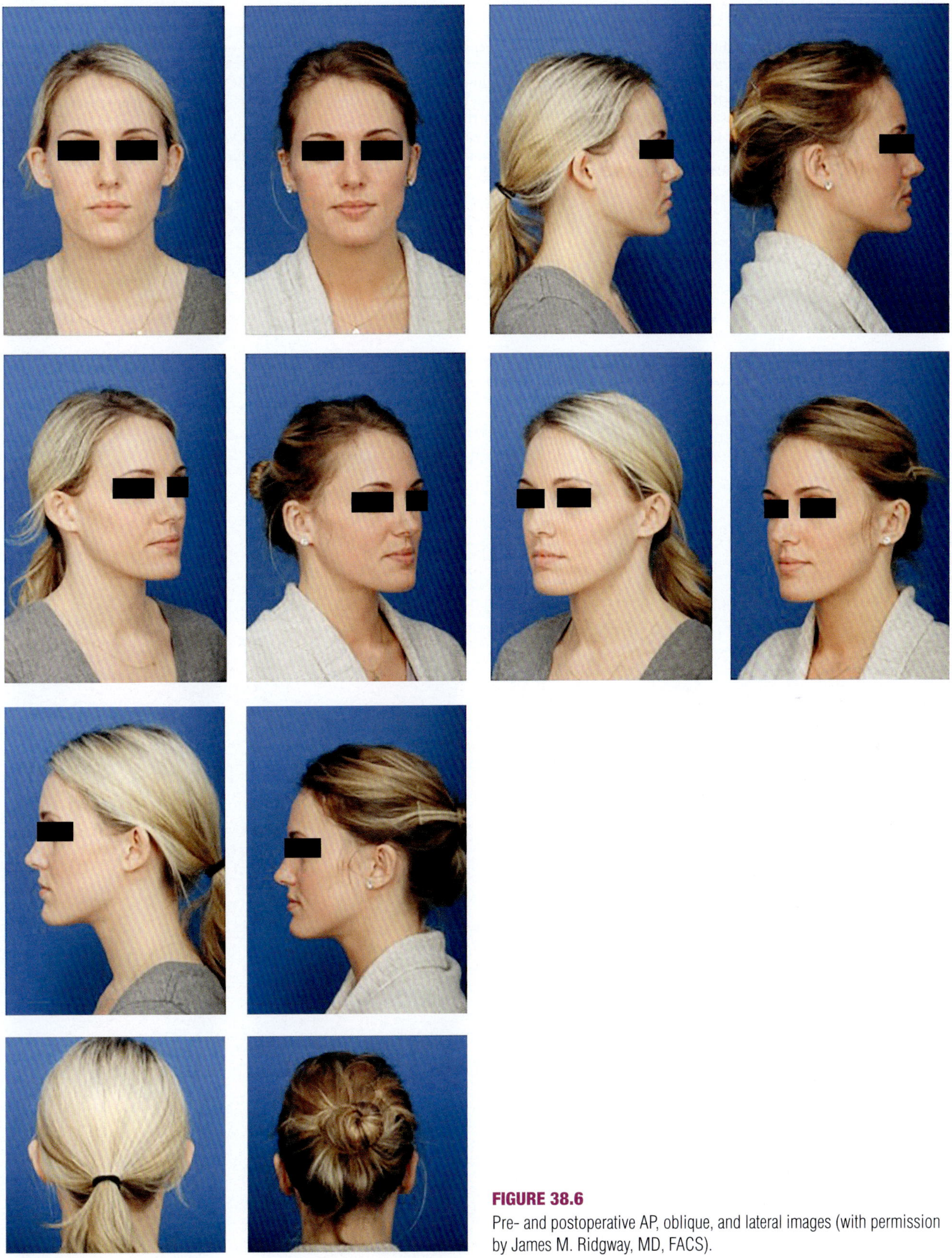

FIGURE 38.6
Pre- and postoperative AP, oblique, and lateral images (with permission by James M. Ridgway, MD, FACS).

SUGGESTED READING

Ducic Y, Hilger PA. Effective step-by-step technique for the surgical treatment of protruding ears. *J Otolaryngol* 1999;28(2):59–64.

Furnas DW. Correction of prominent ears with multiple sutures. *Clin Plast Surg* 1978;5(3):491–495.

Gosain AK, Kumar A, Huang G. Prominent ears in children younger than 4 years of age: what is the appropriate timing for otoplasty? *Plast Reconstr Surg* 2004;114(5):1042–1054.

Owsley TG. Otoplastic surgery for the protruding ear. *Atlas Oral Maxillofac Surg Clin North Am* 2004;12(1):131–139.

Posnick JC, al-Qattan MM, Whitaker LA. Assessment of the preferred vertical position of the ear. *Plast Reconstr Surg* 1993;91(7):1198–1203; discussion 1204–1207.

39 AUTOLOGOUS COSTOCHONDRAL RECONSTRUCTION OF MICROTIA

Kathleen C.Y. Sie

INTRODUCTION

The incidence of microtia ranges from 1:5,000 to 1:10,000. Eighty percent of patients with microtia have unilateral involvement; therefore, this chapter will focus on management of these patients. Infants born with microtia commonly have associated aural atresia and hearing loss. These malformations are obvious at birth, so the families are often eager to understand the abnormality and proceed with treatment of the ear and hearing loss. However, these anomalies are obvious at birth, and the interventions are typically deferred for several years and the otolaryngologist develops a relationship with the child and family. In order to adequately counsel these families, the otolaryngologist must understand the medical and developmental issues related to the ear anomalies, associated medical issues, treatment options, and timing of interventions.

At Seattle Children's Hospital, we have developed a team approach to managing children with microtia. Pediatric audiologists monitor hearing status and make recommendations for amplification. An anaplastologist meets with the families interested in prosthetic management. After the otolaryngologist counsels the families about reconstructive options, our nurse reviews photographs of reconstructed ears with the child and family. Then, the pediatric otolaryngologist and facial plastic surgeon evaluate the child to assess the options for reconstruction.

Craig S. Murakami and I have worked together over the past 20 years to perform microtia reconstruction. Initially, we used the three-staged approach popularized by Brent. In 2010, we started using a modification of the two-staged approach as described by Nagata. More recently, Amit Bhrany has joined our team. Our current technique for microtia reconstruction using autogenous costal cartilage is presented.

HISTORY

Patients with microtia typically come to medical attention during infancy or early childhood. The parents should be asked about the results of newborn hearing screening and their observations of the child's response to sound, speech, and language development. It is important to inquire about ear infections or middle ear effusions in the normally formed ear.

Past medical history should be reviewed to rule out other medical conditions that can be associated with microtia, including renal, cardiac, and vertebral anomalies. Family history may reveal a genetic predisposition for external ear anomalies. A family history of bleeding or anesthetic problems is important in preoperative planning. Social history, including school placement and extracurricular activities, is relevant since microtia reconstruction involves staged elective surgery. Each surgery is associated with postoperative activity restrictions that should be considered before scheduling.

PHYSICAL EXAMINATION

Physical examination should include careful inspection of the abnormal ear with accurate description of the pinna and inspection of the external auditory canal. Some patients with severe microtia may have a patent or stenotic ear canal. Patients with unilateral microtia are also more likely to have relatively minor anomalies of the contralateral "normal" ear.

A complete examination of the head and neck includes assessment of the position of the orbit, symmetry of the mandible, facial nerve function, and soft tissue status. It is helpful to think of the OMENS (ocular, mandibular, ear, nerve, soft tissue) plus (vertebral, cardiac, renal) classification. The position of the hairline and size of the chest should be considered when the plans are being made for surgical reconstruction.

It is also important to assess the overall size of the child, with attention to the chest. While I currently do not use objective measures, some surgeons measure the diameter of the chest several centimeters below the nipples. They use the criteria of 60 cm to proceed with reconstruction. I prefer that the child's height is at least at the 50th percentile for an 8-year-old child. Waiting until the child is closer to the size of a 10-year-old child will provide more cartilage for creation of the framework.

INDICATIONS

Children with microtia should be followed carefully to monitor hearing, speech, and language development. As the child grows, ear-specific behavioral responses should be obtained to assess the hearing status of the microtic ear as well as the contralateral ear. Bone conduction thresholds must be obtained to rule out sensorineural hearing loss. The audiologic management of children with unilateral hearing loss is evolving. With our growing understanding of problems related to unilateral hearing loss, amplification options should be discussed with the family.

While management of the hearing is beyond the scope of this chapter, it is important for the microtia surgeon to consider options for management of the hearing when counseling patients and their families. Ideally, the surgeon, patient, and family will have a clear view of the overall treatment plan before embarking on the first surgical intervention. Children with craniofacial microsomia may benefit from the coordinated services of a craniofacial team.

There are three main options for management of microtia: (1) no intervention, (2) prosthetic management, either adhesive or implant retained, and (3) reconstruction, with either alloplastic or autogenous frameworks. The advantages and disadvantages of these approaches are presented in Table 39.1. It is important for patients and families to review photographs of expected outcomes of reconstruction so that they will have realistic expectations. Hearing management should be considered when formulating a plan for comprehensive management of the ear and hearing.

CONTRAINDICATIONS

The patient must participate in the decision to proceed with autogenous rib reconstruction. This requires that the child be developmentally capable of understanding the process. In order for patients and families to have realistic expectations of surgical outcomes, they should review photographs of reconstructed ears. It is also

TABLE 39.1 Options for Microtia Management

Intervention	Details	Advantages	Disadvantages
Do nothing		No surgery	Appearance and function
Prosthetic management	Adhesive retained	Appearance	Retention less secure Daily maintenance Use restrictions
	Implant retained	Appearance Secure retention	Requires one to two surgeries Appearance of recipient site Daily maintenance Use restrictions
Reconstruction	Autogenous rib cartilage	Autogenous tissue Minimal maintenance Becomes sensate	Donor site Multiple surgeries Appearance
	Synthetic framework	Less donor site morbidity Less variability in carving	Foreign body Multiple surgeries Donor site May be more difficult to integrate with aural atresia repair

TABLE 39.2 Perioperative Management for Patients Undergoing Autogenous Rib Reconstruction of Microtia

Stage	Hospitalization	Out of School	Activity Restrictions	Follow-Up
Stage I	Two nights	7 d	• Protective dressing for 1 wk • No competitive sports, PE, or recess for 2–4 wk • Keep ear dry until the bolster is removed.	1 wk to remove the bolster
Stage II	Outpatient	3–7 d	• Protective dressing for 1 wk • No competitive sports, PE, or recess for 2–4 wk • Keep ear dry for 2 wk	1 wk to remove the bolster

important that the patient and family have a stable social situation. If the patient has significant psychosocial issues, it may not be the appropriate time to embark on elective reconstructive surgery.

Local factors such as the hairline should be considered. A low hairline will result in hair growth over the reconstructed ear. In general, these patients are less favorable candidates for autogenous costal cartilage reconstruction though adjunctive measures such as surgical epilation or postoperative epilation can be considered. Children with severe mandibular asymmetry may be candidates for early mandibular reconstruction. Consideration should be given to associated medical issues.

PREOPERATIVE PLANNING

The goal of ear reconstruction is to create an ear that will be symmetric to the contralateral ear for the patient's lifetime. Therefore, the surgeon must be able to harvest sufficient cartilage to create an appropriate-size framework. Some surgeons require a chest diameter of at least 60 cm. However, chest diameter does not allow the surgeon to determine the thickness of the costal cartilage. The amount of cartilage required is dependent upon the technique for creating the framework. The minimum age of surgical reconstruction using autogenous costal cartilage depends upon the size of the child and the size of the contralateral ear. In general, the ideal age to start autogenous costal cartilage reconstruction of microtia is probably between 8 and 10 years of age. Conversely, the costal cartilage starts to ossify as patients approach skeletal maturity. So the decision to proceed with microtia repair should be made prior to the late teenage years. For patients who are favorable candidates for atresia repair, we prefer to complete microtia reconstruction prior to atresia repair though there is increasing interest in performing atresia repair prior to auricular reconstruction.

A standardized set of preoperative photographs should be taken. The expected postoperative course and activity limitations (Table 39.2) should be reviewed in detail with the family as part of the consent process. See Table 39.3 for complications associated with the procedures. Children who are anxious about surgery may benefit from consultation with a child life specialist.

SURGICAL TECHNIQUE

There are several types of microtia, and each presents the reconstructive surgeon with unique challenges. The techniques presented here will focus on reconstruction of class 3 (lobule-type) microtia. We operate with two surgical teams; one team harvests the cartilage while the other excises the cartilaginous remnant and prepares the recipient bed during the first-stage surgery. At the second surgery, one team harvests the banked rib cartilage and skin graft while the second team elevates the ear and performs local advancement flaps.

Stage 1

Preparation

A template is created from the normal contralateral ear. Unexposed radiographic film is used because it is sufficiently rigid to be placed in the skin pocket and it can be autoclaved.

Preoperative antibiotics are administered intravenously prior to surgery. The patient is anesthetized and an oral RAE tube is inserted. The tube should be secured in the midline so the table can be turned 180 degrees allowing the two surgical teams to work simultaneously on either side of the patient. The face and both ears are included in the surgical field. The desired position of the new ear should be drawn on the patient (Fig. 39.1). Although measurements from the ear to the lateral orbital rim and oral commissure can be compared to the contralateral side, the underlying hemifacial macrosomia may cause some asymmetry in the measurements. We prefer to compare the position of the superior and inferior limits of the ear to be reconstructed with the contralateral ear.

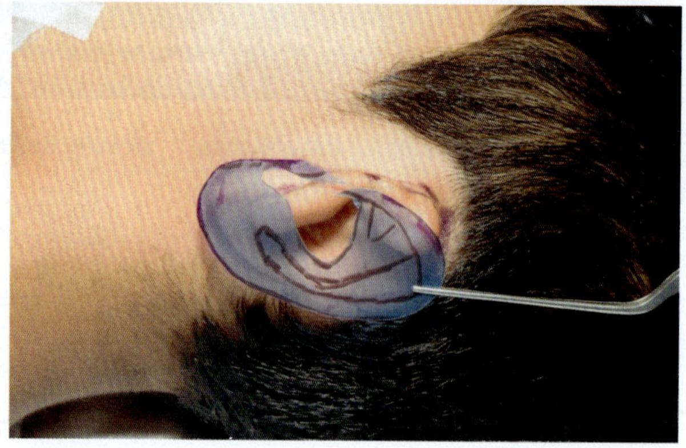

FIGURE 39.1
Determining the position of the ear. A template created from the contralateral ear is used to determine the position of the ear to be reconstructed.

The area around the microtia and the area of the anticipated chest incision on the contralateral side are infiltrated with lidocaine with epinephrine. The placement of the chest incision is important to allow adequate exposure with the smallest possible incision.

Harvest of Costal Cartilage

We have gone to considerable effort to minimize donor site morbidity. With careful placement of the chest incision, we are reliably able to harvest an adequate amount of cartilage through a 2.5-cm incision. The incision should be made just lateral to the genu of the synchondrosis at the inferior aspect of the superior limb of the synchondrosis (Fig. 39.2).

The rectus and lateral oblique muscles are divided beyond the medial and lateral extents of the skin incision. After exposure of the costal cartilages, the floating cartilage with light attachment to the superior cartilage is separated at the point of attachment. The cartilage is dissected laterally, including the surrounding perichondrium. In general, a segment 8 cm in length is desirable though the length is sometimes defined by the location of the bony–cartilaginous junction. The more inferior floating cartilage is also harvested to create the antihelical fold.

The area of the synchondrosis is then addressed. Lidocaine with epinephrine is infiltrated into the intercostal muscles between the two limbs of the synchondrosis. Perichondrial incisions are made at the superior and inferior aspects of the cartilage so that the superficial perichondrium is left adherent to the excised

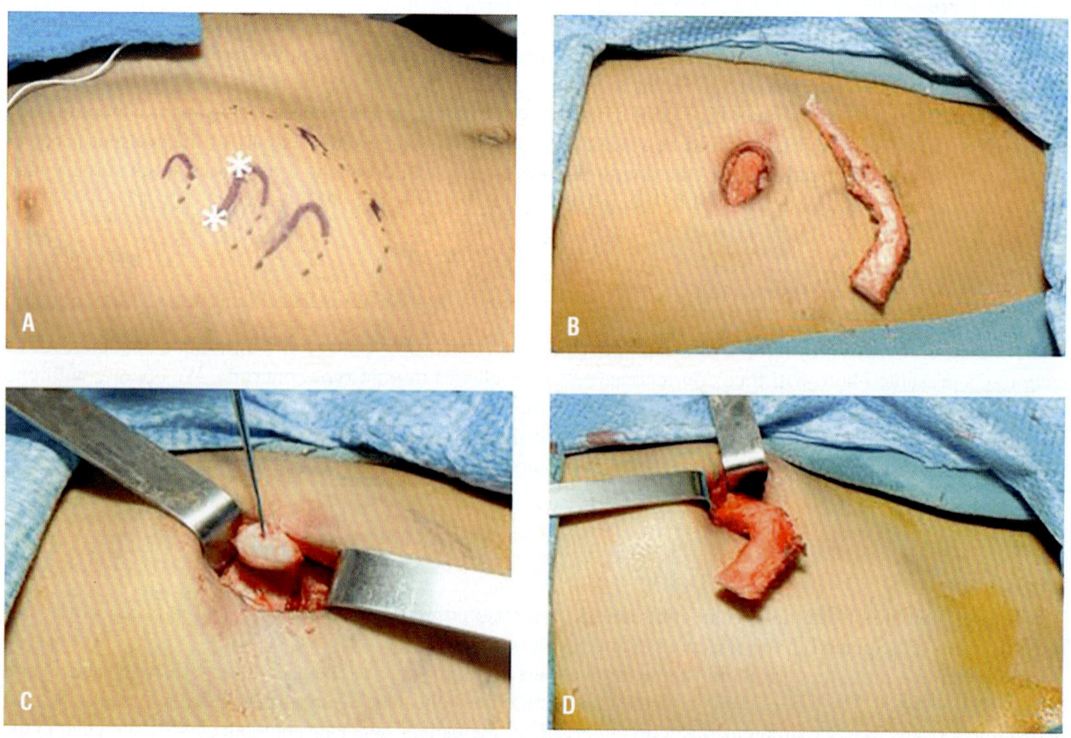

FIGURE 39.2 Position of the chest incision. **A:** Position of costal cartilages drawn on chest. *Asterisks* marking area of anticipated incision. **B:** Attached floater removed. **C:** Lateral aspect of the superior limb of the synchondrosis divided and elevated with single hook. **D:** Inferior limb of synchondrosis elevated and delivered through chest incision.

synchondrosis. The deep perichondrium is separated from the deep aspect of the costal cartilage and left in situ. The inferior limb is defined by making the lateral incision at the bony cartilaginous junction in a beveled fashion to avoid a sharp demarcation at the donor site. Care must be taken to carry this incision through the cartilage only, leaving the deep perichondrium intact. Once the lateral incision is made, the dissection between the cartilage and perichondrium is carried toward the midline under direct vision. When using a small incision, the inferior limb must be replaced into the chest wound so that the superior limb can be defined in a similar fashion. When both limbs are identified, the deep aspect of the synchondrosis must be freed from the underlying soft tissue. The area of attachment should be palpated to ensure that the synchondrosis is free of any soft tissue attachment. The final cut can be performed with placement of heavy Mayo scissors using manual guidance. Care must be taken to maximize the size of the cartilaginous segment removed.

Once the cartilage is removed, hemostasis should be obtained and the wound inspected for evidence of pneumothorax. The wound should be filled with saline and the anesthesiologist is asked to deliver an airway pressure of 30 to 40 cm H_2O to simulate a Valsalva maneuver. There may be initial air bubbles mobilized from the peripheral aspect of the wound. If a pleural defect is identified, a red rubber catheter should be placed through the defect, and it should be repaired with a purse-string suture. The suture is tied down as positive pressure is administered and the red rubber catheter removed. If possible, local soft tissue should be recruited to provide another layer of closure over the repair site.

The edges of the rectus muscle should be approximated with large horizontal mattress sutures. This will prevent the incision from healing to the costal cartilage. We no longer use a drain at the chest site. The wound is left open so that the cartilage remnants from creation of the framework can be banked for use in the second stage. After the remnant cartilage is banked, the chest incision is closed in three layers: Scarpa's fascia, subcutaneous closure, and subcuticular approximation of the skin edges.

Preparation of the Microtia Site

The most important issue with the first stage of the two-stage approach is the placement of the incisions. A modified Z-plasty is designed so that the cartilage remnant can be removed and the lobule transposed. The microtic remnant must be removed and a large subcutaneous pocket is created to accommodate the framework. The extent of the subcutaneous pocket should extend just beyond the outlines drawn at the beginning of the procedure. The flap should be sufficiently thin to accentuate the contour of the framework but thick enough to avoid necrosis, particularly over the most prominent aspects of the framework. An island of soft tissue attachment in the area of the neo-conchal bowl will be preserved (Fig. 39.3). The soft tissue just anterior to the pedicle is removed to increase the depth of the conchal bowl.

The incisions to elevate the lobule should be created first. When designing the incisions, care should be taken to preserve adequate lobule for future piercing. Once the lobule is mobile, the transverse incision is designed to position the lobule symmetrically with the other side (Fig. 39.4).

Creating the Framework

The free-floating cartilage will be used to create the helical root and rim. The cartilage should be inspected to determine the most natural curve of the segment. The cartilage is thinned by gradually shaving either the medial or lateral aspect of the cartilage. The flexibility of the segment is continuously assessed during the shaving. The cartilage should only be thinned enough to allow for adequate bending of the cartilage to create the helix. The helical rim must be substantial enough to withstand the skin pocket.

The synchondrosis is then carved using the template created at the beginning of the procedure. We create a perforated framework so that a single suction drain can be placed deep to the framework. An extra piece of cartilage is carved to accentuate the confluence of the crura of the triangular fossa, and yet another piece is carved to create the antitragus, intertragal notch, and tragus. The three components of the framework are

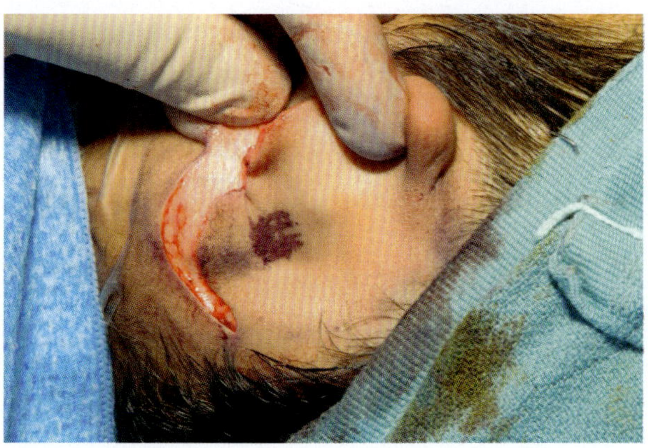

FIGURE 39.3
Skin flap pedicle. Incision with the area of the subcutaneous pedicle indicated with purple marking pen.

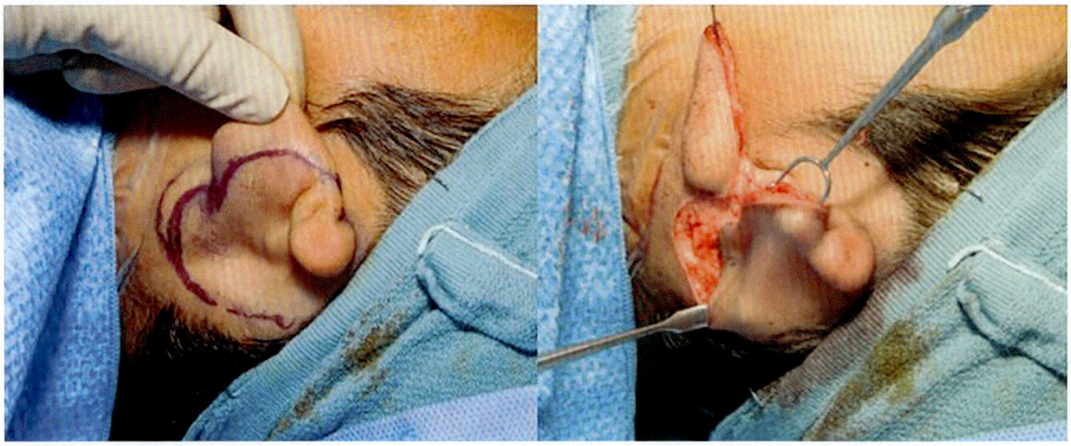

FIGURE 39.4
Lobule transposition. Lobule elevation and transposition.

attached to each other using clear 4-0 nylon sutures placed in a mattress fashion with the knots on the deep surface. We will plan to use the banked piece of cartilage to create the convex aspect of the conchal bowl and improve projection of the reconstructed ear (Fig. 39.5).

Closure

The recipient site is carefully inspected for hemostasis. Any bleeding on the skin flap should be managed with bipolar cautery to minimize the chance of flap necrosis. A stab incision in the hairline and a tunnel to the skin pocket are created to accommodate a 10-French round suction drain. The drain is trimmed and positioned deep to the perforated framework so that it will manage the entire skin flap.

The framework is positioned in the skin pocket and the incisions are closed to create an airtight seal. The apex of the lobule flap is de-epithelialized to create a dermal tag that will be used to prevent notching of the attachment of the lobule (Fig. 39.6). A deep mattress suture starting in the conchal bowl to the mastoid portion of the posteriormost incision delivers the lobule around the tail of the framework (Fig. 39.7). Redundant skin over the microtia remnant often needs to be excised. The posteriormost limb of the Z-plasty is closed with deep interrupted 5-0 polyglactin sutures and a running locked 5-0 plain gut suture. All other incisions are closed with deep 5-0 or 6-0 polyglactin and interrupted 5-0 or 6-0 plain gut sutures to approximate the skin edges. One or two micro Z-plasties are used to break up the incision that lies across the framework. A 6-0 chromic suture on spatulated needles is used for closure of the delicate apices of the micro Z-plasties (Fig. 39.8).

Bolsters are placed in the concavities of the newly reconstructed ear. Three pieces of Xeroform are used to create bolsters for the triangular fossa, the scaphoid fossa, and the conchal bowl. The bolsters are secured with a 4-0 chromic sutures placed through the surrounding skin with care to place the sutures through the cartilage. The skin overlying the antihelical fold remains exposed to allow assessment of the status of the skin flap (Figs. 39.9 and 39.10).

The gauze in a plastic cup dressing is removed and the plastic cup is placed over the newly reconstructed ear. The gauze must be removed to avoid any pressure on the skin flap. A dry dressing is placed over the chest incision. Intercostal blocks may be placed for postoperative analgesia. The drain is placed to bulb suction for transport to the recovery room.

POSTOPERATIVE MANAGEMENT

Patients are admitted for two nights after the first surgery. This allows for pain management and the opportunity to monitor the status of the skin flap. Also, the drain is generally ready for removal by the second postoperative day.

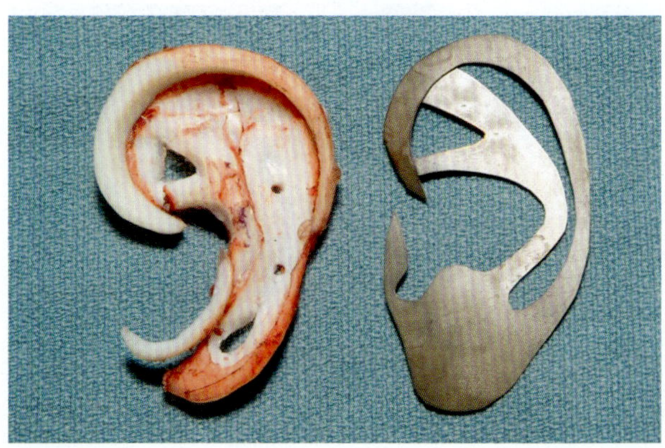

FIGURE 39.5
Framework. The framework is created from four pieces of cartilage. The pieces are attached to each other with interrupted 4-0 clear nylon sutures. Holes are placed in the scaphoid fossa so that a single drain can be placed deep to the framework.

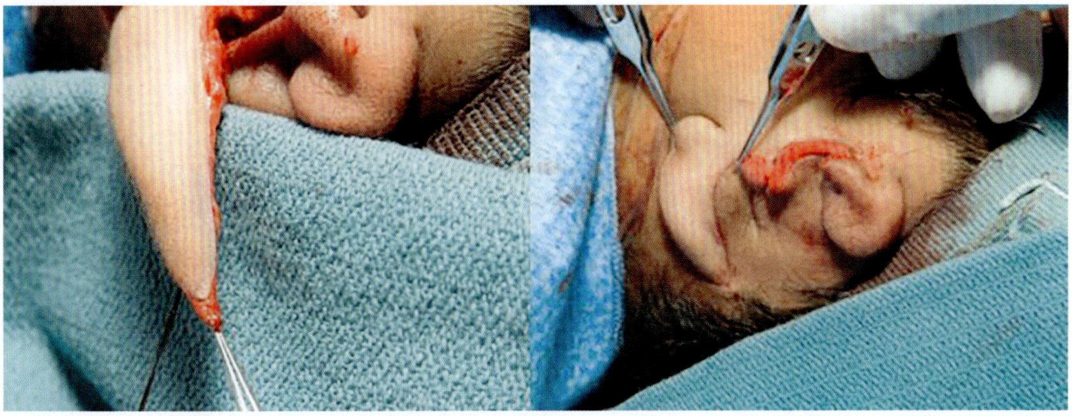

FIGURE 39.6 De-epithelialized apex. The apex of the lobule flap is de-epithelialized so that the dermal tag can be inset into the recipient site to prevent notching at the attachment of the lobule to the superior aspect of the reconstructed ear. The lobule is transposed, and the postauricular aspect of the incision is closed in two layers.

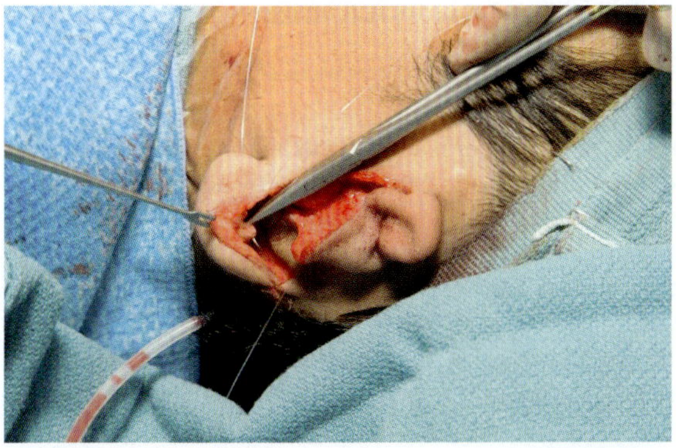

FIGURE 39.7
Lobule delivery suture. The drain has been placed, and the lobule delivery suture is placed to bring the posterior incision superiorly toward the conchal bowl, defining the inferior aspect of the postauricular sulcus.

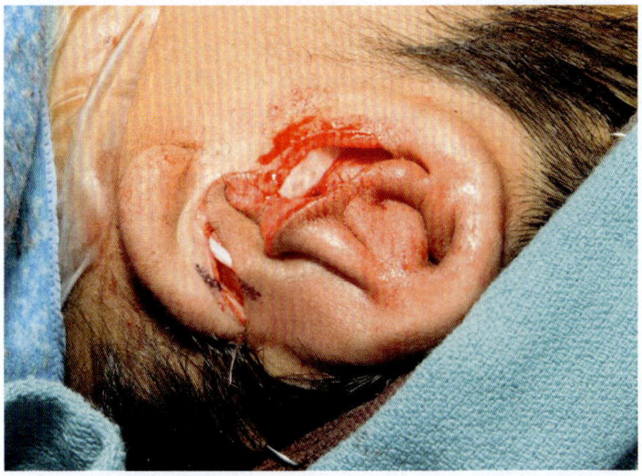

FIGURE 39.8
Micro Z-plasty across transverse incision. One or two small Z-plasties can be placed in the incision that traverses the framework. This can prevent contraction and help to camouflage this incision.

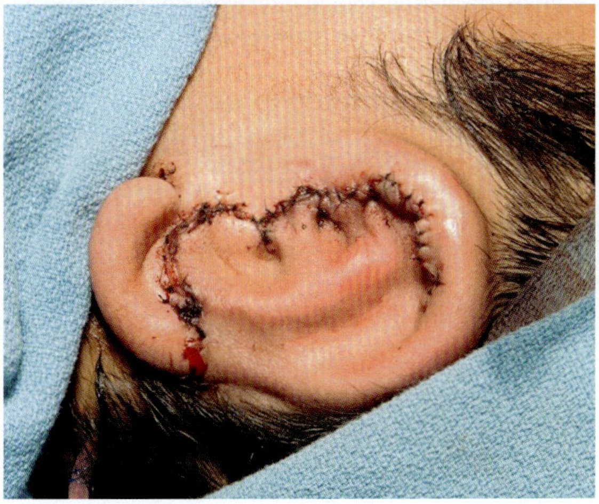

FIGURE 39.9
Closure of the incisions. The redundant skin is removed, and all incisions are closed in two layers to create an airtight closure.

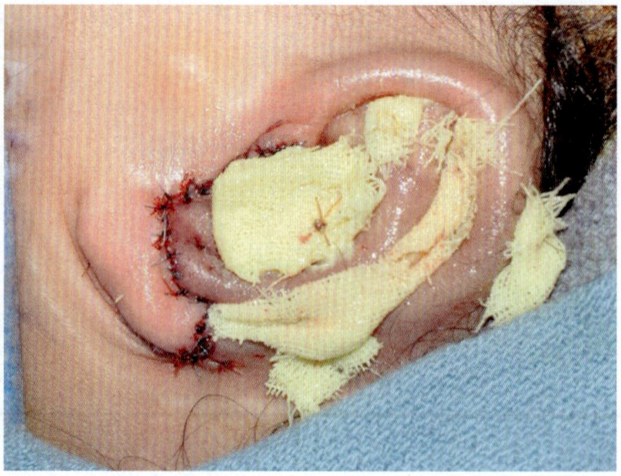

FIGURE 39.10

Bolster placement. Xeroform gauze is used to maintain the concavities of the reconstructed ear. The gauze is secured with 4-0 chromic sutures that are placed through the skin and cartilage framework. The skin overlying the antihelix is exposed for postoperative inspection. These are removed in clinic 1 week after surgery.

The drain is placed to continuous medium wall suction and nurses are asked to check the output every 8 hours. The patients are encouraged to ambulate with the drain on bulb suction. The patients are treated with intravenous antibiotics and analgesics. We have found that placement of topical analgesic cream 30 minutes prior to removing the drain is helpful.

Discharge

The patients are discharged after the drain is removed. They are given oral and topical antibiotics and oral analgesics for outpatient management. They are instructed to wear the plastic cup dressing day and night until they return for follow-up. They are excused from school until after their follow-up appointment. They are scheduled to return 5 to 7 days postoperatively for removal of the bolsters and inspection of the ear. At that point, they are asked to continue to use the protective cup dressing at night time. They may return to school, but they are asked to refrain from physical education and recess for an additional 1 to 2 weeks.

At the postoperative visit, we discuss timing of the second-stage surgery. In general, we plan a minimum interval of 4 months between the first and second stages.

Stage 2

The ear is elevated and the postauricular sulcus is created at the second procedure. Creation of a well-defined postauricular sulcus is important for the function of the reconstructed ear. Specifically, the sulcus will facilitate accommodation of eyeglasses and a hearing aid if atresia repair is performed.

This procedure is performed with the patient under general anesthesia as an outpatient. A skin graft is required. If the patient has a prominent ear deformity on the contralateral side, otoplasty can be performed during the same anesthesia. Postauricular skin can be removed from the otoplasty, thinned, and used as skin graft for the reconstructed ear. Any additional skin graft required is harvested from the left upper thigh.

Skin Graft

We use a freehand harvest technique. An elliptical graft, usually measuring about 9 by 4 cm, is harvested from the upper thigh. The incision is placed in a location to avoid irritation by undergarments. Ideally, the graft should not include hair-bearing skin though this can be difficult to predict as the patients have generally not started puberty at the time of the procedure. The area of the anticipated skin graft is infiltrated with lidocaine and epinephrine. Further expansion of the dermal layer can be achieved with injection of saline.

A 20-blade is used to harvest the thinnest possible graft. The dermis should remain in situ with no exposure of the subcutaneous adipose tissue (Fig. 39.11). The dermal layer is then removed to facilitate closure of

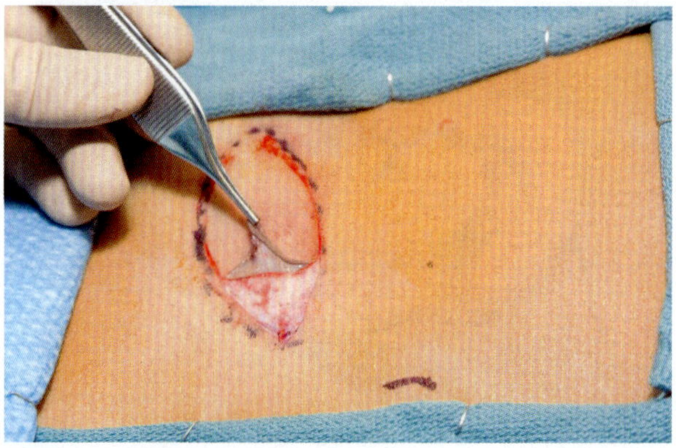

FIGURE 39.11

Harvest of skin graft. A thin full-thickness skin graft is harvested from the upper thigh. The defect is closed in three layers.

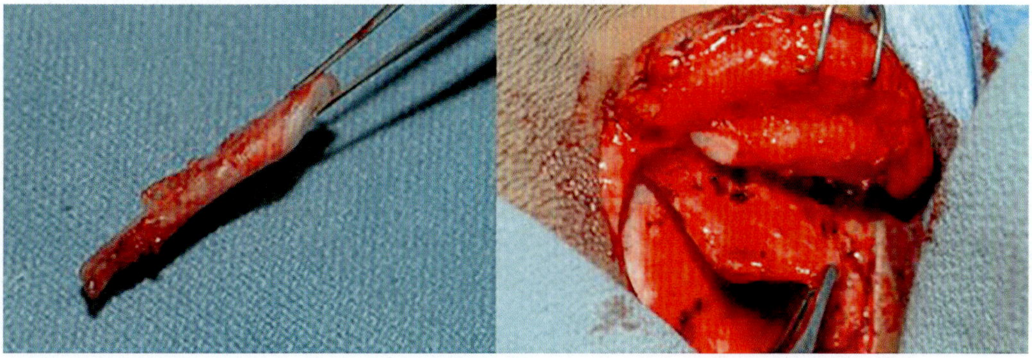

FIGURE 39.12 Banked cartilage and anteriorly based soft tissue flap. The cartilage is retrieved from the chest site and carved to create the posterior aspect of the conchal bowl. It is secured to the posterior aspect of the elevated framework with a semipermanent suture and then covered with an anteriorly based soft tissue flap.

the incision. The wound is not undermined in order to avoid the risk of hematoma or seroma formation. The deep dermal layer is closed with buried 3-0 polydioxanone sutures. 4-0 polydioxanone sutures are used to approximate the dermis and the skin is closed with 5-0 poliglecaprone in a running subcuticular suture. We apply topical cyanoacrylate as a dressing to facilitate wound care.

Elevation of the Ear

An incision is created around the framework and the reconstructed ear is elevated with care to avoid exposure of the cartilage framework. The surrounding scalp is then widely undermined just deep to the hair follicles. The scalp is advanced anteriorly toward the postauricular sulcus. The surgeon is able to determine the superior-most aspect of the sulcus with this maneuver. Care must be taken to position this point as symmetrically as possible with the contralateral side so that glasses will reset symmetrically on the face.

The skin edge is advanced around the helical rim so that the suture line between the skin and skin graft is positioned on the deep aspect of the helical rim. The skin edge is secured to the soft tissue with interrupted 5-0 chromic sutures placed in a horizontal mattress fashion.

The cartilage that was banked in the chest incision is retrieved. Any scar revision required at the chest incision can be performed at this time. The banked cartilage is carved to create a wedge of cartilage that is secured to the deep aspect of the framework to create the convexity of the conchal bowl. An anteriorly based soft tissue flap is elevated and reflected to cover the cartilage wedge (Fig. 39.12).

Advancement of the scalp will result in a standing cone in the hairline. The position of the standing cone will have an impact on the angle of the ear. A towel clip is placed to define the standing cone (Fig. 39.13). A deep 3-0 polydioxanone suture is placed and the towel clip removed. The standing cone is excised and the triangle of skin is thinned to create a small hair-free skin graft that will be used to cover the mastoid aspect of the neosulcus (Fig. 39.14). The incision created by excision of the standing cone is closed with deep interrupted 4-0 polyglactin sutures. The skin edges are approximated with a running locked 5-0 chronic suture.

The skin grafts from the contralateral ear and/or the upper thigh are then used to cover the newly created postauricular sulcus. If a skin graft is harvested from the contralateral ear, it must be thinned as much as possible. The grafts are secured with interrupted 5-0 plain gut and chromic sutures. The triangle of skin prepared from the scalp skin is used to graft the mastoid cortex. Using separate grafts for the posterior aspect of the ear and the mastoid cortex prevents obliteration of the postauricular sulcus.

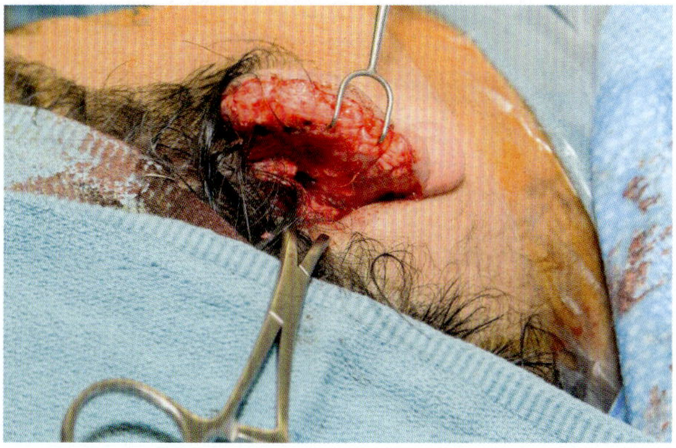

FIGURE 39.13
Defining the standing cone. The postauricular skin is advanced anteriorly often resulting in a standing cone.

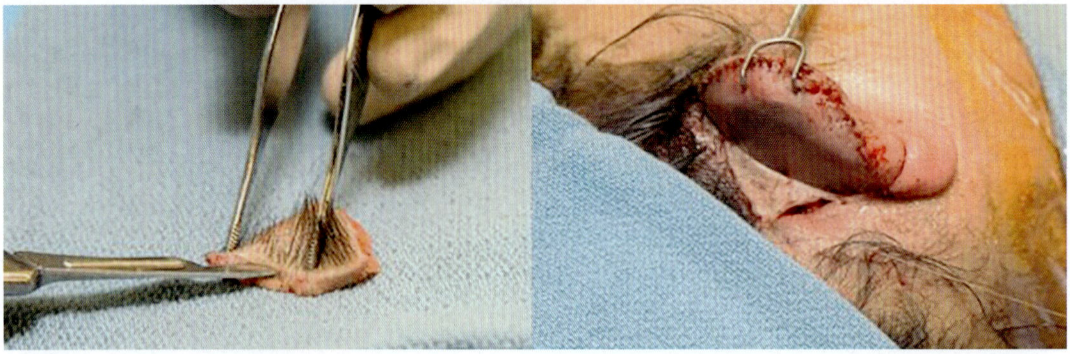

FIGURE 39.14 Excising the standing cone. The excised scalp can be thinned to create a non–hair-bearing skin graft to be placed on the mastoid aspect of the postauricular sulcus. Using two separate skin grafts for the sulcus helps to preserve the sulcus and ensures a non–hair-bearing sulcus.

A bolster is then fashioned from Xeroform gauze and is secured with a running 4-0 permanent suture (Fig. 39.15). A plastic cup dressing is applied, again with the gauze removed to avoid pressure over the reconstructed ear.

POSTOPERATIVE MANAGEMENT

The patients are instructed to use the plastic cup dressing until the first postoperative appointment 5 to 10 days later. They are asked to keep the ear dry until the bolster is removed. They are given oral and topical antibiotics and oral analgesics. At the first postoperative appointment, the bolster dressing is removed. If appropriate, any retained sutures can also be removed.

The patients are advised to use the plastic cup dressing at night and avoid strenuous activity, including physical education, recess, and competitive sports, for an additional week.

COMPLICATIONS

Stage 1

The potential complications associated with first-stage autogenous costochondral microtia reconstruction can be categorized as early and late complications (Table 39.3). Early complications include pneumothorax, hematoma, and poor contour of the framework. Management of pneumothorax was discussed in the description of the surgical procedure. Hematoma formation may be related to inadequate hemostasis or malfunction of the drain. It is important to ensure that there is an adequate seal at the end of the procedure. Hematomas should be evacuated in order to optimize the contour of the reconstructed ear.

Late complications include poor contour and asymmetry of the reconstructed ear and keloid formation. The contour of the reconstructed ear is defined by the framework and thickness of the skin flap at the first stage and the projection of the ear at the second stage. The surgeon can optimize construction of the framework by practicing preoperatively. Symmetry of the ear should be assessed by marking the superior and inferior aspects of the ear to be reconstructed based upon the position of the contralateral ear. Measurements to the lateral canthus and commissure may be less helpful in patients with craniofacial microsomia. Keloid formation should be managed with sequential steroid injections.

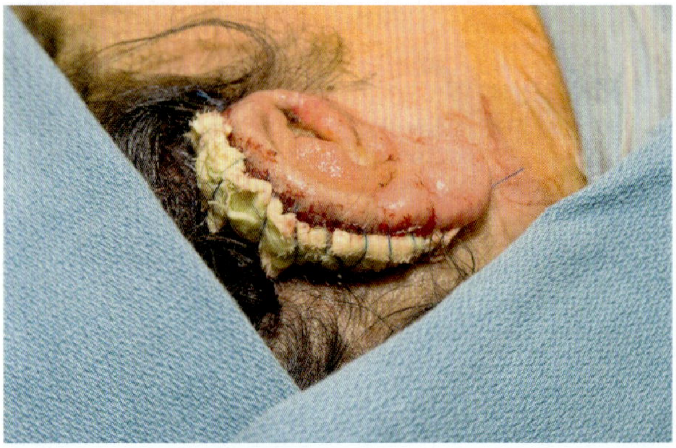

FIGURE 39.15
Postauricular bolster. Xeroform gauze is used to create a postauricular bolster. A permanent suture is used to secure the bolster in place and is removed 1 to 2 weeks postoperatively.

TABLE 39.3 Management of Complications

Complication	Management of Complication
Early	
Pneumothorax	Observation and serial chest radiographs Chest tube
Hematoma	Aspiration Surgical exploration Drain management
Flap ischemia	Monitor Release bolster suture
Late	
Cartilage exposure	Local advancement flap Pedicled delayed flap TPF delayed; skin graft
Keloid	Serial steroid injection Excision

Stage 2

The main complications associated with elevation of the ear are cartilage exposure, inadequate projection of the ear, and poor definition of the postauricular sulcus. Cartilage exposure generally becomes apparent 2 to 4 weeks after the second-stage surgery. Small areas of exposure may heal spontaneously; areas over 10 mm typically require revision surgery. Depending on the size and location of the cartilage exposure, treatment options include local rotation or advancement flaps, delayed pedicled flaps, and temporoparietal fascial flaps with skin grafts.

Inadequate projection of the ear can be addressed by having an adequate piece of cartilage for the wedge. Limited projection of the ear can be made less noticeable by removing skin from the contralateral ear to "deproject" the normally formed ear. This skin can be used to line the postauricular sulcus.

Definition of the postauricular sulcus can be preserved by using separate skin grafts for the mastoid and the posterior auricular surfaces.

RESULTS

Microtia reconstruction is a challenging endeavor. Families are often anxious to pursue reconstructive surgery as early as possible to avoid other children teasing their child during the early childhood years. The surgeon must determine the best time to start reconstruction and help the patients and families to understand.

The main desired outcome of microtia reconstruction is patient and family satisfaction. Therefore, it is important to counsel patients and families about expected results with surgery. We have found it most helpful to have our nursing staff review photographs of reconstructed ears with the patient and family starting when the patient is about 5 years of age. Some families are interested in reviewing photographs earlier. We choose photographs of patients who started with a similar degree of microtia. By having the nurses present the photographs, the patients and families can react honestly. This process helps set appropriate expectations.

The surgeon must continually critique her/his outcomes in order to reliably create an acceptable-looking ear. Since the final appearance of the ear is assessed several months after the initial surgery, it is helpful to keep notes about each surgery so that photographs can be reviewed and the technique continually refined (Figs. 39.16 and 39.17).

PEARLS AND PITFALLS

The main tools the surgeon has to create a natural-appearing ear are the skin flap, the contour of the framework, and the position of the ear. Pearls are often associated with potential pitfalls. Therefore, they will be addressed together.

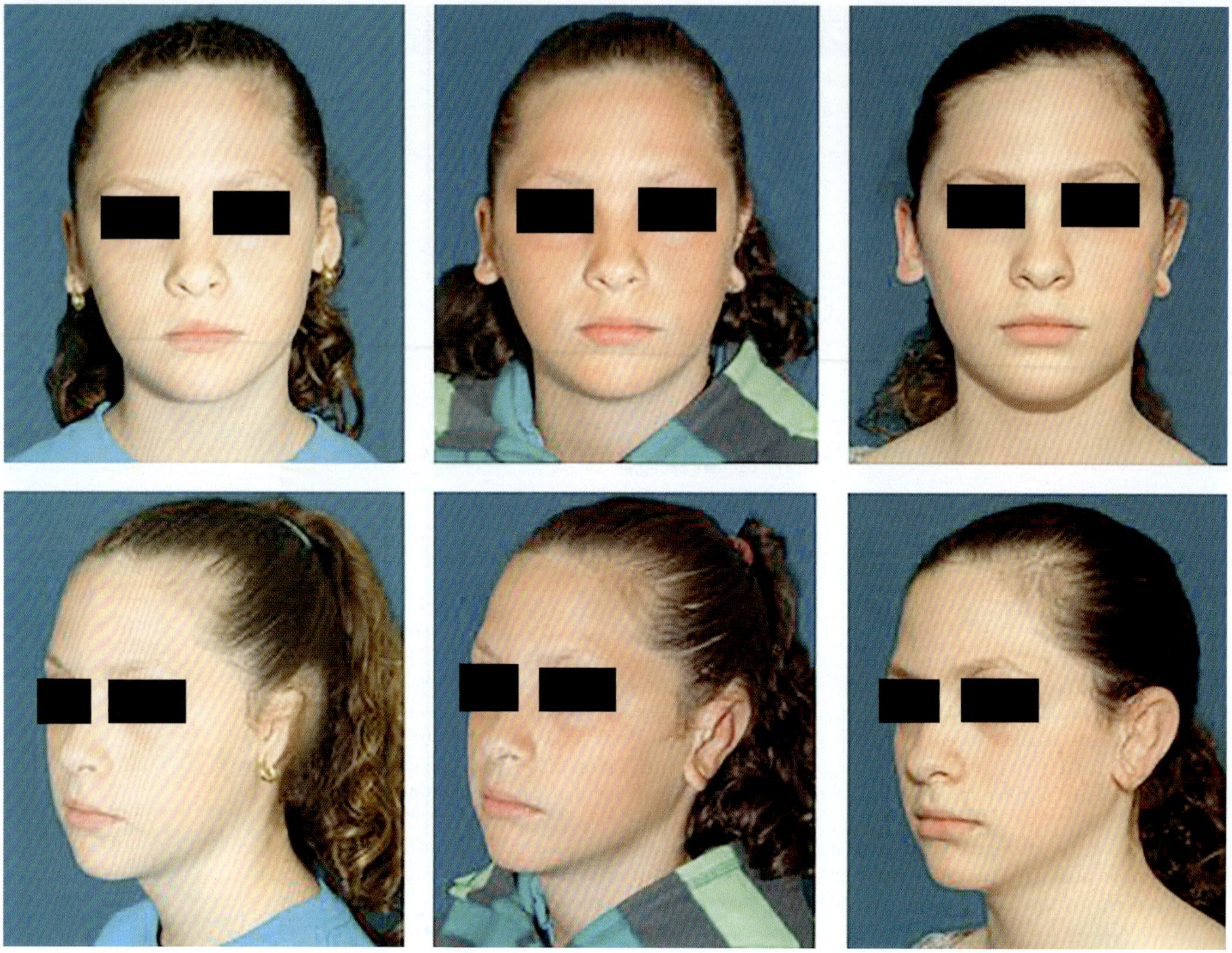

FIGURE 39.16 Stages of autologous costochondral reconstruction. The photos in the left column were taken preoperatively, middle column after first stage and right column after the second stage.

Stage 1 Pearls

- Small incision and beveling of the cartilage harvest site help to minimize the donor site morbidity. In order to minimize the size of the incision to harvest the rib cartilage, the position of the incision is important. It is also necessary to extend the deep incisions well beyond the limits of the skin incision. Retraction of the incision is continuously redirected to expose the area of dissection. The lateral cartilaginous incisions to define the superior and the inferior limbs of the synchondrosis should both be created. This allows direct visualization of the deep dissection toward the midline. The cartilage must be returned into the incision before making the last cut. Careful closure of the muscle layer helps with the long-term healing of the chest incision.
- Careful carving of the cartilage is important. Using a template can help facilitate the definition of the convexities of the ear. The large template should be skeletal in its final form. The concavities of the ear should be cut out so that the surgeon can easily trace the shape onto the cartilage. When carving the cartilage, the concavities should be accentuated so that they are larger than the contralateral ear. This accommodates the skin flap.
- Avoid overthinning of the free-floating cartilage. While a thin free-floating cartilage creates a beautiful curve, it will tend to buckle when placed in the skin pocket. Also, many sutures should be used to attach the helical rim to the body of the framework. This will help maintain the shape of the helical rim. The decision whether to place the free floater around or over the body of the framework is individualized. Placement of the free floater on the lateral aspect of the body will result in improved projection of the ear. However, some children have a relatively small synchondrosis requiring the additional height provided by peripheral placement of the free-floating cartilage.

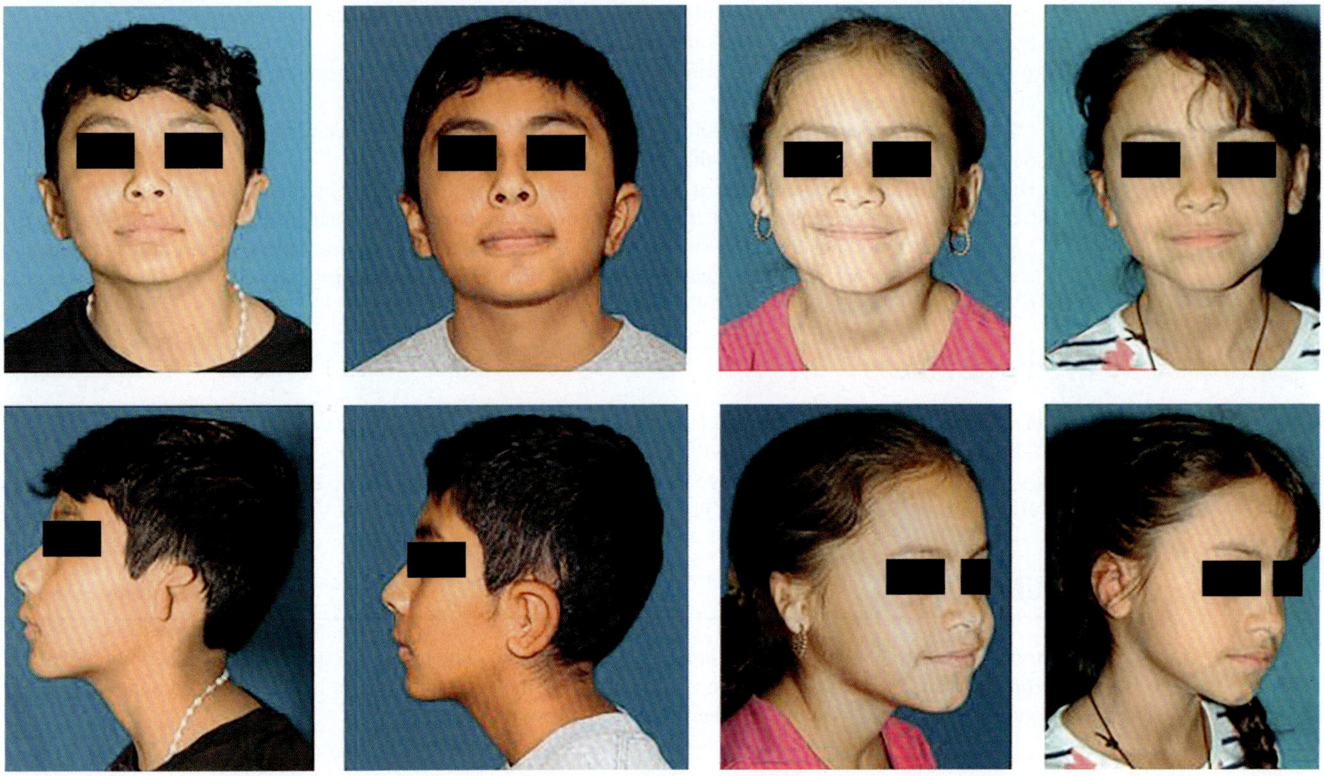

FIGURE 39.17 Before and after autologous costochondral reconstruction of microtia. Photographs taken before and after completion of staged reconstruction.

- Stacking layers of cartilage can help accentuate the contour of the ear. It can be challenging to secure the smaller pieces of cartilage to the body. It may be helpful to bend the needle to create a nearly straight needle.
- The thickness of the flap also contributes to the contour of the ear. The flap should be as thin as possible while maintaining an adequate blood supply. The surgeon should just be able to see the white appearance of the subdermal fat. Also, avoid using monopolar cautery on the skin flap. Hemostasis should be achieved with bipolar cautery.
- The suction drain holds the skin graft adherent to the framework. In order to use a single drain on the deep aspect of the framework, there should be full-thickness perforations in the concavities of the ear. However, the framework needs to be strong enough to maintain its shape under the skin flap. Therefore, the scaphoid fossa can be perforated with a skin punch using a 3- or 4-mm punch.
- We have found that bolster dressings help to maintain the shape of the ear. It is important to place the tacking sutures through the framework itself and avoid excessive pressure when tying the tacking suture.
- The additional cartilage used to define the antitragus and tragus is important.

Stage 1 Pitfalls

- Donor site morbidity is associated with a large incision, palpable or visible cartilaginous defect, and dimpling of the incision with inspiration.
- The reconstructed ear may lack contour.
- There may be notching at the junction of the lobule and newly created helical rim.
- The tragal contour may require accentuation.

Stage 2 Pearls

- In order to minimize exposed cartilage after this procedure, we take care to maintain soft tissue over the framework. The cartilage should never be directly exposed when elevating the ear.
- The position of the ear can be controlled with the scalp advancement. Try different positions of scalp advancement to achieve the most favorable angle of the ear. In addition to controlling the outcome of the

reconstructed ear, the surgeon should consider the position and appearance of the contralateral ear. Otoplasty may be very helpful in the overall appearance of facial symmetry.
- Advancing the scalp skin will help to project the reconstructed ear away from the mastoid cortex, particularly at the superior one-third of the ear.
- Other measures that will help to achieve projection are soft tissue advancement and placement of a crescent of cartilage on the deep aspect of the framework.
- Hair over the reconstructed ear is at least in part defined by the patient's hairline. Hair growth on the superficial aspect of the reconstructed ear may require separate hair removal maneuvers after the ear has healed.
- Inguinal hair in the postauricular sulcus is very bothersome. Harvesting a thin skin graft at the time of the second-stage surgery is the best way to avoid this problem. Once the problem becomes apparent, surgical revision may be required.

Stage 2 Pitfalls

- The main complication to be avoided during this stage is exposure of the cartilaginous framework.
- The position of the elevated ear will be determined at this stage.
- A common problem after this stage is lack of projection of the reconstructed ear.
- Hair over the reconstructed ear is unsightly and can be a nuisance.

SUMMARY

Surgical reconstruction of microtia is a challenging pursuit. The reconstructive surgeon must embrace all the technical nuances of this endeavor to adequately serve these patients. While I have described our current technique, we are always working together to try to improve our outcomes.

INSTRUMENTS TO HAVE AVAILABLE

Stage 1

- Basic soft tissue set
- Periosteal elevators
- Blades: standard 15, 10; Beaver 6700
- Skin punches 2 mm for perforation of the framework; 4 mm for carving the framework

Stage 2

- Basic soft tissue set

SUGGESTED READING

Brent B. Technical advances in ear reconstruction with autogenous rib cartilage grafts: personal experience with 1200 cases. *Plast Reconstr Surg* 1999;104(2):319–334; discussion 335–318.

Horgan JE, et al. OMENS-Plus: analysis of craniofacial and extracraniofacial anomalies in hemifacial microsomia. *Cleft Palate Craniofac J* 1995;32(5):405–412.

Nagata S. Modification of the stages in total reconstruction of the auricle: Part I. Grafting the three-dimensional costal cartilage framework for lobule-type microtia. *Plast Reconstr Surg* 1994;93(2):221–230; discussion 267–268.

Nagata S. Modification of the stages in total reconstruction of the auricle: Part II. Grafting the three-dimensional costal cartilage framework for concha-type microtia. *Plast Reconstr Surg* 1994;93(2):231–242; discussion 267–268.

Nagata S. Modification of the stages in total reconstruction of the auricle: Part III. Grafting the three-dimensional costal cartilage framework for small concha-type microtia. *Plast Reconstr Surg* 1994;93(2):243–253; discussion 267–268.

40 SCAR REVISION AND DERMABRASION

J. Regan Thomas

INTRODUCTION

A scar is the normal result of healing following lacerations, incisions, or tissue loss. They can vary in quality depending on the individual's ancestry, the mechanism of the trauma, and conditions in which the wound healed; all of which are factors beyond the surgeon's control. When a scar involves the face, one of the most prominent parts of the body, it can have significant implications for the patient. These can include psychological as well as social consequences, each with the potential to diminish the patient's quality of life. Factors that the surgeon can control include the favorable repositioning of the scar, proper alignment of the wound edges, and meticulous handling of the tissues.

A discussion with the patient and their family is essential to establish clear expectations for scar revision. Patients should understand that the goal is to improve the scar and not remove it. It is difficult sometimes for the patient to understand that healing is a lengthy process that takes months rather than days or weeks. The final result of the scar depends on a number of factors including the position of the scar, size, location, and the patients' predisposition for appropriate wound healing. The ultimate goal is to modify the scar to a point of maximized camouflage within the junction of facial landmarks and natural facial contour lines that exist within the head and neck.

HISTORY

When evaluating patients with a scar requiring revision, important questions to ask the patient include the following:

- What is the source of the scar?
- How old is the scar?
- Does the patient have a predisposition to forming keloids or hypertrophic scars?
- Is there a history of hyperpigmentation?
- Have there been any prior interventions to improve the appearance of the scar?
- Is the patient taking any medications that would potentially affect healing? Examples include anticoagulants, isotretinoin, chemotherapeutic agents, and radiation therapy.

PHYSICAL EXAMINATION

A detailed analysis of the scar is of the highest importance. A favorable scar is one that is narrow, well positioned along aesthetic subunit borders, and in parallel with relaxed skin tension lines (RSTLs) (Fig. 40.1). Facial scars tend to mature over a period of time and typically continue to improve for at least 1 year. Traditionally, it has been advised to allow scars to completely mature before pursuing any revision techniques. However, if the scar is not exhibiting favorable characteristics, earlier intervention after the first 60 to 90 days may be appropriate. Keloid scar

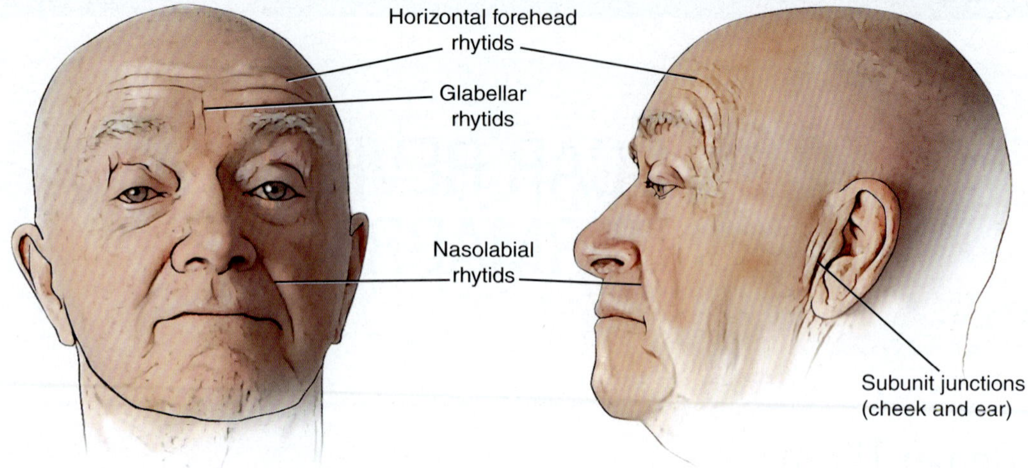

FIGURE 40.1 Relaxed skin tension lines represented in relative anatomic locations: horizontal forehead rhytids, glabellar rhytids, nasolabial, and subunit junctions (cheek and ear).

formation should not be confused with hypertrophic or malpositioned scars. Although keloid scarring resembles hypertrophic scars on a microscopic level, they grow well beyond the wound margin and exhibit a prolonged proliferative phase producing thick hyalinized collagen. The appearance of a hypertrophic scar may improve over the course of a few years. Keloids, however, do not improve with time and frequently require a multimodality approach.

Characteristics of scarring that should be noted on physical examination include

- Width
- Orientation to RSTLs
- Webbing
- Depression
- Hypertrophy
- Interruption of facial aesthetic units
- Proximity to favorable site
- Distortion of facial features or anatomic function

INDICATIONS

The general indication for scar revision is scar improvement, not elimination. Attributes of scar improvement include the following:

- Reduction in size
- Restoration of soft tissue contour
- Reorientation
- Removal of contracture
- Repositioning to a more favorable location

CONTRAINDICATIONS

Contraindications to scar revision include those instances that limit a favorable outcome. Patients who have a history of hypertrophic or keloid scarring are at a higher risk for a poor aesthetic outcome as are patients with thickened or discolored skin because the decreased elasticity may ultimately compromise the final result. Additionally, patients must have realistic expectations and understand that complete restoration to the preinjury state is not possible under any circumstances. Those with unrealistic expectations will likely be dissatisfied with the final results regardless of how excellent the outcome.

PREOPERATIVE PLANNING

When considering the various techniques used for scar revision, the surgeon must consider the specific characteristics of the scar he or she is treating in order to make an appropriate selection in therapeutic treatment.

For example, a contracted scar near the lip is one that requires lengthening to avoid a new contracture after excision. In this instance, a Z-plasty would be the most appropriate as it will add length to the previously contracted scar.

SURGICAL TECHNIQUE

Fusiform Excision

Occasionally, a scar will fall within or parallel to RSTLs but does not exhibit the characteristics of the ideal scar. When evaluating such a scar, all that may be needed is re-excision and closure in a fashion that will allow for a narrow flat scar. Re-excision should be done by use of a fusiform shape, typically with angled ends of 30 degrees or less to avoid standing cone deformities (Fig. 40.2). If the ends of the fusiform excision extend into another aesthetic subunit, an M-plasty may be performed at one or both ends to shorten the end of the ellipse. Closure following a fusiform excision should include appropriate undermining of 1 to 2 cm around the periphery of the wound as this facilitates reapproximation of the skin edges under minimal tension. It is essential to perform multiple layer closure of the wound including absorbable suture closure of the deep and dermal layers as well as everting nonreactive monofilament closure of the epidermis.

Serial excisions can also be performed for a large scar that cannot be primarily closed with a single definitive excision. This takes advantage of the ability of the skin to stretch and slowly accommodate over time.

Z-Plasty

Z-plasty is the classic technique that provides scar interruption while changing the scar direction so that the majority of the length of the scar is aligned with the RSTLs. The classic Z-plasty is a Z-shaped incision using the scar as a central member and two peripheral members of the Z configuration both equal in length, forming equal triangular flaps (Fig. 40.3). These flaps are transposed, which creates a number of changes in the scar including a predictable reorientation and redirection of the central component perpendicular to its original position. Additionally, it lengthens a contracted scar by adding additional intervening tissue. The amount of added length to the scar can be varied by adjusting the angles of the triangle. For example, angles of 30 degrees will

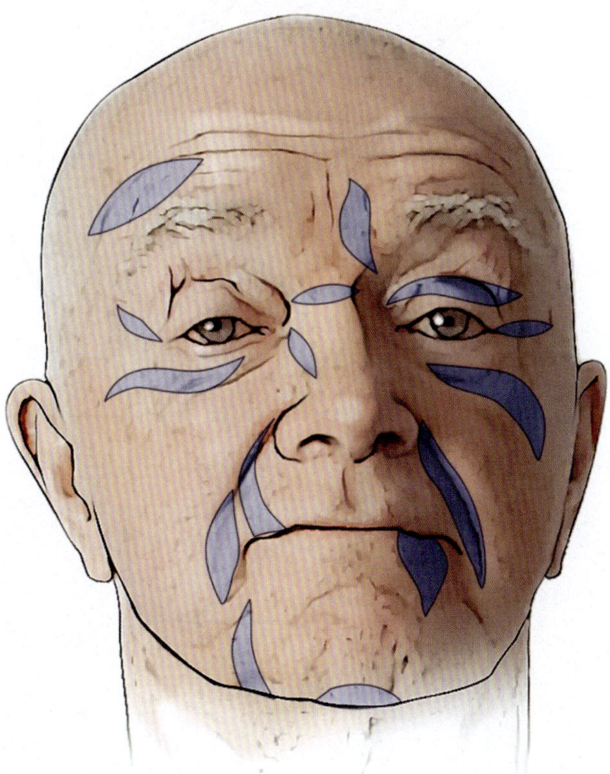

FIGURE 40.2 Examples of proper placement of fusiform excisions with 30-degree angled ends aligned with relaxed skin tensions lines and aesthetic unit boundaries.

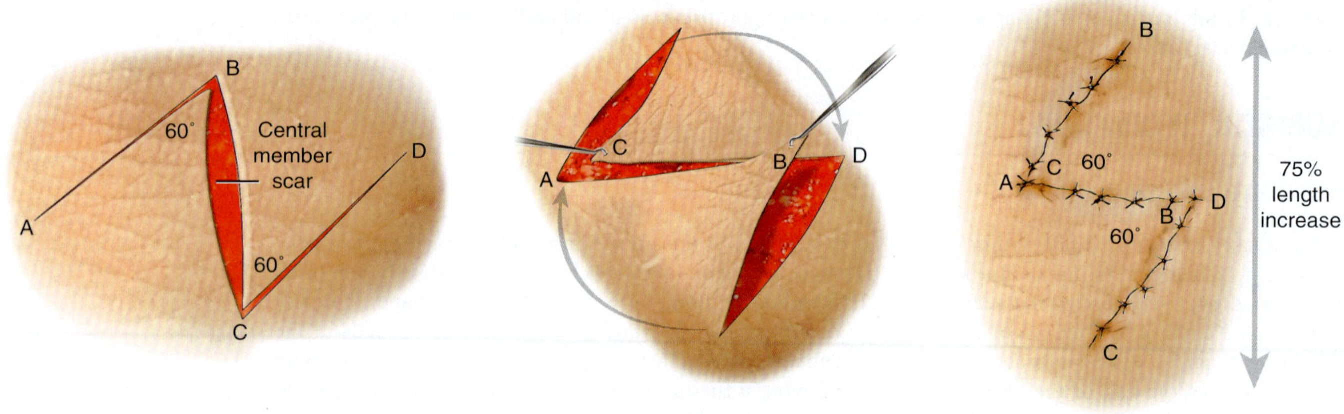

FIGURE 40.3 Classic Z-plasty using the scar as the central member and two peripheral members both equal in length forming equal triangular flaps. Note the resultant increase in length to the scar.

provide lengthening of the contracted area by 25%, whereas 45-degree angles will lengthen a wound by 50%, and 60-degree angles will yield a 75% lengthening. Z-plasty is useful in changing the direction of the scar, increasing scar length, elongating a contracted scar, and shifting malpositioned facial landmarks.

A particularly good use of the Z-plasty is correcting trapdoor scars, also known as pincushion scars. These scars are formed by circular or semicircular scars, which, when they contract, tend to bunch the central soft tissue creating a trapdoor-like flap. Correction of this involves placing small Z-plasties around the perimeter of the wound as this allows for interdigitation of the flap with the surrounding skin and, in effect, lengthens the circular contracted scar (Figs. 40.4, 40.5A–D and 40.6A,B).

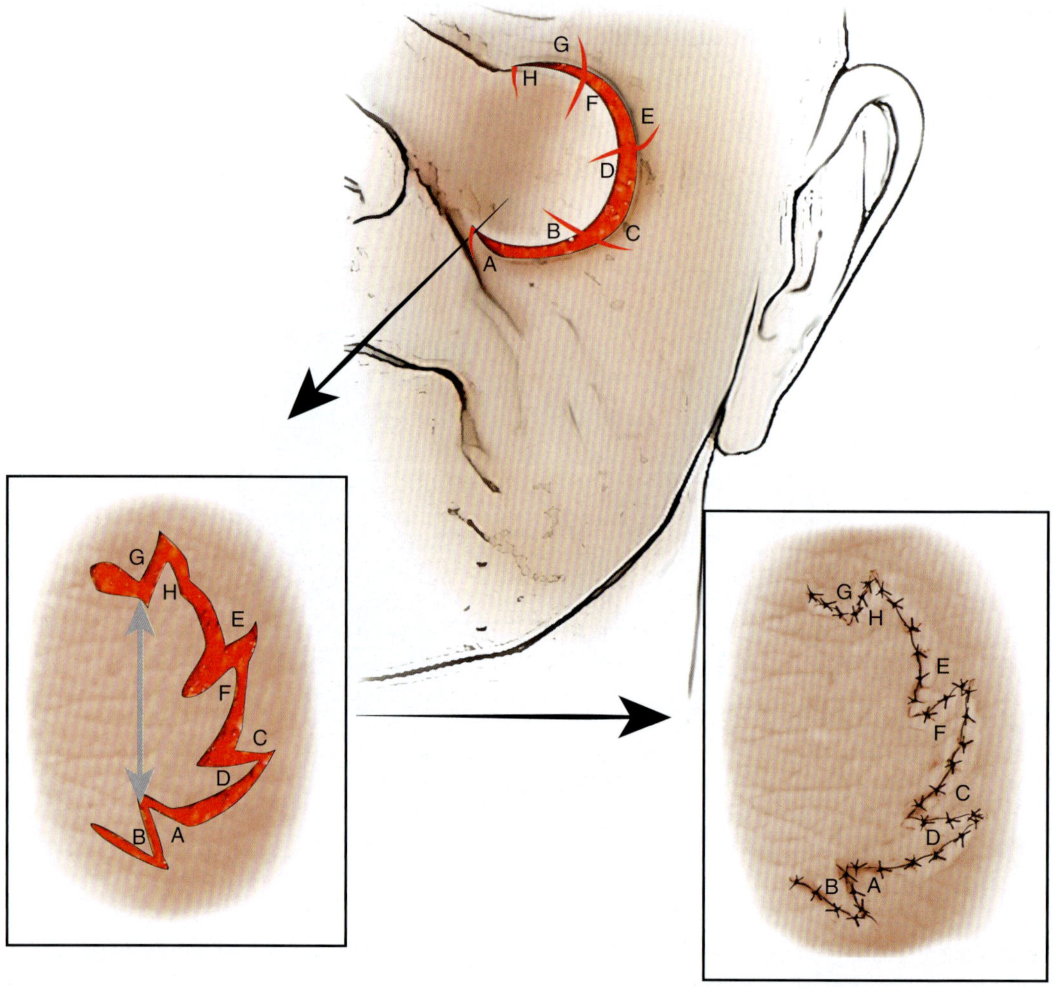

FIGURE 40.4 Trapdoor deformity corrected by placing multiple small Z-plasties around the perimeter of the wound.

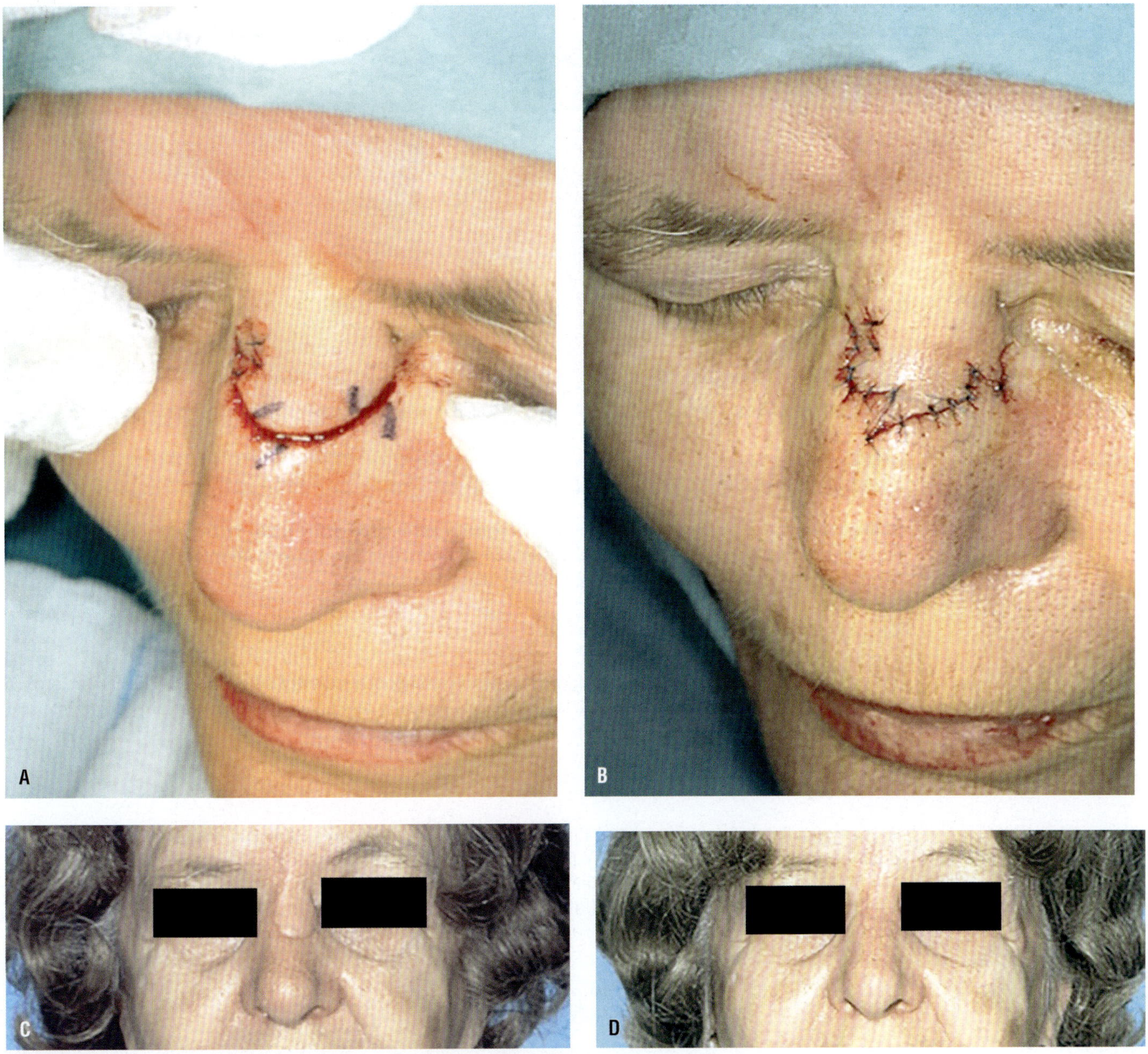

FIGURE 40.5 Use of multiple Z-plasties to correct a "trapdoor" scar deformity. **A:** Excision of scar and placement of Z-plasties. **B:** Following transposition and closure of Z-plasties. **C:** Preoperative appearance. **D:** Postoperative appearance.

Surgical Technique Z-Plasty

The scar is measured, and the proposed elliptical excision and peripheral members of the "Z" configuration are marked with a fine-tip marking pen. The area is infiltrated with 1% lidocaine with 1:100,000 epinephrine and cleansed appropriately. Using a no. 15 blade, the elliptical excision of the scar is performed and the peripheral incisions are made. The flaps are then raised and undermined in a subcutaneous fashion with a no. 15 blade. Once they are widely undermined, the flaps are transposed into their respective positions. They are secured in the dermal layer with interrupted 5-0 PDS suture, and the epidermal layer is closed with a 6-0 prolene suture. The area is cleaned, and triple antibiotic ointment with a semiocclusive dressing is applied to the area.

Multiple Z-Plasties

When multiple Z-plasties are combined along a scar, the same benefits are maintained as one single Z-plasty. However, the resultant scar tends to be less noticeable because the various components are smaller. This is most useful in long scars, which need to have scar interruption as well as the direction of the scar changed where using a single Z-plasty would require a long incision and thus more visible scars.

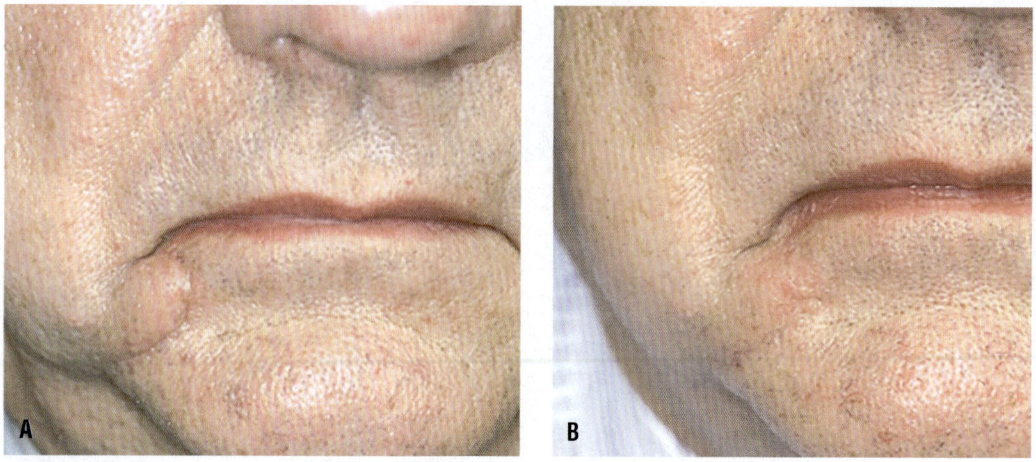

FIGURE 40.6 **A:** Preoperative appearance of "trapdoor" scar. **B:** Postoperative appearance after multiple Z-plasties.

Surgical Technique Multiple Z-Plasties

Multiple running Z-plasties are designed and Z-plasties are incised using a no. 11 blade with the same technique as described above. The flaps are transposed and closed in two layers with interrupted 5-0 PDS in the dermal layer and interrupted 6-0 prolene in the epidermal surface area.

Scar Interruption

The concept of scar interruption is to create a scar whose components ideally fall within RSTLs and are broken up in unpredictable irregular areas. An irregular scar is typically less noticeable than a harsh straight line scar and thus enhances the camouflage effect.

W-Plasty

W-Plasty is a form of scar interruption that tends to make a scar less noticeable and better camouflaged. Unlike Z-plasty, which is a transposed flap, W-plasty is an interposed flap, which does not create lengthening of the scar. W-plasty is created by excising connected triangular units to break up the scar line in a regularly irregular fashion. A series of consecutive triangles are marked out along the wound or scar edge (Fig. 40.7). The arms of the triangles should be approximately 5 to 7 mm in length, with ideally one arm of the triangle drawn parallel

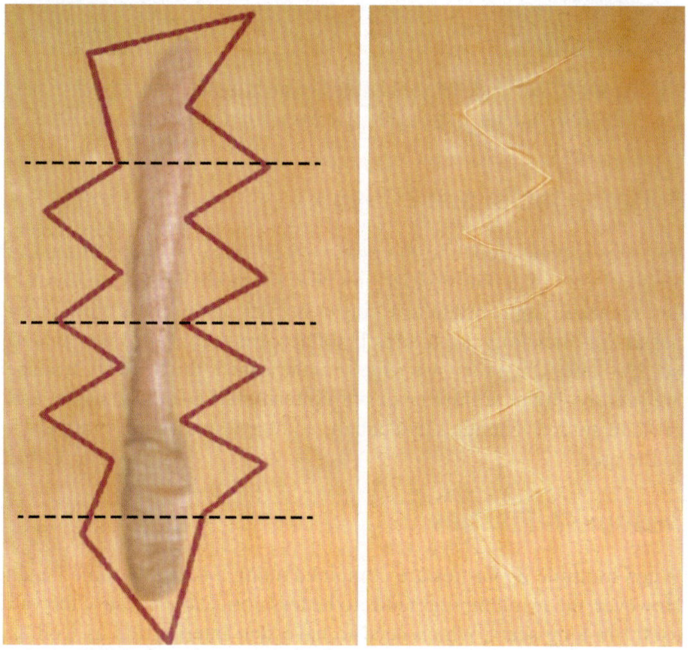

FIGURE 40.7
A W-plasty is performed by excising connected triangular units to break up the scar line.

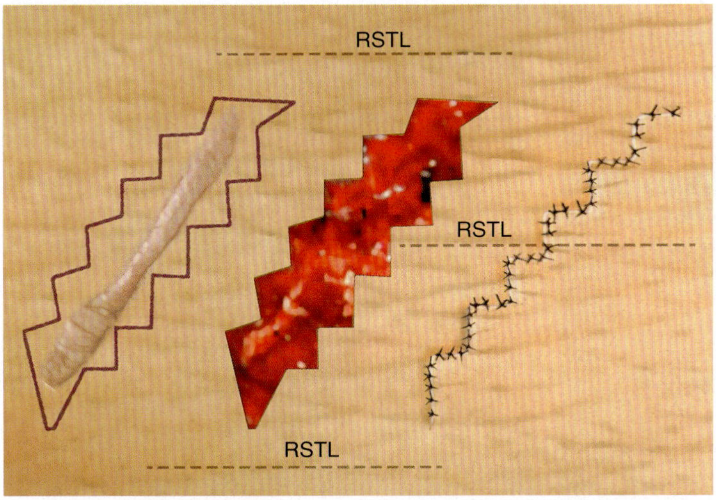

FIGURE 40.8 Running W-plasty with one area of triangle aligned in parallel with relaxed skin tension lines. Note that as scar inclination decreases, the degree of the angles should be increased to ideally maintain one of the arms aligned with the relaxed skin tension lines.

to the RSTL. As scar inclination decreases, the degree of the angles should be increased to maintain one of the arms aligned with the RSTLs (Fig. 40.8). After excision of the triangles, there are mirrored W-plasties on both sides of the wound, which are then advanced and closed. As a result, the W-plasty is a group of interposed flaps as opposed to the transposed flaps of Z-plasty. Frequently, a preplanned second-stage dermabrasion is utilized to further smoothen and camouflage the wound (Fig. 40.9A–F).

Surgical Technique W-Plasty

Careful measurements are made of the scar including the total length and width. The area is then infiltrated with 1% lidocaine with 1:100,000 epinephrine. A precise running W-plasty is then designed with a fine-tip marking pen on the scar with the arms of the triangles 7 mm in length. The scar and W-plasty are excised, and hemostasis is obtained with bipolar cautery. Wound edges are undermined with a no. 15 blade and the wound edges are then advanced, closing the interpolating W-plasty design of the scar repair. The incision is closed with interrupted 6-0 PDS suture in the deep layer and running 6-0 fast-absorbing gut in the epidermal layer. The wound is then cleaned and reinforced with sterile Steri-Strips. The Steri-Strips are removed at 1 week, and the 6-0 fast-absorbing gut is dissolved at this point.

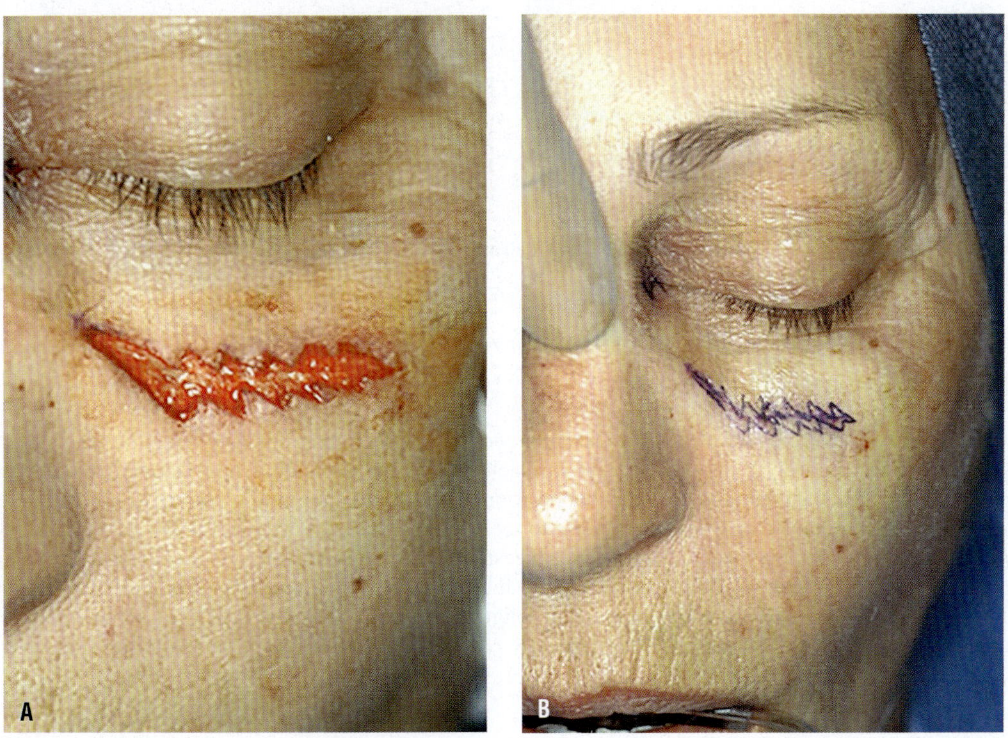

FIGURE 40.9 **A:** Scar excision. **B:** Preoperative plan with W-plasty.

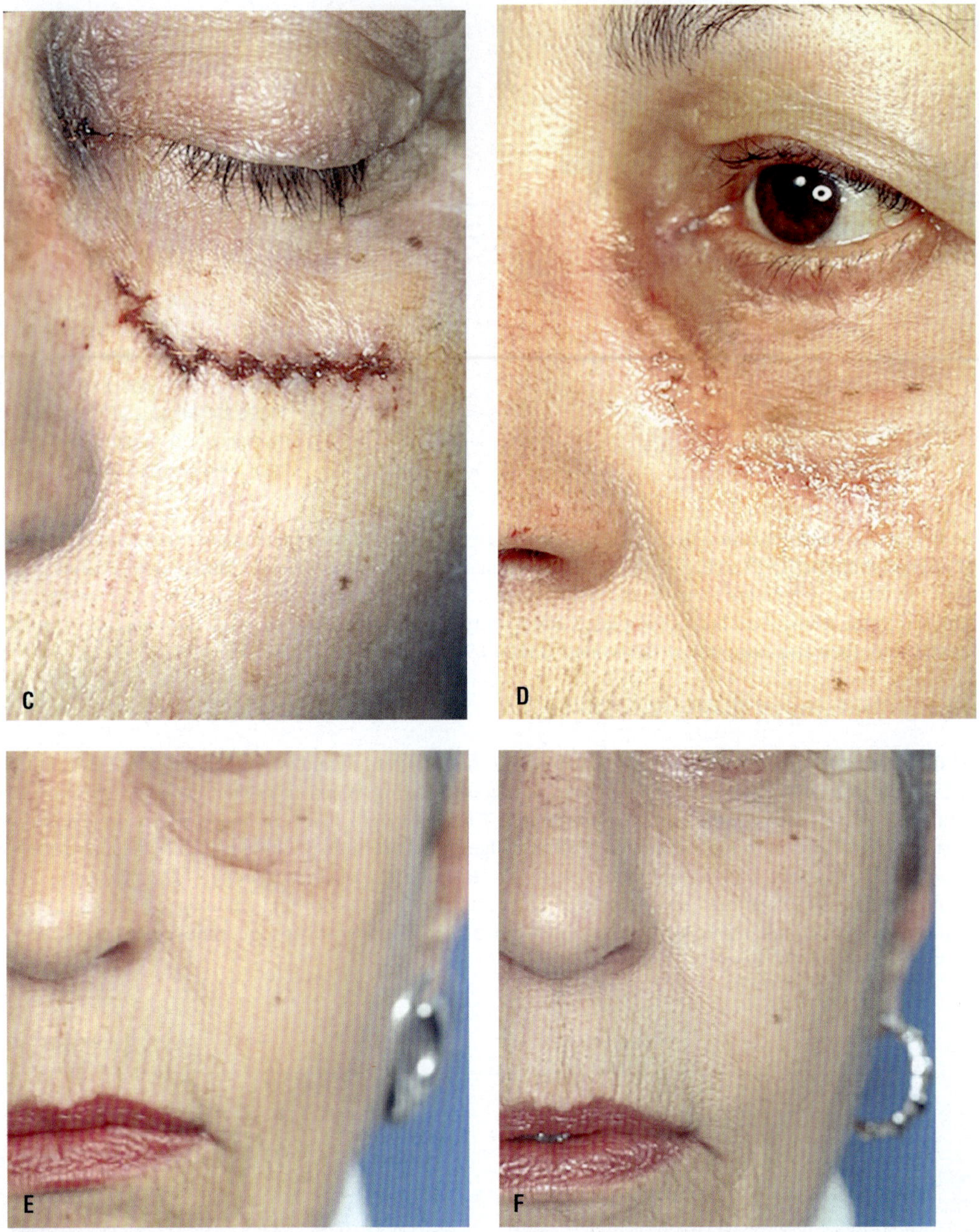

FIGURE 40.9 (*Continued*) **C:** Interpolation and closure of W-plasty. **D:** One week postop and suture removal. **E:** Preoperative appearance. **F:** Four months postop.

Geometric Broken-Line Closure

Geometric broken-line closure (GBLC) is a technique that creates an irregularly irregular scar utilizing random geometric figures as interposed flaps on each side of the excision. These geometric units are a series of squares, rectangles, and various-shaped triangles placed in a random pattern (Fig. 40.10). The geometry of the resultant scar is less detectable to the eye than the more predictable W-plasty. This technique is best suited for longer scars that traverse an aesthetic unit or broad flat surfaces such as the forehead and cheek. Like the W-plasty, GBLC is formed by interposed flaps without affecting length, as opposed to the transposed flaps and resultant increase in length as seen in Z-plasty. GBLC also benefits from a preplanned secondary dermabrasion that is typically performed 6 to 8 weeks after the initial scar revision (Fig. 40.11A–C).

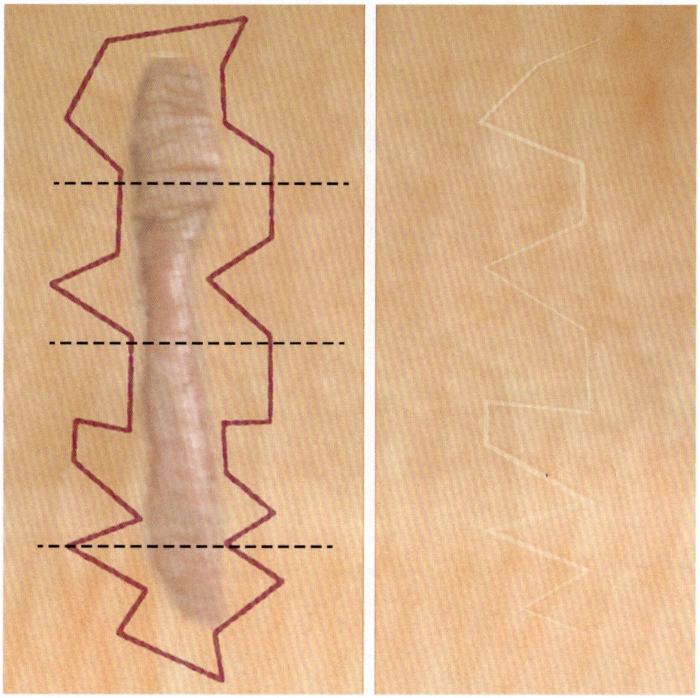

FIGURE 40.10
Geometric broken-line closure creates an irregularly irregular scar with random geometric figures. Certain parts of the geometric shapes are in parallel with the relaxed skin tension lines.

Surgical Technique Geometric Broken-Line Closure

The scar is measured and the design of random, irregular, geometric shapes are drawn on one side of the scar with a fine-tip marking pen with the length of the geometric shapes ranging from 5 to 7 mm. The mirror image of this pattern is repeated on the opposite side of the scar. The marked design and scar are excised using a no. 11 blade. The surrounding area is undermined with the scalpel blade. Two-layered closure is performed with 5-0 PDS in the dermal layer and 6-0 fast-absorbing gut in the epidermal layer. The wound is covered with Steri-Strips, which remain in place for 1 week.

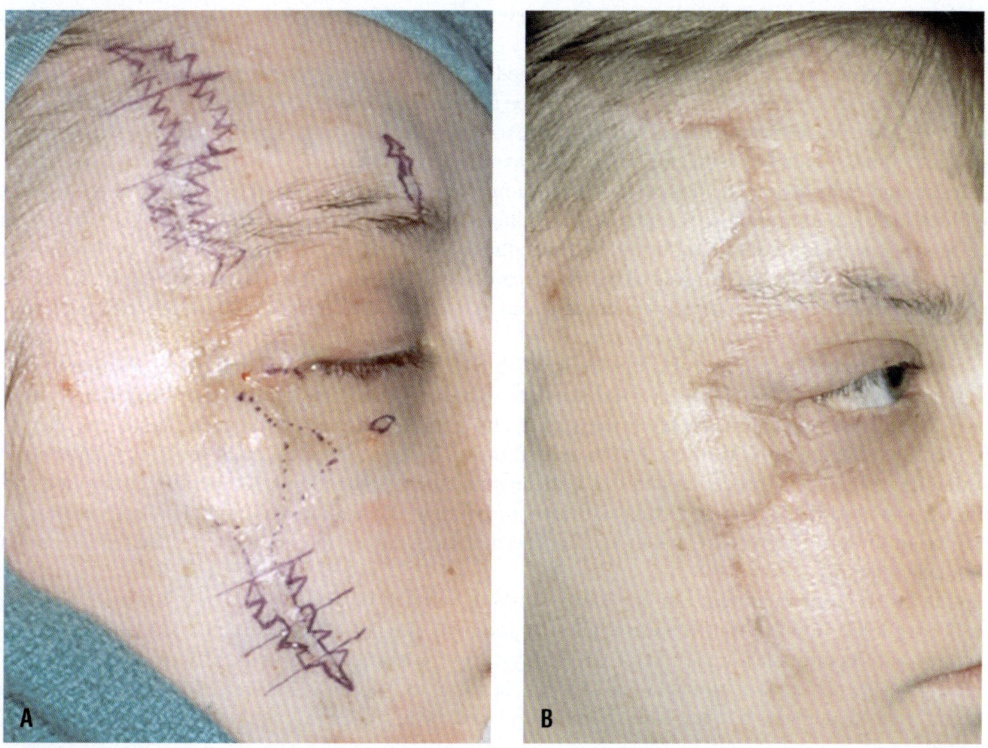

FIGURE 40.11 **A:** Preoperative planning including GBLC to cheek scar. **B:** Preoperative appearance.

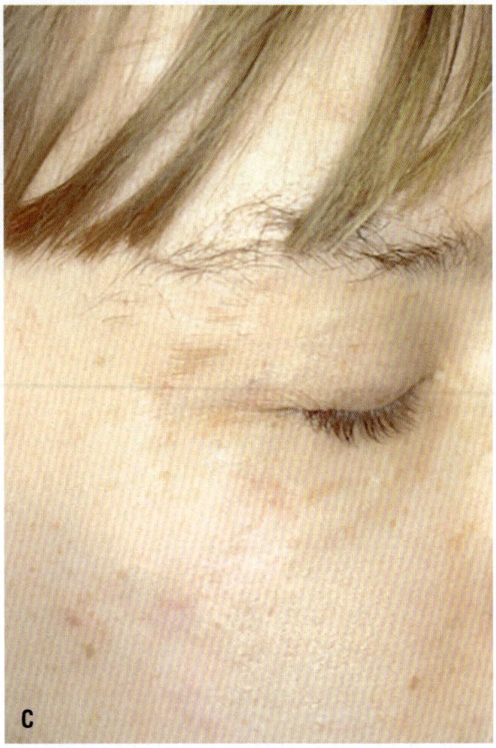

FIGURE 40.11 (*Continued*)
C: A 4-month postoperative appearance.

Dermabrasion

Dermabrasion is a method of controlled superficial skin ablation that is useful for smoothing out elevated scars and other skin contour irregularities. Routinely, dermabrasion is a preplanned second-stage following scar excision or scar interruption techniques. The concept of dermabrasion is that the superficial skin layers, the epidermis and part of the papillary dermis, are removed. This allows the wound to re-epithelialize by the surrounding tissues and underlining adnexal structures. It is best performed at a 6- to 8-week interval as it has been shown that rewounding during fibrillogenesis stimulates more epidermal cells to migrate to the wound leading to an improved appearance of the scar.

Ideal candidates for dermabrasion are fair-skinned patients because there is a lower risk for dyspigmentation following the procedure. Dermabrasion should be avoided in patients with hepatitis or human immunodeficiency syndrome as airborne pathogens pose a risk to health care personnel. Also, patients with a history of herpetic infections should be given antiviral prophylaxis.

Preparation of the area to be dermabraded is accomplished with local anesthesia. This provides not only a nerve block but also infiltration of the area with resultant distention of the skin, which assists in the dermabrasion. The skin surrounding the scar during the procedure is stretched and tightened with 3- or 4-point tension in order to provide an even and firm surface for dermabrasion. A diamond bit is used instead of a wire brush in order to gain greater control of the instrument and also to decrease the chances of abrading too deeply into the reticular dermis, creating an unnecessary scar.

The fraise should be rotating in a clockwise fashion and applied perpendicular and oblique to the axis of the scar (Fig. 40.12). Feathering is appropriate to avoid any demarcation between treated and untreated regions. During the procedure, entering the superficial papillary dermis will reveal small capillary loops easily identified by pinpoint bleeding. As the dermabrasion proceeds deeper, small parallel strands of white-colored collagen can be appreciated and this indicates the appropriate depth. As mentioned previously, proceeding deeper into the reticular dermis will lead to damage of the underlying adnexal structures, which are critical in the proliferation of undamaged epidermal cells across the abraded surface. This can lead to unnecessary scarring.

Immediately after treatment, an occlusive dressing such as polyethylene oxide hydrogel (Vigilon) is applied. This is left in place for 48 hours, and after removal, the patient is instructed to keep the area moist at all times with bacitracin for the next 7 to 10 days. Re-epithelialization is usually accomplished by 5 to 7 days. However, posttreatment erythema can persist for 2 to 3 months before resolution. This is usually less of an issue for females as they can use makeup to cover up the area once re-epithelialization has been completed.

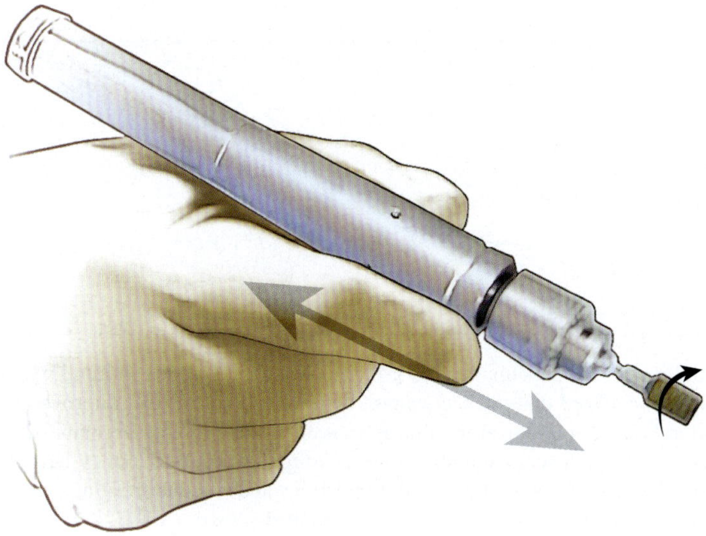

FIGURE 40.12
The handpiece is held 90 degrees to the direction of wheel rotation and is applied perpendicular to the axis of the scar.

ADJUNCTIVE PROCEDURES

Steroids

Intralesional steroids have been used an as adjunctive treatment for healing wounds, hypertrophic scars, and keloids. The injections can be particularly useful when there are areas of persistent tissue edema. Their mechanism of action involves reduction of fibroblast proliferation and collagen synthesis as well as suppressing inflammatory mediators. Triamcinolone (10 mg/mL) is injected into the dermal portion of the scar in the following weeks postoperatively. Repeat injections are often required and are typically performed at 2- to 4-week intervals. Caution should be used when injecting into surrounding tissue as this can cause atrophy and puckering. Additionally, hypopigmentation and telangiectasias can occur when injecting higher concentrations into the dermis.

Silicone Sheeting

The mode of action of silicone gel sheeting remains unclear but is thought to occur through an increased scar hydration effect specifically to the stratum corneum, leading to antikeloidal effects. O'Shaughnessy et al. further explored the theory of occlusion reducing hypertrophic scarring by performing histomorphometric analysis of the epidermis in occluded versus tape-stripped scars. Three occlusion groups were present, one of which was a topical silicone gel. Each of the occlusive treatments were shown to decrease the transepidermal water loss while tape stripping acted to the contrary. Additionally, tape stripping significantly increased the scar elevation index, epithelial thickness, and cellularity while the occlusion group showed reductions in all the former factors. To be effective, the sheets should be applied for at least 12 hours daily for 6 to 12 months. The ease of use of silicone gel sheeting and the lack of morbidity to the patient makes it an attractive alternative to invasive treatments. Adverse events include pruritus, rash, and maceration, all of which can be managed by temporarily stopping treatment and regular washing of the scar.

POSTOPERATIVE CARE

W-plasty and GBLC techniques are covered with Steri-Strips for the first postoperative week. General skin care is used in subsequent weeks. For other scar excisions, in the immediate postoperative period, triple antibiotic ointment is placed along the incision and a semiocclusive dressing with Telfa and tape is applied over this. The patient is instructed to remove the dressing the following day and to continue meticulous and gentle cleansing with soap and reapplication of the antibiotic ointment twice daily until their 1-week follow-up appointment. They are also prophylactically placed on antibiotics for 1 week as well. A first-generation cephalosporin is usually sufficient, or if the patient has an allergy to this class, he or she can be placed on clindamycin as an alternative. The nonabsorbable sutures are removed after 7 days. At this point, the patient is instructed to keep the incision clean and to avoid excessive sun exposure to prevent discoloration and prolonged erythema. After several weeks, if needed, we consider adjunctive procedures to achieve the best cosmetic outcome.

COMPLICATIONS

- Bleeding
- Infection
- Need for additional procedures
- Prolonged erythema
- Recurrence of keloid or hypertrophic scar formation
- Wound dehiscence

RESULTS

A scar on the face can have a substantial impact on self-image, and it is important to keep this in mind when approaching such a patient. It should be emphasized that the scar cannot be removed but instead improved in appearance. In these instances, it is often helpful to counsel the family as well as the patient. Dermabrasion can be extremely useful for smoothing out elevated scars and skin contour irregularities, which may help to camouflage the scar. Additionally, adjunctive procedures such as steroid injections and silicone sheeting can be useful and can ultimately aid in enhancing the final result (Figs. 40.13A,B and 40.14A,B).

PEARLS

- UV protection is important for the best result in the first 6 months after treatment.
- The ultimate goal is to modify the scar to a point of maximized camouflage along the facial aesthetic units and natural facial contours.
- If the ends of the fusiform excision extend into another aesthetic subunit, an M-plasty may be performed at one or both ends to shorten the end of the ellipse.
- A good use of the Z-plasty is in the correction trapdoor scars (pincushion scars).
- Ideal patients for dermabrasion are those who are fair skinned and not at risk for dyspigmentation.

PITFALLS

- Failure to have a thorough preoperative discussion about expectations for scar revision can lead to a disappointed and unrealistic patient response.
- Patients who have a history of hypertrophic or keloid scarring are at a higher risk for a poor aesthetic outcome.
- Patients with darker skin are at a greater risk for dyspigmentation when undergoing dermabrasion.

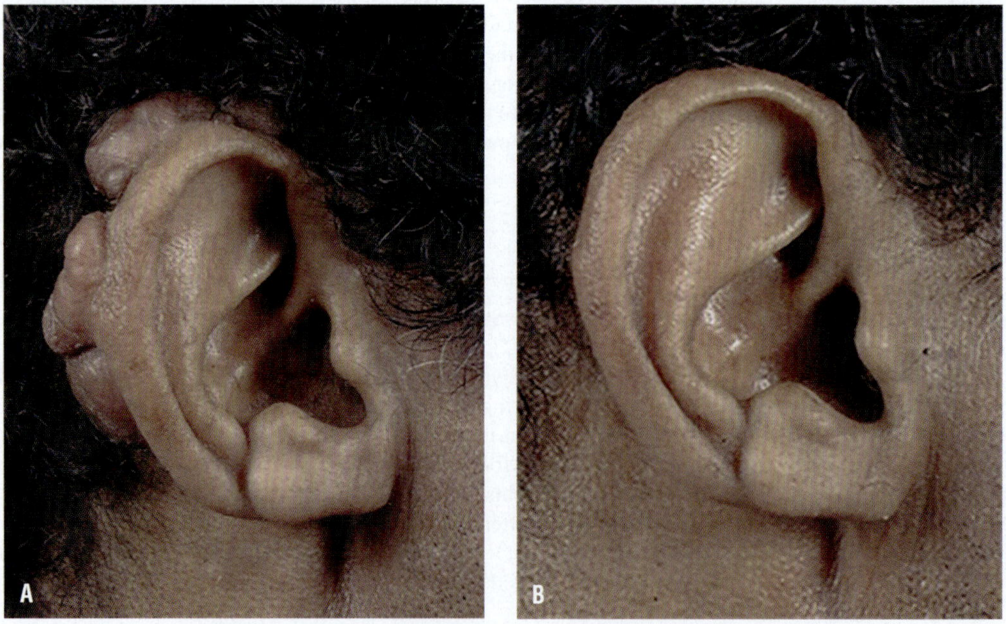

FIGURE 40.13 **A:** Preoperative keloid appearance. **B:** A 3-month postop following excision and serial triamcinolone injection.

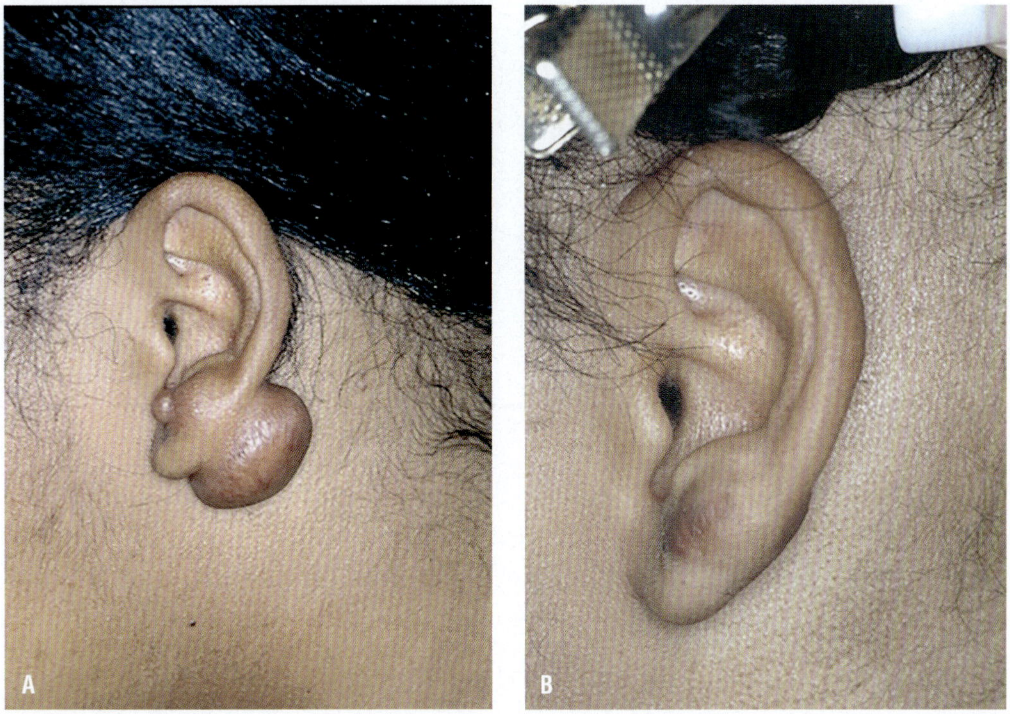

FIGURE 40.14 **A:** Preoperative keloid appearance. **B:** A 3-month postoperative appearance after excision and serial triamcinolone injection.

INSTRUMENTS TO HAVE AVAILABLE

- Standard plastic surgery set

ACKNOWLEDGMENT

My gratitude is extended to Michael Somenek, MD, for his contributions to the writing of this chapter. His work in writing, editing, and figure creation for this chapter is greatly appreciated.

SUGGESTED READING

Kokaska MS, Thomas JR. Scar revision. In: Papel ID, ed. *Facial plastic and reconstructive surgery*. Thieme Medical Publishers, Inc., 2002:55–60.

Thomas JR. Scar revision and camouflage surgery. In: *Advanced therapy in facial plastic and reconstructive surgery*. PMPH Publishers, 2010:687–693.

Thomas JR, Holt GR. *Facial scars: incision, revision and camouflage*. St. Louis, MO: CV Mosby, 1989.

Thomas JR, Mobley SR. Scar revision and camouflage. In: *Cummings otolaryngology head and neck surgery*, 5th ed. St. Louis, MO: Mosby, 2011.

41 BILOBE FLAPS

John A. Zitelli

INTRODUCTION

The bilobe flap is an extremely useful random pattern flap for facial reconstruction. It is a double transposition flap in which both flaps share a common base, the closure of the flap does not cause distortion of surrounding tissues, and the mechanics of the flap allow for the recruitment of redundant tissues from distant sites. The primary flap is used to repair the surgical defect while the secondary flap repairs the original flap donor site. Originally described by Esser in 1918, the bilobe flap, after modifications, has become the flap of choice for reconstruction of small- to medium-sized defects along the lower third of the nose. The original design required that the angle of tissue transfer between each lobe of the flap be 90 degrees, for a total transposition of 180 degrees. Although this design maximizes the distance that skin can be moved, the wide angles also resulted in increased wound closure tension, noticeable pincushioning (trapdoor) of the flap, and prominent tissue protrusion (dog-ears) at the pivotal points of rotation. Excision of this redundant tissue would not be feasible since it would narrow the base of the flap excessively and compromise the circulation and flap survival.

In 1989, I published significant modifications to the original flap design that minimized the risks of pincushioning and dog-ear formation. I emphasized using narrower angles of transfer of 45 degrees between each lobe, so that the total transposition of the flap occurs over no more than 90 to 110 degrees. By reducing the angle of rotation, limitations of pivotal restraint including flap shortening, increased tension of the closure, and cutaneous deformity at the pivot point of rotation were addressed (Fig. 41.1).

The bilobe flap expands the use of the traditional single transposition flap. As a double transposition flap, it transfers the tension of wound closure over a 90 degrees arc, instead of the usual 45 to 60 degrees of a single transposition flap. The addition of the second, tension-releasing lobe allows for the repair of defects that could otherwise not be closed with a single transposition flap due to wound tension and distortion of surrounding structures. This mechanical release of tension offered by the bilobe flap is identical to that of a double Z-plasty, enhancing tissue movement and transposition about the pivotal point (Fig. 41.2). With proper preoperative planning and surgical execution, the bilobe flap is not only useful for reconstruction of surgical defects on the nose, particularly the nasal tip and ala, but can also be used successfully to repair defects involving the eyelids, eyebrows, cheeks, chin, and lips.

HISTORY

Just as every surgical defect is defined by its inherent characteristics, so is each patient who harbors such an infirmity. A comprehensive medical examination is required of all patients undergoing surgery. A detailed medical history, including cardiopulmonary, endocrine, and autoimmune conditions, must be evaluated as each circumstance can compromise wound healing. Details with regard to local trauma, surgery, sun exposure, and radiation therapy are important as well. A list of current medications and allergies is required. The use of tobacco, alcohol, or substance dependence may limit postoperative wound healing

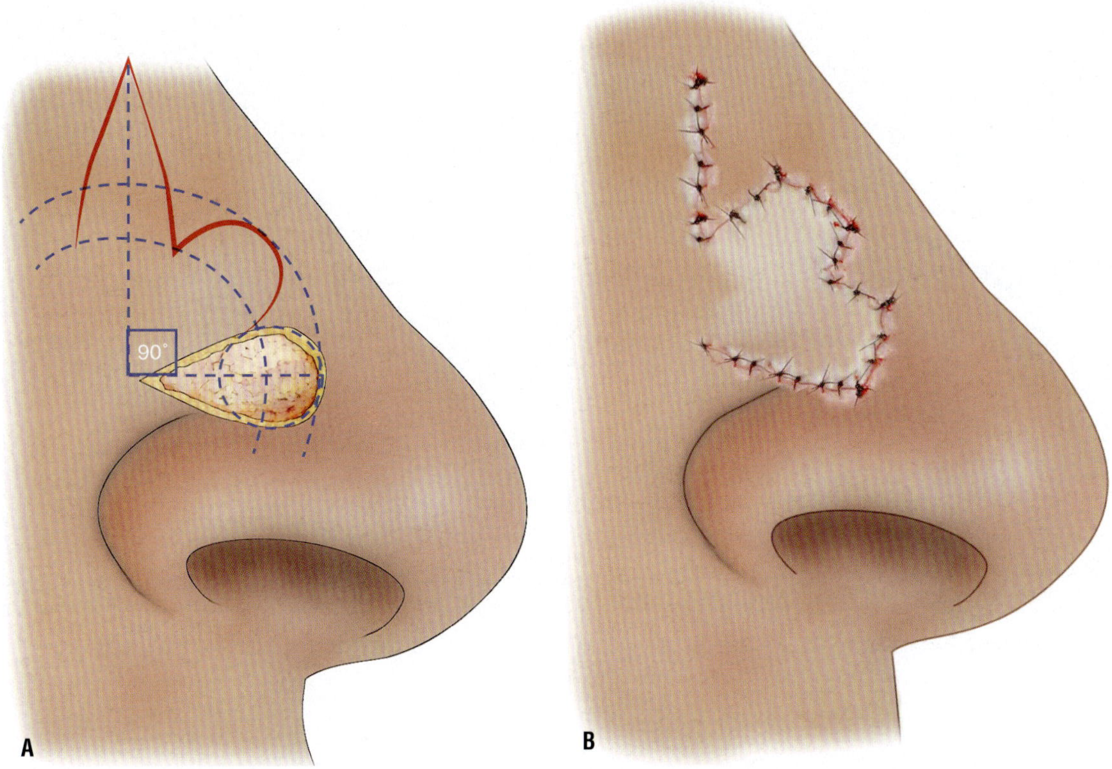

FIGURE 41.1 A and B: Improved design prevents distortion of free margin and minimizes dog-ear and trap-door defects.

as well as postoperative therapies. Finally, medical clearance may require one or more specialist's involvement for medical optimization prior to surgery.

PHYSICAL EXAMINATION

When developing a reconstructive plan, a defect-oriented approach is useful in the determination of what native tissues and resources exist, while also establishing which elements are absent and need to be restored. It is important to consider the quality, quantity, and medical history of the tissues surrounding the current

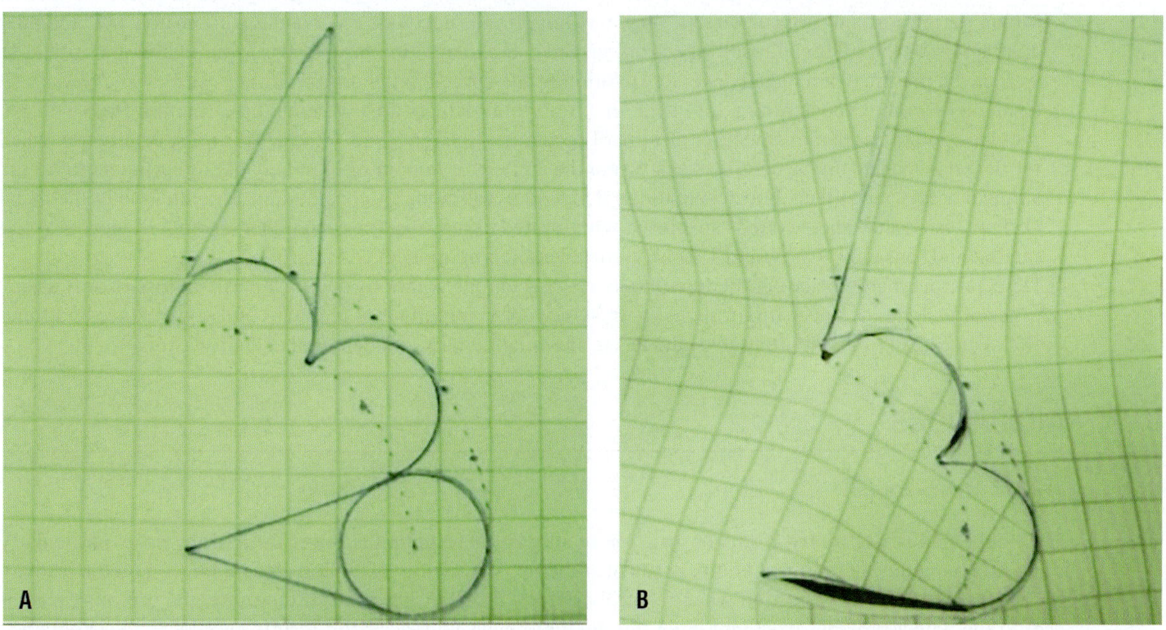

FIGURE 41.2 The effect of a double Z-plasty. **A:** The original design. **B:** The double Z plasty.

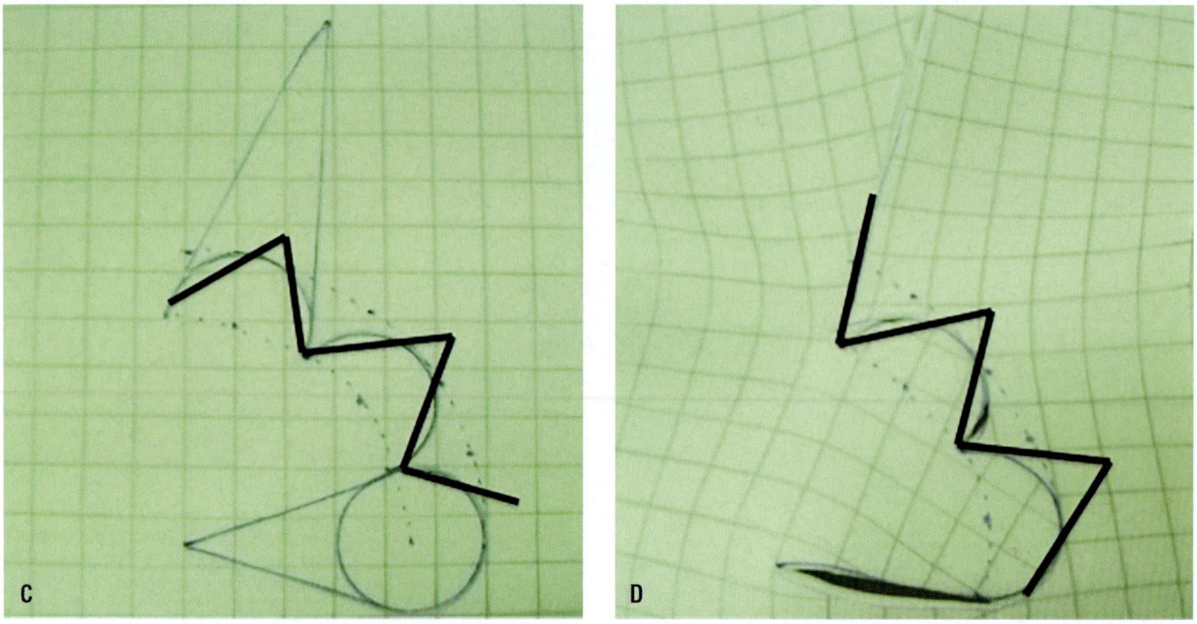

FIGURE 41.2 (*Continued*) **C:** *Lines* demonstrate shortening in the horizontal plane. **D:** The Z-plasty actually lengthens in the vertical plane to prevent upward pull on mobile free margins.

defect as well as the dimension of the facial aesthetic units involved. Specifically, the bilobe flap is best suited for circular defects and has multiple variations that are useful in the closure of defects along the nose as well as the eyelids, cheek, upper lip, and chin. Tissue is taken from one region to restore another. In essence, the defect is transposed to a region that is of less functional and aesthetic priority and has better reconstructive capabilities. For example, the complex anatomy and unique characteristics of the nose make it challenging when planning for reconstruction of surgical defects. Its topography is composed of multiple adjacent convex and concave surfaces that should not be distorted. The free margins of the alar rims are mobile and can be easily displaced. The skin over the lower third of the nose is thick and inelastic making it difficult to recruit for closure of surgical defects. Additionally, the color and texture of the skin is so unique that it can be difficult to match with either distant or nearby skin. Additional considerations during physical examination are as follows:

- The eyelid margin can be easily displaced, and primary wound closure or local flaps used in this area can often result in downward traction on the eyelid. Although full-thickness skin grafts are a good reconstruction option for infraorbital surgical defects, they may not provide adequate color and texture match, and potential contraction of the graft can result in ectropion. Snap and distraction tests of the lower eyelid are critical as well as the presence of a negative vector (relation of the cornea to the orbital rim).
- Challenges in the reconstruction of cheek or infraorbital defects arise when simple rotation flaps will not provide enough tissue movement for closure of moderate- to large-sized defects. This is especially true when the defect is located on the central cheek where the amount of remaining skin may not be sufficient to fill the surgical defect and still enable closure of the donor site. Additionally, considerable accentuation of the facial skeleton can occur when wounds are closed with limited tissue resources and under tension. Review of facial motion and sensation (CN V and VII) is of considerable importance.
- Defects around and including the mouth may require unique solutions due to superficial loss of soft tissue, especially along the upper lip. In such circumstances, it is important to maintain oral competence and function. Once again it is important to evaluate for muscular activity, enunciation, and air wasting.

INDICATIONS

Nasal Defects

The bilobe flap is well suited for reconstruction of surgical defects on the lower third of the nose, particularly those involving the lateral tip, supratip, or ala near the tip. With minimal wound closure tension on the primary flap, there is little or no distortion when repairing defects near the alar rim. Furthermore, the use of skin adjacent to the defect provides excellent color and texture match with aesthetic results exceeding those obtained from the use of full-thickness skin grafts.

Extranasal Defects

Cheek

Bilobe flaps may be used anywhere on the cheek even though the incision lines may not follow the natural wrinkle lines on the face. The advantage of lack of wound closure tension and distortion of surrounding structures outweigh the disadvantage of the final curvilinear scar.

Chin

The bilobe flap can be used to repair large defects on the chin without distortion of the lower lip providing excellent aesthetic results. In this location, the bilobe flap uses skin from the submental and superior neck regions. The first lobe is placed adjacent to the surgical defect in the submental skin and the second lobe is placed in the anterior cervical skin. This allows excellent textural and color match, especially in men with dark terminal hair, while concealing the scars in less cosmetically noticeable locations.

Upper Lip

The cosmetic unit of the cutaneous upper lip has a very restricted surface area, making repair of surgical defects sometimes quite challenging. Most local flaps use the adjacent melolabial fold as a donor site, but movement of these flaps often results in distortion of the upper lip when repairing large defects. The bilobe flap can be used successfully for defects in the lateral upper cutaneous lip by utilizing the skin reservoir of the cheek.

Eyelids

The bilobe flap can be used to repair large surgical defects anywhere in the infraorbital region including the mid and lateral lower eyelid, as well as the medial and lateral canthus. Defects in the lateral canthus take advantage of the skin in the preauricular cheek and temple. Here, the flap can be designed with the pivot point placed caudally where the first lobe is adjacent to the defect, and the secondary lobe lies parallel to the "crow's feet."

Other

In addition to the aforementioned areas, the bilobe flap can be used to repair large surgical defects in the lower forehead, near the eyebrow.

CONTRAINDICATIONS

The successful outcome using the bilobe flap on the nose, as well as in any other location, will depend on proper patient selection (medical, surgical, noncompliance and unrealistic expectations), correct flap design, and good operative technique. It is also important to be thoughtful about which factors may affect the overall outcome in every patient you see. On the nose, for example, cosmetic results are best when the bilobe flap is used in patients with thin lax skin along the nasal sidewall and the design is optimally placed. Patients with thick, sebaceous skin have a higher incidence of flap necrosis, infection, and depressed scars. Defects higher on the nose must recruit skin for the secondary lobe nearer to the medial canthus, where the skin is thin and less mobile. For this reason, although not a complete contraindication, an inferiorly based bilobe flap is not the most suitable reconstruction of defects on the upper half of the nose.

SURGICAL TECHNIQUE (NOSE)

The base of the bilobe flap can be placed laterally or medially, although it is most often designed with a lateral base. In laterally based bilobe flaps, the nasalis muscle is included in the body of the flap providing an excellent blood supply with minimal risk of necrosis. Flaps with a medial base are more useful for repair of alar defects and have also shown to do well, even though the vascular supply is not as rich without a musculocutaneous component.

Bilobe flaps are ideally suited for defects less than 1.5 cm located on the lateral nasal tip or sidewall. These flaps on the nose must be precisely designed as follows (Table 41.1). First, a Burow's triangle is designed with its apex pointing laterally and one side parallel to or along the alar crease. The length of this triangle is approximately equal to the diameter of the defect. The apex of the Burow's triangle serves as a focal point for the rest of the flap's design.

Each donor lobe is designed around two arcs, one arc through the center of the defect and another through the distal end of the defect (Fig. 41.2). The bases of the two flaps are designed to rest on the first arc. The center radius of each flap is positioned at approximately 45 degrees from each other, with the center radius of the first lobe at 45 degrees from the center of the defect. Whenever possible, the axis of this secondary flap should be oriented vertical to the alar rim in order to prevent distortion of the ala. The length of the first lobe extends to the second arc while the length of the second lobe, including its Burow's triangle, is approximately twice that of the

TABLE 41.1 Important Concepts and Consequences of the Bilobe flap for Nasal Reconstruction

Concept	Consequence
Make surgical defect as deep as cartilage	Minimizes the risk of trap-door deformity
Excise a Burow's triangle lateral to the defect	Minimizes tissue protrusion or bulkiness
Orient the secondary defect vertical to the alar rim, especially in patients with large defects or tight skin	Minimizes the risk of alar distortion
The size of the primary flap should be equal to that of the defect	Minimizes the risk of upward retraction of the ipsilateral ala
Widely undermine beyond the base of the flap and the donor site	Minimizes trap-door contraction of the flap
Trim the flap undersurface to the depth of the defect (safe to thin up to 1–2 mm of subcutaneous adipose tissue)	Minimizes fibrosis of adipose tissue and trap-door deformity
Trim excess adipose tissue/muscle under the point of rotation	Minimizes tissue protrusion
Approximate the deep dermal component of the flap with buried vertical mattress sutures	Minimizes the risk of trap-door deformity by eliminating the dead space

first lobe. The width of the first lobe and second lobe should be equal to that of the surgical defect. Undersizing the primary flap replaces less tissue than that of the defect and may result in ipsilateral upward alar retraction.

After incision and elevation of the flap, wide peripheral undermining beyond the base of the flap and along the recipient site is performed. Undermining is done at the level of the perichondrium and periosteum. This is important to maximize blood supply and to minimize the chance of trap-door deformity.

Following elevation of the flap and undermining, hemostasis is obtained. Hemostasis must be precise so that a dry field is obtained without excess char from electrocautery. Closure with buried vertical mattress sutures begins with the donor site of the secondary flap. The primary flap is transposed into the surgical defect, and the secondary flap is transposed into the donor site of the primary flap. If the thickness of the first lobe is greater than the depth of the defect, the undersurface can be thinned to the level of the subcutaneous tissue; moreover, the edge of the flap can be thinned to the dermis, if necessary, to match the thickness of the adjacent skin along the defect. Ideally, the donor flap should be just slightly thinner than the depth of the defect. Next, the primary flap is sutured into place, and finally, the secondary flap is trimmed of its excess length to fit the donor defect of the first lobe before it is sutured.

The suture technique used for closure of the flap is critical in determining the final cosmetic outcome. After elevating the flap, the deep, elastic dermal tissue of the flap tends to retract more so than its superficial, inelastic skin edges. Therefore, the deep dermal component of the flap and wound edges should be approximated with buried vertical mattress sutures in order to eliminate this dead space. If the flap was only supported by superficial sutures, it would heal with an elevated center and a depressed scar along the incision lines. These buried vertical mattress sutures will also provide prolonged wound eversion until healing is complete. Finally, the skin edges of the entire flap are adjusted so they are even with a continuous running suture. Dermabrasion may be performed, if necessary, and is best accomplished at 3 months after surgery. This is most often necessary in patients with thick, sebaceous nasal skin.

POSTOPERATIVE MANAGEMENT

- All dressings are to be kept dry for 3 days and then removed.
- Cold compress is encouraged to the surgical area for 2 to 3 days to help minimize swelling and bruising.
- Incisions are cleaned three times daily with soap and water or hydrogen peroxide 3% diluted 50/50 with water. Reapplication of ointment is performed after washing.
- Bacitracin ointment is applied to the incision three times a day for 1 week.
- Elevation of the head during sleep is recommended for 1 week.
- Keflex antibiotic is prescribed for 5 days.
- All sutures are removed on the seventh postoperative day unless there is a reason for healing delay.
- Restriction in activities: The patient is advised to avoid bending, lifting, or aerobic exercise for 7 to 10 days.
- Avoidance of all NSAIDs (Aspirin, Ibuprofen, Naproxen) is advised for 1 week after surgery.
- Makeup to the incision area is prohibited for 14 days.
- Sun exposure is avoided for 1 month. Use of a sunscreen with SPF 30+ for 6 months after surgery is recommended.

COMPLICATIONS

Complication rates with properly designed and executed bilobe flaps are low. The risk of infection is less than 1%. Slight epidermal sloughing of the flap may occur in up to 10%, although full-thickness necrosis is much less common. If it does occur, it is managed with occlusive dressings until healing is complete. The development of trap-door deformity is extremely rare when careful suturing is performed so that restretching of the deep undersurface of the flap back to the wound edge is accomplished and wide peripheral undermining is done. It quickly responds to treatment with intralesional steroids if needed. Dermabrasion is a complimentary procedure for any scar modification.

RESULTS

The nose is an exceptionally complex structure with multiple soft and hard tissue nuances. Repair of defects along the distal third of the nose uses the skin from the more lax upper nasal dorsum and sidewall, which allows easy transposition of the secondary lobe and primary side-to-side closure of its donor site (Fig. 41.3). When using the bilobe flap for defects on the proximal nose, successful flap mobility can be accomplished by recruiting skin for the secondary flap from the glabella, where skin is more readily available (Fig. 41.4). In other regions of the face, these same principles are applied. In large defects of the central cheek, the bilobe flap recruits cervical skin and is designed with the first lobe on the lateral, preauricular cheek and the second lobe on the infraauricular (cervical) skin (Fig. 41.5). Similarly in the chin, soft tissue from the superior neck is also recruited (Fig. 41.6).

Along the midface, a flap can be designed for an upper lip repair with the first lobe in the medial cheek superior to the defect and the second lobe in the zygomatic cheek. Excellent results can be achieved without displacement of the vermillion border or resulting eclabium (Fig. 41.7). Defects in the midlower or lateral lower eyelid are also successfully repaired with a bilobed flap designed with the first lobe and second lobe in the mid and lower cheek, respectively (Fig. 41.8). Finally, when primary closures cannot be achieved, the bilobe flap can be used in this location utilizing the skin from the mid and upper forehead without causing upward displacement of the eyebrow (Fig. 41.9).

PEARLS

A bilobe flap does not produce scars that lie within the boundaries of the aesthetic facial subunits. However, despite this shortcoming, the surgical results are aesthetically pleasing and often imperceptible. The overstated disadvantage of this flap is the use of multiple curved incision lines that do not follow relaxed skin tension lines. The understated disadvantage of this flap is the unforgiving nature if a flap is too small for defect reconstruction. Other salient points we have found of value include, in addition to Table 41.1, the following:

- The upper limit in size of the defect on the nose to be repaired with a bilobe flap should be not more than approximately 1.5 cm.
- The use of meticulous suturing technique and postoperative dermabrasion can make the scars resulting from these flaps barely noticeable.
- Whenever possible, the axis of this secondary flap should be oriented vertical to the alar rim in order to prevent alar distortion.

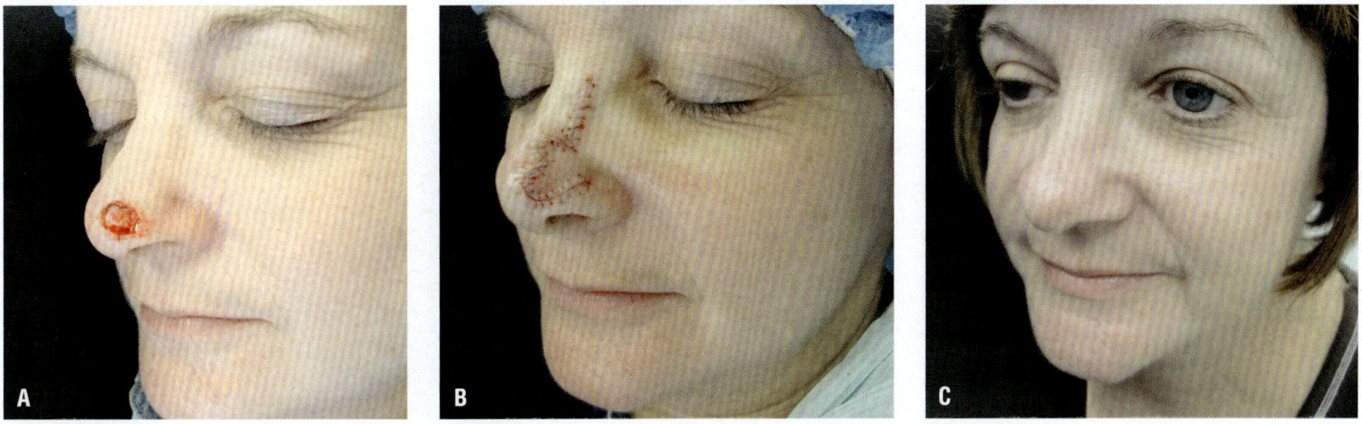

FIGURE 41.3 **A:** A 1.1-cm lateral nasal tip defect after excision of basal cell carcinoma with Mohs surgery. **B:** Laterally based bilobe flap transposed into place. Standing cutaneous deformity excised along the alar crease. **C:** Appearance 3 months postoperative.

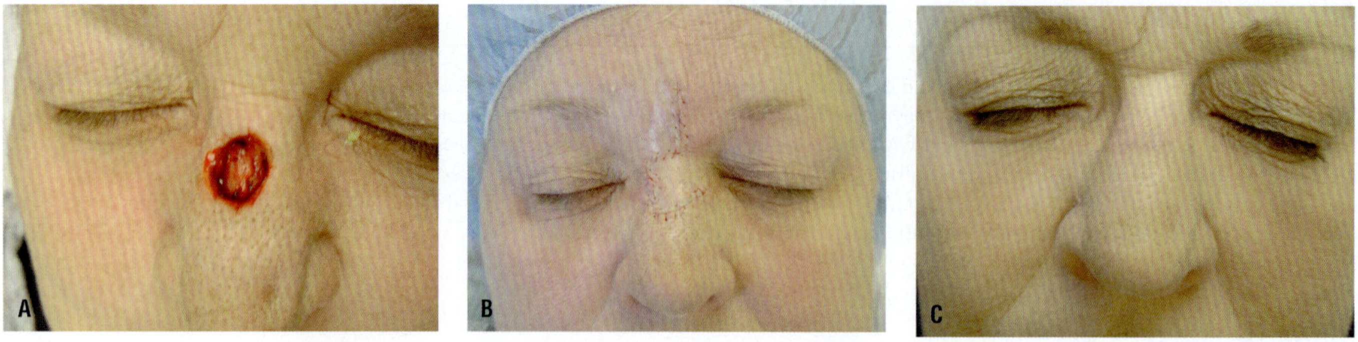

FIGURE 41.4 **A:** A 1.4-cm defect on the proximal nasal dorsum after excision of basal cell carcinoma in two stages with Mohs surgery. **B:** Bilobe flap transposed into place with its secondary lobe donor site in the glabella. **C:** Appearance 3 months postoperative.

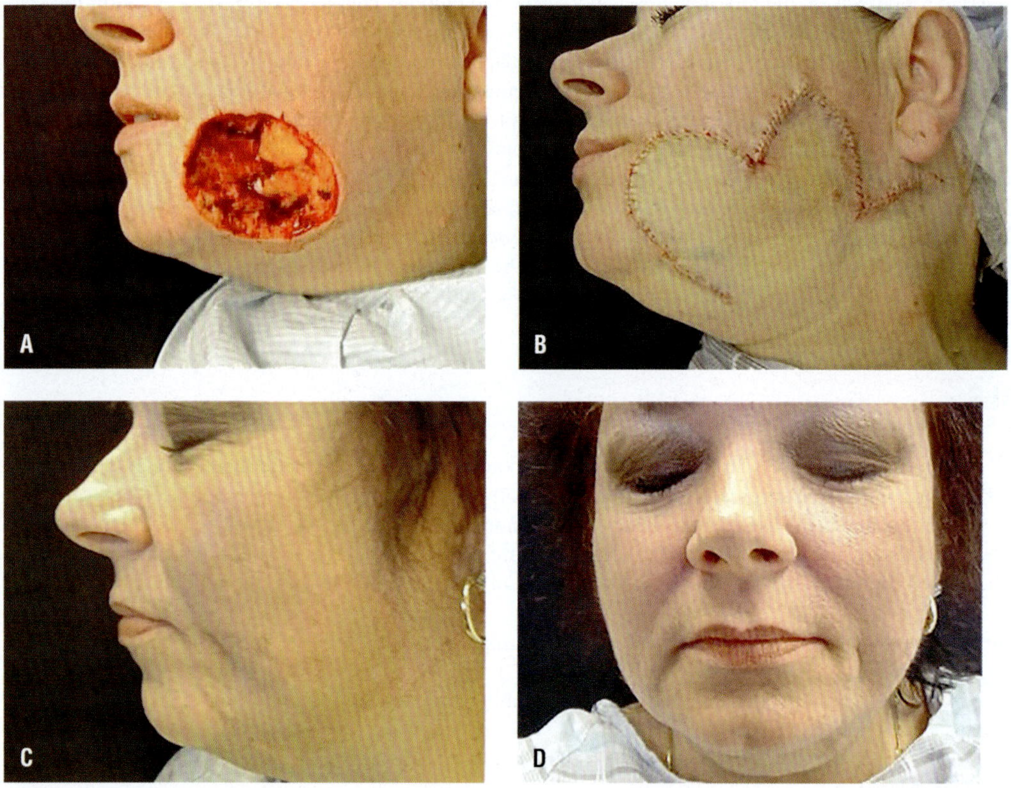

FIGURE 41.5 **A:** A 6.4 × 4.8 cm defect on the cheek after excision of dermatofibrosarcoma protuberans through deep muscle to oral mucosa. **B:** Bilobe flap sutured into place with its secondary lobe recruited from the infraauricular skin. **C and D:** Appearance 6 months postoperative.

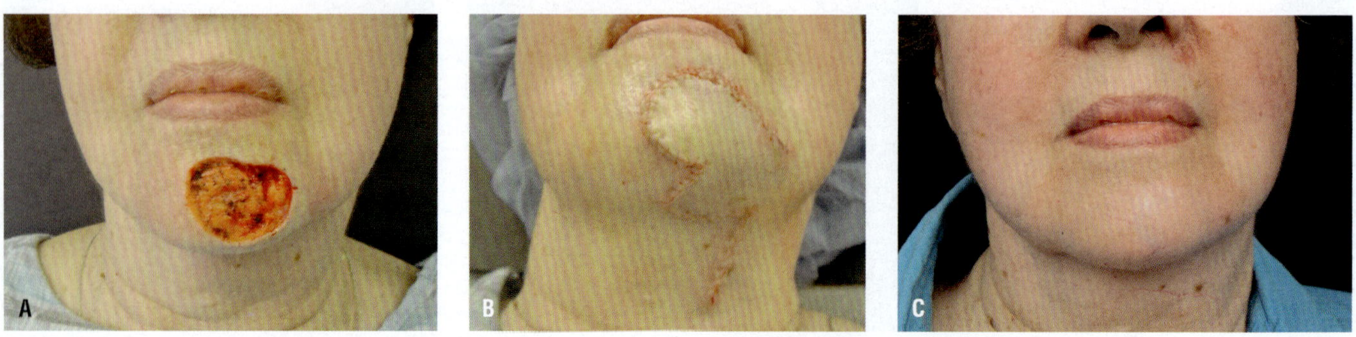

FIGURE 41.6 **A:** A 3 × 4 cm defect on the chin following excision of melanoma in situ after three stages of Mohs surgery. **B:** Bilobe flap transposed into place with its first lobe recruited from the submental skin and the second lobe from the cervical skin. **C:** Appearance 3 years postoperative without distortion of the lower lip.

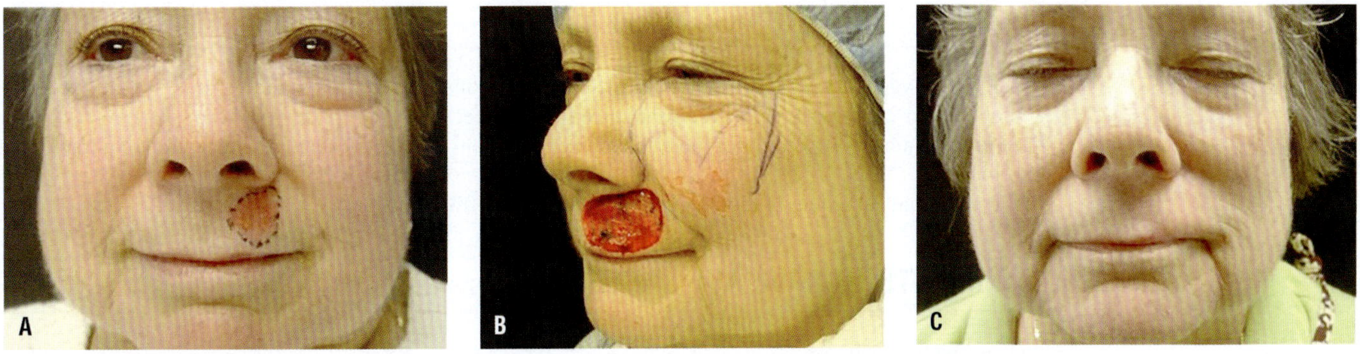

FIGURE 41.7 **A:** CK-7 + squamous cell carcinoma in situ versus extramammary Paget's disease in the lateral upper cutaneous lip. **B:** A 2.8-cm surgical defect following excision by Mohs surgery with the bilobe flap designed in the medial and zygomatic cheek. **C:** Appearance 1 year postoperative with no distortion of the vermillion border.

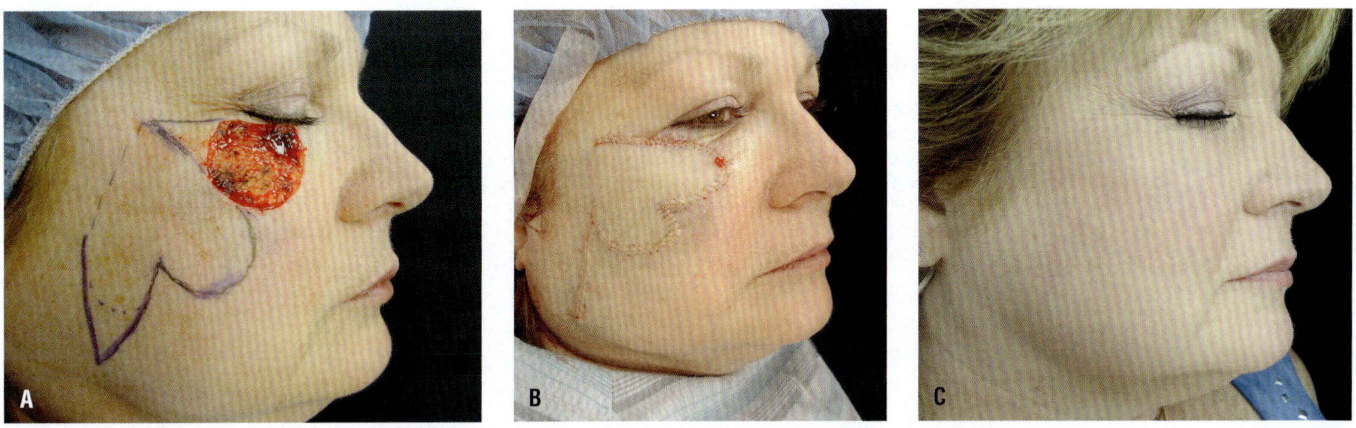

FIGURE 41.8 **A:** A 3.7-cm defect on the lateral lower eyelid following Mohs excision of melanoma in situ. Bilobe flap designed with its first and second lobe in the mid and lower cheek, respectively. **B:** Bilobe flap transposed and sutured into place. **C:** Appearance 10 months postoperative without displacement of the eyelid margin.

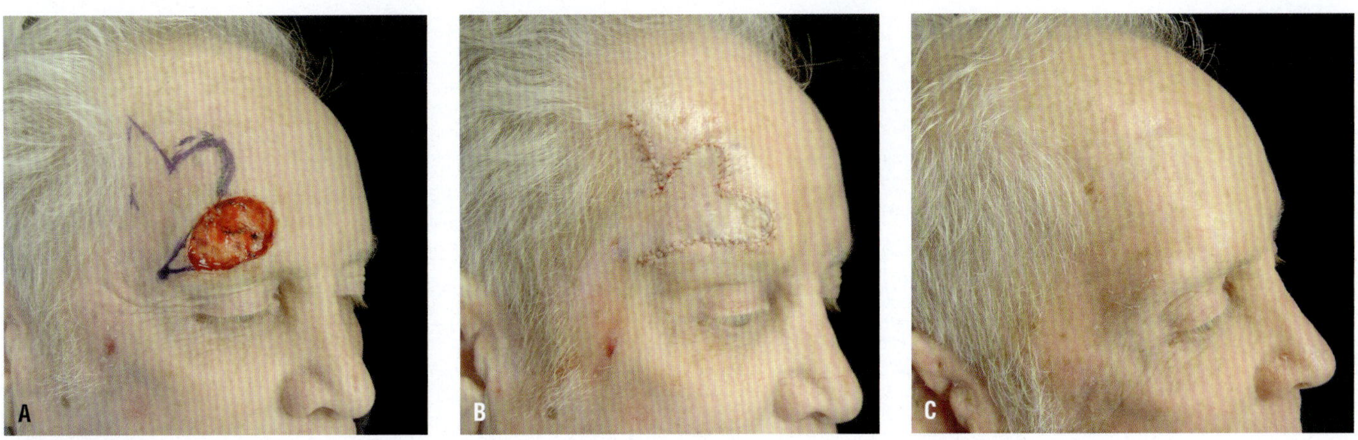

FIGURE 41.9 **A:** A 3.4-cm defect on the right lateral suprabrow after Mohs excision of basal cell carcinoma. Bilobe flap designed with its Burow's triangle placed laterally and the first and second lobe in the mid and upper forehead. **B:** Bilobe flap transposed and sutured into place. **C:** Appearance 20 months postoperative.

PITFALLS

- Hyperbaric oxygen therapy is a viable therapy in the event of substantial flap failure.
- A bilobe flap is not a great reconstructive choice for ear defects.
- Wide undermining is important for the establishment of a tension-free closure and prevention of a trap-door deformity.
- Slight epidermal sloughing of the flap may occur in up to 10% of patients.

INSTRUMENTS TO HAVE AVAILABLE

- Standard facial plastic set

ACKNOWLEDGMENT

My sincere gratitude is extended to Sheila M. Valentín, MD, for her contributions to the writing of this chapter. Her work in the writing, editing, and figure creation for this chapter is greatly appreciated.

SUGGESTED READING

Cook JL. A review of the bilobed flap's design with particular emphasis on the minimization of alar displacement. *Dermatol Surg* 2000;26:354–362.

Ricks M, Cook J. Extranasal applications of the bilobed flap. *Dermatol Surg* 2005;31(8 Pt 1):941–948.

Zitelli JA. Design aspect of the bilobed flap. *Arch Facial Plast Surg* 2008;10:186.

Zitelli JA. The bilobe flap for nasal reconstruction. *Arch Dermatol* 1989;125:957–959.

Zitelli JA, Baker SR. Bilobe flaps. In: Baker SR, Swanson NA, eds. *Local flaps in facial reconstruction*. St. Louis, MO: Mosby, 1995:165–180.

42 FOREHEAD FLAP

Frederick J. Menick

INTRODUCTION

Although some patients may be satisfied with a healed wound, most wish to have their normal appearance and function restored. Traditionally, the emphasis has been on measuring the length, width, and depth of the defect, but the wound may not reflect the actual tissue loss. A fresh wound is enlarged by edema, local anesthesia, gravity, and tension. A wound, which heals by secondary intention, contracts as the defect tissue heals. A defect within an area of a previous reconstruction is often distorted by scar, mismatched quality and dimension of previous grafts and flaps, and the malposition of adjacent residual landmarks. Injury to a three-dimensional landmark presents as a two-dimensional defect. Equally important, clinical experience and skill are finite, while the variety of defects is infinite. Fortunately, the normal never changes and can be employed as a visual guide to formulate principles and a plan. The normal is described by topographic subunits of characteristic skin quality, border outline, and three-dimensional contour.

Although Gillies' principle of "like" tissue is useful, a flat thick forehead, septal, ear or rib cartilage, and most lining materials are very dissimilar to nasal tissues. Only, the quality of the *forehead skin* actually matches what is missing. So, the surgical plan must acknowledge the need to modify "quasi-like" donor tissues to suit the needs of each anatomic layer and the overall requirements of form and function. Tissues must be modified in thickness, outline, and contour to restore the quality, border outline, and three-dimensional contour and function of the nose. Recreating the complex three-dimensional contour of tip and ala—the most aesthetically important parts of the nose—is a special challenge.

Success requires the replacement of thin, conforming cover, which matches nasal skin in color and texture; thin, vascular, and supple lining, which does not occlude the airway; and a three-dimensional hard tissue framework to support, shape, and brace the soft tissues against gravity, tension, and scar contraction. Ideally, the materials and methods available for repair are applicable to varied defects; provide available and well-vascularized donor tissues; are reliable, safe, and predictable; permit intraoperative modification of donor tissues; and provide an opportunity to revise inevitable imperfections or to salvage a complication.

HISTORY

This college student was knocked off his scooter by an automobile (Fig. 42.1A–C). He suffered a fracture of his thoracic spine, grade 1 laceration of the spleen, an injury to the brachial plexus, and a nasal fracture with amputation of tip skin, the right alar cartilage, and full-thickness loss of the right ala and sidewall.

A laminectomy and repair of the brachial plexus were performed. The amputated nose was retrieved and sutured back in place. The 6-cm^2 composite graft failed completely (as most traumatic amputations do). A few weeks later, nasal reconstruction was attempted with a two-stage forehead flap. Cartilage grafting had been recommended to improve the final result.

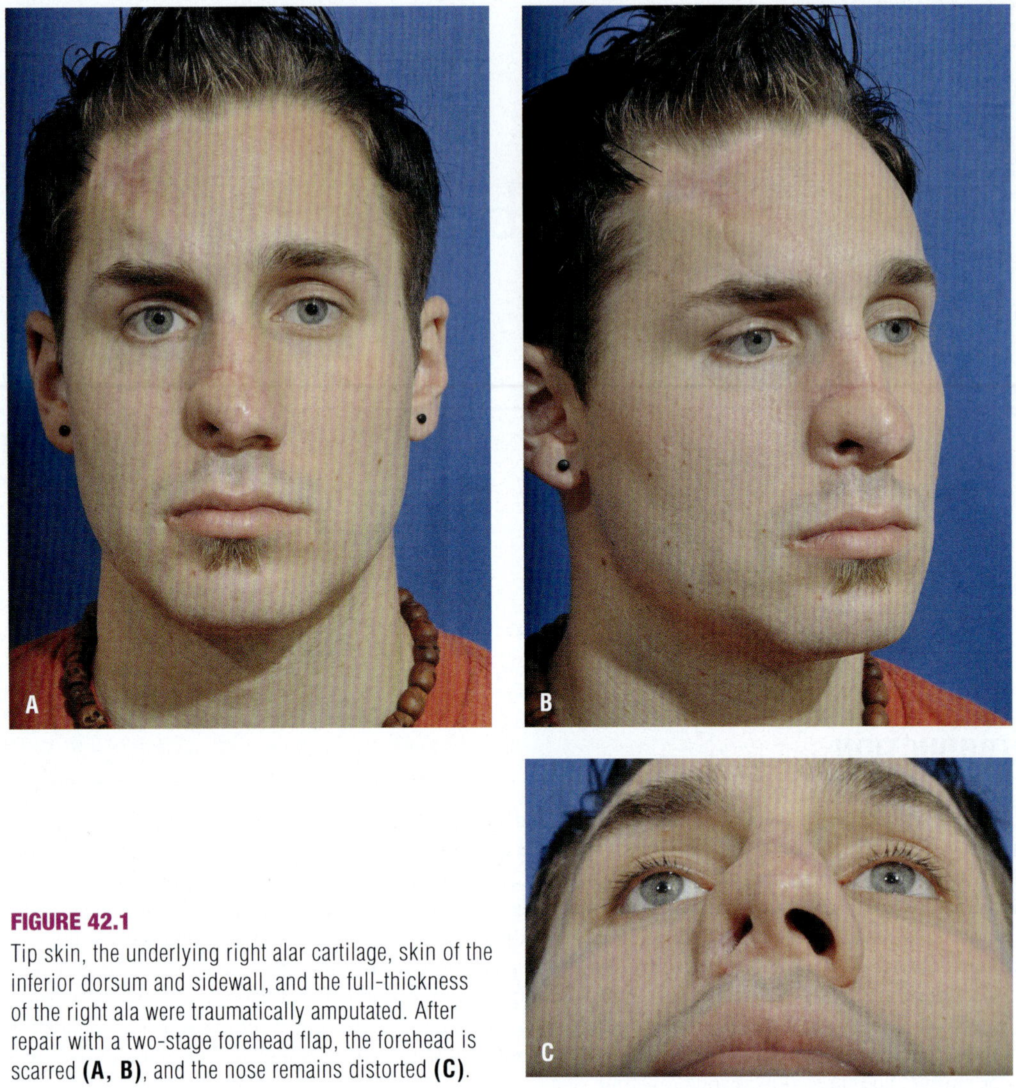

FIGURE 42.1
Tip skin, the underlying right alar cartilage, skin of the inferior dorsum and sidewall, and the full-thickness of the right ala were traumatically amputated. After repair with a two-stage forehead flap, the forehead is scarred **(A, B)**, and the nose remains distorted **(C)**.

PHYSICAL EXAMINATION

Fourteen months after injury, the nose is significantly distorted and obstructed. The forehead flap, although matching in skin quality, appears as a shapeless patch, surrounded by scars. The right alar rim is retracted, and the nasal vestibule is stenotic. A shiny atrophic scar is present under the right hairline in an area of secondary healing. The right oblique forehead flap's pedicle, at least 2½ cm wide, had been replaced within the inferior forehead unit, creating additional scars. The right brow is malpositioned inferiorly.

INDICATIONS

All complex nasal reconstructions will require a revision after pedicle division. The surgeon must evaluate the initial result in dimension, volume, position, projection, symmetry, landmarks, and nostril size. If basic nasal form is correct, modest abnormalities—poorly defined landmarks, a thick rim, or a stenotic nostril—can be improved during a revision. The flap can be reelevated through its peripheral borders, or direct incisions can be made on its surface (disregarding old scars) to reestablish landmarks. Excess soft tissue is sculpted and additional secondary cartilage grafts placed to address the limitations of the initial repair. However, when cover and lining are grossly deficient, the repair must be totally redone with a second regional flap. The normal must be returned to its normal position, the defect recreated, and tissue deficiencies defined and replaced. Occasionally, excess tissue, which would otherwise be discarded, can be used as hingeover lining flaps, for bulk replacement to an area of soft tissue deficiency or other purpose.

Large, deep nasal defects—those greater than 1.5 cm in diameter or requiring cartilage replacement, full-thickness defects, or those adversely located in the infratip or columella where local flaps do not reach, must be repaired with regional flaps. Local flaps will be inadequate.

A two-stage nasolabial flap is best suited for superficial defects of the ala, resurfaced as a complete subunit. A nasolabial flap is precluded, in this case, by the size and depth of the defect, inadequate reach, borderline vascularity, and the risk of severe pincushioning. A nasolabial flap would also add unnecessary scarring and distortion to the central face of this young man with an indistinct nasolabial fold and little excess tissue. A second forehead flap is the only choice because of its reliability, effectiveness, efficiency, and wide application.

CONTRAINDICATIONS

Although multiple stages are required, reconstruction with a forehead flap is a relatively noninvasive procedure and is tolerated by patients of any age, relatively stable health, and appropriate mental disposition.

PREOPERATIVE PLANNING

Taking the time to evaluate the deformity and develop a thoughtful reconstructive plan is vital.

Although the exposure of vital structures may motivate early coverage, a careful evaluation of the patient's overall health and goals and the status of the wound must be performed preoperatively.

A preliminary operation to debride unhealthy tissue, control infection, recreate the defect and return the flap to its normal position, or restore a stable platform by initially repairing the cheek and nasal lip base may be necessary. In this case, the tissues were well healed and the nasal lip and cheek platform was stable. The defect could be recreated and formal nasal repair performed simultaneously.

SURGICAL TECHNIQUE

Operative decisions are guided by principles of aesthetic regional unit reconstruction:

Alter the wound in size, outline, depth, or position, if helpful, to improve the final result.

This may include discarding adjacent residual skin within a subunit (enlarging the wound), the advancement of adjacent skin to the border of a subunit (decreasing the size or outline of the defect), or a combination.

Missing tissues must be replaced in exact dimension and outline. Inaccurate tissue replacement malpositions normal landmarks by pushing or pulling residual tissues outward or inward.

Because the wound does not reflect the true tissue loss, the contralateral normal or ideal are used as a guide to determine the correct dimension and outline of all replacement tissues—cover and lining flaps and cartilage grafts. Operative templates are used to design exact grafts and flaps and to determine the ideal position of important landmarks—such as the alar base inset and alar crease.

Stage 1: Flap Transfer

A three-stage *full-thickness forehead flap* to resurface the nose and septal and ear cartilage grafts for support was planned. The lining deficit would be replaced with an extension of the forehead flap or by hinging over the previous forehead flap for lining.

The hairline, frown lines, and subunits of the nose and lip were marked with ink to identify the outline of the subunits, old scars, the old flap and important landmarks (Fig. 42.2A–C). Once the surgery is underway, they will be very difficult to identify intraoperatively. No local anesthesia is injected into the transferred tissues or the recipient site. All stages are performed under general anesthesia to avoid the tissue distortion and vasoconstriction-associated fluid and epinephrine injection, which make the intraoperative evaluation of contour and vascularity difficult.

Quarter-inch paper tapes, consolidated with collodion, were placed over the intact left nose to create exact templates of the contralateral normal. Foil patterns are made of the left hemitip and left ala and the left upper lip unit (Fig. 42.3). The left hemitip template was flipped over and repositioned on the right lip to ensure the correct position of the right alar base.

The previous forehead flap was elevated thinly and hinged over, based on the retracted alar rim. Although a large amount of tissue was available as a turnover flap, the stenotic nostril could not be opened along the retracted nostril margin without destroying the hingeover flap's vascular base (Fig. 42.4). The previous flap was discarded. The stenotic nasal vestibule was then incised at the alar base at right angles to its margin to open the airway (Fig. 42.5A–C).

The *subunit principle* was applied—if a defect encompasses more than 50% of a *convex* nasal subunit (the tip or ala) and will be *resurfaced with a flap*, residual skin within the subunit is excised to resurface the defect as a subunit, rather than as an incomplete patch.

Because all of the ala and the majority of the tip skin were missing or injured, residual normal skin and scar were excised within the entire tip, planning to resurface the right ala and tip as complete subunits. Although the defect extended into the inferior dorsum and sidewall, the borders of these relatively flat subunits are indistinct so the subunit principle does not apply. Additional normal tissue within the dorsal and sidewall subunits is not excised.

When a convex subunit is resurfaced in its entirety, uniform subunit skin quality is maintained and the scars from the border of the flaps lie in the unions between subunits where their reflected light or cast shadows are relatively camouflaged. Most importantly, scar between the raw surface of the flap and the underlying recipient bed contracts, drawing the surface of the flap above the residual normal adjacent skin. When an entire convex

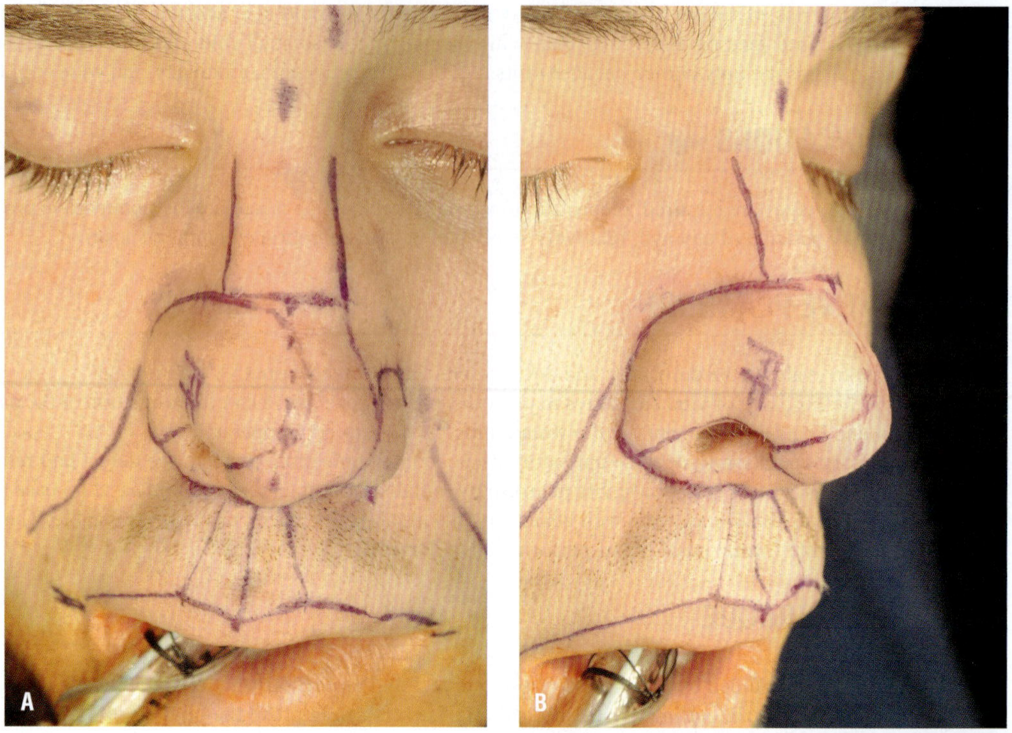

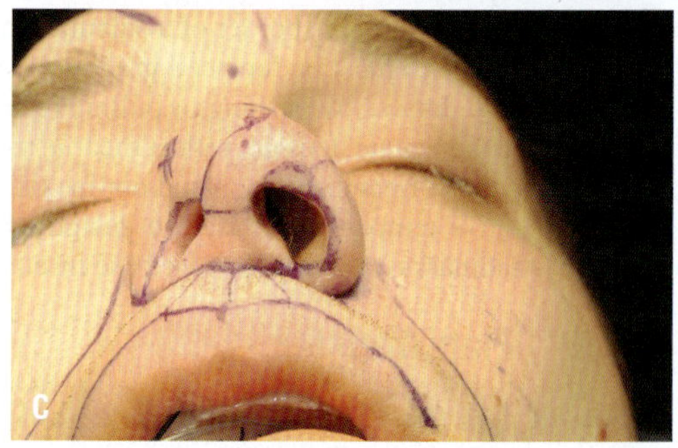

FIGURE 42.2

A–C: A second repair was planned with a three-stage full-thickness forehead flap for cover and lining. The regional units of the nose were marked. The border of the previous forehead flap was outlined. The ideal position of the right alar base was confirmed with a template of the left contralateral upper lip unit.

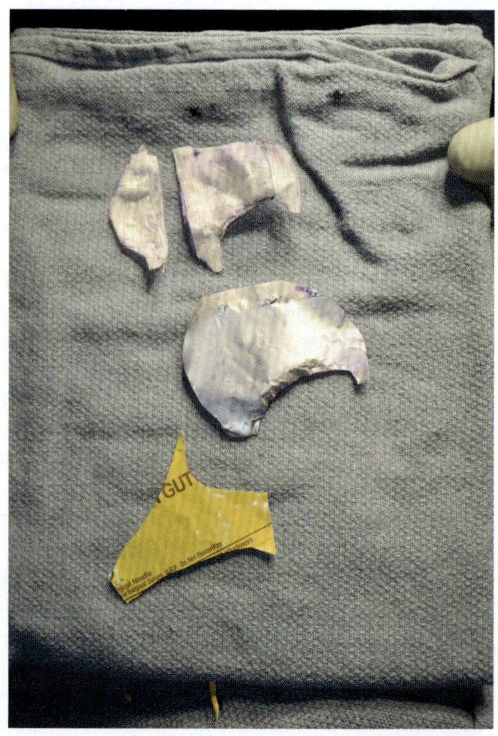

FIGURE 42.3

1/4-inch paper tapes were applied to the nasal surface to design the left hemitip and heminasal templates, based on the contralateral normal nose. The left hemitip template is flipped over and combined with the heminasal template to design a foil template with the exact dimension and outline of the tip and ala subunits. A foil template of the left normal upper lip unit was also created.

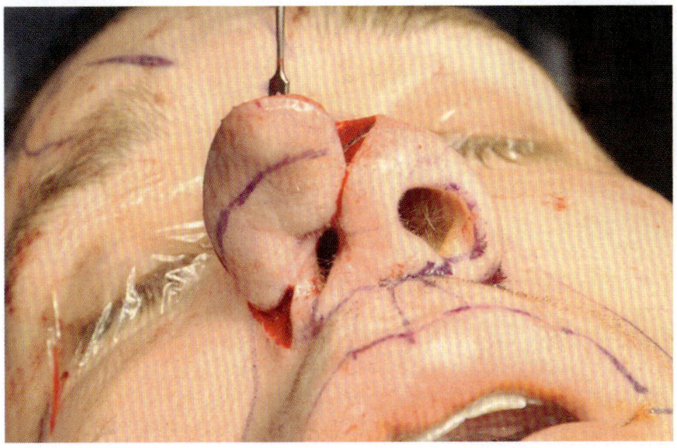

FIGURE 42.4
The previous forehead flap was hinged inferiorly along the healed margin of the nostril. Although vascularized, the airway could not be opened without interfering with its base.

subunit is resurfaced, this inevitable wound contraction is harnessed, in combination with appropriately shaped cartilage grafts, to restore the expected uniform convexity of the tip and ala, rather than a pincushioned patch.

The left alar cartilage was intact, although deprojected. It was advanced and sutured to a septal columellar strut to restore tip projection. A conchal cartilage graft was also fixed to the columellar strut as an anatomic hemitip replacement for the right medial and lateral crura (Fig. 42.6A, B).

A right paramedian *full-thickness* forehead flap was designed to resurface the right tip and ala, based on a template, created by combining the left contralateral alar template with the left hemitip template (which is flipped over to design the complete tip subunit) (Fig. 42.7A–C). The flap will replace the missing external skin of the tip and right alar subunits in *exact* dimension. The lining deficit was estimated by measuring the defect on the contralateral normal nostril. About 1.2 to 1.5 cm of lining was missing along the entire inferior right nostril

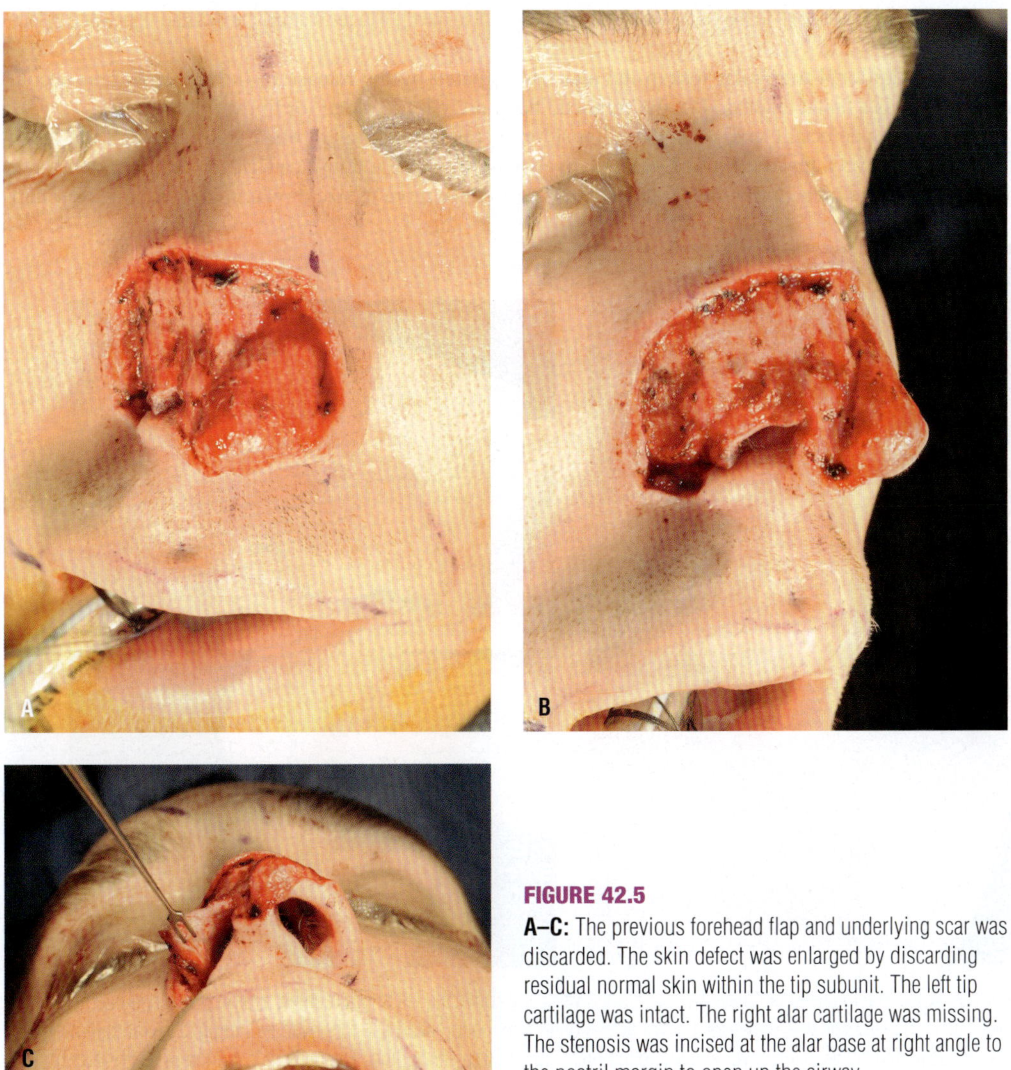

FIGURE 42.5
A–C: The previous forehead flap and underlying scar was discarded. The skin defect was enlarged by discarding residual normal skin within the tip subunit. The left tip cartilage was intact. The right alar cartilage was missing. The stenosis was incised at the alar base at right angle to the nostril margin to open up the airway.

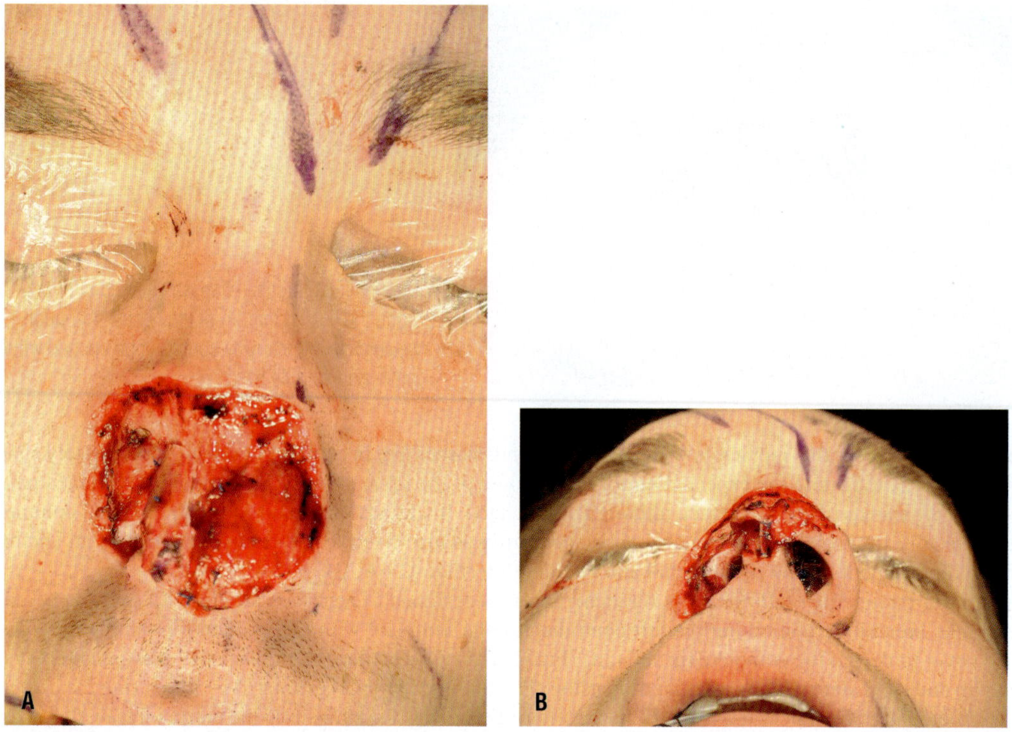

FIGURE 42.6 **A and B:** A septal cartilage columellar strut was positioned and sutured to the left alar cartilage to support the tip. A strip of conchal cartilage was fixed to the columellar strut and then bent to the right to reconstruct the missing right alar cartilage.

margin with an additional triangular loss at the alar base created by the release of the stenosis. This second template is drawn as a distal extension of the forehead flap and will be folded for lining.

In full-thickness defects, the dimension and position of missing lining are often unknown until the defect is defined intraoperatively. Once identified, it is relatively easy to create a lining pattern and add an extension to the forehead flap to line unilateral or bilateral defects up to 3 cm or more in size. Prelaminated or hingeover flaps

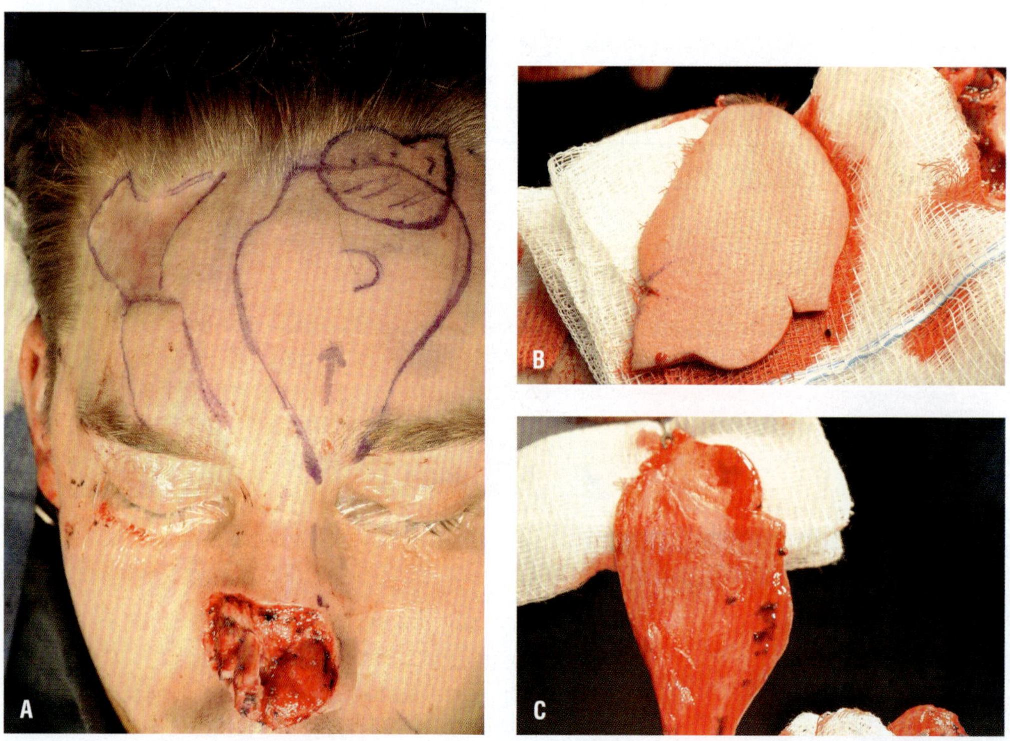

FIGURE 42.7 **A–C:** The forehead template was positioned vertically above the left supratrochlear artery, which had been identified by Doppler. The lining template was drawn as a distal extension to fold the forehead flap for cover and lining. Several millimeters of the extra skin was added between the cover and lining templates to allow easier folding. The pedicle is 1.2 cm in width at its base. The flap is elevated as a full-thickness flap. Frontalis muscle is only excised within the lining extension to permit easier folding.

are often unavailable due to the delay needed to prelaminate the flap or heal cover to lining. Based on the healed margin of the defect hingeover flaps do not permit release of the stenotic nostril, without jeopardizing their blood supply. Intranasal lining flaps are useful but are often precluded by previous vascular injury, limited size, and intranasal/patient morbidity. In this case, prior nasal trauma made their blood supply unreliable. Although useful in salvage situations, skin grafts for lining should be limited to small defects because of their unpredictable "take," risk of contraction, and because they preclude the placement of sculptured cartilage grafts for contour and support. Second flaps, such as a turnover nasolabial flap or a FAMM flap, have limited applicability. Microvascular lining flaps are used for very large or composite defects, often within irradiation injury, when all other options are unavailable.

The cover template was positioned vertically above the left frown crease, typically 2 to 3 mm medial to the supratrochlear artery, identified by Doppler. The axial vessels of the forehead are oriented vertically and are captured by a vertical flap. An oblique design transects these vessels, creating a less vascular random extension.

Although a paramedian flap can be based on either the right or left brow, lateral defects are most easily resurfaced with an ipsilateral pedicle. This contralateral pedicle was farther away from the defect and necessitated designing a longer flap. Midline defects can be resurfaced on either a right or left pedicle.

The cover template was positioned below the hairline. Its pedicle narrows inferiorly to a width of less than 1.2 to 1.5 cm at the brow. It extends through the medial eyebrow. This lowers its pivot point, bringing the flap closer to the recipient site, increasing its reach and limiting needed flap length. The lining template was positioned as a distal extension of the covering flap with a few millimeters of extra skin between the cover and lining flaps to allow easier folding. If necessary, the lining extension can carry a few hair follicles, which may later be visible as "vibrissae" within the nostril. Because the folded extension lies within the area of routine dog ear excision, it adds minimally to the overall donor burden.

The forehead consists of skin, subcutaneous adipose tissue, frontalis muscle, and a thin layer of areolar tissue, which lies over the periosteum. It is perfused by random cutaneous, myocutaneous, and axial blood supplies. A forehead flap is thicker than nasal skin and must be thinned.

Traditionally, a forehead flap is transferred in two stages. At the first stage, soft tissue is excised distally, eliminating the frontalis and some of the axial vessels within the subcutaneous fat. This is not normally significant, but the larger the defect, the wider the area of thinning required, the greater the potential for vascular injury, and the less the flap's ability to tolerate the tension of wound closure.

It is transposed to resurface the inferior aspect of the defect. Weeks later, once healed to the inferior inset, the pedicle is divided, the superior aspect of the recipient site is reelevated and thinned, and the inset completed.

Unfortunately, the inferior most aesthetic parts of the nose cannot be altered without jeopardizing the vascularity of the flap. A poorly designed or malpositioned cartilage graft cannot be shaved, augmented, or repositioned or additional grafts placed. Excessive soft tissue cannot be sculpted. Any imperfection must wait for a later revision. But after pedicle division, wide reelevation of the flap may jeopardize its vascularity and necessitate piecemeal reoperations to improve imperfections.

The two-stage forehead flap is best suited to resurface small defects. Modest defects within the sidewall or dorsum or an isolated subunit alar reconstruction are examples. These defects are small and require a relatively small flap and limited distal thinning. They lie within relatively flat areas of the nose, which require only limited cartilage grafting and modest restoration of the contour.

In contrast, large, deep defects—which require large flaps, extensive primary or delayed primary cartilage grafts and soft tissue sculpting, and lining replacement—are more reliably resurfaced with a three-stage full-thickness forehead flap. It contains all forehead layers, has a maximum blood supply during its transfer, and is better able to tolerate wound closure.

One month later during the *intermediate operation*, the flap is, in effect, physiologically delayed. It can be completely reelevated from the entire nasal inset with 2 to 3 mm of subcutaneous adipose tissue, safely creating uniform, thin, supple covering skin. This exposes the underlying recipient bed in its entirety. Primary cartilage grafts, previously fixed together at the initial flap transfer with sutures over intact or reconstructed lining, are now healed together as a sculptable unit. Excess soft tissue and primary cartilage grafts can be modified by direct excision. Delayed primary cartilage grafts can be added. This permits modification and complete contouring of the distal, most aesthetic part of the nose—the tip and ala—at the initial flap transfer *and during the second intermediate operation*. The pedicle is divided 1 month later (2 months after flap transfer), allowing further sculpting of the superior aspect of the inset.

This three-stage approach also permits a modification of the traditional method of folding a two-stage flap to line a full-thickness defect. Typically, after a two-stage folded flap, the resulting nostril margin is thick, asymmetric, and unsupported because it is impossible to accurately position the nostril rim margin or place cartilage support within the folded flap at transfer or at pedicle division. The three-stage full-thickness flap eliminates these problems. Although the lining is initially too thick and primary support is precluded (as in the traditional two-stage folded approach), excess bulk can be excised, a complete subunit support positioned, and symmetric nostril borders restored during the intermediate operation.

The full-thickness flap was transferred to resurface the entire tip and ala subunits (Fig. 42.8A–E). The distal extension was folded for lining. Each layer was sutured with a single layer of fine suture (the author uses 5.0 Nylon, Prolene or Chromic) to the freshened edges of the defect and short turned up flaps at the nasal base

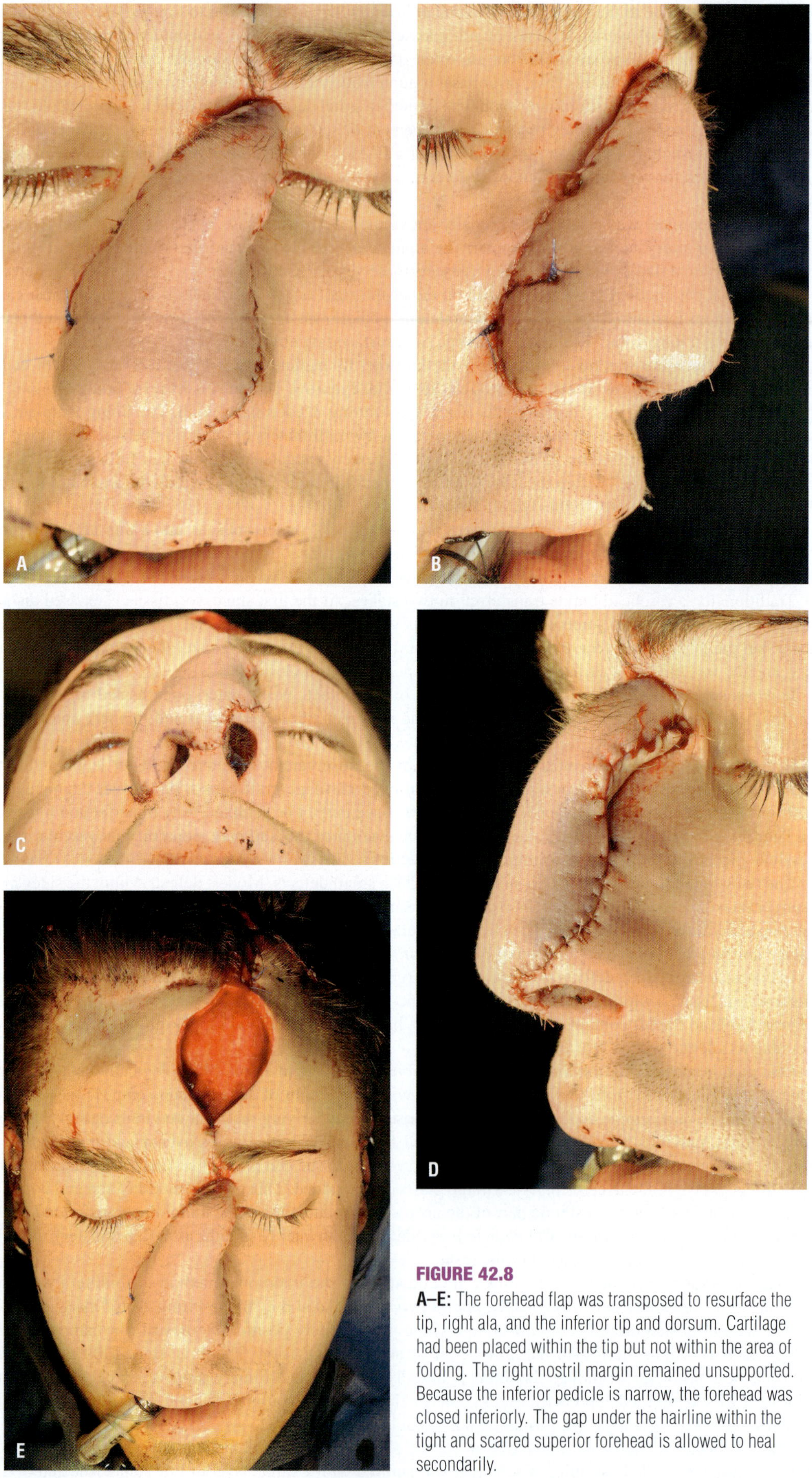

FIGURE 42.8

A–E: The forehead flap was transposed to resurface the tip, right ala, and the inferior tip and dorsum. Cartilage had been placed within the tip but not within the area of folding. The right nostril margin remained unsupported. Because the inferior pedicle is narrow, the forehead was closed inferiorly. The gap under the hairline within the tight and scarred superior forehead is allowed to heal secondarily.

inset. Frontalis muscle was excised into subcutaneous tissue, only along and under the nasal lining portion/extension, to ease its folding. The right nostril margin was left unsupported. An alar batten was not placed. Primary cartilage grafts are routinely placed over residual normal vascularized lining to restore contour and support (in this case, the tip) but are not be placed within the folded lining extension of a forehead flap.

Because the inferior pedicle was less than 1.5 cm in width, the forehead defect could be closed above the brow, leaving a 1-cm gap under the hairline to heal secondarily. The open area was covered with petrolatum impregnated gauze for 1 week and then lubricated daily with petrolatum ointment until second healing was complete in 3 to 6 weeks. The raw pedicle of the flap was resurfaced with a full-thickness skin graft, harvested from the groin crease, to temporary close its deep surface and ease cleansing.

Stage 2: The Intermediate Operation

One month later, nasal shape and airway are bulky (Fig. 42.9A, B). Primary tip cartilage grafts have recreated a basic tip shape, but the right nostril margin remains unsupported. Fibrosis does not occur in a full-thickness flap until the frontalis is excised or the SQ layer injured, so the external skin is completely unscarred and supple. Folded lining has healed to residual adjacent normal lining and is no longer dependent on the forehead pedicle for vascularity (Fig. 42.10).

First, subunits and landmarks are marked with ink (Fig. 42.11A–D). The folded nostril margin is incised along the proposed nostril margin, and forehead *cover skin* is elevated with 2 to 3 mm of subcutaneous fat, based on the superior pedicle (Fig. 42.12A–D). Underlying subcutaneous fat and frontalis (doubled in the area of folding) are excised, exposing a complete thin, healed vascular lining envelope (Fig. 42.13A–C). Accurately designed delayed primary alar support grafts can now be easily positioned to establish complete 3D support.

Although the ala normally contains no cartilage, when significant alar skin is missing, a cartilage graft must be placed along the nostril margin to support, shape, and brace the ala. Because the skin of the forehead flap remains soft and supple at the intermediate reelevation, cartilage grafts are effective whether placed primarily or in a delayed primary fashion. With complete exposure, cartilage grafts can be placed or modified during the intermediate operation.

The forehead flap foil template, which was preserved and resterilized, is used as a guide to design a delayed primary ear cartilage alar batten of correct dimension and nostril border outline. The graft is sutured to the tip structures medially and buried laterally in a subcutaneous pocket at the alar base with a temporary percutaneous suture. 5-0 sutures are passed through the alar batten to catch the superficial raw surface of the lining flap, approximately the lining to the cartilage graft (Fig. 42.14A–C). A lateral crural onlay tip graft was added for additional projection and contour.

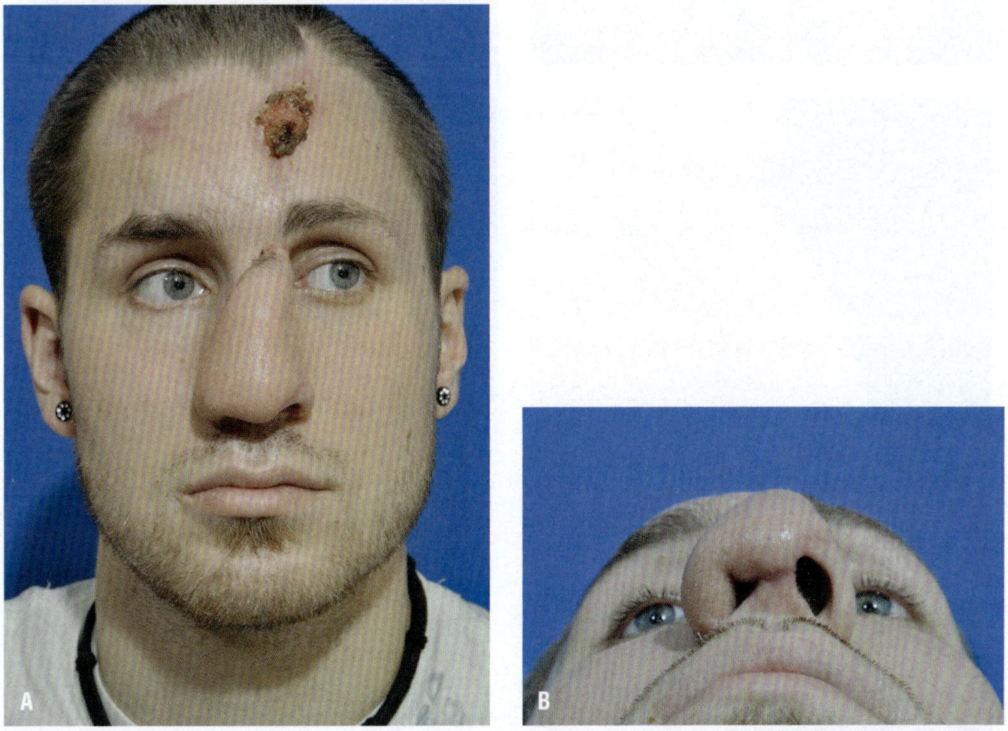

FIGURE 42.9 A and B: One month later, although the nose is bulky and shapeless, the basic nasal form is restored.

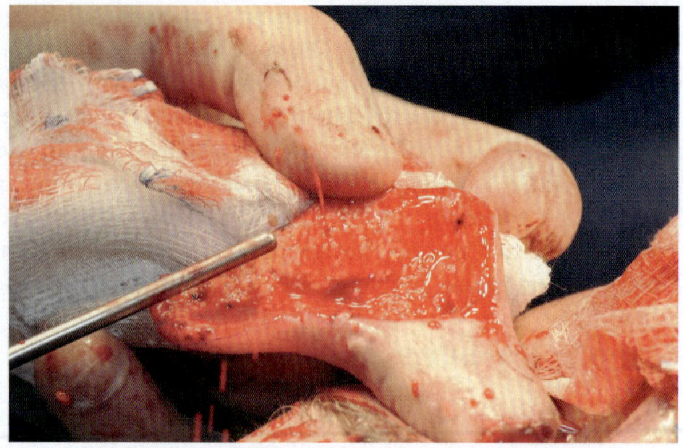

FIGURE 42.10
The flap remains well vascularized with visible pulsatile blood flow after reelevation.

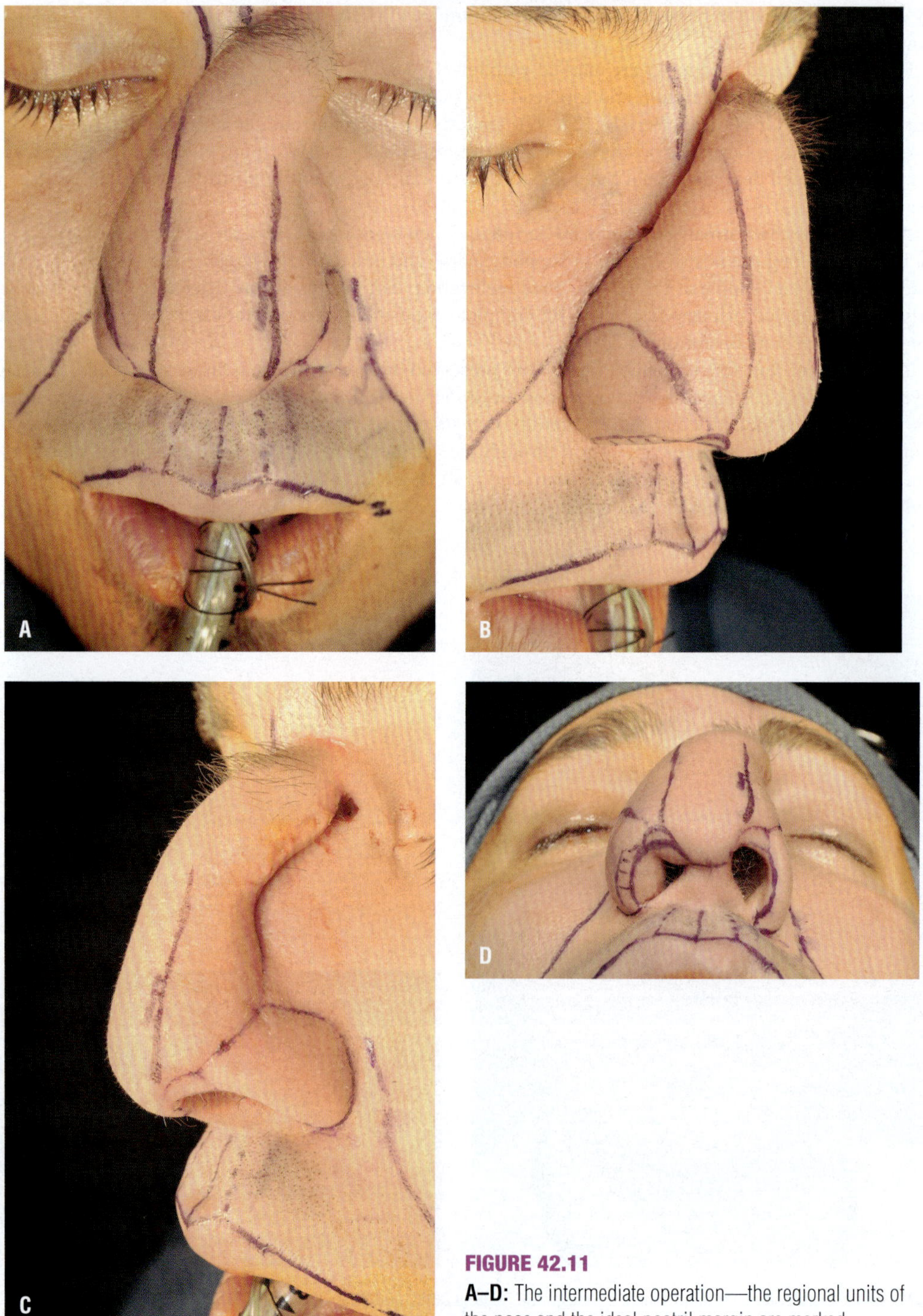

FIGURE 42.11
A–D: The intermediate operation—the regional units of the nose and the ideal nostril margin are marked.

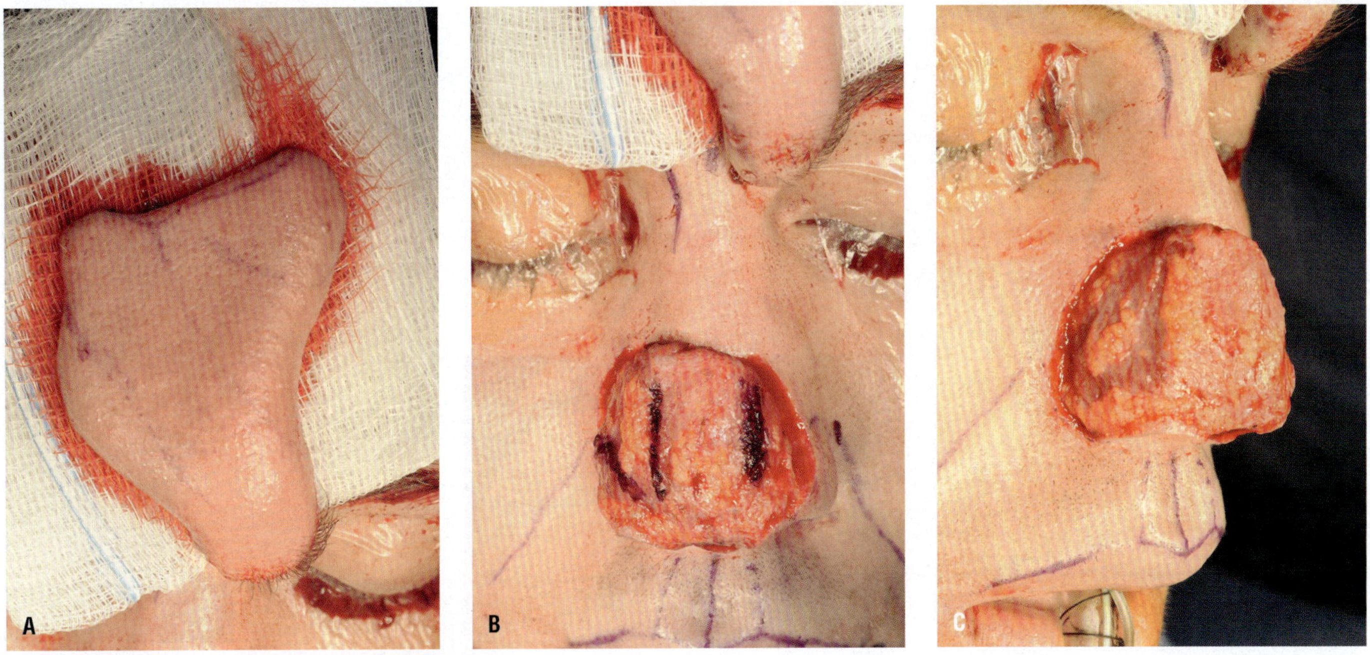

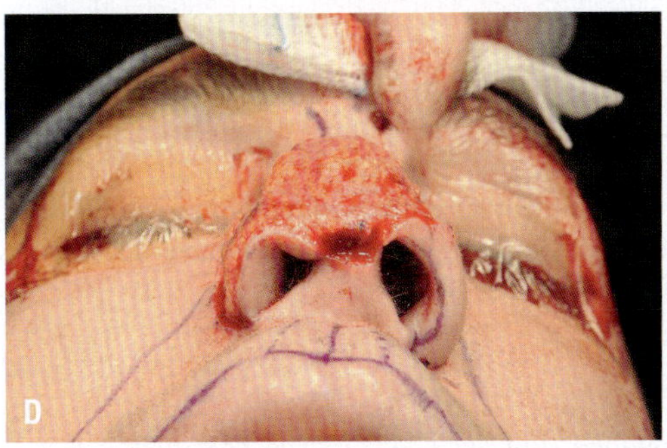

FIGURE 42.12
A–D: The nostril margin was incised, separating the covering flap from its distal extension. Forehead skin is elevated with 2 to 3 mm of subcutaneous fat and the flap and temporarily placed on the forehead, based on its proximal pedicle. The underlying folded excess subcutaneous adipose tissue, frontalis muscle, frontalis muscle, subcutaneous fat, and inner forehead skin lining are exposed. The dorsal lines and alar creases are marked on the recipient site with ink.

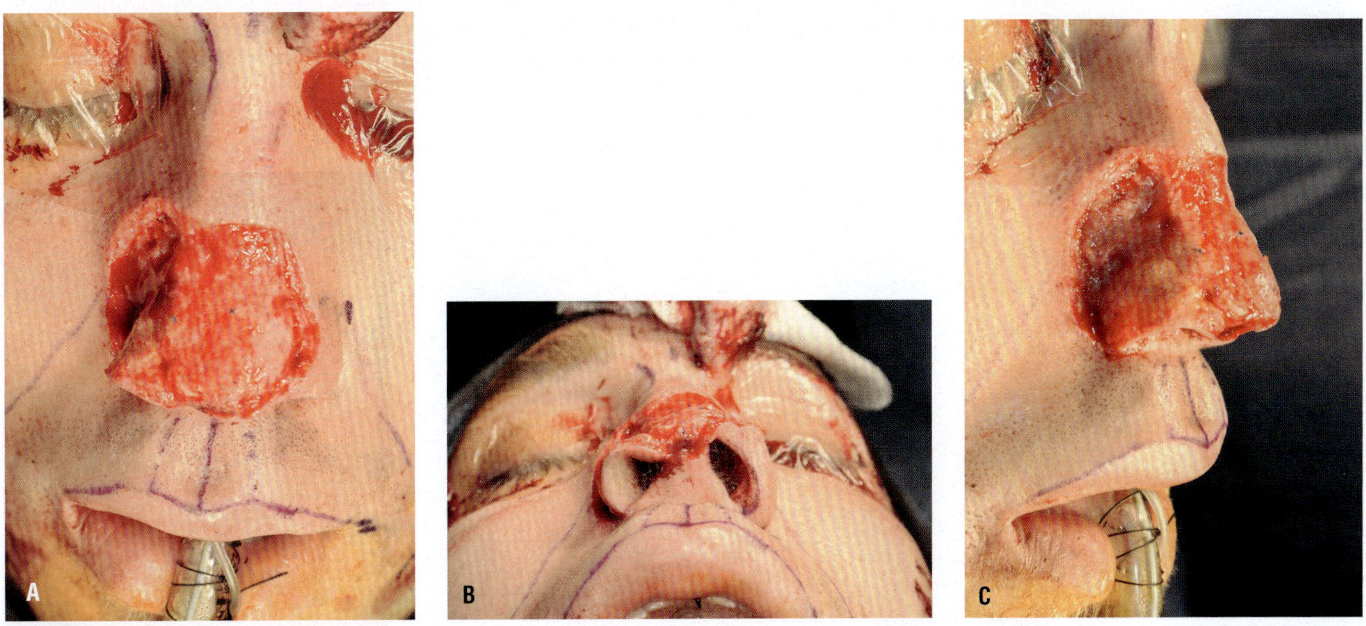

FIGURE 42.13 A–C: Excess soft tissue was excised, exposing the underlying primary cartilage tip grafts and a complete lining envelope. The underlying skin, folded for lining, is integrated into the residual nasal lining and is no longer dependent on the forehead pedicle for blood supply.

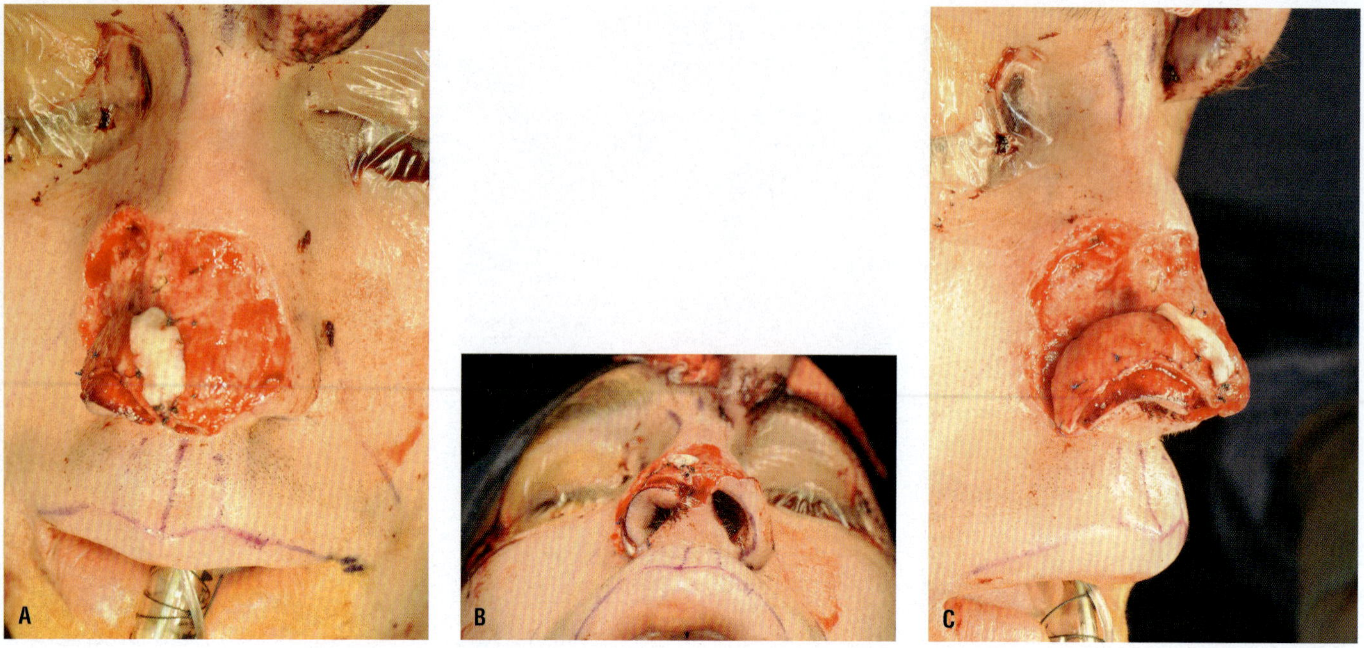

FIGURE 42.14 A–C: Delayed primary conchal cartilage grafts were positioned to support the right alar margin and further augment the right nasal tip.

The same foil pattern is employed as a guide to trim excess cover and lining along the nostril margin and establish symmetry with the opposite normal nostril rim (Fig. 42.15).

Then the uniformly thin cover skin flap is returned to the recipient site. It is sutured with a single layer of fine peripheral sutures, combined with several 5-0 percutaneous quilting sutures to eliminate dead space (Fig. 42.16A–C). The quilting sutures are removed at 48 hours and skin sutures at 5 days.

Stage 3: Pedicle Division

One month later (2 months after transfer), the pedicle is divided (Fig. 42.17A–D). The proximal aspect is trimmed and the medial brow is returned within the eyebrow, as a small inverted "V," where it may be mistaken for a frown line. The residual pedicle is discarded and is not returned to the forehead. Distally, the superior aspect of the recipient site is sculpted to define a flat sidewall, alar crease, and convex superior ala contour (Fig. 42.18A, B). The nasal inset is completed. The hypertrophic forehead scar in the area of secondary healing is excised and the upper forehead readvanced, permitting complete primary closure of the donor site. The single vertical linear scar is permanent but relatively innocuous (Fig. 42.19A–C).

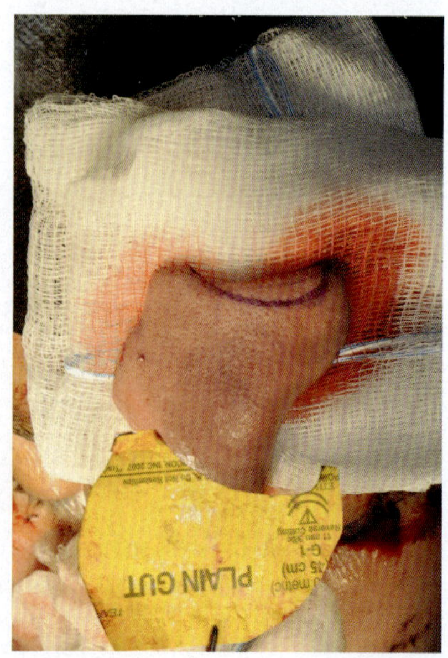

FIGURE 42.15
Using the resterilized template of the contralateral normal as a guide, excess forehead skin in the area of folding was excised to create an exact nostril margin border.

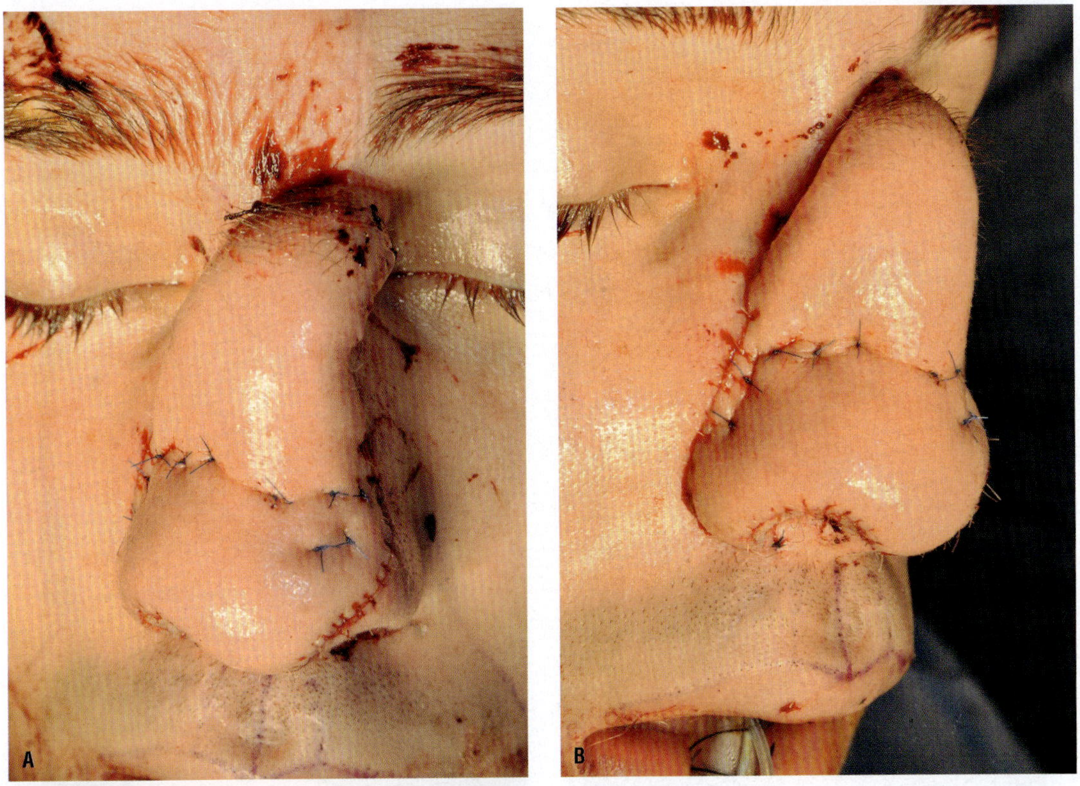

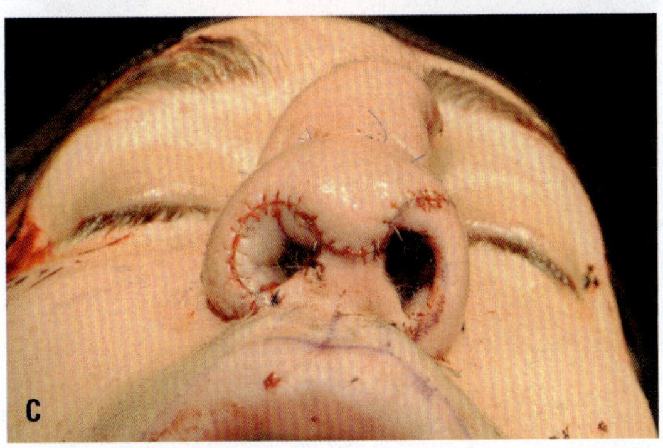

FIGURE 42.16 A–C: The thin supple forehead skin flap was returned to resurface a sculpted and supported nasal framework.

Stage 4: Revision

Almost all significant nasal reconstructions require a revision to refine delicate nasal landmarks and establish ideal symmetry. If present, an area of secondary forehead healing can be revised. Because all surgical stages had been discussed with the patient initially, the revision was expected.

Four months later, the tip and alar landmarks are imprecise. The nostril is small and its margin bulky (Fig. 42.20A–C). The flap's border and the nasal subunits are marked, as well as the ideal nostril diameter, based on templates of the contralateral ala and nostril. The alar crease is recreated by making a direct incision at its ideal position on the surface of the forehead flap, disregarding old scars. The forehead flap skin is elevated with 2 mm of subcutaneous adipose tissue superiorly and inferiorly. Excess bulk is excised to create a flat sidewall, a distinct alar crease, and the expected convexity of the superior ala (Fig. 42.21A–D).

The margin of the nostril was incised, at the ideal nostril margin, elevating the folded lining thinly. Excess subcutaneous adipose tissue and scar was excised between the reconstructed lining and the previously placed delayed primary nostril margin cartilage graft. A small sponge bolus was placed within the nostril for 48 hours to reapproximate the lining against the undersurface of the cartilage graft (Fig. 42.22A, B). Forehead scars were revised in the area of secondary healing from the previous right forehead flap.

POSTOPERATIVE MANAGEMENT

All procedures were performed under general anesthesia without local anesthetic injection. The patient is hospitalized for one night at flap transfer, but all other procedures are performed as an outpatient. Intraoperative prophylactic antibiotics are employed. Petrolatum gauze is used to cover any area on the forehead, which

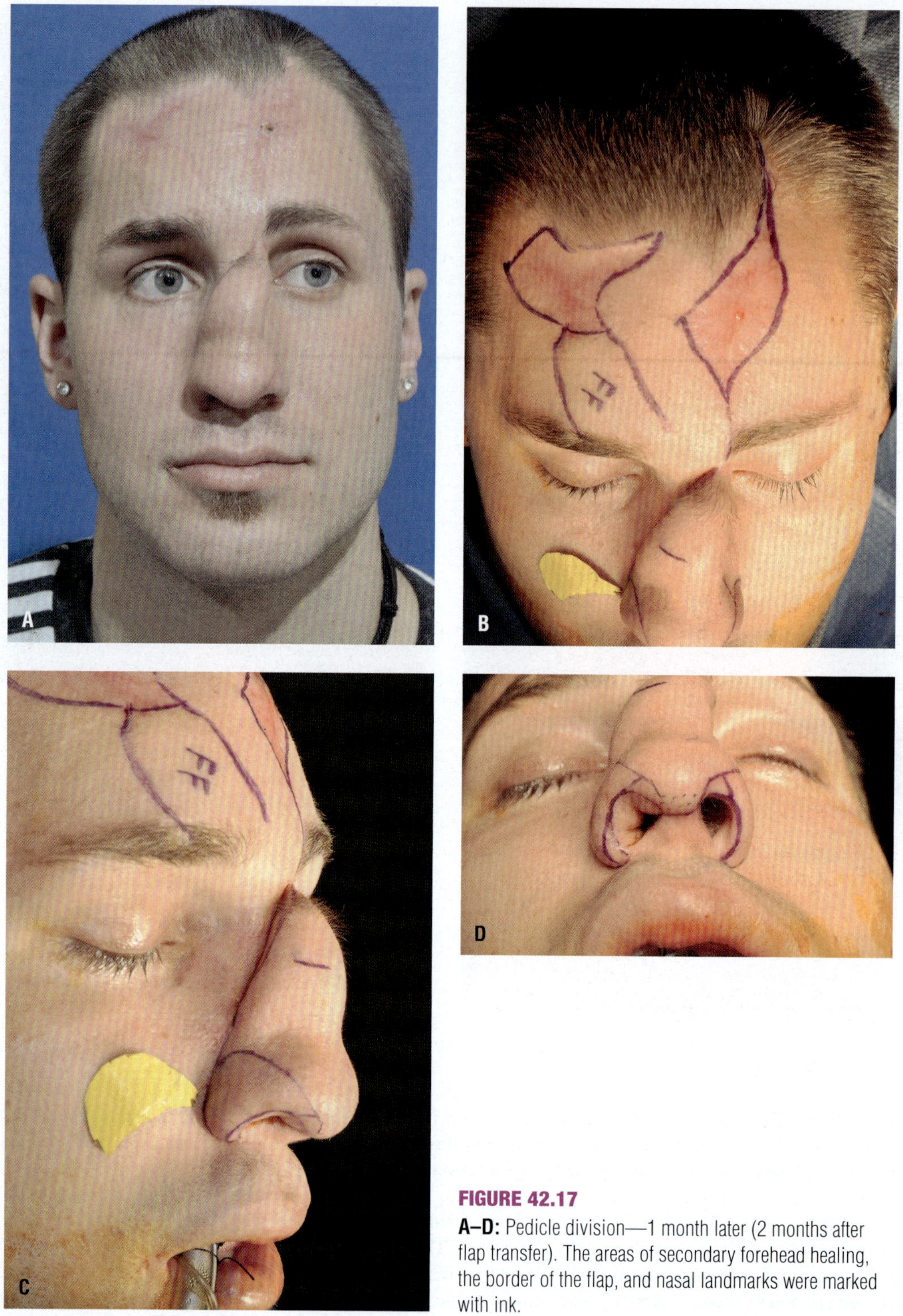

FIGURE 42.17
A–D: Pedicle division—1 month later (2 months after flap transfer). The areas of secondary forehead healing, the border of the flap, and nasal landmarks were marked with ink.

cannot be closed at flap transfer. It is removed at 1 week and the open area is allowed to heal secondarily. Quilting sutures are removed at 2 days, incisional sutures at 5 to 7 days, and sutures within the scalp closure at 10 days. The patient may wash and shampoo their face and scalp the day after each procedure. Dressings cover the nose at the discretion of the patient.

COMPLICATIONS

This patient's postoperative course was uncomplicated.

Flap ischemia is uncommon. It is most often attributable to tension created by designing too small or too short a flap, oversuturing of the lateral border of the flap to the recipient site, wide thinning of a two-stage flap

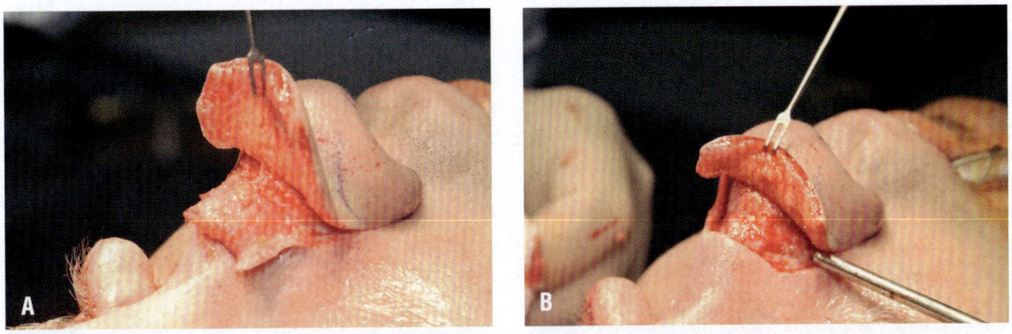

FIGURE 42.18 **A and B:** The pedicle was divided and forehead skin elevated with 2 or 3 mm of subcutaneous fat over the superior aspect of the recipient site. The underlying excess soft tissue was excised and sculpted to recreate the dorsal lines and alar crease.

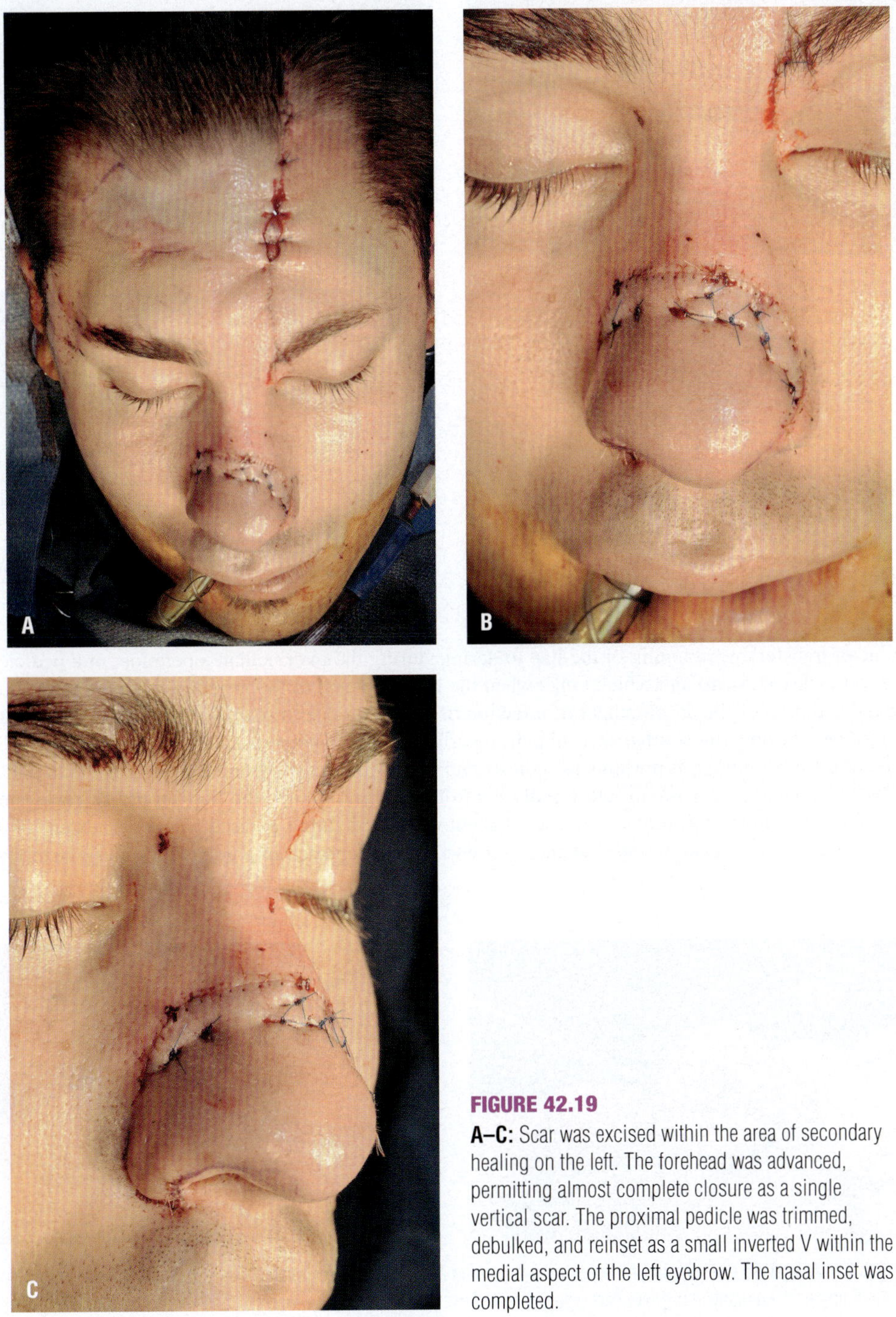

FIGURE 42.19
A–C: Scar was excised within the area of secondary healing on the left. The forehead was advanced, permitting almost complete closure as a single vertical scar. The proximal pedicle was trimmed, debulked, and reinset as a small inverted V within the medial aspect of the left eyebrow. The nasal inset was completed.

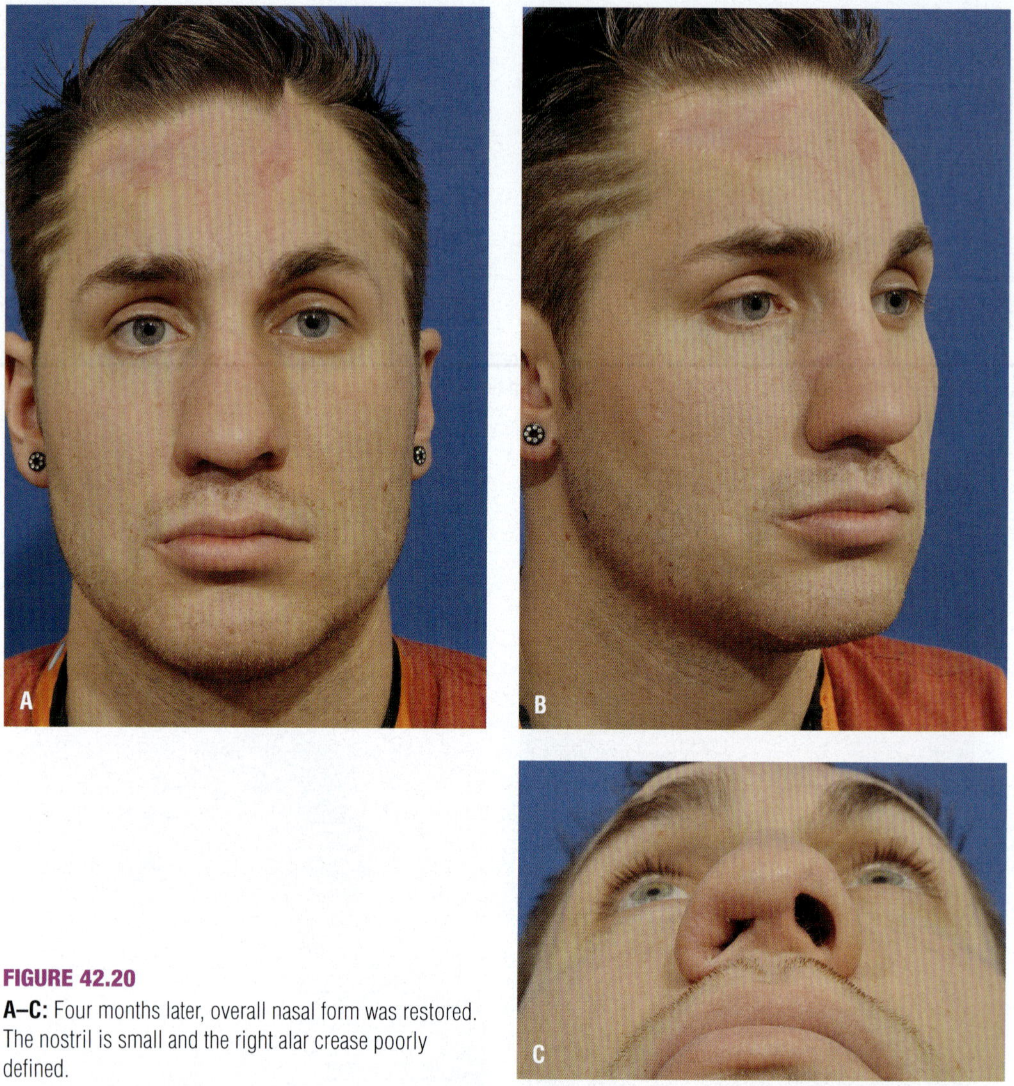

FIGURE 42.20
A–C: Four months later, overall nasal form was restored. The nostril is small and the right alar crease poorly defined.

at the time of transfer, overthinning of the flap to dermis during the intermediate operation, or a pedicle base, which is too wide (>1.5 cm) and which kinks when the flap is rotated to the nose. Once the ischemic area has demarcated and prior to the development of infection or retraction due to scar contraction, dead tissue should be debrided and the area (most often as a subunit) resurfaced with another vascularized flap.

Infection is uncommon. It presents as redness and watery drainage around the edge of the flap at 5 to 7 days after inset. Unless very minor and rapidly controlled by antibiotics, the flap should be reelevated and any cartilage grafts not incorporated into the adjacent cover and lining excised to prevent extension of the infection to the entire reconstruction. Cartilage support can be replaced in a delayed primary fashion 6 to 8 weeks later.

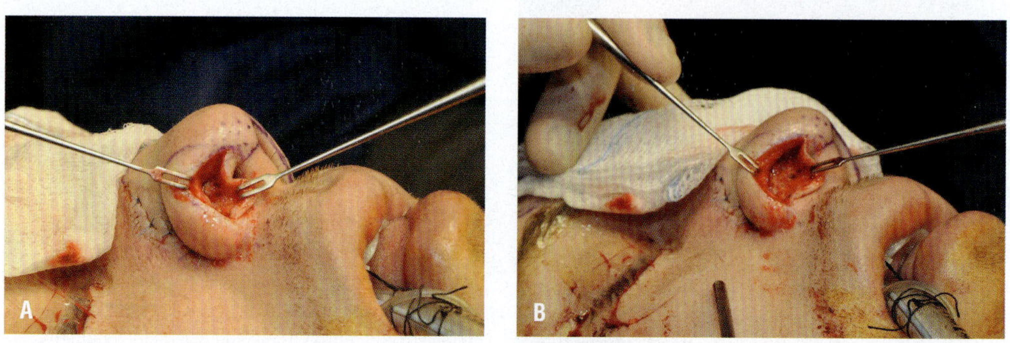

FIGURE 42.21 **A and B:** The margin of the nostril was incised and the lining reelevated thinly. Excess soft tissue and scar between the lining and the delayed primary cartilage graft were excised, thinning the margin of the nostril and opening the airway.

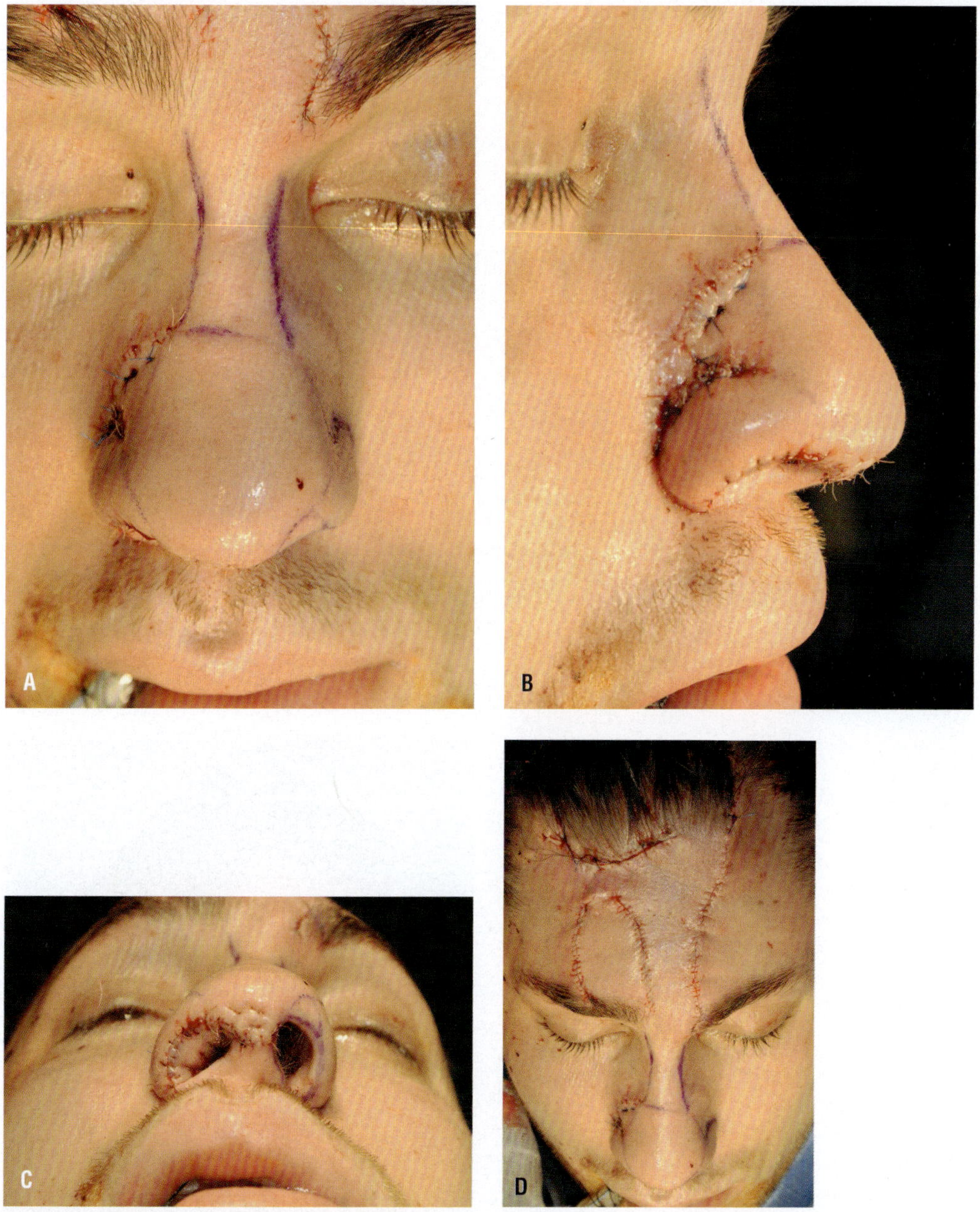

FIGURE 42.22 A–D: The right alar crease was defined at its ideal position by a direct incision. Subcutaneous excision of soft tissue created a flat sidewall, a deep alar crease, and a more convex superior ala. Excess soft tissue in the right infratip was also sculpted. Forehead scars were revised or partially excised within the right forehead.

RESULTS

Postoperatively, a normal nose has been restored. Nasal symmetry, landmarks, proportion, and dimension are good. The left paramedian forehead scar is acceptable. Nasal scars are not apparent. Scarring associated with the first forehead flap will be further revised by serial excision to eliminate the area of secondary healing (Fig. 42.23A–C). A regional unit approach provided principles, which directed the timing, staging, choice of materials, and design.

The repair of large deep defects with a three-stage full-thickness forehead flap has these advantages:

- Maximal blood supply at the time of initial transfer and during complete flap reelevation at the second stage.
- Ideal conformable cover and a complete subunit support framework.
- The use of primary and delayed primary cartilage grafts.
- The opportunity to revise imperfections and maximize contour of the distal most aesthetic parts of the nose prior to pedicle division during the intermediate operation.
- A safe and reliable method of folding a forehead flap to restore vascular, thin, and supple lining and a complete three-dimensional support framework.

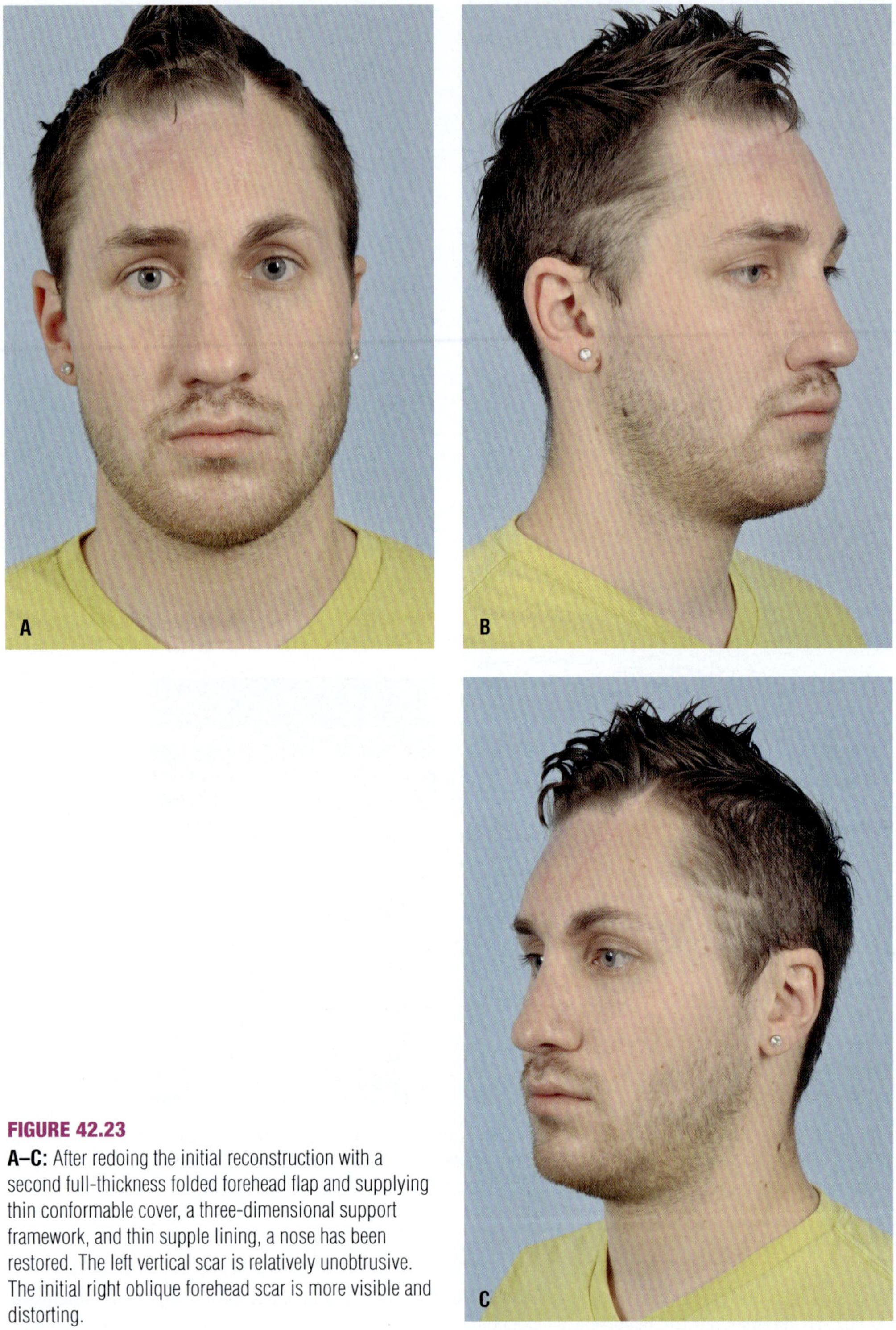

FIGURE 42.23

A–C: After redoing the initial reconstruction with a second full-thickness folded forehead flap and supplying thin conformable cover, a three-dimensional support framework, and thin supple lining, a nose has been restored. The left vertical scar is relatively unobtrusive. The initial right oblique forehead scar is more visible and distorting.

PEARLS

- Determine your surgical goal—a healed wound or the normal.
- Develop an operative plan prior to surgery.
- Envision each stage and perform the operation in your mind prior to going to the operating room.
- The facial subunits, old scars, and areas of tissue deficiency or excess bulk are marked at the start of the procedure.
- Recreate the defect and return the normal to its normal position.
- Identify what is missing and define the true tissue deficiency.
- Alter the wound in site, size, or depth to improve the result, when appropriate.

- Design exact templates based on the contralateral normal or ideal.
- Employ a method that allows you to modify cover and lining flaps and cartilage grafts to establish the dimension, thickness, and quality, which best simulates each missing anatomic layer.

PITFALLS

- Do not assume that any patient of any age does not wish to look normal.
- Replace missing tissues in exact dimension and outline.
- Overaggressive thinning of the flap during the intermediate phase can cause vascular injury.
- After pedicle division, wide reelevation of the flap may jeopardize its vascularity.
- Poor dimensional designing of the flap will create tension, distortion, flap ischemia, and compromise the end surgical outcome.
- A pedicle base greater than 1.5 cm kinks the flap when it is rotated to the nose. This can result in venous congestion and potentially flap loss.

INSTRUMENTS TO HAVE AVAILABLE

- Standard plastic surgery set
- Suture foils for anatomic templates
- Surgical pen

SUGGESTED READING

Menick FJ. Nasal reconstruction: forehead flap. *Plast Reconst Surg* 2004;113:100e–111e.
Menick FJ. "The modified folded forehead flap for nasal lining—the Menick method" in Reconstructive Surgery in Oncology for Surgical Oncology Seminars. *J Surg Oncol* 2006;94:509–514.
Menick FJ. *Nasal reconstruction: art and practice*. Philadelphia, PA: Saunders-Elsevier, 2008.
Menick FJ. Nasal reconstruction CME. *Plast Reconst Surg* 2010;125:135e–150e.
Menick FJ. An approach to the late revision of a failed nasal reconstruction. *Plast Reconst Surg* 2012;129(1):92e–103e.

43 THE MELOLABIAL FLAP

Ritchie A.L. Younger

INTRODUCTION

Dieffenbach, in 1830, popularized the melolabial flap for reconstruction of the nose using superiorly based melolabial flaps to rehabilitate the nasal alae. Von Langenbeck, in 1864, used variations of superior and inferior based flaps depending on the orientation, position, area, and thickness of the flap required for the reconstruction of the nose. Esser, in 1921, employed an inferior based melolabial flap to close palatal fistulae.

The melolabial flap is a versatile technique for functional and esthetic rehabilitation of defects of the central portion of the face. Variations of this flap may be used to reconstruct small- to medium-sized defects involving the chin, upper and lower lip, cheek, nose, and lower eyelid. Because of the relative proximity of this donor site to these areas, not only is the color match of the skin excellent but hiding the donor site incision in a natural crease line (that frequently deepens with age) affords excellent camouflage.

The melolabial area extends from the inferior lateral attachment of the nasal alae to the lateral mouth area, in effect comprised of the volume of tissue surrounding the melolabial crease. The inferior aspect of the melolabial area can be hair bearing in males, with generally less hair in females. This hair variation can be used to advantage occasionally, depending upon whether there is a need to bring hair-bearing or hairless skin into a specific defect.

The surgical literature frequently refers to this region as the nasolabial area, but anatomically speaking, the more accurate descriptor would be melolabial, as the region is in fact bounded by the melum laterally and the labium medially. The superficial musculoaponeurotic system (SMAS) has platysmal fiber remnants extending superiorly and medially, interdigitating with the muscular layers of the orbicularis oris at the melolabial area. The age-defining melolabial crease forms as soft tissue volume depletes at this watershed area where the orbicularis and SMAS fibers meld together. We performed 10 bilateral cadaver dissections at the University of British Columbia Department of Anatomy, which clearly revealed that, for safe elevation of a melolabial flap, the depth of dissection is limited by the orbicularis oris muscle medially and the SMAS fibers laterally. Penetrating these muscle groups reveals the superior and inferior labial arteries in the perioral area medially, indicating that safe atraumatic elevation should preserve these vessels and stay superficial to the perioral musculature. Lateral to this, if one goes as deep as the labial vessel plane of dissection, one could potentially injure the terminal branches of the buccal branch of the facial nerve. The vascular supply to the melolabial flap area is based on the facial artery and the random superficial terminal branches, with venous drainage going to the facial vein. The all-important blood supply to the melolabial flap is not actually based on a specific vessel found in the flap, but rather on a directionally oriented subdermal plexus that courses parallel to the melolabial crease, giving the flap a certain degree of axiality. Essentially, it is a random flap with a directional orientation to the blood flow. Sensory innervation is by way of the infraorbital and mentalis branches of the trigeminal nerve, with motor nerve supply to surrounding musculature via the facial nerve.

HISTORY

Patients that might benefit from the use of a melolabial flap typically fall into one of three categories: a direct referral from a Mohs surgeon (59.3%), a lesion of the central face that I personally excised by using frozen sections to verify margins (31.5%) or patients with a functional or esthetic issue of the central face where a melolabial flap could be used to help resolve the issue (9.2%). Relevant history from the patient that might impact the technical aspects of the planned reconstruction include any microvascular comorbidities (smoking, diabetes, or previous radiation to the donor or recipient site), previous surgery or trauma to the donor or recipient site, and finally systemic hematologic problems (common anticoagulant use in the elderly for atrial fibrillation and cardiac vessel stenting) affecting flow, bleeding, or coagulation in the surgical arena. Pre-Mohs surgery photographs can provide useful information for planning the volume, sizing, and projection of infrastructural grafts for nasal recipient sites, and a careful ophthalmic assessment can help to diminish complications secondary to lower eyelid reconstruction.

PHYSICAL EXAMINATION

A careful examination of the patient is undertaken to determine exactly what is necessary to fabricate an anatomically correct component of the face that is not only functionally accurate but also esthetically balanced and will blend with surrounding facial features. One of the prime tenants of esthetic cutaneous facial reconstruction includes matching color, texture, surface area, and volume of a defect. The location of the melolabial flap donor sites easily affords excellent color matching to most central facial recipient sites. Texture, due to the relative similarity of the melolabial flap surface to potential reconstructed sites, is typically not an issue, except when considering the prospect of mismatching hair-bearing and non–hair-bearing regions. Ideally, I like to see non–hair-bearing donor sites when moving a flap into a non–hair-bearing recipient area (nose and eyelid), and sometimes, I can succeed by taking a hair-bearing flap into a hair-bearing recipient area (upper and lower lip). Current technology with hair epilation lasers allows us to sometimes place a hair-bearing flap into a non–hair-bearing area, but ideally, this can be avoided with judicious planning. The size and volume of the defect is studied so that the best option for reconstruction may be chosen, not only to achieve a superb recipient site result but also to ensure that the donor site can be closed to minimize deformity. Since flap design, volume, and size are limited to the redundancy of available anatomy, medial and superior based flaps are limited not only in width (1 to 5 cm, depending on the laxity of the facial skin) but also in length (1 to 12 cm, depending on the vertical height of the face). Conversely, inferior based flaps are more limited in width and length, as available tissue is more horizontally restricted (substantially less in the upper reaches of the melolabial area) and vertically limited by the nose, medial canthus, and lower eyelid. Pedicle orientation is chosen based on the location of the defect and influenced by whether mostly rotation or advancement will be required to close a resulting defect. Flap thickness at the working end of a pedicled melolabial flap should mirror the thickness of the surrounding recipient site, whereas the thickness of the pedicle itself is somewhat more boundless, although limited by the depth afforded by the presence of the SMAS–orbicularis sheath guarding the neurovascular plexus below.

INDICATIONS

Any reconstructive ladder dealing with defects of the face should in theory mention the possibility of allowing either secondary intention controlled granulation closure of the defect or employing some form of skin or composite graft reconstruction. When we are dealing with easily distorted anatomical structures such as the lower eyelid, lower nose or lip, secondary intention or skin grafting typically remains a poor choice for many reasons. Split-thickness skin grafts not only are a poor color and volume match usually but also can contractually distort some of the fragile anatomy of the lip, eyelid, or nose. Full-thickness grafts can frequently disappoint in volume matching the recipient site, and again, color can be a problem. Composite grafts can be used for small defects in younger individuals with no microvascular comorbidities (smoking, diabetes, or radiation), but surface area and volume limitations can restrict common usage of these elegant grafts.

Choosing a flap for facial reconstruction is invariably determined after weighing the options and figuring out what will give you the best possible result at the recipient site with minimal donor site morbidity. Melolabial flap selection follows the elimination of other flap choices and usually is an easier choice if the patient is perhaps more senior with an already present melolabial crease. For moderate-sized non–full-thickness defects of the upper or lower lip, with dimensions more horizontally oriented, the melolabial flap is a good choice. Superficial or full-thickness defects involving the lower two-thirds of the nose (including the columella) requiring skin, volume, and/or infrastructural support can, in theory, be rehabilitated with primary or staged suprabrow, midline or paramedian forehead, or melolabial flaps (Fig. 43.1). Suprabrow flaps are somewhat limiting due to their donor morbidity and limited potential skin area, whereas forehead flaps provide a possibly massive skin area with modest donor site issues. Melolabial flaps lie somewhere between the two, and where there is already a deep melolabial crease with generous tissue laxity, it becomes the flap source of choice. The melolabial flap has arguably less donor site morbidity (vs. forehead flaps) and normally does not need to be

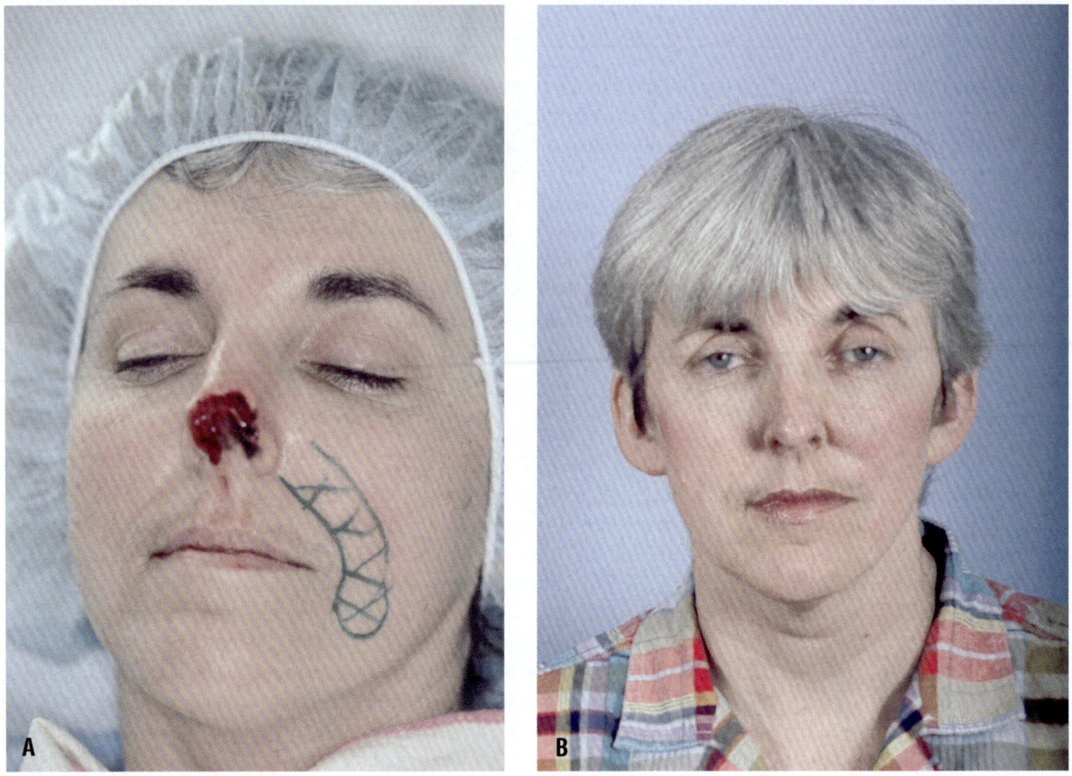

FIGURE 43.1 Superiorly based melolabial interpolated flap for nasal tip, alar, and columellar reconstruction. **A:** Immediate post-Mohs surgery defect. **B:** Twenty-four months postoperative image after four stages of surgery with reconstruction of nasal tip, alae, and superior columella.

delayed (may be necessary with suprabrow flap), but the melolabial flap blood supply is not quite as robust as the forehead sites and must be elevated as atraumatically as possible.

For smaller defects (<2 cm diameter) of the inferior aspect of the nose, local nasal flaps such as transposition or bilobe are a notably better and less invasive option. For larger defects involving the alar rim or a full-thickness loss, the melolabial flap will generally provide surface area, adequate bulk, and a vascular supply, which will support a cartilage graft (Fig. 43.2). Defects of the inferior aspect of the nose or the lips (upper or lower), oriented horizontally, can be more readily covered with a melolabial flap than a forehead

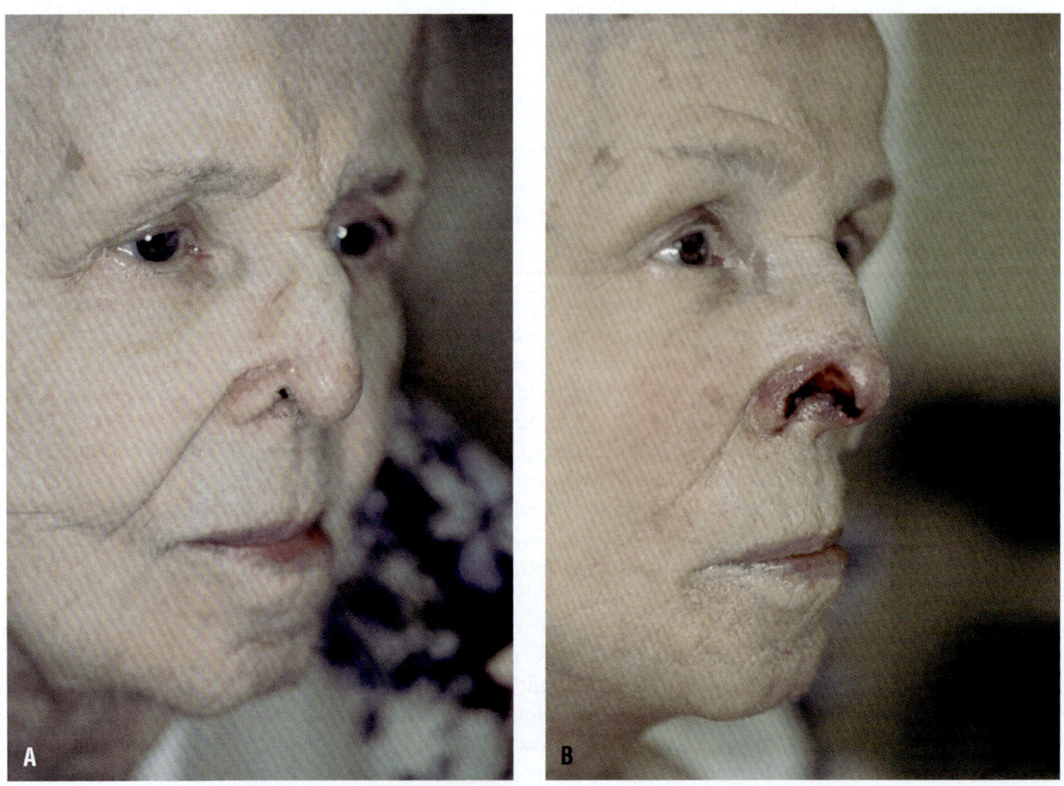

FIGURE 43.2 Superiorly based melolabial transposition wraparound flap. **A:** Skin cancer noted at alar rim prior to Mohs surgery. **B:** Immediate post-Mohs surgery defect.

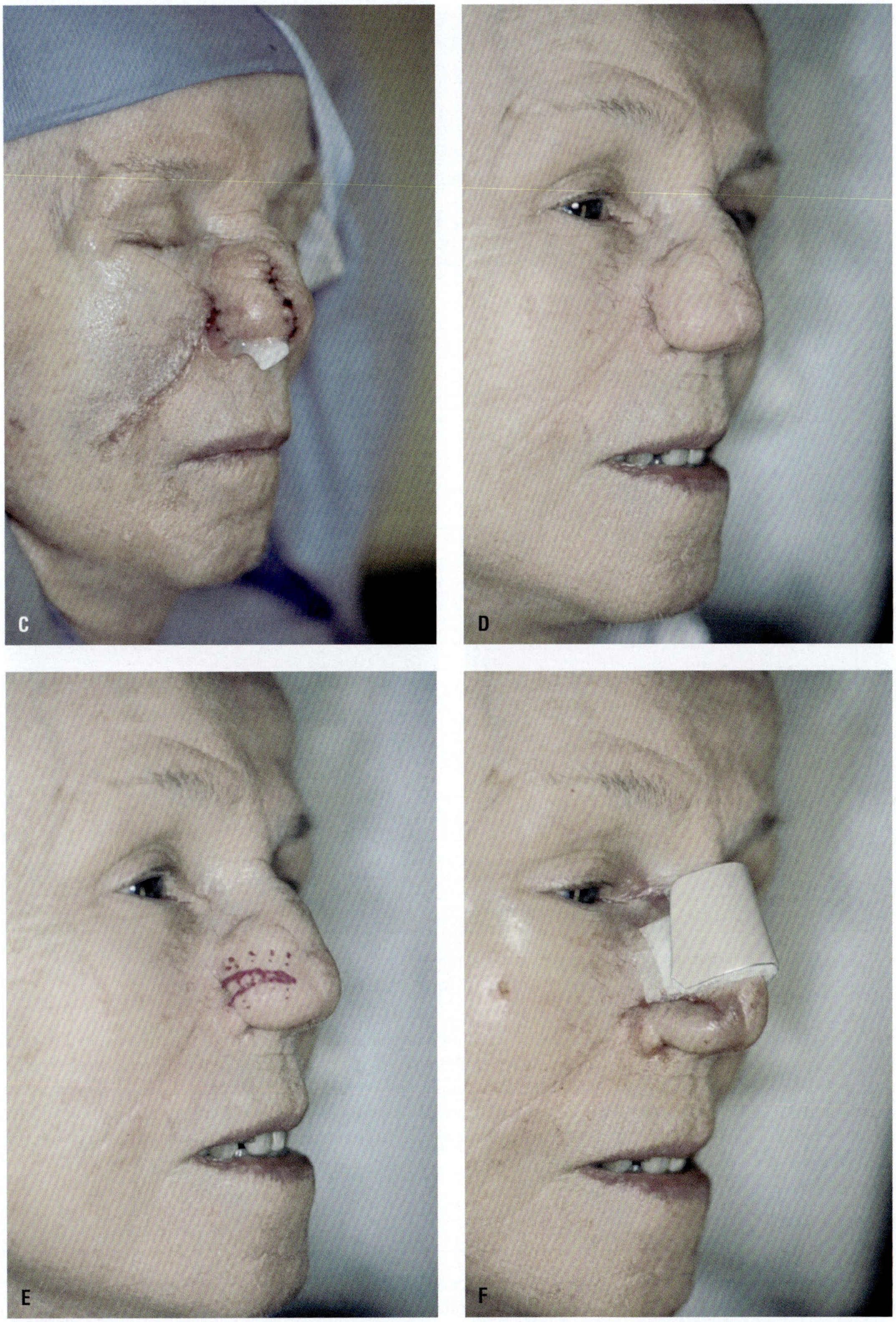

FIGURE 43.2 (*Continued*) **C:** Immediate postoperative wraparound transposition flap with ear cartilage graft for alar infrastructure. **D:** Twelve months postoperative view notable for an absence of a poorly formed supra-alar crease. **E:** Revision surgery to create a supra-alar crease. **F:** Immediate postoperative view after creation of a supra-alar crease.

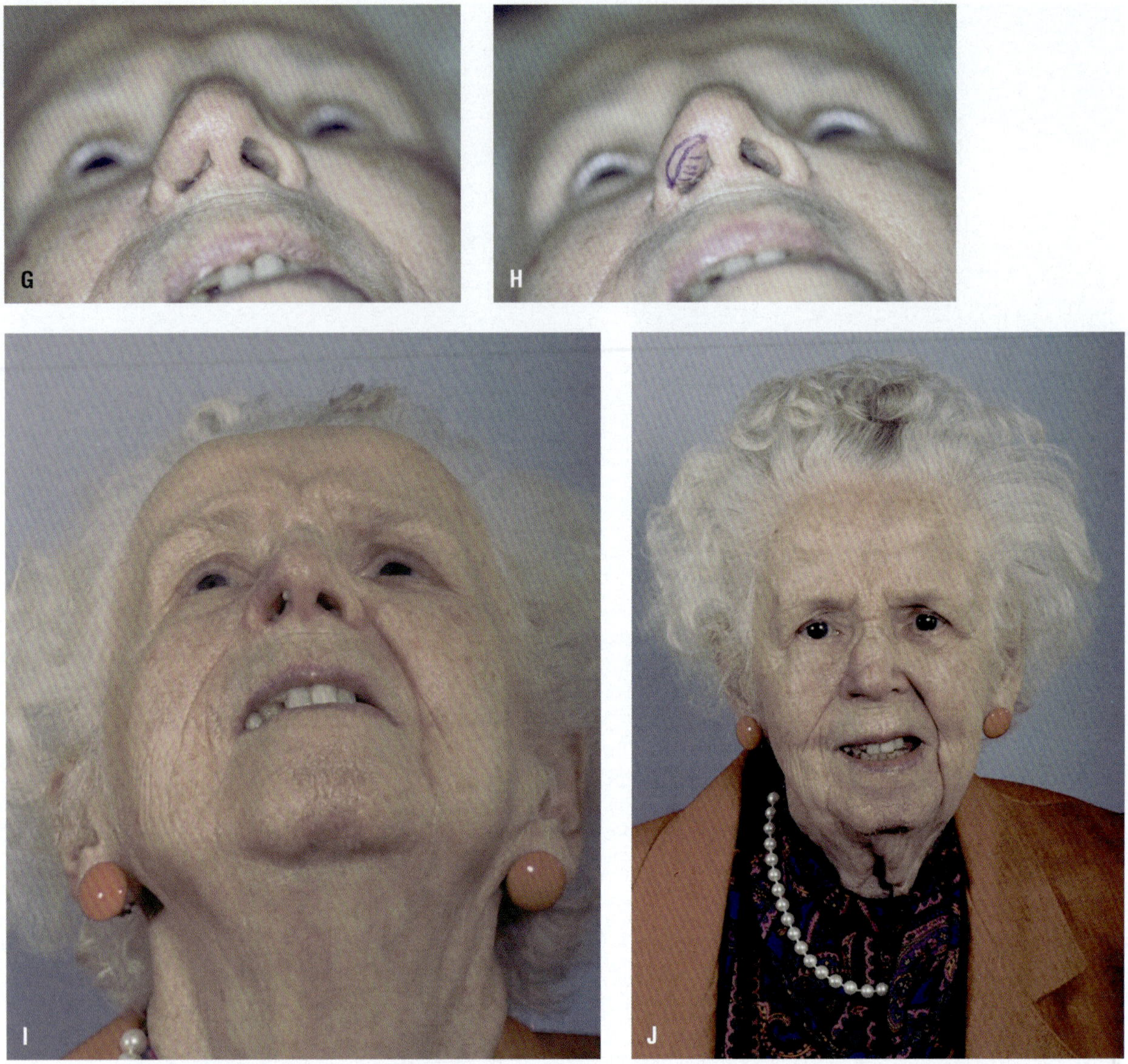

FIGURE 43.2 (*Continued*) **G:** Eighteen months post-Mohs with wide alar rim. **H:** Revision surgery planning to thin alar rim. **I:** Twenty-four months post-Mohs inferior view showing thinned alar rim. **J:** Twenty-four months postoperative result.

flap (Fig. 43.3), while conversely, a vertically oriented nasal defect is better closed with a forehead flap or direct advancement from side to side on the nose (if the nose is rather wide and might require cartilage modifications). Medial cheek, intraoral, and eyelid defects may be reconstructed with a melolabial flap, if other more readily accessible local flaps are not an option. After weighing all of the grafting and flap options, if the melolabial donor site provides the best color match, contour, volume, and functional rehabilitation, with the least donor site morbidity, it remains the best choice.

CONTRAINDICATIONS

Most primary and interpolated two-stage melolabial reconstructions can readily be performed under neuroleptic anesthesia with locally infiltrated anesthetics, eliminating the need for general anesthesia in a patient with multiple comorbidities.

Large lower nasal defects can be a quandary when choosing between a forehead and melolabial flap. Experience with both indicates that when a patient is young and has a very shallow melolabial crease, it may be difficult to camouflage the donor site well, so alternative options might be explored. A Pearson chi-square review of 70 patients who underwent melolabial reconstruction of the central face revealed that there were significantly more complications with the melolabial flap when the patient had received radiation to the face preoperatively or when the patient had a history of smoking. Diabetes was significant at 10%, and there seemed to be no sexual predilection for complications. Based on this report, one would be well advised to avoid the melolabial flap as a method of reconstruction with a radiated smoker who is a diabetic.

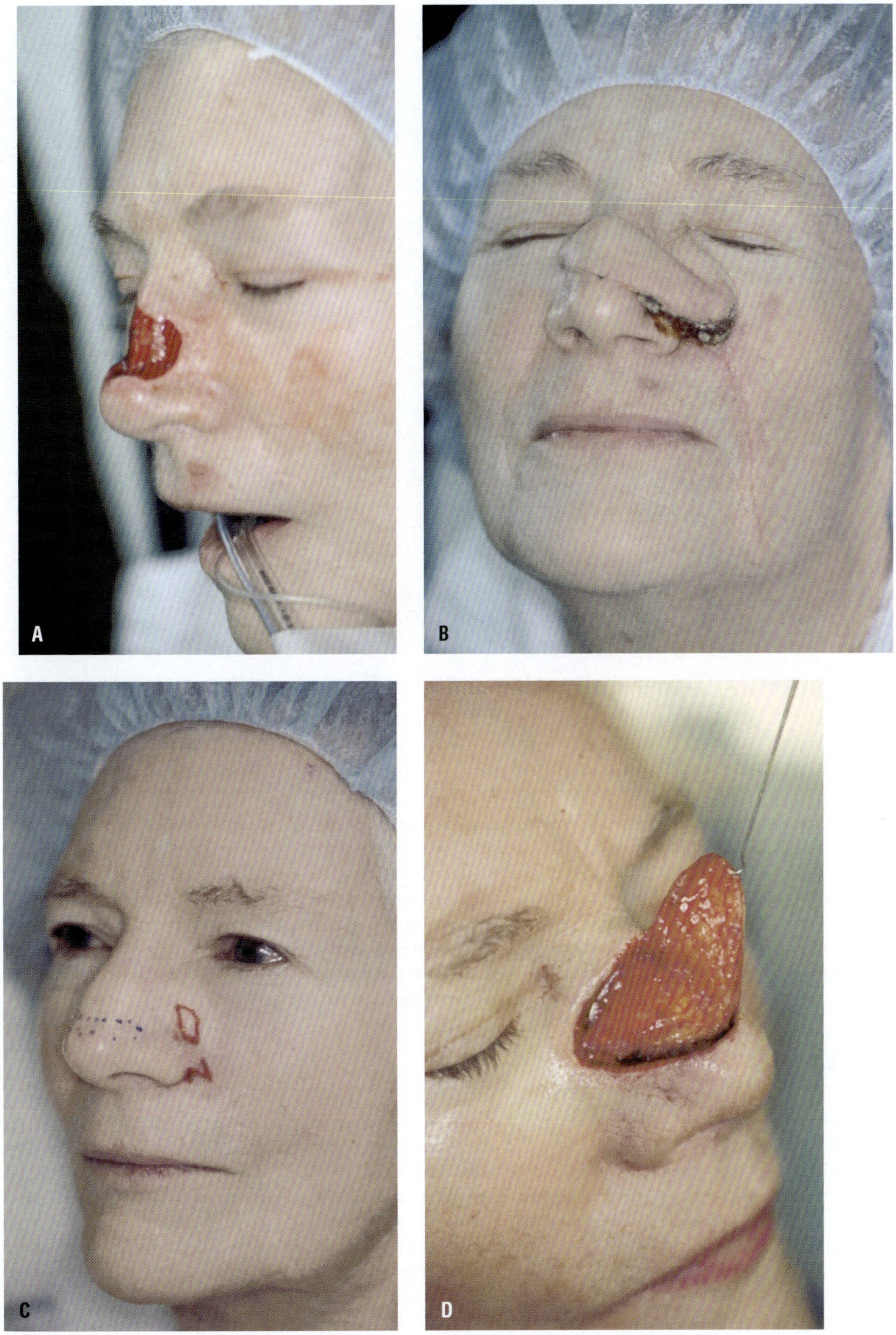

FIGURE 43.3 Superiorly based melolabial interpolation flap for reconstruction of a horizontal nasal dorsal defect. **A:** Immediate post-Mohs surgery nasal dorsal defect. **B:** First-stage interpolation flap after esthetic bisymmetrical equilibration of the Mohs defect. **C:** Twelve months after second stage with a third-stage preoperative plan to improve the operative site by revising the incision lines and debulking of the flap. **D:** Debulking the nasal dorsum.

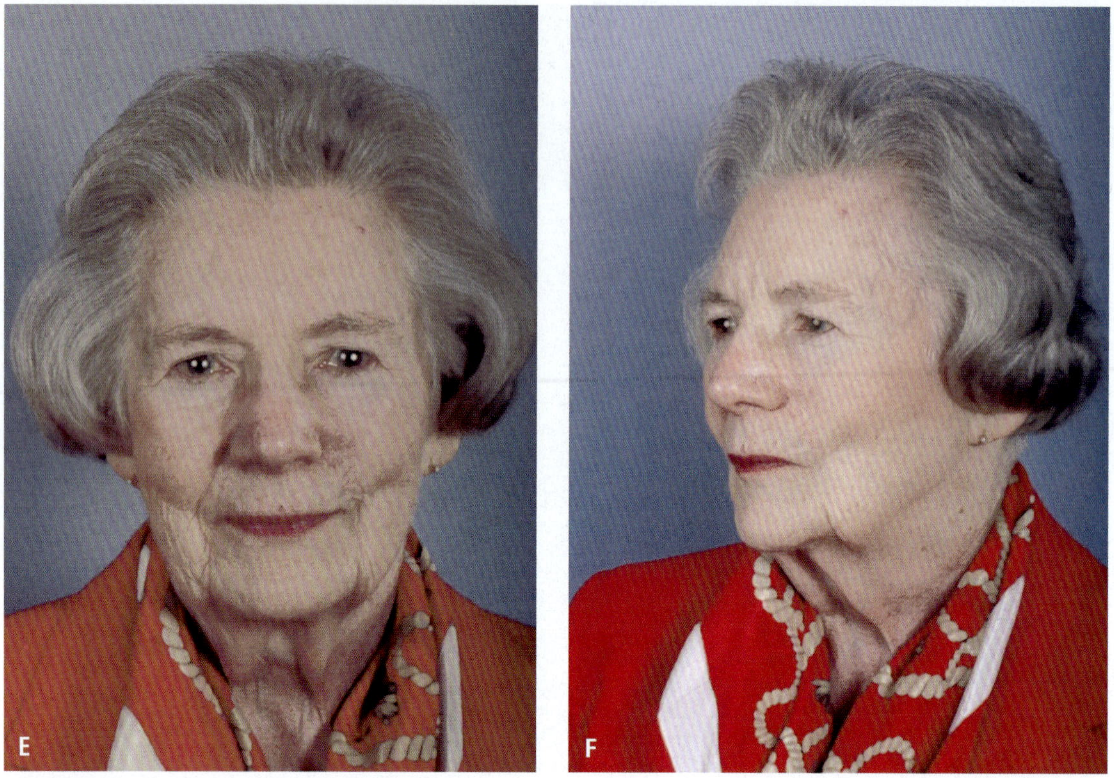

FIGURE 43.3 (*Continued*) **E:** Twenty-four months post-Mohs surgery result. **F:** Twenty-four months post-Mohs surgery oblique view.

PREOPERATIVE PLANNING

A thorough analysis of reconstructive options for reconstruction of the midface will yield the obvious choice in most circumstances. Weighing reconstructive capability against the morbidity of the donor site usually dictates the best option for surgery. A history and physical examination of the proposed patient is undertaken including the appropriate radiologic and endoscopic examinations as deemed necessary. Detailed photographs of the patient are taken (anterior, inferior, close-up, oblique, and lateral views) for review at the time of surgery to assist in infrastructural (if necessary) reconstruction and skin surface area and volume planning. The procedure is outlined to the patient with specifics geared to revealing the number of stages that will be required, donor site morbidity, and details about the expected progress of the recipient area.

SURGICAL TECHNIQUE

In most preoperative circumstances, one of three possibilities will be present if planning to use the melolabial flap.

Situation 1 is receiving a scarred (traumatic, postsurgical or congenital) nose, and as a first step, the surgeon would release the scar and replace the missing or distorted infrastructural support. A template would be made of the skin loss (either at the actual site or the contralateral site to achieve bisymmetrical equality) and exactly transcribed to the melolabial donor site to enable a precision surface area replacement.

Situation 2 is receiving a post-Mohs patient surgery with a bandage on a recent wound. Ideally, the patient would have been assessed pre-Mohs so photos could have been made and thus reviewed when the dressing is removed. Infrastructural compromise is addressed (if the nose is involved) usually with intranasal or auricular cartilage grafts followed by a skin template taken (remember esthetic subunit resection principles) from the actual defect or the contralateral side (Fig. 43.4).

Situation 3 occurs in the outpatient area or operating room when a patient is having a cutaneous lesion removed (malignancy or otherwise), either as a macroscopic resection (if lesion margins are clearly visible) or employing frozen section. The lesion is resected completely (may require additional resection to complete an esthetic subunit removal in the case of a nose or lip), or after the margins are confirmed by pathology, infrastructural support (if needed) is addressed and a template of either the defect or the contralateral unoperated side is taken. This recipient-taken template is transcribed to the donor melolabial site, and melolabial flap elevation commences.

For intraoperative planning for smaller defects of the medial eyelid, the lateral nose, the medial cheek, and the lateral lip, a small transposition or advancement flap from the melolabial area will generally suffice. For larger defects, the presence of a deep melolabial sulcus will facilitate less of a donor site deformity than

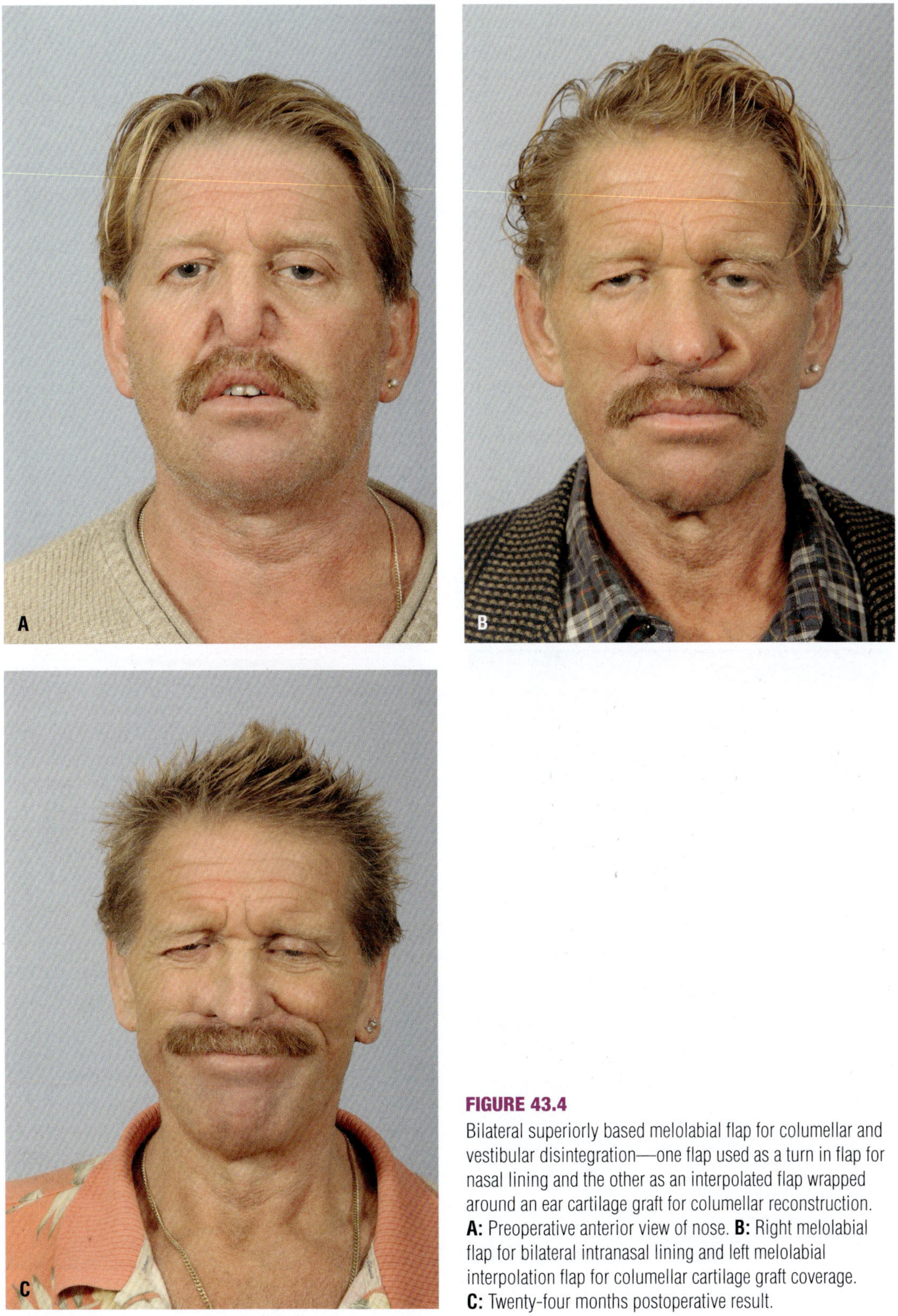

FIGURE 43.4
Bilateral superiorly based melolabial flap for columellar and vestibular disintegration—one flap used as a turn in flap for nasal lining and the other as an interpolated flap wrapped around an ear cartilage graft for columellar reconstruction. **A:** Preoperative anterior view of nose. **B:** Right melolabial flap for bilateral intranasal lining and left melolabial interpolation flap for columellar cartilage graft coverage. **C:** Twenty-four months postoperative result.

forehead flaps or other major reconstructive flaps. The type of melolabial flap required in the operating room is based on the surrounding anatomy, the location and depth of the defect, and the surgeon's observations as to which technique would provide the best long-term result. Larger areas of the nose generally are helped with a superiorly based melolabial transposition flap (if in continuity or close continuity of the melolabial area) or a superiorly based melolabial two-stage interpolation flap (if the recipient site is distant from the donor area). Larger lateral upper and lower lip defects are typically helped with direct advancement melolabial flaps or occasionally transposition flaps (Fig. 43.5).

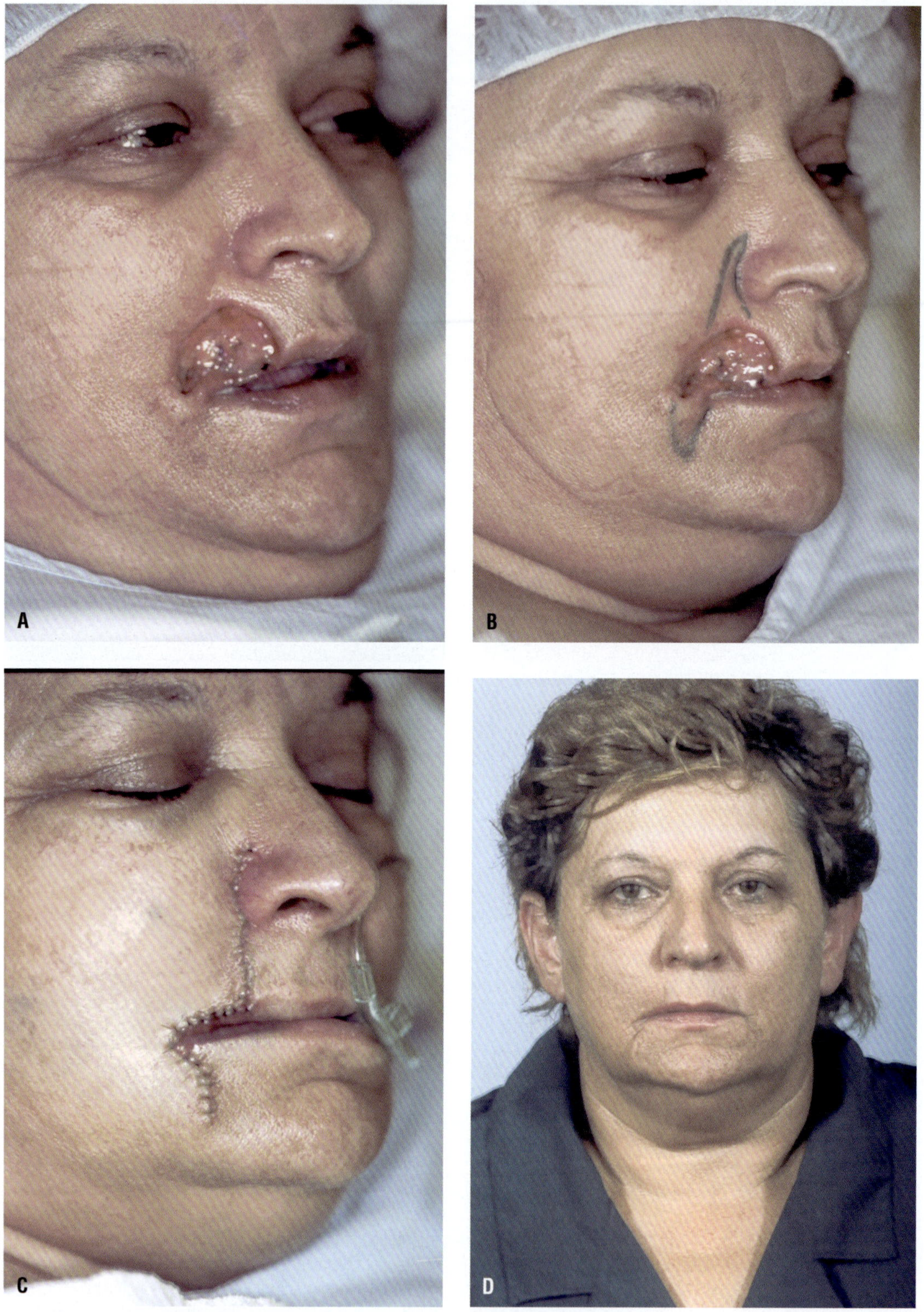

FIGURE 43.5 Laterally based melolabial advancement flap for upper lip reconstruction. **A:** Post-Mohs surgery of morpheaform basal cell carcinoma of the upper lip. **B:** Intraoperative reconstructive plan. **C:** Intraoperative view after reconstruction is complete. **D:** Twelve months postoperative image after the surgery.

The exact type of melolabial flap is determined, lines are drawn on the skin with markers, and a recipient site defect template is transcribed to the flap. Principles of atraumatic tissue handling are paramount when elevating the melolabial flap, since the adipose tissue subcutaneous layer has less fibrous tissue and a more fragile axiality to the blood supply than a more robust forehead flap. Skin hooks are essential for engaging the flap, and compressive tissue forceps are contraindicated during the surgery. The melolabial flap is outlined with a scalpel and elevated with a sharp face-lift scissor dissection, with cautery used sparingly as pinpoint hemostasis control. Cautery is never employed for flap elevation in these melolabial cases, as the distal flap may be prone to vascular compromise. For transposition or interpolation flaps, the dissection should develop a deeper proximal flap, which may go down as far as the investing sheath between the SMAS and orbicularis to maximize the axiality of the blood supply. (Cadaver and patient dissections reveal that the average caliper measurement depth of the flap base is 12 mm). Dissecting the flap proximally to distally, the flap is thinned gradually with the distal flap depth equal to the depth of the recipient defect (as compared to the surrounding tissue and generally ranging from 4 to 8 mm thick distally). To facilitate closure of the donor site, undermining lateral to the melolabial area (out into the cheek) is always done superficial to the SMAS plane, with medial undermining for just a few millimeters to facilitate placement of deep subcuticular sutures. If extensive medial undermining occurs, it can lead to unnecessary distortion of the lip, so it is generally best to minimize medially and maximize lateral dissection to facilitate closure. Closure with deep and skin sutures in a subtle inversion manner frequently allows better camouflage of the melolabial crease donor site. Pincushioning occurs more frequently in melolabial flap reconstruction than forehead flap procedures, and during primary surgery, two technical considerations will minimize this. Undermining widely at the recipient site and employing a few deep subcutaneous sutures peripherally will minimize pincushioning and are essential to ensuring a consistently excellent recipient site esthetic.

POSTOPERATIVE MANAGEMENT

To complete the melolabial flap reconstruction, I apply an antibiotic ointment to the incision line and generally do not employ prophylactic antibiotics unless there is a specific comorbidity that would suggest otherwise. I do not apply wound dressings to the operative site so that I can observe the wound for at least 3 hours, to aid observation of the tip of the flap to ensure an adequate arterial supply and venous drainage. As the adrenalin effect from the local anesthetic wears off, I anticipate a reasonably healthy distal flap, as evidenced by warmth and a good vascular blush that returns with light compression. In the older patient who may be diabetic or a smoker, I anticipate that their potential for healing properly may be limited and generally would try to select a different flap that might have a more reliable vascular supply. If that is not an option, and I have used a melolabial flap that seems to be suffering from some degree of postoperative vascular compromise, my first choice is to return the flap to the respective donor site vascular bed and delay it for 1 to 2 weeks. After the delay, I resume the original surgical plan.

One-stage transposition or advancement flaps are reassessed at 7 to 10 days for suture removal at the donor site and partial suture removal at the recipient site. At 9 to 15 days, the few remaining individual sutures at the recipient site are removed.

Two-stage interpolation flaps again are assessed carefully postoperatively and may be delayed as necessary. Home care nursing evaluates these patients every second day to provide the necessary wound care including a light saline debridement of the bridging pedicle, application of antibiotic ointment, and overall assessment to rule out infection and gauge progress, or lack thereof. Donor site and partial removal of recipient site sutures occur at 7 to 10 days, and then, reassessment at 9 to 15 days facilitates removal of remaining sutures. A tourniquet test at 3 weeks evaluates the viability of the distal flap, and if positive, the second stage is planned for 3 to 5 weeks, dependent on the results of the test. Some patients find it comforting to wear a surgical mask when in public after the first stage and before the second stage is undertaken, which is no surprise as these pedicled patients have a somewhat unusual appearance and the patient should be counseled about this in advance. At second stage, the flap is divided leaving the distal melolabial flap tip attached to the reconstructed area, and the interpolated flap stump is shortened and inset, typically as a straight incision line at the superior aspect of the melolabial sulcus. Antibiotic ointment is applied to the wound daily with a planned revisit at 7 to 10 days to complete suture removal.

COMPLICATIONS

Appropriate preoperative assessment with exacting attention to detail and atraumatic handling of the tissues will invariably lead to an esthetically acceptable result that will function almost as well as the original tissues. Potential complications secondary to melolabial flap reconstruction are listed in Table 43.1. Poor flap design can leave the patient with esthetically undesirable incision lines and tension across the recipient site, which can compromise the end result. Should there be vascular compromise intra- or immediately postoperatively, a flap delay may be in order. Should venous congestion be threatening the flap viability postoperatively, leeches may be helpful to counteract congestive compromise of arterial flow. Infections are few but antibiotics may be necessary when present. Long-term follow-up of 110 patients undergoing a single-stage advancement, transposition, or rotation melolabial flap reconstruction reveals that 65.5% will ultimately undergo a second stage. This second stage is offered to deal with the minor complications associated with minimal shape or contour deficits, the most frequent undertaken to recreate the depth of a supra-alar crease. Long-term follow-up of 52 patients undergoing a two-stage interpolation melolabial flap reconstruction reveals that 28.8% will undergo a third stage. This third stage most frequently seems necessary to deal with either nasal tip contours or positioning of an alae to get absolute bisymmetrical equality. A review of Table 43.2, which itemizes all melolabial flap complications in my experience of 162 flaps, indicates not only

TABLE 43.1 Potential Complications of Melolabial Flap Reconstruction

- Lower eyelid
  - Contour or volume deficits
  - Ectropion
- Lateral nose
  - Alar malposition
  - Blunting of alar-labial groove
  - Comparative melolabial crease asymmetries
  - Contour or volume deficits
  - Ectopic hair growth
  - Loss of nasofacial groove
  - Loss of supra-alar crease
  - Nasal obstruction
  - Skin discoloration (hypo- or hyperpigmentation or persisting erythema)
  - Skin texture mismatch
- Nasal tip
  - Alar height asymmetries
  - Comparative melolabial crease asymmetries
  - Contour or volume deficits
  - Ectopic hair growth
  - Flap detachment
  - Flap tip necrosis
  - Infratip lobule asymmetries
  - Skin discoloration
- Nasal lining
  - Ectopic hair
  - Excessive bulk
  - Flap tip necrosis
- Upper or lower lip
  - Contour or volume deficits
  - Discoloration
  - Hair issues
  - Lip distortion (superiorly, inferiorly, or laterally)
  - Vermilion distortion
- Chin
  - Contour or volume deficits
  - Recipient scar visibility

TABLE 43.2 Complications of Melolabial Flap Reconstruction (162 Patients)

Complication	n
Loss of nasal crease(s) needing revision	37
Noticeable melolabial crease asymmetries postoperative	22
Recipient scar requiring revision	17
Nasal tip contour issues needing revision	8
Partial flap necrosis	7
Ectopic hair growth	6
Recipient site infection	4
Altered lip position needing revision	4
Recipient site pincushioning	4
Donor site scar requiring revision	3
Altered alar position needing revision	3
Nasal obstruction	3
Recipient site hypopigmentation	2
Donor site infection	2
Donor site hyperpigmentation	1
Flap detachment related to psychiatric issues	1

numerous benign issues not requiring any immediate attention but also more serious issues that ultimately may require a revision procedure.

PEARLS

- Consider the melolabial flap in middle-aged or older patients who have a melolabial sulcus that affords donor site camouflage.
- Horizontally oriented defects may be most appropriately reconstructed with the melolabial flap.
- When elevating a transposition or interpolation melolabial flap, employ atraumatic noncompressive handling of the thickest proximal flap possible to ensure flap survival.
- Deeper defects of the nasal tip or alae can readily be approached with various modifications of a melolabial flap, to achieve outstanding results beyond what is realized with skin grafts alone.
- Intraoperative arterial insufficiency or venous congestion can be managed well by one or more salvage techniques: using very deep sutures across the recipient area to reduce tension across the donor flap, using a delay suture technique by placing tagged sutures at the site and tying these 24 hours later, delaying the flap for 10 days, or, post-op, considering the use of leeches.
- Encourage secondary or tertiary revision procedures to maximize outcome.
- Minimize recipient site pincushioning by undermining laterally as needed and using a few deep sutures peripherally.
- Our standard time for flap division of an interpolated flap is 3 weeks. For smokers or other unusual patients with comorbidities, 4 or 5 weeks is safer to optimize recipient site survival.

PITFALLS

- The melolabial flap may not be the best choice for reconstruction in patients who have had radiation to the central face or who are smokers or diabetics.
- When elevating the melolabial flap avoid penetrating deeper than the SMAS or orbicularis oris musculature to prevent neurovascular injury.
- In some male patients with abundant beard growth, a different flap may be more appropriate elsewhere to avoid ectopic hair in the recipient site.
- Placing deep sutures under a narrow transposition melolabial flap, to create depth in anatomical watershed areas or creases (nasofacial, alar-facial, or supra-alar groove) is generally not recommended and best left for a revision procedure—so as to avoid overwhelming the fragile blood supply of the distal flap.

RESULTS

One hundred and sixty-two patients have undergone melolabial flap reconstruction of the central facial area in the last 30 years by me. The average patient age was 58.9 years, with an average follow-up of 3.3 years: 67.9% women, 30.9% men, and 1.2% other. The areas reconstructed are outlined in Table 43.3 and the type of melolabial flap used for the reconstruction is seen in Table 43.4. In my experience, postmicrographic recon-

TABLE 43.3 Anatomical Recipient Sites of Patients Undergoing Melolabial Flap Reconstruction (Total 162)

Site	Number
Nose	
Dorsal	7
Lateral	25
Tip	16
Alar	44
Nasal lining	6
Columellar	15
Lower eyelid	3
Malar	7
Upper lip	27
Lower lip	7
Chin	5

TABLE 43.4 Various Types of Melolabial Flap Used

Transposition	74
Interpolation	52
Advancement	31
Rotation	5

struction was the indication for melolabial flap usage in 59.3%, frozen section removal reconstruction in 31.5%, and 9.2% were required for esthetic and/or functional rehabilitation of varied areas of the central face.

INSTRUMENTS TO HAVE AVAILABLE

- Standard facial plastic surgery reconstruction set
- Single and double skin hooks
- Sharp face-lift scissors for flap elevation
- Fine-point cautery for meticulous hemostasis

ACKNOWLEDGMENT

Dedicated to The Master of Cutaneous Facial Flaps: Prof. Dr. med. Claus Walter 10.3.1927 to 11.9.2016.

SUGGESTED READING

Dieffenbach JF. Die nasenbehandlung. In: Brockhaus FA, ed. *Operative Chirurgie*. Leipzig, 1845.
Esser J. Oben gestielter Arteria-angularis-Lappen ohne Hautstiel. *Arch Klin Chir* 1921;117(3):477–491.
Schmidt BL, Dierks EJ. The nasolabial flap. *Oral Maxillofac Surg Clin North Am* 2003;15(4):487–495.
Younger RAL. The versatile melolabial flap. *Otolaryngol Head Neck Surg* 1992;107:721–726.

44 TECHNIQUES FOR COMPOSITE GRAFTS IN RECONSTRUCTION OF FACIAL DEFECTS

G. Richard Holt

Since this chapter was written, we have lost Dr. Claus Walter, to whom this chapter is now dedicated. Dr. Walter was a pre-eminent, globally recognized facial plastic and reconstructive surgeon, whose contributions to the specialty are reflected in his care of thousands of patients with a wide range of facial disorders, as well as his teaching and publications appreciated around the world. Additionally, on a personal note, Dr. Walter was not just a mentor and colleague to me, but also a friend and father figure, who will be sorely missed. He was a great and wonderful man, an excellent clinician, and a surgical innovator at the highest cognitive level. Abschied, Professor Dr. Walter.

Rich Holt

INTRODUCTION

Composite grafts have been used in the reconstruction of various sites of the face and neck for many decades. In recent years, however, their use has been limited due to the expanding application of composite pedicled flaps and composite free tissue transfer flaps for large defects. Still, there remains ample opportunity for composite grafts to be considered in certain reconstructive requirements for structural support and tissue replacement.

Composite grafts, by definition, are useful in replacing at least two types of tissue in a defect, including internal lining, soft tissue bulk, and hard tissue support. Some defects require multiple tissue type replacement, and the option of composite grafts can be a valuable tool in the reconstruction armamentarium. By leaving perichondrium or dermis attached to the cartilage and adipose tissue, respectively, the grafts have greater stability, ease of fixation, maintenance of size and shape, and increased vascular ingrowth, all of which are important for a successful reconstruction.

HISTORY

Most patients who would need a composite graft will typically have had extirpative cancer surgery resulting in a soft tissue defect; have had a traumatic loss of tissue; or require tissue replacement in functional surgery. Composite grafts can also be used in the reconstruction of the airway, both upper (nasal) and lower (laryngotracheal) where typically there is loss of supportive structure (cartilage) and/or external or internal lining. In some patients, a congenital deformity, such as type I microtia, may be easily improved with a composite graft. For later-onset conditions, as in Romberg's lateral hemifacial atrophy, there is primarily a reduction in the soft tissue bulk of the face, which is amenable to reexpansion with a composite such as a dermis/adipose tissue graft.

Comorbidities of a medical nature, especially those with vascular components such as diabetes, smoking, and vasculitis, may cause the surgeon to be reluctant to use a composite graft, primarily due to the recognition of questionable recipient site vascularity. Patients being treated with chemotherapy, those who have had previous radiation therapy to either the donor or recipient sites, and those with metabolic disorders, including anemia, are usually not good candidates for a composite graft.

PHYSICAL EXAMINATION

In general, the defect will be obvious, whether due to a loss of some tissue layers or due to a reduced functional capacity owing to tissue laxity or degeneration. Composite grafts are most useful in areas where specialized tissues provide complex support and function for a structure. Most commonly, tissue defects of the auricle, eyelid, nose, face, and airway are amenable to the use of composite grafts in their reconstruction. Soft tissue facial defects, whether due to progressive atrophy or from soft tissue resection (parotidectomy), may require soft tissue rebulking that is best managed through the use of a dermis/adipose tissue composite graft. Some laryngotracheal conditions that narrow the airway, such as postintubation cricoid scarring, can be successfully repaired using a composite perichondrium–cartilage graft. In all circumstances, a detailed review of the dimension of the defect, impaired regional function, and available donor site possibilities is obtained. Potential donor sites should be inspected to make certain that previous surgery, trauma, or radiation does not eliminate the donor site from consideration. Certain conditions may downgrade access, for example, previous chest wall surgery or fractures from resuscitation efforts limit access to rib grafts.

INDICATIONS

Defects of the auricle are recognized by a loss of the continuity of the helical rim or a constriction of the auricle in type I microtia. Following a traumatic loss of tissue, there may be sufficient scarring to be of concern for an adequate vascular supply to a composite graft to the auricle. If that is the case, a pedicled flap with cartilage support may be indicated. However, if the tissue is well vascularized, as might be the case following the excision of a cancer of the auricle, the conditions may be conducive to the immediate application of a composite graft to the defect from the opposite auricular helix. Typically, defects smaller than 2 cm have a good chance for survival. In type I microtia, a composite graft (skin and cartilage) from the opposite helix may be inserted in a radial fashion to expand the helix itself to a size that would be more appropriate for the child's face and age. If the region of the external auditory meatus has been compromised due to scarring, then a meatoplasty with a possible composite skin/perichondrium/cartilage graft from the opposite conchal bowl should yield good results.

The use of a composite graft for reconstruction of the eyelid is appropriate after traumatic or surgical loss of the full thickness of the eyelid or the loss of the internal lamella with its tarsal support. In the first situation, the bulbar conjunctiva will be exposed and immediate reconstruction is required to protect the cornea, using an advancement/rotation skin flap in conjunction with a composite cartilage/perichondrium graft internally. In both instances, the cartilage/perichondrium composite graft will provide the structural and antigravity support for the eyelid, as well as the internal lining, in the form of the perichondrium, to renew the conjunctiva. The adjacent skin lateral to the lateral canthus should be examined carefully so that it can be determined whether it is feasible to be used as a flap to reconstruct the outer lamella of the lower eyelid when that tissue is missing. Consultation by an Ophthalmologist is mandatory when reconstructing the eyelid, primarily for their oversight of the protection of vision and the health of the globe.

Generally, the use of a composite graft in the nose is to provide internal lining and structural support of the nasal valve region and vestibular sidewall. In patients who have had a resection of the nasal vestibule or nasal sidewall after extirpative cancer surgery (less commonly from traumatic loss), two or three of the layers will need to be reconstructed (outer lining, inner lining, and structural support). The composite cartilage/perichondrium graft can provide two of the three layers, given that adequate external covering and a healthy vascular supply can be supplied. When the airway diameter has been compromised due to scarring of the nasal vestibular skin and nasal valve region, after the scar is removed, there will be a requirement for both internal lining and cartilage support. Anterior rhinoscopy will reveal the extent of the scar contracture—if it is small, a Z-plasty might be helpful, but for a larger constriction, a composite graft will be required, either conchal bowl skin/perichondrium/cartilage, or if in the region of the internal nasal valve, a mucosal/perichondrium/cartilage graft from the contralateral nasal septum is indicated. Additionally, flexible or rigid nasal endoscopy should be performed to ascertain the general health of the nasal cavity and associated structures and to rule out concomitant pathology.

In patients with lateral hemifacial atrophy, the majority of which are young females, facial muscle function is typically reasonably normal, so unless the atrophy requires the free transfer and reinnervation of facial muscles, rebulking with a composite dermis/adipose tissue graft will be successful. Since the atrophy usually begins after puberty, there is little loss of mandibular and maxillary bone projection. Mastication capabilities and occlusion will be normal. In these patients, there will be a distinct loss of soft tissue substance on one side, both to inspection and palpation, with the loss of tissue primarily of adipose tissue and dermal thickening. Vascularity of the overlying skin should be ascertained, but it will normally be excellent as these are young, healthy patients. The amount of adipose tissue potentially available in the abdomen should be identified by a thorough inspection of that area, including the identification of previous scars and surgical sites. Typically, the left side of the abdomen is used for the composite dermis/adipose tissue graft retrieval since a scar on the right side may be mistaken later for an appendectomy scar.

Some patients with postintubation or posttrauma laryngotracheal airway narrowing may benefit from a composite perichondrium/cartilage graft, either from the nasal septum or more commonly from the cartilaginous portion of a rib. Many of the patients will have a tracheostomy in place, allowing for inspection of the area of narrowing using a flexible scope from both above and below. Imaging studies, as discussed below, will be helpful in determining the extent of the narrowing (circumferential and axial) and its amenability to composite graft reconstruction via laryngotracheoplasty.

CONTRAINDICATIONS

Contraindications to composite grafting lie more in the health of the recipient site than in the donor site itself. The more important consideration for composite grafting is that the recipient bed be adequately vascularized and that the overlying skin covering will be sufficient to decrease the risk of graft extrusion. Obviously, abnormal donor cartilage in the presence of an autoimmune disorder would not lend itself to transfer grafting. Donor adipose tissue abnormalities are rarely seen in patients, although in a very thin person, there may be insufficient adipose tissue to implement a sufficient retrieval; otherwise, the defect would be too obvious. In the case of a composite rib graft, previous trauma, especially resuscitation efforts, or surgery on the anterior chest wall, might be relative contraindications.

Previous nasal surgery, especially with removal of supportive nasal cartilage, or a history of cocaine abuse, might be a contraindication to the use of this tissue owing to insufficient vascularity. Likewise, prior obtaining of auricular cartilage with no obvious available tissue would be a real contraindication. However, in most patients, there is a sufficient "bank" of auricular cartilage that at least a small composite perichondrium/cartilage graft could be obtained.

PREOPERATIVE PLANNING

In the reconstruction of complex facial defects or deformities, in addition to a comprehensive head and neck examination, it may be is helpful to obtain a series of photographic images, which can be used to plan the surgical procedure(s). While not three dimensional, these images can be printed in black and white on regular paper, allowing for the drawing of flaps, site for retrieval of the composite graft, and any additional flaps that might be required. These prints or the color photographs can be shared with colleagues for consultation and for an educational lesson with the medical students and residents in how they would approach the reconstruction. Additionally, the images can be taken to the operating room and used as guidance for the conduct of the surgery.

Imaging studies might be helpful in several situations. In patients with lateral hemifacial atrophy, magnetic resonance imaging (MRI) can assist in determining what general volume of the dermis/adipose tissue composite graft will be required for rebulking. If there is any concern about the development of the underlying osseous framework, then a computed tomography scan will identify a bony discrepancy, as well as providing, through the soft tissue windows, the volumetric reduction in soft tissue. Likewise, fine-cut computed tomography of the laryngotracheal complex will be helpful in identifying the extent of the airway narrowing, both axial and circumferential, and will assist in the determination of whether laryngotracheoplasty using a composite perichondrium/cartilage graft would be appropriate.

SURGICAL TECHNIQUE

Most patients who require a composite auricular or nasal septal composite graft to reconstruct the eyelid, ear, or nose can be operated on under local anesthesia, supplemented by intravenous sedation, and under monitored anesthesia care (MAC). However, for more extensive procedures, pediatric cases, and when the graft is removed from the rib or abdomen, general anesthesia, supplemented by long-acting local anesthesia, will be required.

All of the surgical procedures noted above can be carried out with the patient in the supine position on the operating table. Minimal local anesthesia is used on pediatric patients, injected after general anesthesia has been attained. The use of 1% lidocaine with 1:200,000 epinephrine, volume adjusted for weight and age, is recommended. For adults who are under local anesthesia with sedation, it is helpful to inject the local anesthesia into both the donor and recipient sites before the surgeon scrubs and drapes, to allow sufficient time for both anesthesia and vasoconstriction to occur. A combination of equal volume of 1% lidocaine (10 mL) with 0.25% bupivacaine (10 mL) and 1:1,000 epinephrine (0.2 mL) will give adequate early acting local anesthesia along with a 6-hour prolonged anesthesia. The volumes indicated here will produce a 1:100,000 epinephrine concentration; this can be further diluted, if indicated by reducing the volume to 0.1 mL to produce a 1:200,000 concentration. Additionally, for the nasal septal graft, topical 0.05% oxymetazoline HCl solution applied to the mucosa via cottonoid pledgets will improve the mucosal vasoconstriction. It is important that the surgeon fully understands the risks and untoward effects of local anesthetics.

The patient is normally in the supine position, giving access to the entire face and ears, chest, and abdomen. If one is certain, both from the preoperative physical examination and imaging study (if performed), that there is sufficient nasal septum or abdominal adipose tissue, then the recipient site can be prepared before retrieving the composite graft. Conversely, if one has a good idea of the size of the graft needed for the recipient site, then the graft can be obtained first. It is better to not let the graft be ex vivo for too long. Prepping and draping the patient are performed as required for the exposure of both donor and recipient sites as well as the preference of the surgeon.

Composite Nasal Septal Graft Procedure

The illustrative case for this procedure is a 65-year-old male who sustained a gunshot wound to the right orbit, resulting in loss of the globe and lower eyelid. Following complete enucleation of the globe, an attempt to place an ocular conformer prosthesis was unsuccessful, due to an incompetent lower eyelid support structure (Fig. 44.1). The internal lamella (conjunctiva and tarsus) was absent, and there was no inferior cul-de-sac to receive the conformer. A composite mucosa/perichondrium/cartilage graft from the nasal septum was the graft of choice to reconstruct the internal eyelid lamella.

While in functional septal surgery the cartilaginous septum is exposed by elevating mucoperichondrial flaps through the left nostril, selection of which nasal cavity to conduct the graft removal will depend on the shape of the septum. If the septum is straight, no preference is required. However, because of the bowing of the eyelid over the globe, the ideal graft will have the mucosa located on the concave side of the cartilage graft. The surgical aim for the retrieval of this cartilage graft is to excise a full-thickness section of the septum—mucosa, perichondrium, and cartilage—leaving the contralateral mucoperichondrium intact. Prior preoperative planning will have determined the optimal size of the graft, but the actual size will depend on the anatomy of the patient's septal quadrangular cartilage.

Once the size and orientation of the graft to be retrieved is ascertained, its outline is imprinted in the mucosa with a guarded bipolar cautery, followed by taking the cautery incision down to cartilage with minimal tissue damage. Using a Cottle elevator, the mucoperichondrium around the graft outline is elevated away from the graft for 2 to 3 mm to facilitate exposure of the cartilage. It is important not to elevate the

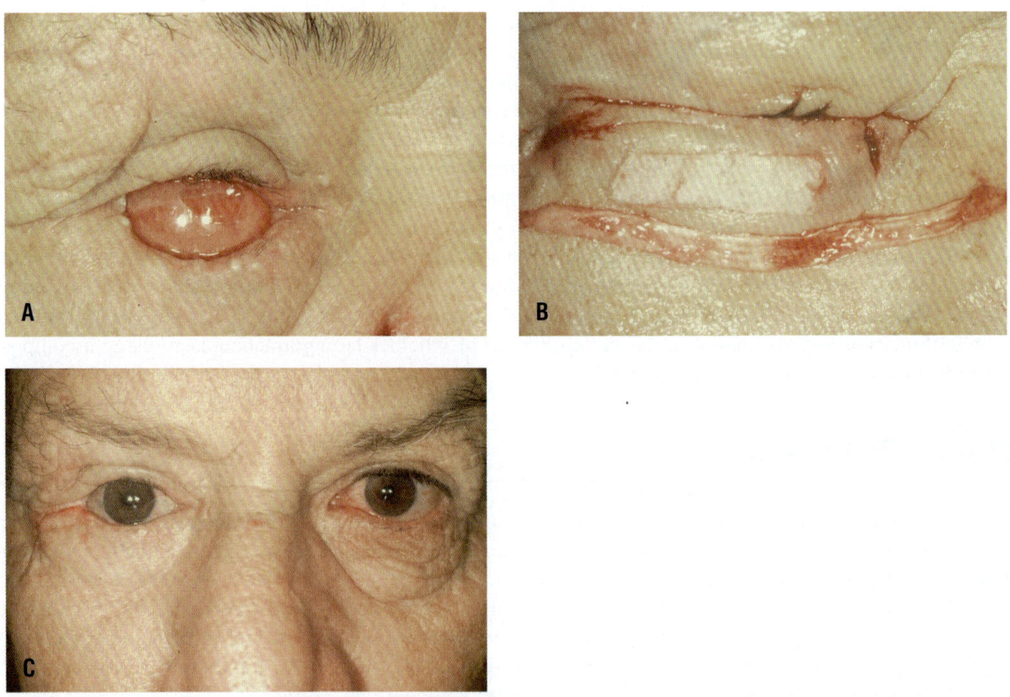

FIGURE 44.1 A: Incompetent right lower eyelid with ill-fitting ocular conformer in an adult male after a gunshot wound to the orbit. **B:** Composite nasal septal graft to reconstruct posterior lamella of right lower eyelid with temporalis fascia sling support. **C:** Patient 3 months after right lower eyelid reconstruction using a lateral Mustarde advancement flap and composite graft with ocular prosthesis in position. (Reprinted from Holt JE, Holt GR. *Ocular and adnexal trauma.* Alexandria, VA: American Academy of Otolaryngology-Head and Neck Surgery Foundation, 1983. With permission from the American Academy of Otolaryngology-Head and Neck Surgery Foundation, Alexandria, Virginia.)

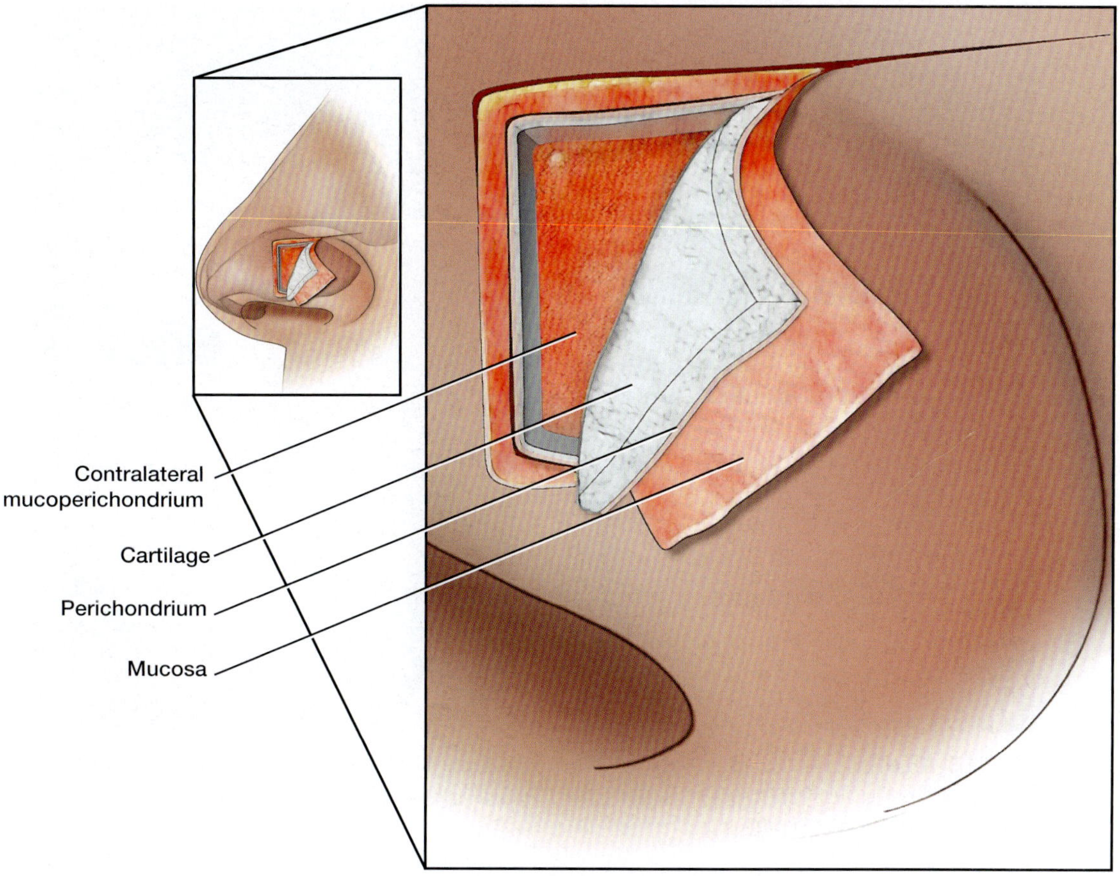

FIGURE 44.2 Artist's drawing of resection of the composite nasal septal graft, including mucosa, perichondrium, and cartilage. Note that the contralateral mucoperichondrium is left intact.

mucoperichondrium from the future graft cartilage. A D-knife is then used to gently incise the margins of the graft cartilage, which is then elevated from the mucoperichondrium on the undersurface of the cartilage to separate it from the rest of the septum (Fig. 44.2). The graft is now free and is placed in a physiologic saline solution. Gentle hemostasis of the remaining mucosal surfaces is carried out with the bipolar cautery. A Gelfoam sponge (absorbable gelatin sponge, Pfizer, New York, New York) coated with 2% Bactroban Nasal antibiotic ointment (mupirocin, GlaxoSmithKline, Research Park, NC) is sized and placed in the septal defect followed by low pressure nasal packing into both nostrils, also coated with mupirocin. The packing prevents the development of a small hematoma in the remaining septum and will be removed in 24 to 48 hours.

If not previously prepared to receive the graft, the eyelid is prepared by releasing scar tissue and exposing the posterior lamellar defect. A corneal protector is applied to the globe prior to preparing the eyelid recipient site. The anterior lamella (skin and orbicularis oculi muscle) is reconstructed primarily by mobilizing inferior maxillary/cheek skin or by performing a Mustarde lateral orbital advancement/rotational flap. The graft is placed posterior to the newly created anterior lamella with the concave mucosal surface placed against the globe. It is often necessary to provide additional antigravity support with a temporalis fascia "sling" placed anterior and sutured to the graft, and suspended from medical and lateral canthi using 4-0 Vicryl® sutures (polyglactin 910, Ethicon, Somerville, NJ). The anterior lamella is also sutured to the canthal bony attachments to give a second set of antigravity suspensions. The eyelid and globe are lubricated with an ophthalmic antibiotic ointment (bacitracin or erythromycin). Do not forget to remove the corneal protector.

Composite Dermis/Adipose Tissue Graft from the Abdomen to the Face Procedure

The illustrative case for this procedure is an 18-year-old female who began developing a left hemifacial atrophy at the age of 14 years (Fig. 44.3). Noted was a mild asymmetry of the left oral commissure, but the facial nerve function was normal. There was no involvement of the ipsilateral facial bones and the disease had been quiescent for 1 year. The patient wished to have some improvement in her appearance before attending college.

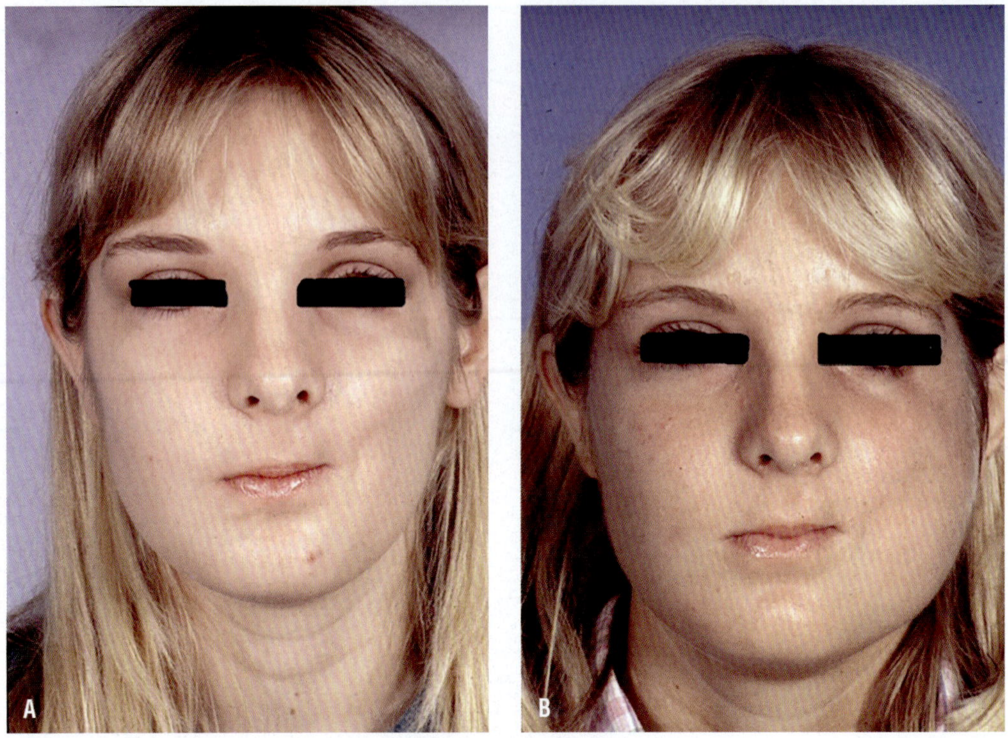

FIGURE 44.3 **A:** Left-sided Romberg's hemifacial atrophy in an adolescent female. Note also elevated left oral commissure. **B:** Patient 6 months after volumetric expansion of soft tissue defect left face after placement of abdominal dermis/adipose tissue graft via a rhytidectomy incision.

Because of the possibility for future disease exacerbation and the possibility of use of free transfer muscle grafts in the future, a simple filler procedure for rebulking the soft tissue of the left face was selected by the patient. A dermis/adipose tissue graft from the abdomen was selected as the graft of choice.

Normally, this procedure will be performed under general anesthesia, supplemented by local anesthetic infiltration and/or infraorbital nerve block. If this composite graft is being used as a filler to reduce the deformity following a parotidectomy or temporalis muscle transfer, the graft can be inserted at the conclusion of the primary procedure. Thus, exposure is already obtained. For the bulking of other facial areas, such as for lateral hemifacial atrophy, the deformity is exposed by either a modified Blair incision, or more favorably, a rhytidectomy incision. Once the area of soft tissue deficiency is exposed and hemostasis has been achieved, a determination of the volume and size of the composite graft can be confirmed using a 3D Gelfoam® template.

Attention is then turned to the left side of the abdomen, which is chosen because an incision in that area would not be confused with an appendectomy scar. Previously injected local anesthetic with epinephrine will have achieved tissue vasoconstriction. The surface area of the template from the face is outlined with a marking pen on the selected abdominal region, taking into consideration such factors as clothing position (swim suit, belt line) and scar camouflage. A horizontal incision is made of the midpoint of the outlined graft dimensions, but its length need only be two-thirds of the axial length of the proposed graft, as exposure for complete excision of the graft will be possible with skin hooks or small retractors. Flaps are elevated on each side of the incision sufficient to expose enough soft tissue to excise a graft. The flap elevation should be at a level that leaves 40% to 50% of the dermis on the flap and the remainder on the composite graft. Using the previous template as a guide, the graft is outlined and excised carefully, using bipolar cautery to achieve hemostasis. It is important to disturb the continuity of the graft as little as possible. The graft should be oversized beyond the template by 10% to 20%, as overcorrection of the recipient site defect is a goal of the procedure. It is helpful to taper or "feather" the margins of the graft to reduce the donor site defect after closure. The graft is washed and stored in physiologic saline while the donor site is closed in layers over a passive ¼″ Penrose drain using 4-0 Vicryl® suture for the deep closure and 5-0 Prolene® (polypropylene, Ethicon, Somerville, NJ) for the skin. Antibiotic ointment of the surgeon's choice is applied to the skin sutures followed by a pressure dressing.

The recipient site is re-exposed and the composite dermis/adipose tissue graft is placed in the defect and trimmed as appropriate to achieve a slight overcorrection of the volume. The graft should be tapered at the margins to create a smooth transition between the graft and the recipient soft tissues. 4-0 Vicryl® sutures are used to secure the graft into position, taking care to avoid the fine branches of the facial nerve and the muscles of facial expression. A final irrigation precedes the closure of the wound in the surgeon's standard fashion. A ¼″ Penrose drain can be helpful to prevent buildup of a seroma or hematoma. Antibiotic ointment is applied to the skin sutures, and a soft pressure dressing is considered if the area of bulking is large.

Composite Auricular Skin/Cartilage Composite Graft to Repair Nasal Stenosis or Collapse

The illustrative case is an adult with nasal vestibular stenosis, unilateral internal valvular collapse, or loss of nasal support at the level of the vestibule. This most commonly occurs after prolonged nasal intubation, extirpative tumor surgery, or trauma. The important features of these nasal conditions include loss of internal lining and loss of cartilaginous support. Thus, a composite skin/cartilage graft is very appropriate for the reconstruction process.

The recipient site can be prepared prior to obtaining the composite graft so that the appropriate-sized graft can be obtained. This may require a lateral alotomy, where the nasal ala is incised at the alar-cheek groove and rotated superiorly to expose the nasal vestibule and caudal septum. Alternatively, if the external nasal alar tissue is intact, but the internal lamella (skin and cartilage) requires the composite graft, the alotomy need not be performed. All scar tissue should be resected as required to re-establish the nasal airway, or the vestibular skin or septum debrided to normal, bleeding tissue to facilitate the graft survival.

Once the required size of the composite graft has been determined by precise measurement, the ear may be exposed for obtaining the graft. Typically for internal nasal vestibular reconstruction, the curvilinear conchal bowl region is an excellent location for the composite skin/cartilage graft as it approximates very nicely the requirement for resurfacing and supporting the vestibule. Following injection of local anesthetic with 1:100,000 epinephrine, the predetermined size and shape of the composite graft is outlined on the conchal bowl. Using sharp scalpel incision and a cartilage elevator to dissect the undersurface of the graft from the posterior soft tissues of the auricle, the graft is carefully excised. Caution is used to maintain the adherence of the anterior conchal skin to the cartilage for perfusion and nutrition, and the cartilage should remain intact during the dissection and elevation (Fig. 44.4A). The composite graft can be placed in a container of sterile saline to remain moist until the reconstruction commences. Repair of the anterior conchal defect is effected by elevating a crescent-shaped pedicled postauricular skin flap, which is then rotated into place through an incision in the conchal defect base (Fig. 44.4B). The skin flap is then loosely sutured into position using absorbable 5-0 Vicryl sutures for the dermis and 6-0 fast-absorbable chromic catgut sutures for the epidermis. An antibiotic saturated cotton ball is placed in the external auditory meatus, both to maintain the meatal opening and to reduce the risk of external canal bacterial pathogen implantation. The postauricular skin defect is closed

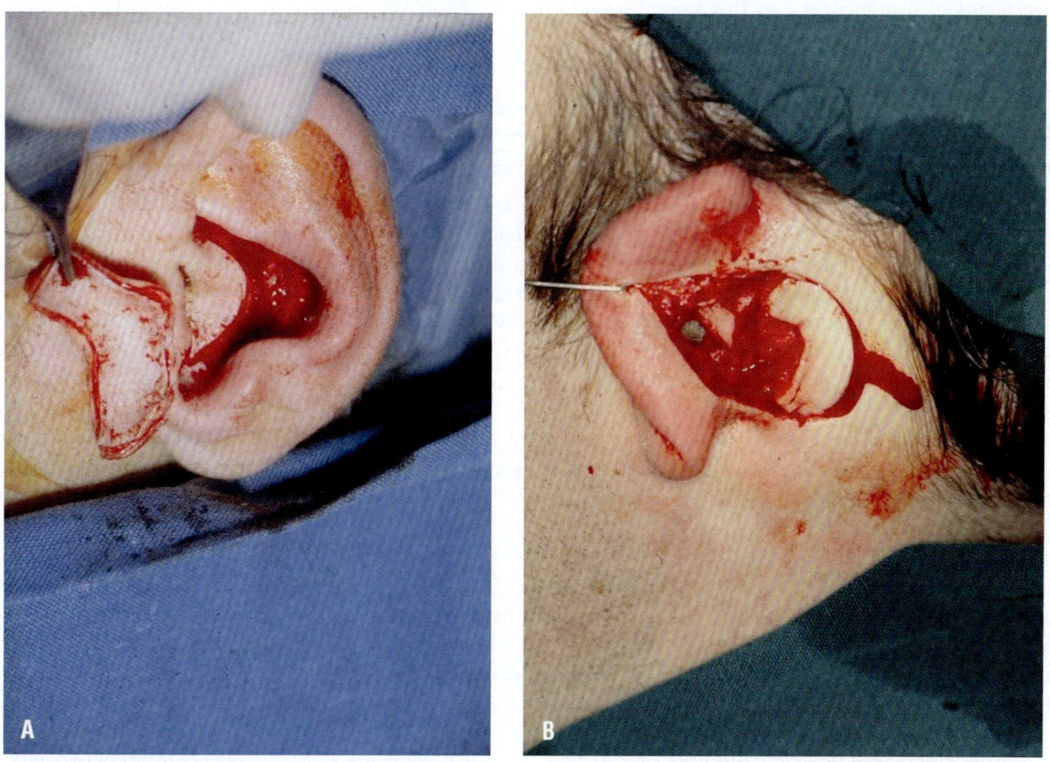

FIGURE 44.4 A: Dissected left auricular conchal skin/cartilage composite graft. **B:** Repair of anterior conchal bowl defect using a pedicled postauricular skin flap.

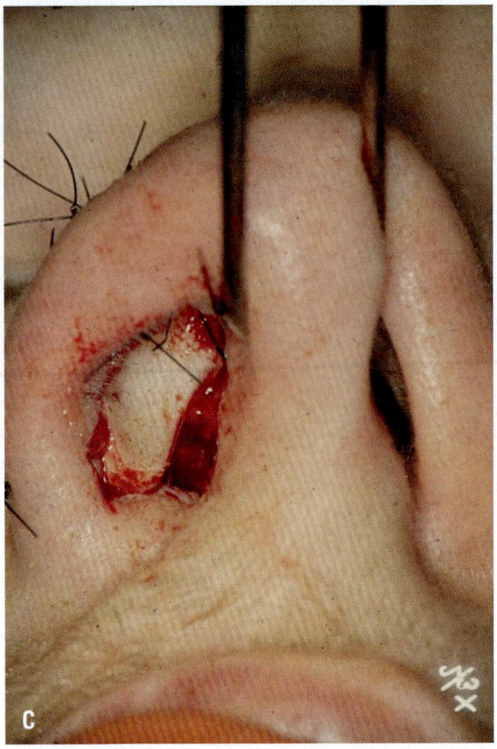

FIGURE 44.4 *(Continued)*
C: Auricular conchal composite graft sutured loosely in right vestibular defect for support and internal lining.

primarily with 4-0 Vicryl sutures in the dermis and 5-0 Prolene for the epidermis. A soft, compressive mastoid dressing is applied at the end of the procedure.

The composite graft is then positioned into the nasal vestibular defect, trimming to proper size and shape as needed. It is sutured into position with loose 4-0 chromic catgut sutures or other absorbable sutures, which are not tight and restrictive (Fig. 44.4C). If needed, several "bolster" sutures of 4-0 Prolene can be used to gently compress the composite graft against the recipient soft tissue so as to close the potential "dead space" and reduce the risk of a hematoma formation. The bolster suture can be tied in a nonrestrictive manner over a small cotton or Gelfoam pledget over the skin of the external ala. Antibiotic ointment is applied both externally and internally, but no internal stent is normally required. There should be no firm compressive forces internally on the composite graft to allow for plasmatic imbibition and inosculation.

POSTOPERATIVE CARE

A dose of broad spectrum antibiotic dose is administered intravenously in the preoperative area and continued in the oral form for 7 to 10 days after the surgical procedure. Generally, composite grafts require a somewhat longer use of perioperative antibiotics than other, nongraft procedures of the face. The soft pressure dressing is removed, if utilized, and both the donor and recipient sites are inspected. The nasal packing can be removed at 24 hours and the septum inspected for bleeding, but the Gelfoam® packing in the nasal septum donor defect should remain in place for at least 48 hours. If necessary, gentle nasal packing or a soft external dressing can be reapplied if the wound inspection requires it. In the case of a nasal composite graft recipient site, it should be gently cleaned with hydrogen peroxide and saline daily, with topical application of antibiotic ointment using a cotton-tipped applicator. When used, the bolster suture should be removed within 72 hours so as not to compromise the overlying nasal skin. The mastoid dressing can be left in place for 48 hours, but should be removed then to inspect the donor site and replaced if edematous. For auricular grafts, it is wise to ensure oral antibiotic coverage for at least 5 to 7 days.

In the case of an abdominal composite dermis/adipose tissue graft, the drains should remain in place until there is no significant evidence of drainage on the dressings, which is usually about 48 hours. The fatty acids released into the tissues from damage to the cell membranes of adipose tissue cells causes an irritative serous transudate, so the drain should not be removed prematurely. For the nasal septal graft, the mucoperichondrium remaining in the septal defect will begin to mucosalize quickly, but the area needs to be kept moist for at least a month with gentle saline sprays. Crusting should be removed in the clinic to prevent local tissue infection and drying.

Skin sutures are typically removed 1 week after surgery, particularly in the region of the abdomen, where movement and irritation from clothing could retard the incision adhesion. If a nasal septal composite graft has been used to reconstruct the inner lamella of the eyelid, a consultation with the ophthalmology colleague should occur at least 1 week after surgery, sooner if symptoms or signs indicate, to observe the status of the cornea. Topical ophthalmic antibiotic ointment can be discontinued by the third postoperative day if the wounds look clean, so as to prevent a topical allergic reaction to the antibiotic. Artificial tears and lubricating nighttime ointment can be applied instead.

COMPLICATIONS

Fortunately, the complications for the use of composite grafts are of low frequency and low grade. Primarily, they involve the following and the patient should be counseled accordingly:

- Collapse of the conchal bowl, particularly at the external auditory meatus
- Corneal abrasion
- Epiphora
- Epistaxis
- Excessive resorption or loss of volume or support
- Hematoma at the donor site
- Hypertrophic scarring
- Infection
- Partial or complete death of the graft
- Septal perforation

RESULTS

Composite grafts are a solid element of the reconstructive armamentarium of the Otolaryngologist–Head and Neck Surgeon. They are a rung in the reconstructive ladder, which also includes primary closure, epithelial or dermis grafts, local or regional flaps, and free flap transfer. There is increasing use of rib cartilage grafts, which if the perichondrium is left on the cartilage, can be considered a form of composite graft. It can be used in nasal and airway reconstruction.

In general, in the absence of infection or hematoma, composite grafts heal very well. Since there will be some lysis of adipose tissue cells in the dermis/adipose tissue graft, it is wise to overcorrect the defect by 10% or more. It may take up to a year for the shrinking process to occur. If the resorption of excess adipose tissue does not occur, one can reduce the bulk using liposuction technique.

Healing of the nasal septum, if the area is kept clean of crusting, is sufficient to provide good epithelialization of the septum. If a septal perforation should occur during the surgery, it would be wise to suture a small piece of human acellular dermis over the rent as a protective covering and scaffolding for healing.

Auricular composite grafts to the nasal vestibule and nasal septum have an excellent chance for survival and maintenance of the stenosed or collapsed airway. Because the grafts are typically 2.0 to 2.5 cm in length, and narrower in width, the survival is normally greater than 90%. The most difficult reconstruction is in the case of nasal vestibular stenosis, which may require multiple composite grafts, including from both auricles, and the application of a soft internal, custom-molded stent for several months. Usually, the conchal donor site assumes a near-normal appearance after the defect closure has healed.

PEARLS

- Composite grafts, in the form of dermis/adipose tissue, mucosa/perichondrium/cartilage, or perichondrium/rib cartilage, can be important elements of the reconstructive ladder for the face and neck region.
- Composite grafts may be obtained from the auricle (conchal bowl and helix), nasal septum, anterior chest wall, and abdomen and can be utilized for structural support and internal lining and as a soft tissue filler.
- Selecting a composite graft will depend on the tissue requirements for the reconstructive procedure.
- If a nasal septal composite graft is used, it can be either mucosa/perichondrium/cartilage or perichondrium/cartilage (if an internal lining is not required). The mucoperichondrium deep to the removed composite graft must be kept intact to prevent a perforation and can be protected with a gelatin/antibiotic dressing as epithelialization of the perichondrium occurs.
- In reconstruction of the posterior lamella of the eyelid, the mucoperichondrium of the composite graft faces the globe and is optimally on the concave side of the graft. An additional antigravity support of a temporalis fascia sling can be salutary. Collaboration with an ophthalmologist is very important.
- Dermis/adipose tissue grafts are taken from the left side of the abdomen, in order not to be confused with an appendectomy scar on the right side, and is oversized by 10% to allow for fat cell lysis over time. The dermis is split between the graft and the skin flaps, in the latter case allowing the wound to be securely closed.

- Composite grafts to the nasal vestibule, typically from an auricular conchal donor site, have excellent healing as long as they are not sutured in place too tightly or compressed with a firm internal stent. A soft, molded internal stent with an airway opening might be required in vexing cases of vestibular stenosis.
- Perioperative antibiotics should be used for up to 10 days, especially with cartilage-containing composite grafts, to decrease the risk of infection and resorption of the graft.
- Large defects, such as with an abdominal donor site and a facial fill, usually require passive drains to reduce the risk of hematoma or seroma, along with a compressive dressing.

PITFALLS

- Failure to adequately assess the adequacy of the nasal septal donor site or abdominal donor site before initiating the procedure and learning too late that there is insufficient tissue for the composite graft.
- Failure to protect the cornea prior to the eyelid reconstruction will likely cause corneal damage.
- Infection or hematoma at the recipient site will likely compromise the integrity of the vascular ingrowth.
- Choosing a composite graft for a reconstructive procedure when another option in the reconstructive armamentarium would have been better.

INSTRUMENTS TO HAVE AVAILABLE

Graft Retrieval

- Standard nasal surgery set

Graft Placement

- Fine-toothed ophthalmic forceps (0.3 or 0.5 mm)
- Castroviejo ophthalmic needle holder with lock (for eyelid grafting)

SUGGESTED READING

Holt JE, Holt GR. *Ocular and adnexal trauma*. Alexandria, VA: American Academy of Otolaryngology-Head and Neck Surgery Foundation, 1983.

Walter C. *Plastisch-chirurgische Eingriffe im Kopf-Hals-Bereich*. New York, NY: Thieme, 1997.

Weerda H. *Reconstructive facial plastic surgery: a problem-solving manual*. New York, NY: Thieme, 2001.

45 CALVARIAL BONE GRAFTS

John L. Frodel Jr

INTRODUCTION

Calvarial bone grafting (CBG) is a well-established technique in the reconstruction of the skull base, midface, orbital, and nasal defects. The treatment of bone defects in a pediatric population, while uncommon, has had noteworthy outcomes as well. However, with continued evolution of excellent alloplastic implants, including sophisticated computer-generated implants for the upper craniomaxillofacial skeleton, the frequency of autogenous reconstruction has been proportionately reduced. The modern developments of alloplastic implants have also highlighted the benefits of autogenous materials in the reconstruction of the facial skeleton. Among the various choices available to surgeons, CBG remains an important and viable resource in facial plastic and reconstructive surgery.

Bone grafts have been an important component of craniomaxillofacial reconstruction for many decades with grafting from various donor sites including calvarium, iliac crest, and rib. Each donor material has been popular at various points in time. The advantages of calvarial bone over other donor sites include direct donor site proximity to the reconstruction site, minimal donor site morbidity, and the observation that there may be less resorption of calvarial bone in comparison to iliac, iliac crest, and rib bone. Conversely, the disadvantage of calvarial bone is the relative lack of cancellous bone and the inability to bend calvarium except in the pediatric population. In this chapter, I will focus on the technique of harvesting calvarial bone grafts and then provide several examples of how such bone grafts can be used.

HISTORY

Each patient should undergo a complete systems-based examination including cardiac, pulmonary, and neurologic. A complete history of all medical conditions, surgeries, medications, and allergies is required. A focused history with regard to the surgical site of interest is performed in a systematic fashion with regard to bone loss, soft tissue compromise, and impaired function. It is particularly important to assess whether the patient has a history of neurologic surgery, scalp surgery, diffuse scalp burns, or radiation therapy to the head. History of head trauma should also be noted. Be sure to note the patient's dominant side, as it is often recommended to take a bone graft from the skull over the nondominant hemisphere. All of the patient's concerns are addressed as well as his or her expectations of surgery.

PHYSICAL EXAMINATION

A complete head and neck examination is performed as many patients have sustained complex injuries. Evaluation and documentation of V1 to V3 and VII is required to consider any deficiencies prior to surgery.

A focus on the size and character of the defect to be reconstructed is documented photographically and in the written record. A careful examination of the scalp is also important to assess for any previous scars, surgical interventions, burns, radiation effects, hair loss, or soft tissue compromise.

INDICATIONS

Indications for calvarial bone grafts include reconstructive cases in which osseous grafting material is essential for recontouring or repair. Anterior skull base trauma, nasal trauma, and defects secondary to extirpative oncologic procedures are several examples. CBG is particularly useful for reconstruction in severe cases of nasal bone and cartilaginous comminution. CBG can also be used in select cases for reconstruction of upper midfacial defects in conjunction with alloplastic material and vascularized tissue. The use of CBG to reconstruct the atrophic maxilla and mandible for facilitating dental implants has also been described.

CONTRAINDICATIONS

Harvesting of a calvarial bone graft is often contraindicated in the younger pediatric patient because of the thinness of the skull and lack of development of the diploic space. Modified soft tissue reconstruction should be planned in patients with severe burn injury or diffuse field effects of radiation treatments due to concerns about delayed wound healing or dehiscence.

PREOPERATIVE PLANNING

Depending on the indication for CBG, consideration of the amount of bone that is required may dictate the type of bone graft that is harvested. In particular, if a large solid piece of bone is required as opposed to smaller strips of bone, it might be advantageous to take advantage of a craniotomy bone segment and split this bone to obtain a larger sheet of calvarial grafting material. The most common situation in which this might exist is for reconstruction of the skull base in either trauma or anterior skull base reconstruction after tumor extirpation. Conversely, for reconstruction of the maxilla and periorbital regions, which are the most common indications for the requirement of grafting material, outer table bone grafts are usually adequate.

Consideration of the precise location of the skull where the grafts are harvested is important. One needs to be aware of the differences in the thickness of the skull and the presence of developmental sutures at which point there is fusion of the inner and outer cortex. The two principal developmental sutures of concern are the coronal suture between the frontal and parietal bones as well as the sagittal suture in the midline. The latter is particularly important due to the presence of the sagittal sinus deep to this area. Accordingly, the midline should be avoided. Other issues include the curvature of the bone as in some cases curvature is desired (e.g., in the zygoma, orbit, or frontal bone), whereas in other areas, a flatter bone graft may be desired (e.g., the nasal dorsum). The most common site for outer calvarial graft harvesting is the parietal bone lateral to the sagittal developmental suture, posterior to the coronal developmental suture, and posterior to the temporal line (or attachment of the temporalis muscle).

SURGICAL TECHNIQUE

Harvesting of the Graft

While exposure to this region is often facilitated by the existence of a coronal approach that may have already been performed, occasionally, direct incisions are required over the parietal region for the sole purpose of harvest for a calvarial bone graft. I favor a geometric incision to best camouflage such incisions just as I favor such geometric designs for coronal incisions. The periosteum over the desired parietal harvest area is exposed and adequate retraction is required. While numerous techniques exist for harvesting the outer table graft, I use the combination of drilling the periphery of the desired graft shape with a cutting burr followed by the use of either a sharp curved osteotome or right-angled sagittal saw to enter the diploic space between the outer and inner cortex as well as to separate the outer table graft from the inner table within this space (Figs. 45.1 to 45.4). Keys to successful harvest of the graft include precise identification of the diploic space with the cutting burr. This is important because on rare occasions, there is very limited or no diploic space and the surgeon must be aware that, in such cases, in an effort to identify this bleeding diploic space, one may actually encounter the dura. Accordingly, it is very important to be observant of the appearance of dura during this process. A similar key is that while cutting horizontally through a diploic space with either an osteotome or saw, the dura may again be encountered. I always make the assumption that when in doubt, the dura may

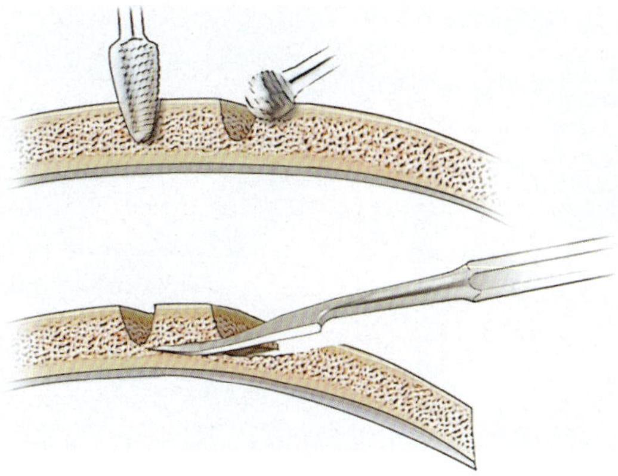

FIGURE 45.1
Top: Cutting burrs are used to identify the diploic space and outline bone grafts. **Bottom:** Using an osteotome to develop graft between inner and outer calvarial cortices.

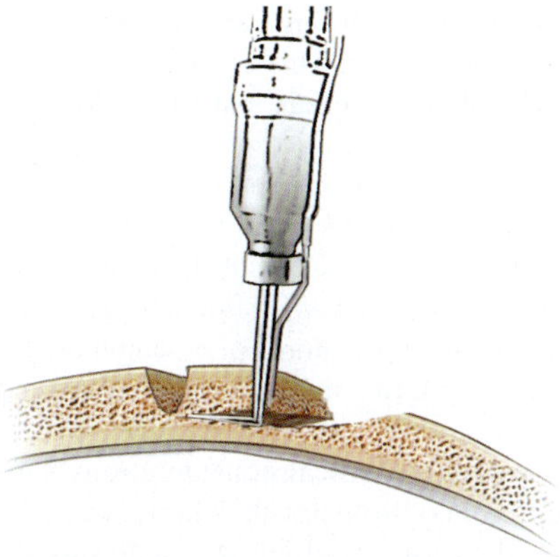

FIGURE 45.2
Using a right-angled sagittal saw to develop graft between inner and outer calvarial cortices.

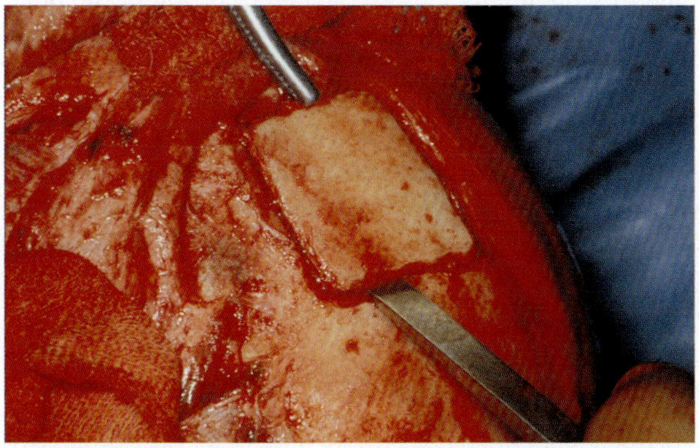

FIGURE 45.3
An osteotome is used to start elevation of the bone graft.

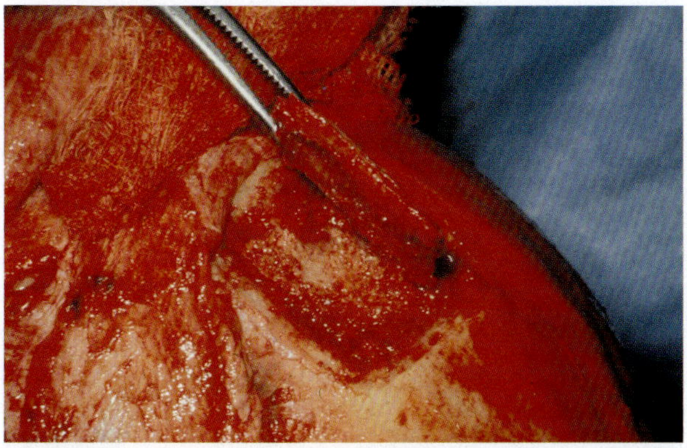

FIGURE 45.4
Bone graft elevated.

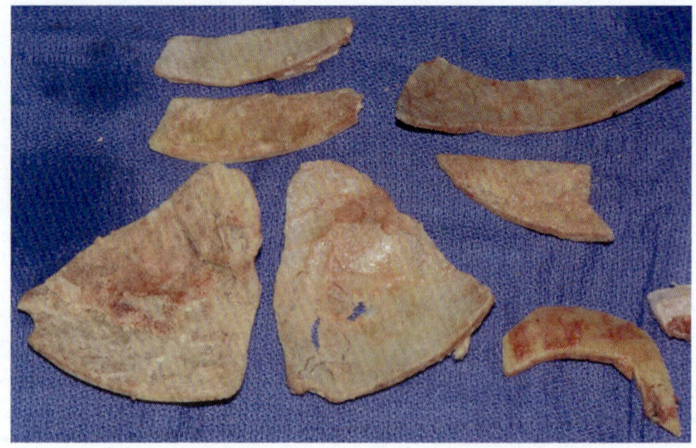

FIGURE 45.5
Multiple inner calvarial cortex grafts after being split with a reciprocating saw and osteotome.

be exposed and I remain diligent in elevating with either the saw or osteotome in a plane and direction that is truly parallel to the inner cortex and the underlying dura. This is facilitated by the use of very sharp and curved osteotomes as well as efficient right-angled saws. It should be noted that during the harvest of outer table grafts, diploic veins may be encountered and significant bleeding may occur. This can be alarming at times and may be requiring packing of the wound with resorbable hemostatic materials, but I have found it has never been a major problem.

When larger amounts of bone are required or a single graft of significant dimensions is required (e.g., >1.5 to 2 cm in width and approximately 4 to 5 cm in length), consideration should be made for the harvest of an inner table bone graft. Fortunately, this situation generally arises during reconstruction of the cranial base and oftentimes when a craniotomy has been performed. In this case, the inner table is meticulously separated from the outer table of the craniotomy bone flap. This can be completed with an osteotome or a combined use of an osteotome and a reciprocating saw (my preference). Large amounts of grafting material can be harvested in this fashion (Fig. 45.5).

Finally, a unique situation exists in pediatric patients. While the philosophical considerations vary between surgeons, I prefer to use autogenous materials for upper craniomaxillofacial skeletal reconstruction whenever possible, particularly in younger children as opposed to use of alloplastic materials. In children under approximately age 8, I have found that split outer cortical grafts can be harvested and actually offer many advantages. Because of the less brittle or softer nature of the relatively underdeveloped pediatric calvarium, one can use a sharp osteotome to sequentially elevate the outer portion of the outer cortex as a graft. This graft will have microfractures within it, appearing similar to a thick "potato chip" but can generally be harvested without much difficulty (Figs. 45.6 and 45.7). While these grafts tend to be quite curved, the indications in these patients often require a curved bone graft, such as in orbital reconstruction.

It should be noted that, while the donor site morbidity is uncommon (see the "Complications" section), an obligatory defect is created at the parietal donor site. Either this can be addressed by smoothing out the surrounding bone ridge with a large cutting burr or the defect can actually be reconstructed. I favor limited reconstruction of such defects commonly using porous polyethylene sheeting with small screw fixation and have found this to be a very useful method to prevent contour deformities in the donor site.

Placement of the Graft

While a number of grafts are placed into defect positions that do not require fixation (e.g., the orbital cavity), the majority of grafts do require fixation for optimal results. One of the controversies surrounding the use of autogenous bone grafting is the understandable concern for bone resorption. I feel that recipient

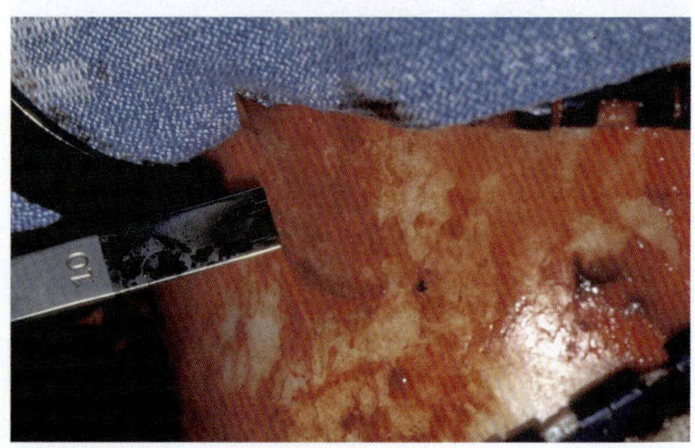

FIGURE 45.6
Using a sharp osteotome, a split outer table graft is harvested in the pediatric patient.

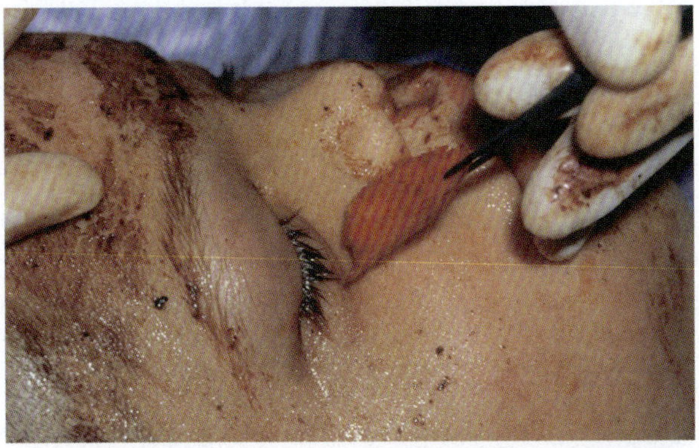

FIGURE 45.7
The curved "potato chip" pediatric bone graft being placed into the orbit.

site preparation and adequate fixation are the keys to retention of the bone grafts. Whenever possible, it is optimal to have overlap of the recipient bone with the inset bone graft. Examples include the orbital rims as well as the frontal bone region. If adequate exposure exists, the surrounding recipient bone can be burred down to allow for overlap of the contoured bone graft. This also facilitates the use of lag screw fixation techniques using small upper craniomaxillofacial screws. I have found this to facilitate excellent retention of the bone graft over time. Figure 45.8 demonstrates the use of a bone graft to reconstruct a right zygomatic arch. Note the graft edges have been burred to underlay the native recipient zygoma and posterior zygomatic arch. Conversely, Figure 45.9 shows the placement of a calvarial bone graft into an infraorbital rim defect, where the medial and lateral recipient areas have been burred to allow for a precise overlay placement of the bone graft also fixated using lag screw fixation. Perhaps the most absolute indication for bone graft placement would be in the situation where bone has been comminuted and/or lost in Le Fort fractures. Figure 45.10 demonstrates an intraoral view of the left maxilla noting plates have been placed across the medial and lateral buttress but with significant bone defects. Figures 45.11 and 45.12 show the placement of contoured bone grafts underneath these plates. I find that after plate placement, if the screws are loosened, the graft can be inset underneath the plate and then is tightly secured by tightening of the screws, noting that no screws actually pass through these grafts. This patient had eventual exposure of the plate in the left lateral buttress of the maxilla, which required its removal. Figure 45.13 shows the healed left lateral buttress 1.5 years after initial placement, at the time of plate removal. Note the solid, contoured healed bone graft.

POSTOPERATIVE MANAGEMENT

Each patient is given an oral antibiotic for 5 to 7 days after surgery. A standardized treatment of all surgical wounds is as follows:

- If a drain is placed, it should be removed once the output of the drain is lower than 30 mL per 24 hours.
- All surgical incisions should be kept dry for 48 to 72 hours postoperatively.
- Each surgical incision is cleaned with ½ strength hydrogen peroxide daily two to three times per day to prevent crusting and accumulation of topical ointment.
- Antibiotic ointment should be applied to the wound four times a day for 7 days.
- Wounds should not be immersed in water for 2 weeks after surgery.

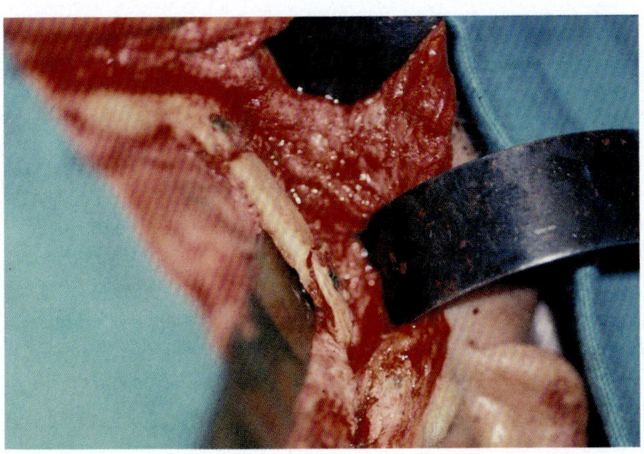

FIGURE 45.8
An underlay bone graft into a zygomatic arch defect, secured with lag screw fixation.

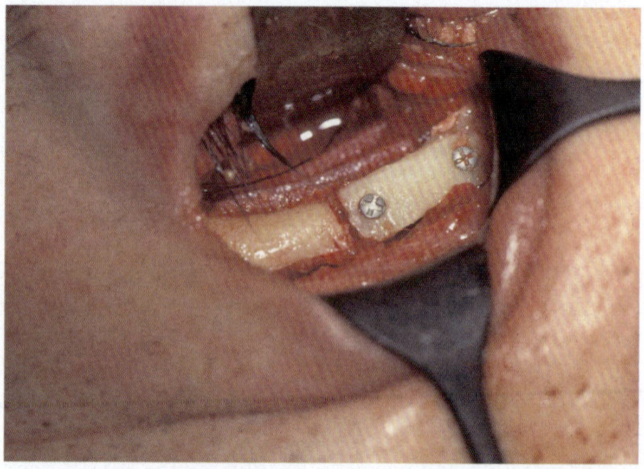

FIGURE 45.9
An overlay bone graft along an infraorbital rim defect, secured with lag screw fixation.

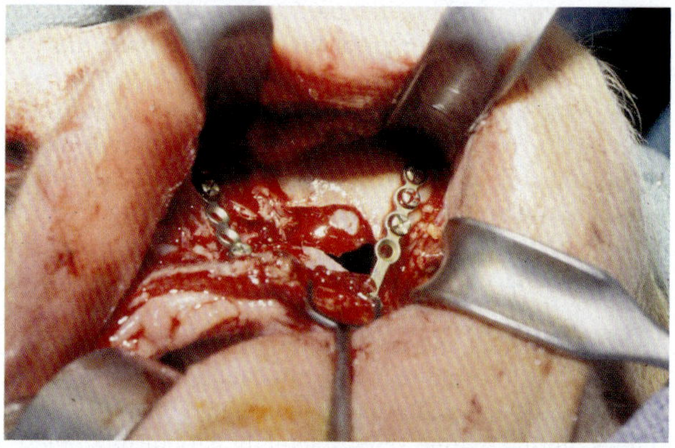

FIGURE 45.10
After reduction and plate fixation of an edentulous maxillary fracture, significant structural defects exist.

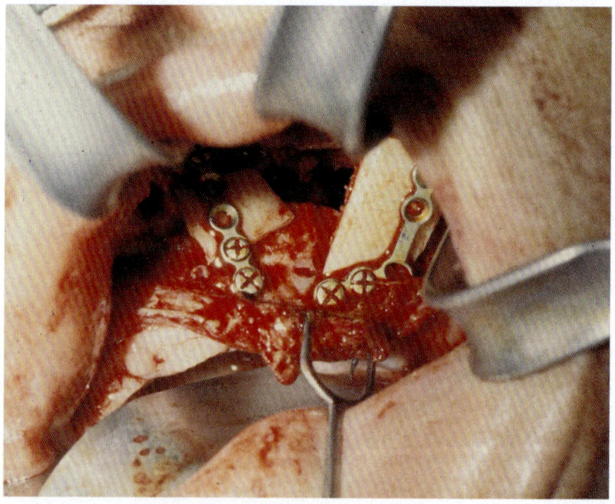

FIGURE 45.11
Placement of calvarial bone grafts under the loosened maxillary buttress plates.

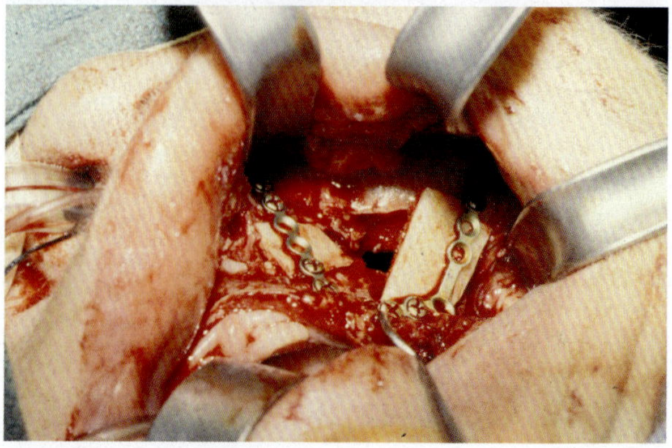

FIGURE 45.12
Final fixation of the maxillary buttress plates.

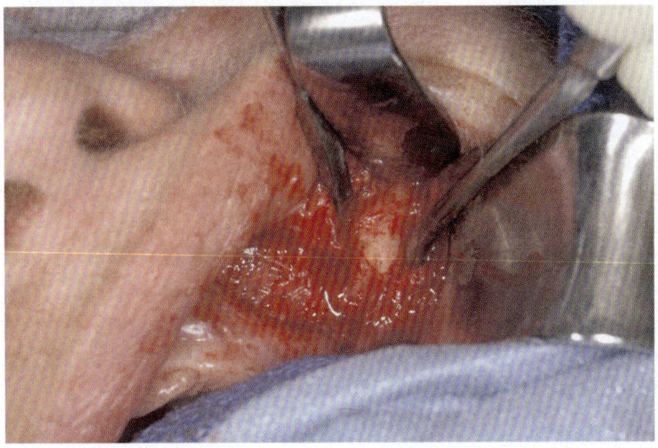

FIGURE 45.13
Healed buttress bone grafts upon plate removal 1.5 years after placement.

COMPLICATIONS

Contour Deformity

Fortunately, bone graft complications are relatively unusual. The most predictable morbidities with calvarial bone graft harvest are the contour deformities that were discussed earlier. Since I switched from burring down the edges around the bone graft, which often left a mild flattening in the parietal region in the area of the bone graft, to reconstructing the defect with porous polyethylene implants with screw fixation, such contour deformities and complaints about the donor site are quite unusual.

Intracranial Injury/CSF Leak

In my experience there have been no intracranial sequelae such as CSF leaks or intracranial infection although these have been reported in the literature. On several occasions, I have had dural exposure and on one occasion had a significant dural tear. This tear was closed primarily and no sequelae were noted. The key is to recognize such dural exposures during the harvest of the bone grafts, which then allows prevention of further injury. When harvesting multiple grafts, not unlike as shown in the diagram in Figures 45.1 and 45.2, I find that meticulous technique in patients during the harvest of the first graft will identify the particular anatomy of the cortices so that one can determine the thickness of the diploic space as well as thickness of the outer cortex. Once this first graft is elevated, it is much easier to harvest such subsequent grafts because of the understanding of the skull anatomy in each particular patient.

Calvarium Integrity

When using inner cortex bone grafts, the risks and complications are more related to the actual elevation of the craniotomy bone segment. One could question whether the resultant placement of a single cortex bone graft might lead to weakness, but we are not aware of reported problems with the replacement of an outer cortex only craniotomy bone segment.

Incisional/Tension Alopecia

Scarring and hair loss along any of the surgical incisions are optimized with low-tension closure of the surgical incision. Attention is given to the meticulous reapproximation of the galea while closure of the hair-bearing skin is performed with staples only. Wounds under excessive tension, due to limited tissue or closure technique, are at risk for hair loss and well-observed scarring.

RESULTS

Long-term outcomes of the CBG have revealed relatively low resorption rates in both animal and human studies. In children, CBG is a reasonable reconstructive option, as I have reported the outcomes of CBG in pediatric patients without significant donor site morbidity, but is recommended for more experienced surgeons in the treatment of this patient population.

PEARLS

- If grafts greater than 2 cm in width × 5 cm in length are required, one should consider inner cranial table bone graft harvest.
- Poor hemostasis can impair visualization and lead to crossing of the inner cortex and possible dural injury.
- Harvest of outer cortex bone grafts is facilitated by identification of the diploic space between the inner and outer cortex, performed with a broad cutting burr.
- Sharp osteotomes are required for the harvest of outer table bone grafts. An alternative use of a right-angled sagittal saw or, in some cases, a reciprocal saw can be very helpful.
- Long-term survival of the bone graft is facilitated by proper preparation of the recipient area and as rigid of fixation as possible, depending on the defect requirements.
- An absolute indication for CBG is in the acute reconstruction of the maxillary buttresses.

PITFALLS

- Patients with advanced age, osteoporosis, or other calcium-depleting conditions may not have suitable bone stock or strength.
- Poor graft fixation and/or compromised surrounding viable tissues can compromise reconstructive results.
- Graft harvesting requires additional operative time and length of general anesthesia.

LIST OF INSTRUMENTS

- Standard plastic surgery set
- Sharp osteotomes (smaller sizes ideal)
- Curved wide-angle osteotome
- 15 blade scalpel
- Right-angled sagittal saw
- Drill and cutting burr
- Miniplates for reconstruction

ACKNOWLEDGMENT

The author would like to thank Prabhat Bhama, MD, for his contributions to the writing of this chapter. His work in the writing, editing, and figure creation for this chapter is greatly appreciated, without which this chapter would not have been possible.

SUGGESTED READING

Baser B, Shahani R, Khanna S, et al. Calvarial bone grafts for augmentation rhinoplasty. *J Laryngol Otol* 1991;105(2):1018–1020.

Frodel JL. Outer table calvarial bone graft harvest in pediatric patients. *Otolaryngol Head Neck Surg* 1999;121:78–82.

Frodel J, Marentette LJ, Quatela VC, et al. Calvarial bone graft harvest. Techniques, considerations, and morbidity. *Arch Otolaryngol Head Neck Surg* 1993;119(1):17–23.

Lee S, Frodel, JL. The use of high density polyethylene implants in facial deformities. *Arch Otolaryngol Head Neck Surg* 1998;124:1219–1223.

Sahoo NK, Rangan M. Role of split calvarial graft in reconstruction of craniofacial defects. *J Craniofac Surg* 2012;23(4):e326–e331.

46 TEMPORALIS MUSCLE TENDON TRANSPOSITION FOR FACIAL PARALYSIS

Kofi Boahene

INTRODUCTION

Facial paralysis can be a devastating injury that results in functional impairment of the eyelids, nose, and lips. Impaired facial expression during communication and the associated blunted emotional exchange significantly affects both the patient and the interactive circle and can lead to depression and strained relationships. The surgical transfer of functional muscle units to the face is presently the only effective option for restoring tone and dynamic animation when the facial muscles are irreversibly paralyzed. Irreversible paralysis of the facial muscle may be the result of prolonged atrophy from chronic denervation, primary muscle disease, extensive scarring, congenital paralysis, and radical surgical resection. Common to these causes is the absence of viable motor units that can respond to neural input. Functional muscle units can be transferred to the face as free neuromuscular units that require reestablishment of neurovascular input using microsurgical techniques. Advantages of free functional muscle transfer include the flexibility in selecting the donor muscle, desired vector of muscle excursion, muscle length and tension, and donor nerve. Recruiting the contralateral facial nerve to drive the free functional muscle provides the potential for achieving a voluntary smile. Free functional muscle transfer is, however, technique intensive and does not provide immediate reanimation. An alternative to free functional muscle flaps for the correction of irreversible facial paralysis is the transposition of regional muscle tendon units (MTU) that maintain their original neurovascular supply. An intact MTU with a given function may be repurposed to perform a new function by releasing and reattaching the tendon from its native insertion site to a new target. Candidate muscles for regional muscle transfer to the paralyzed face include the temporalis, masseter, platysma, and digastric muscles. The major advantage for regional MTU transfer is the potential for immediate restoration of dynamic facial movement in a single-stage procedure. The transfer of the temporalis MTU is the most commonly described regional MTU procedure for facial paralysis and is the focus of this chapter. The transfer of the temporalis muscle as an MTU is distinguished from the transfer of the muscle belly over the zygomatic arch.

In 1952, McLaughlin introduced the concept and technique of mobilizing and transposing the temporalis tendon for facial suspension. This technique was later replaced by the temporalis turndown flap popularized by Rubin, Baker, and Conley. This traditional method had several disadvantages including donor site depression, midfacial widening, and nonanatomic contraction of transposed muscle segment. The temporalis MTU transfer later underwent several refinements to improve functionality and aesthetic appearance. Several authors highlighted the advantages of temporalis transfer in an orthodromic manner. Breidahl modified this technique by approaching the tendon externally, and subsequently, Croxson further modified the procedure by accessing the coronoid–tendon complex through the nasolabial fold. Boahene as well as others adopted a minimally invasive approach for transposing the temporalis MTU through the buccal space sublabial incisions.

The successful application of the temporalis MTU for facial reanimation depends on a fine-tuned adoption and application of the principles and biomechanics of MTU transfer. The principles of MTU transfer have

TABLE 46.1 The Fundamental Principles of Muscle Tendon Unit Transfer
The muscle selected as an MTU donor must be expendable and functioning
Adequate soft tissue bed for the transfer tendon
Full passive range of motion of the involved joints (no fixed deformity)
Adequate excursion and length of donor tendon
Direct line of pull
Suitable insertion technique and firm fixation
Synergy of transfer
Single function for each transferred tendon

evolved over a century through extensive experience in upper extremity reconstruction following injuries of the median, ulnar, and radial nerves. Even though the complexity of coordinated movements of facial muscles poses several challenges in achieving optimal functional outcome, the fundamental principles of MTU transfer and subsequent rehabilitation are applicable to all muscles including facial muscles. Table 46.1 outlines the fundamental principles of MTU transfer in extremities, the basic tenets of which may be applicable to all types of functional muscle transfer procedures including the temporalis muscle tendon transfer.

Of the fundamental principles of MTU transfer, the insertion of the temporalis muscle at the ideal length and tension for adequate excursion is the most important principle necessary for achieving a dynamic smile instead of a mere static suspension.

HISTORY

When selecting patients for a temporalis tendon transfer, a thorough history is necessary to establish the cause and duration of the paralysis. Causes of facial paralysis that allow for potential spontaneous recovery should prompt close follow-up and conservative measures for eye protection. Paralysis from progressive neurologic diseases that may involve multiple cranial nerves including the trigeminal nerve or muscles group as in muscular dystrophy should prompt careful considerations before suggesting a temporalis MTU.

The history taking should also elicit information about previous treatments. Patients who have underdone the classic temporalis muscle transfer procedure in which a segment of the muscle belly was transferred over the zygomatic arch are still candidates for reversal and transfer of the tendon as an orthodromic MTU transfer.

A history of radiation therapy over the lateral face is important to note as secondary fibrosis may modify tissue glide planes and limit the potential excursion that may result from transfer of the temporalis tendon. While not a contraindication for the temporalis MTU, the effects of prior radiation on outcomes should be discussed with the patient prior to the procedure.

PHYSICAL EXAMINATION

The examination of a patient who may be a candidate for a temporalis tendon transfer should be tailored and guided by the principles of muscle transfer previously described. First, is the temporalis muscle functionally intact and expendable? Asking the patient to clench their teeth while palpating the muscle belly can test for contraction of the temporalis muscle. Comparing contraction of the muscle on both sides will help determine whether there is any weakness of the targeted donor muscle. As a principle, weak but functional temporalis muscles should not be transferred as MTU. Patients should also be checked for mouth opening and closing to be certain that there are no premorbid functional impairments that will be made worse with the dissection and transposition of the temporalis tendon. Patients with preexisting trismus may be made worse after a temporalis MTU procedure. On the contrary, a fully functional masticator system will tolerate even a bilateral temporalis MTU procedure without affecting jaw excursion and mastication.

The cheek and perioral regions should be palpated to establish the pliability of the soft tissue bed in the buccal space and passive movement of the lip and oral commissure. When the lip is scarred and stiff, a dynamic temporalis MTU will be ineffective in providing adequate commissure excursion for dynamic smile restoration.

The preoperative examination should also be performed to establish the length of tendon transposition necessary to reach the orbicularis oris from the coronoid. Patients with a broad face and long cheeks with a wide separation between the palpated coronoid and the oral commissure are likely to require measures to lengthen the temporalis tendon to achieve adequate reach. Patients should be counseled about the potential for the harvest of fascia for tendon lengthening or the need for external scalp incisions for the lengthening myoplasty procedure described later in this chapter.

INDICATIONS

Individuals motivated to actively learn the use of the transferred muscle for smiling are ideal candidates for this procedure As a muscle substitution procedure, the temporalis MTU may be considered in the following situations: (1) the transfer can act as a substitute during regrowth of a nerve, which will thereby reduce the time of functional loss, (2) the transfer can act as a helper and add power to normal reinnervated muscle function, (3) the transfer can act as a substitute when the recovery after neurorrhaphy or nerve repair is poor, and (4) the transfer can act as the sole source of muscle movement when the facial muscle is developmentally absent or physiologically nonfunctional from atrophy, scaring, resection, or prolonged denervation.

In clinical practice, a typical candidate for temporalis MTU is a patient who after a radical parotidectomy is scheduled to undergo postoperative radiotherapy. Although the facial nerve is grafted, a temporalis MTU may be performed at the same time to provide facial support. The temporalis MTU transfer procedure can also be considered as an option to upgrade partial recovery after facial paralysis. The indications for the temporalis MTU procedure overlaps with those for free functional muscle transfer such as the gracilis flap. Choosing between the temporalis MTU and the gracilis flap depends upon individual patient features, patient desires, and the surgeon's expertise and success with these techniques.

CONTRAINDICATIONS

On a case-by-case basis, conditions that adversely affect the function of the temporalis muscle should be considered as contraindications for selecting the temporalis MTU procedure. Patients with muscular dystrophy with progressive involvement of the masticator muscle should avoid the MTU procedure. Neurologic processes with present or potential progressive involvement of the trigeminal nerve should temper the selection of the temporalis MTU procedure. Patients with preexisting trismus may be worsened after the temporalis MTU procedure. Other relative contraindications include the patient who has an inadequate soft tissue bed for optimized muscle function.

PREOPERATIVE PLANNING

A full series of preoperative photographs should be obtained. In the preoperative period, patients must visit a physical therapist who plans out a specific exercise program to strengthen the temporalis muscle and to identify isolated attempted movements that will be essential in causing the temporalis muscle to contract. Patients should be motivated to participate in their rehabilitation program.

In the preoperative holding area, the desired vector of smile is determined based on the functional side and marked in the involved side (Fig. 46.1). Anesthesia requirements should be discussed. While nasolabial intubation is ideal, the procedure can be performed with oral intubation with the tube sutured to the teeth to avoid any distorting perioral taping.

Long-acting paralytic agents should be avoided in order to allow intraoperative temporalis muscle stimulation to establish the idea tension–length–excursion relationships for the transferred MTU.

SURGICAL TECHNIQUE

The main surgical steps include an approach to the coronoid process, tendon mobilization, and tendon insertion. The entire face should be prepped including the temporal scalp.

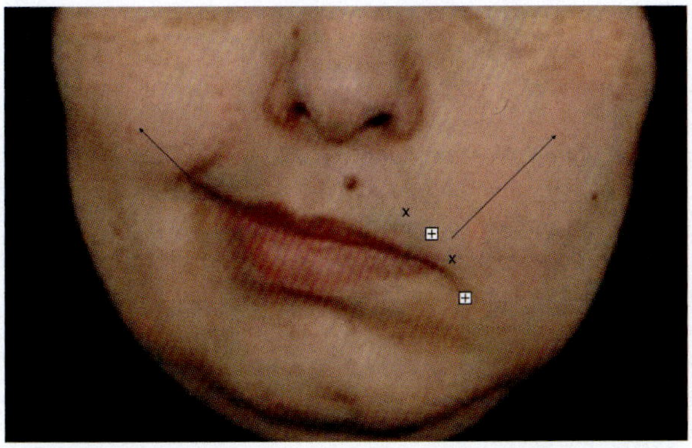

FIGURE 46.1
Marking the site of tendon insertion along the lip margin based on the vector of dominant smile on the functioning contralateral side.

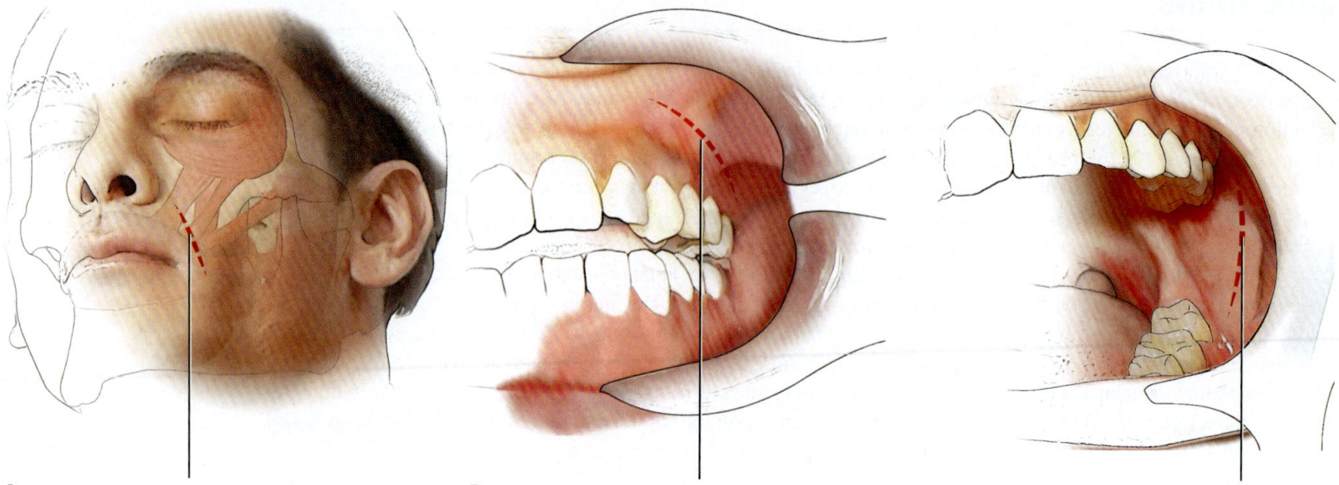

FIGURE 46.2 The coronoid process may be exposed entirely through **(A)** an external melolabial crease incision or **(B)** a sublabial incision alone or in combination with a **(C)** retromolar incision.

Access incision

The incision to access the buccal space and the coronoid may be external or transoral. In patients who have deep melolabial folds, an external melolabial incision may be used with the clear advantage of avoiding oral contamination. In younger patients and those with less defined melolabial creases, an intraoral sublabial incision provides wide exposure of the orbicularis muscle for tendon insertion as well as direct access to the buccal space and coronoid process. The clear advantage of the sublabial approach is the avoidance of facial scars. However, the transoral approach exposes the surgical bed to oral contaminants increasing the risk of infection. Placing a passive drain for a few days may be helpful. For a more direct access to the coronoid, a second intraoral mucosal incision placed along the ascending the ramus of the mandible may be combined with the sublabial incision (Fig. 46.2).

Buccal Space Dissection

The buccal space is injected with local anesthetic to ensure adequate hemostasis. Through the selected access incision, dissection is bluntly carried out through the buccal space. Malleable retractors facilitate exposure of the buccal adipose tissue. The parotid duct should be protected. Buccal adipose tissue should be preserved as a cushion again tendon scarring. As the malleable retractors are advanced deep to the anterior edge of the mandibular ramus and the coronoid process is exposed.

Tendon Mobilization and Coronoidectomy

To protect the temporalis tendon from shredding, subperiosteal elevation of the fascia–periosteum tendon complex is performed on the medial aspect of the coronoid beginning from the retromolar area and extending superiorly to the level of the sigmoid notch. A right-angled hemostat is useful in identifying the sigmoid notch. A Kocher clamp is then placed on the coronoid and a right-angled hemostat passed between the coronoid bone and the elevated tendon into the sigmoid notch. The right-angled hemostat acts both as a retractor and as guide for coronoidectomy. It is important to keep a Kocher firmly secured on the coronoid before detaching the tendon to avoid retraction into the infratemporal fossa. An osteotomy of the coronoid is performed using a small reciprocating saw. The coronoidectomy may also be performed using a sharp osteotome. In performing the osteotomy, it is important to avoid injuries to the surrounding soft tissue including the temporalis tendon and the motor nerves to the temporalis and masseter muscles, which course though the posterior aspect of the sigmoid notch close to the temporomandibular joint. The tendon on the medial aspect of the coronoid is separated from any attachments to the medial pterygoid muscle and the lateral aspect, from masseter muscle attachments (Fig. 46.3). To avoid interference or refusion, the remnant coronoid stump may be further reduced. The tendon is then carefully freed laterally from the masseter muscle and medially from the medial pterygoid muscle. The tendon can now be divided as inferiorly as possible for length and transposed through the buccal space toward the modiolus. If necessary, additional mobilization for length may be achieved by freeing the attachment of the temporalis muscle from the undersurface of the zygomatic arch. This is done carefully staying close to the undersurface of the zygomatic bone in order to preserve a layer of adipose tissue between the arch and the muscle thereby preserving a fatty glide plane.

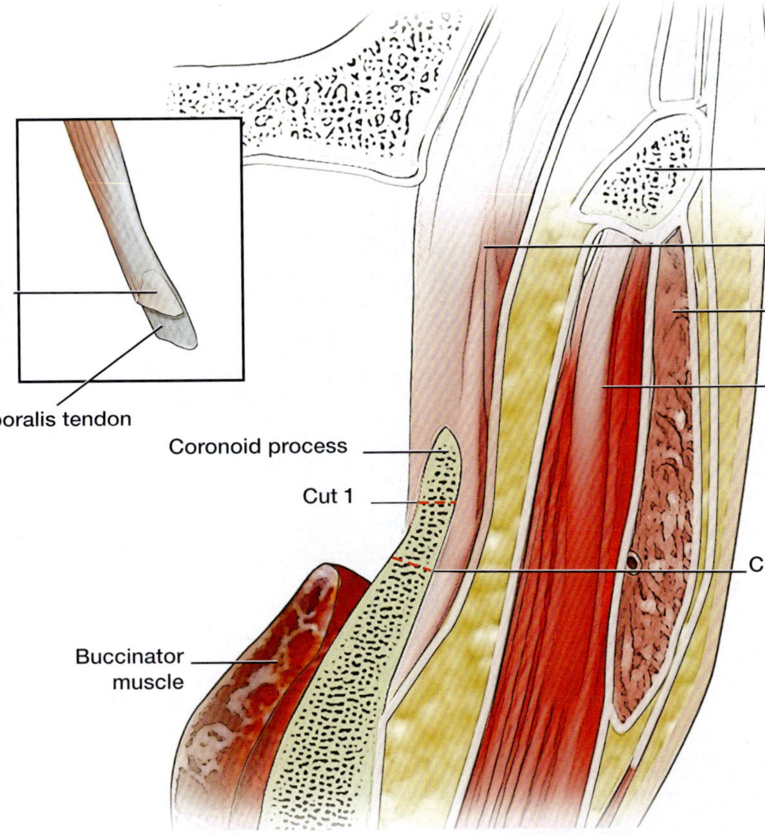

FIGURE 46.3 Steps for segmental coronoidectomy. With the coronoid and the attached tendon exposed, a right-angled hemostat is placed in the sigmoid notch to guide the angle of the desired osteotomy. A segment of the coronoid is removed leaving a gap. With the coronoid clamped, the attached tendon is divided as interiorly as possible to preserve tendon length.

Gaining Tendon Length

Fundamental to the temporalis MTU procedure is mobilization of the temporalis tendon unit from the coronoid and transposing it to the upper lip and modiolus at the optimal tension. This requires the mobilization of an MTU of adequate length to reach the modiolus without overstretch. Labbé originally described the temporalis tendon lengthening myoplasty procedure in which the temporalis muscle is exposed through a scalp incision and elevated off the temporal fossa allowing the entire MTU to slide toward the modiolus following coronoidectomy. With this approach, an osteotomy of the zygomatic arch is carried out to gain access to the coronoid process to release the tendon. When releasing the temporalis muscle, care is taken to avoid injury to the neurovascular supply deep to the muscle. In addition, the released muscle should be refixated at the appropriate tension. A recent modification by Labbé avoids osteotomy of the zygomatic arch and approaches the coronoid through the buccal space similar to the minimally invasive temporalis tendon transfer procedure. In a recent cadaveric analysis of the temporalis lengthening myoplasty procedure, the Labbé group cataloged seven steps in the procedure and quantified the potential length gained by each step. The median maximal total lengthening of all seven steps when performed together was 43.5 mm. The steps that contributed most to this lengthening were coronoidectomy and intraoral temporalis tendon dissection (median, 12.0 mm), incision of temporalis fascia insertion over the orbital rim (median, 6.5 mm), and zygomatic osteotomy with dissection of masseteric fibers (median, 11.5 mm). The extent of incisions, dissection, and temporalis MTU mobilization described in the classic lengthening procedure is extensive, disrupts the multiple glide planes at the level of the muscle belly and transition under the zygomatic arch, and introduces external scars but yields 4 cm or more of tendon for transposition.

Using a minimally invasive approach, adequate temporalis tendon length may be gained by extension with fascia or donor tendon without mobilization of the muscle belly. Brunner studied the effect of tendon extension on muscle force generation. The main disadvantage of tendon extension is the introduction of a passive noncontractile element (extra tendon/fascia) into a dynamic temporalis MTU system with the potential for reducing the effective contraction. The longer the tendon extension, the less the contraction achievable. Therefore, we do not recommend the use of more than 2 cm of fascia tendon extension. When more than 2 cm of tendon extension is needed, the lengthening myoplasty procedure as described by Labbé should be considered (Fig. 46.4).

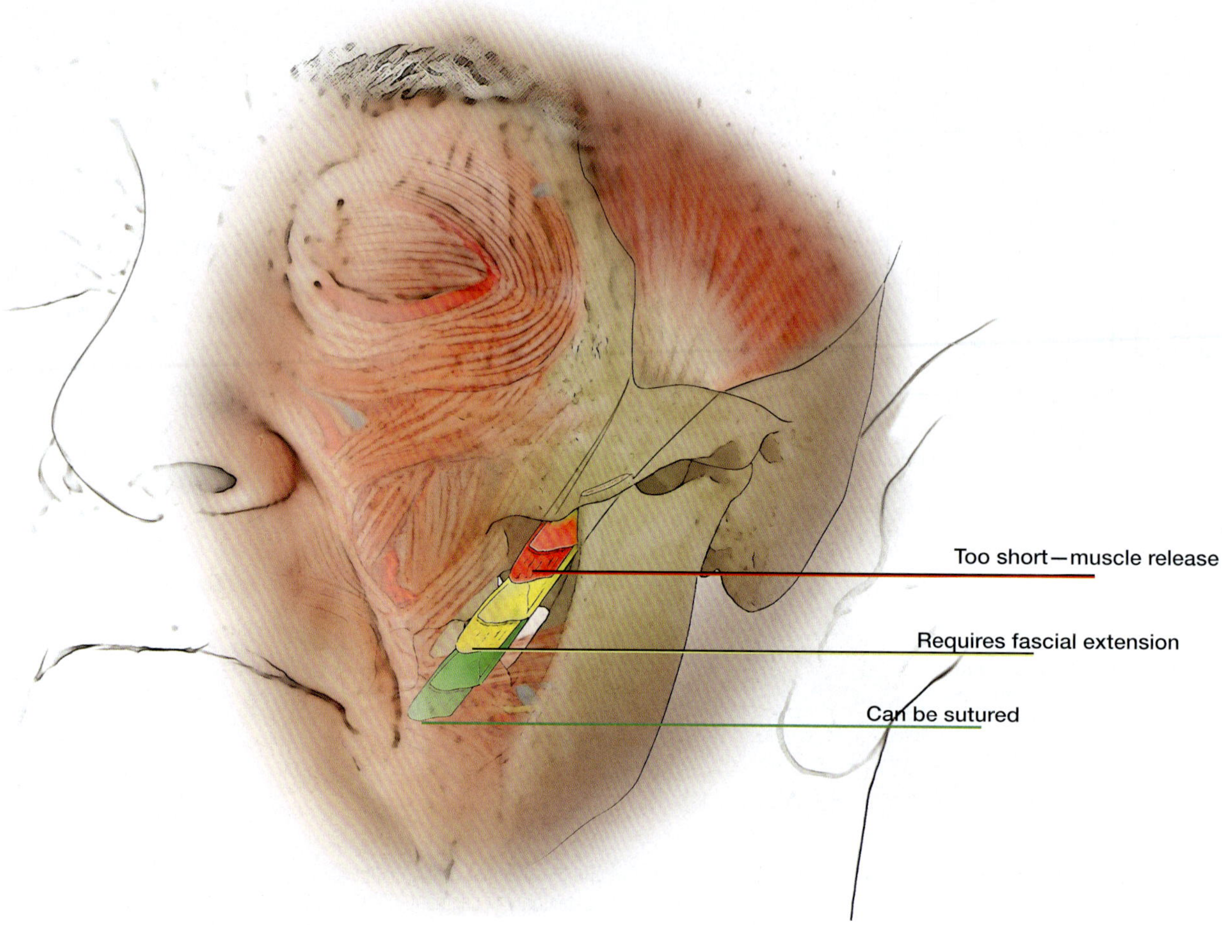

FIGURE 46.4 Guide to the use of fascia extension versus lengthening myoplasty in temporalis MTU procedure.

Generating a Tension–Excursion Relationship for the Temporalis MTU

After transposing the temporalis tendon through the buccal space toward the modiolus, a tension excursion relationship can be generated. The temporalis muscle is electrically stimulated with transcutaneous or needle electrodes placed into the temporalis muscles. The DigiStim II plus stimulator (Neurotechnology), commonly used by anesthesiologists, may be used. With traction of the Kocher clamp, the tension on the released tendon is manually varied while electrically stimulating the muscle. At the point of maximum force contraction, a marker is placed on the Kocher clamp to represent the ideal traction tension and muscle length for maximal excursion. The marked Kocher will be used to guide the degree or traction (tension) needed to ideally position the temporalis tendon for insertion. The tendon is then inserted at the determined optimal length (tension) based on the intraoperative excursion measurements.

Insertion Site

The upper lip elevators including the zygomaticus major insert and interdigitate with fibers of the orbicularis oris around the modiolus. The transposed temporalis tendon should be inserted into the orbicularis oris muscle beyond the nasolabial fold to mimic the insertion of the zygomaticus muscles. In this position, a natural melolabial fold develops and contraction of the temporalis muscle results in excursion of the oral commissure and elevation of the free lip margin for dental show and smile restoration. Insertion of the tendon in the melolabial fold results in a deep fold and muscle contractions that do not translate well into lip elevation and exposure of the teeth when smiling.

POSTOPERATIVE MANAGEMENT

Early postoperative management should ensure stability of the inserted tendon. Patients are placed on soft diet for at least 2 weeks to allow healing of the inserted tendon without the excessive stress of chewing.

Muscle is perhaps the most mutable of biologic tissues, and as such, posttreatment physical therapy is essential for retraining the temporalis muscle for its new function. After transfer of the temporalis tendon from the coronoid to the oral commissure, its mechanical properties change given the altered demands placed on the muscle. In the preoperative period, patients work with a physical therapist who plans out a specific program of exercises to strengthen the temporalis muscle and to identify isolated movements that will be essential in contracting the temporalis muscle. After the first two postoperative weeks, active mobilization of the transposed temporalis MTU should begin. This should be followed by muscle strengthening exercises. The main goal of the therapy is to systematically rehabilitate smile function by transferring labial functions to the transferred temporal muscle. Lambert Prou describes several phases of therapy to acquire a temporal smile. The first phase, termed the mandibular smile, involves mobilization of the mandible by contraction of the transferred temporalis muscle and inducing an elevation of the oral commissure. The second phase, the voluntary temporal smile, is attained by contracting the temporalis muscle without mandibular movement, which remains under voluntary control. The smile produced should be as symmetrical as possible. Finally, the last phase focuses on achieving a spontaneous smile independent of mandibular movement (the spontaneous temporal smile). Biofeedback methods are helpful in this process. The role of electrical stimulation is unclear. As demonstrated by Coulson and colleagues, repeated exercises and practice with the aid of video feedback loops of the best symmetric smile can be powerful tools to achieve a spontaneous smile adapted for social settings.

COMPLICATIONS

Complications from temporalis MTU procedure include infection and hematoma. These occur in the early postoperative period and must be actively managed. Delayed complications include tendon disinsertion, overcorrection with associated inadequate excursion. Overcorrection and insertion of the tendon along the melolabial fold instead of the mobile lip are common reasons for inadequate excursion. When muscles have been inserted under excessive tension, structural and adaptive changes occur within the microstructure on the muscle fibers. These adaptive changes include rearrangement of sarcomere resulting in changes in contractile forces and the length excursion relationship. In revision cases, the tendon should be exposed and isolated. Identifying the tendon within scar tissue may be challenging but is facilitated by electrical stimulation of the temporalis muscle. If the tendon was inserted along the melolabial fold, it should be mobilized, a tension excursion relationship should be determined, and the tendon should be reinserted along the lip margin with or without lengthening as described earlier.

RESULTS

The outcome of the temporalis tendon procedure for a flaccid facial paralysis is immediate and generally satisfactory. Improvement in facial tone, oral commissure symmetry, and redefining of effaced nasolabial folds is consistently achievable. However, restoring dynamic commissure and lip excursion with the temporalis tendon transfer procedure is mixed. Patients should be properly counseled and expected outcomes thoroughly discussed. Below, we have illustrated a case with the potential of restoring both tone and excursion with this temporalis tendon transfer procedure.

Case Sample

A 40-year-old female with right-sided congenital facial paralysis underwent a temporalis muscle tendon using transfer procedure via a sublabial transbuccal approach. Adequate tendon length was exposed and the optimal tension determined with intraoperative muscle stimulation. Two weeks following the procedure, facial retraining exercises were initiated to adapt the transposed muscle for a temporal smile. Results show correction of preoperative lack of right commissure elevation (Fig. 46.5A) with a symmetric smile (Fig. 46.5B) and isolated excursion of the right oral commissure (Fig. 46.5C).

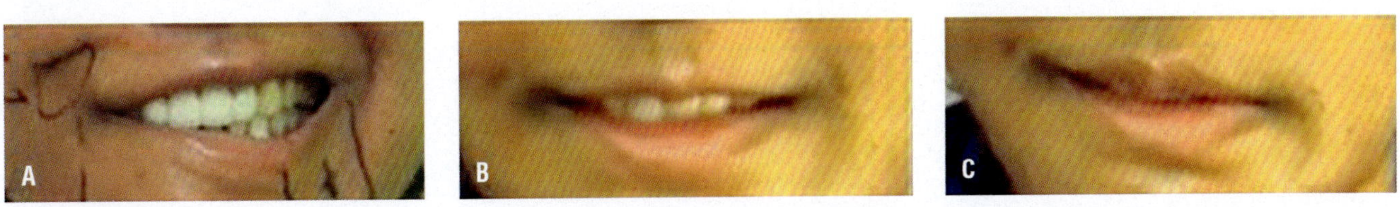

FIGURE 46.5 Case sample for a temporalis MTU in a patient with right-sided congenital facial paralysis. **(A)** Preoperative smile, **(B)** postoperative smile, and **(C)** isolated commissure excursion.

PEARLS

- A detailed history (including previous surgery, injury to the face, history of radiation) as well as physical examination (muscle strength, facial symmetry, functional testing of temporalis if indicated) must be obtained.
- Preoperative consultation with a physical therapist and appropriate discussion of expectations improves patient outcomes.
- The major technical challenge of the temporalis MTU procedure is insertion of the tendon at the optimal tension for lip excursion. The use of intraoperative muscle stimulation is key in establishing the appropriate length–excursion relationship.
- When tendon length is inadequate by less than 2 cm, fascia tendon extension should be considered. When more than 2 cm of extension is needed, the lengthening myoplasty procedure should be considered.
- Facial retraining exercises are key components for optimizing the temporalis MTU procedure for smile restoration.

PITFALLS

- Use of a weak temporalis muscle
- Overstretch of the temporalis MTU
- Insertion of the tendon into the melolabial fold rather than the orbicularis oris muscle

KEY INSTRUMENTS

- Malleable retractors
- Right-angled hemostat
- Periosteal elevator
- Reciprocating saw and drill
- Muscle stimulator and osteotome

SUGGESTED READING

Boahene KD. Principles and biomechanics of muscle tendon unit transfer: application in temporalis muscle tendon transposition for smile improvement in facial paralysis. *Laryngoscope* 2013;123(2):350–355.

Boahene KD, Farrag TY, Ishii L, et al. Minimally invasive temporalis tendon transposition. *Arch Facial Plast Surg* 2011;13(1):8–13.

Boahene KD, Ishii LE, Byrne PJ. In vivo excursion of the temporalis muscle-tendon unit using electrical stimulation: application in the design of smile restoration surgery following facial paralysis. *JAMA Facial Plast Surg* 2014;16(1):15–29.

Coulson SE, Adams RD, O'Dwyer NJ, et al. Physiotherapy rehabilitation of the smile after long-term facial nerve palsy using video self-modeling and implementation intentions. *Otolaryngol Head Neck Surg* 2006;134(1):48–55.

Labbé D, Huault M. Lengthening temporalis myoplasty and lip reanimation. *Plast Reconstr Surg* 2000;105(4):1289–1297.

47

TEMPORALIS TENDON TRANSFER

Patrick Byrne

INTRODUCTION

The treatment options to restore the smile in cases of long-standing complete facial paralysis are limited. A long-standing complete paralysis is generally felt to be one which is present for greater than 1 year. This definition is clinically useful although somewhat arbitrary.

In such cases, in order to restore a dynamic smile, one may perform a regional muscle transfer or free tissue transfer. Free tissue transfer, such as a gracilis free flap, can be an excellent option for many patients. It does, however, require multiple stages, an extended period of recovery prior to movement and has some morbidity at the donor site.

Regional muscle transfer generally comes down to a choice between the uses of temporalis and masseter muscle. The temporalis muscle tends to be preferred due to the ideal vector of pull. Most surgeons have employed a technique that transfers the muscle origin from the temporal fossa to the oral commissure. This requires passing the muscle over the zygomatic arch. The facial morphology is thus adversely affected by the protrusion of tissue around the arch and the depression created in the temple.

An alternative technique instead uses the insertion of the muscle—the temporalis tendon. The temporalis tendon transfer allows effective elevation of the oral commissure without alteration of the facial morphology. The tendon and coronoid process are released and transferred to the oral commissure. I prefer a minimally invasive temporalis tendon transfer (MIT3), in which a single incision is performed for a 1-hour procedure. I have found this a reliable and simple method or restoring oral symmetry and movement (Fig. 47.1).

The causes of facial paralysis are many and beyond the scope of this chapter. It is important to determine via the history if the facial nerve is intact. The facial nerve is often intact in cases of complete facial paralysis after acoustic neuroma resection. The reconstructive surgeon must communicate with the resection team, as well as the patient, about the options for timing of reconstruction. In cases of an anatomically intact nerve, often, the key distinction is the duration and extent of the paralysis. The temporalis tendon transfer is typically considered an option in the case of long-standing complete paralysis. In such cases, alternatives such as nerve transfers are not considered a viable option due to the facial muscle atrophy and fibrosis.

Advantages of the MIT3 procedure include that it is a relatively simple, one stage, minimally invasive procedure that produces results quickly. This is in contrast to free tissue transfer, which is typically a two-stage operation that requires a significant donor site and extended recovery period prior to any dynamic movement being achieved. Disadvantages include the lack of spontaneous mimetic movement and the relatively reduced excursion of the oral commissure in comparison to successful free tissue transfer with gracilis muscle.

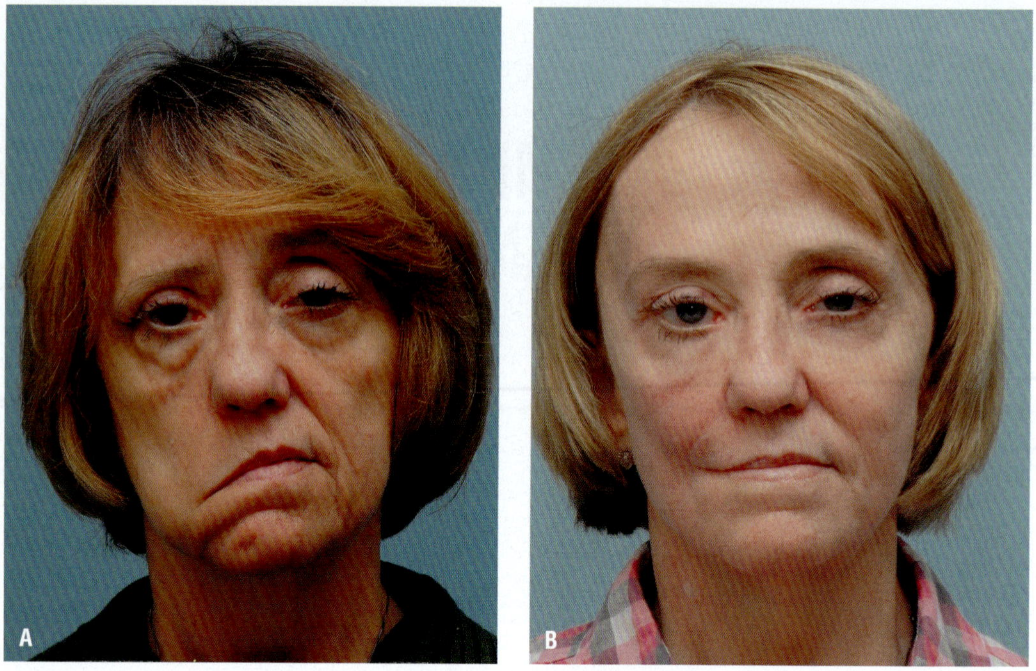

FIGURE 47.1 Pre- **(A)** and postoperative **(B)** example of temporalis tendon transfer.

HISTORY

The patient's age, health status, need for adjunctive treatments such as external beam radiation, and personal preferences for reconstruction all play an important role in the decision-making process. The patient must be provided a realistic portrayal of the available options, which in these cases are limited to free tissue transfer, regional muscle transfer (including the minimally invasive temporalis tendon transfer, or MIT3), or static sling. Each has markedly different expectations and postoperative course, and one must educate the patient fully to help him/her to make the best decision.

PHYSICAL EXAMINATION

A key aspect to the physical examination specific to the temporalis tendon transfer is an evaluation of the temporalis function. I have used EMG in the past to assess this muscle. However, the correlation of electrophysiologic activity does not correlate well with functional results after transfer. I examine the muscle primarily via palpation. The patient is asked to clench their teeth while the belly of the temporalis muscle is palpated. An obvious bulging of the muscle indicates functional muscle activity.

The goal is to minimize asymmetry wherever it is found, both at rest and through the range of facial expression. Therefore, it is important to spend time during the consultation making "small talk" with the patient. I will sit down and spend quite a bit of time asking them about their lives. I attempt to put them at ease and interject humor, as this allows one to observe their own particular use of facial expression, including smiling. These observations are critical in forming the basis for my treatment plan and advice.

INDICATIONS

The temporalis tendon transfer is indicated primarily for patients with long-standing complete facial paralysis. Occasionally, it may be appropriate for cases of incomplete paralysis, but this is uncommon. The gracilis free muscle transfer is an alternative to the temporalis tendon transfer in cases of complete long-standing paralysis. These two options are discussed at length with the patient.

CONTRAINDICATIONS

Paralysis of the temporalis muscle is a contraindication. It is also not typically performed in cases of complete paralysis in which there is a reasonable expectation that the facial nerve may regain function. Doing so, in theory, could transect distal branches of the facial nerve.

PREOPERATIVE PLANNING

It is ideal if the patient can be trained to do the temporalis smile prior to surgery. Most patients have weeks to months to work on the coordination of the temporalis muscle contraction with a contralateral elevation of the oral commissure.

I have the patient stand in front of a mirror, with his/her hand on the temple of the paralyzed side. The teeth are clenched enough to create a palpable bulge of the temporalis muscle as a zygomaticus smile is performed on the contralateral side. The duration is varied, but in each run, the goal is to hold the temporalis in contraction for as long as the contralateral oral commissure is elevated. The patient is advised to perform this in front of the mirror multiple times daily, for as many weeks as possible leading up to the surgical procedure.

The facial anatomy is analyzed carefully to assist in the decision of whether to perform the procedure via a transfacial versus transoral route. It should be noted that I have performed this procedure for over a decade and have found that the melolabial incision is quite favorable if meticulous attention is paid to the tissue handling and closure. I generally prefer to perform the procedure via a transfacial incision when a noticeable crease or fold is present on the contralateral side. If this is not the case, a transoral approach is used.

SURGICAL TECHNIQUE

In the preoperative area, the melolabial fold is marked bilaterally. The vector of the contralateral smile is noted. Marks are placed where the ideal insetting should occur (Fig. 47.2).

Transfacial Approach

General anesthesia is administered and lidocaine with epinephrine is infiltrated into the area. The patient is prepped and draped, with the entire face visible and exposed within the operative field. Steri-Strips are used to protect the eyes.

The incision is made with a #15 blade through the skin. Dissection is performed bluntly through the buccal space directly toward the coronoid process of the mandible. Care is taken to avoid dissection deeply to avoid damage to the buccinator muscle and Stensen's duct (Fig. 47.3). The mouth is opened and closed to facilitate palpation of the ascending ramus. Once identified, two malleable retractors, each 15 to 20 mm wide, are inserted on either side of the ascending ramus of the mandible. These are used to retract the masseter muscle

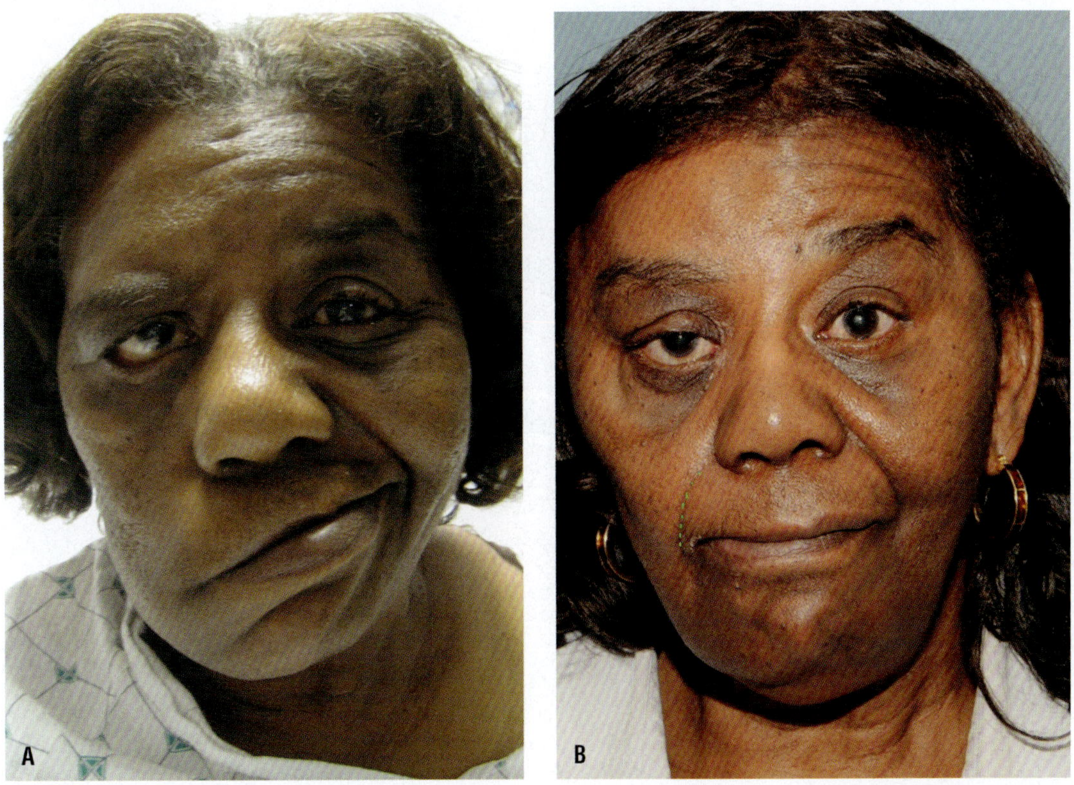

FIGURE 47.2 The vector of the contralateral smile is noted in order to achieve facial symmetry. Pre- **(A)** and postoperative **(B)**.

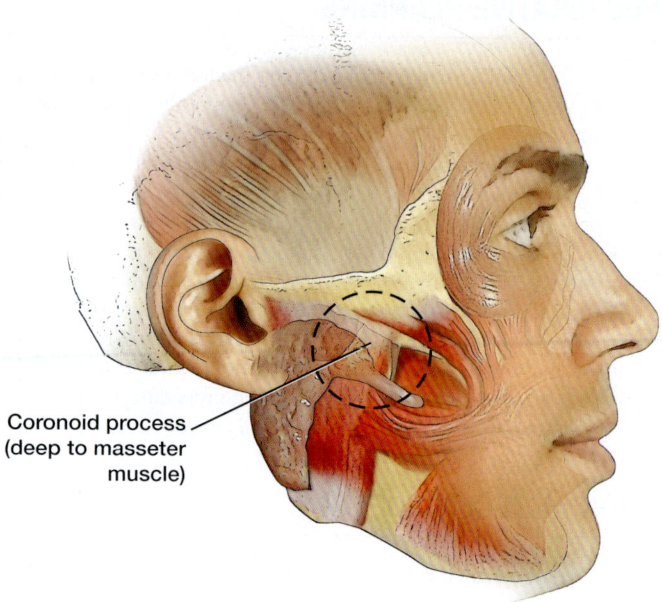

FIGURE 47.3 Anatomic location of the coronoid and surrounding structures of importance.

and buccal adipose tissue from the area of dissection (Fig. 47.4). Additional retractors are often necessary inferiorly and superiorly to prevent adipose tissue from obscuring the visualization. Cummings retractors or small malleables are helpful here.

Using electrocautery, the periosteum is incised, and this along with the temporalis tendon is elevated from the medial and lateral aspects of the ascending ramus. The tendon is kept attached to the coronoid process. Care is taken to isolate the temporalis tendon as medial as possible and down to the buccinator to obtain adequate tendon length. An angled clamp is inserted around the neck of the coronoid process to elevate the mandible toward the surgeon. A reciprocating saw is used to divide the coronoid process in an oblique manner, thus leaving as much of the tendon attached to the coronoid as possible (Fig. 47.5). Before detaching the coronoid, a Kocher clamp is placed to prevent retraction.

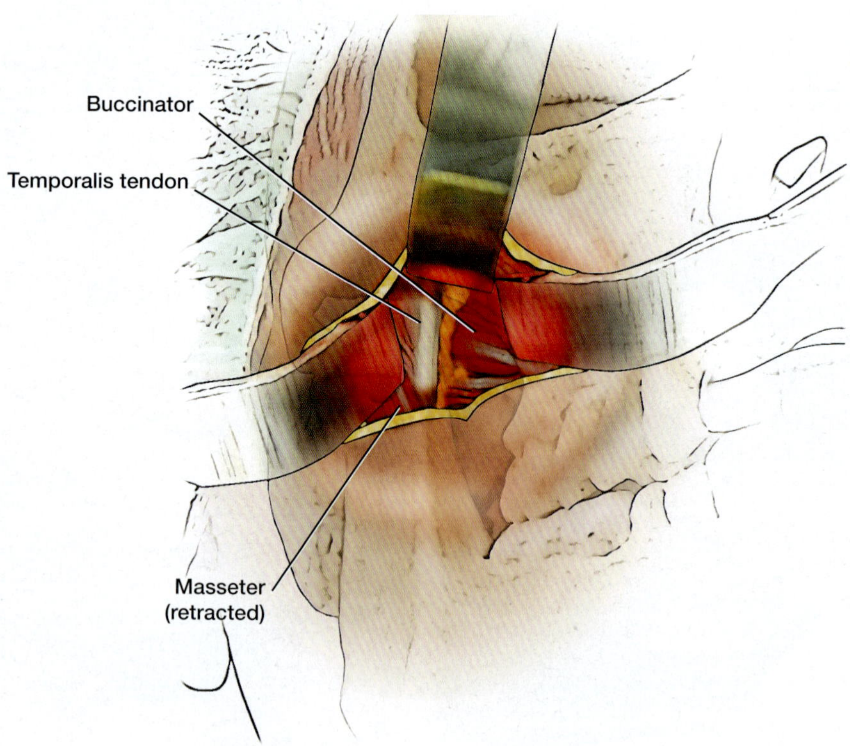

FIGURE 47.4 Isolation of the ascending ramus via transfacial approach.

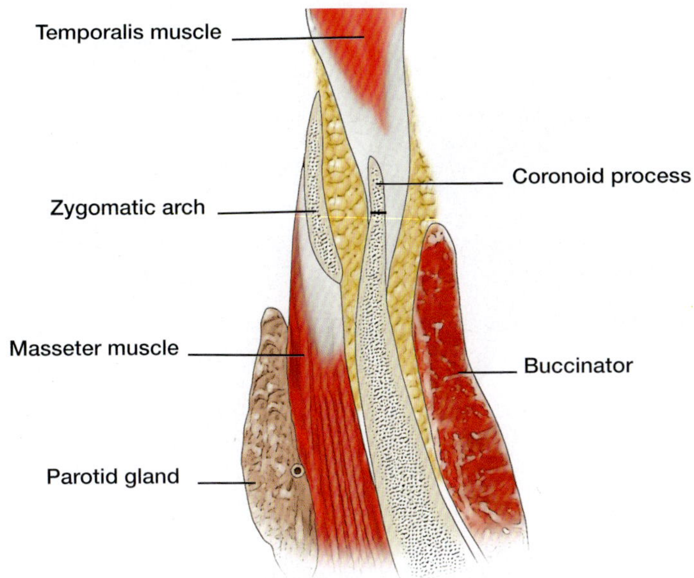

FIGURE 47.5 Illustration of the oblique cut through the coronoid process.

A 2-0 Vicryl suture is then used to "lasso" the coronoid process and attached tendon. This is usually done a second time to ensure that the tendon does not retract in toward the temporal fossa. These two "key" sutures are attached to the oral commissure to recreate the desired pull and contour of the contralateral side (Fig. 47.6). Typically, one is placed just medial to the modiolus, one into the upper lip, the other to the lower lip. Additional 3-0 PDS sutures are then placed where needed to create the desired contour. This usually requires sutures to the modiolus, medial to the melolabial fold, and the upper lip.

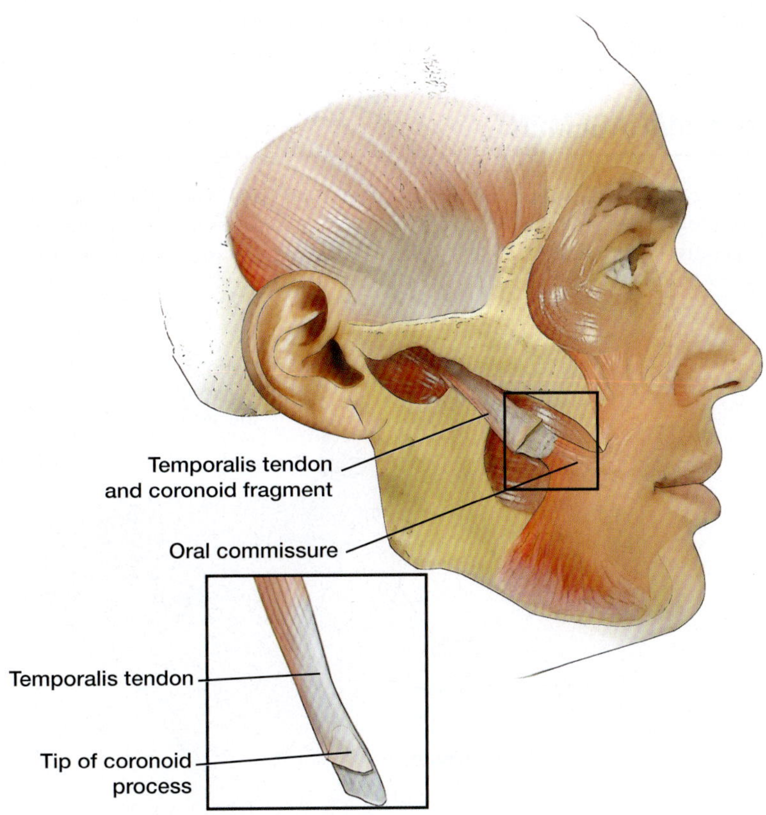

FIGURE 47.6 Illustration depicting the attachment of the coronoid process and attached tendon to the oral commissure.

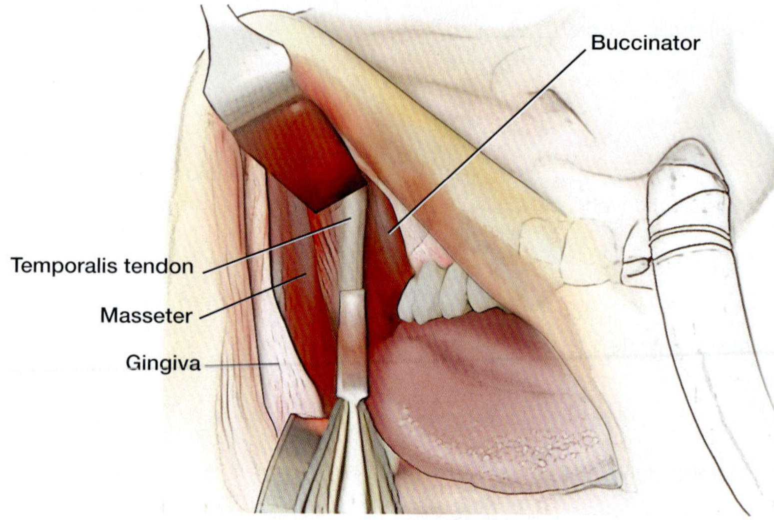

FIGURE 47.7
Transoral approach to the ramus.

The facial incision is then carefully inspected. If the retraction has damaged the skin, then a sharp excision is performed of the edges, with a slight outward bevel, and meticulous multilayered closure is performed. Simple sutures are placed on the skin if there is a desire for a crease to form.

Transoral Approach

Two incisions are placed intraorally. The first is an incision along the ascending ramus of the mandible. The exposure of the ascending ramus is thus very simple. It is easier than the transfacial approach due to the absence of troublesome buccal adipose tissue. Elevation and release are performed as with the transfacial route (Fig. 47.7).

The insetting is more challenging than the transfacial route. A second incision is made adjacent to the oral commissure intraorally, at the point of fixation (Fig. 47.8). Careful dissection is then performed between this second incision and the first. The buccal mucosa is elevated deep to the submucosal glands and buccinator muscle. It is important to note the position of Stensen's duct and avoid injury to this structure. The tendon is then passed through the dissected tissue plane into the second incision. Insetting then proceeds in the same manner as the transfacial approach, except from the inside of the mouth.

POSTOPERATIVE MANAGEMENT

A compressive dressing is applied. A liquid diet is enforced for 7 days. Then, the patient is allowed to chew and begins an active program of physical therapy. The program consists of resuming the exercises that were demonstrated preoperatively. In addition, many patients also require stretching exercises to combat early trismus.

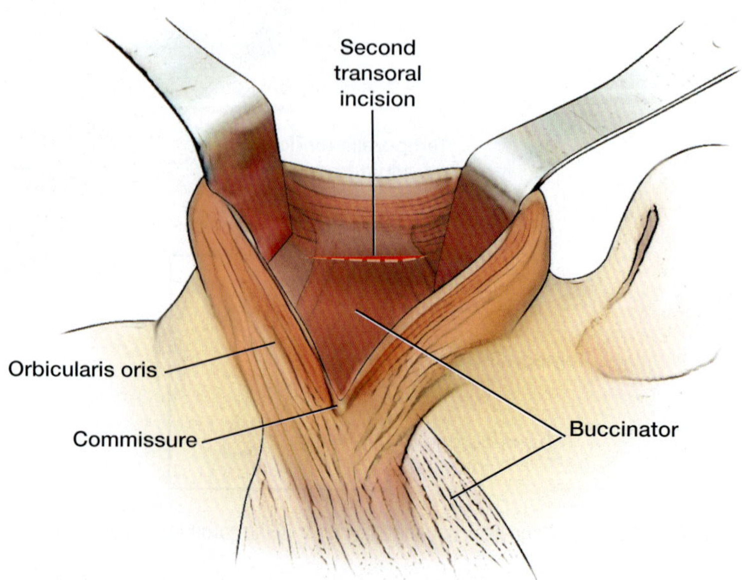

FIGURE 47.8
Second transoral incision for insetting to the tendon to the commissure.

COMPLICATIONS

Complications are rare. I have seen two cases of fluid collections, both of which were likely related to parotid duct injury. These were each managed with wound packing and resolved uneventfully. Patients are advised as to typical surgical risks such as infections, problematic scarring, and the need for further surgery. Both are uncommon.

RESULTS

The temporalis tendon transfer is a fairly simple, quick, and reliable method of facial reanimation. I have found correction of the ptotic oral commissure, with improved symmetry, in all patients. Approximately 85% of patients achieve movement of the oral commissure. Most patients accomplish 5 to 7 mm of elevation, with a range of 2 to 15 mm.

PEARLS

- Nasotracheal intubation is used for all facial reanimation cases, to avoid distortion of the mouth and lips.
- The sutures are placed to overcorrect, as some relaxation is typical. However, the relaxation is not usually as significant as static slings. If necessary, an extender of fascia lata is used. There are two situations in which this may be employed.
  - The first is if the tension on the closure is too great, with excessive elevation of the oral commissure necessary in order to connect the tendon to the oral commissure. Fascia lata may be used to extend the length of the tendon.
  - The other situation is when the point of attachment is made across midline. As described by Sherris, there are some patients with such profound imbalance due to contralateral contraction that the philtrum is markedly deviated away from the side of the paralysis. These patients are best served by making the point of attachment through the upper and lower lip beyond the midline. When this is done, it is important to make a series of stab incisions within the upper and lower lip to place fixating sutures from the fascia to the orbicularis oris. This prevents an "accordion"-like effect once the lip is pulled.
- The "lasso" suture of 2-0 Vicryl is helpful to capture the tendon (and attached coronoid process) and prevent its retraction.
- I have not found it necessary to detach the tendon from the coronoid or to discard the coronoid process.

PITFALLS

- The major pitfall is certainly the poor elevation seen in some patients, perhaps 15%. This does not seem to correlate with the cause of paralysis or the patients' age. It may be more common in patients with a history of radiation therapy.

INSTRUMENTS TO HAVE AVAILABLE

- Malleable retractors
- Sagittal saw
- Osteotomes
- Kocher clamp

SUGGESTED READING

Boahene KD, Farrag TY, Ishii L, et al. Minimally invasive temporalis tendon transposition. *Arch Facial Plast Surg* 2011;13(1):8–13.

Byrne PJ, Kim M, Boahene K, et al. Temporalis tendon transfer as part of a comprehensive approach to facial reanimation. *Arch Facial Plast Surg* 2007;9(4):234–241.

Chan JY, Byrne PJ. Management of facial paralysis in the 21st century. *Facial Plast Surg* 2011;27(4):346–357. Epub Jul 26, 2011;346–357.

Griffin GR, Abuzeid W, Vainshtein J, et al. Outcomes following temporalis tendon transfer in irradiated patients. *Arch Facial Plast Surg* 2012;18:1–8.

48 THE CHAMPY TECHNIQUE FOR ORIF OF MANDIBLE FRACTURES

Andrew H. Murr

INTRODUCTION

Before the discovery of the biocompatibility of titanium spearheaded by Branemark in the early 1980s, open plating techniques to address mandible fractures were fraught with complications. Techniques for fracture fixation usually consisted of intermaxillary fixation (IMF) for prolonged periods of time, usually 6 weeks. Erich arch bars and Ivy loops were in common use as was the use of oral splints and circummandibular wires and suspension wires when midface fractures were present. Alloy plates were adapted from orthopedic surgery for mandibular fixation, but the compound nature of mandible fractures, which are frequently open to the oral cavity with its aerobic and anaerobic flora, created a milieu that favored infection. Nevertheless, engineering principles were developed by many different investigators often in partnership with industry to define the optimal reconstruction method to counteract the massive forces of mastication under which the mandible routinely operates.

The Arbeitsgemeinschaft für Osteosynthesefragen/Association for the Study of Internal Fixation (AO/ASIF) was in the forefront of defining the precise characteristics of plates and screws that are required for open reduction and internal fixation (ORIF) of fractures. The ultimate benefit of engineering a repair properly was the opportunity for immediate function directly after surgery. Without immediate function, patients had their jaws wired shut with subsequent interference with nutrition and substantial weight loss. Compliance with IMF was dismal, especially considering that many patients with mandible fractures had a history of substance abuse. Oral hygiene is challenging when patients are in IMF and dental and periodontal health suffered when closed techniques were used. Finally, temporomandibular joint fixation, especially in the presence of condyle fractures, was a major, though probably under reported, complication of prolonged IMF.

Titanium changed what could be achieved with open techniques. Plates and screws were less likely to become infected or rejected. In fact, bone would encapsulate the screws and the plates over time. Now, surgeons could confidently place titanium implants, and if they adhered to the engineering principles properly, the likelihood of successful ORIF of fractures became an expected rather than an unusual event. New techniques were developed including transoral and endoscopic approaches to the mandible. Instrumentation was developed to support these techniques.

The titanium implants at this time were designed to compress bone fragments as compression was thought to promote beneficial primary bone healing, which obviated the need to develop a callous and progress through secondary bone healing. The plates had countersunk holes and chamfered screw heads to take advantage of the spherical gliding principle whereby the screw head levered the bone fragments into compression when the screw was tightened. This compression could be oriented in several directions depending on the design and orientation of the countersunk hole in the plate. Because the mandible has a nerve running through the center (the inferior alveolar nerve), plates could not be placed in the optimal engineering position, which is right down the center of the jaw. This is partly because in order to gain the compression force generated by the screw, the screw must pass through both the lingual and the buccal cortex (bicortical screw). The need to place a bicortical screw meant that the screw could not be placed in a position where there was the risk of penetrating the neural canal and piercing the nerve. This would risk permanent numbness of the lip from injury to the mental nerve. Therefore, the plate had to be placed on the inferior border of the mandible. However, when the plate is placed on the inferior border of the mandible, it must be either long or thick or both to overcome the tensile forces of mastication generated by chewing. Otherwise, every time chewing occurred, there would be a tensile-type gap occurring at the occlusal surface of the fracture, and this would be detrimental to bone healing.

The concept of the tension band was developed where some sort of fixation was necessary at the upper border of the fracture to counteract this tensile force. Tension bands either consisted of wiring teeth together, usually with an Erich arch bar, or in edentulous areas by placing a four-hole monocortical miniplate to counteract the forces of mandibular function. As a rule of thumb, a six-hole bicortical plate alone on the inferior border was thought to have enough strength to counteract occlusal surface tensile forces. An acceptable alternate approach was to use a four-hole inferior border bicortical plate with an occlusal surface tension band—either an arch bar in dentate areas of the jaw or a four-hole monocortical miniplate. These techniques as outlined were designed to be absolutely rigid and to bear the entire load of mastication. They are therefore referred to as load-bearing fixation techniques. Throughout the United States and much of Europe, this load-bearing technique was considered the standard approach to ORIF of mandible fractures, which had the major benefit of allowing the patient to progress to immediate function directly after surgery.

The above-described "AO standard" technique worked well in the hands of many surgeons for many years. However, the design of the technique was based upon using bicortical screws to obtain enough purchase to compress the fracture to obtain primary bone healing. How vitally important is it to have primary bone healing? If primary bone healing through compression is not needed, might one use monocortical rather than bicortical screws? If monocortical screws are used, can the plate be placed in a more optimal location to counteract tensile force at the occlusal surface of the mandible without the risk of impaling the inferior alveolar nerve? Also, are there situations where compression is not desirable? For instance, in a fracture of the angle of the mandible, the surface area of the bone is narrow in cross section, and fractures, while common, are often oblique. Compression of an oblique fracture could actually distract the fracture creating malocclusion. Michelet and Champy asked these questions and found a different answer than what was being practiced by many maxillofacial trauma surgeons.

Maxime Champy reported the results of stress shielding studies in Araldite models that examined the stress and strain characteristics at play in mandible fractures. What he found was that the tensile force at the angle of the mandible amounted to about 60 decanewtons (daN) and that the tensile force at the mandible anterior to the mental foramen was about 100 daN. A six-hole monocortical miniplate with 6-mm screws just penetrating the buccal cortex could overcome the 60 daN force if placed in an optimal location on the superior border of the mandible. In anterior locations, given the greater amount of force at play and the fact that twist and torsion is more possible, Champy recommended placing two monocortical miniplates in an optimal location derived from the force studies on the Araldite models. Champy also placed the plates via a transoral incision because placement of these small plates did not require as much exposure as placing large bicortical plates and screws. Although originally a short period of IMF was used (7 to 10 days) because the fixation technique is not absolutely rigid, subsequent clinical case series have shown that supplemental IMF is not required when using Champy's technique. Because the Champy technique is not rigid enough to prevent small amounts of movement and because it counteracts tensile forces at the fracture site without addressing compressive forces, it is referred to as a load-sharing nonrigid technique. In short, Champy simplified the ORIF technique of mandible fractures by using miniplates, which did not use the compression which necessitated bicortical screws. This allowed placement of the plates in a more optimal engineered position to counteract the forces of tension at play in a mandible fracture without placing the inferior alveolar nerve at risk. Champy's engineering concept resulted in "Champy's lines of osteosynthesis," which is in effect a blue print for optimal monocortical plate placement to address mandible fractures (Fig. 48.1). However, primary bone healing was lost in the process

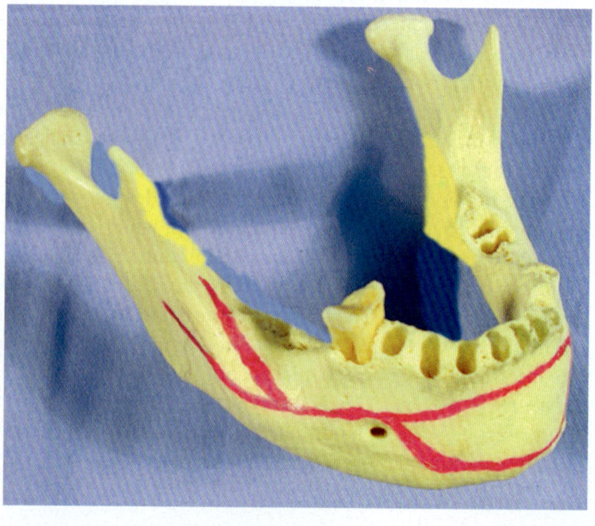

FIGURE 48.1
Champy's lines of osteosynthesis depicted on a skeletal mandible. Two plates are required anterior to the mental foramen to offset torsion loads.

in favor of secondary bone healing through callous formation. Subsequent case series have shown Champy's technique to be the most complication-free technique in the literature. Nevertheless, as a minimalist engineering technique of repair, the Champy technique is unforgiving if attention to detail is not maintained.

HISTORY

Patients with mandible fractures typically present acutely, however, occasionally underlying substance abuse or psychiatric or other factors delay presentation. Patients with mandible fractures may be part of a multiple trauma event and like any patient with multiple trauma should be treated as dictated by good ATLS (advanced trauma life support) practice including assessing the ABCs (airway, breathing, circulation) and clearing the cervical spine. Sometimes patients will relate an accident linked to biking or to other types of sports. Other times, the patient will have had an altercation resulting in interpersonal trauma that results in a fracture. Spousal abuse should be investigated as part of the history of a mandible fracture as protective services may be necessary in cases of battery. Historical information related to previous dental history is sometimes helpful, such as information relating to partial or complete dentures or a history of crown and bridge work or titanium implants. Nevertheless, restorations will usually be apparent after imaging studies are obtained. A thorough social history concentrating upon substance use is important as patients who are alcoholics may be at risk for withdrawal and delirium tremors while undergoing care, and this circumstance can be life threatening. Likewise, the use of heroin, methamphetamines, and cocaine should be elicited to help prevent withdrawal or other problems related to substance abuse. A history of psychiatric intervention is important as continuity of treatment and compliance with medication regimens is important in the postinjury period. The patient should be asked if loss of consciousness occurred either before or after the trauma event as this may impact the type of imaging sought and have importance for calling upon other specialties for consultation. Medical comorbidities, past surgical history, and the presence or absence of drug-related allergies are also important to include in the initial assessment.

PHYSICAL EXAMINATION

A complete examination of the head and neck is performed on all patients with mandible fractures. A general assessment should be made to search for lacerations or concomitant injuries. The forehead should be palpated to search for injury since edema can mask frontal sinus or superior orbital injuries. A thorough eye examination to check for extra ocular motility is helpful to help to screen for orbital injury such as orbital floor fractures as is assessment by palpation of the inferior orbital rim. A screening vision examination should be included. The midface should be evaluated for mobility, which would be found in Le Fort fractures or for step-offs or pain which may accompany zygomatic complex fractures. The nose should be examined and the nasal bridge palpated to screen for a concomitant nasal fracture or nasoethmoidal complex fracture. The oral cavity should be carefully examined with specific attention to lost or missing or injured teeth and to evaluate the occlusion. The occlusion should be characterized as type 1 where the mesiobuccal cusp of the maxillary first molar interdigitates in the mesiobuccal groove of the mandibular first molar, type 2 where the mandible is relatively retruded with respect to the type 1 position, or type 3 where the mandible is relatively prognathic with regard to the type 1 position. An assessment of cross bite whereby the midline of the maxilla and mandible no longer coincide is an important detail to capture on examination. Also, in some types of fractures, especially condyle fractures, the patient may not be able to close the mouth because the posterior molars contact prematurely. This is known as an anterior open bite deformity and should be noted. Intraoral lacerations should be noted and addressed. A neurologic assessment of the first, second, and third divisions of the trigeminal nerve and an assessment of facial nerve function should be recorded. Use of the House-Brackmann scale is an excellent way to record impressions of facial nerve function. Palpation of the neck and larynx, assessment of voice character and quality, and evaluation of the airway for stridor or retractions complete the physical examination.

INDICATIONS

The Champy technique can be appropriate for fractures of the angle, body, parasymphysial and symphysial fractures. This approach is used most commonly in my practice for angle fractures. The reason that the technique is particularly suited for angle fractures is because the surface area of the mandible at the angle is actually less than that of the body and obliquity of fractures of this area is common and is a contraindication to fracture compression. The angle is also well accessed through a transoral incision at its superior border, whereas the inferior border is more of a reach transorally. The Champy technique can be used in cases where more than one fracture is present. However, the Champy technique at one location can be combined with another technique at a second location. As an example, in the case of a right angle fracture and left parasymphysial fracture, one can use a Champy monocortical miniplate on the right angle and a bicortical six-hole inferior border plate at the left parasymphysial fracture. Champy's plates can certainly be used in body, parasymphysial, and symphysial fractures. However, it is often just as easy to place an inferior border plate in the body and parasymphysial area and a lag screw or inferior border plate in the symphysial area so the elegance of the engineering and the swiftness of the Champy approach are not as dramatic as it is in the angle region with its more difficult access.

CONTRAINDICATIONS

- Comminution of a fracture is an absolute contraindication to the Champy technique.
- Loss of bone is an absolute contraindication to the Champy technique.
- Fresh removal of a molar in the line of the fracture at the angle is a relative contraindication to the Champy technique. This is because the molar often contributes to the surface area of contact at the angle and loss of this surface area tips the decision balance toward favoring rigid fixation techniques like those outlined by the AO/ASIF. The Lindqvist study is one that supports this practice.
- Edentulous mandibles with loss of alveolar bone usually have decreased surface contact area and are a contraindication to the Champy technique. This circumstance favors a rigid load-bearing approach.
- Osteomyelitis mandates a load-bearing repair and is a contraindication to the Champy technique.
- The Champy technique is an option for primary surgery but is not usually suitable for revision surgical cases because it is a nonrigid fixation technique.
- Severely displaced fractures requiring transcervical approaches to achieve reduction are better suited to load-bearing repairs rather than the Champy technique.

PREOPERATIVE PLANNING

Patients who have sustained multiple trauma are typically admitted to the hospital, often in a highly monitored setting such as the intensive care unit. However, patients with isolated mandible fractures do not always require hospital admission; rather, the decision to admit or treat as an outpatient depends on the stability of the airway, pain control, medical comorbidities, and social circumstances. Imaging is a mainstay of preoperative decision making. Plain film radiography can help to demonstrate fractures. Specifically left and right lateral oblique views of the mandible and a P–A view can be helpful. A Towne's view can be useful to screen the neck of the condyle. A posterior–anterior oblique view or Waters' view can be useful to visualize the anterior mandible. A panoramic radiograph is useful for evaluation of the fracture and shows the condyles well. In my practice, CT imaging including axial, coronal, sagittal, and 3-D reconstruction views is indispensable and is our standard study. CT can show details such as fractured tooth roots, oblique fractures that would require lag screw placement, and the precise location of the head of the condyle in condyle fractures. This information will have a high degree of influence on the planned operation. Further, the degree of comminution of the fracture can also be assessed, which is a key factor in whether or not the Champy technique can be used. CT imaging also helps the surgeon to plan the approach (transoral or transcervical) and to estimate the amount of operative time that will be necessary to repair the fracture. Timing of repair of the fracture is controversial, but published case series do not necessarily prove that earlier repair decreases postoperative infection rates. It does appear that early repair (defined as repair within the first 72 hours after injury) decreases technical complications from the surgery itself. Yet, patients with substance abuse and psychiatric disease will sometimes not present for treatment until more than 72 hours after injury. As part of preoperative planning, informed consent is obtained from the patient with regard to the steps needed to stabilize the fracture and allow it to heal. Risks such as injury to the nerves or teeth, malocclusion, infection, nonunion, bleeding, scarring, and possible need for revision are typically discussed with the patient and significant others. In addition, the risks and benefits of open repair are compared and contrasted with those of closed repair with approximately 4 weeks of IMF alone if this is thought to be a reasonable option. Patients thus informed are usually able to alert the surgeon as to their preferences for treatment. A plan for the IMF must be made. Options typically include Erich arch bars, Ivy loops, or four-point IMF screws.

SURGICAL TECHNIQUE

The patient is brought into the operating room after adequate informed consent. CT scans and films are immediately available in the operating room. The films are checked to document the side of the fracture or fractures. The patient undergoes nasotracheal intubation, and the operating room table is rotated 180 degrees from the point of intubation. The table is placed into a mild beach chair position (semisitting). The patient is prepped with betadine or green soap and a head drape and split sheet are placed. Chlorhexidine rinse and a toothbrush are used to clean the teeth, and a blue moon retractor is used to retract the lips. The dentition and occlusion are checked with attention to wear facets on the teeth. The gingival buccal sulcus is injected in the area of the fracture with lidocaine 1% with epinephrine 1:100,000 to improve hemostasis. If the fracture is minimally displaced, IMF is then secured. Frequently, IMF screws are used when the fracture is retroocclusal. Examples of retroocclusal fractures include fractures of the condyle, ramus, and angle. The idea is that the fracture is behind the normal interdigitation of the teeth. If the fracture is through the body, symphysis, or parasymphysis, then Erich arch bars are typically placed. However, in severely displaced fractures, Erich arch bars can inadvertently lock the fracture segments into a poorly reduced position. Therefore, in severely displaced fractures, arch bars are typically placed after exposure and reduction of the fracture.

IMF screws come in long lengths (approximately 12 mm) and short lengths (approximately 8 mm). Short IMF screws are usually placed either just mesially or just distally to the maxillary canine tooth root. Meticulous attention must be paid to placing the screw perpendicular to the cortical bone and not to angle the screw toward the tooth root. Also, the screw must be placed so that it does not impale a tooth root. The screws are self-drilling, but a stab incision using a #11 blade may be made to allow smoother placement. IMF screws are placed in the mandibular segment in a similar fashion, but often, a 12-mm screw is used here just mesial to the canine tooth root. It is important to visualize the future plate placement because it is inopportune to have the IMF screw interfere with optimal plate location. Twenty-four gauge stainless steel wire is used to place the mandible into class 1 IMF through the IMF screws.

A gingival buccal incision is outlined with a marking pen. Approximately 1 cm of free gingiva is left on the lingual side of the incision to allow easy closure. The incision is made with a #64 beaver blade or a # 15 blade. A Bovie on coagulation setting is then used to deepen the incision and to approach the periosteum. Sewall retractors and V-notch retractors are used to gain exposure. A Freer elevator is used to dissect the periosteum with masseter muscle off of the angle of the mandible. The angle fracture is identified. The attached gingiva is back elevated to allow complete exposure of the external oblique ridge and the area around the second or third mandibular molar. Reduction of the fracture is then secured. The fracture is inspected to make sure that it is not comminuted, and the exposed molar teeth are checked for viability and to assure that they are not loose or fractured, which would necessitate removal and tip the repair decision making to a load-bearing technique. A 2.0 (or similar) four-hole locking threaded plate is selected. If the plate is to be placed on the external oblique ridge, it is twisted at its midpoint about 90 degrees (Fig. 48.2). If the plate is to be placed on the buccal cortex, it does not usually require much bend. The threaded drill guide is used to act as a handle to hold the plate when checking how it will be placed across the fracture (Fig. 48.3). Typically, a buccal cortex plate is used. After assuring optimal fit and bend, a #11 blade is used to make a 5-mm incision through the skin in a central location that will allow the transbuccal trocar to approach all four screw holes with minimal retraction. A Schnit fine long-angled clamp is used to spread through parotid tissue and masseter in the general direction of the facial nerve fibers and brought through the tougher periosteum until it is visualized in the wound. The trocar with the stylette is placed into the puncture wound and identified in the surgical field. The stylette is removed with the tip of the trocar in the surgical field, and the threaded locking drill guide is placed into the wound through the trocar. The threaded locking trocar is brought into the mouth where it can be reached and the plate is threaded onto the drill guide.

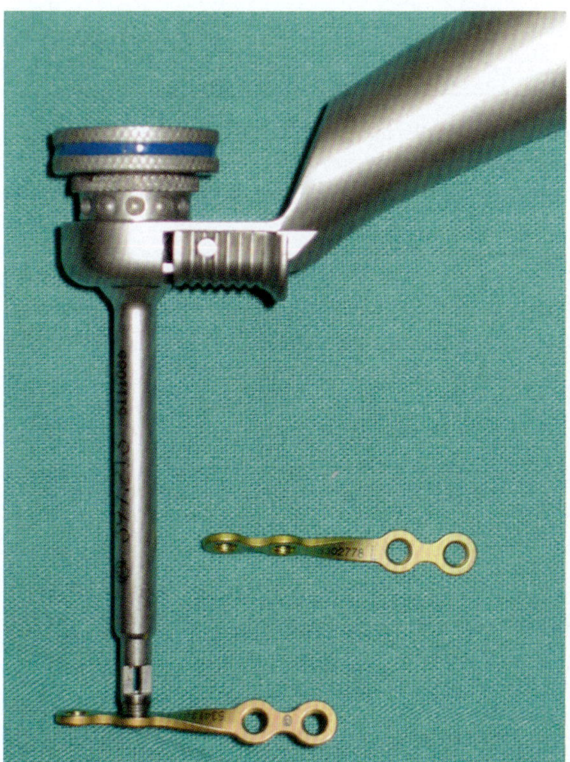

FIGURE 48.2
A transbuccal trocar is shown with a threaded locking miniplate. These plates are manufactured in a bent orientation to be used along the external oblique ridge. The drill guide can be used as a handle to control plate placement.

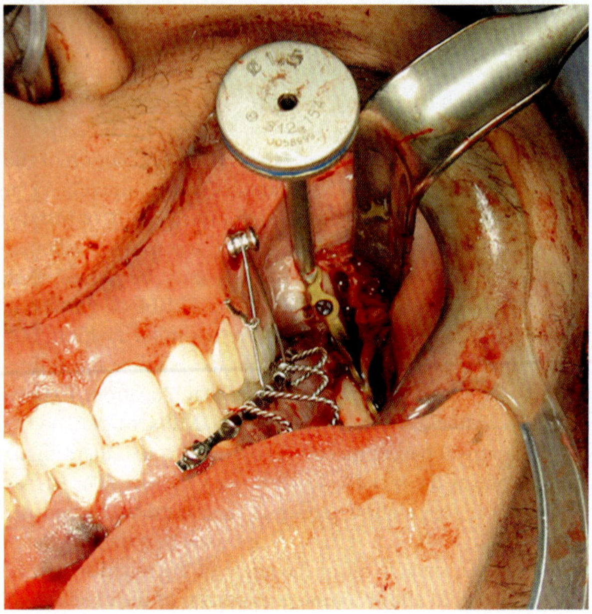

FIGURE 48.3
One prebent miniplate along the external oblique ridge is placed along Champy's lines at the angle of the mandible. The screws along the mesial part of the fracture are often placed using a transbuccal trocar. The distal screws can often be placed through a transoral approach.

The appropriate drill is brought onto the field. I use a 6-mm drill to assure that only one cortex will be drilled. The trocar with drill guide must be placed in the exact optimal position to fixate the fracture along the superior border of the mandible adjacent to the buccal cortex (Figs. 48.4 and 48.5). Irrigation must be used to cool the drill. The 6-mm drill is used to create the hole in the buccal cortex. The plate is unscrewed from the drill guide, and the drill guide is removed from the trocar. A 6-mm threaded or unthreaded screw is loaded onto a screw driver, carefully placed through the trocar, carefully placed through the plate at the intended screw site, and then into the hole drilled into the buccal cortex. The screw is driven home with "two-finger" torsional tension on the screwdriver handle. This screw is the most critical because it sets the orientation of the plate to the fracture. The next three drill holes are placed with the threaded locking drill guide and are less difficult because the plate is fixed by the first screw. Sometimes, two separate trocar puncture wounds are required. A second four-hole plate can then be placed just below the first using the same steps just described. Copious bacitracin irrigation is used. The wound is closed with either running 0-chromic or 2-0 monocryl. The patient may be taken out of IMF at the end of the case. Alternatively, a short period of continued IMF may be recommended, especially if a concomitant condyle fracture is present.

POSTOPERATIVE MANAGEMENT

If the patient remains in IMF, nutritional supplementation is usually indicated. IMF screws are easier on the dentition, gums, and lips as they have less wire projections that can severely annoy the patient. Dental wax available from stores and pharmacies can be used to blunt any remaining sharp edges. Chlorhexidine rinse can

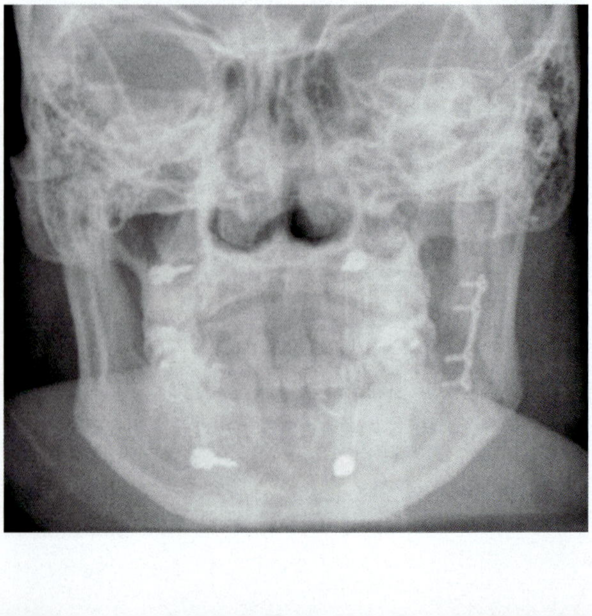

FIGURE 48.4
In this postoperative radiograph, a single plate is placed along the buccal cortex along Champy's line to fix an angle fracture. The screws were placed using a transbuccal trocar.

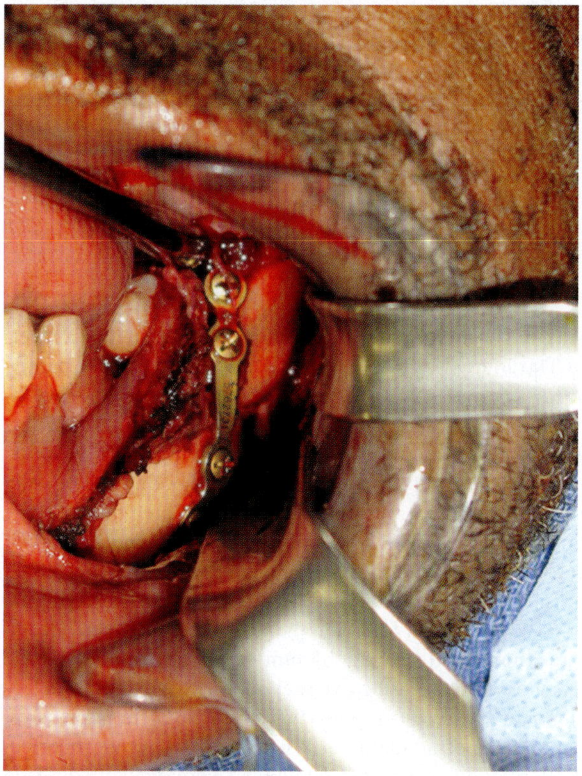

FIGURE 48.5
Transoral view of a single monocortical miniplate bent to conform to the anatomy of the external oblique ridge at the angle of the mandible.

be used to supplement oral care. Antibiotic coverage may be continued in the postoperative period, but this decision is usually made on a case by case basis. If the patient is removed from IMF, instructions encouraging a soft diet are given. At times, all IMF hardware is also removed at the end of the case if the likelihood of complications is felt to be low. Postoperative imaging is obtained as soon as practically possible. This may consist of a panoramic radiograph; a plain film series consisting of a Towne view, P–A view, and left and right lateral oblique views; or in some cases repeat CT imaging. A physical therapy appliance such as the TheraBite device is sometimes recommended in order to improve the ability to open their mouth. This is especially useful in patients with condyle fractures; however, patients often need to purchase the rather expensive device from their own funds. Stacked tongue blades to a height of approximately 4.0 cm are a possible (but inferior) alternative rehabilitation tool if cost issues become a critical factor. The patient can try to stack as many tongue blades as possible between the incisors to improve the opening distance to the usually normal 4.0 cm interincisal opening distance mark. Patients are usually seen at 1 week. If they are in IMF, they are typically encouraged to come in weekly for about 1 month or until the IMF is removed. These patients are also instructed to always carry a wire cutter in the event of nausea and subsequent emesis. Retained IMF hardware is typically removed at about the postoperative week 5 mark. During these postoperative visits, the dentition is inspected, occlusion is assessed, the wound is checked for dehiscence, the mandible is checked for fracture site mobility or infection, and the patient's nutrition and pain control are evaluated. It is optimal to also check on the patient's condition at about the 6-month mark if possible. Referral to a prosthodontist or orthodontist may sometimes be recommended to take care of chipped or cracked teeth or to consider orthodontic adjustments to the occlusion.

COMPLICATIONS

- Malocclusion: When teeth do not interdigitate correctly, this can be disturbing to the patient. It is a potential complication of any mandible fracture and is more common in condylar fractures and fractures through dentate segments of the mandible.
- Malunion: Malunion occurs when the mandible heals in an unfavorable position for function and occlusion.
- Trismus: Scarring and fixation of the temporomandibular joint which limits mouth opening and therefore function.
- Numbness: Stretch injury to the nerve or impalement of the inferior alveolar and mental nerve can lead to temporary or permanent numbness of the lip and cheek.
- Tooth devitalization: Plates and screws driven into tooth roots may cause the tooth to become devitalized and may necessitate further treatment such as root canal therapy or the need for crown and bridge reconstruction or tooth extraction.

- Wound dehiscence: Transoral approaches have a relatively high preponderance of wound dehiscence. Perhaps as high as 25% of transoral wounds will have incisional breakdown. This does not usually mandate hardware removal; rather, local care and antibiotics can often be used to promote good healing.
- Osteomyelitis: This term is generalizable to when the bone itself becomes infected. Revision surgery may be necessary in such cases with conversion to a load-bearing repair. Oral or intravenous antibiotics are recommended, and return of the patient to IMF may be necessary to overcome micromovement at the fracture site from the load-sharing repair.

RESULTS

The original English language paper published by Maxime Champy and his coauthors was presented at a meeting in London in September, 1976, but published in The Journal of Maxillo-Facial Surgery in 1978. Champy described a series of 183 patients treated with "monocortical juxta-alveolar and subapical osteosynthesis, without compression and without IMF, using miniature malleable plates." They recommended repair as soon as possible, hopefully within 6 hours of the trauma, and the main contraindication to the technique was preexisting infection. A four-hole plate was described and attention to proper sizing of the drill, cooling the bit, and assuring no eccentricity of the screw hole was stressed as the screw was only anchored by three threads. The transoral approach to the angle was described, and interestingly formal IMF was not used; rather, an assistant placed the patient into reduction manually. The team also warned against overtightening the screw, which could distort the threads, understanding that the technique is very sensitive to having perfect screw holes relying on minimal fixation. Because of increased torsion anterior to the mental foramen, the team reinforced the need to have two monocortical plates in this area, and they recommended spacing 4.5 mm between the plates. At the angle, two-plate placement areas were described: one twisted plate at the external oblique ridge or alternately on the buccal surface using a transbuccal trocar technique. The results reported by this team were impressive. In the 183 patients who they followed up to 5 years, no cases of nonunion or loss of hardware were reported. All patients began a soft diet on postoperative day 1. Normal diet was achieved on postoperative day 10. "Side effects" including postoperative infection were reported as 3% of a 100 patient cohort. No iatrogenic nerve or dental injury was reported. The overall infection rate in the 183 patient group was 3.8%. Malunion occurred in 0.5% and delayed union in 0.5%. However, 4.8% of patients required disking or grinding of occlusal tooth surfaces postoperatively to achieve adequate occlusion.

These results were spectacular for the era, especially considering that plates were not yet made of titanium when this paper was published. The question was, were the results repeatable by other teams? Fox and Kellman in 2003 published a classic article in Archives of Facial Plastic Surgery. Sixty-eight patients with 70 angle fractures were studied who had at least 12 weeks of follow-up. A two miniplate technique (2.0 noncompression plate; 4, 5, or 6 hole) was used obtaining exposure through a transoral incision and using trans-buccal trocar techniques (Fig. 48.6). IMF was used at the time of surgery but released unless a subcondylar fracture was present after surgery. The time from injury to surgery ranged from less than 24 hours to 18 days with a mean of 7.2 days. No patients had malunion, nonunion, or osteomyelitis. About 18% of patients had some type of complication, however. This included 3% of patients who had a wound infection, occlusal disturbance in 6%, and wound dehiscence in 6%. Nerve injury occurred in about 4.4% (3) patients due to surgical manipulation.

In 2010, Dr. Ed Ellis expanded his examination of the one miniplate angle technique that he classically reported in 1996 in the Journal of Oral and Maxillofacial Surgery where he and Walker reported a 16%

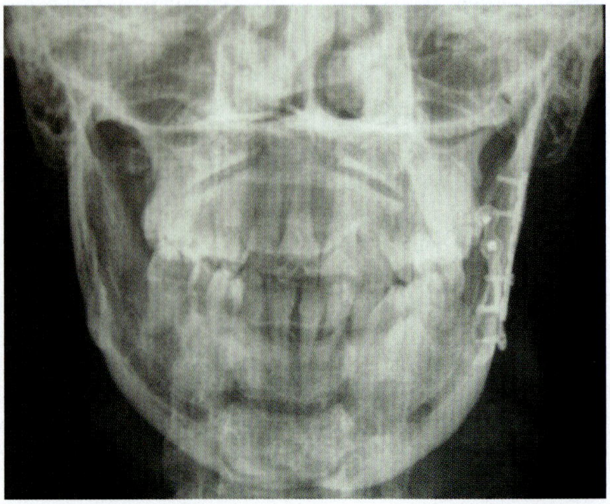

FIGURE 48.6

Some series recommend two plates at the angle along Champy's lines as depicted in the postoperative x-ray.

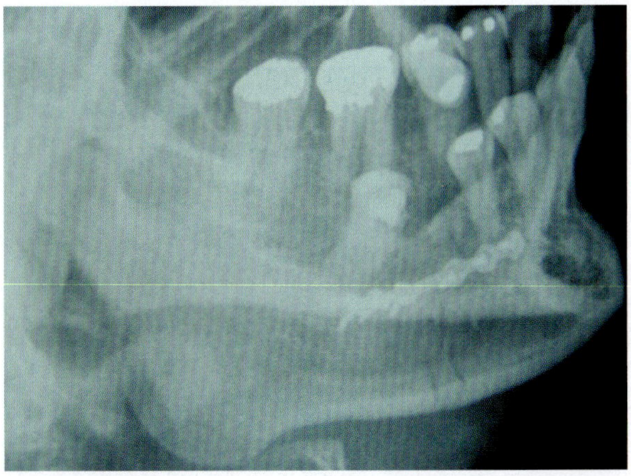

FIGURE 48.7
Body fractures can also be addressed using a single monocortical miniplate placed along Champy's lines. This is usually accomplished through a transoral approach.

complication rate, which consisted of major or minor infection, swelling, and pain. Dr. Ellis reported a prospective (but not randomized) study of 185 patients who met study criteria for follow-up, fracture type, and comorbidities and were divided into three equal groups of about 60 patients each. Group 1 was repaired with nonrigid fixation using maxillary mandibular fixation (MMF) and a wire to approximate the fracture at the angle, Group 2 was treated with a single four-hole titanium noncompression 2.0 miniplate at the medial side of the external oblique ridge. Group 3 was treated with two 2.0 miniplates: one at the medial side of the external oblique ridge like Group 2 and a second plate on the inferior portion of the buccal cortex. Some patients had supplemental IMF. Wound problems were reported in 15% of patients in Group 1, 3.2% in Group 2, and 22% in Group 3. The authors concluded that single miniplate fixation at the angle was the superior fixation technique while understanding that the study was not randomized.

It is obvious that there some selection bias in determining whether a monocortical miniplate can be used to fix an angle fracture. Some of the key issues to consider include lack of comminution, lack of tooth extraction in the fracture line, and avoidance of compression techniques at the angle. Comminution or tooth extraction would tip the balance of decision making toward rigid load bearing reconstruction plate fixation with neutral drilling of screws. Nevertheless, it is intuitive that fractures with tooth loss or comminution are more apt to have associated postoperative complications such as nonunion or osteomyelitis. For this reason, it may not be entirely fair to compare modern reports of complication rates of rigid load bearing fixation to the above monocortical miniplate case series. The Iizuka and Lindqvist publication in the February 1993 Plastic and Reconstructive Surgery emphasized the deleterious effect of molar tooth removal upon mandibular healing. The loss of surface area and the compound nature of such fractures appear to tip the decision process toward choosing a rigid load bearing repair approach.

The Champy repair may also be used in fractures of the symphysis and body, but the results of their use in the dentate areas of the mandible may not be as formidable as when the Champy technique is used at the angle (Figs. 48.7 and 48.8). A study by Ellis published in the Journal of Oral and Maxillofacial Surgery compared the results of 265 patients treated with two 2.0 monocortical miniplates and 417 treated with one thick 2.0 plate using bicortical screws through an intraoral surgical approach. No supplemental IMF was used. The overall complication rate (2.6%) was not statistically significantly different between the two groups; however, wound dehiscence, plate exposure, need to remove plates not related to infection, and tooth root damage were all statistically significantly worse in patients with a two miniplate repair compared to a single larger bicortical 2.0 plate. Malocclusion and nonunion were not different between the two groups. The data on dehiscence showed that 6% of the two-plate technique cases resulted in wound dehiscence, and the usually occurred with exposure of the superiorly based plate. Plate removal was subsequently required in 65% of the wounds that dehisced; however, the need to remove a plate did not necessarily mean that osseous union had not occurred. Nevertheless, Champy's techniques in the dentate portion of the mandible still produce reasonably successful outcomes in fracture repair.

PEARLS

- IMF screws save time and are intrinsically safer for the surgical team than Erich arch bars or Ivy loops. The team must be vigilant about wire stick injuries, which are the most common cause of stick injuries in head and neck surgery.
- The wire holes in the IMF screws line up with the cross hatch of the screw head.
- Use of the Champy technique relies on just a few screw threads to maintain alignment of the fracture. Drills must be sharp and straight. Irrigation should be used to cool the drill bit. Excessive pressure on the drill should be avoided because it can result in an eccentric hole that will not be a perfect match for the screw threads. Overtightening the screw can crack the cortical bone weakening the repair.

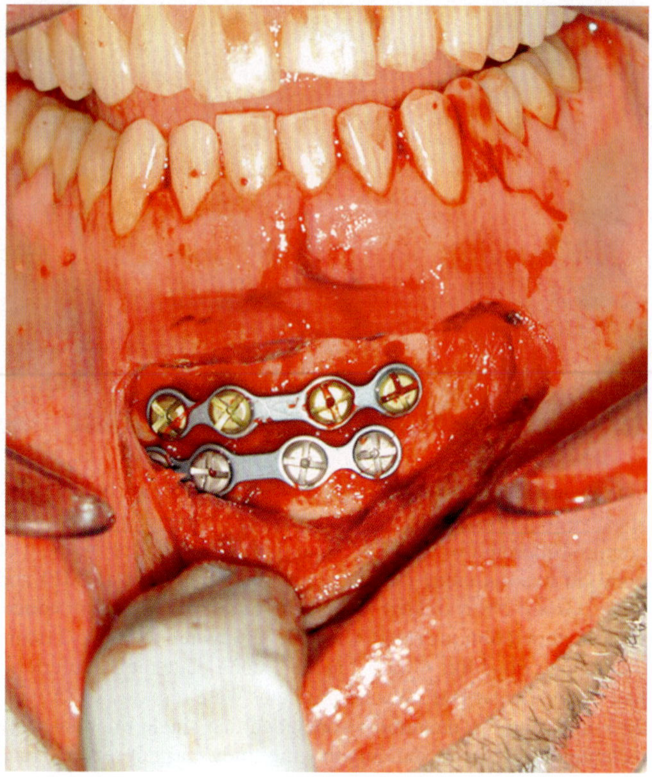

FIGURE 48.8
Anteriorly, two monocortical miniplates are needed to counteract torsional forces.

- When placing a plate on the angle at the external oblique ridge, it may be necessary to take the patient out of IMF to drill holes on the mesial fracture segment. Plates placed on the external oblique ridge are often bent at close to a 90-degree angle in the sagittal plane. Some companies produce prebent plates for this purpose.
- In cases of displaced fractures, we have learned to place IMF hardware after fracture exposure as arch bars can lock a fracture into a suboptimal position if placed before the fracture is reduced.
- A transbuccal trocar drill guide that screws into a threaded locking 2.0 plate can be used as a handle to hold the plate into position. Some companies manufacture right angle screwdrivers and drills in an attempt to obviate the need for transbuccal trocar placement.
- After placement of a stab incision for trocar use, blunt soft tissue dissection is performed with a fine tip clamp, and spreading is performed parallel to the course of the facial nerve.
- Chlorhexidine rinse may help the patient maintain oral hygiene in the immediate postoperative period.
- Transoral incisions are used almost exclusively when accomplishing Champy's approaches to mandible fractures.
- Meticulous closure techniques and stair-stepping incisions are used to help decrease problems with wound dehiscence which is the most common complication of the Champy technique. Wound dehiscence does not mandate the need for plate removal.
- With regard to angle fractures, the lowest complication rate in the reported literature is with the Champy technique.

PITFALLS

- The Champy technique at the angle is not suitable for comminuted fractures nor is it ideal if a tooth has been removed in the line of the fracture. These factors typically tip the balance toward choosing a load-bearing rigid fixation repair.
- The buccal cortex of the anterior mandible is actually quite thin and closely approximated to the tooth roots. This may put tooth roots at risk when repairing anterior mandible fractures using the Champy technique. Torsional forces at play anterior to the mental foramen mandate the need for two Champy plates in this region.
- Edentulous mandibles commonly have loss of alveolar bone and decreased surface contact to support the mechanical forces of this technique.
- Not a rigid fixation technique. In circumstances of active osteomyelitis, revision surgery, severely displaced fractures, or comminuted fracture, a load bearing plate is superior.

INSTRUMENTS TO HAVE AVAILABLE

- Basic maxillofacial trauma set
- IMF screws set with self-drilling screws
- Monopolar cautery with Teflon-coated protected tip
- 2.0 (or similar) miniplate plating system

SUGGESTED READING

Champy M, Loddé JP, Schmitt R, et al. Mandibular osteosynthesis by miniature screwed plates via a buccal approach. *J Maxillofac Surg* 1978;6(1):14–21. PubMed PMID: 274501.

Cornelius CP, Ehrenfeld M. The use of MMF screws: surgical technique, indications, contraindications, and common problems in review of the literature. *Craniomaxillofac Trauma Reconstr* 2010;3(2):55.

Ellis E III. A prospective study of 3 treatment methods for isolated fractures of the mandibular angle. *J Oral Maxillofac Surg* 2010;68(11):2743–2754. PubMed PMID: 20869149.

Ellis E III. A study of 2 bone plating methods for fractures of the mandibular symphysis/body. *J Oral Maxillofac Surg* 2011;69(7):1978–1987. Epub 2011 May 6. PubMed PMID: 21549485.

Fox AJ, Kellman RM. Mandibular angle fractures: two-miniplate fixation and complications. *Arch Facial Plast Surg* 2003;5(6):464–469. PubMed PMID: 14623682.

Murr AH. Mandibular angle fractures and noncompression plating techniques. *Arch Otolaryngol Head Neck Surg* 2005;131(2):166–168. PubMed PMID: 15723951.

49 PERCUTANEOUS APPROACH TO MANDIBULAR ANGLE FRACTURES

Michael A. Carron

INTRODUCTION

Facial trauma is responsible for a substantial portion of injuries seen in the emergency room. The most common cause of injury is physical assault. However, falls, bicycle accidents, industrial accidents, motor vehicle accidents, and sporting injuries are also contributing elements. It is not unusual for victims of facial trauma to have a fracture of the mandible, and about 25% will occur at the mandibular angle. This injury is believed to occur due to the turning of the head upon attack, thereby exposing the angle of the mandible to the brute force. It is further susceptible to fracture because third molars occupy osseous space, thereby weakening the bone stock. Moreover, unique forces can act on the angle because it is a transition zone from the body to the ascending ramus of the mandible.

The region of the mandibular angle is very important as it plays a central role in the functional integrity of the jaw as well as facial aesthetics. Failure to properly reconstruct the mandibular angle may result in malunion or nonunion with resultant malocclusion, chronic pain, facial asymmetry, and impaired mastication. The treatment of these injuries requires expertise and becomes even more difficult and complex when patients have poor dentition, have poor oral hygiene, and are prone to miss appointments for follow-up care.

The repair of fractures of the mandibular angle can be performed through an external submandibular approach or percutaneously through an intraoral incision combined with a transbuccal trocar and screwdriver. The percutaneous approach reduces potential injury to the facial nerve and minimizes external incisions and scarring. However, when drilling holes and placing screws, the technique may be difficult in certain hard-to-reach areas of the mandibular angle.

HISTORY

Patients with a fracture of the mandible usually present to the emergency room with a complex history of trauma. The standard tenants of evaluating the trauma patient (airway, breathing, circulation, Glasgow Coma Scale, IV access) take priority over general patient history. Since the mandible is located in continuity to the floor of the mouth, edema or frank hematoma can displace the tongue posteriorly. Such a patient may present with difficulty breathing and harbor a significant potential for airway obstruction.

Once the trauma evaluation is complete and the patient is stabilized, attention is directed toward the events of the trauma, signs and symptoms related to these injuries, and the patient history. Questions regarding the current event, past surgical interventions, previous trauma, current medications, allergies, family history, and substance use are reviewed and recorded. The patient's general health history is also obtained at this time and includes cardiac, pulmonary, hepatic, and renal systems. Depending upon the patient's level of consciousness, the history may need to be obtained by family or accompanying others. Additional surgical specialists and social services are consulted as necessary.

PHYSICAL EXAMINATION

The physical examination is critical in assessing the fractured mandible. Examination allows the surgeon to determine the location and severity of the injuries. In addition to the standardized "top-down" head and neck examination, particular attention is drawn to the lower third of the face, teeth, lips, tongue, and gingiva. The surgeon should note the presence or absence of swelling over the fracture site, tenderness, and intraoral or external lacerations and possibly exposed bony fragments.

The teeth may be loose, chipped, or avulsed. All teeth and/or dentures need to be accounted for as they may be lodged in the patient's airway. The patient should be questioned as to whether they detect any damage to the teeth or whether their occlusion is abnormal. Teeth create additional stability when repairing mandible fractures, and technical attention is needed in evaluation. Teeth that appear to be carious or devitalized from the injury should be considered for dental extraction to prevent complications. A dental or oral surgical colleague may need to evaluate the patient's teeth if there is a question about their status.

Complaints of loss of sensation of the face, lips, or cheeks may be due to injury of the inferior alveolar nerve, which courses through the body of the mandible or the mental nerve as it exits the mandible between the first and second premolars. Gentle rocking of the mandible will allow the surgeon to evaluate for and document the location of any mobile segments of the mandible. Occasionally, the fracture is "open" with a laceration of the gingiva at the site of injury with bleeding from the marrow space of the bone. Angle fractures often will occur with opposite condylar or parasymphyseal fractures. The examining physician should keep in mind that multiple fractures are often a rule and not the exception.

INDICATIONS

Prompt care of this injury is important as unrepaired mandibular fractures are painful and may also result in malocclusion, open bite deformity, as well as impaired speech, chewing, or swallowing. The goal of internal fixation is to reestablish bony union, prevent nonunion or malunion, and initiate early mobilization of the condyle to avoid ankylosis. For a simple favorable linear fracture of the mandibular angle, the percutaneous approach applying a Champy miniplate should be considered. For unfavorable fractures or fractures complicated by absent teeth, compression, noncompression, or a locking plate would be indicated. The particular plate and screws selected need to ensure neutralization of the functional forces on the angle of the mandible to allow stable bone healing (Fig. 49.1). The percutaneous approach provides minimal morbidity and minimal

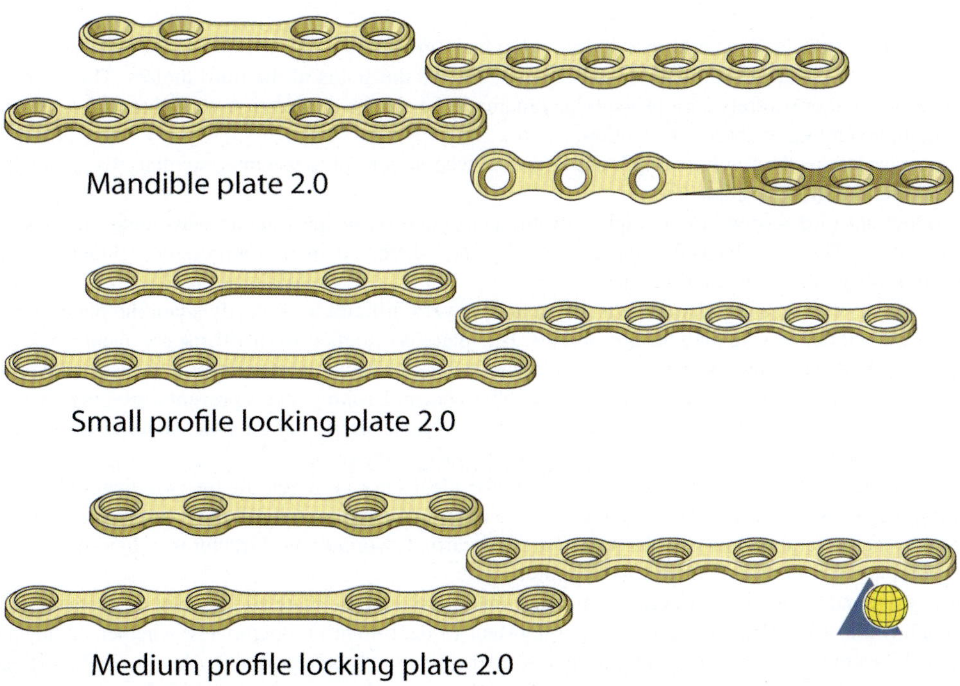

FIGURE 49.1 Plate selection depends on the fracture situation. For minimally displaced fractures of the angle, a Champy plate can be placed across the idea line of osteosynthesis (e.g., Mandible plate 2.0 with near 90-degree twist). For vertical or minimally oblique fractures, a compression plate may be used. For severely oblique fractures, a noncompression fracture plate is suggested. For very irregular bony topography or a high-risk situation of screw back-out or screw failure locking plates are recommended. For severe fractures or highly comminuted fractures, reconstruction plates are suggested.

soft tissue dissection and avoids potential damage to neurovascular and glandular structures of the cheek. Additionally, the intraoral incision used with the percutaneous approach may be advantageous when the surgeon needs to remove a molar tooth from the fracture site.

The extraoral approach is best suited for multiple complicated fractures and comminuted fractures. This approach involves an incision through the neck with a significant dissection to reach the angle of the mandible. The potential for injury to the submandibular gland or to the marginal branch of the facial nerve exists and should not be underestimated.

CONTRAINDICATIONS

The percutaneous technique is not always indicated nor is it always ideal. There are certain trauma situations in which the external approach or an external fixation device should be considered and even used preferentially. On occasion, a large preexisting traumatic laceration to the neck and cheek tissues can be used to access the fracture site, thereby obviating the need for a percutaneous approach. Neglected fractures with abscess formation and/or sequestra necessitate an external approach and drainage of infected material. In cases of severe comminution, a very long reconstruction plate may be needed to bridge a defect. In cases of severe comminution with multiple fractures at the mandibular angle, an external fixation device may be necessary. Essentially, large fragments of bone can be pinned and maintained in a stable manner while the intervening comminuted fragments are stabilized between the large pieces and provide the bone stock for healing the fracture.

PREOPERATIVE PLANNING

Radiographic Examination

The maxillofacial computed tomography (CT) scan is the current standard for evaluation of mandible fractures. The CT scan is very sensitive for demonstrating fractures of the mandible and can be used alone, but limitations have been found in detailing the dental anatomy. The status of the teeth brings an important variable to the management of these injuries. Although posing some limitations at the symphyseal region, a Panorex and complete mandible series provide an excellent view of the mandible from condyle to condyle and yield information about the status of the teeth. This is particularly important for mandibular angle fractures where the examination of the third molar is imperative.

- Identification of the location and severity of all the facial fractures.
- Determine with physical examination and imaging studies the status of the third molars. This is important because nonvital or severely carious teeth may increase the chance of infection with potential osteomyelitis, malunion, nonunion, or abscess formation.
- If the patient has teeth, it will be important to decide whether or not to use intermaxillary fixation with arch bars or intermaxillary fixation screws.
- It is important to determine radiographically the configuration of the fracture (favorable, unfavorable, or comminuted). This will determine the choice of plate, whether it be a compression, Champy miniplate, noncompression, or reconstruction plate.
- If the contour of the mandibular angle is irregular, it is very difficult to perfectly adapt the plate to the bone surface and a locking plate may be appropriate. This plate is designed so that the screw heads lock into the plate acting both as an internal and external fixation device. Locking plates are useful in cases with extensive defects, especially where prolonged healing is likely to occur. Locking plates prevent loosening of the screw heads from the plate or screw back-out and can minimize the resorption of the bone underneath the plate due to direct pressure the screws exert when they pull the bone to the plate.
- For oblique fractures, a compression plate may not be ideal since compressing the two diagonal ends of the fracture may cause one end to slide up and over the other upon compression. In this case, a noncompression plate may be preferable. For very large fractures or partially comminuted fractures, a load-bearing reconstruction plate is usually considered appropriate.
- The severity and extent of the fracture will determine the size of the plate and amount of exposure required for application. If the fracture is old, it is important to determine preoperatively whether or not there is infection, osteomyelitis, or sequestra that requires debridement. It is important to determine the presence of an abscess as this would direct the surgeon toward the external approach where drainage of infection and removal of any sequestra need to be performed.
- If a plate is applied inferiorly, it is important to prevent splaying of the superior border of the fracture. In this case, a two- or four-hole miniplate with monocortical screws can be used as a superior border tension band. An arch bar can also be used provided there is good dentition.

SURGICAL TECHNIQUE

The patient is brought to the operating room, and general anesthesia with nasotracheal intubation is carried out if the patient is awake or has a standard endotracheal tube in place. If plans are for the patient to remain intubated for an extended period of time or the risks of extubation with subsequent nasotracheal intubation are too great, a tracheostomy should be performed at this time. After securing the patient's airway, the operation may proceed.

The initial step is to establish the normal preinjury occlusion for the patient. To achieve this, arch bars are applied to the upper and lower dental arches. However, intermaxillary fixation screws or IV loops can be used to achieve occlusion and intermaxillary fixation. It is important to realize that the arch bar will act as a tension band at the upper mandibular border, while the other two modalities will not provide tension. After intermaxillary fixation is obtained, the patient's entire face and neck is prepared with Betadine solution, which is allowed to dry. The patient is draped in the normal fashion. This is performed in the event that an external approach becomes necessary. The alveolus and retromolar trigone area are injected with 1% lidocaine with epinephrine (1:100,000) and allowed to act for a period of 10 minutes for hemostasis to take effect. A 15-blade scalpel is used to make an incision along the oblique ridge of the mandible, extending into the gingivobuccal sulcus in the second molar. This incision may be extended anteriorly as necessary in order to gain exposure of the fracture (Fig. 49.2). The incision is carried down to the periosteum, and a Cottle elevator is then used to dissect the periosteum off of the posterior body, angle, and proximal ascending ramus to expose the fracture (Fig. 49.3). The fracture may be manually reduced at this point with the patient in intermaxillary fixation.

For the reduced nondisplaced fracture, a Champy miniplate is applied to the oblique line. For more extensive fractures, plates will need to be applied inferiorly for this technique. It is important to choose the site in the skin of the cheek for the trocar that will be used to access the fracture. A blunt instrument can be placed from the medial aspect of the flap outward to indent the lateral skin so the surgeon can judge where to make a stab incision (Fig. 49.4). This site provides access for the percutaneous instruments and the site chosen to allow the instruments to access all aspects of the plate (Fig. 49.5). Care is taken to not place the incision in too superior of a location as the facial soft tissues are not as readily mobile toward an inferior direction if such a position is required. Once a site is chosen, an 11-blade scalpel is used to make a small stab wound in the skin. A fine mosquito clamp can be used to gently dissect into the subcutaneous tissue. The tines of the clamp are spread parallel to the direction of the branches of the facial nerve.

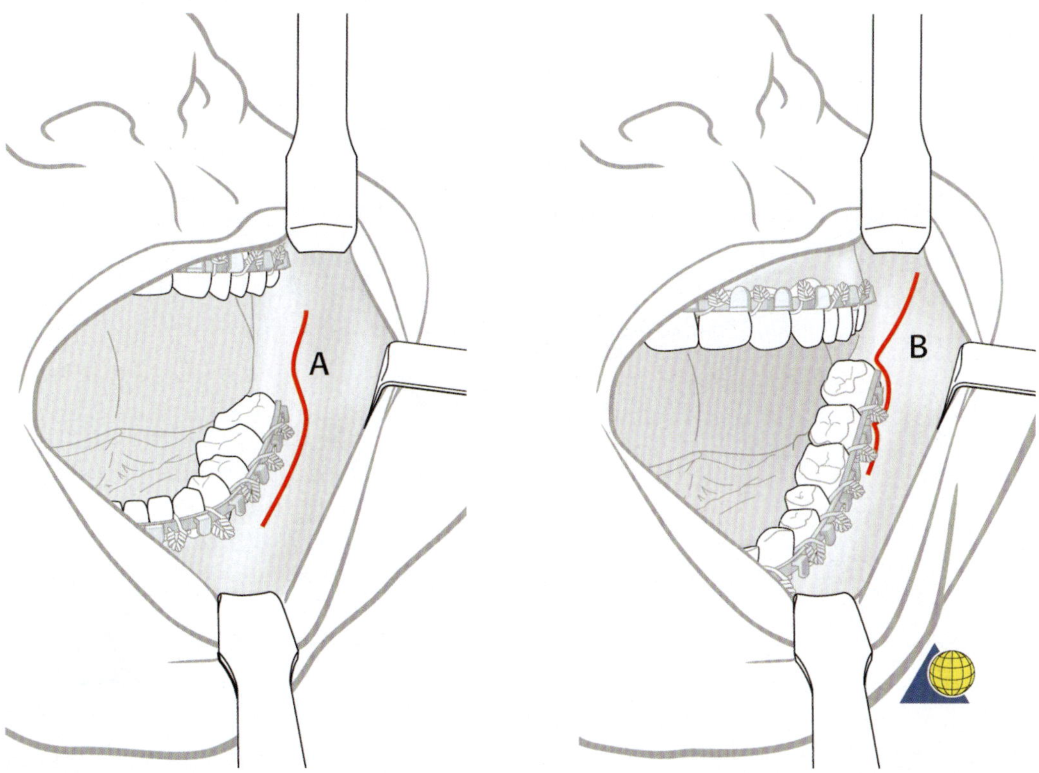

FIGURE 49.2 An intraoral incision is designed so optimal exposure may be obtained to reduce and plate the fracture. The incision is made in the gingivobuccal sulcus from the first molar to the posterior angle (proximal) of the ascending ramus. It is critical that an adequate cuff of mucosa remains to permit a tension-free closure (*A*) versus along the dental line (*B*). The incision may be extended anteriorly as necessary to allow additional exposure.

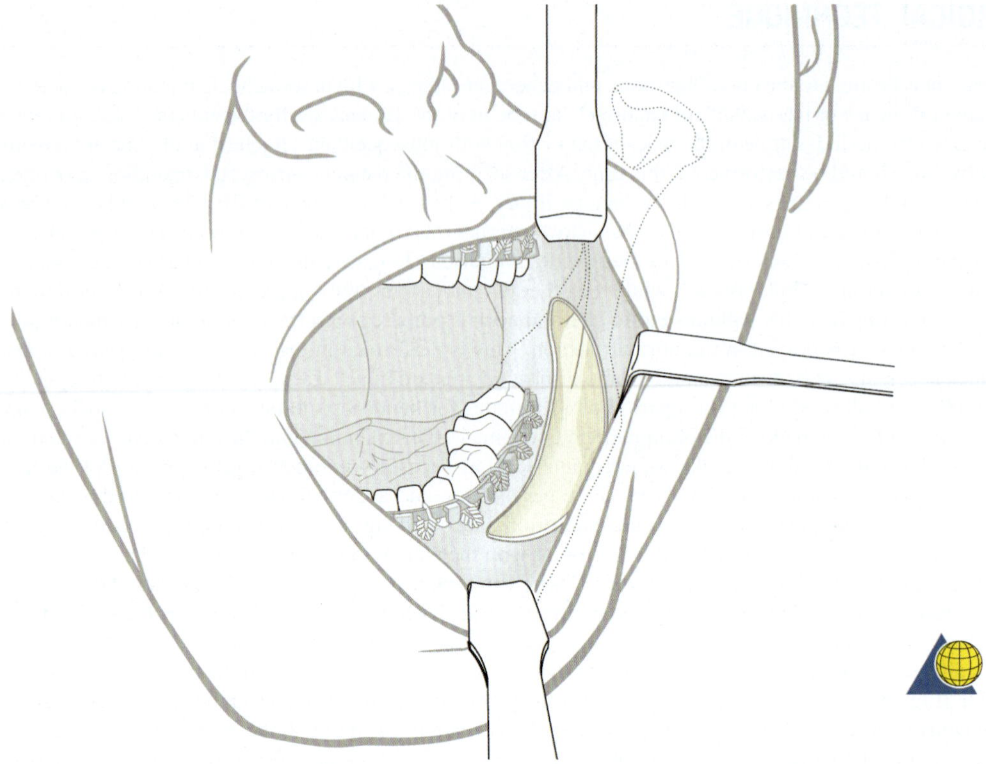

FIGURE 49.3 Exposure of the mandibular angle in addition to the posterior body and ascending ramus is possible with the intraoral incision.

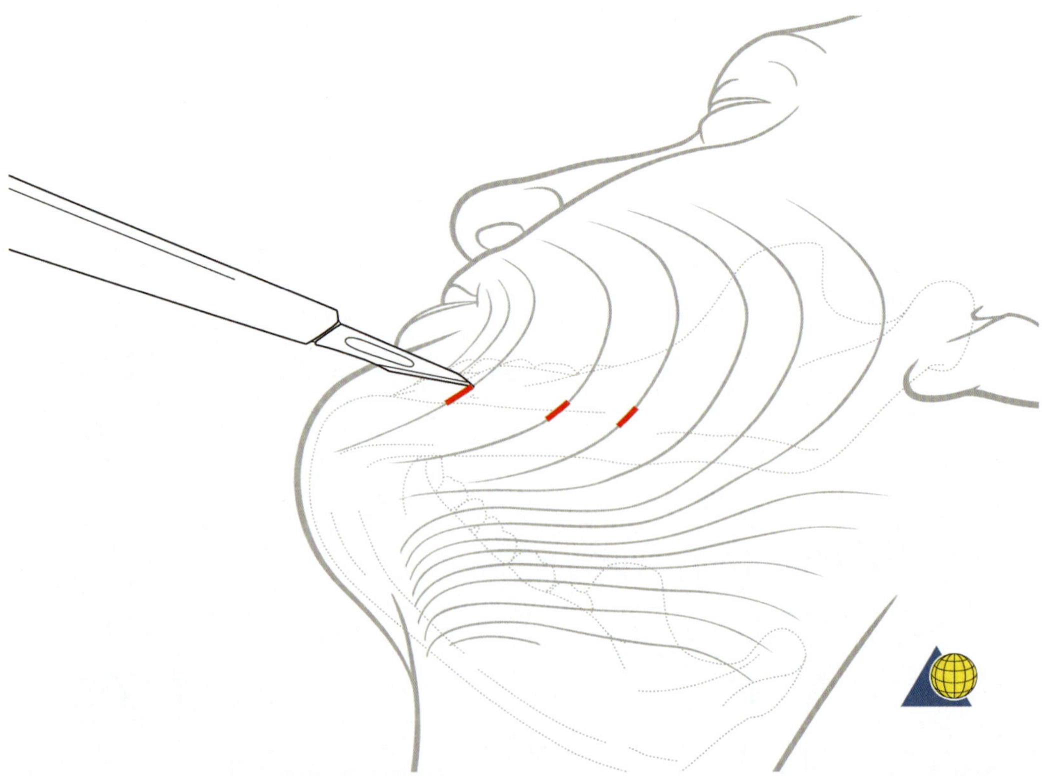

FIGURE 49.4 Stab incisions for the introduction of the trocar to access the region of the mandibular angle should be made in the natural skin creases of the face for cosmetic purposes. The site selected should ultimately allow the drill guide access to all the holes of the plate and allow for "play" with the percutaneous system.

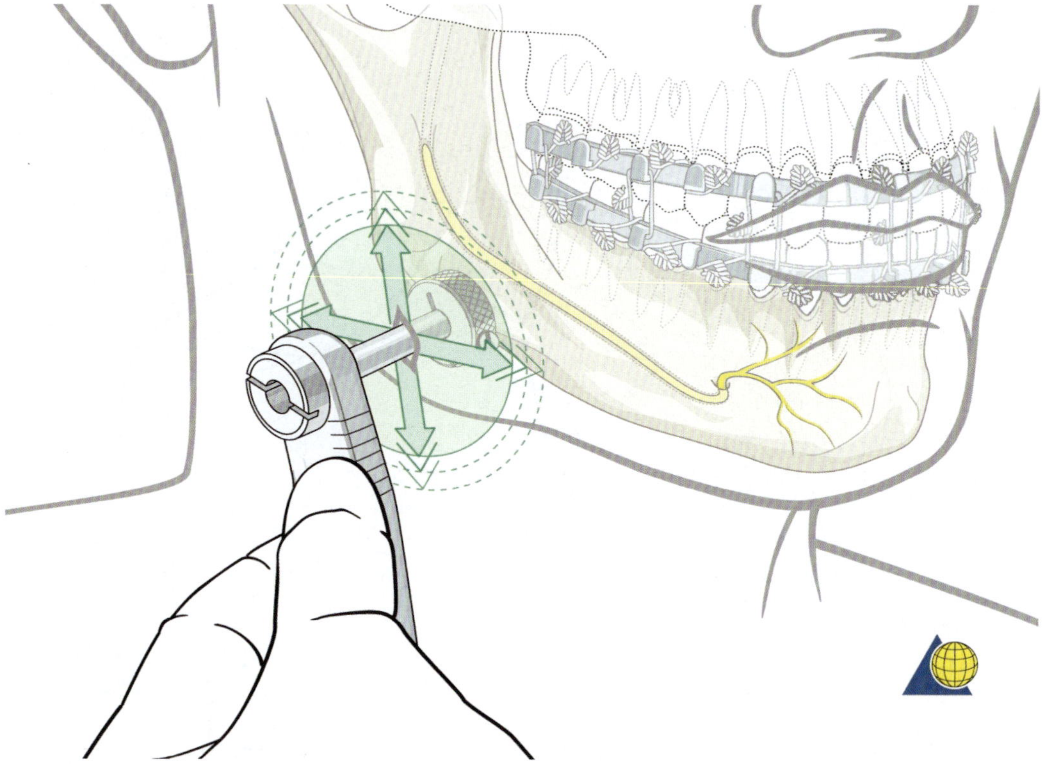

FIGURE 49.5 The percutaneous system should be able to move freely to access all the holes of the fracture plate.

The drill guide, which is attached to the handle of the percutaneous device, and the trocar are placed into the wound (Fig. 49.6). The thumb is used to apply steady but gentle pressure to the trocar as it is introduced into the wound. With gentle pressure, it will pierce the soft tissue at the medial aspect of the cheek flap (Fig. 49.7). The trocar is removed and replaced with the drill guide (Figs. 49.8 to 49.10). The cheek retractor is then attached to the hardware permitting retraction of the cheek flap (Fig. 49.11), which allows the surgeon to

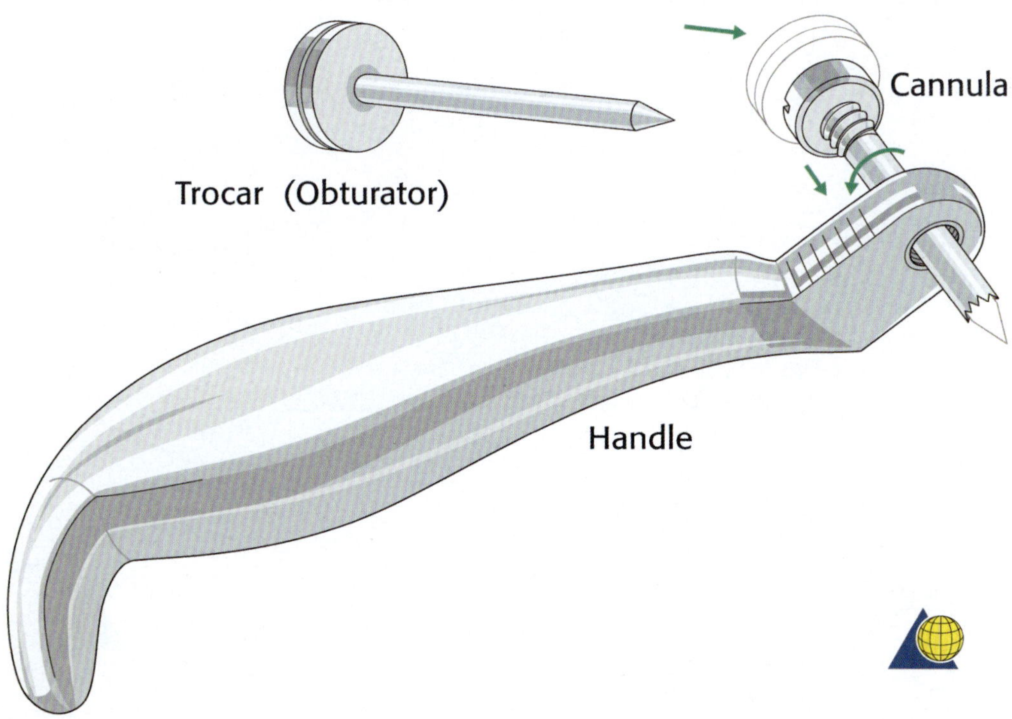

FIGURE 49.6 The percutaneous hardware is comprised of a surgical steel handle with a cannula at its end, trocar, and drill guides. The trocar and drill guides are slid through the cannula.

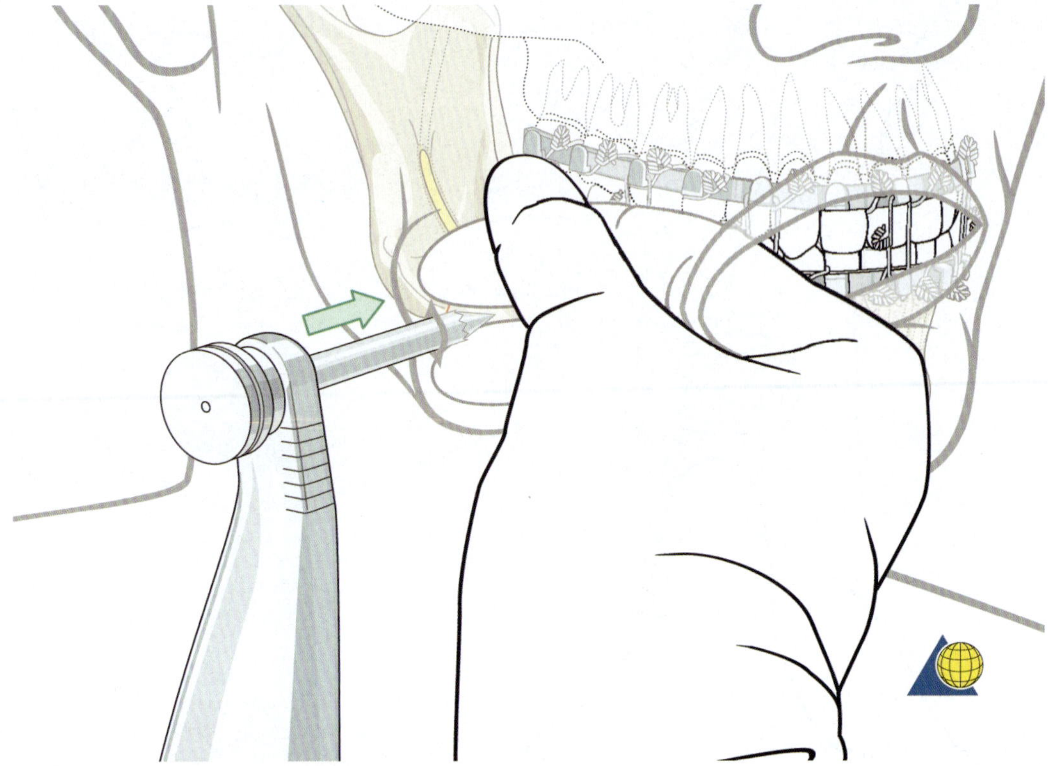

FIGURE 49.7 The trocar is placed through the cannula at the end of the handle, and with firm gentle pressure, it is inserted into the stab wound. The trocar allows access for the cannula through the cheek flap so its open edge does not catch on the surrounding soft tissue. The trocar is slowly inserted so it gently pushes the tissues away as it is advanced through the flap.

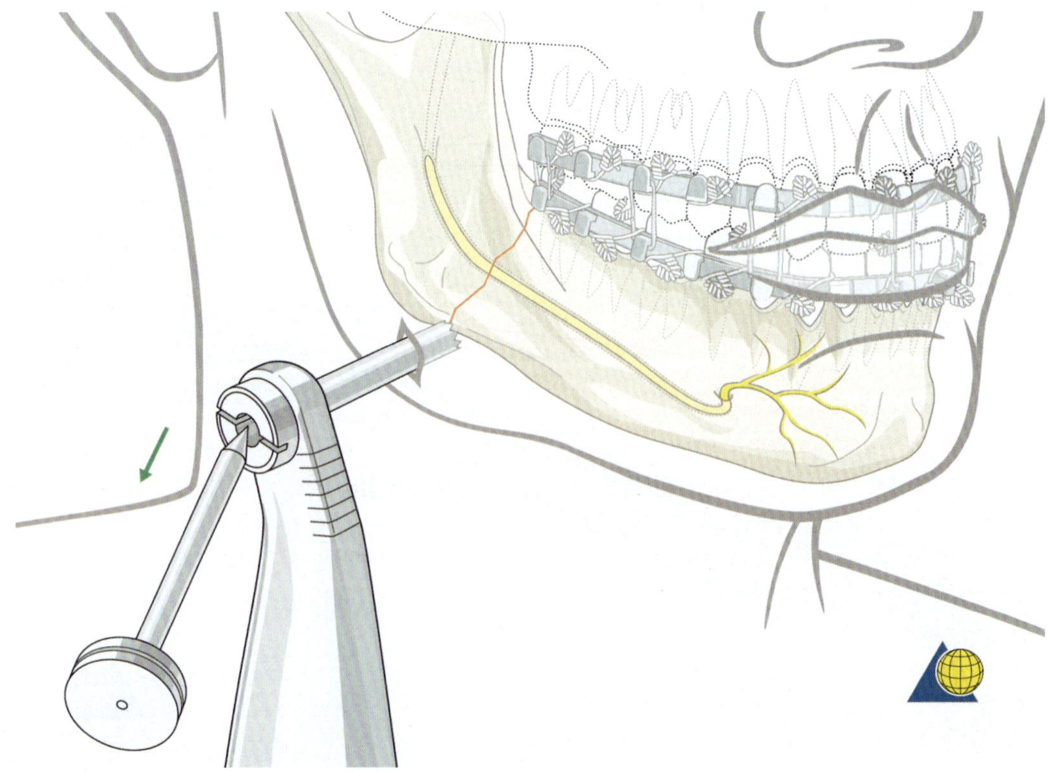

FIGURE 49.8 Once the cannula is successfully advanced through the cheek flap, the trocar is removed allowing the drill guide to be inserted.

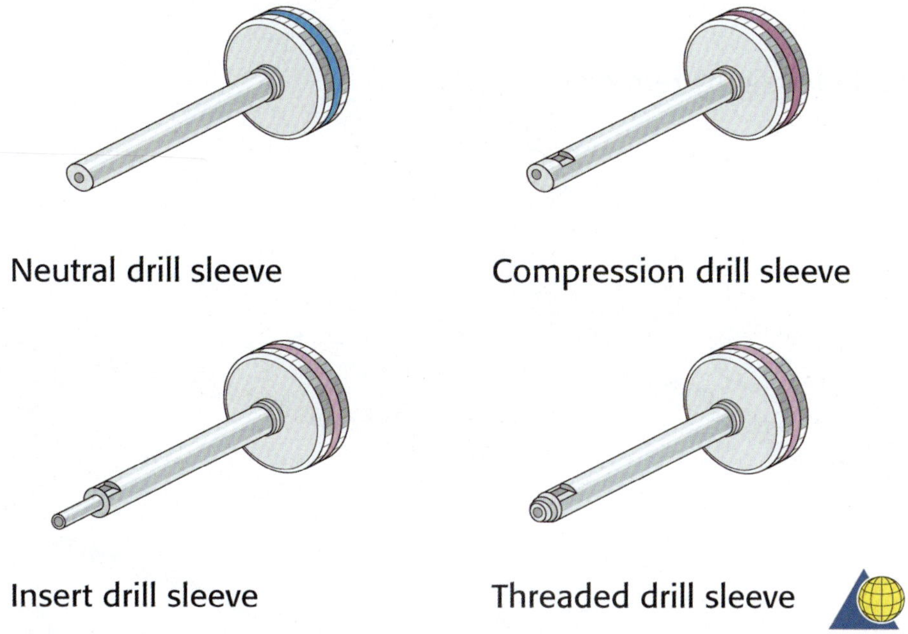

FIGURE 49.9 Various drill guides are available to accommodate your specific choice of drill bit. Some drill guides attach or screw into the plate holes, while others are neutral. When using the compression drill guide, make sure the arrow at the top is facing the fracture line.

maneuver the entire device anteriorly, posteriorly, superiorly, and inferiorly as necessary to access the necessary plate holes for pilot hole drilling and screw placement (Figs. 49.12 and 49.13).

Once the fracture is exposed, the percutaneous instruments are assembled, and the drill guide is placed through the cheek flap so that the fracture can now be reduced with bone clamps or manually. A plate is selected that will bridge the defect with a minimum of two holes on either side of the fracture line. As with any conventional plating situation, the fracture is reduced, the plate is adapted, and the first hole on either side of the fracture is selected to be drilled. The proper drill bit corresponding to the screw that is anticipated

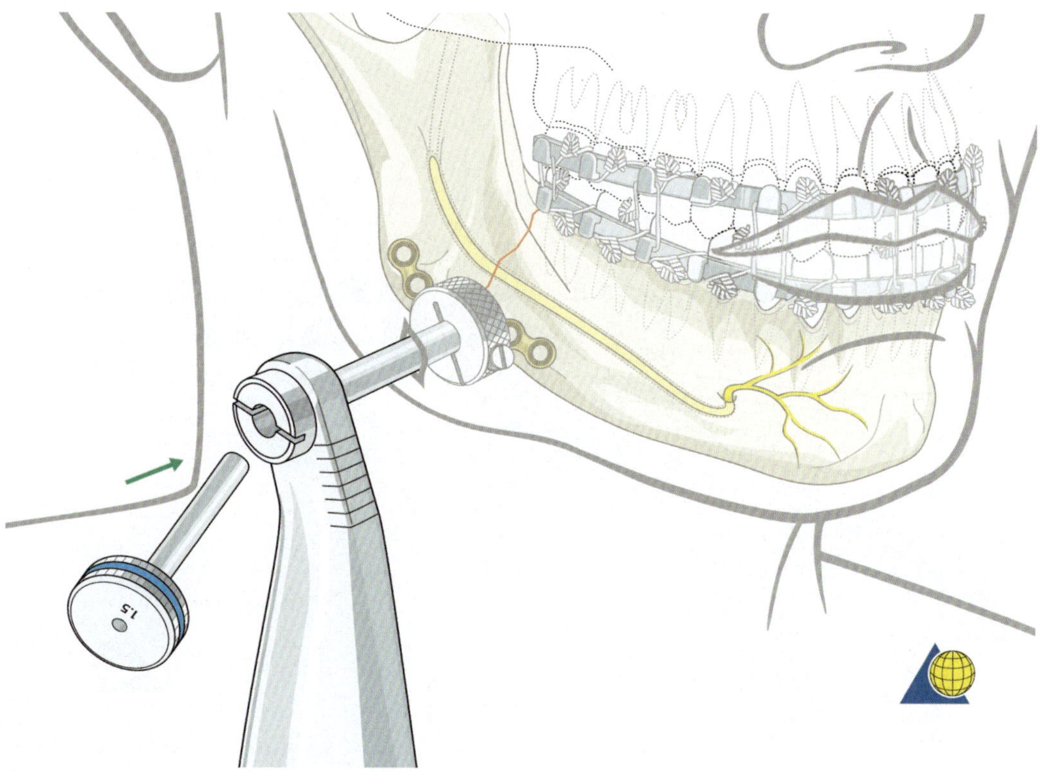

FIGURE 49.10 Drill sleeve is inserted.

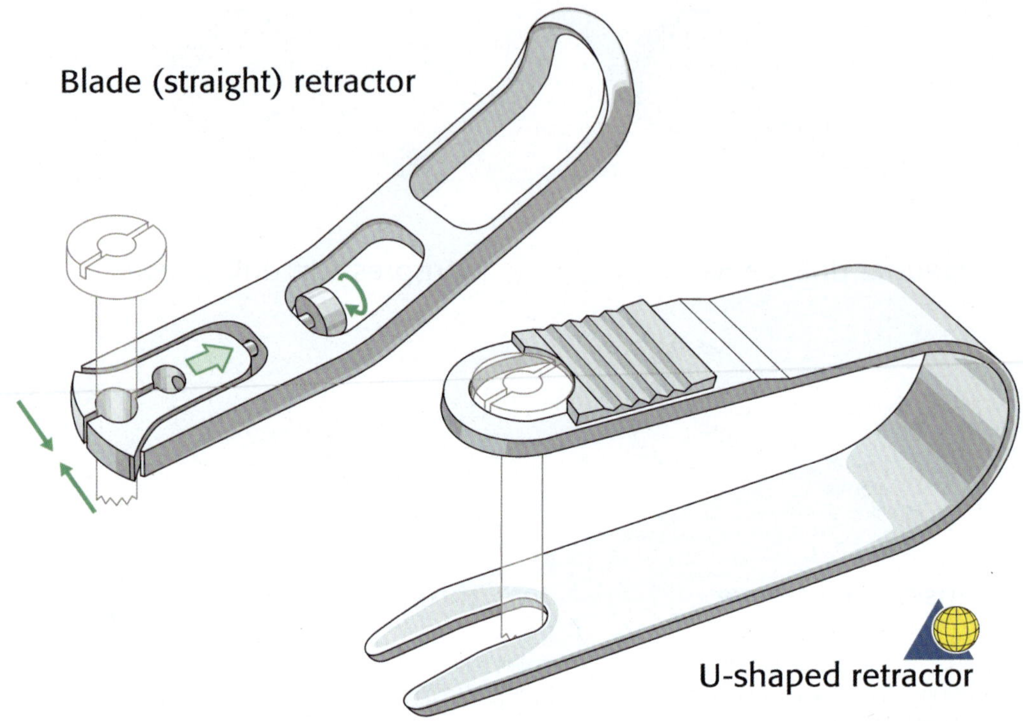

FIGURE 49.11 Two styles of cheek retractor. “Blade” and “U-shaped.” Both attach to the cannula at the end of the handle. This allows retraction of the cheek flap when maneuvering the percutaneous system during the drilling and screw placement steps of the operation.

to be used is placed through the drill guide and seated at 90 degrees to the plate hole. The drilling is to occur with steady pressure, and the operator should first engage the outer cortex and with firm gentle pressure and continue through the inner cortex to the mandible while irrigating copiously to prevent necrosis of the bone secondary to heating (Fig. 49.14). It is important to make sure that the drill guide and drill bit are at 90 degrees to the plate hole to prevent any kind of wobble that will impair placement of the screws. It is also important to realize there are important neurovascular structures medial to the inner cortex of the mandible,

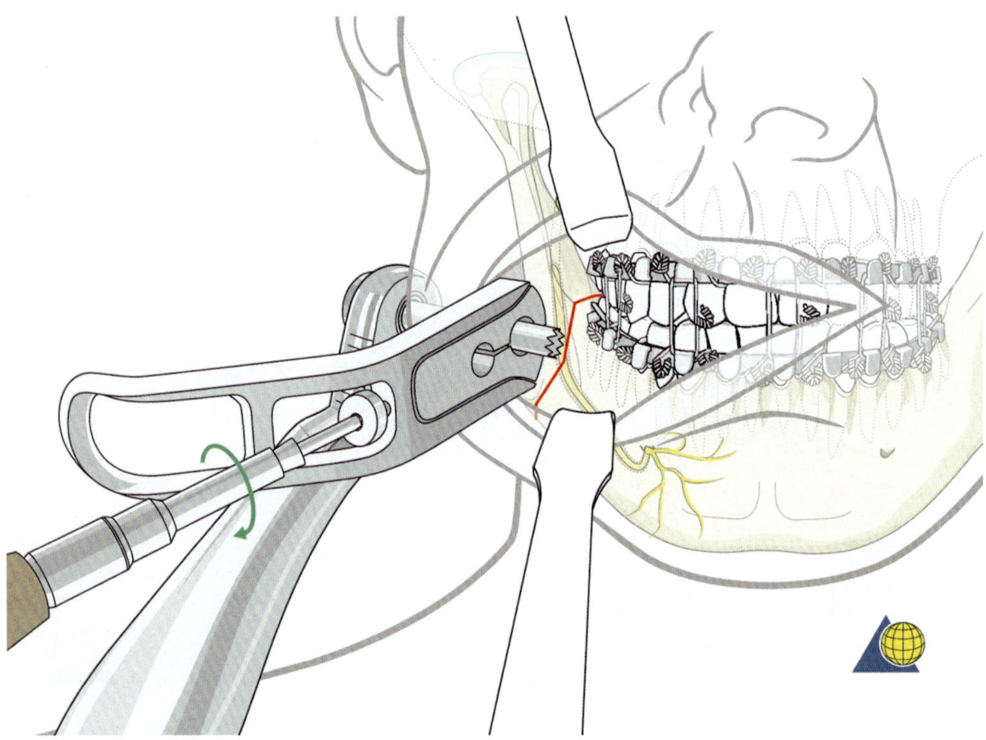

FIGURE 49.12 Demonstration of the “blade” style cheek retractor.

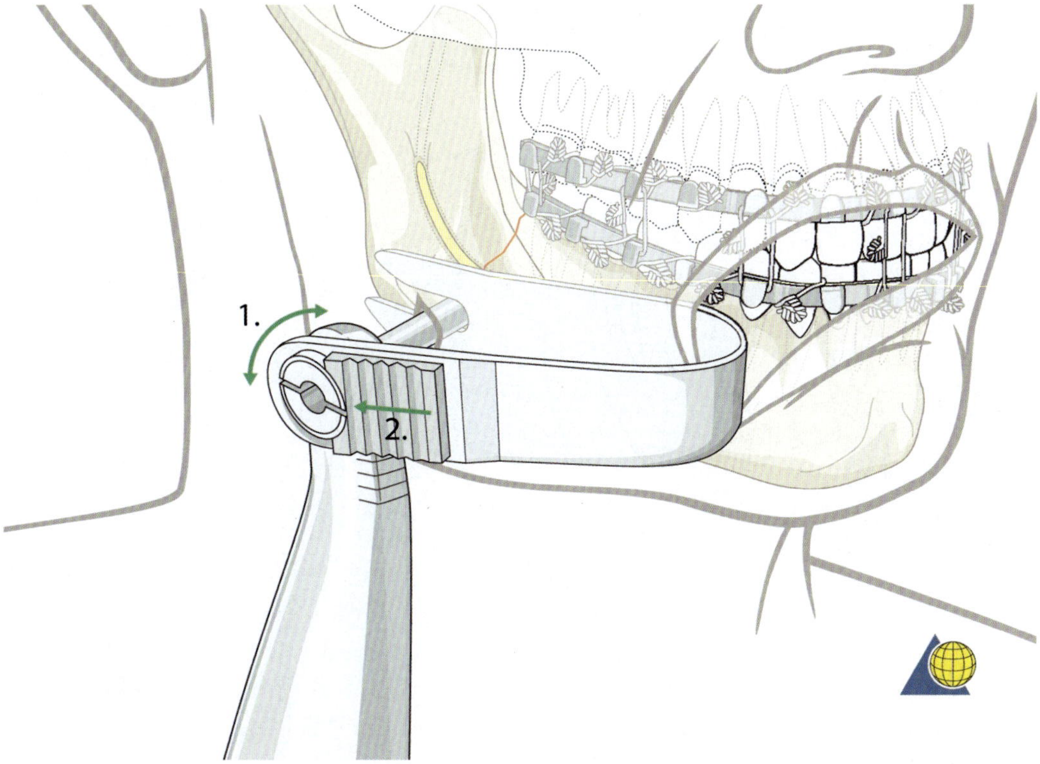

FIGURE 49.13 Demonstration of the "U-shaped" cheek retractor.

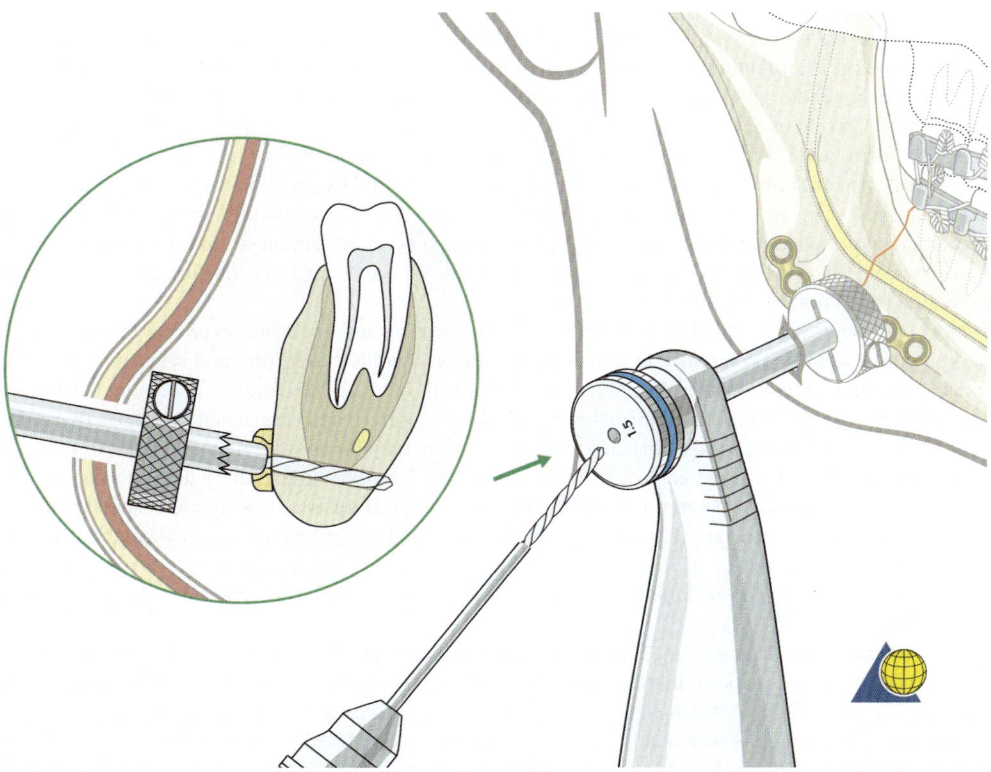

FIGURE 49.14 Insertion of the drill bit through the drill guide. Copious irrigation is necessary to prevent bone necrosis when drilling. The drill bits are usually color coded for the screw diameter and the drill guide to facilitate selection and maintain the proper relationships between the three. When placing the bicortical inferior plate pilot holes, it is important to remain below the tooth roots and the inferior alveolar nerve to prevent injury. Upper border plate pilot holes are unicortical specifically to prevent injury to these structures.

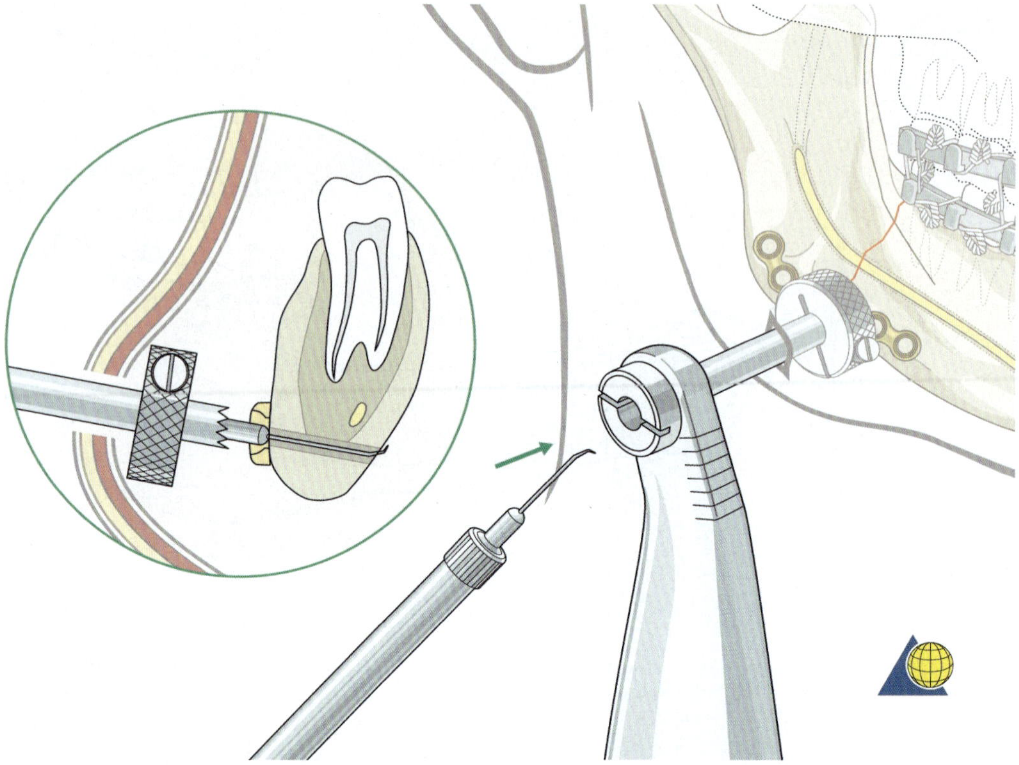

FIGURE 49.15 Depth gauge is used to determine the proper screw length. It is inserted into the pilot hole. A small lip is located on the end of the depth gauge to catch the inner cortex.

so once the second cortex is drilled, the drill should be removed immediately with steady backward pressure while the bit is still spinning. A depth gauge is then placed through the drill guide, the inner cortex of the mandible is gently grasped with the lip of the depth gauge, and the appropriate measurement is taken (Fig. 49.15). A screw of appropriate length is selected, mounted onto the end of the screwdriver, and placed through the drill guide (Fig. 49.16). The first screw is placed at about 90% of maximal tension. The opposite hole nearest the fracture site is then drilled in a similar fashion. However, this screw is placed to 100% of the tension necessary to seat it. Attention is then turned to the first screw that is then torqued completely. The percutaneous system with the cheek retractor can then be manipulated so that the other plate holes can be accessed via the drill guide. The entire process occurs in the exact same fashion until all the necessary screws have been placed (Fig. 49.17).

It is important to periodically check intermaxillary fixation and occlusion to ensure that it is maintained. It is imperative to hold the fracture in reduction at all times while the drilling and screw placement are performed. Once the inferior border plate has been successfully placed, the patient's occlusion is again checked to assure that it is maintained in a normal position. The fracture is also inspected to ensure that it has been maintained in reduction. If an arch bar has been placed, this may be used as a tension band to prevent splaying of the superior border of the angle after reduction of the inferior border. Alternatively, a two- or four-hole miniplate may be used at the superior border as a tension band. Here, a 2-0 miniplate is selected and adapted to the superior border of the angle using the same technique as described above. However, it is important to note that all pilot holes are only monocortical. This is to prevent damage to the tooth roots or the inferior alveolar canal. Four- or five-millimeter screws are then selected and placed on either side of the fracture line (Fig. 49.18).

The wound is then irrigated and any small oozing areas are gently cauterized with a needle-tipped Bovie. The soft tissues are then reapproximated with either 3-0 Vicryl or 3-0 Chromic on a UR-6 urology needle. This needle has a particular curve that makes it very easy to place sutures intraorally in the retromolar, trigone, and gingivobuccal sulcus area. The wound is closed with interrupted buried sutures in order to completely cover the plate (Fig. 49.19). Because there will be some postoperative swelling and fluid accumulation, I elect not to close in a watertight fashion but to leave some space between the sutures to allow the egress of any fluids that may accumulate. The small stab wound in the cheek can be closed with a 6-0 Prolene suture in interrupted fashion.

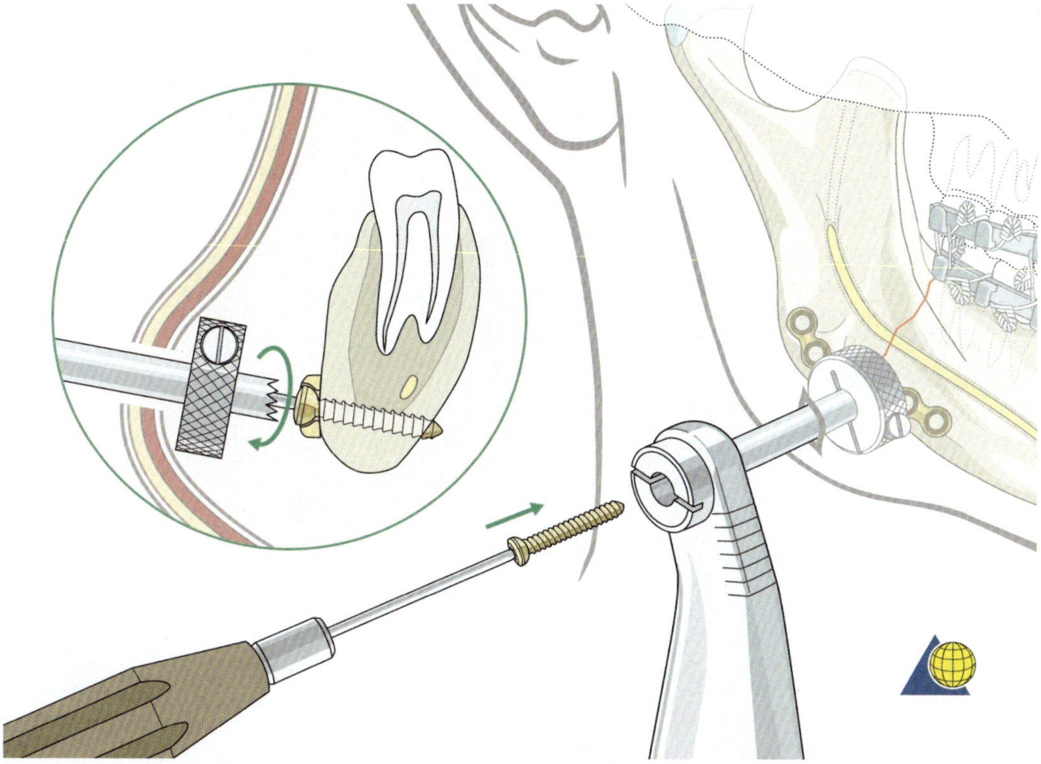

FIGURE 49.16 Screws are inserted sequentially beginning with those closest to the fracture line. The first screw is torqued approximately 90%, while the second screw on the opposite site of the fracture line is torqued completely. The first screw is then completely torqued.

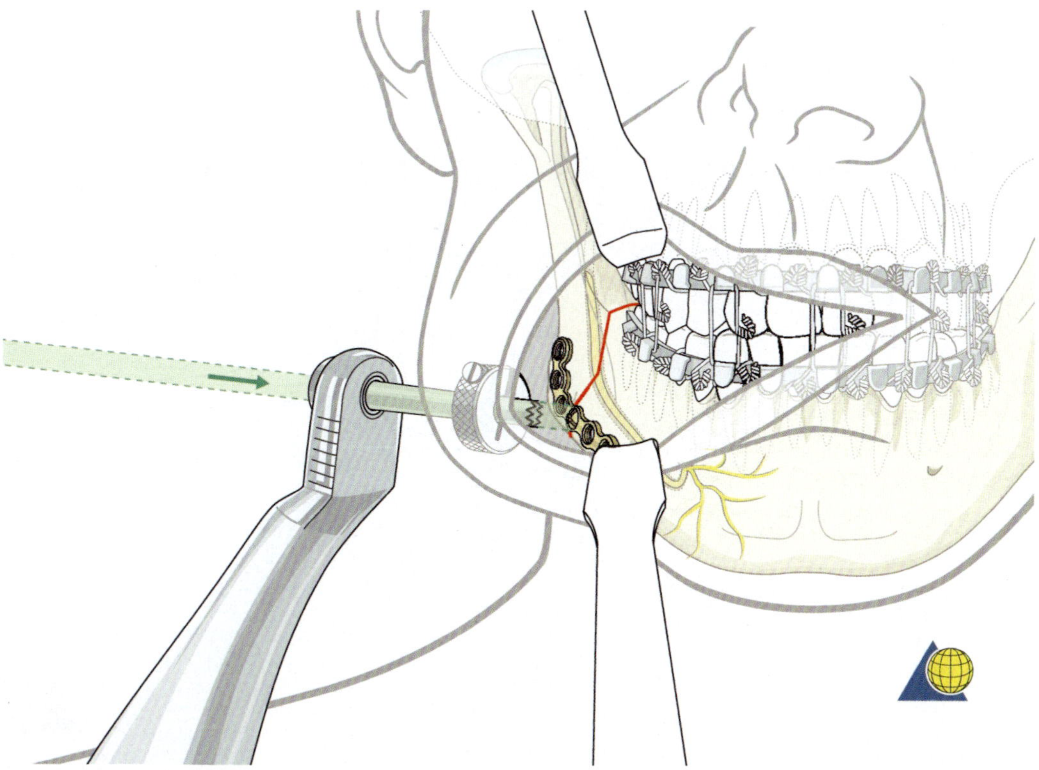

FIGURE 49.17 Once the first two screws are placed closest to the fracture line, the remaining screws are placed with the same technique and in a similar manner.

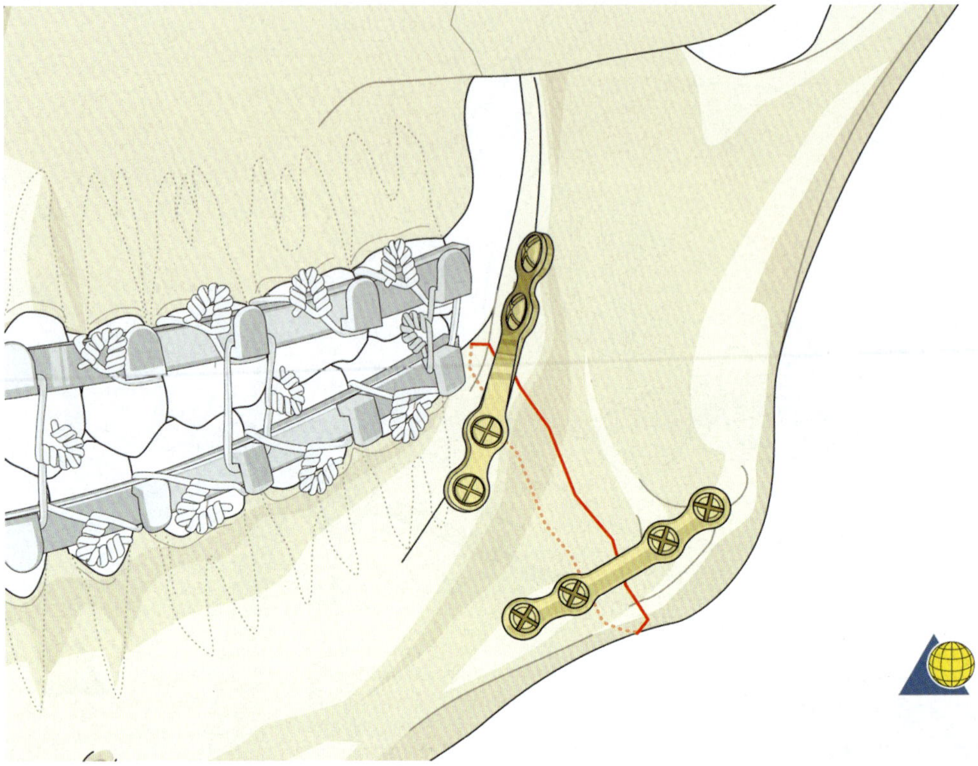

FIGURE 49.18 If the patient is to remain in IMF or to remain with an arch bar, it will act as a tension band preventing splay of the superior border when the inferior border plate is secured. If the arch bars are to be removed, then a superior border miniplate may be used instead. These pilot holes are monocortical to prevent damage to the tooth roots or inferior alveolar nerve.

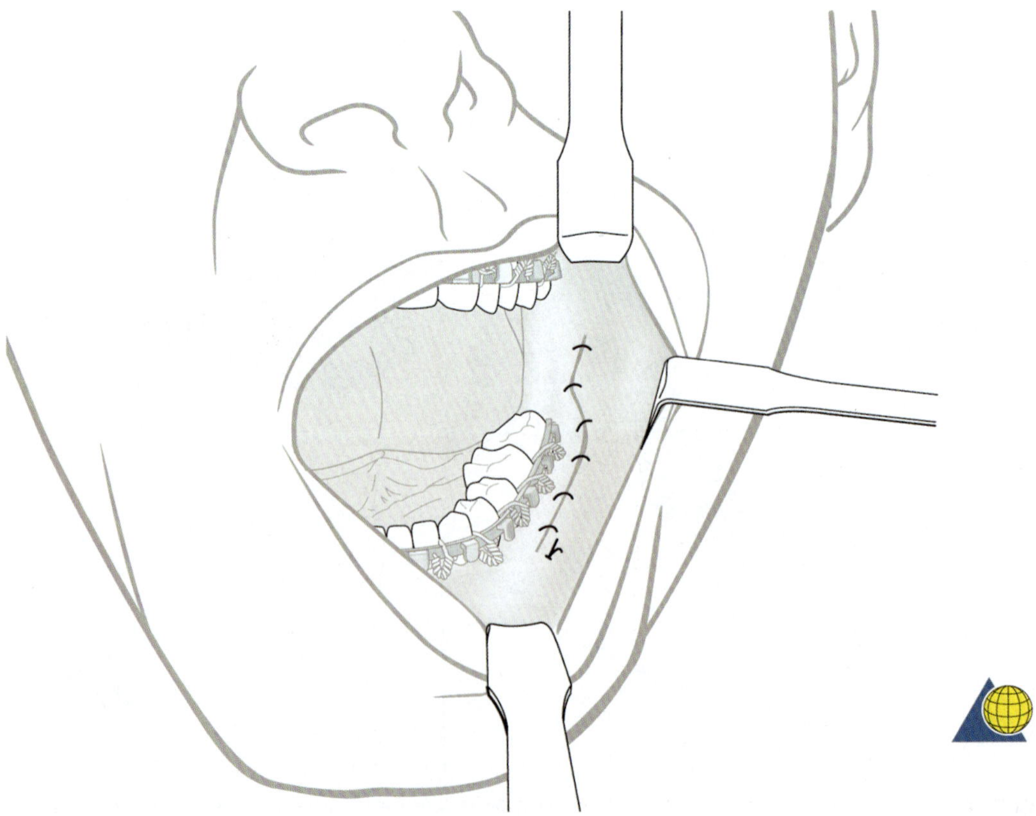

FIGURE 49.19 The wound is closed in an interrupted fashion. A 3-0 Chromic or Vicryl on a UR-6 needle is ideal. The curve of the needle facilitates closure in a relatively compact area. I close the wound in a non–watertight fashion to allow the egress of any trapped fluid. The stab wound on the cheek is closed with a simple 6-0 Prolene suture.

POSTOPERATIVE MANAGEMENT

- If the patient was initially placed in arch bars for intermaxillary fixation, the mandibular arch bar may remain as a tension band, while the IMF wires or bands can be removed at the conclusion of the operation.
- For those who may be at risk of minor postoperative malocclusion, elastic bands may be employed to gently guide the patient back into normal occlusion during healing. The maxillary and mandibular arch bars remain in place, the IMF wires removed, and elastics placed instead.
- Those patients at higher risk of postoperative malocclusion are to remain in formal IMF for approximately 6 weeks while the healing occurs. Some surgeons may elect to take the patient out of strict intermaxillary fixation at 3 to 4 weeks and use guiding elastics and soft diet for the remaining 2 to 3 weeks.
- Considering the degree of contamination of the oral cavity, chlorhexidine "swish and spit" solution can be used to decrease the bacterial load and aid in minimizing infection. If the patient has poor oral hygiene, or a delay in their treatment, or if there is concern about infection, then the patient can be kept on oral antibiotics for 2 weeks.
- If the patient is kept in intermaxillary fixation, it is of critical importance that they carry wire cutters on their person at all times in the event they need to cut the wires or bands to prevent aspiration of any vomited gastric contents. The patient needs to be instructed on which wires need to be cut in the event of an emergency. If the patient is unable to care for himself, the caregiver, either at home or in a hospital setting, needs to be instructed formally on which wires to cut during the event of an emergency.
- The patient should be followed in the office weekly for the first 3 weeks to ensure proper healing is occurring and to look for signs of infection, wound breakdown, or other complications. The surgeon should obtain postreduction radiographs to evaluate the reduction of the fracture.

COMPLICATIONS

The mandibular angle is prone to complications in postoperative healing. This is especially true in the case of inner-city or rural populations with poor oral hygiene and inadequate dental care.

- *Malocclusion*: This is always a potential complication in the repair of mandibular fractures. If the malocclusion is relatively minor, the patient may remain in elastic rubber bands to help guide them back into normal occlusion. On occasion, a dentist or orthodontist will be needed to treat adjustment of the teeth. However, in the setting of severe, major malocclusion, it may be necessary to revise the patient's operation as soon as possible with reestablishment of intermaxillary fixation, maintenance of stable premorbid occlusion, and replating of the fracture. Malocclusion may occur from an improperly reduced fracture or a poorly bent and adapted plate to the mandibular surface. In this situation, the plate actually pulls the bone fragments out of reduction when the screws are placed resulting in malocclusion. In the case of infection and osteomyelitis, malocclusion may occur due to a nonunion. In this situation, the fracture site would need to be explored, any sequestra debrided, occlusion obtained, and a plate replaced. Formal arch bars and intermaxillary fixation can assist in stabilization.
- *Plate Loosening and Screw Back-Out*: On occasion, whether due to improper drilling techniques or inappropriate screw selection, screws not seated properly into the bone may result in screw loosening and back-out. This complication may be revealed if the patient is not healing properly with a delayed union or a nonunion. This tends to be discovered on postreduction radiographs revealing loosening of the screws. The fracture site needs to be reexplored, and the plate may need to be resituated with pilot holes and screws placed in a more stable fashion. The surgeon may elect to employ a locking plate to minimize screw back-out. Meticulous drilling techniques and copious irrigation with proper screw selection decreases the chance of this happening.
- *Inferior Alveolar Nerve Injury*: Screws may, on occasion, be placed through the inferior alveolar canal resulting in pain and hypoesthesia of the teeth or lip. If this occurs, the screws and plates will need to be removed and resituated.
- *Malunion*: The bone may not heal in its preinjury configuration due to operator error when attempting to reduce the fracture. If the fracture is reduced improperly and fixed in poor reduction, a malunion and malocclusion may occur. This would be identified by failure to obtain the premorbid relationship of the teeth or a deformity of the angle of the mandible with potential impairment of mandibular function. In this situation, the fracture would need to be re-explored and proper reduction observed and retained, while the plates and screws are then reapplied.
- *Nonunion*: This is a failure of the bone to heal at the fracture site. This may occur secondary to a number of problems including poor anatomic reduction of the fracture segments or an infection of the plate–screw–bone construct. Nonviable or carious teeth or a previously contaminated fracture site treated without pre- and postoperative antibiotics may result in an infection with nonunion. In this situation, drainage, antibiotic therapy, and removal of any devitalized teeth should encourage healing. If the infection does not respond to these initial maneuvers, re-exploration of the fracture site, removal of the plate, debridement of any sequestra, and external fixation or a reconstruction plate may be needed. Postoperative antimicrobial therapy is essential.

- *Increased Sensitivity*: On occasion, plates may be associated with an increased sensitivity to either heat or cold. Once the healing has declared itself and the fracture has healed properly, the patient may elect for removal of the hardware. Removal may also be indicated for palpable plates.
- *Wound Breakdown and Plate Exposure*: Conservative treatment with antibiotics with possible wound closure in the office under local anesthesia may provide enough coverage to prevent infection and malunion or non-union. However, in this situation, it would be important that the patient have close follow-up for monitoring. If the wound continues to break down and the plate becomes infected, it would need to be removed and either replaced or an external fixation device applied with closure of the mucosa. If the wound continues to break down but healing has occurred, the hardware may be removed followed by wound closure and treatment with oral antibiotics and mouth rinses.
- *Scarring*: Ideally, one single vertically oriented small stab wound is made with an 11-blade scalpel in the cheek skin where the trocar is then placed. This wound usually heals well with simple closure; however, hypertrophic or keloid scarring may arise. Measures should be taken ahead of time to prevent this, including injections of Kenalog to prevent unsightly scarring. On rare occasions, injury of the facial nerve can occur. It is important to gently advance the trocar through the tissues at 90 degrees to the angle of the mandible as the trocar is designed to gently push tissues out of the way. On occasion, salivary fistulas may occur, but these are usually self-resolving.

RESULTS

A percutaneous approach in conjunction with intraoral incision should result in a cosmetically acceptable appearance of the face. There should be one very small stab wound in the cheek skin. This technique has an excellent history in preserving facial nerve and salivary gland function. Selecting this technique is important. Simple fractures, partially oblique fractures, or minimally comminuted fractures are ideal. Using this technique on fractures of these types should allow the surgeon to establish premorbid occlusion with anatomic reduction and fixation of the fracture. If the patient is not left in intermaxillary fixation, early return to oral function and mandibular mobility should ensue.

PEARLS

With every surgery, there are a number of nuances that have considerable ramifications. Below are a few of note for this particular surgery:

- The intraoral, percutaneous plating approach is ideal for the treatment of a simple, favorable linear fracture of the mandibular angle.
- The extraoral approach is well suited for multiple complicated fractures and comminuted fractures.
- Before the start of any mandibular surgery, the airway must be perfectly secured.
- Preinjury occlusion needs to be established prior to surgical correction.
- It is important to periodically check intermaxillary fixation and occlusion to ensure it is maintained throughout the surgical procedure. Early discovery affords early correction and improved outcomes.
- Copious irrigation helps to prevent necrosis of the bone secondary to heating during drilling.
- Precise plate choice, adjustments, and drilling are directly linked to exceptional and poor outcomes.
- The mandibular arch bar may remain as a tension band, while the IMF wires or bands can be removed at the conclusion of the operation.
- Postreduction radiographs are able to reveal a number of complications including reasons for postoperative malocclusion and the loosening of the screws.
- It is critical that the patient in maxillary–mandibular fixation (MMF) carry wire cutters on their person at all times and are trained regarding which wires to cut to prevent aspiration of any vomited gastric contents.
- Weekly follow-up for the first 3 weeks is essential in maintaining patient outcomes and compliance.

PITFALLS

- *Poor Preoperative Planning*: As with any operation, preoperative planning is important. Failure to detect the location and severity of all fractures will compromise the overall rehabilitation of the patient's injuries and likely compromise the proper reduction and internal fixation of the angle fracture. Failure to properly reduce and rigidly fixate all the fractures will likely result in a malocclusion and a malunion. It is important to use all the imaging modalities available, including CT scan, Panorex, and a complete mandible series, to evaluate the mandible and the teeth.
- *Failure to Establish Premorbid Intraoperative Occlusion*: Failure to establish premorbid intraoperative occlusion may result in a malocclusion. It is important to take into consideration the presence or absence and

status of the patient's teeth when establishing occlusion. Though slightly more time consuming, it may be advantageous to apply formal arch bars for intermaxillary fixation and to help ensure proper occlusion. This decision is coincident with the surgeon's experience and judgment.

- *Infection*: Infections can have a serious negative effect on healing. Open reduction and fixation with plating should be delayed until the infection is brought under control. On occasion, patients may need intravenous antibiotics. An abscess must be adequately drained and bony sequestra debrided before formal reduction and fixation.
- *Inappropriate Plate Selection*: Champy plates should be used in favorable nondisplaced simple fractures. Compression plates may not be ideal in severely oblique fractures as the two diagonal ends of the fracture are compressed and slide over each other. This forces the fracture out of reduction. A noncompression fracture plate or a locking plate should be considered in this situation. In severely comminuted fractures, a load-bearing reconstruction plate or an external fixation device may be necessary. Using plates and screws of inappropriate size and strength may result in plate or screw failure with loss of rigid fixation.
- *Failure to Remove Severely Carious or Devitalized Teeth*: Carious or devitalized teeth may act as a nidus of infection potentially jeopardizing the plate/screw/bone construct which may result in a malunion, delayed union, or nonunion. When necessary, consultation with dental or oral surgery colleagues is important to assist with decisions on whether or not a tooth may need to be extracted. In a fracture situation where there is severe comminution of the angle, an external approach with a reconstruction plate or an external fixator may be the best option. Fractures of this severity need longer, larger plates that may not be easily placed through a transoral approach, or the fractures may be so comminuted that a plate cannot be used at all and an external fixator is required.
- *Poor Surgical Technique*: Failure to drill pilot holes perpendicular to the plate, introducing drill bit wobble, or failure to irrigate when drilling may result in eccentric pilot holes where screws fail to purchase properly. Excessive use of electrocautery or failure to leave an adequate cuff of the gingival mucosa may lend itself to a difficulty in wound closure. These errors increase the chance of wound necrosis and breakdown with plate exposure leading to infection of the construct. It is important to maintain meticulous surgical technique as these wound complications may affect the final outcome and healing of the fracture.

SPECIAL INSTRUMENTATION

- 3-0 Vicryl or 3-0 Chromic on a UR-6 urology needle
- Percutaneous instrument set for mandible angle fracture

ACKNOWLEDGMENT

The author would like to acknowledge Professor Robert H. Mathog, MD, whose wisdom, dedication, and insight have guided the development of this chapter, like so many others, to provide a firm educational step from which the physician may serve his fellow man and woman.

SUGGESTED READING

Cole P, Rottgers SA, Cameron H, et al. Improving the minimally invasive approach to mandible angle repair. *J Craniofac Surg* 2008;19(2):525–527.

Ellis E III. Treatment methods for fractures of the mandibular angle. *Int J Oral Maxillofac Surg* 1999;28(4):243–252.

Greenberg A, Prein J, eds. *Craniomaxillofacial reconstructive and corrective bone surgery, principles of internal fixation using the AO/ASIF technique*. New York, NY: Springer, 2002.

Iida S, Hassfeld S, Reuther T, et al. Relationship between the risk of mandibular angle fractures and the status of incompletely erupted mandibular third molar. *J Craniomaxillofac Surg* 2005;33(3):158–163.

Mathog RH, Carron MA, Shibuya T. *Mathog's Atlas of Craniofacial Trauma*, 2nd ed. Philadelphia, PA: Wolters Kluwer/ Lippincott Williams and Wilkins, 2012.

50 FRACTURES OF THE ZYGOMATICOMAXILLARY COMPLEX

Jason H. Kim

INTRODUCTION

Zygomaticomaxillary complex (ZMC) fractures occur frequently, representing the first or second most common facial fracture, depending on the series reported. They are challenging fractures to manage because they may affect the appearance of the face and compromise orbital and/or masticatory function. Depending on the extent of displacement, comminution, and involvement of adjacent structures, ZMC fractures may require either no invasive intervention, limited approaches with or without fixation, or extensive open treatment and internal fixation (OTIF). These fractures may also occur in the setting of other craniofacial injuries. This chapter will focus on methods to restore form and function following a ZMC fracture.

HISTORY

A history of craniofacial trauma is the sine qua non for ZMC fractures. Assaults and automobile accidents are the most common etiologies. Traumatic impact commonly displaces the zygoma in an inferomedial and posterior direction. Displacement of the zygoma can cause considerable anatomic disruption to the inferior and lateral orbital walls. The ensuing volume change of the orbit can result in enophthalmos, diplopia, orbital dystopia, and malar asymmetry.

It is important to ascertain whether the injury was high or low velocity, as high-velocity injuries more commonly will require OTIF. As with any trauma situation, airway, breathing, and circulation (the primary trauma survey) will take precedence. If able to provide a history, patients may complain of pain around the orbit, decreased sensation over the cheek or teeth, or double vision. Pain associated with ZMC fractures is usually not severe. Any severe orbital pain should alert the examiner to the possibility of ocular trauma or bleeding within the orbit, as these are true emergencies requiring immediate intervention with ophthalmologic consultation. For any patient under consideration for surgery, a history of abnormal bleeding should be obtained in addition to a complete past medical history.

Paramount to the successful reduction of ZMC fractures is the restoration of the anatomy of the orbital complex and zygoma. Inadequate treatment with poor three-dimensional reduction can result in the persistence of enophthalmos and hypophthalmos. In addition, late cosmetic deformities can occur from rotational forces of the masseter muscle displacing the zygoma inferiorly resulting in malar asymmetry. Secondary correction after the occurrence of bone healing is exceptionally difficult, and few cases are amenable to further surgical correction.

Anatomy

The ZMC is a significant component of the facial skeleton with important roles in structure, function, and overall aesthetics. The zygoma is bound by four supporting buttresses and attaches to the frontal bone (frontozygomatic suture), the maxilla (zygomaticomaxillary suture), the greater wing of the sphenoid (zygomatico-greater wing of sphenoid suture), and the temporal bone (zygomaticotemporal suture). Each suture line represents one facial buttress with the exception of the zygomaticomaxillary suture, which has two buttresses: a horizontal buttress where the inferior orbital rim/maxilla meet the zygoma and a vertical buttress where the lateral maxillary sinus wall and zygoma meet. Attachment of the masseter muscle to the zygomatic arch provides masticatory capability, while bony structure contributes substantially to the lateral and inferior orbital rim, to the lateral orbital wall, and to the orbital floor.

PHYSICAL EXAMINATION

An accurate history and physical examination will help to determine whether a ZMC fracture is present, how severe the fracture is, and if indications exist for repair. Soft tissue injuries should be closed immediately; they may be reopened at the time of fracture repair to provide exposure. Edema sets in within hours of facial trauma. Bony landmarks are often obscured making it difficult to appreciate malar flattening or displacement of the zygomatic arch. It is imperative to firmly palpate the bony surfaces of both sides of the face in order to elicit tenderness, step-offs, and crepitation. In the setting of a ZMC fracture, there may be tenderness and a palpable step-off over the lateral and inferior orbital rims. The arch is most commonly fractured inward, creating discontinuity as the fingers are swept from the lateral orbital rim toward the tragus. To appreciate malar flattening, the examiner should stand behind the semirecumbent patient and press the index finger of each hand over the infraorbital rims. By observing from a top-down or submental vertex viewpoint, the examiner can appreciate depression of the fractured side. Facial sensation is very often decreased in a V2 distribution due to fracture site involvement of the infraorbital nerve along the orbital floor or at the level of the foramen.

Intraoral examination may reveal ecchymosis in the maxillary gingivobuccal sulcus. Malocclusion is not an expected finding in isolated ZMC fractures. However, some patients may associate numbness of the teeth with malocclusion. Trismus, if present, is indicative of temporalis muscle or coronoid process impingement on the fractured zygomatic arch and is an indication for reduction of the fracture.

It is likewise imperative to examine the eyes for the presence of gaze restriction, enophthalmos, diplopia, globe injury, and loss of visual acuity. In the awake patient, extraocular movements may be elicited in the standard fashion. If gaze restriction is present, it will usually be from edema of the orbital contents, or from inferior or medial rectus muscle entrapment. Forced duction testing is the most accurate method for diagnosing entrapment and differentiating it from orbital edema. This is not a diagnosis made from CT imaging. Enophthalmos is present when the volume of the bony orbit is expanded relative to its contents. ZMC fractures may result in posterolateral displacement of the lateral orbital wall and disruption of the orbital floor. This expansion creates the appearance of a "sunken" eye. The supratarsal crease of the upper lid may become deepened with a hollowed appearance. Enophthalmos following trauma is an indication for repair. Diplopia should be assessed in each cardinal direction of gaze. If present, diplopia must be categorized as monocular or binocular, as the former may be indicative of lens dislocation, retinal tear or detachment, or other ocular pathology requiring ophthalmology consultation. Injury to the globe is not uncommon and, if suspected, must be addressed prior to repair of the fracture. With any bony orbital injury, subconjunctival hemorrhage and chemosis will likely be present (Fig. 50.1). Visual acuity should be assessed and documented using a Snellen chart.

Indications for Ophthalmology Consultation

- Suspected globe injury
- Monocular diplopia
- Loss of visual acuity
- Severe orbital pain

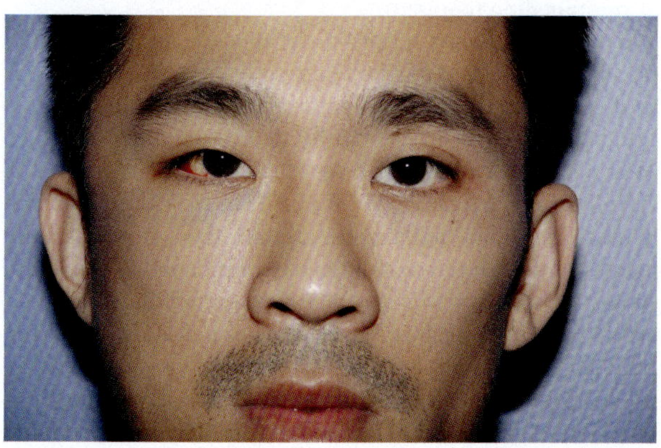

FIGURE 50.1
Right eye with subconjunctival hemorrhage indicative of orbital trauma. Subconjunctival blood will remain bright red long after trauma due to the ease of oxygen diffusion across the thin conjunctival membrane.

- Proptosis/concern for retrobulbar hematoma
- Severely swollen eyelids

INDICATIONS

- Displacement of the zygoma with anatomic disruption to the inferior and lateral orbital walls creating significant volume change of the orbit
- Bony fragments impinging on the optic nerve or musculature
- Hypophthalmos
- Enophthalmos
- Orbital dystopia
- Muscular entrapment with resultant diplopia
- Malar asymmetry
- Orbital rim step-off
- Trismus

CONTRAINDICATIONS

Often, patients with such injuries may also present with a constellation of other injuries requiring attention prior to treatment of ZMC fractures. In such circumstances, the patient must commonly have general medical, anesthesia and neurologic (C-spine) clearance prior to entering the operating theater. In circumstances with suspected or confirmed injury to the globe, consultation must be obtained with an ophthalmologist prior to surgical management.

PREOPERATIVE PLANNING

In the case of multisystem trauma, repair of facial fractures is often delayed by management of life-threatening injuries. It is often advantageous to allow 3 to 5 days for facial edema to subside. Reexamination is then necessary as clinical findings may change. In particular, restriction of gaze may resolve as edema subsides. Systemic steroids may also be given to reduce edema prior to surgery. Prophylactic antibiotics are routinely administered when there is communication between the orbit and the sinus cavities. Patients are reminded not to blow the nose and to sneeze with the mouth open to prevent orbital emphysema. Cervical spine clearance prior to surgery is extremely helpful to avoid bulky cervical collars or immobilization procedures at the time of operation.

Patient consent must be obtained for OTIF of facial fractures via multiple approaches, including sublabial, transcutaneous, and transconjunctival with or without lateral canthotomy and cantholysis. Risks include bleeding, infection, anesthetic complications, malunion or nonunion of fractures, hardware extrusion, scar, development of late enophthalmos, eyelid malposition, damage to the eye including loss of vision, diplopia, gaze restriction, postoperative healing complications, need for additional procedures, and poor cosmetic outcome in spite of optimal treatment.

Imaging

High-resolution CT scanning of the maxillofacial bones with triplanar reconstruction is required for planning of operative treatment of ZMC fractures. We do not routinely obtain plain films. CT images are assessed for displacement of the fracture lines, bony comminution, and involvement of the orbital floor. These three measures will dictate the approaches needed and the extent of rigid fixation required.

CT images: (1) nondisplaced ZMC fracture, nonoperative (Fig. 50.2); (2) arch fracture (Fig. 50.3A–C); and (3) severely displaced fracture (Fig. 50.4A–C).

SURGICAL TECHNIQUE

The preferred surgical technique will depend on the extent of the ZMC fracture. For isolated arch fractures, I will describe the Gilles approach. The technique for OTIF of more complex ZMC fractures is also detailed.

Gilles Approach

With the patient in the prone position, general endotracheal anesthesia is induced. The table is rotated 180 degrees away, and corneal shields with Lacri-Lube ointment are placed to protect the eyes. Examination of the

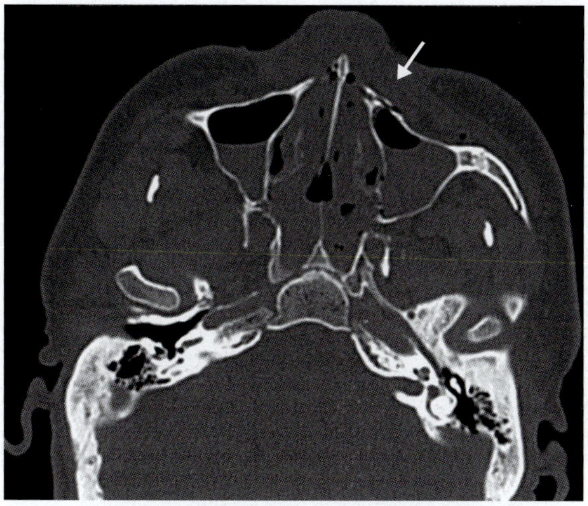

FIGURE 50.2
Left-sided minimally displaced ZMC fracture not requiring OTIF (*arrow*).

zygomatic arch under anesthesia is performed to assess for mobility of fracture segments. The temporal tuft on the fractured side is shaved with surgical clippers in a 2- × 2-cm square over a point 2 cm superior to the root of the helix. The face is prepped including the ears and both temporal regions. The head is draped with a blue towel to cover the hair.

After surgical pause to verify patient, site, and procedure, the superficial temporal artery is palpated. The bifurcation should be at or below the shaved area. It is important that the artery and accompanying vein are not violated during the procedure, as this may add time and cause significant bleeding. 1% lidocaine with 1:100,000 epinephrine is injected in the skin prior to incision with a 15-blade knife. Dissection is carried down through the skin and temporoparietal fascia to the deep temporal fascia, which should appear white and glistening. Ideally, the approach is just superior to the bifurcation of this fascia around the temporal adipose tissue pad. The knife blade is used to make a 1-cm incision in the deep temporal fascia, exposing fibers of the temporal is muscle. A Freer elevator is used to bluntly dissect in an anteroinferior direction toward the zygoma, opening a pocket for placement of the bone elevator. If dissection is carried too far medially, the elevator may perforate the

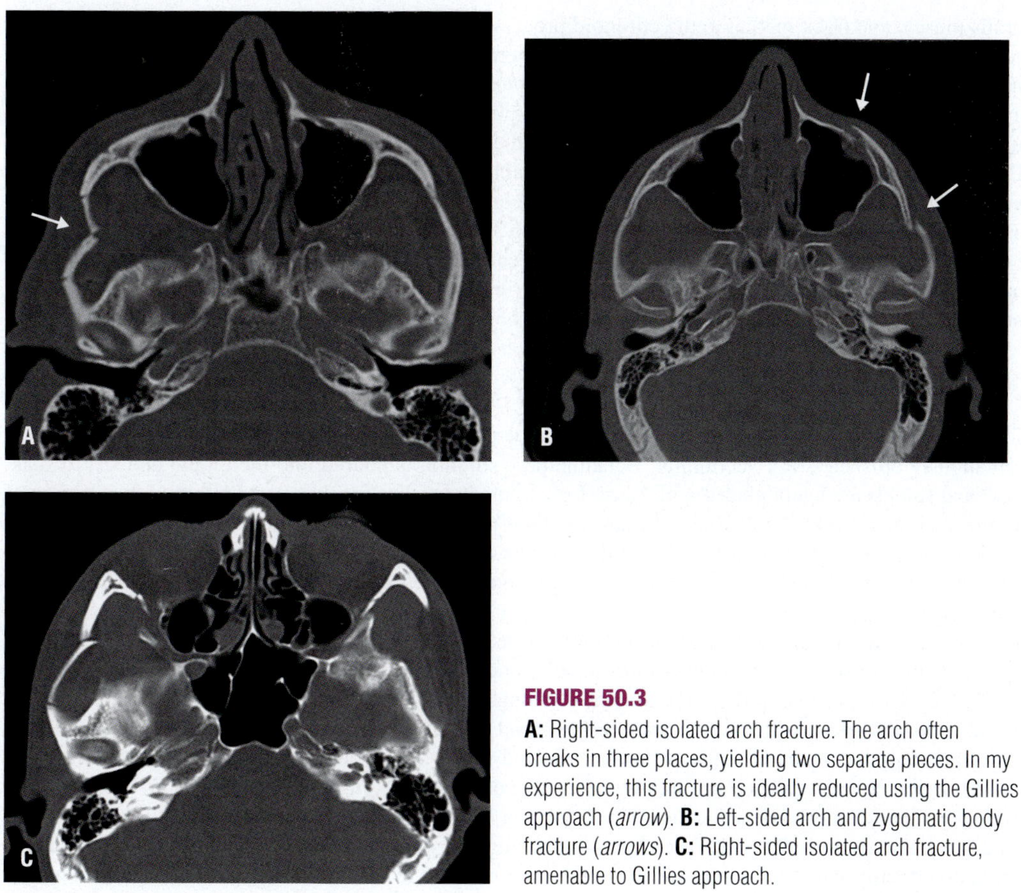

FIGURE 50.3
A: Right-sided isolated arch fracture. The arch often breaks in three places, yielding two separate pieces. In my experience, this fracture is ideally reduced using the Gillies approach (*arrow*). **B:** Left-sided arch and zygomatic body fracture (*arrows*). **C:** Right-sided isolated arch fracture, amenable to Gillies approach.

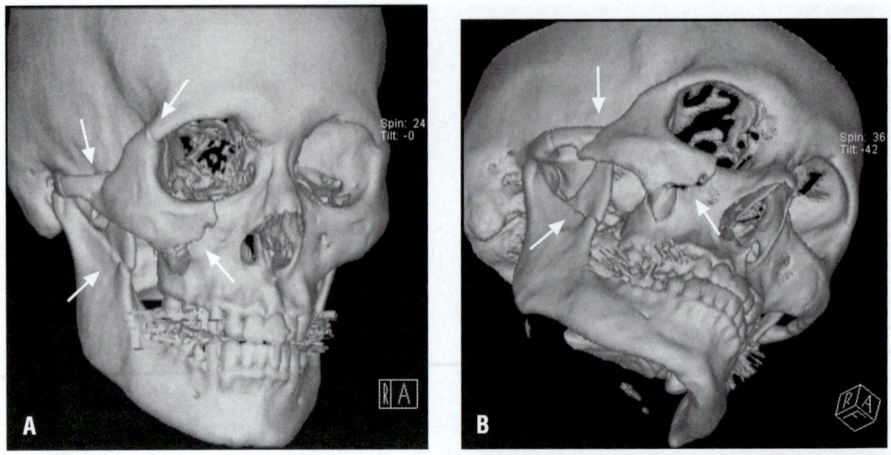

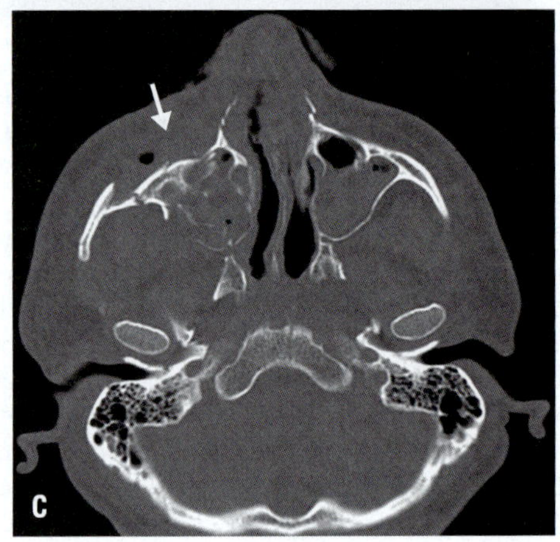

FIGURE 50.4
A: Three-dimensional reconstruction of right-sided classic ZMC fracture with displacement of zygomaticomaxillary, frontal, sphenoid, and temporal buttresses (*arrows*). **B:** Oblique view of the fracture in **(A)** showing associated coronoid process fracture. This combination places the patient at high risk of coronoid impingement or ankylosis to the zygomatic arch if left untreated (*arrows*). **C:** Axial view of right comminuted ZMC fracture showing loss of malar projection (*arrows*).

temporalis muscle and track medial to the coronoid process of the mandible. Lateral dissection may place the Freer elevator over the zygomatic arch, jeopardizing the temporal branch of the facial nerve. Once a sufficient tract has been developed, an elevator may be inserted. I prefer to use the Dingman or Cobb elevator. Measure the length of the elevator against the cheek and place the thumb of the dominant hand at the distal extent of the instrument adjacent to the incision. Insert the elevator in the pocket, and it should advance smoothly into position. Place the fingers of the nondominant hand over the arch. With a movement that is simultaneously twisting and levering, rock the arch back into position. An audible crack may be heard as the fracture is reduced.

The temporal wound is irrigated and closed with deep 3-0 absorbable sutures and 5-0 fast absorbing suture in the skin. An aluminum foam splint is cut to size and secured over the arch with tape to serve as a splint. The corneal shields are removed and the eyes are copiously irrigated with BSS solution to remove Lacri-Lube. The patient is then extubated and transferred to the recovery room.

Combined Approach OTIF

Positioning is similar to the Gilles approach. The mouth is prepped with 3% hydrogen peroxide, and the teeth are meticulously brushed. After suctioning, Betadine prep solution is poured into the mouth and left to soak. Clear corneal shields are again placed with Lacri-Lube ointment to protect the eyes. I begin with exposure of the inferior and lateral orbital rim fracture lines and then proceed with intraoral exposure of the face of the maxilla and zygomaticomaxillary and nasomaxillary buttresses. I then reduce the fractures checking for alignment at three sites. The fractures are then secured with titanium plates. Lastly, the orbit is explored and the floor repaired if necessary.

I begin with forced duction testing of the globe to assess for entrapment. Two 0.5 forceps are used to grasp the conjunctiva several millimeters inferomedial and inferolateral to the iris, and the globe is rotated upward. The forceps are never pulled in a line intersecting the cornea because sudden release could result in corneal laceration. I then proceed with a transconjunctival incision with lateral canthotomy and cantholysis. The lower lid conjunctiva and lateral canthus are injected with 1% lidocaine with 1:100,000 epinephrine. A 6-0 silk retraction suture is placed through the gray line of the lower lid in two passes. A 15-blade knife is used to make a lateral canthotomy incision 1 to 1.5 cm in length, which is continued down to the bone. The lower lid is retracted anteriorly, and Wescott scissors are used to cut the inferior canthal tendon. The scissors are inserted vertically with one tine posterior to the tendon and one tine anterior. The hallmark of a proper cantholysis is a dramatic release of the lower lid away from the orbital rim. Next, the scissors are inserted 2 mm inferior to the tarsal plate and a plane of dissection is created in the preseptal plane along the length of the lower lid up to the plane of the lacrimal punctum. The scissors are then used to release the conjunctiva and lower lid retractors. Bleeding is controlled with needle-point cautery. A small amount of orbital adipose tissue may now be visible especially laterally. A clear Jaeger retractor is used to retain the orbital contents out of the field. Dissection is carried down to the periosteum of the orbital rim, which is incised with the needle cautery. If at all possible, incising the periosteum on the anterior surface of the rim will allow a small cuff of periosteum, which can be used to cover any plates in the region. A Cottle elevator is used to elevate in the subperiosteal plane over the orbital rim to expose fracture lines. There is often a small free-floating bone fragment along the medial third of the rim. If possible, keep periosteal attachments to this fragment to avoid devitalizing it.

Next, I turn my attention to the lateral orbital rim to expose the zygomaticofrontal suture. A Senn retractor is used to elevate the lateral canthotomy incision superiorly. It is nearly always possible to gain exposure of the lateral orbital rim through this approach. It is important not to strip the superior canthal tendon from Whitnall tubercle during elevation. Dissection is supraperiosteal until the fracture line is identified. Then cautery is used to vertically divide the periosteum. Again, incising the periosteum in the lateral part of the rim will allow coverage of the plate at the end. The Cottle elevator is used to elevate periosteum around the fracture line, which is almost always at the suture line. Only enough exposure is needed to allow for two plate holes on either side of the fracture.

After exposing the orbital rims, I proceed with transoral exposure of the zygomaticomaxillary buttress. A plastic cheek retractor is placed. The maxillary gingivobuccal sulcus is infiltrated with local anesthetic solution along its length. Needle-point cautery on cut setting is used to incise the mucosa about 1.5 cm above the teeth, leaving an ample cuff of soft tissue for closure. The incision extends from the upper lip frenulum laterally to the second or third molar. Dissection is then taken directly down to bone along the length of the incision. A #9 dental elevator (Molt elevator) is used to elevate the periosteum over the face of the maxilla and over the piriform aperture. This dissection should be relatively easy. The infraorbital nerve is identified, and care is taken not to traumatize it. The dissection should be carried far laterally, following the contour of the buttress toward the zygomatic arch. Fibers of the masseteric muscle are encountered at the zygoma and arch and may be released with cautery if exposure is required for plating.

I proceed with reduction of the three fracture lines exposed. One method is to use a curved elevator such as a Dingman. The Dingman elevator is inserted transbuccally to rest beneath the zygoma–zygomatic arch junction. At this point, comminuted arch fractures may be reduced by firmly twisting the elevator while palpating over the skin to confirm movement of the arch. By placing the elevator more anteriorly under the zygomaticomaxillary buttress, the entire zygoma can be easily elevated. All three fracture lines are inspected for reduction. I also review the relation of the zygoma to the greater wing of the sphenoid as this is considered the truest point of reduction quality. A Carroll-Girard screw may also be employed to aid in reducing and steadying the body of the zygoma during fixation. Fractures are normally fixated in the following order: (1) zygomaticofrontal (ZF), (2) zygomaticomaxillary (ZM), and (3) infraorbital rim (Fig. 50.5). For the ZF suture, it is important to place the plate at least 2 mm posterior to the rim to reduce the chance that the patient will feel it. The plate, usually 1.5 mm, is placed subperiosteally with two screws on either side of the fracture and an empty hole over it. The periosteum can be used to cover the plate. I place a L-plate, 2.0 mm, over the ZM buttress, taking care to clear the tooth roots inferiorly. Rarely, a plate is placed over the face of the maxilla to stabilize bone fragments. This is typically not necessary due to soft tissue coverage afforded by the cheek and the lack of load-bearing function by this thin bone.

Lastly, I address the infraorbital rim and the orbital floor. With the surgeon standing at the head of the bed, the periorbita is elevated along the floor toward the orbital apex. A malleable retractor is used to hold orbital contents out of the field. The fracture lines are identified and exposed on all sides. It is critical to elevate around the posterior edge of the fracture such that a plate may be placed far posteriorly to support the orbital contents and prevent enophthalmos. Herniated contents are reduced back into the orbit from the maxillary sinus. If a significant floor defect is present, I place a porous polyethylene-coated titanium plate along the orbital floor. The implant is easy to contour and I have not had problems with infection or extrusion. The implant is usually not secured to the rim. The periorbita is then closed at the rim with 4-0 absorbable suture to prevent extrusion. Forced duction testing is again performed to verify the absence of entrapment. Lastly a rim plate, usually 1.0 mm, is placed to span the infraorbital rim fracture. If a free-floating segment of bone is present, I attempt to secure it to the plate with a screw. This can be difficult and is not entirely necessary.

After securing the fracture lines, I observe the face from top-down, again placing an index finger on each infraorbital rim to assess symmetry, and if acceptable, the incisions are closed. The intraoral incision is irrigated and closed in two layers. The deeper layer is approximated with 3-0 Vicryl, and the mucosa is closed with 3-0 running locking Vicryl. Prior to closure of the transconjunctival incision, the midface composite tissue must be resuspended to prevent downward traction on the lower lid and postoperative appearance of malar soft tissue drooping. One or two 3-0 Vicryl sutures are placed in the periosteum over the zygoma and secured to the periosteum of the lateral orbital rim. The cheek should appear overcorrected; with time, it will settle to the appropriate projection. The conjunctival incision can be closed with running 6-0 fast absorbing gut or one

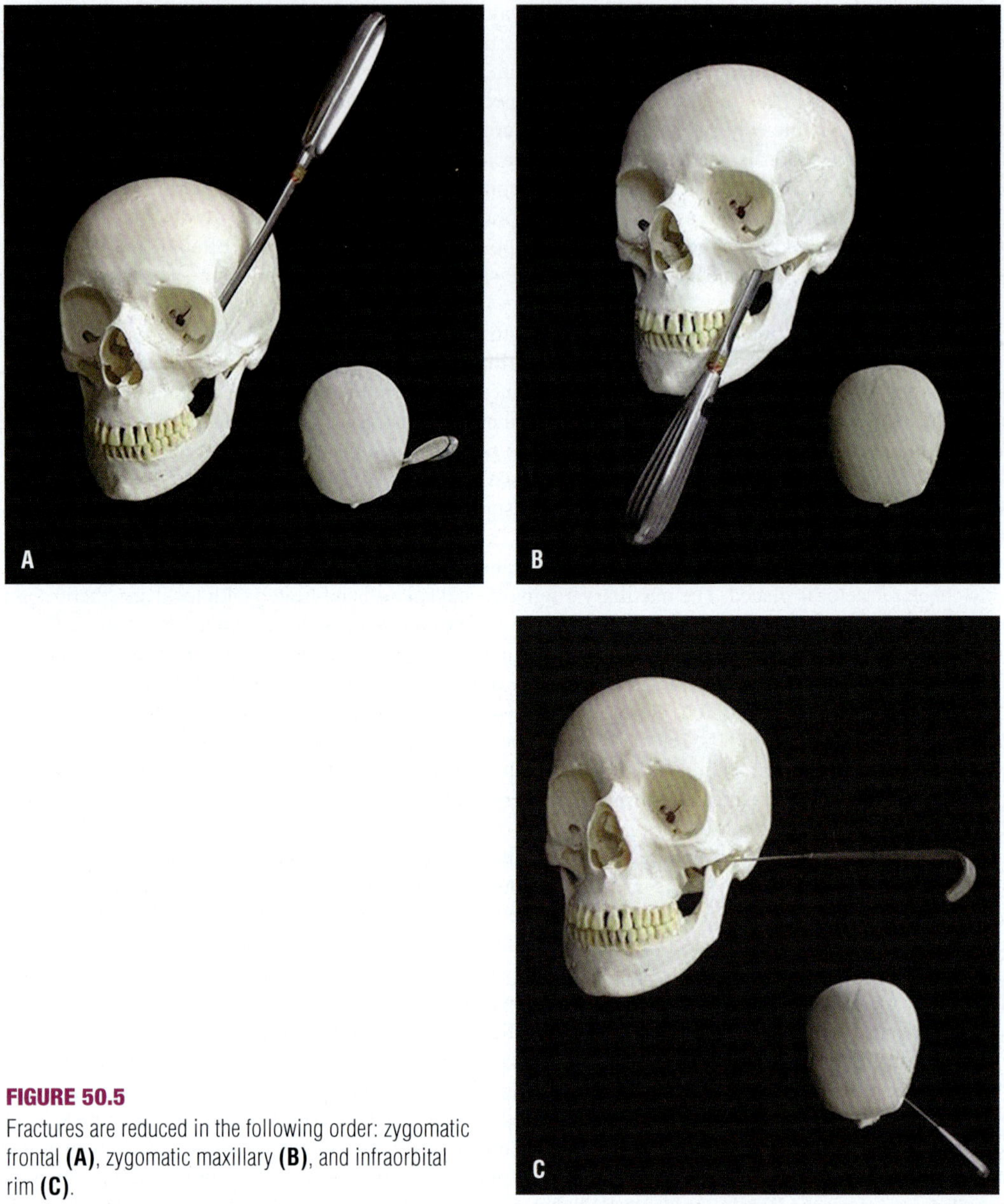

FIGURE 50.5
Fractures are reduced in the following order: zygomatic frontal **(A)**, zygomatic maxillary **(B)**, and infraorbital rim **(C)**.

to two interrupted sutures. The lateral canthal tendon is then sutured to the lateral orbital rim above Whitnall's tubercle to the periosteum inside the lateral rim using an absorbable suture such as 3-0 or 4-0 Vicryl. A horizontal mattress stitch is used. It is critical to approximate the tendon on the inner surface of the lateral rim or the lid will not touch the surface of the globe. Lastly, the lateral canthotomy is closed with 6-0 fast absorbing gut after reapproximating the orbicularis oculi muscle. The lower lid retraction suture may then be taped to the forehead to function as a Frost stitch. This is left in place for 7 days. The tape can be taken down to check the vision or application of antibiotic ointment (Figs. 50.6 to 50.15).

POSTOPERATIVE CARE

Patients who undergo the Gilles approach are discharged the same day with pain medication, soft diet, and antibiotic ointment for the incision site. The temporal wound is evaluated at 1 week follow-up, and healing is assessed at 3 months and 1 year.

OTIF patients are admitted overnight for vision checks and pain control. The nurses should be instructed to assess visual acuity by finger counting every 2 hours; light perception is not sufficient. Oral antibiotics are resumed for 1 week post-op. Ice packs are placed lightly on the face. Maxitrol ointment is placed in the eye and bacitracin ophthalmic ointment is applied to the canthotomy every 12 hours for 5 days. If a Frost stitch was placed, the patient should return in 7 days for removal. Healing takes time, and complications may develop over weeks to months. It is important to schedule follow-up at 1 month, 3 months, and 1 year.

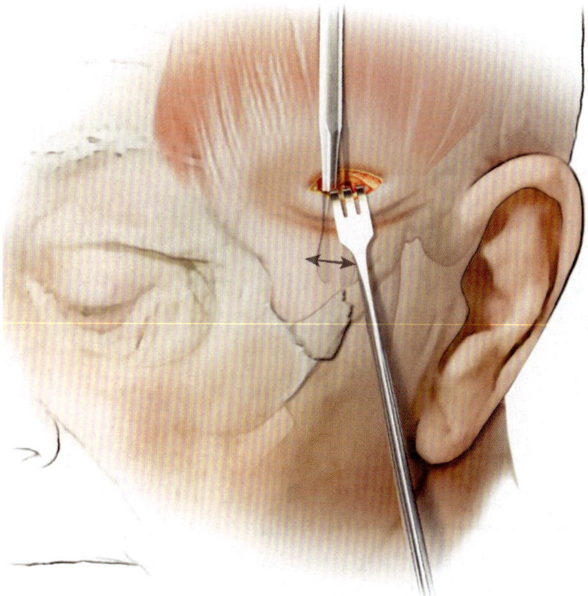

FIGURE 50.6

A Freer elevator is used to bluntly dissect in an anteroinferior direction toward the zygoma, superficial to the temporalis muscle, but deep to the fascia, thereby opening a pocket for placement of the bone elevator.

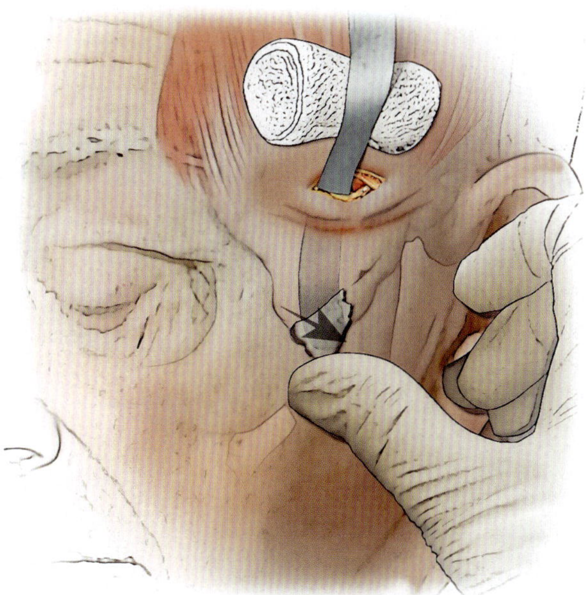

FIGURE 50.7

Insertion the elevator into the pocket. Advancement should proceed smoothly. Place the nondominant hand over the arch with a movement that is simultaneously twisting and levering, rocking the arch back into position. Care is taken to not lever against the temporal bone, creating an iatrogenic fracture.

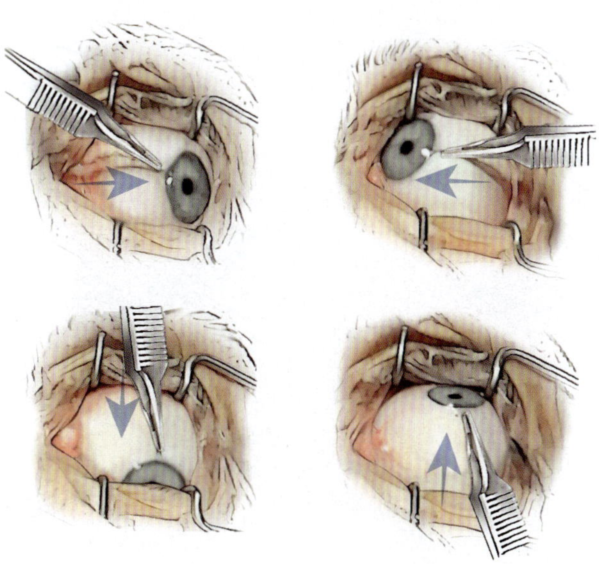

FIGURE 50.8

Forced duction performed in all four directions. Care is taken to avoid any corneal contact in addition to gentle clasping and movement of the eye.

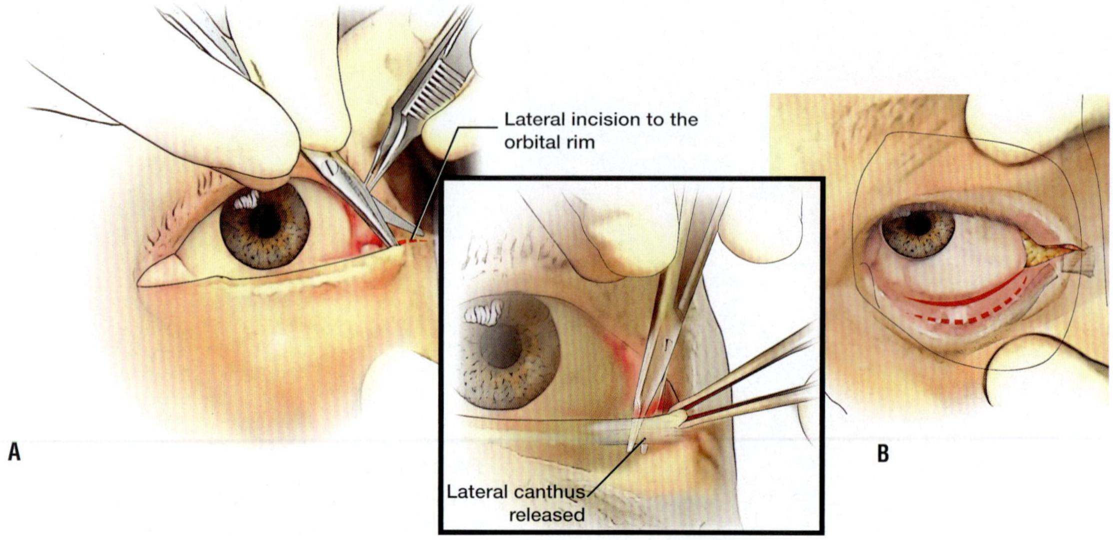

FIGURE 50.9 Lateral canthotomy and subsequent cantholysis **(A)** with dramatic release of the lower lid away from the orbital rim **(B)**.

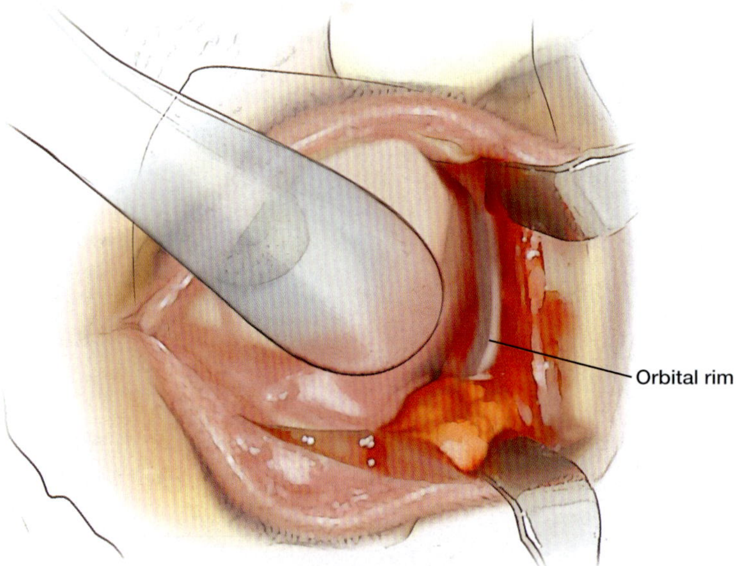

FIGURE 50.10
A clear Jaeger retractor is used to retain the orbital contents out of the field while dissection is taken down to the periosteum of the orbital rim.

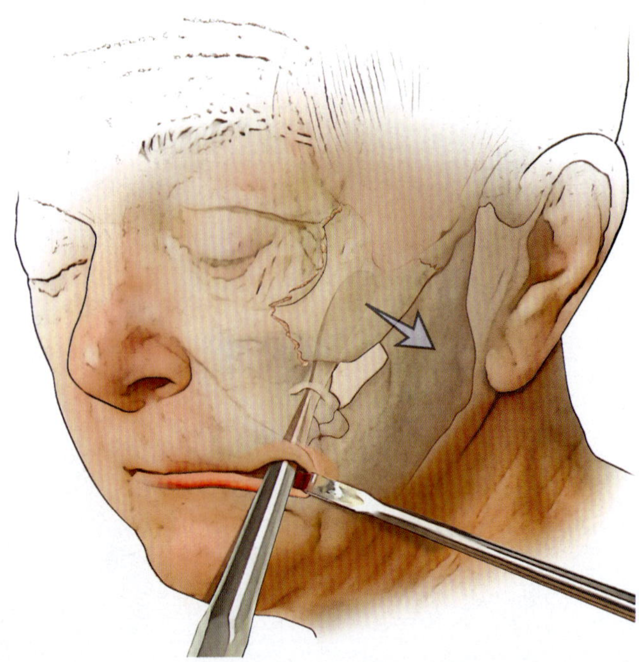

FIGURE 50.11
The elevator is inserted transbuccally to rest beneath the zygoma–zygomatic arch junction. By placing the elevator more anteriorly under the zygomaticomaxillary buttress, the entire zygoma can easily be elevated.

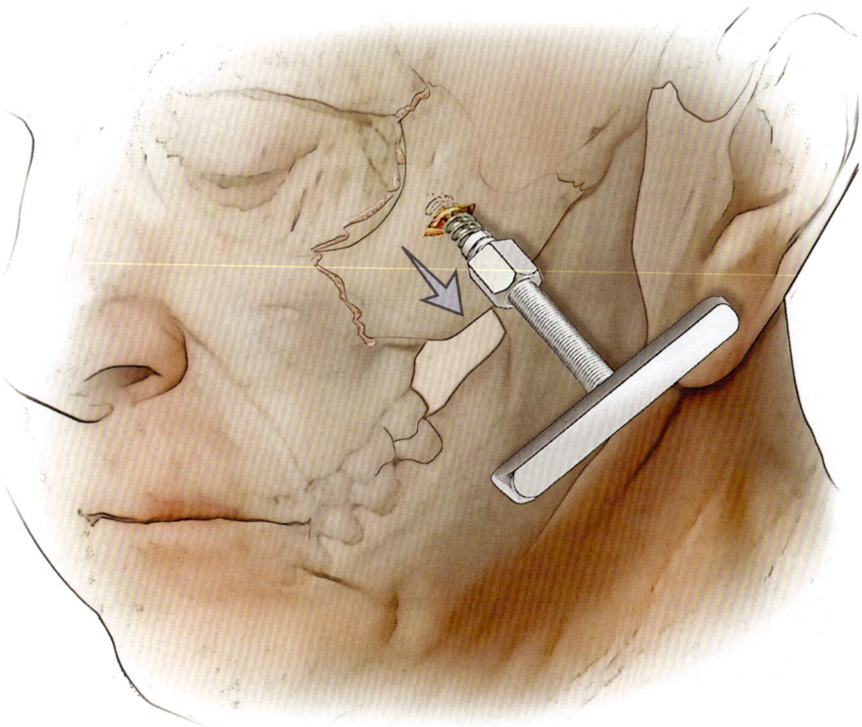

FIGURE 50.12 A Carroll-Girard screw may also be employed to aid in reducing and steadying the body of the zygoma during fixation. This technique allows for forces to be transmitted in multiple vectors thereby affording greater ease in fracture reduction.

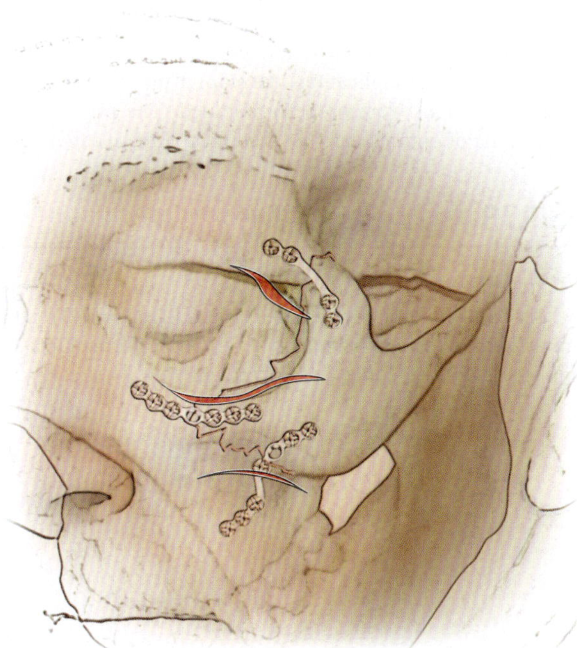

FIGURE 50.13
Fractures are normally fixated in the following order: (1) zygomaticofrontal (ZF), (2) zygomaticomaxillary (ZM), and (3) infraorbital rim.

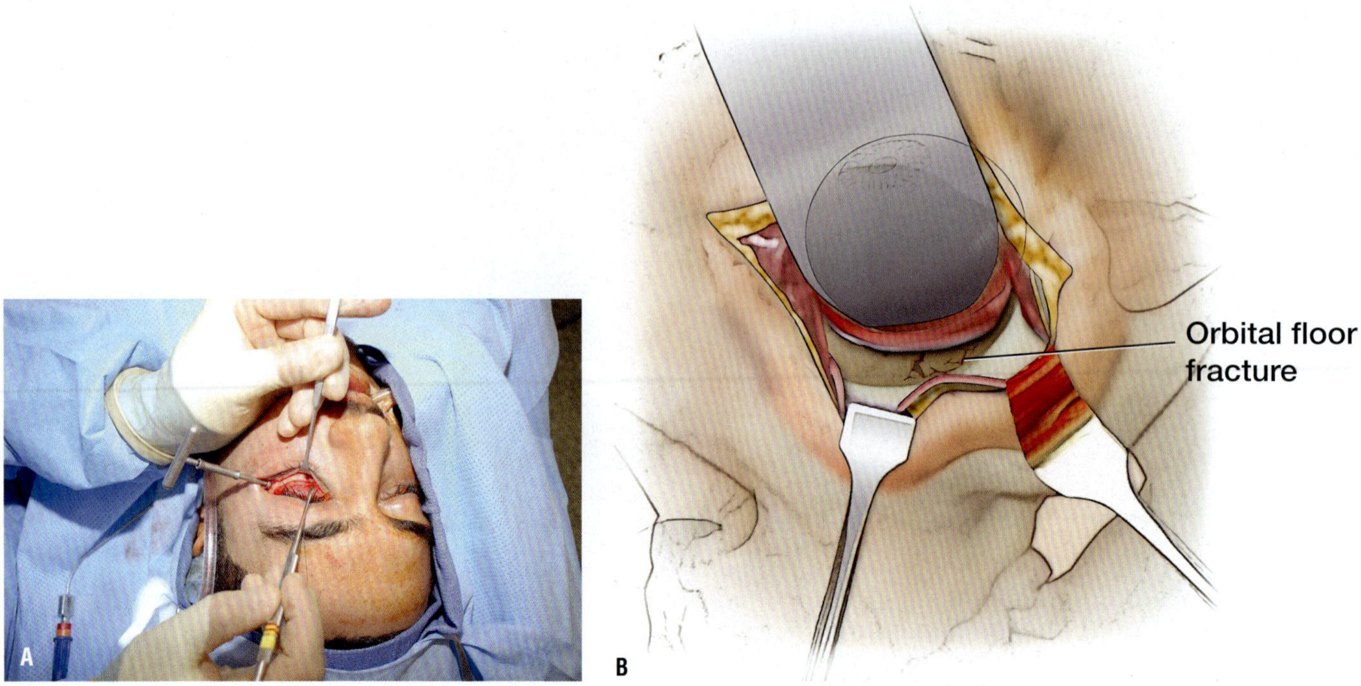

FIGURE 50.14 With the surgeon standing at the head of the bed, a transconjunctival approach is performed with a lateral canthotomy and cantholysis **(A)**. A Carroll-Girard screw placed in the body of the left zygoma for fracture reduction and stabilization. Also shown is exposure of the inferior orbital rim. The periorbita is then elevated along the floor toward the orbital apex for repair of the orbital floor **(B)**.

COMPLICATIONS

Complications are listed in Table 50.1.

Complications can be minimized by excellent exposure, meticulous dissection, and identification of important structures. Preoperative counseling is absolutely necessary to prepare patients for possible complications. In many instances, ZMC fracture repair is undertaken primarily for cosmesis. If lower lid retraction or other unfavorable complications develop, it may be difficult for the patient to justify having had the surgery unless expectations were properly outlined. The physician must inform the patient that complications may result in spite of optimal care but that most of them can be managed satisfactorily.

RESULTS

ZMC fractures are common in craniofacial trauma. Management depends on a focused examination and history, as well as high-quality preoperative CT imaging. Treatment ranges from watchful waiting with soft diet, to minimally invasive reductions, to OTIF. If performed in a stepwise, sequential fashion, operative time can be minimized, while outcomes are optimized.

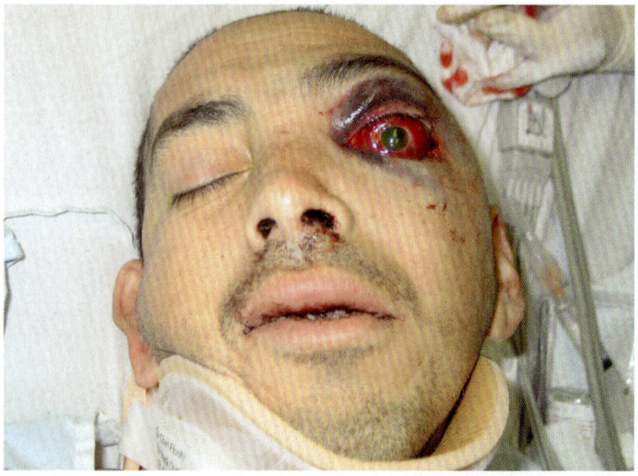

FIGURE 50.15

Appearance of the globe due to retro-orbital hematoma following decompression by lateral canthotomy and cantholysis. Note the proptosis, telecanthus, irregular dilated pupil, and severe chemosis with subconjunctival hemorrhage.

TABLE 50.1 Complications, Causes, and Treatment

Complication	Causes	Treatment
Lower lid retraction/ ectropion/scleral show	Scarring of lower lid to orbital rim	Prevent with meticulous dissection, coverage of plates, Frost stitch Massage, steroid injections, 5-FU injections, repair with grafting
Persistent V2 hypesthesia or facial pain	Nerve impingement	Watchful waiting
Hardware extrusion/ infection/irritation	Postoperative infection, poor wound healing, failure to reapproximate periorbita at rim	Antibiotics Implant removal if persistent
Persistent diplopia	Nerve damage, scar, delay in treatment when entrapment present, present preoperatively	Ophthalmologic consultation
Enophthalmos	Atrophy of orbital adipose tissue, poor implant placement	Reoperation (note that secondary correction is difficult)
Bleeding/retrobulbar hematoma	Poor hemostasis, unrecognized ethmoid artery injury	Lateral canthotomy and cantholysis (Fig. 50.6), urgent ophthalmologic consultation
Blindness	Optic nerve injury, retrobulbar hematoma	Lateral canthotomy and cantholysis, urgent ophthalmologic consultation

PEARLS

- In cases involving severe comminution of the zygomatic arch, or accompanying midface or frontal sinus fractures, a coronal approach to the arch and the lateral orbital rim may be advantageous. For standard treatment of ZMC fractures, I have not found the additional time and risk associated with this approach to be justified.
- Patient education regarding postoperative appearance and possible complications is critical.
- In the event that orbital contents cannot be reduced from the maxillary sinus, widen the floor fracture with an elevator to help with reduction.
- Do not rigidly fix an orbital floor implant to the rim; a separate rim plate should be used instead. In the event that the rim plate is palpable and the patient requests explanation, it will be possible to remove the rim plate only if it is separate from the floor implant.
- I routinely obtain postoperative CT scans for ZMC fracture repairs to assess reduction and implant position.

PITFALLS

- Failure to recognize progressive visual loss. Serial visual examinations are critical in preventing such circumstances.
- Postoperative bleeding and hematoma. This is addressed with serial examinations of the patient and their visual acuity after surgery and surgical intervention when necessary.
- Failure to reestablish appropriate sinus outflow can lead to postoperative infections. Attention is to be directed to not only reestablishing anatomic structure, but anatomic function as well.
- Inadequate operative planning. The complete extent of the facial injury is to be determined prior to the operative procedure and is best established with axial and coronal CT images set for bone windows. 3D reconstruction, if available, is another adjunct that can complement the formulation of an operative plan.
- Incomplete orbital volume correction. This may be seen with postoperative enophthalmos, diplopia, or hypoglobus and often represents inadequate implant size, fracture correction, tissue atrophy/loss, or a combination of the above. Surgical revision is advised.

INSTRUMENTS TO HAVE AVAILABLE

- Clear corneal shields
- 15-blade knife
- Freer elevator
- Dingman or Cobb elevator

- Minnesota retractors
- Army-Navy retractors
- 0.5 forceps
- Adson-Brown forceps
- Cottle retractor
- Senn retractor
- Medium and Large Desmarre retractors
- Guarded bayonet bipolar cautery
- 1.0-, 1.5-, and 2.0-cm malleable retractors
- #9 dental elevator
- Needle-point cautery
- Wescott scissors
- Webster needle holder
- Castroviejo needle holder
- Clear Jaeger retractor
- Carroll-Girard screw
- 7fr and 10fr Frazier tip suction

SUGGESTED READING

Ellis E, Zide M. *Surgical approaches to the facial skeleton*, 2nd ed. Philadelphia, PA: Lippincott Williams & Wilkins, 2006.
Fonseca R, Walker R, Betts N, et al. *Oral and maxillofacial trauma*, 3rd ed. St. Louis, MO: Elsevier, 2005.

51 LE FORT I AND LE FORT II FRACTURES

Jacob O. Boeckmann

INTRODUCTION

Fractures of the midface account for up to 20% of facial fractures presenting to the emergency department. When fractures of the midface occur, significant functional problems and aesthetic deformities can result. Much of the understanding of midface trauma is attributed to Rene Le Fort's work published in 1901. Le Fort studied the impact of low-velocity blunt force to cadaver facial skeletons and noted three distinct fracture patterns based upon inherent lines of weakness (Fig. 51.1). The original descriptions were represented as symmetric and occurring in isolation. In today's society, Le Fort fractures are rarely seen in their pure form and can present as a unilateral fractures, combined fracture patterns, or comminuted fractures. Timely diagnosis and treatment of these injuries is important in order to optimize patient outcomes and minimize long-term sequela. The goals of management are directed toward the reestablishment of preinjury structure and function. Advances in implant technology have allowed the reconstructive surgeon the ability to perform a single-stage repair with rigid internal fixation. This provides the patient more rapid bone healing, improved cosmesis, enhanced nutrition, and earlier return of preinjury function.

HISTORY

In the United States, Le Fort fractures typically are sustained as a result of motor vehicle accidents, physical assault, and occupation-related, sport-related, or gunshot injuries. The majority of these injuries occur in males during their 3rd and 4th decade of life. However, the elderly remain an at-risk group due to a higher incidence of falls in this population. Rarely do children sustain these injuries due to their developing craniofacial anatomy.

The mechanism of injury, including the velocity, direction, and location of the force, can help the physician anticipate the fracture pattern. Le Fort I fractures typically occur following blunt force directed in an anterior to posterior direction to the midface. Le Fort II injuries can result either from a horizontal force directed across the midface or from a transmitted force from the mandible following forces directed to the chin. Due to the amount of force needed to fracture the midface, it is not uncommon for patients to present with coexistent complex fractures to the surrounding facial skeleton, cervical spine, central nervous system, and/or orbit.

The treating physician must have a high index of suspicion for associated injuries. Critical components of the history should focus on the status of the dentition, cranial nerve defects, vision changes, and rhinorrhea. Malocclusion is common following fractures of the craniofacial skeleton and, in some instances, may be the only clue in a patient without obvious signs of injury. Cranial nerve defects may accompany these fractures, particularly the second branch of the trigeminal nerve (V2). Any change in vision reported by the patient raises the possibility of an orbital fracture or orbital trauma. Finally, anosmia, rhinorrhea, or otorrhea may be indicative of a skull base injury with potential cerebrospinal fluid (CSF) leak.

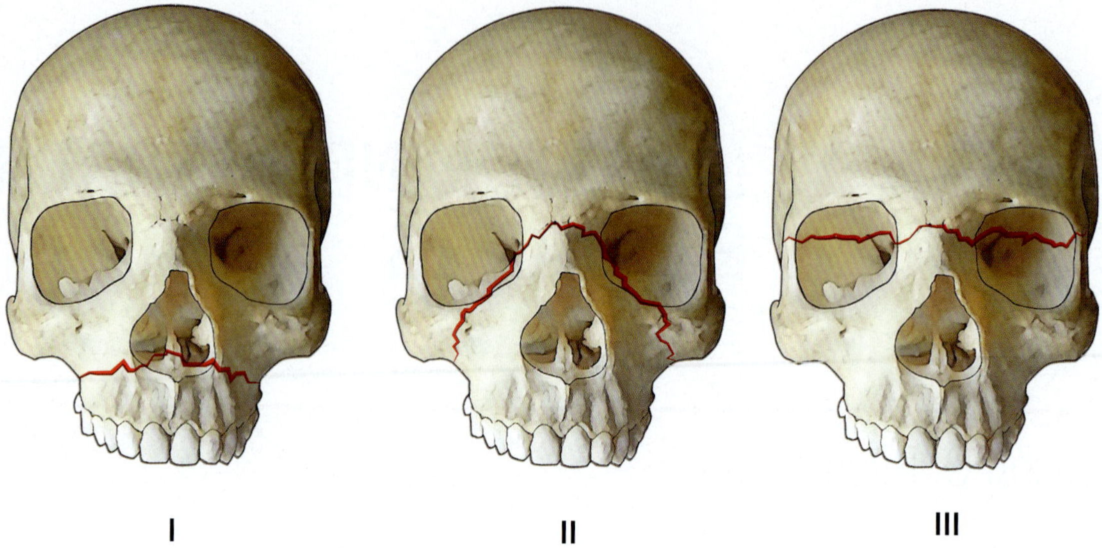

FIGURE 51.1 Le Fort fracture patterns.

PHYSICAL EXAMINATION

Frequently, the evaluation of these patients occurs in an emergency room setting. As in all trauma situations, initial assessment and resuscitation using the ABCDE primary survey and immediate treatment of life-threatening injuries take precedence. Airway assessment takes priority, as the potential for obstruction exists secondary to posterior dislocation of the fractured segment into the airway. Bleeding can also result in obstruction if the patient is unable to control his or her airway secretions.

When airway compromise exists, the preferred method for airway management is orotracheal intubation by a skilled responder. This may not always be possible due to impaired visualization from blood and secretions, coexistent cervical spine trauma, or altered anatomy. One must therefore always anticipate the need for an alternate airway. If coexistent cervical spine injury is suspected or present, the airway can be obtained via fiberoptic or nasotracheal intubation. When these options are unsuccessful, a surgical airway can be established in an emergent or planned situation via a cricothyroidotomy or tracheostomy.

It is not uncommon to encounter epistaxis following midface trauma due to disruption to the delicate nasal and sinus mucosa. Bleeding of this nature is typically self-limited but occasionally requires control with nasal packing, a 30-mL Foley balloon, or temporary fracture reduction. Epistaxis can also be the source of life-threatening hemorrhage from disruption of the distant branches of the external carotid artery (e.g., internal maxillary artery) or the skull base. When this occurs, timely awareness and intervention is warranted to minimize significant morbidity and mortality from hypovolemic shock. This scenario requires advanced techniques for control, which may include ligation of the external carotid artery, or intravascular control with coils and/or embolization.

Once the patient is stabilized, a detailed physical examination is possible. Examination of facial symmetry is an important first step in evaluating trauma patients. Unfortunately, this can be challenging to identify in the acutely injured patient due to soft tissue edema and ecchymosis overlying the facial skeleton. Once the acute edema subsides, the surgeon can easily note the facial asymmetry.

Assessment of occlusion is essential for all patients with facial fractures because malocclusion sometimes may be the only evidence of a fracture. Frequently, the disrupted premaxilla leads to premature contact with the molars and a resultant anterior open bite deformity. A palate or alveolar fracture can also complicate the occlusive relationship by widening the dentoalveolar arch resulting in a posterior cross-bite deformity. Any dental gaps and avulsed teeth must be accounted for to ensure that the airway is clear. A patient with avulsed teeth should have a chest radiograph to rule out aspiration of dental fragments.

Palpation of the bony skeleton often reveals step-off deformities and tenderness overlying the fracture lines. Crepitus involving the soft tissue or gingivobuccal sulcus may be present if an associated fracture of the paranasal sinus is present. Mobility should be assessed with bimanual palpation from the thumb and index finger. With Le Fort I injuries, mobility of the palate will be present while those with Le Fort II injuries will have movement of the maxilla and nasal complex. Absence of mobility does not always exclude a Le Fort injury as impaction can impair mobility of the fractured segment. Any lacerations should be noted as these can be associated with underlying bony defects and may be used as potential routes of exposure for reduction.

A complete ocular examination is important when any concern exists for periocular trauma. Periorbital edema, ecchymosis, chemosis, and subconjuctival hemorrhage frequently are present when an orbital fracture is present. Ocular motility should be assessed as impingement of bony fragments may restrict extraocular motility. When a disturbance is present, forced duction testing should be performed to distinguish between entrapment and neurologic impairment. Epiphora can result from a disruption of the nasolacrimal duct drainage system.

Finally, a complete head and neck neurologic evaluation should be performed, with particular emphasis on the level of consciousness, cranial nerve examination, and cervical spine status. Frequently, patients have paresthesia of the midface along the second branch of the trigeminal nerve due to direct injury, bony impingement, or neural edema. If a CSF leak is suspected, it can be confirmed with collection of a fluid sample for beta-2 transferrin testing or further imaging.

INDICATIONS

These injuries are not life threatening, but left unrepaired, they can result in significant cosmetic and functional sequela. The vertical buttress system is composed of paired zygomaticomaxillary (lateral), nasomaxillary (medial), and pterygomaxillary (posterior) buttresses and functions to resist the forces of mastication and establishes midface height. The horizontal buttress system is composed of the frontal bone and supraorbital rims, the infraorbital rims and zygoma, and the alveolus and palate. The horizontal buttress establishes facial width and projection and further supports the vertical buttresses. Le Fort injuries often disrupt one or both buttress systems, resulting in a vertical shortening of the face and a flattened appearance.

For Le Fort injuries, the goals of treatment are threefold:

1. Restoration of preinjury occlusion
2. Restoration of facial height and width
3. Restoration of soft tissue integrity

Not all patients require open reduction and internal fixation. If the patient is reliable and has a nondisplaced Le Fort I with easily restorable occlusion, closed reduction with MMF for 4 to 6 weeks can be considered. For all other patients, repair with open reduction and internal fixation is indicated.

The proper timing of repair remains debatable with few studies available to provide definitive evidence supporting early versus late repair. Advocates for early repair report improved outcomes in function, cosmesis, and decreased rates of infection. However, not all patients are candidates for early repair due to coexistent injuries and medical instability from other life-threatening injuries. Any patient with periorbital trauma should undergo preoperative examination by an ophthalmologist to rule out an orbital injury or other condition that may preclude repair. A ruptured globe, retrobulbar hematoma, or extraocular muscle entrapment may require urgent intervention while findings of a hyphema or traumatic optic neuropathy may delay or alter the treatment strategy. Those patients with closed head injuries, significant frontal or skull base fractures, or CSF leak should be evaluated by a neurosurgeon and cleared for surgery prior to intervention. These patients must await medical stability prior to fixation.

When delayed repair is indicated, most surgeons agree it is best to address these fractures within 2 weeks of injury to avoid the potential need for bone grafting or osteotomies. Ultimately, the reconstructive surgeon must exercise judgment as to the optimal timing of repair for each individual patient.

CONTRAINDICATIONS

Contraindications for surgical repair of midface fractures generally are related to coexistent life-threatening injuries that have not been stabilized from the initial trauma or those at high risk of general anesthesia due to coexistent medical comorbidities and instability.

PREOPERATIVE PLANNING

High-resolution computer tomography (CT) of the facial skeleton with axial and coronal thin cut (1.5-mm) imaging has become the standard imaging modality in the evaluation of a patient with facial trauma. CT provides superior characterization of the facial fracture segments and overlying soft tissue compared to traditional plain film radiography. It also allows the reconstructive surgeon the opportunity to evaluate the degree of injury and the potentially involved adjacent structures such as the optic canal, skull base, carotid canal, and integrity of the globe.

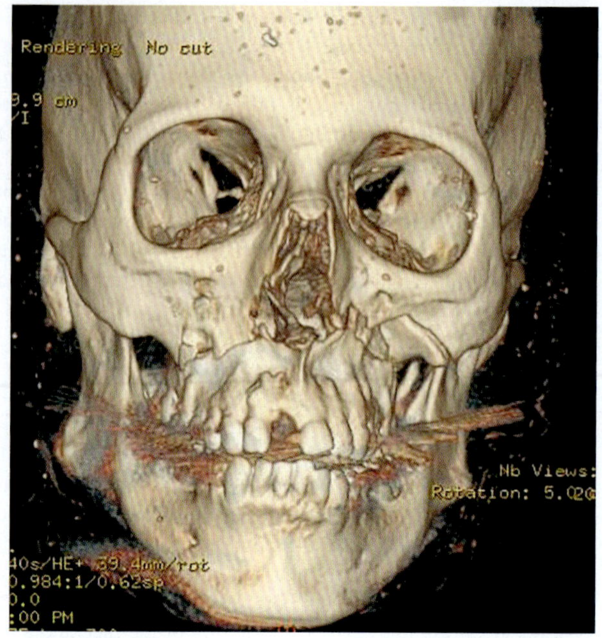

FIGURE 51.2
3-D reconstruction of Le Fort I.

One should develop a systematic method for evaluating imaging so that nothing is overlooked especially in the setting of panfacial fractures. Combined fracture patterns, unilateral injuries, and comminuted patterns are typically present, and one should assess for concomitant injuries, especially the status of the cervical spine. As a general rule, vertical structures are best noted on coronal imaging, while horizontal structures are best viewed on axial imaging. All Le Fort fractures involve fractures of the pterygoid plates. Once the pterygoid plate fracture is identified, the physician can work on determining the remaining fracture patterns. Le Fort I fractures are low transverse fractures cephalic to the dentition spanning the lower lateral walls of the zygomaticomaxillary buttress, the medial nasomaxillary buttress at the pyriform aperture, the posterior maxillary wall, and septum. These fractures are best visualized on coronal plane. Le Fort II fractures are pyramidal shaped in nature, with involvement of the zygomaticomaxillary buttress, nasomaxillary buttress superiorly, inferior orbital rim, orbital floor, and nasofrontal junction. These fracture patterns are best viewed on coronal views.

Three-dimensional reconstructed images should be obtained if possible because they provide the reconstructive surgeon further understanding of the spatial relationships and are useful for determining the overall treatment plan (see Figs. 51.2 and 51.3).

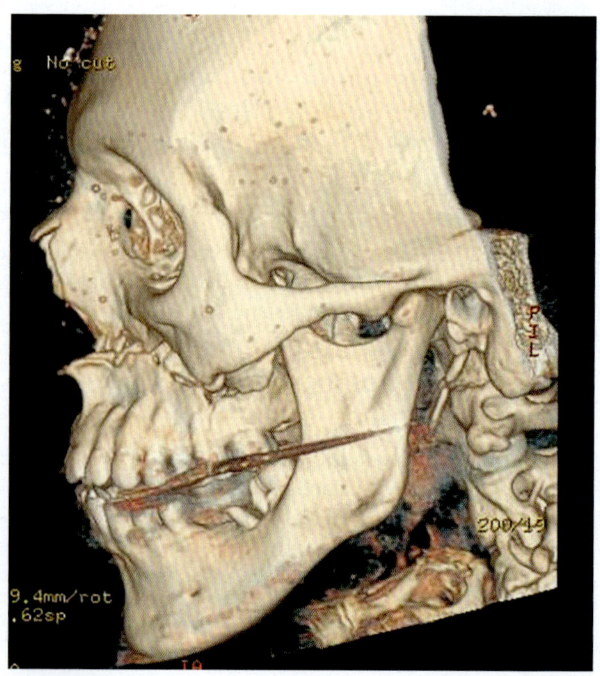

FIGURE 51.3
3-D reconstruction of Le fort I.

SURGICAL TECHNIQUE

Surgical correction of Le Fort fractures is performed under general anesthesia. Due to the need for maxillomandibular fixation (MMF), nasotracheal intubation is necessary if a tracheotomy is not present. In order to appropriately restore the midface, the reconstructive surgeon must reestablish the integrity of the buttress system. The approach to the patient with Le Fort fractures is dependent upon the injury pattern. The sublabial incision provides access to the lower lateral and medial buttresses and is the preferred approach for midface fixation. Injecting local anesthetic with epinephrine (e.g., 1% lidocaine 1:100,000 epinephrine) into the incision site helps to minimize bleeding and improve visualization. Chlorhexidine gluconate oral rinse is used to reduce the bacteria load of the oral cavity. A self-retaining lip retractor or appropriately sized cheek retractor is used to better visualize the oral cavity.

The sublabial incision is made along the gingivobuccal sulcus from first molar to first molar with Bovie electrocautery, taking care to leave behind an adequate cuff of mucosa for closure. The fractured segments are widely exposed to enable the placement of a titanium plate with two to three holes on either side of the fracture line. Subperiosteal elevation of the overlying soft tissue is performed with a Cottle or Freer elevator in order to widely expose the nasomaxillary buttress, zygomaticomaxillary buttress, pyriform aperture nasal spine, and anterior maxilla. The infraorbital nerve, which exits the infraorbital foramen 6 to 7 mm below the infraorbital rim, must be protected during dissection. Care should be taken when dissecting along the medial buttress and pyriform aperture to avoid inadvertent entry into the nasal cavity.

Once all the fractures are adequately exposed, the integrity of the bone is assessed. If fibrous in-growth and granulation tissue is present in the fracture line, it is debrided prior to reduction. When significant comminution of the fracture site is present or bone gaps greater than 5 mm are encountered, one should consider bone grafting. Bone grafting provides stability to the repair and restores the vertical height of the midface. Grafts can be harvested from the calvarium or costal framework, depending upon the surgeon's preference.

Once the fracture line is clear, reduction of loose fragments is performed using a bone hook, screw, elevator or Carroll-Girard device. When significant impaction prevents appropriate alignment, the Rowe forceps can be used to apply greater force for reduction. This should be done with care to avoid injury to the orbit, infraorbital nerve, and nasolacrimal duct.

After reduction of the fracture site, the occlusion is reassessed and the patient is placed into MMF. At least four miniplates are required to appropriately stabilize Le Fort I fractures. Plating of the lateral buttress is performed first using a 1.5-mm or 2-mm titanium miniplate with 4-mm or 5-mm self-tapping screws. It is important to place the plate so that at least 2 screws can be secured on either side of the fracture line along the load-bearing segment of the maxilla. An L-shaped plate works well along the lateral buttress and avoids violation of the tooth roots, but other plate shapes may be utilized (Figs. 51.4 and 51.5). After precisely contouring the plate to the configuration of the maxilla, the plate is secured to the zygoma with the placement of a screw adjacent to the fracture line. The second screw is then inserted on the opposite side of the fracture line along the alveolar segment. If reduction is satisfactory, the remaining screws are then placed. The medial buttress is then fixed in a similar fashion with the optimal plate design dependent upon the fracture pattern. When plating the medial buttress, it is important to position the plate along the weight-bearing segment of the maxilla, adjacent to the pyriform aperture for maximum stability of the reconstruction (Fig. 51.6). Once plated, occlusion should be rechecked to ensure satisfactory position.

After reduction is complete, resuspension of the soft tissue should be ensured. If extensive subperiosteal dissection of the soft tissue and skeletonization of the midface was performed, attempts should be made to resuspend the tissue to the zygoma to limit the possibility of postoperative scar contracture, deformity, and ectropion. This is easily performed by passing a strong braided suture through a bone tunnel or a miniplate hole. Prior to closure, copious irrigation with sterile normal saline is performed to further minimize bacterial

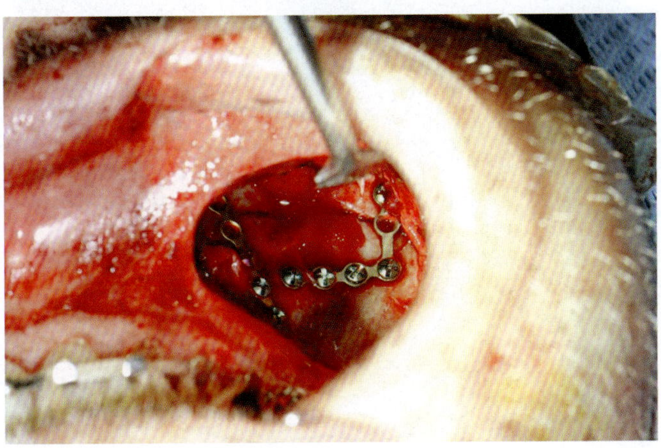

FIGURE 51.4
Intraoperative photo demonstrating the sublabial approach with L-plate application for reestablishment of the lateral buttress. Also noted is a linear plate for reestablishment of the medial buttress.

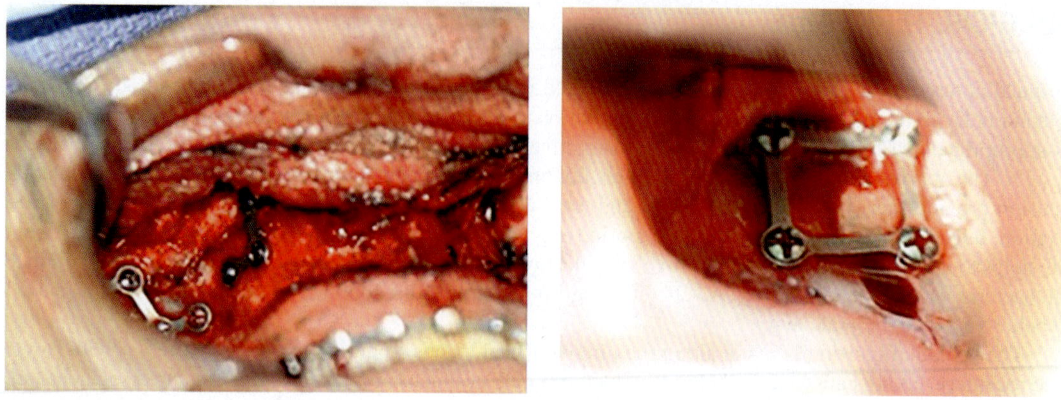

FIGURE 51.5 Intraoperative photo demonstrating the sublabial approach and various plating configurations for stabilization of the midface.

contamination in the surgical site. Closure of the sublabial incision is then performed using 3-0 or 4-0 Vicryl® (polyglactin 10) or Chromic Gut suture in a running or interrupted fashion.

If the surgeon is confident in the anatomical reduction and occlusion, the patient can be taken out of MMF and the arch bars can be removed. However, if there is a question of correct intraoperative occlusion or if the fracture is comminuted, continuation of the arch bars with wire fixation or elastic guidance is maintained for 4 to 6 weeks postoperatively until occlusion concerns are corrected.

Patients with Le Fort II fractures may require additional fixation along the infraorbital rims to correct step-off deformities and to stabilize the segment.

There are a number of ways to approach the orbit. The transconjunctival and subciliary approaches are the most commonly used techniques for access to the infraorbital rim and floor. I prefer the transconjunctival approach, due to the avoidance of a facial incision and the reduced risk of ectropion. If needed, this approach can be combined with a lateral canthotomy for increased lateral exposure. Alternatively, an existing laceration can be used for access to the orbital rim if it is in a favorable position.

For the transconjunctival approach, a corneal shield is placed and a small amount of local anesthetic with epinephrine is placed along the lower fornix and lateral canthus. A Desmarres retractor is used for the lower lid and a malleable Ribbon retractor is used to gently retract the globe. The transconjunctival incision is performed

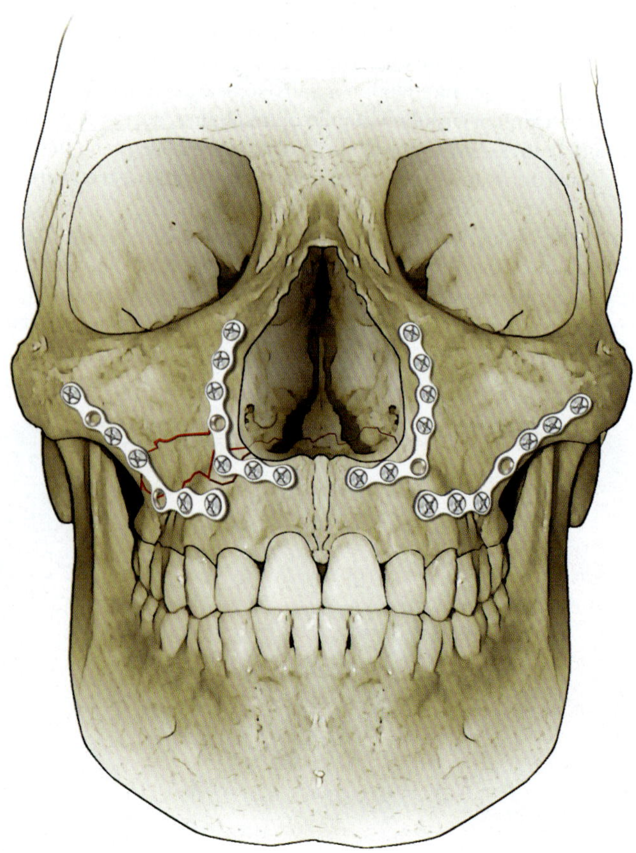

FIGURE 51.6
Illustrated representation of Le Fort I fracture status post reduction and fixation.

at the base of the fornix in a medial to lateral direction using a fine-tip Bovie cautery. A traction suture can be placed along the inferior aspect of the transconjunctival incision to improve tissue retraction and exposure. The surgeon can access the orbital rim in a preseptal or postseptal plane.

Once the orbital rim is reached, Bovie cautery can be used to incise through the periosteum and a Freer elevator is used to elevate the periosteum off of the bone. With the orbital rim exposed, the fracture can be reduced and fixation can be accomplished using a 1.0-mm or 1.3-mm titanium miniplates with 4-mm self-tapping screws. When stabilizing the plate into position, it is best to place the screw into the stable segment first. Larger plates are to be avoided in this area due to their potential to cause postoperative soft tissue retraction, palpability, and prominence. After the orbital rim is reduced, an exploration of the orbital floor can be performed if indicated.

After completing the periorbital reduction, the surgeon should make an attempt to cover the plate with periosteum to minimize postoperative palpability. Meticulous care is necessary when approximating the layers to avoid inadvertent approximation of the orbicularis oculi muscle to the periosteum of the orbital rim. After periosteal closure, two to three conjunctival sutures can be placed in an interrupted manner using 6-0 fast gut chromic sutures. Finally, a Frost suture can be placed for several days if there is a significant concern for ectropion.

Rarely does the nasofrontal fracture line need plating, but if it is deemed appropriate, access can be obtained via a bicoronal approach and fixation can be achieved using 1.0 or 1.3 miniplates.

Palate Fractures

A palatal fracture may also complicate the establishment of preinjury occlusion and must be addressed to establish the width of the lower central midface.

For a large, sagittal palate fracture or one with significant instability, rigid fixation of the hard palate and anterior pyriform can provide precise arch reduction and correct a widened arch from posterior splaying. This can be accomplished with a 2.0-mm titanium plate with 4-mm monocortical screws placed via a longitudinal palate and sublabial incision. Care must be taken not to devascularize the hard palate mucosa with extensive lateral dissection in order to minimize the risk of a flap breakdown and resultant plate exposure.

When a comminuted or complex palate fracture is present, a palatal splint can be used as a guide to establish preinjury occlusion and secured with an arch bar to stabilize the palatal segment. Once the palate width is restored, the repair of the midface can proceed.

Edentulous Mandible

The edentulous patient with a Le Fort injury provides additional challenges when attempting to recreate the relationship between the maxilla and the mandible. Without MMF, inadequate reduction of these fractures can result in inferior displacement of the posterior maxilla secondary to gravity and the pull of the pterygoid musculature. This results in narrowing between the upper and lower arch, which can complicate postoperative use of a denture. This posteroinferior displacement can be avoided with MMF. The establishment of MMF can be achieved with dental splints or dentures secured to the maxilla and mandible with screw fixation or circummandibular and circumzygomatic wiring. The repair can then proceed along in a similar fashion as the dentulous patient. If the patient is not a candidate for MMF, the lateral and medial buttresses are stabilized after clinical reduction of the fractured segments (Fig. 51.7).

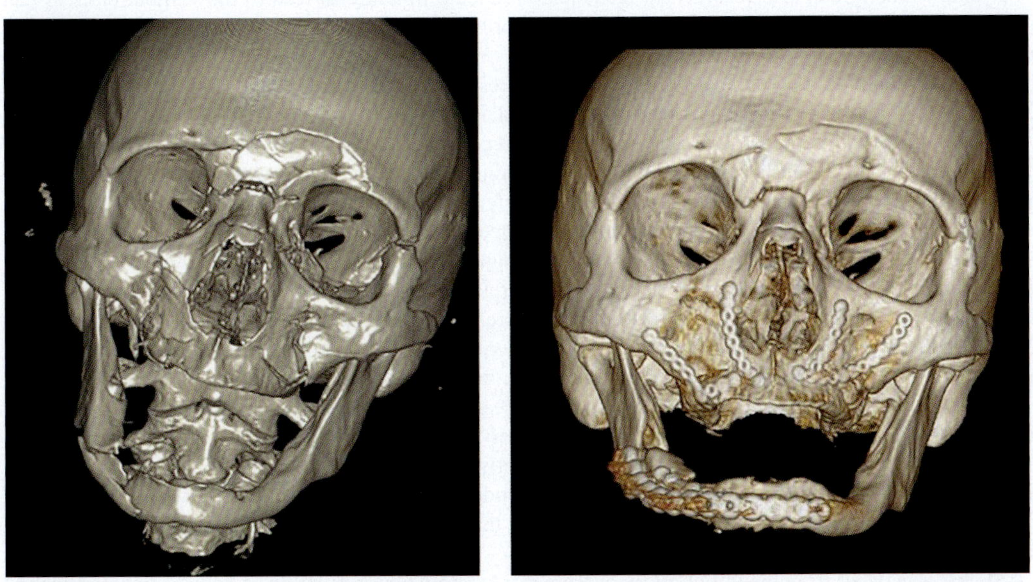

FIGURE 51.7 Preoperative and postoperative imaging of edentulous right-sided Le Fort II and left-sided Le Fort III fracture. Open reduction and internal fixation was performed to stabilize the medial and lateral buttresses.

Resorbable Plating Systems

Resorbable plating systems composed of polylactic acid have expanded in popularity and use over the last two decades especially in the pediatric population. Their biodegradable properties are advantageous in this population due to the limited potential for growth disturbances and the reduced need of a second operation for removal. Early studies in orthognathic surgery report similar outcomes compared to those undergoing fixation with titanium plating systems. However, widespread adoption of resorbable plating systems remains limited due to the increased learning curve with the material, longer operative time, and cost.

POSTOPERATIVE MANAGEMENT

Patients are observed following repair for any airway issues, bleeding, pain control, and nausea control. If the patient was kept in MMF, wire cutters or scissors need to be immediately available in the event of an airway crisis or vomiting. Upon discharge, the patient must have an understanding of how to cut and remove the wires or bands in case any of the above mentioned issues arise.

Antibiotics are given perioperatively. These fractures are considered contaminated, due to the involvement of the oral, nasal, and sinus cavities. The optimal duration of antibiotic use remains undefined and is dependent upon patient characteristics and the surgeon's preference. Typically, a 5- to 10-day course of a penicillin or cephalosporin is given for coverage against gram-positive organisms and anaerobes. Alternatively, clindamycin may be given for penicillin-allergic patients. Chlorhexidine gluconate (Peridex™) mouth rinse is also used until the intraoral sutures dissolve and the oral cavity is healed.

All patients are maintained on a soft diet for 6 to 8 weeks postsurgery. Follow-up is 1 week postdischarge to ensure appropriate wound healing and oral hygiene. Patients are then seen every 2 weeks to ensure stability of the fracture site with particular attention to the occlusion. Guiding elastics may be necessary for subtle malocclusion, and adjustments may be needed. MMF can be released at 6 weeks if the fracture site is stable, but arch bars are left in place for an additional 2 weeks to ensure stability of the occlusion. The patient is slowly transitioned to a regular diet, and if occlusion remains stable, the arch bars can be removed.

COMPLICATIONS

The majority of complications are associated with inadequate reduction of the bone fragments. Therefore, all attempts should be made by the reconstructive surgeon to minimize this complication with early repair when possible, meticulous attention to occlusion intraoperatively, and the appropriate use of bone grafting.

One of the most common consequences of inadequate reduction is malocclusion. This frequently results from failure to establish occlusion prior to bony fixation or from an unrecognized palate and alveolar fracture. Guiding elastics can help treat subtle malocclusion; however, it is unable to overcome situations where inadequate or improper reduction was rigidly fixed. In this situation, one must return to the operating room to remove and replace the plates after appropriately reducing the bone fragment. When discovered late, advanced treatment with orthodontic appliances or osteotomies and advancement may be needed to correct malocclusion.

Facial asymmetry can also result from inadequate reduction. Failure to restore the vertical buttress can result in a shortened midface, while failure to restore the horizontal buttress can result in midface flattening and alteration of the facial width.

Malunion, nonunion, and delayed union can be the result of inadequate reduction, infection, failure of immobilization, or hardware failure and needs to be treated appropriately.

Hardware infection is a rare occurrence in midface reconstruction due to the excellent blood supply of the face. When this occurs during the healing process, maintenance of the plates while treating the infection with culture-directed antibiotics, and local drainage is preferred. Once 6 to 8 weeks has elapsed to allow for osteosynthesis, the plates can be removed and replaced if needed.

Osteomyelitis can occur in the setting of a long-standing, untreated infection associated with the hardware. When this occurs, incision, drainage, and debridement of retained hardware and involved bone are necessary. If instability of the fracture line is present, stability can be restored with replating, MMF, or external fixation.

Plate exposure, while unusual, can occur with inadequate closure over the fracture line. This can be avoided by preserving adequate mucosal cuffs for closure, meticulous attention to technique, and appropriate oral hygiene. If dehiscence and exposure occur, maintenance of oral hygiene is recommended with avoidance of irritants such as smoking. If exposure persists despite conservative measures, the hardware should be removed.

Paresthesia, either temporary or permanent, is frequently present along the second division of the trigeminal nerve. This can be consequence of the injury or secondary to trauma or traction injury intraoperatively. It is important to counsel the patient preoperatively about this expected finding, with the majority of injuries improving with time.

CSF leak can occur from the initial injury or from intraoperative manipulation of bony segments attached to the skull base. Conservative management with elevating the head of the bed, stool softeners, acetazolamide, and lumbar drainage is employed as first-line treatment. For those leaks lasting longer than 2 weeks, closure is indicated to reduce the risk of meningitis.

Additional complications may occur including sinusitis, mucocele formation, enophthalmos, epiphora, extraocular muscle entrapment, ectropion, diplopia, and nasal obstruction.

RESULTS

Unfortunately, due to the heterogeneous patient profile, few long-term outcome studies are available for this treatment population. Long-term, patients with complex Le Fort injuries are more likely to experience ongoing disability. Le Fort patients have more somatic complaints compared to the general trauma population, with ongoing visual disturbances, disturbances of smell, mastication difficulties, disrupted breathing, and epiphora. Therefore, the reconstructive surgeon must be aware of the potential ongoing needs of this patient population.

PEARLS

- The goals of treatment are the restoration of preinjury occlusion, the facial height and width, and soft tissue integrity.
- CT with thin cut axial and coronal imaging is the gold standard for preoperative identification of the fracture pattern.
- Restoration of the horizontal and vertical buttress is critical to regaining preinjury function and form to the midface.
- Rigid internal fixation with or without MMF allows for accurate approximation of bony fragments and is the superior choice for midface stabilization.

PITFALLS

- The majority of complications result as a consequence of inadequate reduction of the fracture line.
- Always take care to preserve an adequate cuff of mucosa to minimize the risk of postoperative hardware exposure.
- Poor oral hygiene, smoking, and diabetes can contribute to delayed wound healing and should be managed accordingly.

INSTRUMENTS TO HAVE AVAILABLE

- Standard plastics set (Mayo-Hegar needle holder, suture cutting scissors, Adson's tissue forceps, Debakey forceps, Cottle elevator, Freer periosteal elevator)
- Internal fixation system (wire holder, wire cutter, 24-gauge and 26-gauge wire, bone plate and screws, Erich's arch bars)
- Drill
- Saw
- Rowe maxillary disimpaction forceps
- Asch nasal bone reduction forceps
- Osteotomes
- Bone hooks
- Army–Navy retractors
- Self-retaining cheek retractors
- Desmarres lid retractor
- Ribbon retractors

SUGGESTED READING

Crawley WA, Azman P, Clark N, et al. The edentulous Le Fort fracture. *J Craniofac Surg* 1997;8(4):298–307.

Gruss JS, Mackinnon SE. Complex maxillary fractures: role of buttress reconstruction and immediate bone grafts. *Plast Reconstr Surg* 1986;78(1):9–22.

Janus SC, MacLeod PR, Odland R. Analysis of results in early versus late midface fracture repair. *Otolaryngol Head Neck Surg* 2008;138:464–474.

Le Fort R. Experimental study of fractures of the upper jaw Parts I and II. *Rev Chir Paris* 1901;23:208; translated by Tessier P, and reprinted in *Plast Reconstr Surg* 1972;50:497.

Manson PN, Clark N, Robertson B, et al. Subunit principles in midface fractures: the importance of sagittal buttresses, soft-tissue reductions, and sequencing treatment of segmental fractures. *Plast Reconstr Surg* 1999;103:1287–1306.

52 NASOETHMOIDAL AND LE FORT III FACIAL FRACTURES

Robert M. Kellman

INTRODUCTION

The fractures discussed in this section are typically described as high-energy or high-velocity or high-impact injuries to the facial skeleton. The nasoethmoid complex (NEC) fracture is also known as the naso-orbital ethmoid (NOE) fracture, both names being attempts to describe the clinical and anatomic components of the bone injuries involved. These types of fractures occur when a force is directed primarily to the area of the root of the nose. The solid nasal root may or may not fracture, but frequently, the thin medial orbital wall bones behind the nasal root will be compromised (Stranc described this fracture as an "ethmoid crush"), allowing the nasal root to "telescope" inward into the area of the ethmoid sinuses. The loss of support of the lacrimal bones often results in disarticulation of the medial canthal ligaments (with or without bony attachments), thereby often resulting in lateral displacement of the medial canthal ligaments or "telecanthus." The injury creates the appearance of hypertelorism, often called "pseudohypertelorism," since the orbits themselves are not actually displaced laterally as the term hypertelorism implies. The term NEC fracture or NOE fracture refers to the fractures of the bones involved (Fig. 52.1).

The Le Fort III fracture refers to the most serious level of the Le Fort fracture series, otherwise known as the "craniofacial separation." The Le Fort I, II, and III fractures were described by Rene Le Fort in 1901. They refer to primarily horizontal fractures that traverse the facial skeleton between the maxillary dentition and the upper face or cranium. The Le Fort III fracture breaks through the lateral and medial orbital walls, crosses the nasal root and nasal septum, and is completed by extending across the posterior floor of the orbits and the zygomatic arches, as well as the pterygoid plates posteriorly. This results in a complete separation of the midfacial bones from the cranial portion of the skeleton (Fig. 52.2).

The NEC fractures may occur together with or independently from the Le Fort III fractures.

HISTORY

In civilian life, most NEC and Le Fort III fractures are the result of high-velocity injuries as might typically be seen in motor vehicle accidents (particularly when seat belts are not worn and/or air bags are not deployed), industrial accidents, and direct assaults to the central face using heavy instruments, such as a pipe or baseball bat. Intracranial injuries may be associated, and a complete history, including loss of consciousness, should be elicited. Symptoms and/or signs of neurologic injury are common, and changes in vision may be present as well. Though difficult to determine when the nose is filled with blood, the possibility of anosmia should be considered.

Of course, other comorbidities should be considered as well. It is important to determine if drugs and/or alcohol played a role in the patient's condition, as it may impact medical management and the timing of surgery. These issues may also affect the patient's ability to cooperate with postoperative care.

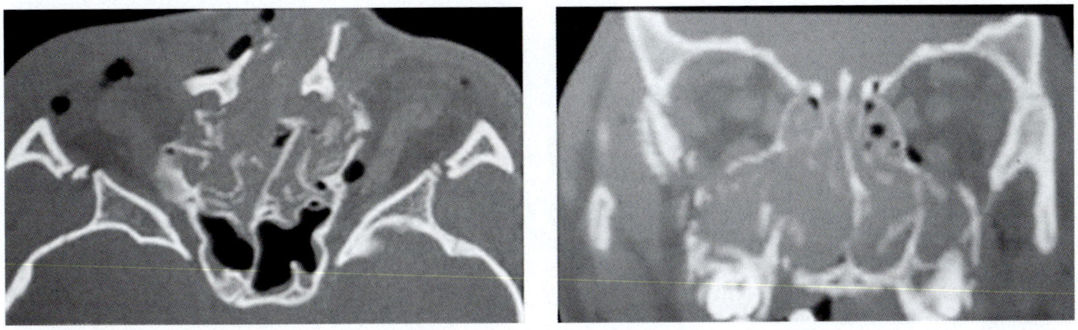

FIGURE 52.1 Axial and coronal CT demonstrating the telescoping of the nasal bones posteriorly with damage to the lacrimal bones and medial orbital walls.

PHYSICAL EXAMINATION

The ABCs of trauma must first be addressed. It is of course important to assure that the patient is neurologically stable and that there is no impending loss of vision due to increasing intraocular pressure or other cause of pressure on the optic nerve(s).

The tell tale findings of an NEC (NOE) fracture include telecanthus (widening of the intercanthal distance) and depression of the nasal root, which may or may not be associated with the appearance of nasal shortening (Figs. 52.3 and 52.4). Telecanthus may not be obvious initially due to edema as well as the possibility of slow lateralization of the medial canthal ligament. Typically, it is stated that the distance between the medial canthi should be about half the interpupillary distance or equal to the horizontal palpebral fissure length (Fig. 52.5). Also, the midline between the brows should be marked, and the distance to each medial canthus should be equal. Note that the midline of the nose is often difficult to use due to trauma-associated alterations. An epicanthal fold may sometimes develop as well. Lateral distraction of the medial canthus may be attempted to assess for detachment. Additionally, some surgeons advocate performing bimanual palpation of the bone underlying the medial canthal attachment using an instrument placed inside the nasal cavity and a finger outside. Note that the detached tendon tends to drift laterally, inferiorly, and anteriorly over time, creating a most unsightly deformity.

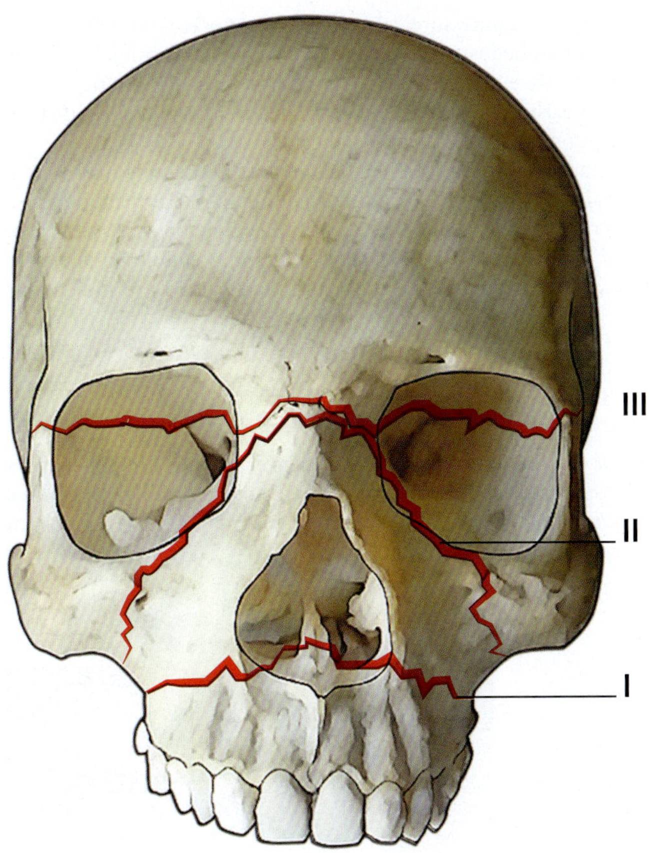

FIGURE 52.2
Drawing of the Le Fort I, II, and III fracture lines, as classically depicted.

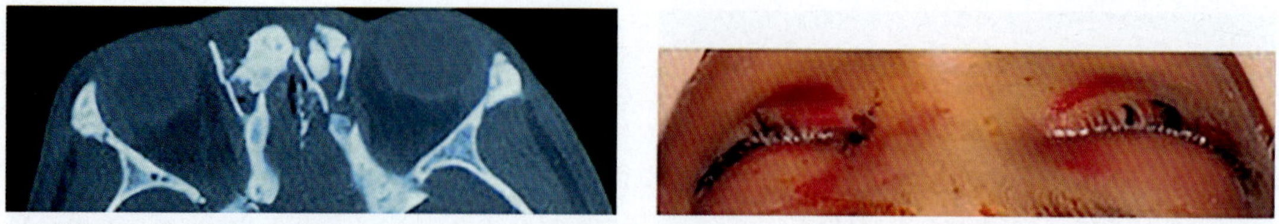

FIGURE 52.3 An axial CT demonstrating marked telescoping of the nasal root posteriorly, actually causing lateral displacement of the bones to which the medial canthal ligaments attach. Note the anterior and lateral displacement on the clinical photo as seen from above.

In a complete (bilateral) Le Fort III fracture, the midface may be freely mobile relative to the frontal skull. If possible, the anterior maxillary alveolus is grasped firmly in one hand, while the other hand is placed on the frontal bone and an attempt is made to gently rock the maxillary alveolus. If motion is detected relative to the frontal bone, a Le Fort fracture is present. Depending upon the level at which the movement takes place, it is often possible to clinically assess the level of a Le Fort fracture. In a Le Fort III fracture, the movement includes the entire midface relative to the frontal skull.

It is important to evaluate visual acuity and motion of the globe. A complete retinal examination should be completed by an Ophthalmologist. A retinal tear or globe rupture may require delaying the repair of the periorbital bones, and of course, a significant rupture of the globe may require enucleation. The presence of a hyphema may preclude proper visualization of the retina and should be documented if present. The position of the globe should also be evaluated, looking for both the anterior–posterior position (enophthalmos, exophthalmos) and vertical position (hypophthalmos, hyperophthalmos).

If there is any nasal discharge, the possibility of cerebrospinal fluid (CSF) leak should be considered, and appropriate steps are taken to assess and manage this. A complete examination of the cranial nerves is essential and should be performed in all trauma patients.

Appropriate consultations should be obtained. Since these fractures involve the bones of the orbit, there is significant potential for ocular and periocular injury, so evaluation by an Ophthalmologist is important. Similarly, if there is concern for intracranial injury, a Neurosurgeon should be consulted. It is important to note that concussion tends to be underdiagnosed in facial trauma, so this possibility should be entertained.

INDICATIONS

Fractures involving the NEC (NOE fractures) as a rule require surgical repair. When the medial canthal ligament is either detached or if the bone to which it is attached is fractured and freed from the surrounding bone, the natural tendency is for the medial canthus to lateralize. It also tends to move anteriorly and inferiorly over time. This creates an unsightly appearance, and the earlier that it is repaired, the better the outcome is likely to be. Therefore, so long as there are no contraindications, surgical repair is indicated.

Le Fort III fractures generally create instability of the midfacial complex. Left unrepaired, these typically lead to malocclusion and midface malposition (typically either lengthening or foreshortening). Posterior displacement often results in lateral protrusion of the convexity of the zygomatic arch with associated midface widening. Therefore, proper repair is generally indicated, including stabilization of the occlusion and fixation of the bones. Similarly, globe malposition and/or orbital dystopia are indications for repair.

CONTRAINDICATIONS

Contraindications may be related to the injury, or they may be due to other patient problems. First the patient has to be medically/hemodynamically stable for surgery. Repair of these fractures typically involves a coronal flap and a sublabial exposure and may also require orbital exploration, so hemodynamic stability is important for surgery of such magnitude. Coagulation issues may also pose a problem as well.

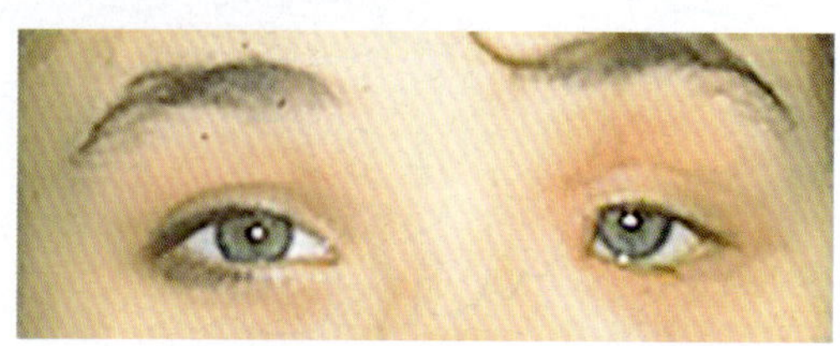

FIGURE 52.4

Photo of a patient with a unilateral injury that has been allowed to heal without surgery. Note the obvious lateral and inferior displacement, with less apparent inferior displacement of the medial canthus.

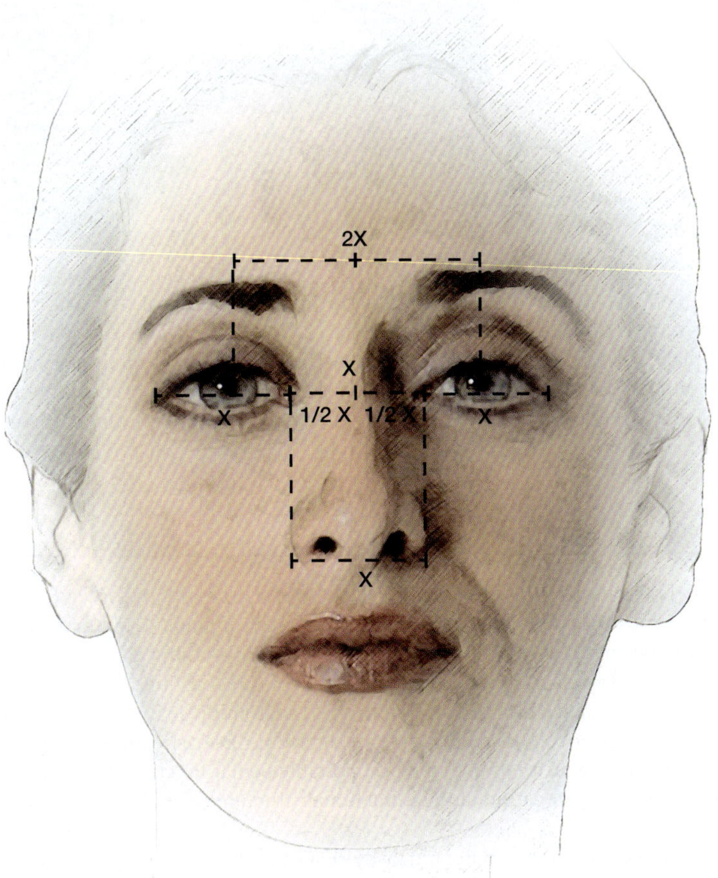

FIGURE 52.5
Illustration depicting the "typical/expected" relationships.

Ocular injury may be a contraindication to surgical manipulation of the orbital bones, particularly if there is a repaired globe rupture or a retinal injury. A hyphema may preclude evaluation of the retina and may mandate delay of surgical repair.

Brain injury may also be a contraindication, particularly if there is significant edema.

In general, Ophthalmology and Neurosurgical clearances are a good way to assure that the patient is ready for surgery. Injury to the cervical spine must be thoroughly evaluated and requires precautions at the time of surgery.

PREOPERATIVE PLANNING

The Le Fort III fracture is actually separate and distinct from the NOE fracture. When they occur together, the Le Fort fracture is typically repaired first, so that a stable facial skeletal structure is created, allowing for repositioning of the central structure of the nasal root and medial orbital walls. However, when the frontal sinuses and/or the floor of the anterior fossa are involved in these fractures, it is wise to assess and repair these areas in concert, so as to completely stabilize the midface and avoid disrupting the skull base repair later. The need for management of a disrupted posterior wall and/or floor of the frontal sinuses will also affect the surgical plan and approach. Thus, careful assessment of the computerized tomographic (CT) scans and surgical planning are of the utmost importance when repairing these injuries.

Furthermore, the status of the dentition and the occlusion is critically important in the repair of a Le Fort fracture, so this must be carefully planned as well.

Imaging

CT imaging is standard for injuries of this type. With high-resolution helical CT scans, both coronal and axial images are easily created from a rapidly obtained data set. Three-dimensional reconstructions may help the surgeon visualize the three-dimensional relationship of the injuries, but it should be kept in mind that the computer algorithms that create these images may insert inaccuracies as well (Fig. 52.6). The scan should of course include both the cranial vault to assess for skull fractures and brain injuries as well as the entire facial skeleton. Cervical spine imaging can also be carried out to assure that no injuries are overlooked. Additional studies may include magnetic resonance imaging (MRI).

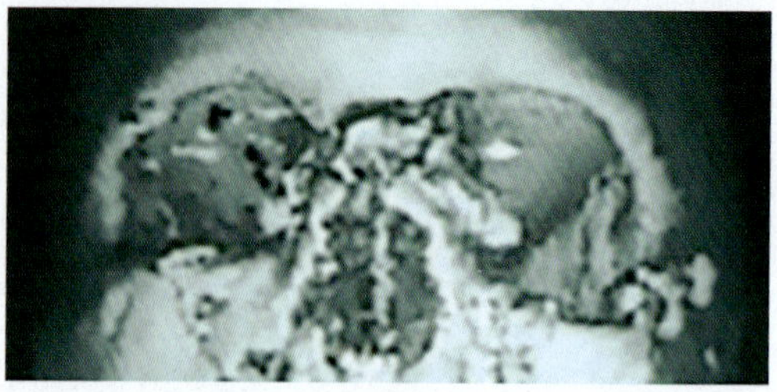

FIGURE 52.6
A three-dimensional CT reconstruction of a patient with marked fracturing and telescoping of the nasal root with lateral displacement of the medial orbital walls anteriorly.

The NEC fracture is best seen on the axial scans, as these clearly show the relationship of the nasal root to the ethmoid sinuses. The axial scans will also nicely demonstrate the vertical structures such as the medial and lateral orbital walls and pterygoid plates, as well as the zygomatic arches (Fig. 52.7). The orbital floors and roofs, on the other hand, are best seen on the coronal scans, as is the cribriform plate and roofs of the ethmoid sinuses (floor of the anterior fossa). These structures should be carefully assessed to determine the need for surgical repair.

SURGICAL TECHNIQUE

While the precise pattern of a Le Fort III fracture of the craniofacial skeleton is fairly straightforward, this precise pattern is rarely seen clinically, as most fractures are more complex, often comminuted and may vary in location and involve the orbit(s), maxilla(e), nasal bones, zygomas, and maxillary alveoli in ways other than the classical pattern. Nonetheless, the overall approach is the same. The goal is to reconstitute the original, preinjury, three-dimensional skeletal shapes as is possible. In addition to this "anatomic" goal, there are also the functional considerations of assuring a proper occlusal relationship of the teeth for mastication, restoring nasal function for breathing and smell, and assuring restoration of the best possible ocular function. In addition, it is important, as noted above, to assure a proper segregation of the intracranial structures and CSF space from the nose and sinuses.

While there remains controversy as to whether to begin the repair by securing the midfacial bones to the cranium or to begin either centrally or peripherally, this is really the choice of the individual surgeon, so long as the surgeon is able to achieve satisfactory results. My preference is to start by attempting to secure the proper occlusal relationship between the mandibular and maxillary dentition. Obviously, this may not always be possible, especially when the patient is completely or partially edentulous, as well as when the injury includes severe mandible fractures and possibly significant alveolar and palatal fractures. Nonetheless, it is still my preference, in general, to at least attempt to re-establish the patient's occlusion first. Often this will require an approximation of the bone fragments.

Unless establishing the occlusion is quite straightforward once the arch bars have been applied, the fractures will often be exposed surgically prior to fixing the patient in occlusion. The lower midface is typically exposed using a sublabial exposure from first molar to first molar. The upper face, in most cases, is exposed using the coronal incision. An irregular incision is preferred (sine wave or running "w") in patients with hair, since this allows the incision to be hidden within the hair once the hair has regrown (Fig. 52.8). Great care should be taken using the surgeon's preferred method to avoid injury to the temporal branches of the facial nerves and the V1 branches of the trigeminal nerves. Occasionally, a midface degloving approach may be needed for superior access to the medial maxillae, but this does risk the development of later nasal stenosis and is used only when absolutely necessary. Approaches to the orbital floor(s) are beyond the scope of this chapter.

Once the above is accomplished, I turn my attention to the skull base. If this requires repair, the transglabellar, subcranial approach is often used, as this provides generous access to the anterior fossa floor without requiring any retraction of the frontal lobes. It also allows maximum access to the medial canthal ligaments and repair of this region in the NEC/NOE fracture (Fig. 52.9). If the skull base is intact, attachment of the zygomas to the frontal and temporal bones will stabilize a true Le Fort III fracture and will convert the more typical mixed Le Fort fractures from a Le Fort III to a Le Fort II.

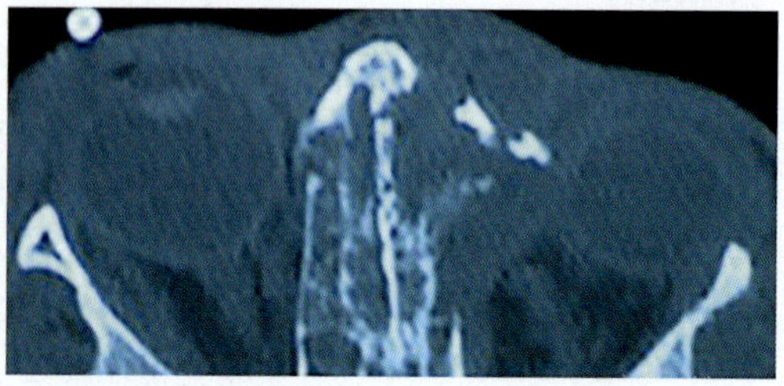

FIGURE 52.7
Axial CT of a unilateral NOE fracture, with marked lateral displacement of the bones to which the medial canthus attaches.

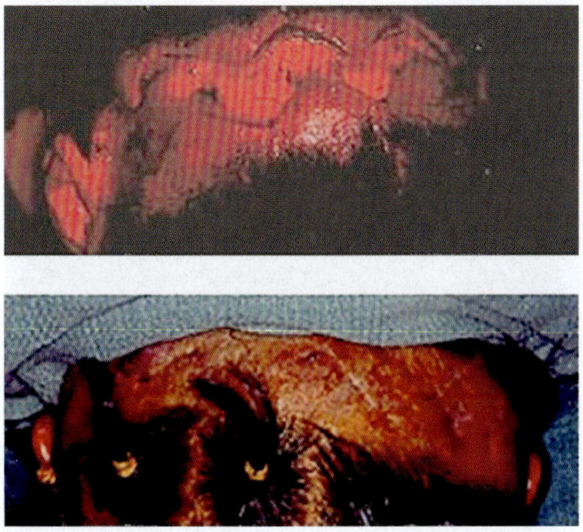

FIGURE 52.8
Clinical photo of a "running w" incision on the scalp. The patient had to return to the operating room, and the second photo depicts the healing of the incision prior to reincision.

In severe injuries, there is often comminution and telescoping of the zygomatic arches. Such an injury requires direct exposure and repair to re-establish the anterior–posterior dimension of the face. Keep in mind that the zygomatic arch is not a true "arch," but rather, the anterior portion is typically a bit straighter as it connects to the malar eminence. This is important as creating too much of a curved shape will lead to lateral facial widening and shortening in the anterior–posterior dimension. Plates on the zygomatic arch will often create lateral prominence in this anatomically sensitive area with thin skin. Even a comminuted arch can often be recreated in "chain-link" fashion using wires to attach the fragments to each other. In severe injuries, it is often necessary to wire all of the bones together (i.e., including the lateral orbital rims and the inferior orbital rims) to re-establish the three-dimensional position of these complex bones in space prior to rigidly fixing them in position with plates and screws (Fig. 52.10). This seemingly extra step may save time later, if removal and reapplication of plates can be avoided.

In Le Fort III fractures, the nasal root is usually separated from the anterior skull base. In this situation, there may be significant rotation of the midface upward, with the nasal root rotated posteriorly relative to the frontal bone and the upper dentition elevated, creating an anterior open bite. If this is not carefully assessed, it can be missed, even if the patient is in maxilla–mandibular fixation (MMF), as proper MMF may occur due to forward and upward distraction of the mandible with malpositioning of the condylar heads in their fossae. Failure to recognize this will result in an anterior open bite when the MMF is released. Sometimes, the midface is impacted and may require disimpaction. If this is needed, it is generally accomplished using the Rowe disimpaction forceps. If these are used, it is important to be careful to pull downward and forward to avoid creating an injury to the skull base.

Completion of the Le Fort repair is carried out at the zygomaticomaxillary level (lateral buttresses) as needed, as well as along the pyriform apertures (medial buttresses), to complete the stabilization of the maxillary alveoli and dentition to the skull. Ellis suggests that when all attempts to reposition the midfacial bones

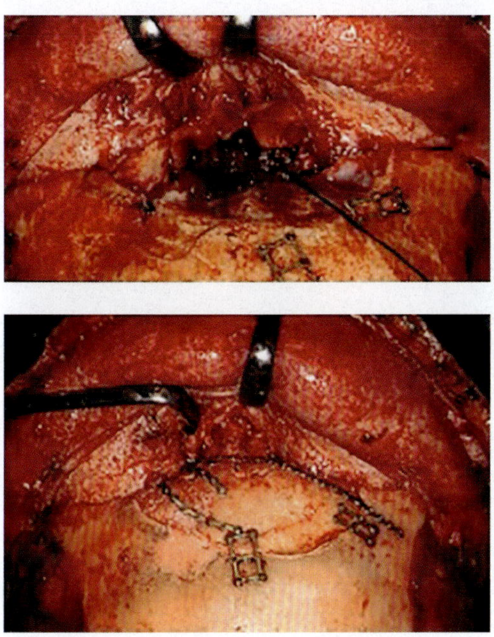

FIGURE 52.9
The nasal bones have been repositioned, but these photos of a "subcranial" exposure demonstrate the broad access that this exposure provides for placement of medial canthal sutures.

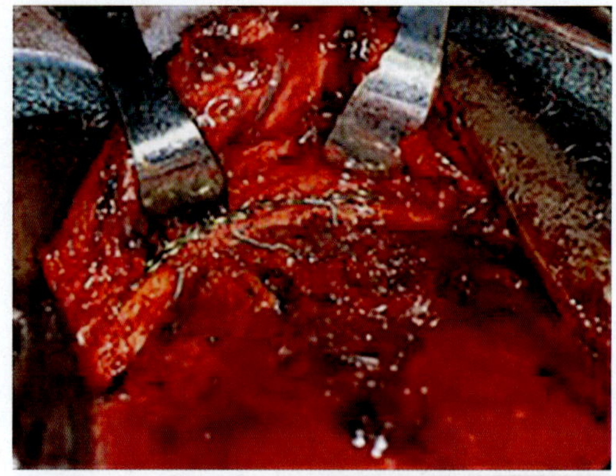

FIGURE 52.10
An example of approximation of the zygomatic arch with wires prior to plating.

seem to be unable to succeed in re-establishing the proper occlusion, advantage can be taken of fractures at the Le Fort I level (which can even be carried out or completed if not already present and mobile) to allow creation of the proper occlusion prior to fixating the bones at this level.

Repair of the NEC/NOE fracture is focused on repositioning and fixation of the medial canthal ligaments/tendons. While there are typically three levels of severity used to classify these fractures, for repair purposes, it is most important to distinguish between the minor (type I) fractures and the more severe (types II and III) fractures. In type I fractures, the medial canthal tendons remain firmly attached to large fragments of bone. Stable plate fixation of the fractured fragments will therefore adequately stabilize these fractures and assure that the tendons will stay in their proper positions (Fig. 52.11). For the more severe (types II and III) fractures, the tendons are either attached to small, unstable bone fragments (type II) or completely detached (type III). In either of these situations, the re-establishment of the stability of the medial canthal tendon and position requires transnasal fixation. This can be accomplished either by fixing the tendons to each other transnasally using surgical wire or by fixing each tendon across the nose (using either wire or permanent suture) to a plate, screw, or hole in the bone on the contralateral side (Fig. 52.12). It is important to assure that the tendon(s) is(are) positioned posteriorly, medially, and superiorly to counteract the tendency for them to drift anteriorly, laterally, and inferiorly, which occurs naturally when they are detached. The most difficult part of repairing these injuries is the proper passing of the wire/suture across the nose in the proper position.

First, the tendon must be captured. In type II fractures, if there is a significant piece of bone attached to the tendon, a wire may be passed through two holes drilled in this piece of bone, passing the wire first medially and

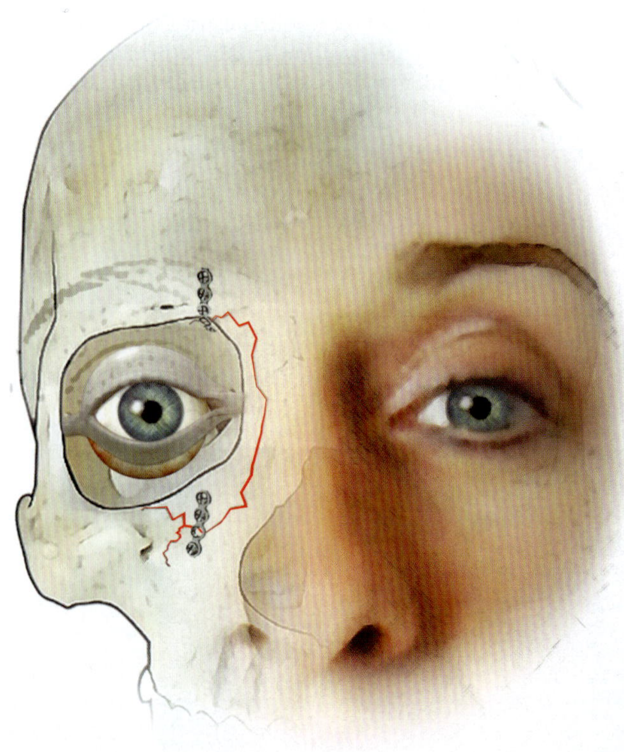

FIGURE 52.11
Cartoon depicting the repair of a type I NOE fracture, which requires only restabilization of the bones holding the ligaments.

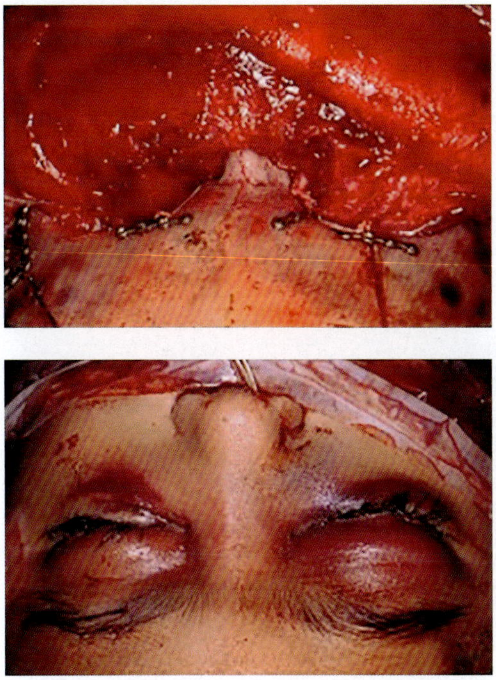

FIGURE 52.12
A clinical example demonstrating bilateral, independent repair of the detached ligaments (as seen in type II or III NOE fractures) using permanent suture fixed to the contralateral frontal bones.

then laterally. However, if the bone shatters or is too small (effectively a type III fracture), it is best to free the tendon and capture it with the wire or a suture. Passing the wire or suture transnasally first requires reduction of the nasal root anteriorly, which is completely removed in the subcranial approach and makes this technique much easier. Then a hole must be made in the nasal septum, which is generally present and bony in this area. This is best approached using a drill. The wire/suture is then passed through this hole and brought out on the other side. Great care must be used to protect the contralateral globe during this maneuver, and a sterilized "tea spoon" works well for this purpose. If a wire has been used, it is generally fixed to the contralateral medial canthal tendon and tightening of the wire should bring the two canthi together. A suture may be tied similarly, though it is commonly fixed to the contralateral frontal bone.

When the medial orbital wall is significantly deficient, it can be reconstructed using calvarial bone. The tendon can then be fixed by passing the wire or suture through holes drilled in the bone graft (Fig. 52.13). Some surgeons advocate placing percutaneous bolsters which are wired transnasally to fix the skin anterior to the medial canthus firmly in position, though this remains controversial.

Wounds are closed as appropriate. For the coronal incision, it is important to reapproximate the galea. Finally, it is important to assure that the temporalis fascia is resuspended superiorly prior to closure to avoid a midfacial droop (a "reverse midface lift").

POSTOPERATIVE MANAGEMENT

Wounds are treated with antibiotic ointments; drains, if used, are managed per the surgeon's preference. It is important to monitor visual function and neurologic status during the postoperative period. A postoperative CT scan will allow assessment of the adequacy of the reduction. Some surgeons advocate use of intraoperative CT scanning to assure reduction prior to waking the patient.

COMPLICATIONS

The most common complication is inadequate or imprecise repositioning of the fractures. These are difficult fractures to repair, and it is important to assess the adequacy of the repair as soon as possible since a poor reduction may require a return to the operating room. Of course, in some cases, it may be the surgeon's determination that a return to the OR would be fruitless since the best repair possible may have been obtained. This is a clinical judgment that only the operating surgeon can make.

Visual problems seen during the postoperative period require urgent assessment by an Ophthalmologist. Increasing intraocular pressure is a surgical emergency that must be evaluated and addressed before permanent injury results. Neurologic issues should be urgently evaluated as well.

It is difficult to assess the clinical outcome with the typical postoperative edema so it may take several weeks before the surgical result is apparent.

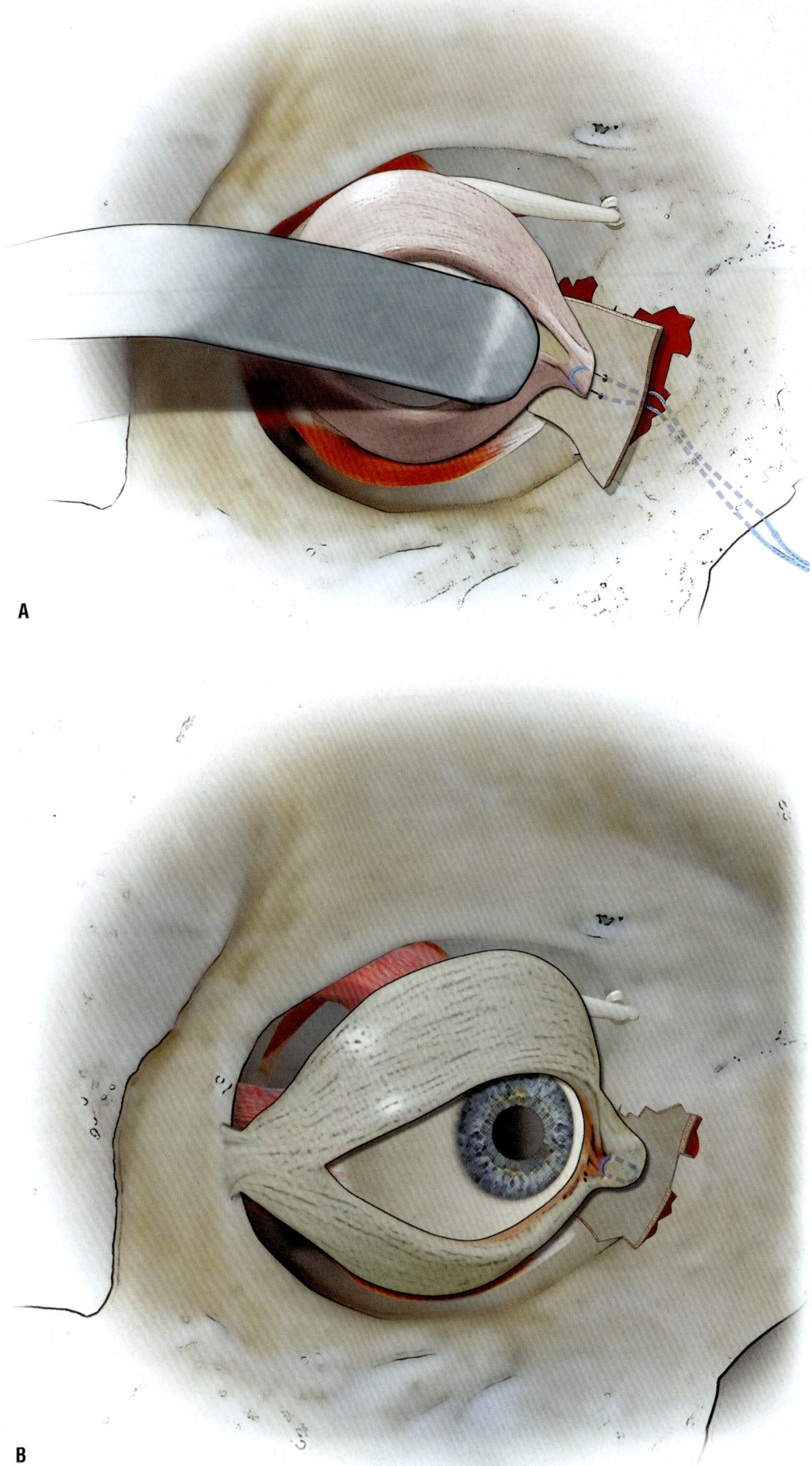

A

B

FIGURE 52.13 This diagram depicts the use of calvarial bone to replace a severely deficient medial orbital wall **(A)**. This bone is then used for fixation of the medial canthal tendon **(B)**.

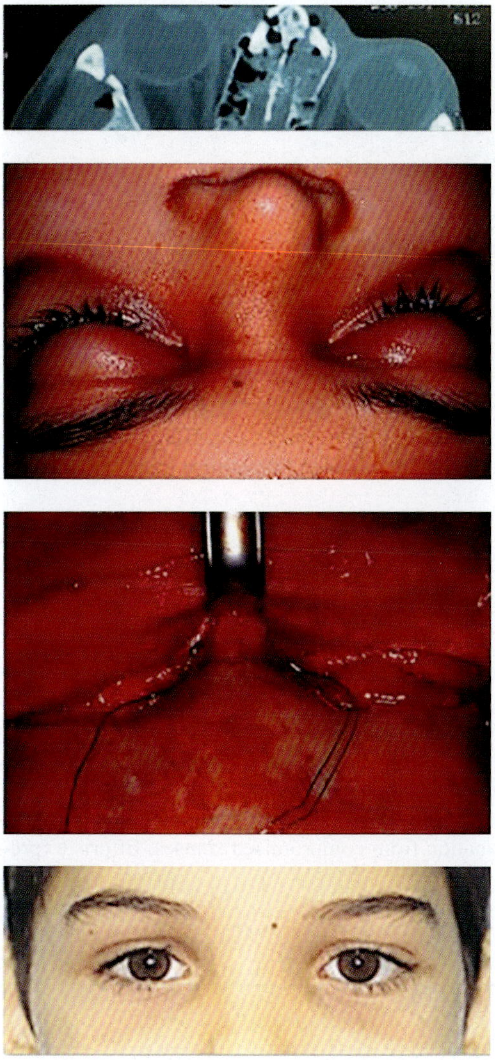

FIGURE 52.14
This is a case demonstrating the degree of intraoperative tension that can be applied using the independent contralateral fixation, along with the clinical outcome.

The patient should be asked about the correctness of the occlusal result. However, keep in mind that it may be difficult for the patient to recognize subtle variations initially due to alterations in sensation and neuromuscular feedback.

RESULTS

Repair of the NEC/NOE and Le Fort III fractures represents a significant surgical undertaking in extensive facial trauma. Central to the reconstructive outcome is a dedicated and uncompromising repositioning and refixation of the facial skeleton and associated structures (Figs. 52.14 and 52.15). A comprehensive understanding of anatomic and surgical options is essential in the restoration of the facial skeleton and orbital complex. Additional surgeries may be necessary and asymmetries may exist—but these are only observed with appropriate postoperative and long-term follow-up care.

PEARLS

- Remember that in any fracture involving the occlusion, it is quite important to assure that the proper occlusion has been re-established (so long as this is possible).
- For complex and comminuted fractures, do not hesitate to wire the fragments together initially. Although the repair is not stable at this point, it helps re-establish the proper three-dimensional position of the bones, after which rigid fixation should be easier and be likely to provide a better outcome.
- Do not settle intraoperatively for a suboptimal result if you believe that it can be improved. Once rigidly fixed, the result will not change, and a poor outcome will be made permanent. Consider an intraoperative CT scan if necessary, but it is always wisest to replate poorly positioned fractures during the initial procedure whenever possible.

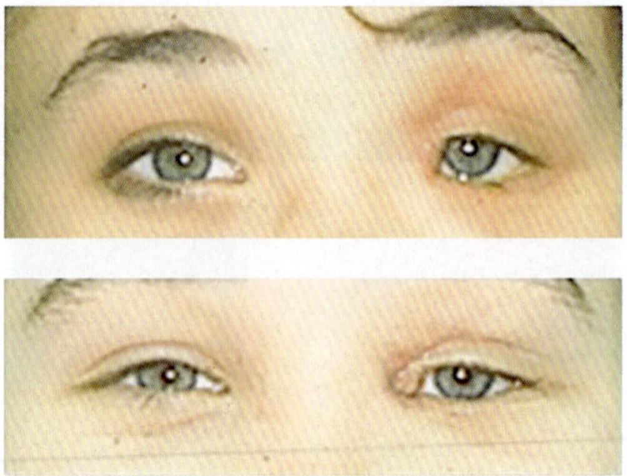

FIGURE 52.15
This is the result obtained after delayed repair of the lateralized and scarred left medial canthus.

- If there is difficulty in obtaining the correct occlusion with repositioning of the Le Fort III fractures, keep in mind that the occlusion can be repaired at the end of the case by completing or creating a Le Fort I fracture/ osteotomy to compensate.
- The midface must be resuspended before closing the coronal incision.

PITFALLS

- Failure to disimpact a rotated midface will result in an anterior open bite later, even if the patient appears to be in proper occlusion using MMF during the procedure.
- Failure to identify the severity of fractures prior to observing them intraoperatively. Detailed studies with CT in coronal, axial, and three-dimensional reconstruction are helpful tools.
- Undetected increase of orbital volume may lead to enophthalmos after swelling has resolved. Posttraumatic loss of adipose tissue can be causative in well-reduced fractures. Postoperative follow-up is essential.
- Postsurgical infections may be a consequence of contamination from compromised sinuses. Efforts to preserve and re-establish normal outflow are of importance.

INSTRUMENTS TO HAVE AVAILABLE

- Standard head and neck set
- "Fish hooks"
- Rubber bands
- Raney clips
- Malleable retractors
- Small osteotomes
- Arch bars (standard or hybrid)
- Rigid fixation system
- Rowe midfacial disimpaction forceps

SUGGESTED READING

Ellis E. Passive repositioning of maxillary fractures: an occasional impossibility without osteotomy. *J Oral Maxillofac Surg* 2004;62(12):1477–1485.

Kellman RM. Maxillofacial trauma. In: *Cummings Otolaryngology Head and Neck Surgery*, 5th ed. Philadelphia, PA: Mosby Elsevier. 2010:318–341.

Manson PN. Dimensional analysis of the facial skeleton: avoiding complications in the management of facial fractures by improved organization of treatment based on CT scans. *Plast Reconstr Surg* 1991;1(2):213–237.

Manson PN, Hoopes JE, Su CT. Structural pillars of the facial skeleton: an approach to the management of Le Fort fractures. *Plast Reconstr Surg* 1980;66(1):54–61.

Markowitz BL, Manson PN, Sargent L, et al. Management of the medial canthal tendon in nasoethmoid orbital fractures: the importance of the central fragment in classification and treatment. *Plast Reconstr Surg* 1991;87(5):843–853.

53 MANAGEMENT OF FRONTAL SINUS FRACTURES

Paul J. Donald

INTRODUCTION

Fractures of the frontal sinus have become less common due to the introduction of the seat belt in modern automobiles. The frontal sinus is contained within the frontal bone and is particularly vulnerable to violent trauma due to its position in the anteroinferior skull. Fortunately, there are a number of anatomical features that make it the strongest structure in the facial skeleton. The thick bone of the anterior skull coupled with its arch configuration is also reinforced by a series of septations that act as trusses rendering it highly resistant to fracture. It takes about 800 to 1,600 ft-lb of pressure to fracture the anterior wall of the frontal sinus compared to 550 to 900 ft-lb to fracture the mentum of the mandible and 200 to 650 ft-lb to fracture the body of the zygoma. In contrast, the posterior wall and floor of the sinus are thin and fragile. The posterior wall forms the anterior wall of the anterior cranial fossa. The floor is in common with the roof of the orbit.

Each frontal sinus has a funnel-shaped duct located in the anteromedial aspect of floor of the sinus adjacent to the intersinus septum located vertically in the midline of the sinus. The mucosa of the sinus has a characteristic and unique response to injury. Damaged mucosa tends to form cysts which as they expand fill the sinus cavity. These frontal sinus mucoceles erode bone and can become secondarily infected forming a mucopyocoele.

Fractures of the frontal sinus can be classified in a number of ways. Initially, they are classified according to the wall or walls involved:

- Anterior wall
- Posterior wall
- Nasofrontal duct.

They are also classified according to type:

- Linear
- Displaced
- Comminuted
- Compound
- "Corner"
- "Through and through"

The utility of this classification system is that each specific type of fracture demands a specific treatment, and in so many instances, the fractures will be of multiple walls and multiple types; therefore, the treatment plan will need to incorporate all of the appropriate modalities that are specific to each site and type of fracture.

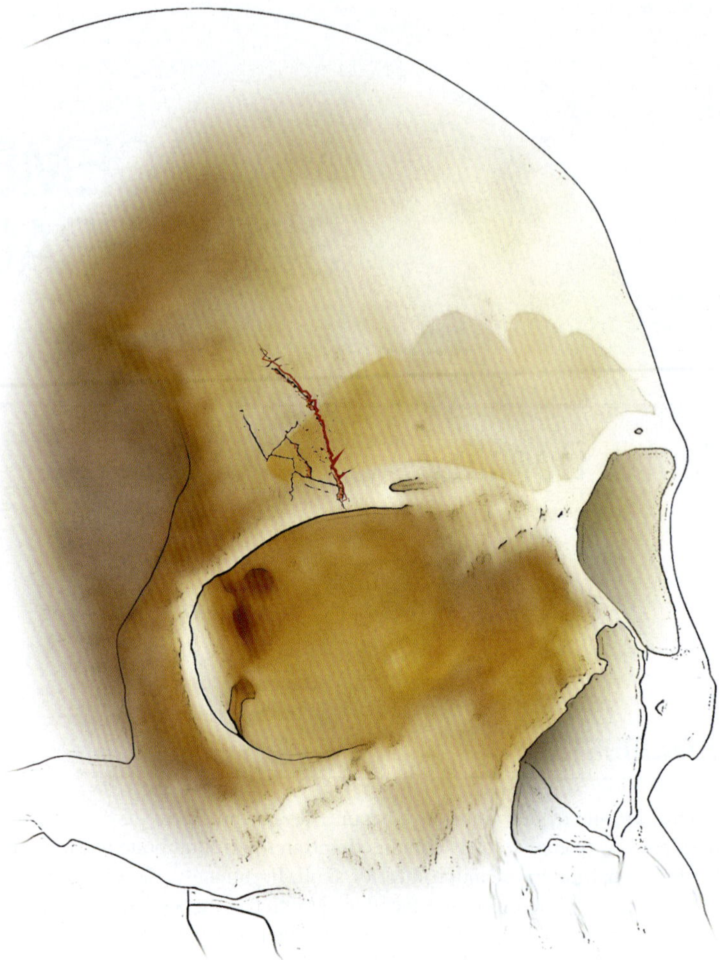

FIGURE 53.1
Corner fracture.

The two classification types requiring further explanation are the "corner fracture" and the "through-and-through" fracture. The corner fracture (Fig. 53.1) is basically a skull fracture that goes through the lateral extremity of the frontal sinus usually including the anterior and posterior walls and the floor. It is undisplaced and does not require operative treatment. The "through-and-through fracture" is the most severe of all the fractures and usually accompanies a more severe type of skull fracture that is compound and comminuted. The injury includes a compound, comminuted fracture of the anterior and posterior walls of the frontal sinus. The dura is torn and the underlying brain lacerated and contused (Fig. 53.2). Most patients with through-and-through fractures are victims of polytrauma and 50% die at the scene of the trauma or in the hospital.

HISTORY

The force required to fracture the frontal sinus is considerable such that a history of violent trauma followed by a variable period of unconsciousness is generally the rule. The most catastrophic of these injuries, a through-and-through type of fracture, is often first encountered when the Otolaryngologist enters the operating room following a call from a Neurosurgeon who has the patient draped on the table, has stopped the intracranial bleeding, patched a dural defect, and is puzzled about how to manage the wide open frontal sinus.

Most of the fracture types will be found in patients who have recovered consciousness and commonly complain of severe frontal headache. There may be numbness over the forehead if the injury to the branches of the supraorbital nerve that supplies the sinus periosteum and mucosa occurs. The patient with fractures of the anterior wall may complain of a depression or a swelling in the forehead. The swelling could be a hematoma masking an underlying depressed fracture.

Epistaxis may occur, and in fractures of the posterior wall if there is a dural tear, the drainage from the nose may be a mixture of CSF (cerebrospinal fluid) and blood. A halo sign when a drop of fluid from the nose is captured on a towel and the halo surrounding the clot is wider than the width of the clot will denote a CSF leak.

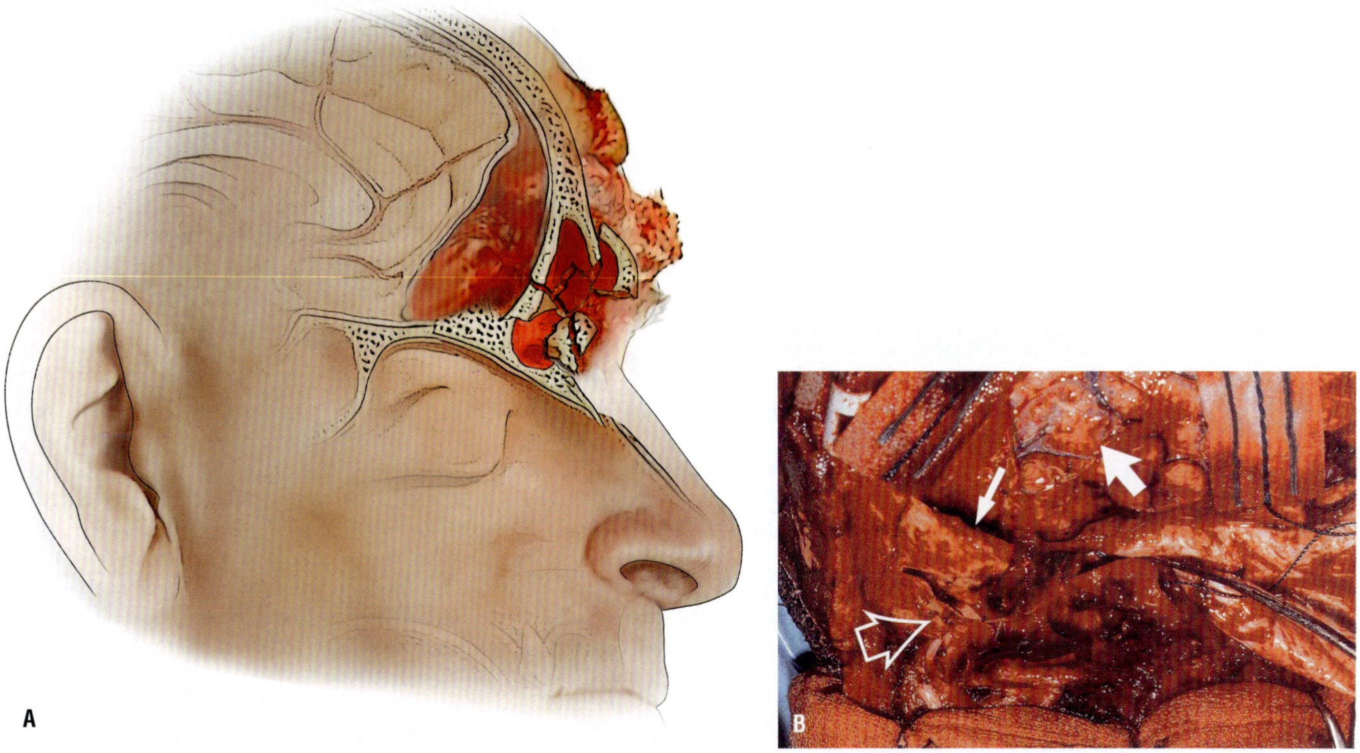

FIGURE 53.2 **A:** Illustration of a through-and-through fracture. **B:** Patient with through-and-through fracture (*arrows*). (From Donald PJ. Frontal sinus fractures. In: Donald PJ, Gluckman JL, Rice DH, eds. *The sinuses*. New York, NY: Raven Press, 1995:389.)

PHYSICAL EXAMINATION

The patient with an undisplaced fracture of the anterior wall fracture will probably have no abnormal physical findings other than edema of the forehead over the site of trauma. Care must be taken to not mistake a subgaleal hematoma for a displaced fracture. To palpation, the subgaleal hematoma may feel like a displaced fracture, but a CT scan of the skull will reveal no evidence of bony displacement.

An isolated fracture of the posterior wall is usually accompanied by a companion fracture of the anterior wall. The only situation when an isolated fracture of the posterior wall is seen is when it is part of an extensive adjacent skull fracture especially when it is displaced. A nondisplaced fracture of the posterior wall of the sinus cannot clinically be differentiated from a displaced fracture. A nondisplaced fracture without a dural tear is not only difficult to detect clinically but even on a CT scan especially if it is thick cut. When such a fracture lacerates the underlying dura, it is often accompanied by CSF rhinorrhea, or in the case of an overlying laceration, leakage through the lacerated skin.

Fractures of the nasofrontal duct are difficult to diagnose clinically but may be suspected by nasal endoscopy. The clinician should have a high index of suspicion in cases of an accompanying Le Fort III fracture or a naso–fronto–orbital fracture especially when it is displaced. The through-and-through fracture is usually very obvious on clinical examination. The anterior wall is usually fragmented. Blood, CSF, and even brain may be seen oozing onto the forehead. There is common association with polytrauma especially in a motor vehicle accident or in a combat or terrorist situation.

INDICATIONS

Undisplaced fractures of the anterior wall usually do not require repair. The vast majority of depressed fractures should have an open reduction and internal fixation to avoid a depression in the forehead, as well as the possibility of entrapped mucosa forming a mucocele later on. The biggest dilemma surrounds the management of a nondisplaced fracture of the posterior wall. The problem is to be certain that there is no entrapment of sinus mucosa in the fracture line that has the serious potential of developing a mucocele which will expand into the anterior cranial fossa. Modern fine cut CT scanning has reduced the chance of misinterpretation but such patients require close follow-up.

The most difficult fracture of the frontal sinus to detect is that of the nasofrontal duct. Except in circumstances mentioned above, a degree of watchful waiting is the most conservative approach. If there is radiographic evidence of retained secretions within the sinus cavity, the sinus should be further investigated.

CONTRAINDICATIONS

The only contraindication to surgery in a patient with a through-and-through fracture of the sinus would be fragility of the patient's condition. The Otolaryngologist must strongly persuade the Neurologic surgeon not to pack the sinus cavity with methacrylate or bone wax.

PREOPERATIVE PLANNING

Prior to operative treatment, the patient must be stabilized and cleared by Neurological Surgery and, when relevant, Ophthalmology.

The through-and-through type is the only fracture that requires emergency surgery. There is usually bleeding from the brain and a CSF leak. A fine cut CT scan will delineate the type of fracture and the extent of displacement of the fragments for a final diagnosis.

The most difficult fracture of all to delineate is the fracture of the nasofrontal duct. Even a fine cut CT scan may not reveal this fracture. The sagittal view is the best to define this injury. If after a 2- or 3-week waiting period and repeating the scan to see if the sinus is still opacified by fluid, a functional test may be done to detect a possible fracture. A trephine is drilled in the medial aspect of the roof of the orbit lateral to the trochlea. A cannula is placed through the opening, and the fluid in the sinus is suctioned away through the trephination. The sinus is then irrigated with a mixture of saline and cocaine or epinephrine. Methylene blue is placed in the sinus cavity, the patient is placed in a sitting position, and a nasal endoscope is inserted into the nasal cavity to see if the dye appears in the middle meatus. Alternatively, radiopaque dye can be introduced into the sinus and a plain radiograph made to visualize the course of the duct and any obstruction. Another way to assess patency is to visualize the duct from the frontal sinus cavity by passing an angled telescope through the trephination. This unfortunately only reveals the status of the internal meatus of the duct. More information can be gleaned by adding an endoscopic examination of the middle meatus.

One of the problems encountered when an osteoplastic flap procedure is required is predicting the size and shape of the sinus. A 5-foot Caldwell view of the sinuses taken in the AP projection will be of great help in predicting the outline of the frontal sinus. Many radiology technicians are untrained in plain radiographs of the sinuses so this may not be an option. An alternative method is to attempt transillumination of the sinus and then map it.

If a coronal scalp flap is planned, the site of incision must be cleared of hair by braiding the hair so as to clear a path, a limited shave of the track of the planned incision is usually done. A Mayfield head rest helps with exposure and ease of access to the operative field.

SURGICAL TECHNIQUE

Fractures of the Anterior Wall

Undisplaced isolated fractures of the anterior wall generally do not require treatment. Periodic observation with a yearly CT scan for several years is usually sufficient follow-up. A caveat regarding physical examination of undisplaced fractures is that a fresh injury to the frontal area may feel through the skin as if there is an underlying sharp fracture line. This sensation can be created by a subgaleal hematoma. Re-evaluating the CT scan will reveal the true nature of the fracture which is actually nondisplaced. On the other hand, a hematoma overlying a depressed fracture of the anterior wall may give the appearance of a normal contour of the forehead.

Displaced fractures must be reduced because of the residual deformity that will evolve as the overlying hematoma of the forehead resolves, but more importantly, because of the possibility of developing a mucocele in the future because of entrapment of mucosa in the fracture line.

There are three types of incisions which may be used to access the fracture: the coronal scalp incision, the so-called butterfly incision, and an extension of a forehead laceration in the case of a compound anterior wall fracture (Fig. 53.3). The coronal scalp incision is the most useful. If the patient is male and has all his hair, the incision is made about 2 or 3 cm. behind the hairline and curves forward at the widow's peak. Xylocaine 1% with 1:100,000 epinephrine is injected along the proposed incision line and the actual incision delayed for at least 5 minutes in order to maximize the vasoconstrictive effect. Raney clips and bipolar cautery are used to ensure hemostasis.

The "butterfly" incision is used when the patient has a very low frontal sinus and in the bald patient. The incision is made through both brows and connected across the midline in a natural glabellar crease line. Care is taken to slant the knife blade at an angle in order not cut across the hair follicles of the eyebrow thus producing the "split brow" appearance. In most instances, the cosmetic result is quite good, but the exposure is limited.

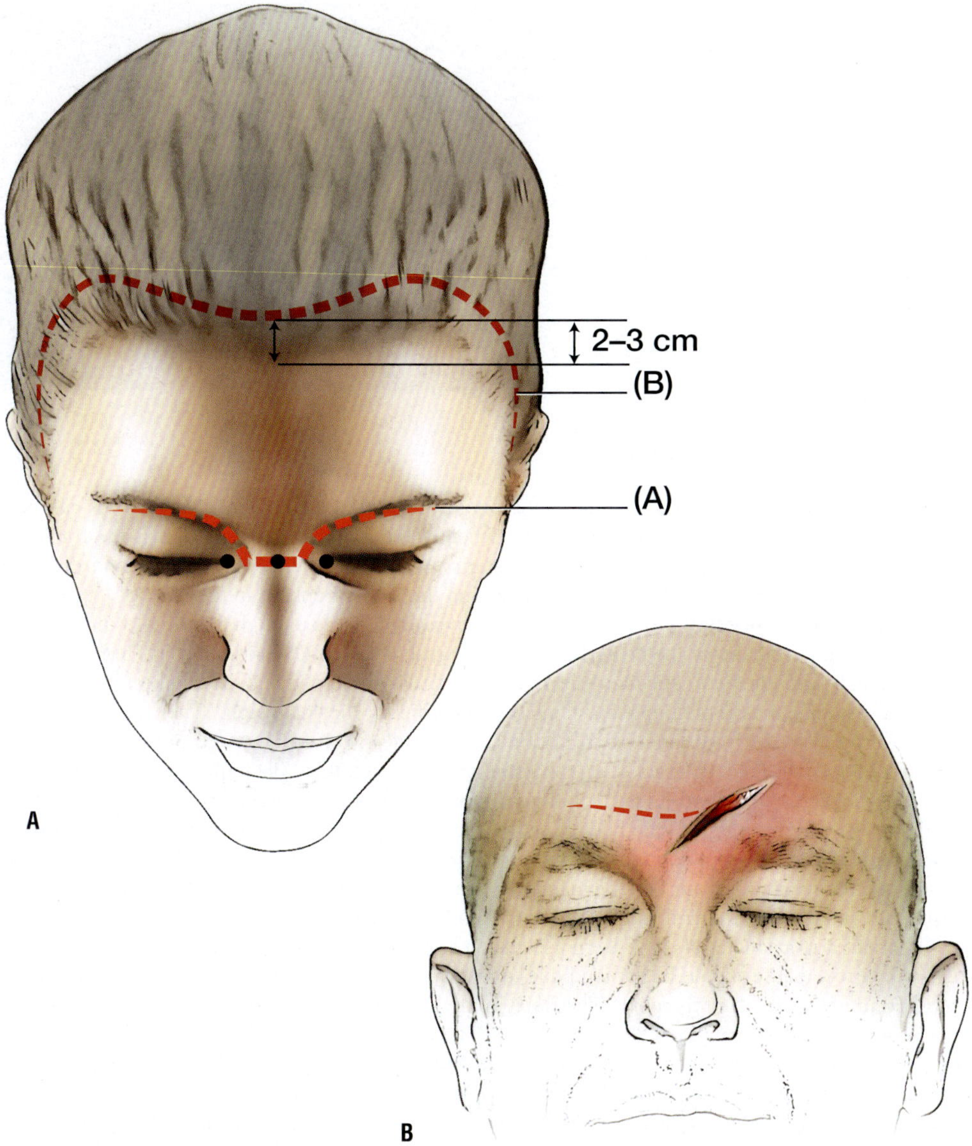

FIGURE 53.3 Incisions for open frontal sinus surgery. **A:** (B) Coronal scalp incision and (A) Butterfly incision. **B:** Extension of existing laceration in a natural crease line in forehead skin.

Existing lacerations can be a useful approach to underlying fractures and can be combined with endoscopic techniques to offer excellent exposure for evaluation of the sinus. However, this approach may prove more restrictive than either of the former incisions and should be disregarded if exposure is inadequate through the laceration or if expansion of the existing laceration would create an unfavorable cosmetic result.

The incision for the coronal flap is made through the skin, subcutaneous adipose tissue, and galea aponeurotica. The periosteum is left undisturbed. As the flap is elevated, care must be taken to include the superficial layers of the temporalis fascia with the scalp flap in order to avoid injuring the temporal branch of the facial nerve. The scalp flap is elevated to identify the fracture. Once the fracture is identified (if there is any doubt concerning the integrity of the frontonasal duct or the presence of a posterior wall fracture), then an endoscope can be inserted between the depressed fragments, and these areas are carefully examined.

The periosteum is sufficiently elevated around the fracture fragments to accommodate a miniplate to provide fixation for the fracture fragments. A bone hook is used to reduce the fragments and hold them into position, while either holes are drilled for nontapping screws or self-tapping screws are placed to secure the plate. Prior to plating the fragments into position, it is wise to elevate and remove strips of mucosa around the major fragments in order to prevent mucosal entrapment and the possible future formation of a frontal sinus mucocele. At least two screws should be placed in every major fragment and at the anchor points in the intact portions of the skull (Fig. 53.4). Absorbable suture is used for closure of the periosteum. The scalp is closed in layers over a Penrose drain and a light pressure dressing applied.

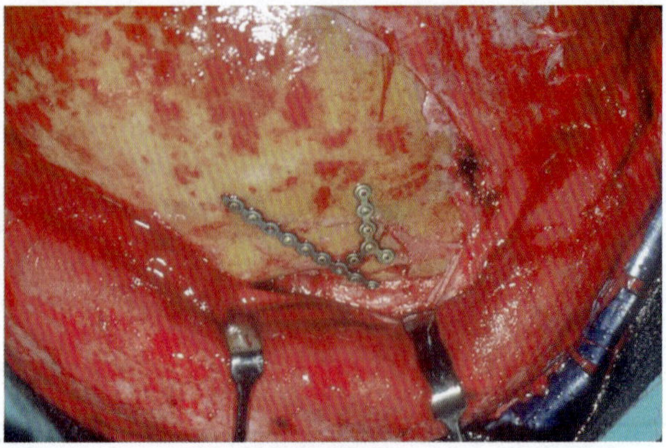

FIGURE 53.4
Miniplates applied to provide fixation of a depressed fracture of the anterior wall.

Fractures of the Posterior Wall

Management of fractures of the posterior wall is the biggest challenge for repair. The fractures can be either linear or displaced. The dilemma lies in establishing whether there is displacement across the fracture. New generation CT scanning is very accurate, but the posterior wall is a curvilinear structure and displacement cannot always be established correctly. Direct visualization through a trephine in the floor of the frontal sinus requires a small incision just inferior to the brow and drilling a hole large enough to admit a sinus endoscope.

The patient with a fracture of the posterior wall may present with a CSF rhinorrhea. This will usually be noticed immediately after the traumatic incident. It may be mixed with blood and the quickest way to differentiate it from blood-stained mucus or simple epistaxis is by looking for the "halo sign." The "halo sign" is elicited by allowing a drop of blood from the nose to fall onto a surgical towel. If the width of the clear area around the periphery of the central clot is larger than the diameter of the clot, then this indicates a CSF leak. The halo sign is not specific, and other clear fluids (including rhinorrhea) may also yield a positive result. At least 30% of the fluid must be CSF prior to the halo becoming noticeable, so a negative "halo sign" should not discourage further evaluation if clinical suspicion remains high for injury to the posterior table and dura.

The most effective and certain way of managing the displaced fracture of the posterior wall is with an osteoplastic flap and obliteration with adipose tissue taken from the subcutaneous area of the anterior abdominal wall. Other autologous materials have been used, such as bone pate, muscle, and fascia, but synthetic materials such as hydroxyapatite should be avoided due to resorption and higher infection rates. The coronal scalp flap is most commonly used for this repair. The steps in the operation were well described by Montgomery.

The coronal scalp flap is made as described above. The flap is elevated to the brows and to the glabella. A template of the sinus is cut from the 5 Foot Caldwell view radiograph, applied to the corresponding calvarium and the sinus outlined with a needle dipped in methylene blue. The periosteum is incised about 2 cm away from the markings previously made and then carefully dissected to the points where the methylene blue marks have been made on the skull.

A bone-cutting needle such as the Midas Rex B5 is used to make a series of obliquely directed openings into the sinus cavity. These small openings are then connected and taken down to the brow. An osteotome is then placed consecutively in the brows at each lateral extremity of the sinus and driven through the hard bone at this site. The next osteotomy is made in the midline just below the glabella. A broad flat osteotome is then placed at the superior border of the midline intersinus septum. It is gently tapped inferiorly using a surgical mallet staying close to the posterior wall of the osteoplastic flap. When the floor of the sinus is reached, the osteotome is gently pried anteriorly to produce a fracture through the roof of both orbits. The osteoplastic flap is now created pedicled on the periosteum of the brows.

The interior of the sinus is inspected with special attention to the posterior wall. All displaced fragments of bone are removed and the entire sinus denuded of mucosa, first with an elevator such as the Woodsen and then with a diamond bur. The key to a successful procedure is the complete removal of all of the mucosa and ensuring the drilling of all the superficial layer of bone in the sinus cavity. The mucosa of the frontonasal duct is inverted on itself and displaced into the frontal recess. While the bone is being drilled, a second surgical team harvests adipose tissue from the subcutaneous area of the abdominal wall. Care is taken to be gentle with the graft and to place it in the sinus cavity as soon as possible after harvesting. All the empty space in the sinus is obliterated as much as possible. The difficult areas to obliterate are the very narrow extremities of the sinus. The adipose tissue will be hard to place in the lateral recesses, but fortunately, this is of little consequence as long as all the mucosa is removed from these sites.

The problem that arises in these cases is when a large amount of the bone of the posterior wall bone must be removed. This is especially true in the cases in which there is a CSF leak from a tear in the dura. Often a considerable amount of bone must be removed from the posterior wall to reach the limits of the dural tear so that it can be sewn shut. In addition, the repair may have to be bolstered by a fascia graft in order to achieve a safe watertight closure. This means that the adipose tissue graft will be exposed to a poorly vascularized tissue, such as the dura, or an avascular tissue in the case of a fascia graft. This carries a serious risk of absorption of the adipose tissue graft and the subsequent migration of mucosa up the frontonasal duct and the formation of a mucopyocoele.

Once the adipose tissue is carefully trimmed and placed into the sinus, then the osteoplastic flap is returned to its anatomic position and fixed to the adjacent calvarium with square plates. The periosteum of the flap is sutured to the periosteum of the calvarium and the coronal flap returned to its anatomic position and the wound closed and drained.

If the sinus is not suitable for an adipose tissue graft, then the frontal sinus is cranialized as described in the management of "through-and-through" fractures.

Fractures of the Frontonasal Duct

Fractures of the frontonasal duct are the most difficult to diagnose and may not be immediately apparent on imaging of the sinuses. If a fluid level in the frontal sinus fails to resolve in 2 weeks, then one can assume the duct is fractured. Often a CT scan in the sagittal plane will reveal the fracture. If not, and suspicion of an injury exists, then a small trephine can be placed in the anterior part of the floor of the frontal sinus. The sinus is then irrigated with a solution of saline + xylocaine with epinephrine. Methylene blue is then instilled within the sinus cavity. Observation with a sinus endoscope in the middle meatus will reveal the presence of the dye if the duct is patent. An alternative plan is to place, via the trephination, a radio opaque dye in the sinus and detect radiographically whether there is patency or not by the dye entering the nasal cavity.

Fractures of the nasofrontal duct can be managed in a number of ways. If an osteoplastic flap has been used for another fracture, such as that of the posterior wall, the adipose tissue obliteration of the sinus will also obliterate the nasofrontal duct.

Another open procedure that can be performed is the removal of the floor of the frontal sinus using the Lothrop procedure and then the turning up a septal flap like a Sewell Boyden flap to line the tract into the sinus.

A Draf III procedure, which is simply an endoscopic Lothrop procedure, can accomplish the same goal with an endonasal endoscopic approach. This provides the necessary drainage and is conducted in a less traumatic fashion than the open Lothrop procedure and probably improves success rates.

The osteoplastic flap and adipose tissue obliteration will have a more reliable result in the patient who may not return for follow-up.

The Through-and-Through Fracture

The most serious of all frontal sinus fractures is the through-and-through fracture. The Otolaryngologist often first encounters the patient at the operating table summoned by the attending Neurologic Surgeon. The fracture of the frontal sinus will be just one component of a more devastating open skull fracture.

The coronal scalp flap or equivalent has already been done and the central bleeding stopped, devitalized brain removed, and the dura repaired. There are two options in the management of the fracture of the frontal sinus: simple resection of all the walls of the sinus or cranialization.

The cranialization procedure is relatively simple. The basic principle is to enlarge the volume of the anterior cranial fossa by the removal of the posterior wall of the frontal sinus. The anterior wall, if it has been removed, is replaced and the nasofrontal duct obliterated. This will expand the anterior fossa volume such that the edematous brain has room to expand. The sinus is essentially eliminated as a source of infection to the exposed brain, and the forehead is allowed to maintain its normal esthetic appearance.

The first step is to locate the anterior wall of the frontal sinus. Dirt and debris are scrubbed from its surface, and the mucosal lining of the inner portion is elevated and discarded. The cortical bone of the inner surface is drilled away. The bone flap is left soaking in Betadine until the end of the case. A double-action rongeur is then used to eliminate the entire posterior wall of the frontal sinus (Fig. 53.5). The edges are smoothed out with a cutting bur so the side walls of the anterior cranial fossa are flush with that of the sinus. Great care is taken to remove all of the bone of the posterior wall, especially the feathered extremities along the floor of the anterior fossa that can extend almost all the way to the lesser wing of the sphenoid. The mucosa of the sinus floor which makes up the roof of the orbit is gently polished with a diamond burr.

Obliteration of the nasofrontal duct is now carried out by burring away some of the thin wall of the duct and then plugging the duct with a small block of temporalis muscle (Fig. 53.6). The frontal bone that made up the anterior wall of the sinus is now replaced and fixed to the calvarium with miniplates and screws or square plates (Fig. 53.7). If the frontal bone was discarded at the time of craniotomy, a split calvarial bone graft can readily be obtained from the craniotomy bone flap and used to reconstruct the anterior wall of the frontal sinus.

The scalp flap is returned to its anatomic position and the wound closed and drained. Often the neurosurgeon does not use a suction drain for fear of possible suctioning away of CSF. Multiple Penrose drains should be placed as needed and a light craniotomy dressing applied.

Usually, the dead space in the anterior aspect of the anterior fossa will initially fill with blood, and the brain will expand to fill the space. Even if this does not occur right away and some air is present in the anterior

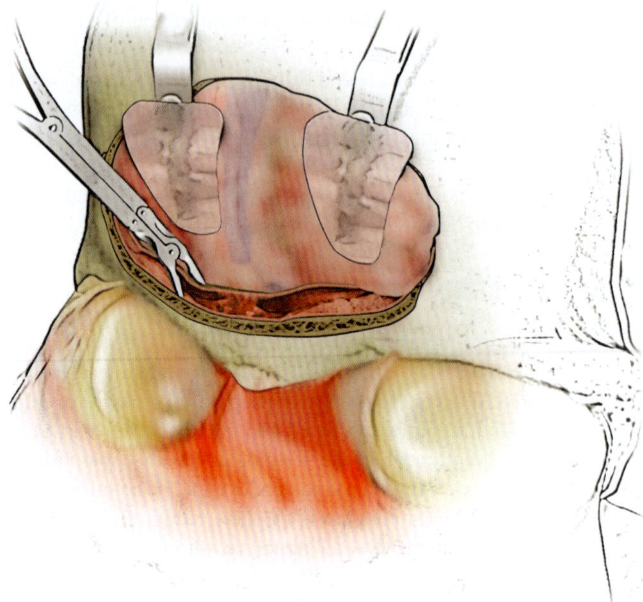

FIGURE 53.5
Removal of the posterior wall of the frontal sinus during cranialization.

fossa, it is of no concern unless it is expanding, thus becoming a tension pneumocephalus. In my experience, rarely is there absorption of the anterior bone flap with loss of frontal contour.

POSTOPERATIVE MANAGEMENT

Suction drains are placed especially if a scalp flap has been raised. When the drains are removed once there is minimal drainage, the wound should be covered by a light craniotomy type of dressing. If prophylactic antibiotics are used, they should be stopped 1 to 2 days after the operative procedure. Patients are instructed not to blow their nose. If not limited by concomitant injuries, the patient should be ambulated on the day of surgery. The dressing can be removed 2 to 3 days after the drains have been removed.

The postoperative care in patients with the through-and-through fracture will be administered by the neurologic surgical service. Postoperative CSF leaks are rare. Initial treatment using a head-up position possibly with a lumbar drain and careful observation. If the drainage does not stop, surgical intervention should be employed. The use of prophylactic antibiotics is controversial.

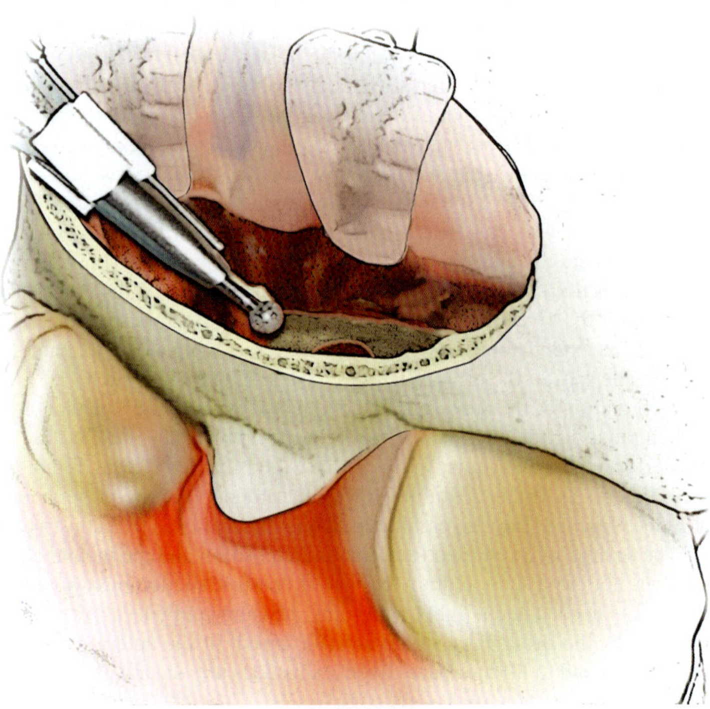

FIGURE 53.6
Removal of all mucosal remnants from the sinus cavity.

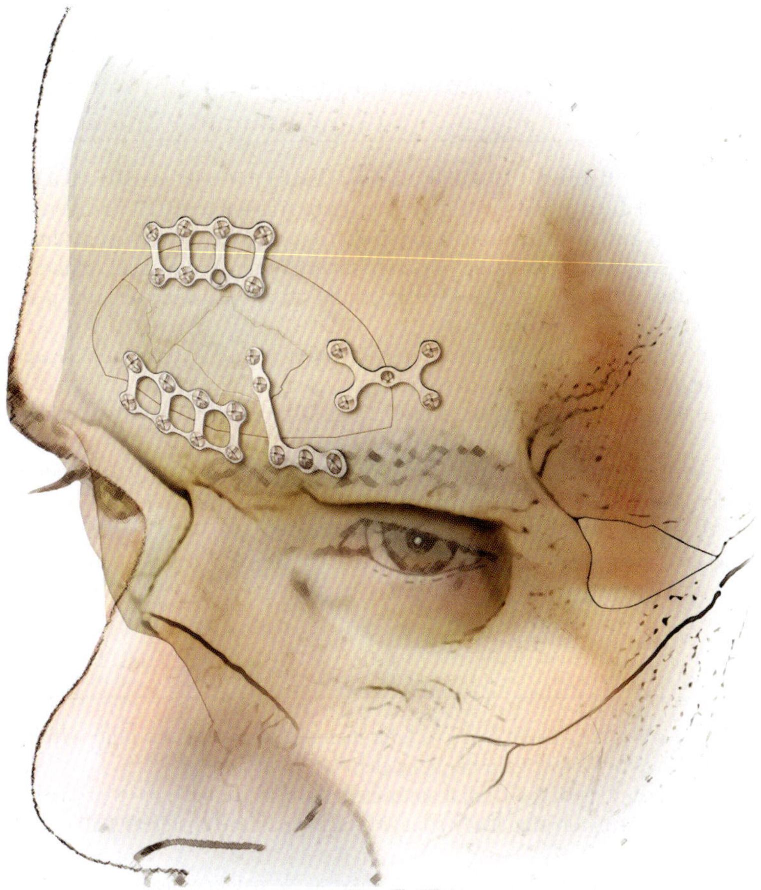

FIGURE 53.7
Frontal bone fragments reduced and fixed with miniplates.

Any patient who refuses surgery or has equivocal findings on the CT scan especially regarding the posterior wall or nasofrontal duct should be carefully observed for at least 3 years.

COMPLICATIONS

In fractures of the anterior wall if intraosseous wire is used to stabilize the fragments, the forehead needs to be protected to prevent prolapse of the fragments with resultant deformity. This is seen rarely when rigid plate fixation is used.

When an osteoplastic flap and obliteration with adipose tissue are used, there may be complications secondary to the coronal scalp flap. Loss of hair at the incision line may occur. Part of the scalp may necrose especially if a subcutaneous rather than a subgaleal approach is used. Other factors may be excessive pressure on the flap during the procedure or the injudicious use of cautery.

Wound infection is uncommon and is treated by local care and antibiotics. The most dreaded complications of these procedures are CSF leak, meningitis, and brain abscess which may occur in patients who have had a fracture of the posterior wall with a dural tear and through-and-through fractures. Fortunately, these complications have been rare in my experience. Late in the follow-up a cosmetic deformity may be seen in those patients who have had an osteoplastic flap. Because of the obliquity of the bone cut in the anterior wall of the sinus, there may be some absorption of the thin bone near the incision which leaves a linear depression along this track.

The most avoidable of the complications is the late formation of a frontal sinus mucocele or mucopyocele. These are usually the consequence of inadequate removal of the mucosa lining the sinus cavity or rapid and excessive absorption of the adipose tissue graft used to obliterate the cavity.

RESULTS

Since the beginning of the use of miniplates, the results of repair of a depressed fracture of the anterior wall have been excellent. Fractures of the posterior wall and those of the nasofrontal duct were mostly treated by the osteoplastic flap and obliteration with an abdominal adipose tissue graft. The only mucoceles seen in this group were those who had been treated by this method but had a significant area of bone missing in the posterior wall and the adipose tissue graft abutted the fascia graft used to seal the CSF leak. No mucoceles have developed when such patients were treated primarily by the cranialization technique.

In over 30 cranializations for through-and-through fractures, no mucoceles, late CSF leaks, or bone resorption have occurred. There were three calvarial deformities and one small area of osteomyelitis over the nasion.

PEARLS

- In preparation to preforming an osteoplastic flap, a 5-foot Caldwell view radiograph may not be available to map the outline of the sinus. An estimate of the size and shape may be made by transillumination of the frontal sinuses through the roof of each orbit. It is best to underestimate the size of sinus the size than to overestimate.
- Care must be taken to ensure that the image is taken in the posterior–anterior direction instead of anterior posterior to prevent magnification of the image of the sinus. The superimposition of a penny over the penny image on the film will avoid any confusion.
- When using an existing laceration to access a depressed fracture of the anterior wall, it is important to extend the incision horizontally in a so-called frown line to minimize scarring.
- Starting the penetrating bur holes, a little to the inside to the sinus outline will prevent inadvertent perforation of dura.
- The penetrating openings made to outline the frontal sinus must be slanted for two reasons. The important one is that if the size of the sinus has been overestimated, then the obliquely aligned bur hole will enter the sinus cavity rather than the anterior cranial fossa. The second reason is that the flap, when returned to its prior position, will rest against the shelf created by the cut and accurate reconstruction can be assured.
- Sturdy square plates should fix the flap securely when it is returned to its site.

PITFALLS

- If there is absorption of adipose tissue when the patient loses weight, then the adipose tissue graft will prolapse into the cavity or conversely in cases of weight gain the bone flap will protrude.
- When drilling out the mucosa in the extremities of the frontal sinus cavity, the space becomes very narrow. It is important to enlarge these tight crevices by drilling away some of the bone of the posterior wall or thinning the bone of the orbital roof.
- It is essential to be extremely gentle with the adipose tissue graft at harvest. No cautery should be used and only fine forceps employed to handle the graft.
- The graft may need to be inserted piece meal, but they should be as large as possible.
- The graft will take its blood supply from the drilled bone. Absorption of the adipose tissue will be only about 15% to 25% in a carefully handled graft.
- The graft will not survive in a poorly vascularized bed such as subcutaneous tissue, a dural graft, and even the dura itself.
- In performing the cranialization procedure, it is essential to remove all mucosal elements.
- The nasofrontal duct is best eliminated by a muscle plug and not a fascia graft.
- If no frontal wall had been preserved, large fragments of posterior wall bone can be used instead of a split calvarial graft.

INSTRUMENTS TO HAVE AVAILABLE

- Sinus surgery set
- Padded Mayfield horseshoe head rest without spikes
- Rainey clips
- Midas Rex drills with B1 and B5 perforating burs, both cutting and diamond down to 1 mm in diameter
- Houk osteotomes
- Freer, Woodson, and Penfield elevators
- Bipolar cautery
- Standard soft tissue set for harvest of abdominal wall adipose tissue graft:
  - Scissors
  - Forceps

SUGGESTED READING

Donald PJ, Bernstein L. Compound frontal sinus injuries with intracranial penetration. *Laryngoscope* 1978;88:225–232.

Draf W. Endoscopic micro-endoscopic frontal sinus surgery: the Fulda concept. *Oper Tech Otolaryngol Head Neck Surg* 1991;2:234–240.

Dula DJ, Fales W. The 'ring sign': is it a reliable indicator for cerebral spinal fluid? *Ann Emerg Med* 1993;22(4):718–720.

Ettin M, Donald PJ. The safety of frontal sinus fat obliteration when sinus walls are missing. *Laryngoscope* 1986;96:190.

Montgomery WW. *Surgery of the upper respiratory system*. Philadelphia, PA: Lea & Febiger, 1971:141–160.

(Note: Page numbers in *italics* denote figures; those followed by 't' denote tables.)

D

E

U

V

W

X

Z